PHILIP L. HILLSMAN, M.D.

BURNSIDE's
MEDICAL
EXAMINATION
REVIEW

BURNSIDE's
MEDICAL EXAMINATION REVIEW

Edited by

John W. Burnside, M.D.

Professor of Medicine
The Milton S. Hershey Medical Center
Pennsylvania State University College of Medicine
Hershey, Pennsylvania

Churchill Livingstone
New York, Edinburgh, London, Melbourne   1986

Acquisitions Editor: *Gene C. Kearn*
Copy Editor: *Kamely Dahir*
Production Designer: *Michiko Davis*
Production Supervisor: *Joe Sita*
Compositor: *Progressive Typographers, Inc.*
Printer/Binder: *The Maple-Vail Book Manufacturing Group*

Accurate indications, adverse reactions, and dosage schedules for drugs are provided in this book, but it is possible that they may change. The reader is urged to review the package information data of the manufacturers of the medications mentioned.

Distributed in the United Kingdom by Churchill Livingstone, Robert Stevenson House, 1–3 Baxter's Place, Leith Walk, Edinburgh EH1 3AF and by associated companies, branches and representatives throughout the world.

First published in 1986

Printed in U.S.A.

ISBN 0-443-08265-0

9 8 7 6 5 4 3 2 1

Library of Congress Cataloging in Publication Data

Main entry under title:

Burnside's medical examination review.

Includes bibliographies and index.
1. Medicine—Examinations, questions, etc. 2. Medical sciences—Examinations, questions, etc. 3. National Board of Medical Examiners—Examinations—Study guides.
4. Federation of State Medical Boards of the United States—Examinations—Study guides. 5. Educational Commission for Foreign Medical Graduates—Examinations—Study guides.
I. Burnside, John W., date. II. Title: Medical examination review.
[DNLM: 1. Medicine—examination questions.   W 18 B967]
R834.5.B87 1986   610′.76   85-17439
ISBN 0-443-08265-0

Manufactured in the United States of America

CONTRIBUTORS

John J. Botti, M.D.
Associate Professor of Obstetrics and Gynecology, The Milton S. Hershey Medical Center, Pennsylvania State University College of Medicine, Hershey, Pennsylvania

John W. Burnside, M.D.
Professor of Medicine, The Milton S. Hershey Medical Center, Pennsylvania State University College of Medicine, Hershey, Pennsylvania

William E. DeMuth, M.D.
Professor Emeritus of Surgery, The Milton S. Hershey Medical Center, Pennsylvania State University College of Medicine, Hershey, Pennsylvania

L.J.A. DiDio, M.D., D.Sc., Ph.D.
Chairman and Professor of Anatomy, Medical College of Ohio at Toledo, Toledo, Ohio

Mychelle Farmer, M.D.
Assistant Professor of Pediatrics, Division of Adolescent Medicine, University of Maryland School of Medicine, Baltimore, Maryland

Thomas D. Flanagan, Ph.D.
Professor of Microbiology, State University of New York at Buffalo School of Medicine, Buffalo, New York

Lois W. Forney, M.S.
Research Administrator, The Milton S. Hershey Medical Center, Pennsylvania State University College of Medicine, Hershey, Pennsylvania

Stephen A. Geller, M.D.
Director, Department of Pathology and Laboratory Medicine, Cedars-Sinai Medical Center, Los Angeles, California

Joseph S. Gonnella, M.D.
Professor of Medicine; Dean and Vice President, Jefferson Medical College of Thomas Jefferson University, Philadelphia, Pennsylvania

Igor Grant, M.D.
Professor of Psychiatry, Veterans Administration Hospital, San Diego, California

Donald A. Kennedy, Ph.D.
Vice President and Director of Research, Xicom Inc., Sterling Forest, Tuxedo, New York

Alberto Marchevsky, M.D.
Associate Professor of Pathology, Mount Sinai School of Medicine of the City University of New York, New York, New York

Rodrigue Mortel, M.D.
Professor and Chairman of Obstetrics and Gynecology, The Milton S. Hershey Medical Center, Pennsylvania State University College of Medicine, Hershey, Pennsylvania

Evan G. Pattishall, Jr., Ph.D., M.D.
Professor of Behavioral Science and Dean, College of Human Development, Pennsylvania State University, University Park, Pennsylvania

Cara-Lynne Schengrund, Ph.D.
Associate Professor of Biological Chemistry, The Milton S. Hershey Medical Center, Pennsylvania State University College of Medicine, Hershey, Pennsylvania

Dennis W. Schneck, M.D., Ph.D.
Associate Professor of Medicine and Pharmacology, Indiana University School of Medicine; Clinical Pharmacologist The Lilly Laboratory for Clinical Research, William N. Wishard Memorial Hospital, Indianapolis, Indiana

John H. Straus, M.D.
Assistant Professor of Pediatrics, Johns Hopkins University School of Medicine; Senior Pediatrician, Primary Care Center, Sinai Hospital of Baltimore, Baltimore, Maryland

J. Jon Veloski, M.S.
Instructor of Psychiatry and Human Behavior; Director, Division for Research in Medical Education, Jefferson Medical College of Thomas Jefferson University, Philadelphia, Pennsylvania

Charles W. Whitney, M.D.
Assistant Professor of Obstetrics and Gynecology, The Milton S. Hershey Medical Center, Pennsylvania State University College of Medicine, Hershey, Pennsylvania

PREFACE

The purpose of *Burnside's Medical Examination Review* is to help you prepare to take a medical licensing examination. Few such resources exist as the task of compiling them is difficult. The need for both brevity and completeness has challenged the contributors of this text; they have however, succeeded in preparing distillates of their respective disciplines which will allow you to prepare for a variety of certifying and/or licensing examinations.

The text is also written for those responsible for preparing examinations in medical schools and elsewhere. The book will assist instructors with the design of didactic sessions for those studying for examinations. Medical students can study sections prior to or as a review of basic science courses or clinical clerkships. The practicing physician, too, with a modest investment in time, will find "state of the art and science" in each chapter. This becomes increasingly important as more specialty disciplines are establishing recertification examinations and more states may soon be requiring relicensing examinations.

Four major examinations have for years comprised the majority of testing devices for licensure. The National Board of Medical Examiners prepares the National Board Examinations I, II, and III. Part I, given at the conclusion of preclinical studies, tests basic science competence in anatomy, physiology, biochemistry, microbiology, pathology, behavioral sciences, and pharmacology. Part II tests clinical knowledge in medicine, obstetrics and gynecology, pediatrics, preventive medicine and public health, psychiatry, and surgery. This test is given in the 4th year of medical school. Part III, given during the first postgraduate year, assesses clinical competence.

The second major examination which has been given is the Federal Licensing Examination (FLEX). It is prepared by the Federation of State Medical Boards. In order to encourage standardization and facilitate reciprocal licensing among states, because of the variations among states in licensing requirements, the Federation in cooperation with the National Board of Medical Examiners offers the FLEX exam to states wishing to use it. This test is given twice yearly and is 3 days long. Many states are again reviewing their testing procedures and it is likely that changes will be forthcoming.

One major change in 1983 by the Educational Commission for Foreign Medical Graduates has been the replacement of two examinations, the Educational Commission for Foreign Medical Graduates (ECFMG) examination and the visa qualifying examination (VQE), by the new Foreign Medical Graduate Examination in the Medical Sciences (FMGEMS). Both of the old examinations were designed to test graduates of foreign medical schools and the VQE was specifically designed to test foreign nationals from foreign medical schools. With an agreement with the National

Board of Medical Examiners, the new examination enables all graduates of foreign medical schools to meet the medical science examination requirement for ECMFG certification. Such certification is required for entry into residency or fellowship programs accredited by the Accreditation Council for Graduate Medical Education. The Secretary of Health and Human Services has recognized the FMGEMS as equivalent to the National Board Examinations Part I and II.

The FMGEMS consists of a 1-day test in basic medical sciences and a 1-day test in clinical sciences. This program began in 1984 and is offered twice a year in worldwide locations.

This book begins with a review of the procedures for these examinations as a surprise in format of the examination could prohibit a fair expression of your competence. Important to your satisfactory performance is a full understanding of testing techniques or knowing how to take the tests.

Subsequent chapters review basic medical science material followed by a section on clinical sciences. There is a brief bibliography at the end of each chapter. This includes the author's judgment of the best additional reading. Finally, each chapter includes sample questions. These questions serve two purposes. First to acquaint you with the range of information tested, and second, to give you additional learning material.

Contributing authors were carefully selected for this difficult assignment. They are all medical educators. Each commands respect for mastery of the topic material and each writes well. In their labors to help you, they have made judgments regarding what is important and what is superfluous. Each sentence contains valuable material. Where some controversy exists, the authors commit to a position. The information is there; highly concentrated, pertinent, and up to date. Like good tennis players, they make it look easy.

Use this text according to your individual needs. First, what examination are you preparing for? Second, what is an accurate judgment of your strengths and weaknesses? Look at the contents page and pencil in a numerical score; rate the chapters from those you feel comfortable with through those you need to work on. If you feel uncertain about a given area, try the sample questions at the end of that chapter.

Begin with an area in which you feel weak. If this is your first exposure to the subject matter, read it through at moderate speed. List the subheadings with which you find the greatest difficulty and use the bibliography for additional material. Then return to this book and reread carefully and slowly. You should move to another chapter before working on the questions. Return to the questions a bit later for both a test of your retention and for additional material. Lest you feel discouraged, intersperse a few chapters of material that you are comfortable with.

Let me conclude with a note of thanks to the chapter authors. They took this assignment with enthusiasm. Review material for them is not the most rewarding use of their time. It contributes little to their research or to recognition from their peers. They do it because they are dedicated teachers and because they are challenged to distill material to the essence. I would also like to thank Gene Kearn of Churchill Livingstone for his patience with delays and difficulties and Kay Cassel and Ann Espenshade, secretaries to our division, here at Hershey.

John W. Burnside, M.D.

CONTENTS

CONTENTS

SECTION 2
CLINICAL SCIENCES

Preparing for the Examination: Principles to Remember

J. Jon Veloski and Joseph S. Gonnella

Some readers may be tempted to skip over this chapter. Such inclinations are understandable because the selection procedures used at many medical schools, as well as their typical internal and external examinations, often rely heavily on objective testing formats. Most of you who have earned the privilege of taking medical certifying examinations have already demonstrated your ability to prepare for, and to take formal written examinations. Why then should you review this chapter?

The examination that you are about to take is likely to be much more stressful than most of the examinations you have encountered before. Anticipating one of the major, standardized examinations in such a vast field as medicine can overwhelm many otherwise confident examinees. Not only are these examinations longer and more comprehensive than most other written tests, but the consequences of not doing well may be substantial. A failing score on any of these examinations may disrupt your medical career or may even be catastrophic. Performance at a level below the national average might limit your career plans, or prevent you from being accepted into the postgraduate training program of your choice.

We believe, and will try to demonstrate in this chapter, that your approach to the examination should be guided by certain principles. We feel that you should consider these principles before reviewing the material within each discipline. Unless your preparation is carefully and efficiently planned, you may be overwhelmed by the enormity of the task.

Besides the abilities that they are designed to measure, standardized tests also reflect an individual's prior test taking experience. Your performance on any examination is not simply a function of your specific knowledge of the disciplines being tested. Your score on a test is also influenced by other factors. Some of these factors are under your control and some are not; for example, your understanding of the test's unique formats and scoring methods, your level of anxiety, your motivation, your physical and mental health, and whether or not the testing environment is physically comfortable, all affect your score. In this chapter we emphasize those variables which are under your control and provide suggestions to help you manage them.

Although many students think of examinations as unwanted hurdles, a test should be approached positively.

It is most likely that the examination that you are about to take will not be the last written examination in your professional life. Subsequent examinations will most likely be similar in format and, although the content may be different, they may very well require that you integrate what you are studying now with what you will learn later in postgraduate education and practice. The present use of recertification examinations, for example, by the American Board of Family Practice, and the possibility of the introduction of similar requirements by other specialty boards makes this even more certain. Therefore, by approaching the examination you are about to take with a positive attitude and by developing or refining your test taking skills, you will strengthen your base of medical knowledge and be better prepared to face the next challenge.

How effective are written tests in measuring and predicting the competence of physicians? Even though there is careful attention directed to the quality of certifying examinations, debate continues as to the validity of these instruments. Many critics assert that paper and pencil tests are artificial hurdles which must be passed merely to satisfy certifying or licensing authorities, or to comply with questionable rules imposed for promotion by the faculty of medical schools. Others argue that performance on a written examination does not necessarily assure that good medical care ultimately will be delivered to patients. This position has been documented by empirical studies that show little correlation between scores on tests and later measures of the performance of physicians in practice. But physician performance should not be confused with physician competence. The latter is a complex entity which includes medical knowledge, a wide array of technical abilities, interpersonal skills, and personal qualities. It is obvious that without an essential component of knowledge one cannot be competent. Unfortunately, having knowledge or competence does not always guarantee clinical performance. The latter is influenced by variables other than competence. Some of these factors are the reward system in the practice setting, institutional and environmental elements, the expectations of patients, and community factors. Nevertheless, written examinations do measure a minimal but essential component of the competence of physicians.

DIAGNOSIS

There are a number of simple and concise guidelines which will apply to almost any examinee who wants to improve his or her chances of performing well on an examination. While it is not useful to outline one complete set of recommendations which will apply to every

candidate, we will focus on the following three groups of examinees in this chapter.

The student or physician who is taking a particular comprehensive examination for the first time and who sincerely is worried about *failing* the test. Even if you think you are in this category you must first determine whether your perceptions are accurate. It may be that your concern is inappropriate in view of your past performance on similar examinations and the expected rate of failure on the test you are about to take. This chapter will aid you in determining whether you do in fact fall into the category of examinees who are truly in danger of failing.

The examinee who is taking an examination for the first time and who is appropriately confident about being able to pass the test, but who also wants to achieve the *maximum* score of which he or she is capable. If you have consistently performed above the average on objective examinations and have done well in recent, relevant course work then you may place yourself in this category with confidence.

The examinee who is *repeating* a particular test after having failed one or more times.

Before you begin to prepare for the examination you should evaluate your present status and set realistic goals for the process of review. The following will provide clues to help you determine into which category you fall.

Only a small percentage of those who take Part II or Part III of the National Board Examinations are expected to fail based on the past performance of the candidate reference group (Table 1-1). The expected failure rate for Part I is somewhat higher; however, even it is only about 11 percent. The differences between the failure rate for the candidates and noncandidates on the National Board Examinations may be attributed to the differences in motivation and intensity of preparation between the two groups. It would be assumed that the candidates seeking certification by the National Board of Medical Examiners would have a greater fear of failure than other examinees. The actual failure rates in 1982 for Part I are higher than the theoretical long-term rate because they include examinees who were repeating the examination. The failure rates for the Federation Licensing Examination (FLEX) and the previous examination for Foreign Medical Graduates are higher, partly because of the diversity of the premedical background and the medical education of the examinees who take these examinations.

You may have imagined yourself as being in one of these failing minorities. Fortunately, history tells us that the majority of examinees need not be overly anxious about passing most of the tests. These gross failure rates

Table 1-1. Estimated Rates of Failure in Standardized Comprehensive Medical Examinations

Examination	Estimated Rate of Failure (%)
National Board Examinations[a]	
Part I	
Candidates	14
Noncandidates	27
Part II	
Candidates	2
Noncandidates	7
Part III	
Foreign Medical Graduate Examination in the Medical Sciences[b]	67
Federation Licensing Examination (FLEX)[c]	
Graduates of United States and Canadian medical schools	20
Graduates of other medical schools	61

[a] Data reported are for all examinees in 1984 including those taking the examinations for the first time and also those repeating. The long-term failure expected failure rates are 11 percent for Part I, and 2 percent for both Part II and Part III.

[b] The first administration of this examination was July, 1984. The failure rate reported is the overall failure rate for the previous ECFMG Examination. Source: Results of 1982 ECFMG Examinations, Educational Commission for Foreign Medical Graduates (ECFMG).

[c] The use and interpretation of FLEX scores vary in some states. These rates are approximate.

will provide the general odds. But to obtain a better estimate of your true chances of failing you must adjust the overall failure rate by taking into account your own experience in related courses and on standardized examinations, and the recent track record of students at your medical school or other peers. For example, if you are about to take Part I of the National Board Examinations and are worried about failing, first inquire about the historical rate of failure at your own medical school over the past years. This rate provides an even better approximation of your risk of failure than does the national rate. Your odds of failure will be further predicted by your relative level of performance in the corresponding courses in medical school and your scores on previous standardized tests such as the Medical College Admissions Test (MCAT). Research has even shown that scores on the Scholastic Aptitude Test (SAT) taken earlier during high school will be related to performance on medical certifying examinations.

Consider a sophomore student who has performed at the average level in a medical school in which the historical failure rate has been, for example, 15 percent on Part I of the National Board Examinations. This student would therefore be expected to have approximately the same chance of failure. However, if this hypothetical student had performed at a below average or marginal level in the basic science courses at that medical school, he or she would have a much greater chance of failure. Consistent performance in the lower fifth of the class in the majority of courses would raise concerns. If this particular student had also recorded below average (less than 8) scores on one or more of the science scales (Biology, Chemistry, Physics, or Science Problems) of the MCAT, or below average (less than 500) on either the SAT Verbal or Quantitative scales, then the chances of failure would be even greater. These rules of thumb are based on a number of studies published in the literature and studies prepared by the National Board of Medical Examiners which show positive correlations between medical school grades and scores on subsequent comprehensive examinations.

As you evaluate your earlier performance on various examinations and extrapolate your record of achievement into the future, there is one critical assumption which must be kept in mind. Remember that the accuracy of any prediction you make is based on the assumption that you continue to perform at least as well as you have done in the past. Even if all the prior data suggest that you will probably do well in the coming examination, it is important for you to guard against complacency or overconfidence which might lower your score.

The concept that past performance is predictive of the future is sometimes discomforting to students. Those students who are already having difficulty in the early years of medical school feel especially uneasy when they discover that their scores on the next examination may be closely related to their last set of scores. Over the past 15 years the prediction of performance on examinations in addition to other issues related to the competence of physicians has been studied as part of an intensive longitudinal study of over 4,400 medical students and graduates at the Jefferson Medical College of Thomas Jefferson University. We are including a few representative findings and figures which illustrate the strength of the predictions which can be obtained. The relationship between performance in selected basic science courses during the first year of medical school and later performance on Part I of the National Board Examinations is summarized by a scatter diagram (Fig. 1-1).

In this study a statistical prediction of each student's total score on Part I was calculated at the end of the freshman year for every entering class between 1975 and 1980 using a weighted composite of grades in anatomy, biochemistry, physiology, pathology, and selected scores on the MCAT. After actual total scores on Part I were obtained almost 1 year later, a strong relationship was found when each student's predicted score was plotted against his actual score. The Pearson product-moment correlation is .78 for this sample of 1,260 students. This evidence supports the notion that your performance in a particular examination will be closely related to your performance in the relevant courses, all other things being equal.

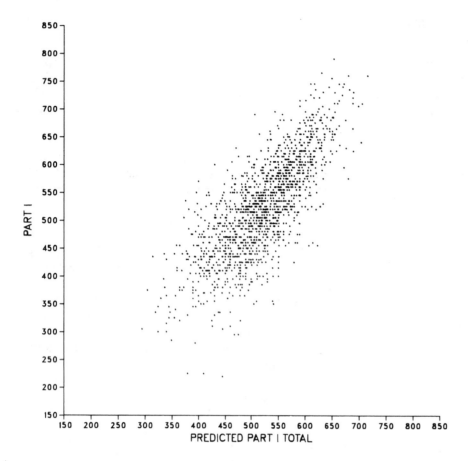

Fig. 1-1. Scatter diagram of predicted total scores on Part I of the National Board Examinations calculated from a composite of grades in the first year of medical school and the MCAT, v actual total scores obtained 1 year later for 1,260 students at the Jefferson Medical College of Thomas Jefferson University between 1975 and 1980.

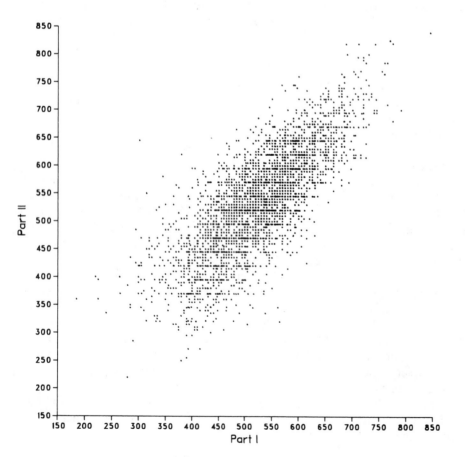

Fig. 1-2. Scatter diagram of total scores on Part I of the National Board Examinations v total scores on Part II for 3,210 students at the Jefferson Medical College of Thomas Jefferson University between 1966 and 1982.

There is a similar relationship between students' total scores on Part I and total scores on Part II which was taken by these students 1 year and 3 months after Part I (Fig. 1-2). Although the data show that a few students improved their scores remarkably, and some scores actually fell below the predicted level, the majority of students tended to score at about the same level in both examinations. The product-moment correlation is .78 for these 3,210 students.

A word of caution is needed concerning what these data suggest. They do provide solid evidence that the level of performance on Part II will be similar to the level of performance on Part I, but they should not be interpreted to mean that your scores will be necessarily equal on both tests. In Figure 1-2 the mean for this sample on Part I is 521, but the mean for Part II is 531. Thus, if a current student were using these data to predict his total score on Part II he would need to add 10 points to his Part I score. If you want to predict your Part II total score from your Part I score find out what the comparable difference is at your medical school.

Another similar but somewhat weaker relationship is described when scores on Part II are plotted against scores on Part III (Fig. 1-3). The product-moment correlation is .69 for 1,805 graduates of the classes of 1970 through 1981. In the following section on special issues

in medical certifying examinations we will discuss one of the possible explanations for this lower correlation.

If you are repeating an examination after having failed you will have a clearer idea of your strengths and weaknesses, and you will be already knowledgeable about the actual format of the examination. If your failure can be attributed to an atypical cause such as physical distress which you have never before experienced with standardized tests, or some emotional upset which distracted you, simply plan on a general review before the retest. Even if you failed because of gaps in your knowledge your chances of passing the next time will be better than on your first attempt, but you should have three major concerns. First, you should concentrate on improving your subtest scores in the areas in which you fell below the passing level. Your second problem will be time. If more than a few months elapse before the retest you will probably forget some of what you knew. Finally, you may be subject to a higher level of anxiety when you repeat the examination because you will not be taking it with most of your peers and a second failure may block your medical education or postgraduate training.

If you have had consistent difficulty with examinations, it will be important for you to find out why. The previous findings and discussion of relationships between scores on the different parts of the examinations

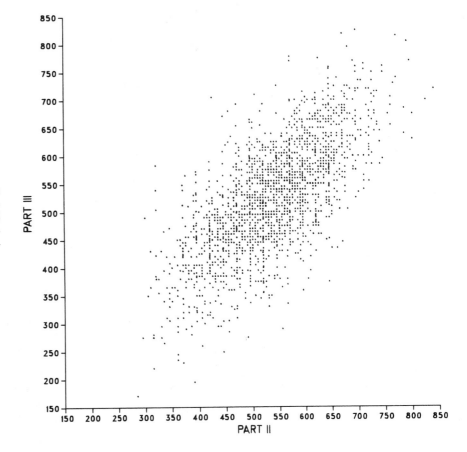

Fig. 1-3. Scatter diagram of total scores on Part II of the National Board Examinations v total scores on Part III for 1,805 graduates of the Jefferson Medical College of Thomas Jefferson University between 1970 and 1981.

suggest that, although the content is somewhat different in the three parts of the National Board Examinations, there may be enduring characteristics in examinees which affect their approach to standardized tests and the scores they achieve. The examinee who is afraid of standardized tests is often his own worst enemy. In many cases it is the nature of the multiple choice test and the testing situation that presents difficulty, not the content. By preparing for the examination in advance and doing practice tests you may be able to control your anxiety in the testing situation and improve your scores.

The second phase of your diagnostic work will require that you answer self-assessment examinations in order to gain a deeper understanding of your own strengths and weaknesses. There are many sources of objective type questions which can be used in addition to those pro-

vided in this book; for example, your own personal files, and the library of your medical school. Review as many questions as possible and make notes about questions you miss. One easy way to keep notes is to write problems on 3 × 5 index cards and then sort and group them into broader categories.

Having a better idea of your strengths and weaknesses in various disciplines and topics may lead to a dilemma. Should you concentrate on filling in the gaps of your knowledge identified as weaknesses, or should you try to build on your strengths, which might actually be closer to your long-term career interests? Whether one passes or fails on most of the examinations is determined solely by the total score. For example, in Part I of the National Board Examinations you may receive failing scores in one or more of the seven basic science subtests and nev-

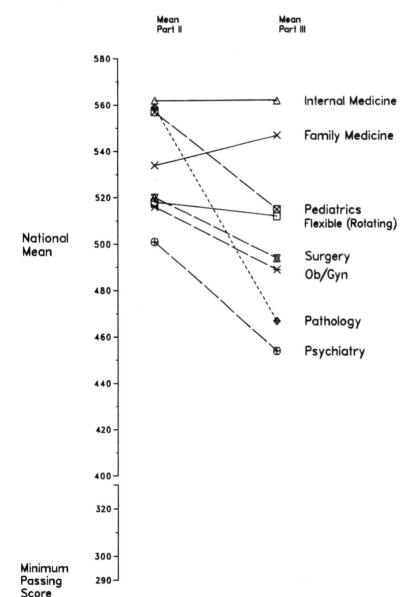

Fig. 1-4. Mean levels of performance for total scores on Part II and Part III of the National Board Examinations for 1,805 graduates of the Jefferson Medical College of Thomas Jefferson University. The numbers of graduates in each group are as follows: Internal medicine (n = 626), family medicine (n = 221), pediatrics (n = 121), flexible/rotating (n = 320), surgery (n = 341), obstetrics/gynecology (n = 83), pathology (n = 42), and psychiatry (n = 51).

ertheless pass the entire test by offsetting these failures with sufficiently strong scores in other areas. We recommend that you first concentrate on your weaknesses and fill in any gaps of knowledge by relearning what may have been forgotten since you first studied the discipline. This approach will also have long-term benefits as you build a sounder base of knowledge for professional practice and subsequent learning.

In conclusion, you should honestly and objectively review your past performance. By assessing your present strengths and weaknesses you will be able to define goals to prepare for the examination. Determine whether you are trying to *pass* the examination or *maximize* performance and set realistic goals. Nevertheless remember that the *past* is predictive of the future, but the odds can be changed if you are willing to work hard and modify your behavior.

SPECIAL ISSUES

The Impact of Early Specialization

One major effect of the changes in medical knowledge, science, and technology that has occurred in recent years is an increase in the pressure placed on students to specialize earlier in their careers. Some curricula now permit students to begin limiting their experiences through the selection of electives in the last year of medical school. Although there may be broad long-term effects of this early specialization on the overall clinical competence of these graduates, there are also very pragmatic issues which should be addressed when preparing for an examination such as the FLEX, Part II, or Part III of the National Board Examinations.

In a study of the potential impact of early specialization on general clinical competence, we analyzed the performance of graduates of the Jefferson Medical College of Thomas Jefferson University on Part III of the National Board Examinations which is taken near the end of the first year of residency. Data on 1,805 graduates from 1970 to 1981 are now available. The mean level of performance for the graduates who completed first year residencies in internal medicine, family medicine, or the flexible program (rotating in earlier years) did not decrease over the 1½ years between Part II and Part III (Fig. 1-4). The means for graduates who entered other programs, especially pathology and pediatrics, decreased sharply. The average scores for the graduates in obstetrics/gynecology, surgery, and psychiatry decreased by moderate amounts. It is likely that the changes between performance on Part II and Part III are due both to the programs themselves and to the characteristics of the groups of graduates who chose the pro-

grams. The relative contribution of these two factors will vary from one physician to another.

If you are planning to take FLEX or Part III, the implications of these findings seem clear. If you have spent most of your time in a residency which emphasized one particular specialty and if you have not reviewed general medicine and other specialties since your required clerkships in medical school, you will need to pay particular attention to these broader and sometimes neglected disciplines as you prepare for the examination. Do not let your intensive knowledge and expertise in one or two disciplines lead to overconfidence in other areas.

The Effects of Time on Knowledge

Special problems arise as the interval increases between your studies in medical school and the time of the comprehensive examination. In order to clarify these effects we studied the performance of senior medical students at the Jefferson Medical College of Thomas Jefferson University who took Part II of the National Board Examinations in their senior year.

We see the mean level of performance for 1,963 students between 1975 and 1983 on five subtests of Part II plotted according to the block of their junior year in which they completed the corresponding required clerkship (Fig. 1-5). For example, the students who took psychiatry during the summer (group SU) immediately preceding the beginning of their senior year in which they took Part II, performed at a level about 30 points higher on the average than those who had completed the clerkship 1 year earlier (group F). Similar patterns are observed in obstetrics/gynecology, pediatrics, and surgery where the difference is over 20 points. In internal medicine the difference between the fall and summer groups as well as the difference among the four blocks is small and was not found to be statistically significant by analysis of variance ($P < .05$).

This phenomenon of decay of knowledge has implications if you must choose the time to take a particular examination; register for the examination as soon as possible after the completion of the relevant courses or clerkships. For example, Part I of the National Board Examinations should be attempted as soon as possible after completion of the basic science courses *before* you become involved in the rigors of clinical work, and Part II should be completed as soon as you have finished your required clerkships. A second implication is obvious. Even if you performed well in a course or clerkship taken many months before the examination you will need to review that material even more carefully than recent course work if you want to do well on all parts of the examination. This point seems to be trivial, but the results shown in Figure 1-5 suggest that many medical

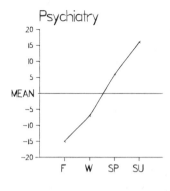

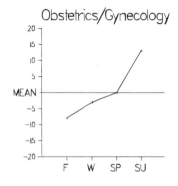

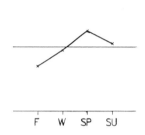

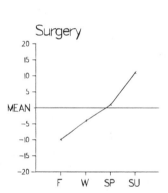

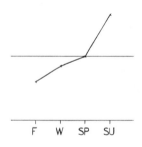

Fig. 1-5. Variations in mean level of performance on five subtests of Part II of the National Board Examinations related to the elapsed time between completing the relevant clerkship and taking the examination. Students completed each clerkship in either one of four groups: fall (F), winter (W), spring (SP), or summer (SU). Variation is reported as deviations in score point units from the overall mean for the four groups.

students either do not recognize this, or do not take action in order to review material from the clerkships completed early in the clinical year.

Pass/Fail Grading Systems

If you have studied in a medical school which uses pass/fail grading exclusively, you may face a number of unique problems as you approach a major examination such as the National Board Examinations or FLEX. Inexperience with fairly large objective examinations will put you at a distinct disadvantage in relation to many other examinees at other medical colleges who regularly have taken 2 or 3 hour final examinations in many disciplines. Nor does a pass/fail grading system always pro-

vide students with adequate information about their standing relative to their classmates. Students who are actually performing at a level of "marginal pass" may not realize this until it is too late. Finally, there is evidence that some directors of residency programs are relying more heavily on scores from the National Board Examinations as indicators of achievement for students who provide only pass/fail grades on their medical school transcripts. The uncertainty and pressure resulting from all of these problems may increase your degree of anxiety.

If you really do not have a good idea of how you stand make greater use of self-assessment tests. Find many sample multiple-choice questions in libraries and review books, and try to answer them. Make notes about difficult questions and search for patterns both within and across disciplines.

Commercial Review Courses

Many examinees wonder whether they should invest the time and money to take one of the proprietary test preparation courses which are available in most large cities. The large professional testing agencies such as the National Board of Medical Examiners, the Association of American Medical Colleges which administers the MCAT, and the Educational Testing Service (ETS) have been concerned about the influence of these courses on all standardized test scores. The effects have been studied in many different disciplines including medicine. The majority of findings seems to suggest that the coaching courses have been somewhat effective. Naturally, many variables, such as the self-selection of students in commercial review programs and the differing motivation of these students, have not been controlled in these studies.

One article did report an analysis of the effects of a commercial review course on students' performance on Part I of the National Board Examinations. A comparison of 55 medical students who had enrolled in a commercial review course and 55 other students with comparable records of academic performance before the examination who had not taken a review course revealed higher (about 27 points) mean scores on Part I for those who took the course. When asked in a questionnaire why they thought the review course was effective, the majority of the responding students mentioned the organization of the material. The students said that they had been overwhelmed by the volume of material to be covered in the examination, but the commercial review program provided a much needed framework for systematic study. The students pointed out that it would be counterproductive to rely exclusively on the review questions provided by the preparation course, but that the concepts presented in the course were valuable.

Are these courses worth the time and money? If you are in serious danger of failing, or if you already failed an examination and are repeating it, a review course might be one option. There may be, however, an additional price you must pay. If you become dependent on commercial review courses to manage your time and rely on such a mechanism to assign your priorities for study, you may not develop the skills you need to handle future examinations and to become a professional. By abdicating responsibility for preparation you are admitting defeat. If you do choose to use a review course it is important that you try to improve your skills in the process and learn about proven study techniques so that you will be able to prepare for future examinations without outside assistance.

Difficulty with the English Language

The graduate of a foreign medical school who continues to have difficulty with the English language will be confronted with two problems when taking the Foreign Medical Graduate Examination in the Medical Sciences (FMGEMS). The Educational Commission for Foreign Medical Graduates (ECFMG) will continue to administer an English test with each administration of the new FMGEMS. In 1982 of 3,616 examinees who took only the English test, 1,925 failed. You must be able to pass this test. Furthermore, difficulty with English will undoubtedly interfere with your performance on the medical sciences portion of the FMGEMS. If you feel that you are weak in English you will need to concentrate especially on reviewing sample questions and on becoming familiar with the instructions for each format of question which will be used. You should pay special attention to the test outline for the FMGEMS, and look for topics that may have been either deemphasized or ignored in your medical education.

THE TECHNOLOGY AND RELEVANCE OF TESTING

One common belief held by medical students is that the questions used for standardized medical examinations are prepared by professional writers at testing agencies such as the National Board of Medical Examiners. These same students are surprised to learn that the majority of questions actually have been written by a wide array of teachers, research scientists, and clinicians who are faculty members chosen from representative medical schools such as their own throughout the country. This section will briefly describe how the standardized examinations are constructed, scored, and analyzed, and what an examinee needs to know about this process in order to attain the best possible score.

Each form of a standardized examination is assembled from a subject outline which is similar in appearance to a very detailed table of contents for a book. Using this outline a carefully selected test committee of six to eight faculty members from appropriate disciplines in medical schools selects the questions to be used on the administration of a particular test. Each of the separate disciplines on an examination such as Part I of the National Board Examinations is the responsibility of a separate committee of specialists in that field. Questions, or more accurately items as they are referred to by specialists in testing, may be selected from a large database of properly calibrated items which have been used in previous examinations. Properly calibrated items have several objective characteristics. In addition to measuring content which has been deemed relevant by one or more test committees, such items will be of appropriate *difficulty* for the level of student or physician being examined. The difficulty of an individual item on an examination is computed as the percentage of a defined group of examinees who are able to answer the question correctly. Easy items will yield high values for this index. If an item has a high value for this difficulty index (e.g., 90 or 95 percent correct), generally it will not be used in a medical examination. The average level of difficulty for test items used by the National Board of Medical Examiners is typically about 60 or 65 percent correct. A properly calibrated question also *discriminates* between competent examinees and less competent examinees (i.e., the "good" students can answer it and the "poor" students cannot). This property of an item is measured by a second index which estimates the degree of correlation between responses to the item and performance on the total test, or subtest. It is assumed that if the test as a whole measures an important competency, then each item should contribute to this measurement. If it is found that examinees who generally did well on the entire examination tended to answer a particular item *incorrectly,* while those who did not do well on the examination answered the item *correctly,* the item will be reviewed carefully for possible defects.

If appropriate, calibrated items are not available in the pool of old items, new items may be written to examine topics recently added to the test outline. Examinations may also include a few items which are being pilot tested, and which will not count toward the examinees' total scores. The blueprint for each test, which is available in abbreviated form, should serve as your study guide, but you cannot be absolutely sure which topics will be emphasized or ignored in a particular form of the test.

It is important to keep in mind that all the items on each examination are meticulously screened by the panel of experts on the test committee as well as professional editors before they are actually used in the examination. After the examination has been administered, the same standard psychometric indices are calculated based on the answers given by the current group of examinees. As described previously, the mean percentage of correct answers as well as the distribution of responses for all items are tabulated. Coefficients of the correlation between the responses to each item (correct or incorrect) and the total test score are computed and monitored carefully after the examination to spot inaccurately keyed or ambiguous items. It is an accepted practice in standardized testing to retrospectively delete any examination items that are either too difficult for the pool of examinees or do not correlate with the total test scores. If items are rejected, the examination is scored without counting the responses to these defective items whether you answered them correctly or incorrectly. The implication here for the examinee is that you should not waste time trying to unravel what seems to be an item with a printing error, an exceedingly difficult option, a poorly worded phrase, or an ambiguous question. Make your best guess, make a note to review the question if you have time at the end of the test, and move on to the next question.

The style and content of items written by discipline based authors, however, may be less familiar to those students who learned the material using the body systems approach. For example, if you studied antibiotics in a multidisciplinary curriculum under the direction of a microbiologist, a pharmacologist, and an internist specializing in infectious diseases, you might not be acquainted with the level of specificity of separate items prepared by pharmacologists and microbiologists for an examination in the basic sciences. Pay careful attention to the test outline presented and use it as your study guide rather than the curriculum of your medical school.

In most standardized medical examinations the minimum passing level is determined by the performance of a previously tested criterion group rather than on the distribution of the current group of examinees. In theory, therefore, the failure rates can vary widely from year to year, but the rates for most tests actually have remained fairly constant over a number of years.

MULTIPLE CHOICE QUESTIONS

Many different types of objective, multiple choice questions have been developed to test examinees' abilities beyond rote memorization and simple recall. Complex question formats enable examiners to probe subtler abilities such as recognition, discrimination, interpretation, or reasoning. Some students perform poorly on objective examinations simply because they do not appreciate the purpose and mechanics of the different formats. Familiarity with these structures and a thorough understanding of the reasons for their use will probably lower your anxiety when you encounter them, and improve your efficiency during the examination. For those who have not had routine experience with a wide variety of multiple choice tests in all disciplines in medical school, or those who have difficulty with English as a second language, a review of this section is essential.

One Best Answer

You are likely to be familiar with the conventional "one best answer" multiple choice question. In this format a stem consisting of a statement or question is followed by four or five options identified by letters (A, B, C, D, E). The examinee is instructed to select the single best (correct) answer, but in practice more than one choice may appear to be reasonable or at least partially correct. The recommended approach to any type of multiple choice question is to read the stem first and temporarily *ignore* the options given. After you understand the question being asked you should *anticipate* the correct answer *before* reading any of the options presented. Keeping the author's question in mind search for your answer among the options. Though you will not always anticipate the precise answer that is called for, the answer that you construct may contain some of the logical characteristics or thought processes of the correct answer provided by the writer of the question. Even if you find the anticipated answer among the choices, carefully consider each of the other options. Remember that the questions in these examinations have been carefully constructed, edited, and revised to discriminate between the best examinees and those who are not competent. The most effective questions will almost certainly include distractions intentionally written to be attractive to an examinee with a superficial understanding of the discipline being tested.

In any multiple choice examination, feel free to write in the test booklet, underscore key phrases, and draw diagrams or make notes concerning specific facts which you might have difficulty recalling later. This is especially appropriate for those few difficult questions which you may need to leave blank and reconsider at the end of the examination.

Many students have successfully used several traditional hints for taking tests which exploit flaws in the construction of questions. These include choosing the longest option, searching for specific determiners (the use of the same word in the stem and the correct option), grammatical flaws in wrong answers, and the likelihood that the correct answer will be near the top of the list of choices. These tactics are often quite helpful when taking tests which have been written by medical school faculty under the pressures of time restrictions, but such methods are not recommended when taking one of the large standardized tests. You will recall from the previous section that, although these questions are written by faculty members, they are also scrutinized by other experts and professional editors. Furthermore, the patterns of responses are reviewed after each use of the questions in an examination, and the distractions are sometimes revised to make the questions better discriminators. Although you may occasionally find a defective question in one of the tests, we feel that you can use your time more effectively by concentrating on the content of the items.

Matching

Another variety of the objective question is the one best answer matching question. You might encounter this format with, for example, a list of drugs followed by a list of questions or statements about their use, contraindications, or side effects. Some examinees become confused and use the wrong set of options when answering questions; therefore be careful. As you answer the items based on a set of matching items treat each question independently. Do not look for trends or patterns in your responses. Remember, also, that an option may be used as a correct answer more than once in a sequence of matching questions unless you are directed not to do this.

Multiple True False

Many examinees feel that the multiple true or false questions are the most difficult. In this type of question four numbered choices are presented with the following directions:

A	1, 2, 3 only
B	1, 3 only
C	2, 4 only
D	4 only
E	All are correct

If you are familiar with this format and understand the logic of the pattern of responses you will be able to work much more quickly and efficiently during the examination, and you will avoid the anxiety of trying to decipher what, on first impression, appears to be an unnecessarily complicated coding scheme. Remember the name of these questions, "multiple true false," and approach them as such. First read the stem of the item and anticipate the possible correct answers. If at first you think of only one, try to think of other possibilities. Then proceed to the numbered options and note any of those which correspond to your anticipated correct answers.

The logic of multiple true false items implies a strategy you can use if your answers do not correspond exactly to those of the author (Table 1-2). The coding of the responses is designed to reward you for your appropriate use of partial information. As you can see if you know only one of the four numbered options you will be able to narrow your choice (or guess) to only three of the five lettered choices.

Table 1-2. Pattern of Options in Multiple True False Questions Utilized in Standardized Medical Examinations

	Numbered Option			
Responses	1	2	3	4
A	T	T	T	
B	T		T	
C		T		T
D				T
E	T	T	T	T

T represents "true." For example, if an examinee believes that options 1, 2, and 3 are true he or she would choose response A.

If you feel comfortable with the format you will be able to cope with the uncertainty of knowing only a few of the numbered options presented. The following strategies are obvious, but you must be sure to use them if you know only two of the choices.

If you are certain that both 1 and 2 are true, or if you are certain that 2 and 3 are true then it is necessary to choose only between A and E according to whether you think that 4 is true or false.

If you are certain that 1 and 3 are true then you must choose between A, B, or E depending first on whether 4 is true or false. If your best guess is that 4 is true then choose E. If you think 4 is probably false then you will choose between A and B depending on whether 2 is true or false.

If you are certain that 1 and 4 are true, or if you are certain that 3 and 4 are true then you know immediately that the correct answer is E.

Many examinees panic when they see the multiple true false questions, however if you use these rules when you administer your self-assessment and practice examinations you will find these questions to be no more difficult than the conventional multiple choice questions.

Items Based on Pictorials and/or Case Histories

Most of the examinations will include groups of questions that require you to interpret photographs of patients' abnormal physical signs, photomicrographs, roentgenograms, electrocardiograms, and other diagnostic tests. To make the best and most efficient use of your time, read the question or questions; then analyze the pictorial. If you know what you are searching for you will not waste time making interesting observations or inferences which will not be examined on the test.

PATIENT-MANAGEMENT PROBLEMS

Patient-management problems (PMPs) make up a large portion of Part III of the National Board Examinations as well as one clinical portion of the FLEX exam. In this section we will describe the format of these unique examination items, the special scoring method which is generally used, and some logical strategies that may help you to achieve the best score.

PMPs were first used in 1961 by the National Board of Medical Examiners following a 2 year study that defined nine major areas of clinical competence necessary for certification. The areas of clinical performance measured were history taking, physical examination, tests and procedures, diagnostic acumen, treatment, judgment and skill in implementing care, continuing care, the physician-patient relationship, and other responsibilities of a physician. Before the advent of PMPs these attributes had been measured by oral examinations administered in addition to the written portion of the Part III examination. However, there was great dissatisfaction with this technique because of a lack of standardization of the cases used for examining candidates. PMPs are designed to measure a broad set of clinical capabilities while trying to achieve an accurate measurement of the competence of physicians.

Presented in a manner resembling real clinical encounters, PMPs are printed simulations of medical problems. Through a latent printed image exposed only by a special pen this format will give the results of information selectively gathered from the patient's history, physical examination, diagnostic, and management evaluations so that you will be able to build and record a logical approach to the solution of the problem. The score for the PMP is determined by an analysis of whether you select appropriate options and reject inappropriate ones. More will be said about this scoring technique in the following paragraphs.

Since the pacing is somewhat different in PMPs you will not be concerned primarily with the total number of questions being asked. When you begin a section of the examination which includes PMPs, consider the total time allowed for an examination period and divide this by the total number of PMPs, not the number of questions asked in the section. Check your time at the end of each PMP and adjust your pace accordingly. Resist the temptation to deliberate on what seems to be an unusually challenging case. When answering PMPs it is very important to avoid being caught short of time because there is no sensible way to mark responses randomly in order to take advantage of chance success if you are not finished when time is up.

There are two general approaches to PMPs which have

been used successfully. Some prefer to complete the problems sequentially as they appear in the examination booklet; others scan all the PMPs in the section being tested and pick those of which they are most knowledgeable, which look most familiar, or simply prove to be the most interesting. The latter strategy has the advantage of building confidence and possibly stimulating your ability to recall appropriate diagnostic strategies which may be useful in other PMPs in the same section.

Each case begins with a description of a clinical problem designed to guide a competent examinee toward an appropriate differential diagnosis. After the introduction the PMP is divided into a series of decision points where options are offered concerning history, physical examination, and diagnostic procedures such as laboratory studies or management of the patient. It is important for you to remember that the options are deliberately presented at random so there is no implied importance according to their order on the page. Read through the options and make your selection in what you think is a logical sequence.

Approach each PMP as if it were a real patient and proceed systematically. Take advantage of the introductory information provided (i.e., history of present complaint, other illnesses, allusion to changes in life style, etc.) and read each very carefully. Underscore important information or note it in the margin of the page. Select each option very carefully since each area you expose will earn or deduct points from your score. First, choose the relevant options. Avoid making stray marks or partial exposure of the latent image. Since these will be counted as responses and reduce your score.

Next, scan all sections or decision points of the PMP, but do not try to guess the diagnosis by reviewing in detail all the available options at each decision point. The authors will try to set traps for you with irrelevant treatment options such as surgical or radiation therapy when the problem should be treated medically. They may also include options which are completely irrelevant to the case in order to make the simulation seem as real as possible.

As you begin each section of the PMP, analyze all prior information available, decide which options to choose, expose the information you need, reevaluate, and reconsider the available options. You will face a dilemma if you are midway through the PMP and begin to suspect that you have been pursuing the wrong diagnosis. Should this occur, check the time remaining in the examination and do not go back to the beginning of the problem unless you are ahead of schedule. If you are not ahead of schedule proceed through the case and choose options relevant to your latest, more accurate diagnosis. If time remains after you have finished all the PMPs in

the section, return to the case with which you had difficulty to determine if you should have exposed other options. Be very cautious if you decide to go back to the beginning because valuable time needed for subsequent problems may be lost and, of course, the responses already made cannot be changed.

Do not be naive and try to guess the content of the latent image by its surface area on the page. Ignore the size of the response area. The authors will try to disguise this factor by occasionally using verbose, multisentence reports of "normal findings" or very brief summaries of "abnormal findings." Options are generally presented randomly. Keep in mind that the number of appropriate options within a section might range from none to all, so do not confuse this type of examination with a conventional multiple choice format.

Remember that you are being tested on your methods of making as well as your ability to make an accurate diagnosis. Some critics have challenged the validity of PMPs as tools for measuring physician competence because they place too great an emphasis on the process of diagnostic reasoning without assigning equal or greater weight to the results. The examinee who makes accurate diagnoses by means of creative shortcuts will not earn as many points as the skilled test taker who chooses the conventional, proven options. If you want to maximize your scores on PMPs you must choose the latter, conventional strategy. Avoid a tendency to try to solve a problem by choosing the smallest number of choices. There is no reward or bonus for taking shortcuts. You are not being evaluated only on accuracy, but also the steps you take in solving the PMPs.

Order all tests and procedures which you feel are appropriate, routine, relevant, or important to the diagnostic possibilities being investigated. The feedback you receive in the problem will not always suggest the correct line of reasoning. Do not waste time trying to understand how the specific case is being scored.

The PMPs are scored based on a concept of total possible points. The authors of a PMP assign points to each option in accordance with their opinion of its overall utility in solving the case presented. You begin at zero and earn varying numbers of points by choosing correct options. If you select options which the authors feel are inappropriate because of cost ineffectiveness, discomfort to the patient, or unnecessary risk, you will lose points. For this reason do not become preoccupied with finding the precise diagnosis. Do not request unnecessary lab tests to "rule out" a possible diagnosis.

PMPs are unique. Because of their complexity and cost of production most medical students have not had extensive experience with them. There is no easy method of studying for them in advance since they attempt to measure a wide array of competencies. Familiarity with the format and the strategies we have outlined should enable you to record accurately what you do know.

APPROACHING TESTS IN GENERAL

This section covers the tactics that can improve your performance when taking any examination. We could assume that an examinee who has reached the postbaccalaureate level of education, or who is already a physician in practice, is very likely to be an expert test taker. However, we feel that it is appropriate to remind you of some of these tactics for one reason. Since you are taking an unusually long certifying examination which will be used as a milestone in your medical career you may be subject to unusual anxiety, particularly if you are actually in danger of failing. A formal review of these tactics may increase your chances of applying them in a situation of high stress.

Six to Twelve Months Before the Test, or Earlier

Ideally, you should be reading this book far in advance of the actual examination date. Your planning for certifying examinations should begin very early in medical school. Your approach to the examination and your strategy for studying should be planned early. There is evidence, from studies of long-term memory and research in test taking techniques, that shows that last minute cramming is useless and in some cases may even be counterproductive. Preparation should be based on a systematic review and directed toward an understanding of basic principles in the disciplines on the test. Avoid trying to memorize minutiae. View your study for the examination as a learning opportunity and concentrate on integrating your knowledge in long-term memory.

Obtain a copy of the test outline from your medical school or from the test publisher. The National Board of Medical Examiners prepares booklets of twenty to thirty pages for each of their examinations. These booklets include sample directions, sample questions, and some hints for taking the examinations. Consider carefully the test outline, rather than the curriculum followed in medical school, remembering that the questions are written by discipline based faculty members from many schools. Use the test outline as a guide in planning a study schedule for the next 6 to 12 months.

Self-assessment tests can be much more effective if used *before* reviewing the content of the examination. Individuals preparing for an examination are often given a false sense of security (e.g., studying the biochemistry materials in a review book and immediately attempting a set of sample questions). You will naturally do well by answering questions immediately after study! A much sounder technique is to try to answer the questions before your review. This measure of performance provides a better estimate of your recall of the original course. These self-assessment tests can be used as a diagnostic tool to clarify perceptions of current strengths and weaknesses. To anyone but the most confident and knowledgeable examinee it may be upsetting to take a test before reviewing the material, but the results of the test will provide valuable information about your strengths and weaknesses. Sometimes there is a tendency to overestimate strengths and underestimate weaknesses. You should, of course, allocate more time to strengthing your weaknesses.

It is important that you select a strategy based on whether it is necessary to pass each part of the test or achieve only an overall passing score. The use and interpretation of the examination scores from the FLEX exam varies in some states. Interpretations of the National Board Examinations are usually based on the total score. Many examinees in danger of failing ignore the way in which their performance will be graded, and spend a great deal of time reviewing the things that are easy to review because they already know them.

If an examination has more than one section, should you review each section separately or study more than one discipline simultaneously? Should you review microbiology before pathology or the opposite? Some students find it helpful to try to integrate disciplines across body systems or topics (e.g., oncology) rather than to review course material exactly as it was taught. Alternatively, you may find it helpful to review the material by discipline if you were taught by the body systems or topic approach.

When studying, especially clinical material, remember that textbook material is probably more important than current literature. Examinees who are sufficiently confident about passing the examination and who have generally done well in earlier examinations may profit from reading current literature. Remember, since examination questions review fundamental competencies and are often drawn from item pools, most questions will not be based on contemporary issues.

The Month Before the Test

Begin to arrange your personal affairs to eliminate the chance of any crisis developing on the day of the examination. If it is necessary to travel more than a routine commuting distance to the testing center, it is probably worthwhile to arrive the day before and stay overnight.

During the final month you may be especially susceptible to increased anxiety unless you are sufficiently confident about your preparation for the test. Research in test taking behavior suggests that a moderate amount of anxiety is not necessarily undesirable and can actually improve your performance. This is sometimes referred to as the "inverted U hypothesis" which describes a graphical model of the quantitative relationship between an examinee's performance and anxiety. Too little or too much anxiety can hurt performance, but a moderate amount will optimize performance. It is doubtful that you will experience too little anxiety, but care must be taken to guard against debilitating worry.

The Night Before the Test

By this time your studying should be complete. The night before the test should be one of relaxation and rest. Go to the movies or visit a friend! Avoid last minute cramming.

The Morning of the Test

Although it seems obvious and unnecessarily pedantic, you are reminded to be punctual. Wear loose, comfortable, seasonal clothing, but plan for the worst possible climate in the testing center. During cold weather the heat may be too high or too low, and conversely in the summer the air conditioning may be uncomfortably cool. Plan for the worst case with a flexible wardrobe including a sweater or light jacket. Being physically comfortable will help you to concentrate and reduce your anxiety. Arrive at the examination center early.

During the Examination

Relax. Read the directions carefully. If you have prepared adequately you will recognize every format. At the beginning of each section scan the questions, being careful to note the format and total number of questions.

If the questions are of uniform format you can pace yourself by allocating a standard amount of time to each question (total time – 10 minutes) ÷ (number of questions). Allocate 10 minutes as a buffer just in case you lose track of the time or need to go back and check some of your answers. When questions require more reading or are of a more complicated format, such as multiple true false, adjust your time accordingly. Pace yourself and check your watch periodically.

Most examinees complete the questions sequentially within a section, but others choose to scan the entire section and attack the most difficult formats first. By using the latter strategy energy will be used effectively at the beginning of the examination period. Also separate the tasks of answering the questions and transcribing the answers. Be sure to leave adequate time to transcribe them during the last 15 minutes of the examination period, and you are less likely to be distracted by examinees leaving and the pressure to finish.

Read every question very carefully and try first to answer it before reading the list of choices provided. Remember that the distractors (wrong answers) have been very carefully written, edited, and pilot tested to appear reasonable to all but the most competent examinees. If you cannot answer the question reread it. If you depend on the choices to guide your search of your memory you will be likely to fall into a trap. When you look at the choices and find the answer you recalled it is very likely that you are correct. At this point look at the other options and reason why each is wrong.

If you are not able to answer a question do not waste time on it. Make a small mark on your answer sheet or test booklet and go back to it at the end of the test. If you find that you are behind schedule, try to avoid having to skip questions since you may not have time to return to them or if you do, rereading and analyzing them again will waste valuable time. If you become overwhelmed and fall behind schedule be sure to go over your answer sheet before the end of the examination and fill in any unanswered questions with random responses. Mark your answers on the answer sheet carefully. Do not lower your score by making simple clerical errors.

Do not panic. Most examination questions are difficult for examinees and an average score about 60 or 65 percent correct. You will recall, from the previous section of this chapter, that defective questions which are either too difficult or do not contribute to the psychometric quality of the examination will probably be eliminated from scoring. Remember also that the examination may include pilot questions which are experimental in nature. There is always the possibility that you are wasting time trying to answer a question which eventually will not count toward your score.

Each session of an examination usually lasts at least 2 hours. Some examinees find it worthwhile to leave the room after an hour or so for a short break.

Take as much time for the examination as possible and avoid being distracted by those who leave early. We have observed a significant number of examinees who leave $\frac{1}{2}$ to 1 hour early especially in the afternoon session on the last day of an examination. Do not feel discouraged when you see other people leaving even if you have completed only three-quarters of the test. Every point you earn is to your advantage.

After the Examination

It is natural to want to celebrate with your friends or family at the end of the examination, but if a fear of failure remains, you may want to make a special effort and spend a few minutes reviewing mentally what happened during the test. Assess objectively your strengths and weaknesses just in case the test has to be repeated. Be honest with yourself and make a list of areas in which you need improvement. Remember, the test is a learning experience too!

THE DISTINGUISHING FEATURES OF EACH EXAMINATION

The trend in medical examinations during the 1970s and 1980s has been marked by greater uniformity in both the format and content of the major standardized examinations. The maturation of the psychometric and computer technology needed to generate uniform examinations of high quality has enabled the test committees to assemble examinations from large databases or pools of items (questions). To a large extent the examinations described in the following section are interchangeable where knowledge related to the same disciplines is being measured. Generally, only variations in the length and relative weights of components distinguish one from another. An item which measures a fundamental concept in biochemistry may just as likely appear on a form of the FLEX as on Part I of the National Board Examinations. We will try to emphasize the unique features of each examination rather than repeat their obvious similarities. Further, as a result of great concern over the differential effects of proprietary test preparation and coaching services, those responsible for each test are currently providing examinees with much more preliminary information about the format and types of items used as well as the content of the examinations. Carefully read the materials sent to you before the examination, and request any other booklets or pamphlets offered.

National Board Examinations

The National Board of Medical Examiners is an independent, nonprofit organization which prepares and administers qualifying examinations in a variety of subject areas. The medical examinations are recognized by most states as meeting the requirements for licensure. These examinations are taken by over three quarters of the medical students in the United States. To be eligible to take these examinations, one must be a medical student/graduate of either a United States or Canadian medical school accredited by the Liaison Committee on Medical Education (LCME).

The examinations are scored according to the highest available standards of psychometric technology. The scores on each of the three examinations are reported on a scale which can range from 5 to 995 with a mean of 500 and a standard deviation of 100. In practice nearly all scores fall in the interval between 200 and 800. Scores are computed based on a criterion group of examinees relevant to each examination. For example, on Part I the criterion group consists of the last 4 years of examinees who were second year medical students at the time they took the test, who were candidates for certification by the Board, and who took Part I for the first time at a June administration.

Part I is a 2 day examination consisting of about 1000 multiple choice questions in anatomy, behavioral sciences, biochemistry, microbiology, pathology, pharmacology, and physiology. Each subject area contributes approximately the same number of questions. Questions are constructed to test not only knowledge, but also the ability to interpret, discriminate, and reason. Some questions deal with interdisciplinary topics such as molecular biology, cell biology, or genetics. The examination is separated into six books, each consisting of between 150 and 175 questions. Although the questions are grouped by format (e.g., multiple choice, multiple true false, matching) with appropriate directions, the presentation of questions from the seven individual disciplines is mixed.

The Part II examination is similar in format to Part I, and includes questions in internal medicine, obstetrics/gynecology, pediatrics, preventive medicine and public health, psychiatry, and surgery. In addition to simple objective questions, more complicated questions are included which require the examinee to interpret photographs of patients' abnormal physical signs (e.g., skin lesions), roentgenograms, photomicrographs of pathological specimens, electrocardiograms, electroencephalograms, or computer assisted tomographs. A portion of Part II requires interpretation of clinical data including values of clinical laboratory tests. As indicated in the *Guidelines and Sample Items* published by the National Board of Medical Examiners, the ranges of normal values are included in the examination booklet. Therefore, there is no need to be concerned about memorizing these.

Part III is a 1 day examination consisting of three sections. The test is designed to measure clinical competence with particular emphasis on the use of medical knowledge to solve a variety of clinical problems. The first section is a multiple choice examination dealing with the indications, contraindications, and risks associated with pharmacotherapy, life support measures, and other forms of management. The second section is a multiple choice examination that evaluates the candidate's understanding of the indications and interpretations of diagnostic tests and results. This format incorporates a variety of pictorial and graphic materials. Section three comprises a large part of the test and consists of PMPs.

Federation Licensing Examination

The Federal Licensing Examination (FLEX) is a 3 day test covering seven basic science areas (anatomy, behavioral sciences, biochemistry, microbiology, pathology, pharmacology, and physiology) and six clinical science disciplines (internal medicine, obstetrics/gynecology, pediatrics, preventive medicine and public health, psychiatry, and surgery). The examinee's ability to apply this knowledge to simulations of clinical problems is also tested. Although the examination is constructed and scored nationally its administration and interpretation are regulated at the state level. Most states require only an overall passing score, but some states establish other standards.

Approximately one-half of the FLEX program is designed to measure the examinee's knowledge and understanding of the basic and clinical sciences. The principles and mechanisms underlying disease, and modes of therapy are emphasized. This component of the examination includes approximately 630 standard multiple choice questions in four books, with 2 to 2½ hours allowed for each book.

The second half of the examination consists of 15 to 20 PMPs in one book and approximately 500 standard multiple choice questions. Examinees are allowed approximately 4 hours to complete the PMPs and approximately 6 hours to take the multiple choice questions.

Scaled scores for the two parts of the examination are computed by taking into consideration the performance of the examinee and the level of difficulty of the items (questions) used in the examination. Although a recommended passing score on each component of the test is 75, this scaled score is not a percentage. Generally, a score of 75 can be achieved by answering correctly fewer than 75 percent of the questions. It is also important to recognize that although the passing requirements may vary from state to state, the examinations are not scored on a state-by-state basis. Differences in the passing rates for the examination among states are not due to different methods of scoring.

Foreign Medical Graduate Examination in the Medical Sciences

Since 1977 there have been two examinations for assessing the medical knowledge of graduates of medical schools outside the United States. The Visa Qualifying Examination (VQE) for alien physicians needing a visa

for entry in the United States and the ECFMG Examination for all other graduates of foreign medical schools who did not require a visa. In 1983 the Educational Commission for Foreign Medical Graduates (ECFMG) announced that a new examination would be developed to take the place of both the earlier ECFMG medicine examination and the VQE. The new 2 day FMGEMS is designed to assess the readiness of graduates of foreign medical schools to enter accredited residency training programs in the United States, including Puerto Rico.

The FMGEMS is administered twice each year in a large number of centers throughout the world. Examinees are eligible to take the basic science test after completing at least 2 years of medical school and will be able to take the clinical science test later after completion of medical school. This provides a valuable opportunity and we suggest that you register for the examination at the two separate times rather than waiting until the end of medical school to attempt both examinations. A passing score on the test will enable any graduate of a foreign medical school to meet the ECFMG medical science examination requirement and will also help alien physicians who wish to enter the United States to meet the requirements for a visa. For this purpose the government of the United States has recognized a passing score on the new examination as being equivalent to passing Parts I and II of the National Board Examination.

The multiple choice English test includes questions in three sections dealing with comprehension of spoken English, vocabulary, and sentence structure. All applicants are required to take and pass this test, although it is graded separately from the medical portion. If a candidate fails this portion of the test, but passes the medical part, scores on the Test of English as a Foreign Language (TOEFL) administered by the ETS may be substituted.

The medical component of the new examination is constructed by a test committee using calibrated items (questions) drawn from the extensive pool of items used for Parts I and II of the National Board Examinations. Passing scores are determined based on the previous performance of the graduates of United States medical schools on the items. The 2 day examination includes approximately 500 items from the basic science disciplines of anatomy, behavioral sciences, biochemistry, microbiology, pathology, pharmacology, and physiology. Another 450 items are drawn from the clinical science disciplines of internal medicine, obstetrics/gynecology, pediatrics, preventive medicine and public health, psychiatry, and surgery. The 13 disciplines are represented in the examination by approximately equal numbers of items.

An overall designation of pass or fail is reported together with a numeric score for the basic sciences and clinical sciences. Further breakdowns of scores into specific disciplines are not routinely reported. Examinees are required to pass *both* the basic science test and the clinical science test in order to achieve an overall passing score on the examination. The relatively high level of emphasis placed on the basic science disciplines and the establishment of a level of pass or fail based on the performance of the graduates of United States medical schools suggest that the FMG Examination in the Medical Sciences is as difficult as Part I and Part II of the National Board Examinations.

SUMMARY

The following are key points which you should remember as you prepare for the examination.

1. Start early (at least 6 to 12 months before the examination) and plan your strategy for preparation.

2. Large, standardized examinations measure not only the abilities they are designed to assess, but also test taking skills. Master the skills that will help you with the test.

3. Examinations should be approached positively because they can serve important functions for the examinee as well as the faculties and licensing groups who use them for decision making.

4. The past performance on examinations by you and your peers will provide an important clue in predicting your score on the next examination.

5. Administer self-assessment examinations to yourself *before* you begin to review the content being examined.

6. Concentrate on and improve your areas of weakness. Be honest with yourself.

7. Early specialization during residency training will tend to lower performance on examinations of general clinical competence.

8. Register to take the examination as soon as possible after completion of the relevant courses or clerkships.

9. A pass/fail grading system may not provide you with adequate detailed information regarding your strengths and weaknesses.

10. Use a commercial review course only as a last resort.

11. The questions in medical examinations are actually written by teachers, research scientists, and clinicians who are faculty members at a variety of medical colleges.

12. Do not waste time trying to unravel exceedingly difficult questions. Mark them and return if you have time, or make your best guess.

13. Become familiar with the standard formats used for multiple choice questions.

14. If your examination will include PMPs, become well acquainted with that format since the scoring differs from multiple choice tests.

15. Use the test outline provided by the publisher as your overall study guide. Concentrate on your areas of weakness.

16. In most cases do not be concerned with the current literature in your preparation for a written examination.

17. Relax during the examination. Schedule your time and monitor it carefully.

18. Assess objectively your strengths and weaknesses after the examination as insurance in case you must repeat it.

19. Learn about the unique features of the examination you will be taking, especially the types of items used, the scoring methods, and the interpretation of subtest scores.

REFERENCES

Gonnella JS, Veloski JJ: The impact of early specialization on the clinical competence of residents. N Engl J Med 306:275, 1982
> Differences in the level of performance on Part III of the National Board Examinations for residents in flexible programs, family medicine, internal medicine, obstetrics/gynecology, pediatrics, psychiatry, and surgery are reported.

Hubbard JP: Measuring Medical Education: The Tests and the Experience of the National Board of Medical Examiners. 2nd Ed. Lea and Febiger, Philadelphia, 1978
> This is a thorough presentation of the technology behind the National Board Examinations, including a few sample questions and a PMP.

Millman J, Pauk W: How to Take Tests. McGraw-Hill, New York, 1969
> Representative of many general books on test taking, this or a similar book will be useful if you have had limited experience with large multiple-choice examinations.

Resident and Staff Physician, each October issue since 1980.
> Each year a number of articles in the October issue are devoted to hints on taking examinations, directories of information on standardized tests, and the personal anecdotes of successful examinees.

Sarnacki RE: Test Taking Skills: A Programmed Text for Medicine and the Health Sciences. University Park Press, Baltimore 1981
> If you are inexperienced with multiple-choice questions this book of programmed instruction or a similar text should be reviewed.

Scott LK, Scott CW, Palmisano PA, et al: The effects of commercial coaching for the NBME Part I Examination, J Med Educ 55:733, 1980
> If you are debating whether or not you should take a commercial test preparation course reading this study of 55 second year medical students from the University of Alabama in Birmingham may help you to decide.

Weinberg E, Bell A: Performance of United States Citizens with Foreign Medical Education on Standardized Medical Examinations. N Engl J Med 299:858, 1978
> This article summarizes data on the performance of foreign medical graduates on examinations.

Zeleznik C, Hojat M, Veloski JJ: Long range predictive and differential validities of the scholastic aptitude test in medical school. Educ Psychol Measurement, 43:223, 1983
> This article provides evidence that performance on the SAT is related to performance on the National Board Examinations.

Section 1

Basic
Medical Sciences

2

Anatomy

L. J. A. DiDio

INTRODUCTION

Anatomy is a branch of morphology, the "study of form." The two terms are occasionally used synonymously. Human anatomy, the study and description of form, structure, and organization of human beings, consists of cytology and subcellular structure, embryology, histology, gross anatomy, neuroanatomy, physical anthropology, and history (of anatomy), thus, including all levels of organization from subcellular particles to man and human groups, including the development of this knowledge as well.

Human anatomy is the foundation of medical sciences. It also has significant relationships with most human endeavors in many areas, such as esthetics, philosophy, theology, art, history, and sports.

The study of medicine and of health sciences includes:

1. Subcellular structure
2. Cytology or cell biology
3. Histology or tissue biology
4. Organology or organ biology
5. Embryology
6. Fetology
7. Neonatology
8. Nepiology (anatomy of the infant who "does not speak" yet)
9. Anatomy of the child
10. Adult anatomy
11. Gerontologic anatomy
12. Applied anatomy (surgical and clinical anatomy)
13. Living anatomy
14. Surface anatomy
15. Constitutional (biotypologic or somatotypic) anatomy
16. Artistic anatomy (the evaluation of form or beauty for esthetic or plastic surgery)
17. Radiologic anatomy
18. Comparative anatomy
19. Systemic anatomy or system biology
20. Topographic or regional anatomy

ANATOMICAL NOMENCLATURE

Nomina anatomica (anatomic names or nomenclature), *Nomina embryologica, Nomina histologica, Nomina medica,* and *Nomina anatomica veterinaria* are lists of official internationally accepted terms for use in the health sciences and related fields. Human anatomic nomenclature is the basis for the technical language used in anatomy, medicine, dentistry, and all biologic sciences dealing with the morphology of man. It is divided into general and special terminology.

General Anatomic Nomenclature

To indicate the parts of the body, a conventional "anatomic position for description" is assumed; the individual is standing, the superior members extended at each side of the body, the eyes are looking straight ahead, the face, palms, and tips of the toes are directed forward. For teaching purposes, the body is compared to a parallelepiped, a solid geometric figure defined as a rectangular prism having parallelograms as its base, sides, and top.

A. Main divisions of the body
    Head
    Neck
    Trunk
        thorax
        abdomen
        pelvis
    Back
        nuchal region
        thoracic dorsum
        gluteal region
    Members
        superior
            shoulder
            axilla
            arm
            elbow
            forearm
            wrist
            hand
            fingers
        inferior
            hip
            thigh
            knee
            leg
            ankle
            foot
            toes

B. Axes (imaginary lines, one in each direction)
Each major axis is drawn from the center of one limiting plane to the opposite.
  1. Vertical, longitudinal, superoinferior, craniocaudal, cephalopodalic, cephaloplantar, cranioplantar
  2. Horizontal, transverse, transversal
    a. Anteroposterior, ventrodorsal
    b. Laterolateral, right, left

C. Limiting planes
  1. Horizontal or transverse planes
    a. Superior, cephalic, cranial
    b. Inferior, podalic, plantar, caudal (tangential to tip of coccyx)
  2. Vertical or longitudinal planes
    a. Anterior, ventral
    b. Posterior, dorsal
    c. Lateral, right, left

D. Planes of section
Fundamental sections are longitudinal, transversal, and oblique.
  1. Longitudinal sections

    a. Median anteroposterior or sagittal section resulting in right and left halves of the body. There are infinite paramedian planes of sections.
    b. Median frontal or coronal section and infinite parallel planes of section, resulting in anterior and posterior portions of the body and its parts.
  2. Transversal sections (almost all horizontal)
  Median transversal and infinite parallel planes of section, resulting in superior and inferior portions of the body or its parts.
  3. Situation, position, and directional terms
  Each organ is compared to a solid geometric figure where faces, margins (borders), extremities (ends), and center may be recognized. The following adjectives are commonly used:
  Medial: An organ or its parts facing the median anteroposterior plane
  Lateral: Opposite to medial
  Median: Structures situated in the sagittal plane
  Mesial: A tooth, its margin or face nearer to the sagittal plane
  Distal or lateral: Opposite to mesial
  Proximal: In the proximity or nearer the center (used for locomotor, respiratory, circulatory, urinary, reproductive, and nervous systems; not used for the digestive system)
  Medius, mid- or middle: An organ between two others (superior and inferior, anterior and posterior, internal or external to it)
  Internal: Toward the cavity (for head, trunk)
  External: Opposite to internal
  Superficial: Nearer to the surface or external to the muscular fascia
  Deep: Opposite to superficial
  Oral: Near the mouth (for digestive system)
  Aboral: Opposite to oral
  Preaxial: Corresponding to thumb or hallux
  Postaxial: Opposite to preaxial
  Ulnar: Same as medial in superior members
  Radial: Opposite to ulnar
  Tibial: Same as medial in inferior members
  Fibular: Opposite to tibial
  Palmar: Anterior in the hand
  Plantar: Inferior in the foot
  Rostral: Relating or toward the rostrum (beak, snout) or anterior end of an animal (for nervous system).
  Central: Near or toward the center (for circulatory, nervous system)
  Peripheral: Opposite to central

Special Anatomic Nomenclature

To name each structure and its parts.

ARCHITECTURE OF THE HUMAN BODY

The body is built with subcellular particles or organelles, cells, tissues, supracellular units, anatomicosurgical segments, organs, and systems or apparatuses.

Man has characteristics of mammals, trichozoa, and vertebrates. These characteristics include mammary glands, hair, vertebral column, amnion, and placenta.

In each body, a gross bilateral symmetry (with several morphologic and physiologic exceptions), metamerism, pachymerism or tubulation, and stratification are observed. In fact, the median anteroposterior plane divides the body into "similar" but not identical right and left portions, as is apparent on the surface or deep within structures.

The body shows, especially in the trunk and better seen in the embryo, similar portions that are arranged longitudinally and separated by transversal planes, called metameres (spinal nerves, ribs).

In the body a frontal plane isolates an axial, dorsal, posterior, or neural tube (pachymere or canal) and a large ventral anterior or visceral tube (pachymere, canal, or cavity).

The body and its parts are made up of concentrically arranged layers or strata (skin, intestine, vessel).

NORMAL INDIVIDUAL

A normal individual or structure is defined in medicine as healthy, in physiology as the one that is best suited for optimal performance, and in anatomy as the most frequent (statistically). Variations are slight deviations from the normal morphologic pattern of the body or its parts; they are so frequent that "variation is the most *constant* finding" (there is no man, there are men; there is no disease, there are diseases). Anomaly, abnormality, deformity, or malformation is a congenital or acquired deviation from the normal morphology and physiology. A severe anomaly incompatible with life is a monstrosity, studied in teratology. When these slight or severe deviations occur in 1 to 2 percent of the cases, they are considered rare and called rarities.

FACTORS OF VARIATION

Factors responsible for the appearance of variations are general and individual.

General Factors

General factors include:

Age (e.g., in addition to size, the presence of a relatively large thymus in children; newborn infants are not merely miniatures of adults).

Sex (e.g., in addition to genital organs, the prominentia laryngea is usually better seen in men than in women).

Race (e.g., in addition to common racial somatic characteristics, such as skin color, type of nose, hair, lips, and eyelids, the vermiform appendix is longer, thicker, and wider in blacks than in whites and the termination of the spinal cord reaches the level of the 2nd lumbar vertebra more frequently in blacks than in whites).

Biotype, body build, physique, body constitution, or somatotype is the morphologic facet of the constitutional type of the individual; the others are the biochemical, physiologic, pathologic, psychologic, and psychopathic. The morphologic patterns of the biotype are the longitype (members relatively more developed than the trunk), the brachytype (opposite features), and the many transitional mediotypes intermediary to the preceding two types (e.g., the hook-shaped stomach is more frequent in longitypes and the steer-horn shape is more frequent in brachytypes).

Evolution (e.g., cranial capacity and stature have increased from caveman to modern man).

Environment (e.g., men living in equatorial, tropical, or polar regions exhibit differences).

Biorhythms (e.g., periodic alternation of function causing morphologic changes, such as those of the uterus and pineal body).

Sport (e.g., muscular "hypermorphisms" occur according to the different modality of sports practiced by individuals).

Gravity, though classifiable under environment, space travel experiments have shown structural changes under weightlessness.

Individual Factors

Each individual presents certain variations that are responsible for special morphologic features. For example, fingerprints, utilized for purposes of identification and in forensic medicine, as well as many other variations, can be detected by means of radiology.

Postmortem Changes

After death morphologic changes occur. Some are caused by rigor mortis and others by other phenomena, such as muscular relaxation or loss of tonus (e.g., the intestinal length is greater after than before death). The action of formaldehyde, used during embalming, obviously produces changes (e.g., the ileal papilla, at the termination of the small intestine in the living individual, becomes a postmortem valvelike frenulated structure).

CYTOLOGY

Cells are biologic units that are usually grouped in tissues. The three major components of the cell are the plasmalemma, the cytoplasm, and the nucleus.

The plasmalemma or cytolemma is the outermost limiting membrane made up of a lipid bilayer coated on either side by proteins (the unit membrane). Globular proteins are also scattered between lipid molecules, and they may be gliding in the plasmalemma. Glycocalyx, the cell coat, is made up of polysaccharides, some are protein-bound and others are synthesized by the cells.

The three types of plasmalemma specializations are of the free cell surface (e.g., microvilli), of contact surfaces (e.g., desmosomes), and of the cellular base (e.g., infoldings).

1. Microvilli are found in proximal convoluted tubules, in epithelial cells of the gallbladder, of the intestine, and of the uterus, and in hepatic and mesothelial cells, among many others. Other specializations at this level are stereocilia, cilia, and flagella.
2. Between cellular contact surfaces there are areas of firm attachment. Tight junction (zonula occludens), intermediate junction (zonula adherens), and desmosomes (maculae adherentes); the first two beltlike and the latter a discontinuous buttonlike structure. The nexus or gap junction is called the "macula communicans" or communicating spot.
3. Specializations of the basal plasmalemma are found in cells involved in water transport and appear as infoldings which penetrate the cytoplasm.

Interdigitations of the Plasmalemma of Adjacent Cells

The cytoplasm is made up of a cytoplasmic matrix or cytosol containing organelles and inclusions (International Anatomical Nomenclature Committee, 1983).

Organelles and inclusions comprise the following structures:

Cytocentrum, possessing centriole and diplosome

Mitochondrion, having a membrane and mitochondrial cristae (with elementary particles), tubules, matrix, inclusions, granules, and filaments

Golgi's complex, containing vesicles, lamellae, vacuoles, and sacculi

Endoplasmic reticulum, comprising lamellae, tubuli, sacculi, cisternae, and of two forms (granular or agranular endoplasmic reticulum)

Ribosomes and polyribosomes (polysomes)

Annulate lamellae

Cytoplasmic and pinocytotic vesicles

Lysosomes, peroxysomes, phagosomes, phagolysosomes, microbodies

Autophagic and heterophagic vacuoles

Corpora cepiformia or onionoid bodies

Residual corpuscles

Cytoskeleton (microtubules, microfibrils, microfilaments)

Multivesicular bodies

Granules, such as secretory, protein, glycogen, and pigment

Crystalloid inclusions

Lipid droplets

Kinetosomes, in the cilia rootlets

The nucleus is enclosed in a bilayered envelope, the outer layer belonging to the endoplasmic reticulum (ER). The nuclear envelope shows many pores through which contact is established between the nucleoplasm and the cytoplasm.

The nucleus contains the following structures:

Karyo- or caryotheca. It has an outer and an inner nuclear membrane, an intervening caryothecal cisterna, and nuclear pores.

Nucleoplasm (caryoplasm). It has chromatin (granules, eu- and heterochromatin).

Sexual chromatin corpuscle.

Nucleolus (nucleonema, pars filamentosa, and pars granulosa).

Cells reproduce or divide by mitosis, amitosis (direct), or meiosis. Mitosis takes place in phases: pro-, meta-, ana-, and telophases. During meiosis, the chromosomes of the prospective gametes are reduced to half or one set (haploid), while during mitosis each cell receives the diploid number (two sets) of chromosomes. Meiosis occurs in spermatogenesis and oogenesis.

Cell cycle comprises mitosis and interphase (i.e., periodus intervalli primi (G_1 for gap-preduplication), periodus synthesis (S), periodus intervalli secundi (G_2 postduplication) periodus mitotica (M)).

HISTOLOGY

Histology deals with general microscopic features of tissues, structures, or materials that constitute organs. Tissues are a collection of morphologically and physiologically similar cells with their interstitial substance.

For teaching purposes, tissues can be classified according to their intercellular substance and the form of their cells, as follows:

1. Tissues without (or very little) intercellular substance (epithelial)
2. Tissues with intercellular substance
   Semifluid intercellular substances
      Connective
   Solid intercellular substance
      Cartilaginous
      Bone or osseous
   Fluid intercellular substance
      Blood
      Lymph
3. Tissues with elongated cells
   Partially elongated
      Nervous
   Totally elongated
      Muscular

Epithelial Tissue

Epithelium is made up of one or more layers of epithelial cells and is subdivided into the following types:

1. Simple (single-layered)
Squamous (e.g., in pulmonary alveoli, mesothelium (lining serous cavities), and endothelium (lining vessels)
   Cuboidal
      Ovary, certain renal tubules
   Columnar
      Small intestine
2. Stratified
Squamous
   Keratinized: skin
   Nonkeratinized: mouth, epiglottis, esophagus, vagina
   Cuboidal
      Ducts of sweat glands
   Columnar
      Olfactory mucosa
3. Pseudostratified (ciliated and nonciliated)
Respiratory passages
4. Transitional
Urinary bladder
5. Glandular (cells specialized for secretion)
Uni- or pluricellular glands

The presence or absence of ducts leads to exocrine glands (e.g., parotid gland – saliva), endocrine or ductless glands (e.g., thyroid gland – hormones), and amphicrine glands (e.g., pancreas – pancreatic juice and insulin).

According to the type of secretion discharged, exocrine glands are subdivided into the following:

1. Holocrine glands, which have cells that disintegrate and become part of the secretion (e.g., sebaceous glands).
2. Merocrine glands, which have cells that expel the secretion without any other structural loss (e.g., salivary glands).
3. Apocrine glands, which have cells that lose their apex to become mixed with the secretion (e.g., mammary gland).

Pluricellular glands are subdivided into mucous, serous, and seromucous. They may also be divided into simple or compound; or into tubular, acinous or alveolar, and tubuloalveolar glands.

Connective Tissue

Connective tissue is composed of cells and intercellular substance that is made up of ground substance, fibers, and tissue fluid. Connective cells are fibroblasts, fibrocytes, reticular cells, pericytes (perivascular cells), pigment cells, adipose or fat cells, histiocytes, mast cells, lymphocytes, plasma cells, monocytes, and granulocytes.

The intercellular substance has a fundamental or ground substance (containing polysaccharides and nonesterified mucopolysaccharides, such as hyaluronic acid), and collagenous, elastic, and reticular fibers.

Varieties of connective tissue are:

Mesenchyme: unspecialized
Mucoid connective tissue (e.g., in umbilical cord and vitreous humor)
Reticular tissue: lymph nodes, bone marrow, and liver
Loose fibrous connective tissue: almost everywhere in the body
Dense fibrous connective tissue: fasciae, dermis, capsules, periosteum, perichondrium, tendons, and ligaments
Adipose tissue: tela subcutanea
Elastic tissue: intervertebral (yellow) ligaments
Hematopoietic tissue: lymphoid structures and bone marrow
Reticulohistiocytic (macrophagic) system: suprarenal, hypophyseal, splenic, and hepatic sinusoids

Cartilaginous Tissue

Cartilaginous tissue is a specialized connective tissue, made up of chondroblasts, chondrocytes, and a prevailing solid but flexible intercellular substance, which contains fibers and chondromucoid, a glycoprotein, rich in chondroitin sulfuric acid. Cartilage forms the preosseous skeleton of the body, and, in the adult, organs, such as the ears, respiratory passages, and joints. There are three varieties of cartilage:

1. Hyaline cartilage, containing numerous collagenous fibers (e.g., in the nose, larynx, trachea, ribs, and on articular surfaces of bones).
2. Elastic cartilage, containing many elastic fibers (e.g., in the epiglottis, auditory tube, and external ear).
3. Fibrous cartilage, containing dense fibrous connective tissue and hyaline cartilage (e.g., the intervertebral discs and pubic symphysis).

Osseous Tissue

Bone is a specialized connective tissue, made up of osteoblasts, osteocytes, osteoclasts, (eroding cells), and a prevailing solid nonflexible matrix or intercellular substance, which contains fibers and ground substance impregnated with inorganic salts (calcium phosphate as hydroxyapatites, calcium carbonate, calcium fluoride, and magnesium fluoride).

As in connective and cartilaginous tissues, in bone tissue the intercellular substance prevails upon the cellular component. Bone matrix is arranged in concentric lamellae, whose lacunae contain osteocytes. The lamellae surround a capillary on an arteriole, a venule, and a lymphatic vessel in a central (Havers') canal, thus constituting a supracellular functional unit (the smallest portion able to function as the entire organ) called osteon (or Haversian system). Perforating transverse (Volkmann's) canals originate from the peri- and endosteum to reach the central canals.

Bone can be compact or spongy (trabecular) such as the spaces filled with bone marrow. Long bones contain a medullary cavity also filled with bone marrow. Periosteum is made up of a fibrous and an osteogenic layer. Collagenous fibers originating from the periosteum and reaching the periosteal lamellae are the perforating (Sharpey's) fibers. Endosteum lines the bone marrow cavities.

Bone formation, called osteogenesis, leads to the development of membranous or cartilaginous bone. Reconstruction, remodeling, erosion, and deposition of bone in different areas occur in undifferentiated mesenchyme. Membranous osteogenesis starts in a membrane of mesenchyme due to an ossification center (e.g., in the cranial vault). Mesenchymal cells differentiate into osteoblasts, which lay down trabeculae of collagenous fibers and ground substance. Osteoblasts become osteocytes surrounded by the bone matrix and the tissue is called osteoid (ossification without calcification).

After impregnation with mineral salts, the tissue becomes osseous and the flat bone is surrounded by periosteum. Cartilaginous osteogenesis takes place in a hyaline cartilage that represents the model of the future (short or long) bone by peri- and endochondral ossification. Replacement (and no transformation) of cartilage by bone takes place. The primary ossification center grows longitudinally from the diaphysis toward the epiphyses where a secondary ossification center later appears and expands radially.

Growth occurs as long as active cartilage remains, except at the level of joints where articular cartilage persists to perform other functions. However, at the level of the metaphysis (the portion of the diaphysis adjacent to the epiphysis), is the epiphyseal cartilage, which is responsible for growth in length until early adulthood. It is made up of the capping or resting, proliferative (growth), hypertrophic cartilage, calcified, and ossification zones.

Bone is continuously being remodeled (formed and destroyed) and bone resorption takes place by osteocytic and osteoclastic lysis (osteolysis).

Blood Tissue

Blood can be described as the tissue made up of elements separated by a fluid intercellular substance. The elements of the blood are cells or corpuscles (erythro- and leukocytes) and platelets; all are suspended in the fluid blood plasma.

Erythrocytes (red blood cells) are biconcave discs (7.2 μm in diameter). They do not possess a nucleus when mature. Their number is 5,000,000/cu mm on average, whereas that of leukocytes is 8000/cu mm. All cells together are approximately equivalent in bulk to the plasma. The volume of blood in the adult is 5 L (10 percent of the body weight). The red color of erythrocytes is due to a colloidal complex (lipoid plus a protein, mainly hemoglobin). Hemoglobin, responsible for O_2 transport, appears as HbO_2 or after releasing O_2 and combined with CO_2, as carbaminohemoglobin. Agglutination is the aggregation into clumps of erythrocytes, and may occur under pathologic conditions.

Leukocytes are formed in the lymphoid, myelopoietic, and reticular components of the reticuloendothelial system. They may have a myeloid, a lymphoid, or a monocytic line of evolution from primitive cells. Leukocytes are classified as follows:

1. Agranular
   Lymphocytes
   Monocytes
2. Granular
   Neutrophils
   Basophils
   Eosinophils

In a blood smear the average percentages of leukocytes are:

Lymphocytes	22%
Monocytes	5%
Neutrophils	68%
Basophils	2%
Eosinophils	3%

The degree of activity (tissue migration, ameboid movement, and phagocytosis) is highest in neutrophils, followed by monocytes and basophils, and lowest in lymphocytes, which migrate as a rule to sites of chronic inflammation. Eosinophils increase in number in cases of allergy and in those of parasitic infestations.

Blood platelets (thrombocytes) are groups of granular protoplasmic discs, exhibiting a variety of shapes, and having neither nucleus nor hemoglobin. Their size is $\frac{1}{2}$ to $\frac{1}{3}$ that of an erythrocyte (2 to 4 μm in diameter), and their number ranges from 200,000 to 300,000/cu mm of blood. Their function in blood clotting is indicated in the thrombocytes. The life span of erythrocytes is 4 months and that of leukocytes is approximately 1 day.

Hematopoiesis, or hematocytopoiesis, occurs in bone marrow (for erythro- and granulocytes) and in lymph nodes (for lymphocytes) in the adult. It includes erythrocytopoiesis, granulocytopoiesis, megakaryocytopoiesis, thrombocytopoiesis, lymphocytopoiesis, plasmacytopoiesis, and monocytopoiesis.

Blood plasma may diffuse through vascular walls, and is then named tissue fluid. Plasma is a solution of colloids (proteins, such as albumin and fibrinogen) and crystalloids, being 90 percent water and 10 percent solutes (55 percent of the blood volume).

Lymph Tissue

Lymph is a tissue made up of cells, mostly lymphocytes, suspended in a fluid intercellular substance (lymph plasma). The composition of lymph in lymphatic capillaries is almost the same as the tissue fluid and only differs in afferent and efferent vessels (to and from lymph nodes). Lymph in the thoracic duct contains more lymphocytes and more fat globules than the lymph of other vessels, especially if the sample is taken postprandially (lymph known as chyle). Lymph in the thoracic duct is 3 percent protein while in peripheral vessels is only 0.6 percent protein. Peripheral lymph contains 450 leukocytes/cu mm (85 percent are lymphocytes) and several hundred erythrocytes. Lymph coagulation is slower and its coagulum is softer than blood coagulation and coagulum, respectively.

Nervous Tissue

Nervous or neural tissue is made up of partially elongated cells, namely neurons (morphofunctional units), specialized for irritability and conductivity, and neuroglia, (gliacytes or gliacells, supporting cells).

NEURONS

A neuron comprises a cell body (perikaryon) that has branched processes (dendrites) and an axon. Dendrites and axons are called nerve fibers, and their branches are called collaterals and terminal arborizations.

The contact between neurons is termed a synapsis or synapse (interneuronal junction), which is axodendritic or axosomatic (when the axon is related directly to a perikaryon).

Dendrites are afferent processes to the perikaryon, and the axon is efferent (i.e., it transmits neural impulses away from the perikaryon). Neurons may be uni-, bi-, or multipolar. Unipolar (pseudounipolar) neurons have one process that bifurcates into an afferent (dendritic) peripheral branch and an efferent (axonic) central branch. Bipolar neurons have a single dendrite and an axon, where as, multipolar neurons have several dendrites and an axon. Unipolar neurons are found in spinal ganglia, bipolar neurons in sense organs, and multipolar neurons in the central nervous system (CNS). Dendrites present many branches that in turn ramify profusely.

The cytoplasm of the cell body contains granular ER, the nucleus (and nucleolus), and the chromophil or tigroid substance (Nissl bodies), the latter extending into the dendrites and into only an area adjacent to the origin of the axon (axon hillock). Neurofibrils are found in the cell body, the dendrites, and the axon. The Golgi complex is situated in the cell body. Mitochondria are more abundant in the axon terminals, microtubules in the cell body, and inclusions (melanin, lipofuscin) in the cell body of certain areas of the CNS.

Each axon possesses an axolemma and an axoplasm. Axons may or may not be surrounded by myelin (phospholipids and neurokeratogenic protein), a layered white substance responsible for the color of the white matter of the CNS. Remak's or nonmyelinated fibers are found in the autonomic nervous system (ANS), and are covered by neurolemma or Schwann's Sheath (made up of neurolemmocytes or Schwann's cells). Myelinated fibers have both neurolemma and myelin, and their axons present narrowings (nodi neurofibrae or Ranvier's nodes). Fissures (incisurae myelini or Schmidt-Lantermann's clefts) in the myelin sheath extend to the axon. Bundles of nerve fibers make up nerve fascicles, groups of nerve fascicles constitute nerves, and groups of nerves form a nerve trunk. Each nerve is surrounded by the connective tissue, epineurium (collagenous and elastic fibers), each fascicle by a thinner layer of connective tissue called perineurium, which sends partitions (endoneurium) to separate individual fibers (Henle's or Key and Retzius' sheath).

Motor endings are terminations of efferent fibers (e.g., motor end-plate and end-bulb), of small loops, nodular thickenings, for muscles or glands. Sensory (afferent) endings include free endings, encapsulated endings, genital, lamellar (Pacini's), bulbous (Krause's), and cylindrical corpuscles, and muscle spindles.

NEUROGLIA

Neuroglia is one of the accessory elements of the nervous system, the others being connective tissue, neurolemma, and capsular cells of ganglia. Gliacytes protect and support neurons and connect them with blood vessels.

Gliacytes. These cells intervene between neurons and basal lamina of blood capillaries, at the level of the blood-brain barrier. Gliacytes are divided into two groups: central and peripheral.

Central gliacytes comprise ependymocytes (from ependyma), the lining of the primitive neural tube, encephalic ventricles, and central canal. Protoplasmic astrocytes (from ectoderm) are found in gray matter and fibrous astrocytes (from ectoderm) are found in white matter. Oligodendrocytes (from ectoderm) are found in gray and white matter and are related to capillaries. Microglia (from mesoderm) are phagocytic cells that move to areas where there is pathologic nervous tissue.

Peripheral gliacytes include ganglionic and terminal gliacytes and neurolemmocytes.

Muscular Tissue

The muscular tissue consists of myocytes (i.e., totally elongated cells (fibers) for contraction (shortening) and thus movement). Each muscular fiber has a sarcolemma, a sarcoplasm containing myofibrils, and sarcoplasmic reticulum, among other organelles, and a nucleus. A sarcomere is a cylindrical segment limited by two successive Z lines and can be considered a contractile unit. A

myon, comparable to a neuron, corresponds to the functional unit of muscular tissue (i.e., the minimum amount of tissue able to function as the organ). There are three types of musculature:

Skeletal: Cross and longitudinally striated; voluntary; innervated by the CNS
Cardiac: Cross and longitudinally striated; voluntary; innervated by the ANS.
Smooth: Only longitudinally striated; involuntary; innervated by the ANS.

SKELETAL MUSCLE

Skeletal muscle derives from mesoderm and its myocytes present sarcolemma (covered by glycocalyx) and myofibrils that are thicker than those of smooth muscular cells, and of the eccentric nucleus. Myofibrils show successive bands of periodically alternating refractive indexes (anisotropic dark disk or A stria or band, and isotropic light disk or I stria or band). The dark A band is intersected by a thick light H band, which in turn is bisected by a thin M line (mesophragma). The light I band is bisected by a thin Z line (telophragma). The bands of adjacent myofibrils are in register (at the same level).

Myofibrils ($2\,\mu$m in diameter) comprise longitudinally parallel thick ($100\,\text{Å}$ in diameter) and thin ($50\,\text{Å}$) myofilaments. Thick myofilaments occupy the A band (the central portion of the sarcomere) whereas the thin ones have midpoints at the level of the Z line (where they are attached, interdigitating with the thick myofilaments). The A band contains both types of myofilaments whereas the H band contains only the thick ones. The I band consists only of thin myofilaments, since its width is limited by the ends of the thick myofilaments.

Thin myofilaments contain the three proteins actin, tropomyosin, and troponin; the thick myofilaments contain myosin.

A triad of sarcolemmal tubules (T system) transversely encircle the myofibrils at the level of the A bands in amphibia, and two T tubules per sarcomere in mammals, in which there is better stimulus transmission. Mitochondria are large and numerous, having closely packed parallel cristae. The Golgi complex is near one of the poles of the nucleus, and glycogen granules are abundant.

Cohnheim's areas are muscular columns of groups of fibrils separated by sarcoplasm when seen in cross section.

Connective tissue fibers insert into the sarcolemma at the level of the myotendon junction.

Skeletal muscle is divided into red (richer in sarcoplasm), intermediate, and white, depending on the amount of pigment (myoglobin) and density of vascularity. Endomysium surrounds single myofibers, perimysium encircles muscular fascicles, and epimysium covers groups of fascicles. Blood vessels reach the endomysium (where capillaries intervene between muscular fibers) through the epi- and perimysium. Lymphatic vessels are limited to epi- and perimysium.

A motor unit is made up of a muscle fiber and its neuron (somatic motor neuron). The area of contact between the end of an axon and the myofiber is called the motor- or end-plate or myoneural junction. Acetylcholine is liberated at the myoneural junction, thus, increasing the permeability of the plasmalemma.

CARDIAC MUSCLE

The myocardium has some of the characteristics of the skeletal and the smooth muscle, but its function differs from both since its contractions are rhythmic and automatic.

Cardiomyocytes possess central nuclei, have more sarcoplasm, mitochondria, and glycogen than skeletal muscle cells, and present an additional special striation (the intercalated disks) to maintain cell cohesion. Actin myofilaments insert in specialized areas of cellular contact, which thus become equivalent to intercalated disks. Gap junctions are found along the sides of intercalated disks, corresponding to areas of low electrical resistance; in each nexus (gap junction) the spread of excitation impulses from myocyte to myocyte occurs easily.

Cardiomyocytes exhibit the same striae (bands) and lines of the skeletal myocytes. The sarcolemmal T tubular invaginations, located at the level of the Z line, are larger in ventricular cardiomyocytes than in skeletal myocytes. The T tubules are in close contact with the branched sarcoplasmic reticulum.

SMOOTH MUSCLE

Myocytes of smooth musculature are fusiform and possess sarcolemma covered by glycoprotein and a central nucleus with a nucleolus. They derive from loose mesenchyme and vary from 15 μ to 0.5 mm in diameter. Their myofibrils are extremely thin. Fibers are packed together in bands, layers, or sheets. The sarcoplasm contains thin longitudinal myofilaments, most of the organelles near the nuclear poles, and the micropinocytotic vesicles in subsarcolemmal position. These myocytes are surrounded by a network of reticular fibers, by capillaries and nerve fibers, in the walls of viscera. Smooth muscle cells are able to contract and to synthesize elastic and collagenous material as well as proteoglycans (e.g., in arterial and uterine walls).

EMBRYOLOGY OR PRENATAL DEVELOPMENT

Embryology in a narrow sense is the study of the embryo, (i. e., the organism from the second to the eighth week after fertilization or conception; formation of the ovum). In a broad sense it includes the oology or ovology (the study of the fertilized ovum) and fetology (the study of the fetus, from the ninth week to birth; the prenatal development) until neonatology (the study of the newborn).

In the male and female the formation of spermatozoon and egg cell (ovum), respectively, is called gametogenesis (spermatogenesis and ovogenesis), and is characterized by meiosis, causing a chromosomal reduction from diploid to haploid number. Spermatogenesis is followed by spermiogenesis, the conversion of spermatids into spermatozoa. Semen volume must be above 1 ml and sperm concentration above 20,000/ ml, with less than 15 percent abnormal sperm to be fertile (below these minimum figures the male is sterile).

Fertilization (in the ampulla or in the lateral $\frac{1}{3}$ of the uterine tube) is followed by the ovum transport to the uterus, then preimplantation and implantation. With fertilization, the diploid number of 46 chromosomes is restored, and cleavage (series of mitoses) of the zygote takes place, resulting in blastomeres or daughter cells by the seventh day postfertilization. This mass is termed successively morula and blastula (blastocyst, containing the embryoblast and the trophoblast). The embryoblast then makes up a bilaminar germinal or embryonic disk (ectoderm and endoderm). The trophoblast in turn divides into cytotrophoblast and syncytiotrophoblast (eighth day). The amniotic cavity (the roof of which is the amnion) appears between the ectoderm and the cytotrophoblast. Around the amnion and the primitive yolk sac, the extraembryonic mesoderm and coelom develop (eleventh to twelfth day), followed by the primordial structure corresponding to the umbilical cord. Primary chorionic villi develop from the trophoblast and the somatopleure and the splanchnopleure are formed from the splitting of the mesoderm. The syncytiotrophoblast forms lacunar networks, the primordial intervillous spaces of the placenta. The endometrial erosion ceases when the placenta is formed.

During the third week, the primitive streak appears and the bilaminar disk becomes trilaminar, with the addition of the mesoderm, between the ecto- and the endoderm (gastrulation). The primitive knot forms the notochordal process, canal, and plate; the latter forms the notochord. The neural plate, groove, and folds lead to the neural tube (neurulation) and, at the same time, the neural crest appears. Somites, coelom, blood, blood vessels, and secondary chorionic villi are then formed.

At the end of the embryonic period, the development of the systems of the new organism has begun, having originated from the primitive germ layers.

The derivatives of the ecto-, meso-, and endoderm are the following:

1. Ectoderm
   Integumentary system
     Epidermis
     Hair
     Nails
     Mammary glands
     Sweat glands
     Sebaceous glands
   Nervous system
     Central nervous system (except meninges, vessels, and microglia)
     Peripheral nervous system
     Neural crest (i.e., cells of spinal, cranial, and autonomic ganglia), neurolemmocytes (Schwann's cells), melanocytes, and suprarenal medulla
     Hypophysis
   Sensory system (sense organs)
     Sensory epithelium of the olfactory mucosa
     Sensory epithelium of the inner ear and external epithelium of the eardrum
     Lens and corneal anterior epithelium
   Digestive system
     Enamel of the teeth
     Epithelium of the anterior portion of the oral cavity and its glands, and of the anal portion
   Respiratory system
     Epithelium of the vestibular and nasal cavities, and paranasal sinuses
   Reproductive system
     Epithelium of the distal portion
   Urinary system
     Epithelium of the distal portion
2. Mesoderm
   Connective tissue
   Cartilaginous tissue
   Bone tissue
   Dermis
   Striated and smooth musculature
   Urinary system
   Reproductive system, gonads
   Pleurae, pericardium and peritoneum
   Alimentary tube

Circulatory system, blood cells, lymphatic vessels, hematopoietic organs
   Suprarenal cortex
   Microglia
   Dentine and cementum of teeth
3. Endoderm
   Digestive system
     Lining epithelium (except of the mouth, part of the pharynx, and of the anal canal)
       Pancreas, liver, and remaining glands
       Tonsils
   Respiratory system
     Lining epithelum of larynx, trachea, bronchi, and lungs
   Urinary system
     Lining of bladder (portion), and male (portion) and female urethra and urethral glands
   Endocrine system
     Thyroid, parathyroids, thymic reticulum, and corpuscles
   Sensory organs
     Inner epithelium of eardrum, tympanic cavity, and tube

GROSS ANATOMY

Head

The head is the superior portion of the trunk. It is connected to the thorax by the neck. The inferior limit of the head corresponds on the surface to the inferior border of the mandible, to a horizontal line that extends it posteriorly until it reaches the anterior border of the sternocleidomastoid muscle, where it follows this border up to the mastoid process, then to the superior nuchal line.

On the surface, the head is divided into skull and face by a line that begins at the root of the nose, runs along the superior orbital margin, follows the zygomatic arch, the tragus, and reaches the apex of the mastoid process. The head contains the encephalon, most of the sensory system (sense organs, such as those of sight, hearing, smell, taste, and part of touch), and the initial portions of the digestive and respiratory systems.

The skull (cranium) may be subdivided into superficial regions and cranial cavity. The superficial regions include the frontal, parietal, occipital, and temporal regions, corresponding to the area occupied by each bone in the calvaria. The cranial cavity comprises the anterior, middle, and posterior regions (fossae). The skull is made up of a neurocranium, for the encephalon, and the viscerocranium (aplanchnocranium), for the face. According to the type of bone formation, one may recognize in the skull a chondrocranium (bone replacing cartilage) and desmocranium (membranous bones developing directly from connective tissue).

Neurocranium
Occipital, sphenoid, temporal (squamous and mastoid portions), parietal, and frontal bone

Viscerocranium
Ethmoid, inferior nasal concha, lacrimal, nasal, vomer, maxilla, palatine, zygomatic, temporal (tympanic and styloid processes), mandible, and hyoid bone

Chondrocranium
Occipital (most), sphenoid (most), temporal (most), ear (ossicles), ethmoid, inferior nasal concha, and hyoid bone

Desmocranium
Occipital (part of squama), sphenoid (concha and medial lamella of pterygoid process), temporal (tympanic and squama), parietal, frontal, lacrimal, nasal, vomer, maxilla, palatine, zygomatic bone, and mandible

The newborn skull shows bilateral frontal and parietal eminences and possesses fontanelles such as the anterior (closes by the 36th month) and posterior (closes by the 3rd month), both unpaired, sphenoidal (closes by the 6th month) and mastoid (closes by the 18th month), both paired. The formula of the closure order is 3P, 6S, 18M, 36A (using the number of months and the initial letter of the fonticulus). The fontanelles are also known as bregmatic (anterior), lambdoid (posterior), pteric (sphenoidal), and asteric (mastoid), which correspond to landmarks for anthropologic and obstetric purposes (i.e., bregma, lambda, pterior, and asterior, respectively).

Sagittal, coronal (frontoparietal), sphenofrontal, sphenosquamous, squamous, petrosquamous, lambdoid, sphenoparietal, parietomastoid, and occipitomastoid are the sutures that are found in the young and adult individual.

The acronym "scalp" is the mnemonic procedure by which the order (outward to inward) of the layers of the coverings of the scalp can be remembered. The layers are *s*kin, *c*onnective tissue (dense), *a*poneurosis (galea aponeurotica, between frontal and occipital muscles), *l*oose connective tissue, and *p*ericranium. The skull cap is the calvaria.

The head will be described in superior, posterior, anterior, lateral, inferior, and interior views.

SUPERIOR VIEW OF THE HEAD

The arteries of the scalp are the occipital, posterior, auricular, superficial temporal, supraorbital, and supratrochlear. The veins are the frontal, temporal, posterior auricular, and occipital. The superficial lymphatic vessels form a plexus that drains into the submandibular, preauricular, parotid, mastoid, and occipital lymph nodes. The motor nerves belong to the facial nerve (VII) and the sensory nerves are the supraorbital, frontal, supratrochlear, auriculotemporal, greater auricular, lesser occipital, and greater occipital.

The tela subcutanea contains an outer areolar layer of fat and connective tissue, an intermediate fascia superficialis that corresponds to the epicranial muscle (galea aponeurotica, frontal muscle and occipital muscle), and an inner lamellar layer of adipose and connective tissue. The pericranium is the external periosteum of the skull. The bones consist of two tables (external and internal) of compact substance and the intervening diploë of spongy substance, containing diploic veins. The periosteum lining the internal table is the endocranium (endosteal layer of the dura mater), in turn covering the meninges and the encephalon. The sutures are the interparietal (sagittal), frontoparietal (coronal), and occipitoparietal (lambdoid). The vertex is the highest point of the cranial dome, situated in the midline, behind the bregma.

POSTERIOR VIEW OF THE HEAD

The occipital region corresponds to the occipital bone and to portions of the parietal and temporal (mastoid) bones. The region contains the lambda, the asterion, the external occipital protuberance (inion), and the superior and highest nuchal lines. Vessels and nerves are branches or trunks of those mentioned in the preceding view, of those from adjacent areas, and from the nuchal region.

ANTERIOR VIEW OF THE HEAD

The anterior view of the head comprises the forehead, the orbits, the cheeks, the nose, the mouth, and the chin. The frontal bones are united in the midline (sometimes a metopic suture may persist in the adult) and form the skeleton of the forehead, where the frontal sinuses are found. In this region, the glabella and the superciliary arches are seen. The major structures of the face are the orbits (made up of several bones), the prominence of the cheeks (formed by the zytomatic bone), the nose (the skeleton of which is both bony and cartilaginous), the mouth (corresponding to the maxilla and mandible), and the chin (mandible).

The regions of the face are nasal, orbital, oral, mental,

infraorbital, buccal, and zygomatic. Organs will be mentioned at times combining a few of these regions.

Nasal Region. The nasal region contains the nose, the nasal cavity, and part of the paranasal sinuses. The nose presents the nostrils, separated by the nasal septum. The form of the nose constitutes a racial characteristic (leptorrhine, mesorrhine, and platirrhine). The muscles (or portions of muscles) found in this region are the procerus, nasal, depressor septi, levator labii superioris alaeque nasi, and dilator naris. The vessels in the nasal region are the dorsal artery of the nose and the septal artery, the veins that drain into the angular and the facial, and the lymphatics, which follow the arteries and drain into the submandibular nodes. Motor nerves originate from the facial (VII) and the sensory nerves are branches of the trigeminal (V). The skeleton of the nose is made up of the nasal bones and cartilages (lateral, major, and minor alar, accessory, septal, and vomeronasal). The septal cartilage joins the perpendicular lamina of the ethmoid and the vomer to form the nasal septum, which includes a pars membranacea and a pars ossea. The nasal septum may be deviated. The inferior, mobile, and membranaceous portion of the septum is the clumella.

The nasal cavity is divided by the septum into two fossae (right and left), the apertures of which are the nostrils, the choanae, those of the paranasal sinuses, and those of the nasolacrimal canal.

Each nasal fossa begins with a nasal vestibule, lined by skin, whereas the remainder of the cavity is lined by the tunica mucosa. The vestibule contains hair and its lateral wall presents a prominence, the limen nasi. The paranasal sinuses are extensions of the nasal cavity into neighboring bones (i.e., maxillary, ethmoidal, sphenoidal, and frontal).

In the lateral wall of each fossa three nasal conchae (superior, middle, and inferior) limit three nasal meatuses, where the paranasal sinuses and the nasolacrimal duct open.

Superior meatus: posterior ethmoidal cells
Middle meatus: frontal and maxillary sinuses, anterior ethmoidal cells
Inferior meatus: nasolacrimal duct

The sphenoethmoidal recess, superior and posterior to the superior concha, contains the opening of the sphenoidal sinus.

The nasal fossa is divided into a respiratory and an olfactory region, the latter corresponding to the superior concha and the superior $\frac{1}{3}$ of the septum.

The arteries that supply the nasal area are the ophthalmic, sphenopalatine, anterior, and posterior ethmoidal, ascending palatine, infraorbital, and superior labial. The

veins follow the arteries and drain into the facial, the maxillary plexus, and the ophthalmic. The lymph is drained into the submandibular, retropharyngeal, and jugular lymph nodes. The nerves belong to the trigeminal (V) and to the olfactory (I).

Orbits. The orbits are four sided pyramidal cavities, on each side of the nasal root. They contain the eyes and are related to the anterior and middle cranial fossae, temporal fossa, frontal, sphenoidal and maxillary sinuses, and ethmoidal cells. Near to or at the margins of the base of the orbit there are the supraorbital foramen, the infraorbital foramen, and the fossa for the lacrimal sac. The superior wall (roof) is made up of the frontal and sphenoid bones, presenting the fossa for the lacrimal gland, the trochlear pit, and the optic canal. The lateral wall (zygomatic and sphenoid bones) shows the orbital eminence, palpable in the living, the superior orbital fissure (leading to the middle cranial fossa), and the inferior orbital fissure (leading to the infratemporal and pterygopalatine fossae).

The inferior wall (maxilla, zygomatic, and palatine bones) shows the infraorbital groove and canal.

The medial wall (ethmoid, lacrimal, and frontal bones) presents the anterior and posterior ethmoidal foramina.

The superior orbital fissure transmits cranial nerves III, IV, and VI, the ophthalmic (V) nerve (and its branches) and veins.

The inferior orbital fissure transmits the infraorbital (V) nerve and artery and the zygomatic nerve.

The ophthalmic nerve divides into lacrimal, frontal (supraorbital and supratrochlear nerves), and nasociliary branches (branch to ciliary ganglion, long ciliary, infratrochlear, and anterior ethmoidal nerves).

The ophthalmic artery gives off the central artery of the retina, long and short posterior ciliary arteries, lacrimal (recurrent meningeal branch), muscular branches (anterior ciliary arteries), supraorbital, anterior ethmoidal, palpebral arteries, and two terminal branches (supratrochlear and dorsal nasal arteries). Vorticose veins drain into the ophthalmic veins (superior and inferior), which end in the facial vein, pterygoid plexus, and cavernous sinus. Oculomotor (III) nerve supplies all muscles of the eyeball except the superior oblique (innervated by the trochlear or IV nerve) and the lateral rectus (innervated by the abducent or VI nerve).

The ciliary ganglion is lateral to the optic nerve and has three roots from the nasociliary nerve, nerve III and the internal carotid plexus (to the dilator pupillae). It gives the short ciliary nerves for the ciliary muscle and sphincter pupillae.

The muscles of the eyeball are four recti (superior, lateral, inferior, and medial), and two oblique (superior and inferior).

The optic (II) nerve is the tract from the retina to the chiasma; it is surrounded by sheaths, which are meningeal extensions, and is contained in the cone of the recti muscles, closely related to the ophthalmic artery, nasociliary nerve internal carotid, and hypophysis. The optic (II) nerve contains the central artery of the retina and passes through the optic canal to reach the optic chiasma.

The eyelids or palpebrae are located in front of each orbit to protect the eyeball and to spread the tears on the cornea. The superior and inferior eyelids limit the palpebral fissure and meet at the lateral and medial canthi. The eyelids present eyelashes, ciliary glands, and lacrimal punctum, lake, and caruncle, the latter lying on the plica semilunaris. The levator palpebrae superioris muscle is innervated by nerve VI and inserts into the skin of the eyelid and the superior tarsal muscle (supplied by the ANS) which, in turn, inserts into the superior tarsal plate. The tarsal plates (related to the tarsal glands) are connected to the medial and lateral palpebral ligaments, the latter being inserted into the orbital eminence of the zygomatic bone.

The orbital septum is the limit between the deep contents of the orbit and the superficial structures.

The palpebral conjunctiva is the tunica mucosa that lines the eyelids, and the bulbar conjunctiva covers the anterior aspect of the eyeball, both limiting the conjunctival sac. Their reflections are called superior and inferior fornices. The muscles of the eyelids are the orbicular, lacrimal, and ciliary. The conjunctiva is innervated by the ophthalmic nerve and receives branches from the anterior ciliary arteries and the peripheral palpebral arcade (lateral and medial palpebral arteries). The veins drain into the superficial temporal, angular, anterior facial, and ophthalmic veins. The lymphatic vessels are tributaries of the submandibular and parotid lymph nodes. The innervation of the orbicular muscle is the VII. The innervation for the superior eyelid is provided by the frontal and supraorbital, and for the inferior eyelid by the infraorbital nerve.

The lacrimal apparatus consists of the lacrimal glands, ducts (12), canaliculus (beginning at a punctum on a papilla), and the nasolacrimal duct (ends in the inferior meatus).

The orbital cavity contains the eyeball, muscles, nerves, and abundant adipose tissue. The vagina bulbi or bulbar fascia (Tenon's capsule) divides the cavity in an anterior compartment (for the eyeball) and a posterior compartment (for the vessels, nerves, and fat).

The eyeball comprises an external fibrous tunica (sclera and cornea), a vascular tunica (choroid, iris, and ciliary body), and an internal nervous or sensory tunica (retina).

The transparent cornea is continuous with the sclera at the level of the limbus, where the sinus venosus sclerae is seen. The sclera is pieced posteriorly by the fibers of the nerve II at the lamina cribrosa. The choroid lines the sclera and is connected to the iris by the ciliary body, which contains the ciliary muscle and processes. The 60 ciliary processes secrete the aqueous humor. The iris is a pigmented disc with a central hole, the pupil. The iris divides the space between the cornea and the lens into an anterior and a posterior chamber, both filled with aqueous humor. Near the pupil are a sphincter and a dilator muscle. The lens is biconvex, located behind the iris, in front of the vitreous body, and anchored by the suspensory ligament to the ciliary body. The refractive organs are the cornea, aqueous humor, lens, and vitreous body.

Mouth. The mouth corresponds to the oral region, which is made up of the lips, the vestibule, and the oral cavity. The superior and inferior lips are cutaneomusculomucosal folds that limit the oral fissure. The superior lip presents the philtrum and the tubercle, and is united to the inferior lip at the level of each oral angle by labial commissures. The inferior lip is separated from the chin by the mentolabial sulcus. Labial morphology is a racial characteristic. The musculature of the lips shows circular, radial, and anteroposterior fibers, the latter constituting the cunaneomucous muscle. The whole makes up a mechanism for partially or totally opening and closing the oral fissure. The mental region presents the mental muscle and bundles of adjacent muscles. The labial glands found in the submucous layer open into the vestibule. The mucous layer shows the prominence of the glands and frenula, which divide the superior and inferior vestibular sulci into right and left halves.

Vessels of the mentolabial area are the labial arteries (and arcades), mental artery, and submental artery. The veins follow the arteries and drain into the facial, submental, and anterior jugular. The lymphatics drain into the submandibular and submental nodes. The nerves for the muscles are branches of the nerve VII and the sensory nerves are the infraorbital (superior lip) and mental (inferior lip).

The vestibule is the cavity between lips, cheeks (externally) and gums and teeth. It communicates with the exterior and oral cavity. The parotid duct opens on a papilla in the vestibule at the level of the second upper molar tooth (M^2). Labial and buccal glands join the parotid in secreting into the vestibule. The oral cavity stands between the vestibule and the fauces. It has a floor (tongue and gingivolingual sulcus), a ceiling (palate), and walls (gingivodental arches). The gingivolingual sulcus presents the sublingual folds, ducts, and caruncle. The gingivodental arches are formed by gingivae and teeth.

The tongue has a body and a root for implantation.

The body presents a dorsum and an apex. The dorsum is divided into a pars presulcalis (in front of the sulcus terminalis) and a pars postsulcalis, corresponding to the oral and pharyngeal portions, respectively. The inferior aspect of the tongue shows the plica fimbriata. The oral portion, which sometimes has a median sulcus, presents lingual papillae (filiform, conical, fungiform, vallatae, lentiform, and filiatae). Vallate and foliate papillae possess taste buds that may be found also in fungiform papillae, soft palate, and epiglottis. The pharyngeal portion has the foramen caecum (just behind the sulcus terminalis), the lingual tonsil, and the glossoepiglottic folds. The lingual mucosa covers muscles and is supported by connective tissue. The muscles are extrinsic (genio-, hyo-, chondro-, stylo-, and palatoglossus) and intrinsic (superior and inferior longitudinal, transverse, and vertical). The connective tissue has a median, a paramedian, and a lateral septum. The tongue has mucous, serous, and seromucous glands. The lingual artery originates the hyoid artery, dorsal lingual arteries, sublingual artery, and deep lingual artery. The veins follow the arteries and drain into the internal jugular veins, and the lymphatics drain into the submental, submandibular, and superior deep cervical nodes.

The gingivae (gums) surround the alveolar processes of the maxillae and mandible and the neck of each tooth. Their surfaces are called vestibular and lingual.

Teeth appear in two sets or dentitions, namely, primary (deciduous) and permanent. The three parts of the tooth are the root, neck, and crown. Enamel surrounds the crown, and cement surrounds the root. In addition, there is a middle layer or dentin and an inner tissue, the pulp, which is contained in the dental (pulp) cavity. The latter comprises a pulp chamber in the crown and root canals. Each canal has an apical foramen through which vessels and nerves enter or exit. Periodontium is a modified alveolar periosteum between the cementum and the alveolar wall. The aspects of each tooth are labial, buccal, or vestibular, mesial, lingual, and distal. Teeth are classi-

fied into incisors (I), canines (C), premolars (PM), and molars (M) (Table 2-1).

"Milk" or deciduous teeth appear approximately in the following order:

Inferior I	6 months
Superior I	7 months
C	16 months
First M	13 months
Second M	20

Permanent teeth erupt approximately in the following order:

I	6 years
C	9 years
First PM	10 years
Second PM	11 years
First PM	7 years
Second M	11 years
Third M	18 years

The arteries that supply the teeth are the posterior, middle, and anterior superior alveolar branches of the maxillary, and the inferior alveolar. Blood is drained by corresponding veins and lymph is drained to submandibular and submental nodes. Nerves from the superior teeth belong to the maxillary (V) and from the inferior belong to the mandibular (V). The gingiva is innervated by branches of the V nerve.

The mouth receives the secretion of salivary glands, which can be classified as majorvestibular (parotid), oral (submandibular and sublingual), and minor (labial, buccal, palatine, lingual, incisive, and molar).

The palate (oronasal septum) is the roof of the oral cavity and the floor of the nasal cavity. It is divided into hard (anterior two-thirds) and soft palate. The skeleton of the hard palate is made up of the palatine processes of the maxillae and the horizontal plates of the palatine bones; it is covered by mucoperiosteum and, above, by nasal mucosa. The soft palate (velum palatinum) is the myofibrous extension of the hard palate, presents the palatine uvula and continues with palatoglossal and palatopharyngeal arches. The muscles of the soft palate are the muscles of the uvula, levator and tensor veli palatine, palatoglossal and palatopharyngeus. Blood is supplied by the greater palatine artery and drained by accompanying veins. Lymph is drained into adjacent nodes. The innervation is provided by the palatine and nasopalatine nerves (to pterygopalatine ganglion).

The fauces (throat) is the term that designates the area of the lateral wall of the oropharynx, which lodges the palatine tonsil, limited by the palatoglossal and palatopharyngeal arches. The area is the transition between mouth and pharynx.

Table 2-1. Formulas for Dentitions

	Primary		Permanent	
---	Maxilla	Mandible	Maxilla	Mandible
M	2	2	3	3
PM	—	—	2	2
C	1	1	1	1
I	2	2	2	2
I	2	2	2	2
C	1	1	1	1
PM	—	—	2	2
M	2	2	3	3

LATERAL VIEW OF THE HEAD

Included are parts of the occipitofrontal, temporal, and auriculomastoid region and, in the face, the parotidomasseteric, the infratemporal, the pterygopalatine, and the cheek. The temporal region corresponds to the temporal fossa of the skull. The skin is covered by hair. The tela subcutanea contains the superficial temporal artery and vein, accompanied by the auriculotemporal nerve, branches of the VII for the auricular muscles, and lymphatic vessels, which are tributaries of the parotid and posterior auricular nodes. The temporal fascia is inserted into the zygomatic arch. This fascia transforms the temporal fossa into a cavity, which contains the temporal muscle, middle temporal artery, anterior and posterior deep temporal arteries, deep temporal nerves, and adipose tissue. The skeleton is represented by the parietal, frontal (part), and sphenoid (part) bone.

The auriculomastoid region comprises the area of the auricle and the mastoid process. The skin contains hairs at the entrance of the external acoustic meatus. The subcutaneous tela presents the auricular (anterior, superior, and posterior) muscles, branches of the superficial temporal and posterior auricular arteries and veins, lymphatic vessels that drain into adjacent nodes, and nerves from the VII, auriculotemporal and great auricular. Inserted into the mastoid area are the sternocleidomastoid, the splenius muscle of the head, and the longissimus muscle of the head. The elastic cartilage of the auricle continues with that of the external acoustic meatus; the latter is lined by skin that contains many sebaceous and ceruminous glands. The external acoustic meatus extends from the auricle to the tympanic membrane, which separates the external from the middle ear.

The middle ear is divided into the tympanic cavity, adnexa mastoidea, and auditory tube. The tympanic cavity is situated in the thickness of the temporal bone, under the middle cranial fossa, and above the jugular fossa. The tympanic cavity has six walls and contains the auditory ossicles. The walls are superior or tegmental (roof, tegmen tympani), inferior or jugular (floor, jugular fossa), anterior or carotid (carotid canal, auditory tube, ostium), posterior or mastoid (aditus leading to mastoid antrum, pyramidal eminence for stapedius muscle), lateral or membranaceous (tympanic membrane, epitympanic recess), and medial or labyrinthic (prominences of lateral semicircular canal and of facial nerve canal, fenestra vestibuli or oval window closed by stapes, cochleariform process, promontory formed by cochlea basal turn and related to the tympanic plexus, and fenestra cochleae or round window, closed by mucous membrane). The auditory ossicles are the hammer (its handle is inserted in the tympanic membrane), incus, and stapes, articulated by incudomalleal and in-

cudostrapedial joints. The muscles are the tensor tympani and the stapedius.

The inner ear, contained in the petrous portion of the temporal bone, is constituted by a fluid-filled membranous labyrinth covered by a bony labyrinth. The osseous labyrinth consists of continuous cavities containing a fluid, perilymph. The cavities are semicircular canals, vestibule, and cochlea. The semicircular canals (anterior, posterior, lateral) contain the homonymous ducts of the membranous labyrinth (filled with endolymph). The vestibule contains utricle and saccule of the membranous labyrinth and the endolymphatic duct. The cochlea has a core, the modiolus, for the cochlear nerve and spiral ganglion. The cochlear duct (of the membranous labyrinth) extends from the osseous spiral lamina to the wall of the cochlea, dividing the space in the cochlea into a scala vestibuli and a scala tympani. The scala vestibuli begins in the vestibule and reaches the apex of the cochlea (helicotrema) where the scalae communicate with each other. The scala tympani ends at the fenestra cochleae (closed by the secondary tympanic membrane). The perilymphatic duct (aqueduct of the cochlea) is found in the cochlear canaliculus, possibly connecting the scala tympani with the subarachnoid space.

Each semicircular duct shows an ampulla having a neuroepithelial ampullary crest. Utricle and saccule intercommunicate by utricular and saccular ducts. As the anterior and posterior semicircular ducts have a common opening, the utricle has five openings. A ductus reuniens connects the saccule to the cochlear duct. Both saccule and utricle have a macula. The cochlear duct has $2\frac{1}{2}$ turns, begins in the saccule and ends blindly in the apex of the cochlea; it extends from the osseous spiral lamina to the cochlear wall and presents the vestibular (anterior) and basilar (posterior) membranes (walls). The spiral organ (of hearing) lies on the basilar membrane and comprises the tectorial membrane and neuroepithelial hair cells.

The facial (VII) nerve is closely related to several structures of the middle ear and the vestibulocochlear (VIII) nerve is made up of afferent fibers from the inner ear (vestibular part and ganglion for balance and cochlear part and spiral ganglion for hearing).

The parotidomasseteric region is the lateral area of the face that includes the parotid and the masseter muscle and related structures.

The parotid gland is located in front of the external acoustic meatus and behind the mandible. It is enclosed in the parotid fascia, is divided into superficial and deep portions, and may present an accessory gland. The base of the parotid gland is related to the superficial temporal vessels and auriculotemporal nerve, the apex to the mandibular angle, the lateral aspect to lymph nodes, the anterior aspect to the mandible, masseter, maxillary, and transverse facial arteries, branches of nerve VII, and the posterior aspect to the mastoid and styloid processes (and related muscles), sternomastoid and digastric muscles. The facial nerve and plexus, the superficial temporal, maxillary and retromandibular veins and the external carotid artery are found within the gland. The parotid duct (4 mm thick and 6 cm long) emerges from the anterior surface of the gland, runs forward below the zygomatic arch on the masseter muscle and the buccal fat pad, pierces the buccinator muscle and opens into the oral vestibule on top of the parotid papilla opposite to M^2.

The masseter is one of the muscles of mastication, situated laterally to the ramus of the mandible, which separates the muscle from the infratemporal region; it is divided into superficial, middle, and deep portions. The parotidomasseteric fascia (continuation of the cervical fascia that covers the sternocleidomastoid muscle) di-

vides into a superficial and a deep parotid fascia, and extends forward to cover the masseter.

The infratemporal fossa is limited by the maxilla, the greater wing of the sphenoid bone, the lateral pterygoid plate, and the mandibular ramus. It contains the two pterygoid muscles (both masticatory), the maxillary artery, the pterygoid venous plexus, the mandibular nerve, and the chorda tympani.

The pterygopalatine fossa is the space (height 2 cm, width at the base 1 cm) bounded anteriorly by the tuberosity of the maxilla and posteriorly by the anterior surface of the pterygoid process. It contains the posterior superior alveolar vessels and nerves, mandibular nerve, pharyngeal nerve, pterygopalatine branch of the sphenopalatine artery, sphenopalatine ganglion, vessels, and nerves, and the vessels and nerve of the pterygoid canal.

The cheek is limited by the orbit, the inferior border of the mandible, the masseter muscle, the nasolabial sulcus, and a vertical line that from this sulcus reaches the inferior margin of the mandible. This region contains the parotid duct, the buccinator muscle, the adipose body (buccal fat pad), and is covered by a beard in adult males.

Table 2-2. Cranial Fossae of the Cranial Cavity

Cranial Fossa	Foramina and Contents
Anterior cranial fossa	
Lamina cribrosa	Olfactory nerves
Anterior ethmoidal foramen	Anterior ethmoidal nerve and vessels
Posterior ethmoidal foramen	Posterior ethmoidal nerve and vessels
Middle cranial fossa	
Optic canal	Optic nerve and ophthalmic artery
Superior orbital fissure	Nerves III, IV, V (ophthalmic), VI, sympathetic nerves, ophthalmic veins
Round foramen	Nerve V (maxillary)
Oval foramen	Nerve V (mandibular) accessory meningeal artery
Spinous foramen	Middle meningeal artery
Hiatus for greater petrosal nerve	Greater petrosal nerve, petrosal branch of middle meningeal artery
Posterior cranial fossa	
Foramen magnum	Spinal cord, nerve XI, vertebral arteries, anterior and posterior spinal arteries
Jugular foramen	Nerves IX, X, XI, inferior petrosal and transverse sinuses, meningeal branches of occipital and ascending pharyngeal arteries
Hypoglossal canal	Nerve XII, meningeal branch of ascending pharyngeal artery
Internal acoustic meatus	Nerves VII, VIII, labyrinthine (internal acoustic) artery

INFERIOR VIEW OF THE HEAD (SKULL AND FACE)

The inferior view of the skull (base) comprises the occipital, the temporal, and the sphenoid bone, the choanae, the vomer, the horizontal plates of the palatine bones, and the palatine processes of the maxillae and the mandible.

INTERIOR VIEW OF THE HEAD (CRANIAL CAVITY)

The cranial cavity is divided into three fossae (anterior, middle, and posterior) (Table 2-2). The limit between the anterior and the middle cranial fossae is the posterior margin of the lesser wing of the sphenoid bone and the limit between the middle and posterior cranial fossae is the superior margin of the petrous portion of the temporal bone. The vault of the skull covers the three fossae and its inner aspect shows digital impressions (from cerebral gyri), sagittal groove (for superior sagittal sinus), and granular pits (for arachnoid granulations).

Anterior cranial fossa
    Crista galli
    Cribriform plate
    Jugum sphenoidale
    Orbital plate (sphenoid)
    Anterior clinoid process

Table 2-3. Divisions of the CNS

Divisions	Vesicles	Derivatives	Cavities
Encephalon	Prosencephalon (forebrain) Telencephalon	Cortex Corpus striatum Rhinencephalon Thalamus dorsalis	I, II, and rostral part of third ventricle
	Diencephalon Mesencephalon (Midbrain) Rhombencephalon (hindbrain)		
Medulla spinalis[a]			

[a] In the vertebral column.

Middle cranial fossa
    Sphenoid bone
    Sella turcica
    Posterior clinoid process
    Carotid groove
    Superior orbital fissure
    Foramen rotundum (maxillary nerve)
    Foramen ovale (mandibular nerve)
    Foramen spinosum (middle meningeal vessels)
    Trigeminal impression
    Arcuate eminence (anterior semicircular canal)
    Hiatus for the greater petrosal nerve
    Tegmen tympani
    Foramen lacerum
Posterior cranial fossa
    Foramen magnum
    Hypoglossal canal
    Clivus
    Internal occipital crest
    Internal occipital protuberance
    Groove for the transverse sinus
    Groove for the sigmoid sinus
    Jugular foramen
    Internal acoustic meatus
    Aqueduct of the vestibule
    Cochlear canalicular

Contents of the Cranial Fossae
    Anterior
        Frontal lobes of the brain
    Middle
        Temporal lobes of the brain, the hypophysis cerebri
    Posterior
        Hindbrain (cerebellum, pons, medulla oblongata)

The cranial cavity also is divided into a cerebral fossa (anterior and middle cranial fossae), rhombencephalic fossa, under the tentorium cerebelli (posterior cranial fossa), hypophyseal fossa, and trigeminal fossa (for the trigeminal ganglion).

The cranial cavity contains the encephalon, one of the divisions of the CNS the other being the medulla spinalis (Table 2-3).

The coverings of the CNS are the dura mater (pachymeninx), the arachnoid, and the pia mater (leptomeninges). The dura mater forms the falx cerebri, the tentorium cerebelli, the falx cerebelli, and the diaphragma sellae. The subarachnoid space, between the arachnoid and the pia mater, is filled with cerebrospinal fluid (CSF) or liquor (120 ml) and communicates with the ventricles by means of the median foramen (Magendie) at the roof of the fourth ventricle and the lateral foramen (Luschka) at each lateral recess of the fourth ventricle. The arachnoid and pia mater are separated by large subarachnoid cisterns: cerebellomedullary (cisterna magna), pontine, superior, interpeduncular, chiasmatic, of the lamina terminalis, and of the corpus callosum.

The rhombencephalon comprises the medulla oblongata, the pons, and the cerebellum.

The medulla oblongata (bulb, myelencephalon) presents the following:

    Anterior median fissure, decussation of pyramids
    Pyramid
    Anterolateral sulcus, ventral roots of C1, nerve XII, and nerve VI
    Olive (inferior)
    Posterior medial sulcus
    Posterolateral sulcus, roots of nerves XI, X, IX, VII
    Posterior intermediate sulcus, gracilis, and cuneate tubercles
    Tuberculum cinereum
    Restiform body
    Fourth ventricle (floor of inferior portion)

These grooves divide the bulb into ventral, lateral, and dorsal areas. The pons is part of the metencephalon (in front of the cerebellum) and presents:

Basilar sulcus
Superior and inferior pontine sulci
Middle cerebellar peduncle
Nerves VIII, VII, VI (inferior pontine sulcus)
Nerve V (sensory and motor roots)
Fourth ventricle (floor of superior portion)

The cerebellum is the dorsal portion of the metencephalon and occupies most of the posterior cranial fossa. It is attached to the brain stem by three pairs of cerebellar peduncles (inferior to the bulb, middle to the pons, and superior to the midbrain). The fourth ventricle is interposed between the cerebellum and, in front, the medulla oblongata and the pons. The cerebellum presents:

Hemispheres, connected by the vermis
Transverse sulci or fissures
Gyri or primary cerebellar folia
Cranial lobe
    Lingula
    Lobulus centralis
    Culmen
    Ala lobuli centralis
    Lobulus quadrangularis
First fissure
Caudal lobe
    Declive
    Folium vermis
    Tuber vermis
    Pyramis vermis
        Fissura secunda
    Uvula vermis
    Lobulus simplex
    Lobulus semilunaris cranialis
        Fissura horizontalis
    Lobulus semilunaris caudalis
    Lobulus paramedianus
    Lobulus biventer
    Tonsilla cerebelli
Dorsolaeral fissure
Flocculonodular lobe
    Nodule
    Flocculus
        Peduncle of flocculus
    Paraflocculus

Functional areas of the cerebellum are the vestibular (flocculonodular lobe) or archeocerebellum, spinal (cranial lobe and part of the caudal lobe, such as tonsil, declive, and uvula) or paleocerebellum, and cerebral (caudal lobe except the tonsil, declive, and uvula) or neocerebellum.

The cerebellum contains a cortex (gray matter), subcortical nuclei (dentate, emboliform, globose, and fas-

tigial), and white matter. The cortex consists of the molecular, piriform, and granular layers.

The mesencephalon or midbrain is limited inferiorly from the pons by the superior pontine and continues superiorly with the diencephalon. It consists of the cerebral peduncles and, dorsally, the tectum. The right and left peduncles are separated by the interpeduncular fossa, where the tuber cinereum and the infundibular stem of the hypophysis, the mamillary bodies, and the posterior perforated substance are found. Nerve III emerges at the inferior margin of the mesencephalon and medial border of the cerebral peduncle. The dorsal aspect of the mesencephalon has two superior and two inferior colliculi and the rootlets of nerve IV.

The inferior brain stem includes gray and white matter and the central canal.

Gray Matter. From the midline to each side the somatic motor, branchial motor, visceral motor, visceral sensory, and somatic sensory columns of nuclei are seen.

1. Somatic motor column: nerves III, IV, VI, XII
2. Branchial motor column: nerves V, VII, ambiguus, nerve XI
3. Visceral motor column: nerve III, superior and inferior salivatory, nerve X
4. Visceral sensory column: nucleus tractus solitarus
5. Somatic sensory column: nerve V

Nuclei for special sense organs are hearing, dorsal and ventral cochlear nuclei on each side; balance, superior, lateral, medical, and inferior vestibular nuclei on each side; and taste, nucleus of tractus solitarius.

White Matter. Tracts are the following:

1. Descending tracts
    Corticospinal and corticobulbar fibers
    Vestibulospinal tract
    Medial longitudinal fasciculus
    Reticulospinal tracts
    Tectospinal tract
    Rubrospinal tract
    Olivospinal tract
2. Descending autonomic pathways
    Lateral tectotegmentospinal tract
3. Ascending tracts
    Spinothalamic tracts
        Lateral
        Anterior
    Trigeminal, medial, and lateral lemnisci
    Spinocerebellar tracts
        Posterior
        Anterior

The brain stem presents the reticular formation

(caused by the numerous decussating fibers through its gray matter), the substantia nigra, and the red nucleus.

At the level of the mesencephalon, the fourth ventricle narrows down to become the mesencephalic aqueduct. The prosencephalon or forebrain consists of the diencephalon and telencephalon and includes the first, second, and third ventricles.

The diencephalon comprises the thalami, the epithalamus, the metathalamus, and the hypothalamus. The thalami include the ventral (subthalamus) and dorsal; the epithalamus is made up of the pineal body, the habenula, the subfornical and subcomissural organs; the metathalamus consists of the medial and lateral geniculate bodies; and the hypothalamus comprises the optic chiasma, the tuber cinereum, the hypophysis (neurohypophysis), and the mamillary bodies.

The telencephalon consists of the cerebrum (cerebral hemispheres), an organ characterized by an extensive peripheral cortex (gray matter), subcortical nuclear masses (basal ganglia), and fibers (white matter) to and from lower centers and fibers connecting portions of the cortex (corticocortical fibers). It contains the lateral (first and second) ventricles.

The cerebral hemispheres have a superolateral aspect, are separated by the longitudinal fissure, which contains the falx cerebri (dura mater), and are united by the corpus callosum (rostrum, genu, trunk, and splenium). Each hemisphere is made up of lobes (frontal, parietal, temporal, occipital, limbic, and insular) and is divided into frontal, temporal, and occipital poles that are situated in the anterior, middle, and posterior cranial fossae, respectively.

The cerebral cortex is folded into gyri, which are separated by sulci. The lateral sulcus has three rami (anterior, ascendens, and posterior) and separates the frontal and parietal lobes from the temporal lobe. The insula is found deep in the lateral sulcus. The central sulcus separates the frontal and parietal lobes; the parietooccipital sulcus limits the parietal and occipital lobes; and the sulcus cinguli limits the limbic lobe. The calcarine sulcus is on the medial surface of the occipital lobe. The cortex in front of the central sulcus (precentral gyrus or area 4 of Brodmann) is the motor area and the postcentral gyrus is a general sensory or primary receptive area (areas 3, 1, 2, and 5). A few others, among the 52 Brodmann's areas, are as follows:

Premotor cortex area: 6
Parietal association area: 7
Eye motor area: 8
Visual cortex: 17
Auditory cortex: 41
Auditory association area: 42 and part of 22 and 52
Gustatory area: 43

Cortical representation of speech is usually placed in the dominant (usually left) hemisphere (areas in the frontal, parietal, and temporal lobes). The rhinencephalon (olfactory brain) includes the olfactory nerve, bulb, tract, striae, anterior olfactory nucleus, anterior perforated substance, subcallosae (paraolfactory) area, hippocampal formation, prepiriform cortex, and rostral portions of the hippocampal gyrus.

Basal ganglia comprise the caudate nucleus, the putamen, the globus pallidus, the claustrum, and the amygdaloid body. They can be grouped as corpus striatum (caudate nucleus, putamen, and globus pallidus) or as lentiform nucleus (putamen and globus pallidus).

Most of the caudate nucleus is separated from other nuclei by the internal capsule (white matter). The lentiform nucleus is located between the insular cortex and the thalamus, being separated from the thalamus and caudate nucleus by the internal capsule. Laterally, the external capsule, the claustrum, and the extreme capsule are interposed between the lentiform nucleus and the insula. The lentiform nucleus is divided by the lateral medullary lamina into the putamen (lateral) and the globus pallidus; the latter is subdivided by the medial medullary lamina into lateral and medial portions. The putamen and caudate nucleus are similar (small perikarya) and quite different from the globus pallidus (large perikarya). The amygdaloid body is located on the roof of the inferior horn of the lateral ventricle, where the tail of the caudate nucleus ends.

The white matter of the cerebral hemispheres is divided into projection, commissural, and association fibers. Projection fibers connect the cerebral cortex and structures outside the telencephalon. Except for the extreme and external capsules, all projection fibers form the internal capsule. Rostrally the fibers to and from the internal capsule make up the corona radiata and caudally they are divided into several bundles (the largest enters the cerebral peduncle).

The internal capsule has an anterior limb (between caudate and lenticular nuclei), a genu, and a posterior limb (between the thalamus and the lenticular nucleus). Functional groups of fibers within the internal capsule are thalamic radiations (anterior, superior, posterior) with corticothalamic and thalamocortical fibers, in the three portions (both limbs and genu); auditory and optic radiations through the sub- and postlenticular portions of the posterior limb; corticofugal fibers (corticobulbar fibers in the genu and corticospinal fibers in the posterior limb); corticopontine fibers; and corticorubral fibers.

Commissural fibers (between the hemispheres) comprise the corpus callosum, the hippocampal, and the anterior commissure. Association fibers connect different areas of the same hemisphere.

The cerebral cortex has an area of 200,000 sq mm ($\frac{2}{3}$ in the depths of the sulci), a thickness varying from 1.3 to

4.5 mm. It holds 15 billion perikarya distributed in molecular, external granular, external pyramidal, internal granular, internal pyramidal, and fusiform layers. The cortex contains a network of afferent, efferent, and intracortical fibers:

1. Afferent from thalamus, commissural fibers from opposite hemisphere, association fibers from same hemisphere
2. Efferent: projection, commissural, and association fibers
3. Intracortical: short ascending and descending, horizontal association fibers

The cranioencephalic topography is variable but it is possible to consider the following landmarks:

1. The cerebral hemispheres are above and the cerebellum below the level of the orbitomeatal plane.
2. The inferior limit of the hemispheres corresponds approximately to the eyebrow, zygomatic arch, external acoustic meatus, and external occipital protuberance.
3. The central sulcus (Rolando) corresponds to a line that begins 1 cm posterior to the vertex (or the midpoint, the nasioinion line) and runs for 10 cm to reach the middle of the zygomatic arch.
4. The lateral sulcus (Sylvius) corresponds to a line that begins at the pterion, runs backward, and ends at the parietal eminence.

Ventricles and Cerebrospinal Fluid. The ventricles are filled with CSF and consist of two (first and second) lateral ventricles (one in each hemisphere), and the diencephalic (three) ventricle (in the diencephalon) united to the rhombencephalic (fourth) ventricle by the cerebral aqueduct. The fourth ventricle continues with the central canal of the spinal cord. These cavities are lined by ependyma and, in the four ventricles, portions of the ependyma are invaginated by pial vessels to form the chorid plexuses, which produce CSF.

Circumventricular organs are the pineal body, subcommissural organ, hypophysis, vascular organ of the lamina terminalis, subfornical organ, paraphysis, and area postrema.

There are 12 pairs of cranial nerves, as follows:

Nerve I	olfactory, sensory
Nerve II	optic, sensory
Nerve III	oculomotor, motor
Nerve IV	trochlear, motor
Nerve V	trigeminal, mixed
Nerve VI	abducent, motor
Nerve VII	facial, mixed
Nerve VIII	vestibulocochlear, sensory
Nerve IX	glossopharyngeal, mixed
Nerve X	vagus, mixed
Nerve XI	accessory, motor
Nerve XII	hypoglossal, motor

Nerve I (from the nasal mucosa) enters the cranial cavity through the cribriform plate, is special visceral or somatic afferent, and functions in the sensation of smell.

Nerve II (from the retina) enters the skull through the optic canal, is special somatic afferent, and functions in vision.

Nerve III originates from the mesencephalon (at medial border of cerebral penduncle), leaves the skull through the superior orbital fissure, is somatic and visceral motor (efferent), and functions in movements of the eye (most ocular muscles), miosis, and accommodation (intrinsic muscles).

Nerve IV originates from the mesencephalon (below the inferior colliculus), leaves the skull through the superior orbital fissure, is somatic motor, and supplies the superior oblique muscle of the eye.

Nerve V is attached to the encephalon on the side of the pons; its branches pass through the superior orbital fissure, the foramen rotundum, and the foramen ovale. The branches originate from the sensory nuclei and from the motor (masticatory) nucleus of the trigeminal nerve. Nerve V is special visceral efferent or branchial motor and general somatic afferent or sensory; it functions in mandibular movements and sensation of the head.

Nerve VI originates from its nucleus beneath the floor of the fourth ventricle, is attached to the inferior margin of the pons, leaves the skull through the superior orbital fissure, is somatic motor (afferent), and innervates the lateral rectus muscle of the eye.

Nerve VII originates from the nucleus in the lower portion of the pons, the superior salivatory and solitarius nerve, and the geniculate ganglion. It is attached to the inferior margin of the pons and passes through the stylomastoid foramen. The nerve is special visceral efferent or branchial motor, general visceral efferent (parasympathetic), and special visceral afferent (sensory). It functions in facial expression (movements), secretion of tears and saliva, and taste.

Nerve VIII (from spiral and vestibular ganglia) is attached to the inferior margin of the pons, is special somatic afferent, and comprises the vestibular nerve (for equilibrium) and the cochlear nerve (for hearing).

Nerve IX originates from the nucleus ambiguus, inferior salivatory nucleus, superior and inferior ganglia, is attached to the bulb (medulla oblongata), laterally to the olive, and passes through the jugular foramen; it is special visceral efferent or branchial motor, general visceral efferent (parasympathetic) or motor, general somatic, general visceral, and special visceral afferent (sensory). The nerve functions in swallowing, secretion of saliva, taste, and sensation of tongue, pharynx, and external and middle ear.

Nerve X originates from the nucleus ambiguus, dorsal motor nucleus, superior and inferior (nodosum) ganglia, is attached to the bulb (medulla oblongata), laterally to the olive, and passes through the jugular foramen. It is special (branchial), general visceral (parasympathetic), efferent (motor), general, special visceral afferent, and general somatic afferent (sensory). The nerve functions in taste, movements of larynx, movements and secretions of viscera (thorax and abdomen), and sensation in external ear, pharynx, larynx, and viscera (thorax and abdomen).

Nerve XI originates from the nucleus ambiguus and spinal cord, is attached to the bulb (medulla oblongata), laterally to the olive, and leaves the skull via the jugular foramen. It is special visceral (branchial) and general visceral efferent (motor), and functions in movements of the pharynx, larynx, head, and shoulder, and movements and secretion of viscera (thorax and abdomen).

Nerve XII originates from the hypoglossal nucleus, is attached to the bulb (medulla oblongata) between pyramid and olive, and leaves the skull via the hypoglossal canal. It is somatic efferent (motor) and functions in lingual movements.

There are parasympathetic (vegetative) ganglia related to cranial nerves, as follows:

1. Ciliary ganglion, between the lateral rectus muscle and nerve I, having three "roots" (parasympathetic from nerve III, sympathetic from the internal carotid plexus, and sensory from (to) the nasoociliary nerve). It is distributed to muscles (ciliary, sphincter and dilator pupillae, and tarsal).
2. Pterygopalatine ganglion, in the homonymous fossa, having a parasympathetic root from the greater petrosal nerve and nerve of pterygoid canal, and a sympathetic root from the internal carotid plexus. It is distributed to the lacrimal gland.
3. Otic ganglion, located below the oval foramen, having a parasympathetic root from the lesser petrosal nerve and a sympathetic root from the middle meningeal artery plexus. It is distributed to the parotid gland.
4. Submandibular ganglion, adjacent to the hyoglossal muscle, having a parasympathetic root from the chorda tympani (lingual nerve) and a sympathetic root from the facial artery plexus. It is distributed to the submandibular and sublingual glands.

The branchial arches are the following:

1. Mandibular (mandibular nerve from V, facial artery, masticatory muscles, mandible, malleus, and incus Meckel's cartilage).

2. Hyoid (facial or nerve VII, external carotid artery, facial muscles, stapes, styloid process, stylohyoid ligament, hyoid horn Reichert's cartilage).
3. Thyrohyoid (glossopharyngeal or nerve IX, internal carotid artery, stylopharyngeus muscle, hyoid body, and greater horn).
4. Unnamed (external branch of superior laryngeal nerve, cricothyroid muscle, larynx).
5. Unnamed (recurrent laryngeal nerve, laryngeal muscles, larynx).

Blood Supply and Drainage of the Encephalon. The brain receives blood from two internal carotid and two vertebral arteries. At its origin, the internal carotid artery presents a dilation, the carotid sinus, which is a pressoreceptor area (supplied by nerve IX) that promotes reflex slowing of the heart and peripheral vasodilation when blood pressure rises. Near the carotid sinus, the carotid body, a chemoreceptor organ, is found. It is supplied by nerve IX and causes reflex increase in respiration as blood oxygen tension decreases. The internal carotid artery enters the cranial cavity through the carotid canal and changes direction six times (carotid siphon) within a short distance; an arrangement that protects the cerebral tissues from the pulsating force of the blood pressure. After traversing the cavernous sinus, the artery emerges laterally to the optic chiasma and divides into two terminal branches, the anterior and middle cerebral arteries (for the rostral $\frac{2}{3}$ of the brain). The anterior cerebral arteries are anastomosed by the anterior communicating artery.

The anterior cerebral artery is subdivided into pars pre- and pars postcommunicalis. The branches of the pars precommunicalis are anteromedial central arteries, short and long central arteries anterior communicating artery, and anteromedial central branches. The branches of the pars postcommunicalis are medial frontobasal artery, callosomarginal artery, paracentral artery, precunial artery, and parieto-occipital artery. In short, the anterior cerebral artery supplies the anteromedial and superolateral aspects of the hemisphere and small areas of the basal ganglia and internal capsule.

The middle cerebral artery is subdivided into pars sphenoidalis, pars insularis, and pars terminalis. The pars sphenoidalis gives off the anterolateral central arteries; the pars insularis gives off the insular arteries, lateral frontobasal artery, anterior, intermediate, and posterior temporal arteries; and the pars terminalis gives off the central sulcus artery, precentral sulcus artery, postcentral sulcus artery, anterior and posterior parietal arteries, and angular gyrus arteries. In short, the middle cerebral artery supplies the basal ganglia, the internal capsule, and most of the lateral aspect of the hemisphere.

Prior to its bifurcation, the internal carotid artery provides the ophthalmic artery (branch, central artery of the retina), anterior choroidal artery, inferior and superior hypophysial arteries, and posterior communicating artery, which anastomoses the internal carotid artery with the posterior cerebral artery (branch of the vertebrobasilar artery).

The pars intercranialis of the vertebral artery has the following branches: anterior and posterior meningeal branches, anterior and posterior spinal arteries, and inferoposterior cerebellar artery. The two vertebral arteries form the basilar artery, the branches of which are inferoanterior cerebellar artery (its branch is the labyrinthine artery), pontine arteries, mesencephalic arteries, and the superior cerebellar artery. Near the superior margin of the pons, the basilar artery divides into two posterior cerebral arteries.

The posterior cerebral artery is subdivided into a pars pre-, a pars postcommunicalis, and a pars terminalis. The pars precommunicalis presents the posteromedial central arteries. The past postcommunicalis gives off the posterolateral central arteries, thalamic branches, medial and lateral posterior choroid branches, and the peduncular branches. The pars terminalis branches are the lateral and the medial occipital arteries. The lateral occipital artery has anterior, medial intermediate, and posterior temporal branches. The medial occipital artery has the dorsal branch of the corpus callosum, parietal, parietooccipital, calcarine, and occipitotemporal branches.

The vertebrobasilar arteries supply the caudal structures of the encephalon and the inferior and medial surfaces of the temporal and occipital lobes of the hemisphere.

The two vertebral and the two internal carotid arteries are anastomosed by the circulus arteriosus cerebri. This arterial ring is formed by the posterior cerebral, posterior communicating, internal carotid, anterior cerebral, and anterior communicating arteries. The circulus arteriosus is situated at the base of the brain and surrounds the optic chiasma, infundibulum, tuber cinereum, mamillary bodies, and interpenduncular fossa.

The cranial leptomeninges receive blood supply from plexuses derived from vessels of the brain. The cranial dura mater is mainly supplied by the middle meningeal artery (a branch of the maxillary artery), the anterior and posterior meningeal arteries, and posterior meningeal branches of the vertebral and occipital arteries.

The venous drainage of the encephalon is accomplished by the (1) superior cerebral vein, which drains into the superior sagittal sinus; (2) superficial middle cerebral vein, and superior and inferior anastomotic veins, which are tributaries of the superior sagittal, transverse, and cavernous sinuses; (3) inferior cerebral veins, tributaries of the sinuses near the inferior surface of the cerebral hemispheres; (4) basal vein, which drains into the great cerebral vein; and (5) great cerebral vein, formed by the two internal cerebral veins, draining into the straight sinus. The veins of the brain make up a plexus in the pia mater and lead to two groups of large cerebral veins; the external cerebral and cerebellar veins, superior, middle, and inferior cerebral, and cerebellar veins, which are tributaries of adjacent sinuses; and the right and left internal cerebral vein united at the level of the splenium, resulting in the formation of the great cerebral vein, joining in turn the inferior sagittal sinus to lead to the straight sinus.

The venous sinuses of the dura mater are the superior and inferior sagittal sinuses, confluence of the sinuses, transverse (lateral) sinuses, sigmoid sinus, and superior and inferior petrosal sinuses.

Lateral lacunae are found in the vault of the skull, near the superior sagittal sinus, and receive emissary, meningeal, and diploic veins.

Liquor (CSF) is also drained into the sinuses, chiefly into the superior sagittal sinus, through the arachnoidal granulations.

The blood from the encephalon is drained ultimately into the internal jugular veins.

Neck

The neck is the portion of the body that connects the head to the thorax. Its superior limit was given (see Head Section), and its inferior limit corresponds to a line that begins in the jugular incisure, follows the superior aspect of the clavicle to the acromioclavicular joint, then runs dorsally along a transverse line that reaches the tip of the spinous process of C7.

The cervical regions are the following:

Anterior cervical region
    Suprahyoid
        Submental triangle
        Submandibular triangle
    Infrahyoid
        Carotid triangle
        Muscular (omotracheal) triangle
Sternocleidomastoid region
    Minor supraclavicular fossa
Lateral cervical region
    Major supraclavicular fossa
Posterior cervical (nuchal) region

ANTERIOR CERVICAL REGION

The anterior cervical region is limited by the line drawn from the median point of the chin down to the middle of the jugular notch, by the anterior margin of the sternocleidomastoid muscle, and by the inferior mandibular margin extended horizontally to the mastoid process. It can be subdivided into supra- and infrahyoid portions, and contains small regions, as follows.

Suprahyoid portion

Submandibular or digastric triangle, so named because the largest structure is the submandibular gland and because it is limited by the bellies of the digastric muscle against the inferior margin of the mandible.

Submental triangle, bounded by the anterior belly of the digastric muscle, by the body of the hyoid bone, and by the median plane of the neck; the mylohyoid muscle is the floor of the triangle.

Infrahyoid portion

Carotid triangle, limited by the anterior margin of the sternocleidomastoid, by the omohyoid muscle, and by the posterior belly of the digastric muscle. It contains parts of the carotid artery, internal jugular vein, nerves X, and XII, and cervical sympathetic trunk.

Muscular, inferior carotid or omotracheal triangle, limited by the median plane of the neck, by the omohyid muscle, and by the anterior margin of the sternocleidomastoid muscle. It contains the infrahyoid muscles, the thyroid, the trachea, the inferior portions of the carotid artery and jugular vein, and oral portion of the esophagus.

STERNOCLEIDOMASTOID REGION

The sternocleidomastoid region is limited by the borders and extremities of the corresponding muscle. The minor supraclavicular fossa is found between the sternal and clavicular bundles of the same muscle.

LATERAL CERVICAL REGION

The lateral cervical region (posterior cervical triangle, not to be confused with the posterior cervical region or nuchal region) is limited by the posterior margin of the sternocleidomastoid muscle, the anterior margin of the trapezius muscle, and, inferiorly, by the intermediate $\frac{1}{3}$ of the clavicle. The inferior belly of the omohyoid muscle subdivides the region into two triangles, namely, the occipital triangle (superoposterior) and the omoclavicular triangle, major supraclavicular fossa, or subclavian triangle. The floor of the posterior cervical triangle is the prevertebral lamina of the cervical fascia, on the splenius, levator scapulae, scaleni medius, and posterior muscles. The external jugular vein pierces the fascia in this triangle to open into the subclavian vein.

POSTERIOR CERVICAL (NUCHAL) REGION

The posterior cervical (nuchal) region comprises the cervical vertebrae and the soft parts that cover them posteriorly. The limits of the region are a curved line that starts at the external occipital protuberance and follows the superior nuchal line, an inferior horizontal line at the level of the acromion and spinous process of C7, and the anterior margins of the trapezius muscle. The region presents the median and superiorly located nuchal fossa, the nuchal ligament, the dorsal extension of the fascia cervicalis superficialis, and the trapezius, splenius, levator scapulae, rhomboid, posterior superior dentate, semispinalis capitis, longissimus capitis and colli, major and minor posterior rectus, superior and inferior oblique, transverse spinous, and posterior interspinous muscles. The arteries are occipital, deep cervical, cervical transverse, and vertebral. The veins are tributaries of the occipital, posterior auricular, and posterior jugular vein. The lymph is drained into suboccipital, cervical, and subclavian nodes. The nerves are the posterior branches of the eight cervical nerves, the largest being the suboccipital and the greater occipital nerves.

The skin of the neck, made up of epidermis, dermis, and tela subcutanea, presents the platysma muscle in the thickness of the latter. In fact, deep to the dermis, the areolar layer of fat, the most superficial layer of the tela subcutanea, precedes the fascia superficialis (second layer of the tela subcutanea), which contains the platysma muscle. The lamellar layer of fat, the third layer of the tela, is found deeper to the fascia superficialis and contains the cervical branch of nerve VII, the transverse cervical nerve, and the external jugular vein.

The superficial vessels of the neck are the external jugular, posterior external jugular, suprascapular, transverse cervical, and anterior jugular veins. The cutaneous nerves derive from dorsal rami of cervical nerves and ventral rami of C2, C3, and C4 from the cervical plexus. The dorsal rami include the greater occipital nerve and the occipitalis tertius. The cutaneous branches of the cervical plexus comprise the lesser occipital, the greater auricular, the transverse cervical, and the supraclavicular (medial, intermediate, and lateral) nerves.

The fascia cervicalis is divided into superficial, pretracheal, and prevertebral laminae and the carotid sheath. The superficial lamina or investing layer encloses the sternocleidomastoid and trapezius muscles, covers the anterior and posterior triangles, and limits the suprasternal space. The pretracheal lamina is infrahyoid, surrounding the thyroid gland, infrahyoid muscles, trachea, and esophagus. The prevertebral lamina is inserted in the base of the skull and transverse processes of cervical vertebrae, covering the prevertebral, scaleni (and phrenic nerve), and deep muscles of the back; it is the floor of the posterior triangle and has an extension, the axillary sheath. The carotid sheath or vagina surrounds the common and internal carotid arteries, the internal jugular vein, and nerve X.

The retropharyngeal space is found between the buccopharyngeal fascia (surrounding the superior portion of the digestive tract) and the prevertebral lamina. The alar fascia, between the pretracheal and the prevertebral laminae, is attached to the carotid sheath and to the buccopharyngeal fascia.

The infrahyoid muscles are divided into superficial (sterno and omohyoid) and deep (sternothyroid and thyrohyoid). The sternohyoid, omohyoid, and sternothyroid are supplied by the ansa cervicalis and the thyrohyoid by nerve XII.

The thyroid gland is surrounded by its capsule and by a sheath provided by the cervical fascia; it has two lobes and an isthmus at the level of the third tracheal ring. The gland is supplied by the superior and inferior thyroid arteries and by the accessory thyroid (thyroidea ima), and drained by the superior, middle, and inferior thyroid veins. The lymph is drained to the deep cervical, paratracheal nodes, prelaryngeal and pretracheal nodes.

The four parathyroid glands (superior and inferior) are found outside the thyroid capsule, on the posterior aspect of each thyroid lobe.

The short cervical portion of the trachea is related to the infrahyoid muscles, the thyroid isthmus, and vessels. The cervical portion of the esophagus is related to the trachea, the long muscle of the head, and the cervical region of the vertebral column.

The common internal carotid arteries are related to the cervical vertebrae and their muscles, the pharynx, esophagus, larynx, trachea, thyroid gland and sternocleidomastoid muscle. The common carotid artery can be compressed at the level of the transverse cervical vertebrae. The external carotid artery is found in the carotid triangle branches the superior thyroid, lingual, facial, occipital, posterior auricular, ascending pharyngeal, superficial temporal, and maxillary. The cervical portion of the internal carotid artery has the carotid sinus and body.

Nerve IX is found between the internal jugular vein and the internal carotid artery, curves around the stylopharyngeus muscle and runs between the superior and middle constrictors muscles of the pharynx. Its branches are the tympanic nerve and plexus, lesser petrosal nerve, communicating branch to nerve X, branch to carotid sinus, pharyngeal branches, branch to stylopharyngeus muscle, and tonsillar and lingual branches.

Nerve X is enclosed in the carotid sheath, between the internal jugular vein, and the internal and common carotid arteries. It is joined by the internal branch of nerve XI. The branches of nerve X are meningeal, auricular, pharyngeal, superior laryngeal, depressor, cardiac, and right recurrent laryngeal nerves.

Nerve XI, above the middle of the sternocleidomastoid muscle, which it supplies, crosses the posterior triangle of the neck on the levator scapulae muscle and supplies the trapezius muscle.

Nerve XII descends between the internal carotid artery and the internal jugular veins, and lies on the hyoglossus muscle, deep to the digastric and mylohyoid muscles. Its branches are meningeal, superior root of ansa cervicalis, thyrohyoid, and lingual.

The subclavian artery passes behind the scalenus anterior muscle and branches into the vertebral, internal thoracic, thyrocervical, costocervical, and descending scapular arteries. The subclavian vein passes in front of the scalenus anterior muscle and joins the internal jugular to form the brachiocephalic vein.

The cervical pleura (cupola) is the pleura surrounding the pulmonary apex. It is covered by the suprapleural membrane and the scalenus minimus muscle. The cervical part of the sympathetic trunk consists of three ganglia connected by a cord; superior, middle, and inferior (cervicothoracic or stellate) ganglion.

The internal jugular vein is enclosed in the carotic sheath and covered by the sternocleidomastoid muscle. Its tributaries are the inferior petrosal sinus, the pharyngeal, lingual, superior, and inferior thyroid veins.

Deep cervical lymph nodes lie along the internal jugular vein, the right lymphatic duct, and, on the left side, the thoracic duct opens into the internal jugular vein near its angle with the subclavian vein. Groups of lymph nodes that form the pericervical collar and receive the lymph from the superficial vessels are the occipital, retroauricular, parotid, submandibular, buccal, and submental nodes. There are also the jugulodigastric and the juguloomohyoid nodes, which are superficial and deep cervical nodes.

The cervical plexus is made up of the ventral rami of C1–C4 and the brachial plexus is made up of C5–T1.

The branches of the cervical plexus are the following:

    Superficial branches
        Lesser occipital
        Greater auricular
        Transverse cervical
        Supraclavicular
    Deep branches to muscles
        Sternocleidomastoid
        Trapezius
        Levator scapulae
        Scalene
            Anterior, middle, posterior, smallest

Prevertebral
> Longus (capitis and colli), recti (anterior and lateralis)

Infrahyoid
> Sterno-, omo-, thyrohyoid, and sternothyroid

Diaphragm

The cervical portion of the thymus is located anteriorly and laterally to the trachea, and posteriorly to the sternohyoid and sternothyroid muscles.

The hyoid bone is suspended from the base of the cranium by the stylohyoid ligaments (inserted into the lesser horn) and is located at the level of the superior limit of the larynx. It has a body, and on each side a greater and lesser horn.

The pharynx is a viscus common to the digestive and respiratory systems. It is a 13 cm long tube, extending from the cranial base to C6, and the ventral wall communicates with the nasal cavity (choanae), the fauces, and the larynx, corresponding to the naso-, oro-, and laryngopharynx. The roof presents the pharyngeal tonsil and the pharyngeal bursa. The lateral walls have the pharyngeal orifice of the auditory tube, the tubal torus, the tubal tonsil, the salpingopharyngeal and the salpingopalatine folds, the torus levatorius, and the deep pharyngeal recess. The posterior wall is separated from the prevertebral fascia and muscles by the retropharyngeal space (containing loose fibrous connective tissue).

The laryngopharynx presents the aditus of the larynx, the piriform recesses (each having the prominence of the laryngeal nerve), and the pharyngoepiglottic fold.

The mucosa is lined with pseudostratified columnar ciliated squamous epithelium (nasopharynx) or stratified squamous epithelium (oro- and laryngopharynx); it is surrounded by the pharyngobasilar fascia.

The muscular layer consists of the external coat, made up of the superior, middle, and inferior constrictor muscles and the internal coat (elevators), made up of the palato-, salpingo-, and stylopharyngeal muscles. All muscles, except the stylopharyngeal (nerve IX), are supplied by nerve XI (via nerve X).

There is a mechanism for deglutition, and its main components are the following:

Sphincter component
> Muscular
>> Pharyngeal: Constrictors
>> Esophageal: Circular and spiral fibers
> Vascular (submucous venous plexus)

Dilator component
> Pharyngeal: Stylopharyngeal muscle
> Esophageal: Longitudinal fibers

Blood is supplied to the pharynx by the ascending palatine, ascending pharyngeal, and thyroid arteries, and is drained by veins leading into the pterygoid plexus and by the internal jugular vein. Lymph is drained into retropharyngeal and deep cervical nodes. Innervation is provided by nerves IX and X and by sympathetic nerves.

The larynx connects the pharynx and the trachea; it is a 5 cm long tube, made up of a chondral skeleton, membranes, ligaments, and muscles.

The cartilages are the thyroid (having two plates, each having a superior and an inferior horn), cricoid, arytenoids (having vocal and muscular processes), corniculate (on the apex of each arytenoid), cuneiform (in the aryepiglottic fold), and the epiglottis.

The membranes are thyrohyoid and fibroelastic, the latter consisting of a superior quadrangular membrane and an inferior elastic cone.

The ligaments are the vocal, at the superior margin of the elastic cone, vestibular, at the inferior margin of the quadrangular membrane, cricothyroid, and cricotracheal.

The muscles are divided into extrinsic and intrinsic, and each group is subdivided into subgroups according to its main function, as follows:

Extrinsic
> Elevators
>> Thyro-, stylo-, and milohyoid, digastric, stylo-, and palatopharyngeus
> Depressors
>> Sternothyroid, omo-, and sternohyoid

Intrinsic
> Sphincters
>> Cricothyroid, thyro-, lateral, transverse and oblique arytenoid, thyro-, and aryepiglottic, and vocal
> Dilator
>> Posterior cricoarytenoid

The cavity of the larynx presents the following:

1. The vestibule or supraglottic cavity (from the aditus to the vestibular folds).
2. The right and left ventricles (from the vestibular to the vocal fold), lined by stratified cylindrical epithelium. Each extends into a ventricular appendix and its walls have the laryngeal tonsil. The right and left vestibular folds limit the rima vestibuli. The right and left vocal cords limit the rima glottidis (located below the rima vestibuli). These cords and their rima make up the glottis. Each vocal fold contains vocal muscle and ligament, and is lined by nonkeratinizing stratified squamous epithelium. The rima glottidis is divided into an

intermembranous and an interchondral (interarytenoid) portion.

3. The infraglottic cavity, limited by the cricothyroid ligament and the inner aspect of the cricoid cartilage, continues with the trachea.

The larynx is supplied by the superior and inferior laryngeal arteries, accompanied by veins and lymphatic vessels, the latter leading to the deep cervical nodes. The innervation of the larynx above the vocal folds is supplied by the internal laryngeal branch of the superior laryngeal nerve, and the remaining by the recurrent laryngeal. The cricothyroid muscle is supplied by the superior laryngeal nerve and the other intrinsic muscles by the recurrent laryngeal.

Thorax

The thorax is the portion of the trunk connected superiorly with the neck and inferiorly with the abdomen. The superior limit is given by a plane drawn from the spinous process of C7 to the jugular notch; laterally, the thorax is superficially separated from the superior members by a plane drawn from the midpoint of the clavicle to the axillary fossa. The axillary region can be studied with the thorax or with the superior member. The inferior limit follows the inferior margin of the thoracic cage from the base of the xiphoid process, to the costal cartilage, to the last rib to T12. The deep inferior limit corresponds to the diaphragm.

The regions of the thorax are the presternal region, infraclavicular fossa, clavipectoral triangle, pectoral region, mammary region, inframammary region, axillary region, and axillary fossa.

In order to take advantage of bony landmarks, the skeleton of the thorax will be mentioned first. It consists of sternum (manubrium, body, and xiphoid process), ribs, and thoracic vertebrae.

The manubrium corresponds to T3–T4 and the body to T5–T10. The manubrium and the body form the sternal angle, which corresponds to T4 and to the second costal cartilage. The xiphosternal joint corresponds to T10 and is at the apex of the infrasternal angle. The 12 ribs are divided into true (1–7), false (8–10), and floating (11, 12). Each rib has a head, neck, and shaft. At the neck-shaft junction there is a tubercle (for articulation with transverse process of vertebra). The shaft has an angle and inferiorly the costal groove (for insertion of the internal intercostal muscle and for intercostal artery, vein, and nerve). The superior aspect of rib 1 presents the groove for the subclavian artery and the brachial plexus, the tubercle for insertion of the anterior scalene muscle, and anteriorly the groove for the subclavian vein.

The head of each rib articulates with two thoracic vertebrae (superior and inferior costal facets) and the intervening intervestebral disc.

Vertical lines are commonly used as landmarks for the topography of thoracic organs, such as median sternal, parasternal, mammary (midclavicular), anterior, middle and posterior axillary, scapular (apex of inferior angle of scapula), median dorsal, and, between the latter two, the paravertebral.

The skin of the thorax has a variable amount of hair according to the region, age, sex, race, and biotype. It contains the anterior and lateral branches of the intercostal nerves (ventral rami of the spinal nerves) except in the dorsum, supplied by the dorsal rami of the thoracic spinal nerves, and in the superior portion, supplied by the supraclavicular nerves.

The skin presents the breasts (rudimentary in the male) in the anterior aspect of the thorax (mammary regions), overlying the pectoral major, anterior serratus, and external oblique muscles, and projected within an area limited by the second and sixth ribs, and by the sternal and anterior midaxillary line.

The mammary gland is located in the fat areolar layer or superficial layer of the tela subcutanea, in front of the superficial fascia and the deeper fat lamellar layer, followed by the pectoral major muscle and the anterior dentate muscle. The glandular parenchyma extends into the axilla (axillary tail) and is made up of 15–20 lobes, each drained by a lactiferous duct on the nipple. The body of the breast presents a more pigmented area, areola (papilla mammaria), which contains acessory mammary, sweat, and sebaceous glands and, in the center, the prominence called the nipple, at the level of the fourth intercostal space. The mammary gland is supplied by the internal thoracic, axillary, and intercostal arteries and is drained by the corresponding veins. Its lymph is drained by the pectoral and apical nodes of the axillary nodes, the internal thoracic nodes, and contralateral nodes, and the subperitoneal and the subhepatic plexuses.

The thoracic wall shows the pectoral major and minor muscles, the subclavian muscle, the serratus anterior muscle, the levatores costarum muscles, the intercostal (external, internal, and innermost muscles), the subcostal muscles, the transverse thoracic muscle, and, occasionally, the sternal muscle. Inferiorly, the diaphragmatic muscle corresponds to a thoracoabdominal septum.

The external intercostal muscles are replaced anteriorly by the homonymous membranes, the same occurring posteriorly to the internal intercostal muscles. The internal and the innermost intercostal muscles are separated by the intervening intercostal vessels and nerves. The innermost intercostal muscles and the thoracic skeleton are lined by the endothoracic fascia, which is in contact with the costal pleura.

The diaphragm has sternal, costal, and lumbar portions inserted into the centrum tendineum. A (right and left) sternocostal triangle separates the sternal and the costal portions. Each lumbar portion originates from a lateral arcuate ligament (over the quadratus lumbar muscle), a medial arcuate ligament (over the greater psoas muscle), and a crus dextrum and a crus sinistrum (from vertebrae 11-13). The right crus joins the left crus anteriorly to the aorta, the thoracic duct, the greater splanchnic nerves, and the azygos vein, forming the median arcuate ligament (aortic hiatus). The right crus is subdivided into two bundles, which form the esophageal hiatus; and it is connected to the suspensory ligament (muscle) of the duodenum. In the centrum tendineum there is the inferior vena caval foramen, which also includes the right phrenic nerve and lymphatic vessels.

Each thoracic nerve (12) has a meningeal branch and divides into a dorsal and a ventral branch. The ventral branch is subdivided into a lateral and a median cutaneous branch. The superior 11th ventral branches are called intercostal and the 12th is subcostal. Each of these branches gives off an anterior cutaneous branch and a lateral cutaneous branch. Intercostobrachial nerves lateral cutaneous and anterior cutaneous branches of intercostal nerves VII-XI supply also the abdominal wall, thus named thoracoabdominal nerves.

The thoracic wall receives blood supply from the subclavian artery (internal thoracic artery and highest intercostal artery), axillary artery, and aorta (posterior intercostal artery and subcostal artery).

The internal thoracic artery splits into the superior epigastric artery and musculophrenic artery, the former anastomosing with the inferior epigastric artery and the latter with the deep circumflex iliac artery.

The highest intercostal artery (branch of the costocervical trunk of the subclavian artery) originates posterior intercostal I and II arteries, whereas intercostal arteries III-XI are originated from the aorta. There are important anastomoses between the internal thoracic, the posterior intercostal, and the inferior epigastric arteries, and also between the intercostal arteries and branches of the internal thoracic or musculophrenic artery.

The blood is drained by the internal thoracic, posterior intercostal, and subcostal veins, ultimately into the brachiocephalic, vertebral, azygos, hemiazygos, and accessory hemiazygos veins.

The lymph is drained to parietal nodes, such as the parasternal, phrenic, and intercostal, and to phrenic and intercostal nodes. The position of the vessels and nerve in each intercostal space is usually indicated by the acronym VAN (vein, artery, nerve).

Joints of the thorax
   Costovertebral
      Head of rib with body of vertebra
      Costotransverse
   Costochondral
      Ends of costal cartilage and bone
   Sternocostal or sternochondral
      Manubriosternal
      Xiphosternal

THORACIC CAVITY

The thoracic cavity includes the mediastinum and the pleuropulmonary regions.

The mediastinum (quod in medio stat, that which is in the middle) corresponds to a median region, septum, or interval between the pleuropulmonary regions. It is divided into superior and inferior mediastinum, above and below a horizontal plane, passing through the disk between C6, C7, and T5. The inferior mediastinum is subdivided into anterior, middle, and posterior mediastinum. The subdivision of the mediastinum is the following:

Superior: Above level of pericardium, contains thymus, great vessels, trachea, and esophagus
Inferior
   Anterior: Between sternum and pericardium, contains thymus
   Middle: Above diaphragm, behind anterior mediastinum, contains pericardium and main bronchi
   Posterior: Behind pericardium, anterior to vertebral column (C7-C12, T5), above diaphragm, contains esophagus and aorta

The thoracic portion of the esophagus is the longest, between the cervical and the abdominal portions. In addition to the narrowing at the level of C6 (i.e., still in the cervical portion), the esophagus presents others at the level of the aortic arch (T4), the left bronchus (T5), and the diaphragm (T11). The mnemonic technique is the formula C6, T4, T5, T11.

The esophagus wall is constituted by the mucous, submucous, muscular, and adventitia (serous, in the abdominal portion) layers. The tunica mucosa is lined by squamous stratified epithelium on a lamina propria; the latter having many papillae and the muscular mucosae. The tela submucosa contains tubuloalveolar glands, blood and lymph vessels, lymph nodules, and the nervous submucous plexus. The musculature is striated in the oral portion and smooth in the aboral ($\frac{2}{3}$ of the length to $\frac{1}{2}$), being made up of spiral, inner circular, outer longitudinal, and a few innermost oblique. The longitudinal fibers are connected to the cricoesophageal tendon (in the dorsal aspect of the cricoid cartilage). Broncoesophageal and pleuroesophageal muscles are extensions of the musculature of the esophagus.

The phrenoesophageal membrane maintains the relationship between the esophagus and the diaphragm. the esophagus is supplied by the inferior thyroid, esophageal, intercostal, inferior phrenic, and left gastric arteries. The blood is drained by veins leading to the thyroid, azygos, and left gastric (portocaval communication). The lymph is drained into the inferior deep cervical, posterior mediastinal, and superior gastric nodes.

The nerves of the esophagus are nerve X and the nerves of the sympathetic trunks, which form the submucous and myenteric plexuses. The X nerves make up the periesophageal plexus, from which an anterior and a posterior vagal trunk emerge.

The trachea is a 15 cm (average) long tube that connects the larynx to the main bronchi, from the level of C6, to T5, where it usually bifurcates. It is divided into the cervical and thoracic parts. The trachea is a median mediastinal, preesophageal organ but just before its bifurcation into main bronchi, deviates to the right, causing the left main bronchus to relate anteriorly to the esophagus. The trachea is made up of hyaline cartilaginous arches united by annular ligaments and completed posteriorly by a fibroelastic membrane containing the smooth tracheal muscle. The tracheal epithelium is pseudostratified cylindrical ciliated and the mucous layer contains longitudinal elastic fibers. The submucous tela presents mucous and serous glands. The tracheal bifurcation has a ridge called the carina of the trachea, a landmark for bronchoscopy.

The blood is supplied by the interior, internal, and superior thyroid and bronchial arteries, and is drained by the inferior thyroid veins. The lymph is drained into the cervical, tracheal, and tracheobronchial nodes.

The innervation is supplied by preganglionic parasympathetic fibers; the postganglionic fibers stimulate the smooth muscle and glands, which are inhibited by postganglionic sympathetic fibers.

The main bronchi, resulting from the tracheal bifurcation, are tubes that, having reached the hilus of each lung, form a tree in the pulmonary parenchyma. They are lined with pseudostratified ciliated columnar epithelium, and their walls contain collagenous, elastic, and muscular tissue, cartilage, and glands.

The main bronchi are divided into lobar, segmental, and subsegmental bronchi, and subdivided into bronchioles. The wall of the bronchioles is lined by columnar ciliated epithelium and contains collagenous, elastic, and muscular fibers. Respiratory bronchioles and alveo-

lar ducts have a cuboidal epithelium instead, and the alveoli possess squamous epithelium, and collagenous and elastic fibers. A summary of lobar and segmental bronchi follows:

Right main bronchus
  Right superior lobar bronchus
    Apical segmental bronchus   (B I)
    Posterior segmental bronchus   (B II)
    Anterior segmental bronchus   (B III)
  Right middle lobar bronchus
    Lateral segmental bronchus   (B IV)
    Medial segmental bronchus   (B V)
  Right inferior lobar bronchus
    Superior segmental bronchus   (B VI)
    Medial basal segmental
bronchus   (B VII)
    Anterior basal segmental
bronchus   (B VIII)
    Lateral basal segmental
bronchus   (B IX)
    Posterior basal segmental
bronchus   (B X)
 Left main bronchus
  Left superior lobar bronchus
    Apicoposterior segmental
bronchus   (B I + II)
    Anterior segmental bronchus   (B III)
    Superior lingular bronchus   (B IV)
    Inferior lingular bronchus   (B V)
  Left inferior lobar bronchus
    Superior segmental bronchus   (B VI)
    Medial basal segmental
bronchus   (B VII)
    Anterior basal segmental
bronchus   (B VIII)
    Lateral basal segmental
bronchus   (B IX)
    Posterior basal segmental
bronchus   (B X)

The lungs are bilateral thoracic organs that are separated by the mediastinum or interpulmonary region. Each lung is surrounded by a double-layered serous sac, the pleura.

The pleura consists of an outer layer, lining the endothoracicfascia, called the parietal pleura, and an inner layer, in contact with the lung, termed the visceral pleura. Both layers limit the pleural cavity, which contains a very small amount of pleural fluid. The parietal pleura has a cupola, and costal, mediastinal, and diaphragmatic aspects. At the level of the reflection of the visceral to the parietal pleura, the costodiaphragmatic, costo- and phrenicomediastinal, retroesophageal, and right infrapericardial recesses are found. The mediastinal pleura extends downward from the root of the lung and constitutes the pulmonary ligament.

The lung has a base, an apex, a diaphragmatic aspect or surface, a costal aspect, and a medial aspect. The latter is divided into a vertebral portion and a mediastinal portion, which has the cardiac impression. The anterior margin in the left lung presents the cardiac incisure and the lingula is found between this incisure and the oblique fissure. The inferior margin separates the diaphragmatic surface from the costal and medial surfaces.

The concavity in the medial aspect is the pulmonary hilum, containing the root of the lung (i.e., the peduncle, or pedicle, formed by the bronchi, nerves, blood, and lymphatic vessels. The left hilum presents in front and above the branches of the pulmonary artery, below the branches of the pulmonary vein, and behind the main bronchus. In addition, the right hilum shows the eparterial bronchus. The three lobes of the right lung are separated by an oblique and a horizontal fissure, whereas the two of the left are separated by an oblique fissure (Table 2-4). The interlobular surfaces limit the fissures. The right oblique fissure begins at the level of rib 5 (the left at a higher level), follows rib 4, and ends at chondrocostal joint VI. The horizontal fissure begins at the oblique fissure, where the midaxillary line crosses rib VI and follows costal cartilage IV.

The aortic arch passes over the left root of the lung (radix pulmonis), and the azygos vein passes over the right root of the lung (radix pulmonis).

Branches of the pulmonary arteries accompany the bronchi, and their venous blood is oxygenated in the alveoli. Pulmonary veins collect the oxygenated (arterial) blood from the alveoli and venous blood from bronchial walls and pleura. Bronchial arteries (one right and two left) supply the nonrespiratory structures of the lungs. Blood from the first branches of the bronchi is drained by bronchial veins to the posterior intercostal, azygos, and hemiazygos veins. Lymph is drained to the bronchopulmonary nodes, then to tracheobronchial nodes. Lymph of the parietal pleura is drained into nodes of the thoracic wall, then into axillary nodes.

Innervation is provided by nerve X and the sympathetic trunks, forming anterior and posterior pulmonary plexuses (at the root of the lung), which contain parasympathetic ganglion cells.

The pericardium is the double-layered serous sac that encloses the heart and part of the great vessels. It is surrounded by the fibrous pericardium and connected to the sternum by the sternopericardial ligament. An infracardiac bursa may be found between the pericardium and the esophagus just above the diaphragm. The outer layer of the serous pericardium is the parietal lamina and the inner layer is the visceral lamina (epicardium), both lined by mesothelium and limiting the pericardial cavity, which contains a few drops of pericardial fluid. The transverse sinus is a canal between the aorta and pulmonary trunk (in front) and the superior vena cava and the atria (behind). The recess between the inferior vena cava and the pulmonary veins is the oblique sinus.

The phrenic nerves and the pulmonary root (peduncle or pedicle) are closely related to the pericardium and can be used as landmarks for its division, as follows:

1. Prephrenic area and retrophrenic area
2. Suprapedicular zone, pedicular zone (prepedicular and retropedicular portions) and infrapedicular zone

The heart consists of two atria (each having an appendage, termed auricle) and two ventricles. The heart can be compared to a cone or inverted pyramid, having a basis, an apex (having the apical notch), three surfaces (sternocostal or anterior, diaphragmatic or inferior, and pulmonary or lateral), and a right margin (surface or aspect). On the surface, the coronary sulcus separates the atria from the ventricles, and the anterior and posterior (inferior) interventricular sulci indicate the limit between the ventricles. Internally, the atria are separated from the ventricles by atrioventricular valves, the right or tricuspid (anterior, posterior, and septal cusps), and the left or bicuspid or mitral (anterior and posterior cusps). The right and left atria are separated by the interatrial septum (containing the oval fossa and its limbus). The interventricular septum is interposed between the ventricles.

The heart is a modified and twisted vessel and as such is made up of the epicardial, myocardial, and endocardial layers. It contains a fibrous skeleton, which surrounds the tricuspid and the mitral valve, the roots of the aorta and pulmonary trunk, and contains the pars membranacea of the interventricular septum. The fibrous skeleton is made up of anuli fibrosi, the left and the right fibrous trigones, the conus tendon, and part of the membranous septum. The atria have thinner walls than the

Table 2-4. Segments of Pulmonary Lobes

Lobes	Right Lung	Left Lung
Superior	Apical (S I)	Apicoposterior (S I + II)
	Posterior (S II)	
	Anterior (S III)	Anterior (S III)
Middle	Lateral (S IV)	Superior lingular (S IV)
	Medial (S V)	Inferior lingular (S V)
Inferior	Superior (S VI)	Superior (S VI)
	Basal medial (S VII)	Basal medial (S VII)
	Basal anterior (S VIII)	Basal anterior (S VIII)
	Basal lateral (S IX)	Basal lateral (S IX)
	Basal posterior (S X)	Basal posterior (S X)

ventricles and the left ventricle has a wall three times thicker than that of the right.

The right atrium presents the pectinate muscles, the terminal sulcus and crest, the intervenous tubercle, the foramens of the minimal veins, of the superior and of the inferior vena cava, and of the coronary sinus (the latter two guarded by valves). The left atrium shows the oval fossa, the valve of the oval foramen (falx septi), and the four foramens of the pulmonary veins.

The right ventricle has the supraventricular crest, the arterial conus (infundibulum), the septomarginal trabecula (moderator band), the papillary muscles (anterior, posterior, and septal) the chordae tendineae (for the cusps), the valve of the pulmonary trunk (made up of anterior, left, and right semilunar valvulae having noduli and lunulae). The left ventricle has the aortic valve (made up of posterior, right, and left semilunar valvulae noduli and lunulae), papillary muscles (anterior and posterior), and chordae tendineae.

The cardiac conducting system (or elements) is constituted of specialized nodal myocytes and Purkinje's conducting myofibers. It is divided into Keith-Flack or sinoatrial node (pacemaker), anterior, middle, and posterior internodal (atrial) tracts, Aschoff-Tawara or atrioventricular node, His fascicle (bundle), and trunk (right branch and its ramus, and left branch and its anterior and posterior rami).

Blood is supplied to the heart by the left and right coronary arteries and is drained by the coronary sinus (60 percent) and the minimal cardiac veins. The coronary arteries possess atrial, ventricular, ventriculoatrial and atrioventricular branches. The main branches of each coronary artery are as follows:

    From the right
        Branch of the arterial conus
        Branch of the sinoatrial node (60 percent of the cases)
        Branch of the right margin
        Intermediate atrial branch
        Posterior interventricular branch and its posterior septal branches
        Branch of the atrioventricular node (90 percent of the case)
        Right posterolateral branch
    From the left
        Anterior interventricular branch and its branches
            Branch of the arterial conus
            Lateral branch
            Anterior septal branches
        Circumflex branch and its branches
            Anastomotic atrial branch
            Left marginal branch

        Intermediate atrial branch
        Left posterior ventricular branch
        Branch of the sinoatrial node (40 percent of the cases)
        Branch of the atrioventricular node (10 percent of the cases)

The blood is drained from the heart by anterior cardiac veins, which empty into the right atrium, and by the minimal cardiac veins, which open directly into the cardiac cavities. The major vein is the coronary sinus, which ends in the right atrium after receiving the great, middle, and small cardiac veins; left posterior ventricular vein; and oblique vein of the left atrium.

The heart is innervated by sympathetic and parasympathetic cardiac nerves, which form a ganglionated cardiac plexus, providing nerves that follow the cornary arteries directed to their walls and the myocardium. The autonomic and sensory fibers are provided by the vagus nerve and sympathetic trunk. The cardiac nerves are classified according to their origin (i.e., cervical, cervicothoracic, and thoracic). The lymph of the heart is drained into vessels that accompany the coronary arteries and are tributaries of a right or a left collecting trunk. The right trunk leads to superior mediastinal nodes and the left to the caval node of the superior tracheobronchial group.

The vessels and nerves of the thorax are the pulmonary trunk arteries and veins, the aorta, the brachiocephalic veins, the cava veins, the azygos and vertebral veins, the lymph nodes and vessels, the phrenic and vagus nerves, and the sympathetic trunks, nerves, and autonomic plexuses.

The pulmonary trunk (5 cm long) begins in the conus arteriosus of the right ventricle and ends by dividing into right and left pulmonary arteries, for the right and left lung, respectively. The left artery is linked to the aortic arch by the fibrous, obliterated remains of the arterial ducts, the arterial ligament. The four pulmonary veins originate from the five lobar veins after the right superior and middle veins join to form a single trunk before entering the left atrium. The pulmonary trunk and veins and the ascending aorta are invested with pericardium.

The aorta begins at the left ventricle and supplies the entire body. It is divided into ascending aorta (5 cm long), arch of the aorta, and descending aorta. The root of the aorta, part of the ascending aorta, presents the sinuses of the aorta, each corresponding to a semilunar valvula of the aortic valve. The arch of the aorta (T4) causes a narrowing of the esophagus just above the constriction caused by the left bronchus (T5). The arch prominence, seen in radiograms, is called aortic knuckle. The branches of the arch are the brachiocephalic trunk, the left common carotid artery, and the left subclavian artery. Just after giving off the left subclavian artery the aorta shows a narrowing called isthmus aortae. The descending (thoracic) aorta is found in the posterior mediastinum, extending from the arch to the aortic orifice of the diaphragm (T12), where it continues to descend as the abdominal aorta. Its branches are the 3rd to the 11th posterior intercostal arteries and the subcostal arteries, superior phrenic arteries, two left and one right bronchial arteries, and two esophageal, pericardial, and mediastinal arteries.

The main veins are the right and left brachiocephalic (each formed by the internal jugular and subclavian veins), which join the superior vena cava. The latter receives the azygos vein and terminates in the right atrium. The inferior vena cava, ascending from the abdomen, pierces the orifice of the central tendon of the diaphragm and, after a short course (3 cm), ends in the right atrium. The main azygos veins are the azygos, hemiazygos, and accessory hemiazygos. The azygos receive the hemiazygos and the accessory hemiazygos and ends in the superior vena cava. The vertebral veins form plexuses that drain the dorsum, the vertebral column, and the organs contained in the vertebral canal; they anastomose with intracranial portal, intercostal, lumbar, and sacral veins. Parietal thoracic veins, such as the superficial thoracoepigastric veins, establish communication between the superior and inferior vena cavae (collateral circulation).

The lymph nodes are paramammary, parasternal, intercostal, prevertebral, superior phrenic, prepericardial, lateral pericardial, anterior mediastinal and, among the posterior mediastinal, the pulmonary juxtaesophageal, hilar bronchopulmonary, superior, and superior tracheobronchial, and paratracheal. The lymph is drained ultimately to the bronchomediastinal and descending intercostal trunks and the thoracic duct; the latter begins in the abdominal cisterna chyli, penetrates in the thorax through the aortic orifice of the diaphragm, runs in the osterior mediastinum, reaches the neck and ends in the angle between the left internal jugular and subclavian veins. Among tributaries of the thoracic duct are found the left jugular, subclavian, and bronchomediastinal trunks. On the right, these trunks unite into a short (1 cm) right lymphatic duct, which ends in the right internal jugulosubclavian venous junction.

The right and left phrenic nerves, which innervate the diaphragm, originate from C3, C4, and C5, run in the neck in front of the anterior scalene muscle and in the thorax in front of the pulmonary pedicles, giving branches to pericardium, pleura, peritoneum, vessels, and diaphragm. The right and left vagus nerves contribute to the ipsilateral pulmonary plexus, form the anterior and posterior esophageal trunks, and present a recurrent laryngeal branch and cardiac branches. The right recur-

rent laryngeal nerve forms a loop below the subclavian artery and the left forms a loop below the aortic arch. The thoracic portion of the sympathetic trunks, located in front of the neck of the ribs, have 12 ganglia (the first is united to the inferior cervical ganglion and is called stellate ganglion). Rami communicants link the trunks and ganglia to the ventral rami of the thoracic nerves. The main branches are cardiac, pulmonary, and the greater, lesser, and lowest splanchnic nerves. The latter three enter the abdomen through the crura of the diaphragm and end in the celiac and renal plexuses and ganglia. Cardiac, aortic, pulmonary, and esophageal plexuses are formed by the vagus and sympathetic trunks.

The thymus has a cervical and a thoracic portion. The lobes of the thymus are those in front and on the sides of the trachea, and behind the sternal manubrium. The organ develops until puberty, when it regresses and is replaced almost competely by fibrous and fatty tissue.

Abdomen

The abdomen is the portion of the trunk between the thorax and the pelvis. Its superior limit superficially is the inferior margin of the thorax (base of the xiphoid process, costal cartilages, last rib to T12), and deeply is the diaphragm. Its inferior limit is the horizontal plane at the level of the terminal lines of the pelvis, (i.e., the pelvic superior limit). There is, then, a "thoracic" portion of the upper abdomen (protected by the lower ribs) and there is ample communication with the pelvis.

Drawing vertical lines at midinguinal points and two horizontal lines, one tangential to the rib cage (subcostal), and the other at the level of the anterosuperior iliac spine, the anterolateral wall of the abdomen can be divided into three stages (epi-, meso-, and hypogastrium) and nine regions, as follows:

1. Right hypochondriac
2. Epigastric, containing the epigastic fossa
3. Left hypochondriac
4. Right lateral (lumbar)
5. Umbilical, containing the umbilicus (L4)
6. Left lateral (lumbar)
7. Right inguinal
8. Pubic

Using the median plane (lines alba) and a horizontal plane at the level of the umbilicus, the anterolateral abdominal wall is divided into quadrants (right and left superior, right and left inferior).

The abdomen has walls (parietal regions) and a cavity, which is lined by a serous sac (peritoneum) and contains viscera. The abdominal wall is made up of skin, fasciae, muscles (or bone), extraperitoneal tissue, and parietal peritoneum.

The skin comprises epidermis, dermis, and subcutaneous tela, the latter constituted of areolar layer (fat), superficial fascia, and lamellar layer (fat). The abdominal surface contains hair, especially in the pubic region, where distribution of hair in the adult is triangular (with a superior base) in the female and is rhomboid (with the superior angle near the umbilicus) in the male.

In the subcutaneous tela, there are superficial vessels and nerves, as follows:

1. Superior arteries originate from the superior epigastric artery (terminal branch of the internal thoracic artery, branch of the subclavian artery); inferior arteries originate from the inferior epigastric artery (branch of the external iliac artery), from the superficial epigastric artery, and from the superficial circumflex iliac artery (the latter two branches of the femoral artery); lateral arteries originate from the intercostal arteries and some are cutaneous branches of the lumbar arteries.

2. The veins are tributaries of the superior and inferior epigastric veins. The superior epigastric veins anastomose with the internal thoracic vein; thoracoepigastric veins run laterally uniting the inferior epigastric to the superior epigastric, ultimately, to the axillary vein; the network formed by all these veins is connected to deep veins and to rootlets and roots of paraumbilical veins (usually two), which follow the round ligament of the liver to drain into the portal vein. In the periumbilical area the anastomoses among the superior and inferior caval and the portal systems are established.

3. The two territories for lymph drainage are the supraumbilical, leading to the axillary nodes; and infraumbilical, leading to the inguinal nodes.

4. Nerves originate from the lateral and anterior branches of the last six intercostal nerves and from the iliohypogastric and ilioinguinal nerves.

The muscular fascia follows the subcutaneous tela and covers the external oblique muscle (Table 2-5).

The inguinal ligament (from the anterosuperior iliac spine to the pubic tubercle) is the inferior margin of the EO muscle. It is fused with the iliopubic ligament and medially both extend to the pectineal fascia and ligament (lacunar ligament). The EO aponeurosis is split into medial crus and lateral crus, both crura forming the superficial inguinal ring. Intercrural fibers exist, as the name implies, between the crura.

The lumbar triangle is limited by the posterior margin of the EO muscle, the lateral margin of the latissimus dorsi muscle, and the iliac crest.

The transversal fascia lines the internal aspect of the

Table 2-5. Muscles of the Anterolateral Abdominal Wall, Their Origins, and Insertions

Muscle	Origin	Insertion
Rectus abdominis (RA)	Pubic symphysis Pubic crest	Xiphoid process Ribs 5–8
Pyramidalis (P)	Pubic body	Linea alba
External oblique (EO)	Ribs 5–12	Linea alba Pubic tubercle Iliac crest
Internal oblique (IO)	Thoracolumbar Fascia	Linea alba
	Iliac crest	Ribs 10–12 Rectus sheath Pubis
Transversus abdominis (TA)	Ribs 7–12	Linea alba
	Thoracolumbar Fascia Iliac crest	Pubis

TA muscle and of the RA muscle, and is continuous with adjacent fasciae throughout the abdominal cavity.

The right and left aponeuroses of the EO muscle pass in front of the RA muscle of the corresponding side, and meet in the median plane with those of the IO and TA muscles to form the linea alba.

The linea semilunaris correspond to the line along which the aponeuroses of the IO and TA muscles meet at the lateral margin of the RA muscle.

The superior portion of the TA aponeurosis runs posteriorly to the RA muscle (the lower limit is the arcuate line) but inferiorly it runs anteriorly to the RA muscle.

The aponeurosis of the IO muscle is split into anterior (to the RA muscle) and posterior (to the RA muscle) laminae; the anterior lamina fuses with the EO aponeurosis and the posterior fuses with the TA aponeurosis.

The 4 cm long (in the adult) inguinal canal is located just above the inguinal ligament. Above the midpoint of the inguinal ligament the deep inguinal ring is found, whereas laterally to the pubic tubercle there is the superficial inguinal ring. The oblique inguinal canal has a floor represented by the inguinal ligament and at its medial extremity the lacunar ligament (fibers of the inguinal ligament inserted into the pecten of the pubis, its lateral continuation being the pectineal ligament). The EO muscle aponeurosis is superficial to the canal, and the transversal fascia, the TA, and the IO muscles form the posterior wall. The IO muscle originates from the inguinal ligament in front of the deep ring (lateral) and inserts posteriorly to the superficial ring (medial), arching over (ceiling) the spermatic cord in the male and the (uterine) round ligament in the female.

The inguinal canal contains the spermatic cord (or the

round ligament) which components are the ductus deferens, joined by nerves and vessels (differential artery and vein, testicular artery, venous pampiniform plexus, lymphatics, and autonomic nerves). In addition, the ilioinguinal nerve, the genital branch of the genitofemoral nerve, and the cremasteric artery (from the inferior epigstric artery) should be mentioned. The spermatic cord is surrounded by the internal spermatic fascia, by the cremaster muscle and fascia, and by the external spermatic fascia.

Components of the spermatic cord, the epididymis, and the testis are contained in the scrotum, which is divided by the scrotal septum into right and left cavities.

The layers of the wall of the scrotum correspond to those derived from the abdominal wall, as this was "pushed" by the descending testis:

1. Epidermis and dermis: Epidermis and dermis of abdominal wall
2. Dartos: Subcutaneous tela
3. External spermatic fascia: EO muscles
4. Cremaster muscle and fascia: IO and T muscles
5. Internal spermatic fascia: Transversalis fascia
6. Connective tissue: Extraperitoneal connective tissue
7. Tunica vaginalis testis: Peritoneum (vaginal process)

The posterior abdominal wall is made up of the lumbar vertebrae; the diaphragm with its right and left crura, median (in front of the aorta), medial (over the major psoas muscle), and lateral (over the quadratus lumborum muscle) arcuate ligament; the iliopsoas (iliacus and major psoas muscles); and the minor psoas muscle.

ABDOMINAL CAVITY

The abdominal cavity is lined by the peritoneum, a serous sac that surrounds the abdominal viscera or organs.

The peritoneum, like the pericardium, the pleura, and the tunica vaginalis testis, is a sac formed by parietal and visceral laminae, which limit the peritoneal cavity and contain a few drops of peritoneal fluid. The peritoneal cavity is closed in the male and open in the female (at the level of the abdominal orifice of the uterine tubes). The main folds, omenta (epiploons), mesos, and ligaments of the peritoneum can be classified according to the embryogenesis:

1. From the ventral mesogastrium
Lesser omentum
  Hepatoesophageal ligament
  Hepatogastric ligament
  Hepatoduodenal ligament
  Hepatocolic ligament

Falciform ligament
Round ligament of the liver
Coronary ligament
Right triangular ligament
Left triangular ligament
2. From the dorsal mesogastrium
Greater omentum
  Gastrophrenic ligament
  Gastrosplenic ligament
  Gastrocolic ligament
Splenorenal (splenophrenic) ligament
Phrenicocolic ligament
3. From the dorsal common mesentery
Mesentery (mesojejunoileum)
Mesoappendix
Mesocecum (only in the embryo)
Ascending mesocolon (only in the embryo)
Transverse mesocolon
Descending mesocolon (only in the embryo)
Sigmoid mesocolon
  Iliac mesocolon
  Pelvic mesocolon
4. From the urachus*
Median umbilical ligament
5. From the obliterated umbilical artery*
Medial umbilical ligament
6. From the inferior epigastric vessels*
Lateral umbilical fold

The abdominal cavity, then, contains the peritoneal cavity, the anteperitoneal structures, and the retroperitoneal organs, such as the kidneys.

The peritoneal cavity is divided into a greater and a lesser sac. The greater sac is found between the thoracoabdominal diaphragm and the pelvic diaphragm. It extends through the omental or epiploic foramen (limited by the hepatic pedicle, the duodenum, the inferior vena cava, and the caudate lobe of the liver) into the vestibule of the omental bursa (lesser sac), located posteriorly to the lesser omentum, and extends further, beyond the arch of the left gastric vessels, at the level of the lesser curvature of the stomach, into the omental bursa or lesser sac. The latter is, thus, mainly retrogastric and presents a superior omental recess, an inferior omental recess, and a splenic recess.

The abdominal cavity is divided into a supra- and an inframesocolic region; the latter is subdivided by the root of the mesentery (mesojejunoileum) into a right and a left area, each presenting a parietocolic sulcus or recess (right and left), adjacent to the ascending and descending colons, respectively.

---

* These structures raise low folds of parietal peritoneum in the inner aspect of the ventral abdominal wall.

In the supramesocolic region, the subphrenic, subhepatic, and hepatorenal recesses are related to the liver and/or diaphragm.

At the level of the duodenum, there are the superior and inferior duodenal folds, and the paraduodenal fold, related to the homonymous recesses. In the ileocecolic area, the superior and inferior ileocecal recesses, the ileocecal fold, and the retrocecal recess are found. The sigmoid mesocolon limits the intersigmoid recess, the vertex of which is related posteriorly to the left ureter.

The anterior parietal peritoneum presents the para- and the supravesical fossa (between the median and the medial umbilical ligaments), the medial inguinal (between the inferior epigastric vessels and the umbilical artery) and the lateral inguinal fossa (lateral to the epigastric vessels), and the inguinal trigone.

The urogenital peritoneal includes the broad ligament (of the uterus), comprised of mesometrium, mesosalpinx, and mesovarium; the suspensory ligament of the ovary; and the rectouterine fold. In the pelvis, it is possible to recognize the rectouterine, the vesicouterine, and the ovarian fossa in the female. In the male, there is a rectovesical fossa, and in both sexes, the paravesical fossae.

ABDOMINAL VISCERA

The abdominal portion of the esophagus, the stomach, and the intestines is the continuation of the alimentary canal.

The abdominal esophagus is short and its aboral end presents the esophagogastric orifice (or cardia), surrounded by a muscular mechanism for opening and closing, although less prominent than that found around the gastroduodenal orifice. Since the word sphincter means only closing (constriction) or obliteration, and since there is also an active opening or dilator component, it was suggested that it also be called esophagogastric pylorus (as pylorus means doorman, implying the existence of a closing or sphincter component and an opening or dilator component).

The submucous veins of the esophagus and stomach constitute a portocaval anastomosis (by means of the left gastric and azygos veins). At the level of the abdominal esophagus, the vagus nerves can be sectioned surgically (vagotomy and vagectomy). Through the esophageal hiatus of the diaphragm, hiatal herniae can occur. The vessels and nerves of the abdominal esophagus are as follows:

Arteries: Phrenic and left gastric
Veins: Esophageal
Lymphatics: Superior gastric nodes
Nerves: Vagus nerves and sympathetic trunks

The stomach has an anterior and a posterior wall, the lesser (right) and greater curvature, the angular and the cardiac notches, and two orifices, (i.e., cardiac or esophagogastric and the gastroduodenal). It is divided into a cardiac portion, fundus or fornix, body, and pyloric portion (the latter subdivided into pyloric antrum and canal). The wall of the viscus is made up of a serous coat, subserous tela, muscular coat (longitudinal and circular layers, and oblique fibers), submucous tela, and mucous coat.

The serous coat covers the stomach, except its bare area (limited by the gastrophrenic ligament) and connects the viscus to adjacent organs by means of the gastrohepatic, gastrophrenic, gastrosplenic, and gastrocolic ligaments.

The muscular coat contributes the gastric component of the esophagastric mechanism for opening and closing the junction with the esophagus, and of the gastroduodenal pylorus, which shows a well developed dilator muscle and sphincter muscle.

The submucous tela contains many arteriolovenular anastomoses or shunts. The mucous coat presents gastric folds and areas, foveolae, and glands, classified into cardiac, gastric proper, and pyloris. The epithelium is sharply demarcated from stratified squamous and the esophageal, and appears as a simple column. The vessels and nerves of the stomach are as follows:

Arteries: Right, left, and posterior gastric, right and left gastroepiploic, and short gastric.
Veins: Right and left gastric, right and left gastroepiploic, and short gastric.
Lymphatics: Vessels and nodes named after the artery.
Nerves: Celiac plexus, left phrenic, and vagus nerves. The fibers are sympathetic, parasympathetic, and sensory.

The intestines begin at the gastroduodenal orifice and end at the anus. They are divided into the following portions:

1. Small intestine
   Duodenum
   Jejunum
   Ileum
2. Large intestine
   Cecum
   Vermiform appendix
   Colons
      Ascending colon
      Transverse colon
      Descending colon

Sigmoid colon
   Iliac colon
   Pelvic colon
Rectum
Anal canal

The duodenum is the first, shortest, and almost entirely fixed portion of the small intestine; it is about 12 fingerbreadths long. The duodenal loop may appear as the letters C, U, or V, and it embraces the head of the pancreas; it is usually divided into superior, descending, inferior (horizontal), and ascending (oblique) portions. The duodenal bulb or cap is mobile and is connected to the liver by the hepatoduodenal portion of the lesser omentum. The duodenum is hidden behind the root of the transverse mesocolon, the coalescent ascending mesocolon, and the root of the mesentery (pars tecta duodeni). It is then divided into supra- and inframesocolic portions. The duodenum, the left renal vein, and the pancreatic uncinate process are contained in the mesenterico-aortic forceps. The duodenojejunal flexure is united to the right crus of the diaphragm by the suspensory ligament and muscle.

The peritoneum forms recesses adjacent to the aboral portion of the duodenum. The musculature continues that of the stomach at the gastroduodenal pylorus. The mucous coat presents the greater duodenal papilla for the openings of the common bile duct and the main pancreatic duct, which may open together in the hepatopancreatic ampulla; and the lesser duodenal papilla for the accessory pancreatic duct.

The vessels and nerves of the duodenum are as follows:

Arteries: Right gastric, gastroduodenal, superior and inferior pancreaticoduodenal.

Veins: Follow the arteries.

Lymphatics: Anterior and posterior collecting vessels and nodes (in front and behind the pancreas), then into celiac and superior mesenteric nodes, and into the thoracic duct.

Nerves: Autonomic and sensory fibers from the celiac and superior mesenteric plexuses.

The duodenum receives the exocrine fluids from the liver and pancreas.

The liver occupies the right hypochondriac and the epigastric region. It has a diaphragmatic (right and left lobes) and a visceral aspect (right, left, quadrate, and caudate lobes). The latter shows the hilum (hepatic portal), and contains the hepatic pedicle (hepatic ducts and artery, and branches of the portal vein) at the cross bar of the letter H, represented by the fissures for the round

ligament, the venous ligament, the inferior vena cava, and the gallbladder.

The arrangement of the branches of the portal vein and of the hepatic artery as well as the biliary ducts is the same; it interdigitates with the distribution of the hepatic veins. It is then possible to divide the liver into right and left hemilivers (by plane from fossa of gallbladder to fossa of the inferior vena cava), and into portobilioarterial segments and hepatic venous segments.

The official terminology of the lobes and segments is as follows:

Right hepatic lobe
   Anterior segment
   Posterior segment
Left hepatic lobe
   Medial segment
     Pars quadrata
   Lateral segment
Quadrate lobe
Caudate lobe
   Papillary process
   Caudate process

The venous hepatic segments or venous drainage segments are left, intermediate, right, and caudate (each having its tributaries to the inferior vena cava).

The peritoneal connections of the liver are coronary, right, and left triangular, hepatorenal, falciform, and round (teres) ligaments, and lesser omentum.

The liver is a modified compound tubular gland. Except for the bare area, most of its surface is covered by a serous coat, a subserous tela, and a fibrous capsule, which enters at the hilum, investing each segmental pedicle and penetrates within the parenchyma. The hepatic cells form perforated interconnected plates, which appear as cords in transverse sections. The bile flows in biliary capillaries, which are intercellular canals that join to form biliary ducts. The plates are surrounded by venous sinusoids. The hepatic acinus or glandular unit contains branches of the bile system, portal vein, and hepatic artery; the polygonal hepatic lobule contains the central vein. Each lobule is composed of several acini and the venous sinusoids which drain into a central vein. The interlobular veins, arteries, nerves, and lymphatics, as follows, accompany the bile ductules:

Artery: Hepatic.

Veins: Portal and hepatic (caudate, right, intermediate, and left).

Lymphatics: Deep and superficial networks, which join at the hilum, and the resulting vessels run in the lesser omentum to end in nodes near the neck of the pancreas as well as in celiac, gastric, and mediastinal nodes.

Nerves: Sympathetic and parasympathetic fibers from the hepatic plexus.

The extrahepatic biliary passages begin with the common hepatic duct, formed by the right and left hepatic ducts, one from each hemiliver. The common hepatic duct continues as the common bile duct (choledochus) after it joins with the cystic duct. The gallbladder contains the fundus, body, and neck, and the vesicular wall is made up of serous, subserous, muscular, and mucous layers. The neck of the gallbladder and the cystic duct contain a spiral fold. The common bile duct is joined by the main pancreatic duct and both form the hepatopancreatic ampulla, surrounded by sphincter (circular) and dilator (longitudinal) musculature, as a diminutive "pylorus." The nerves and vessels of the extrahepatic biliary passages are as follows:

Arteries: Cystic, supraduodenal, and posterosuperior pancreaticoduodenal.

Veins: Cystic, venous plexus leading to the liver, duodenum, and pancreas.

Lymphatics: To liver and pancreas.

Nerves: From the hepatic plexus.

The pancreas is the amphicrine (both exo- and endocrine) extraparietal gland of the duodenum. It is divided into head (embraced by the duodenum), neck, body, and tail (next to the splenic hilum). The head shows the uncinate process, the top of which is contained (along with the duodenum and the left renal vein) in the mesenterico-aortic forceps, and the body has the omental tubercle. The pancreas is divided into the supra- and inframesocolic portions.

The pancreas combines the structures of an exocrine and an endocrine organ. The exocrine corresponds to a compound tubuloacinar gland; secreting cells form the walls of the acini and tubules. The endocrine organ is represented by (Langerhans') pancreatic islets, which form cords next to capillaries. There are A, B, and D cells (C cells in guinea pigs). Glucagon is secreted by A cells and insulin by B cells.

The vessels of the pancreas are as follows:

Arteries: Superior and inferior pancreaticoduodenal, dorsal pancreatic, pancreatica magna, and arteries of the tail.

Veins: Follow the arteries.

Lymphatics: Drain to splenic, gastric, mesenteric, hepatic, and celiac nodes.

The spleen develops in the dorsal mesogastrium, and in the adult is located in the left hypochondriac region. It is the largest lymphoid organ, surrounded by a fibrous capsule, from which septa penetrate the parenchyma. The spleen has diaphragmatic and visceral aspects, superior and inferior borders, and posterior and anterior extremities. The visceral aspect is subdivided into renal, gastric, and colic areas, and contains the splenic hilum, where the splenic pedicle (splenic vessels and nerves) is found. The viscus is made up of tunica serosa, tunica fibrosa, trabeculae, and pulp. The latter is comprised of white and red pulp. The white pulp corresponds to splenic corpuscles (lymphatic follicles) and the red pulp has reticular fibers, venous sinuses, erythrocytes (which are responsible for the red color), and reticuloendothelial cells. The vessels and nerves of the spleen are as follows:

Artery: Splenic, ultimately giving off four segmental arteries, one for each splenic segment (almost independent anatomicosurgical territory).

Vein: Splenic, usually formed by four segmental veins that drain the blood to the portal vein.

Lymphatics: Lead to splenic nodes. The lymphocytes directly join the bloodstream.

Nerves: From the celiac plexus. The splenic plexus contains postganglionic sympathetic and sensory fibers.

The jejunoileum consists of the jejunum (midportion of the small intestine) and the ileum (aboral portion of the small intestine), both making up the mesenterial portion of the adult intestine. It begins at the dudenojejunal flexure and ends at the ileal papilla (formerly called the ileocecal valve) in the cecocolic junction. The demarcation between the jejunum and the ileum is not distinct and, as a consequence, several criteria are used: (1) the junumum ends at the eighth loop of the small intestine; (2) the length of the jejunum is the oral two-third or one-half, or two-fifths of the small intestine; (3) the jejunum ends at the insertion of (Meckel's) diverticulum ilei, which appears only in 1 to 2 percent of the cases (at approximately 60 cm orally to the cecum); (4) the jejunum ends at the point where the extension of the superior mesenteric artery reaches the small intestine; and (5) the ileum begins where the first Peyer's patches (aggregated follicles) appear. The jejunum is often empty and wider, and has a thicker wall than the ileum; it appears feathery in radiograms, whereas the ileum is homogeneous.

The average length of the small intestine is circa 3 m in the cadaver, while it is shorter and variable in the living adult individual. The superior left and right (all jejunal), and inferior left (jejunal and ileal), and right (ileal) are the four groups of coils of the small intestine.

The jejunoileum is attached to the posterior abdominal wall by the mesentery, the root of which (15 cm long) runs from L2 to the right sacroiliac joint. The mesentery contains fat, vessels, nerves, and lymph nodes (circa 150).

The terminal ileum is the distal portion (3 cm long), which usually has a dilation or ileal ampulla. In the living and in cadavers embalmed soon after death, the ileum ends in the large intestine with a conical papilla having a star-shaped orifice (ileal papilla), containing a muscular mechanism to control the flow of the intestinal contents (ileal pylorus). The opening and closing of the orifice is caused by longitudinal and circular (sphincter) musculature, respectively.

The nerves and vessels of the small intestine are as follows:

Arteries: Celiac trunk, superior mesenteric artery, through jejunal and ileal arteries, forming arches and giving off straight arteries.

Veins: Superior mesenteric vein (portal vein).

Lymphatics: Central lacteals, intramural networks, mesenteric lymphatic vessels, interrupted by lymph nodes, and thoracic duct.

Nerves: Celiac and superior mesenteric plexuses, autonomic fibers (sympathetic and parasympathetic) and sensory fibers that accompany the arteries.

The large intestine consists of the cecum (and vermiform appendix), colons, rectum, and anal canal. It is wider and shorter than the small intestine.

The cecum is a pouch separated inferiorly from the vermiform appendix by the appendicular orifice and continues with the ascending colon at the horizontal plane crossing the middle of the ileal papilla. The ascending colon ends at the right or hepatic colic flexure, where the transverse colon begins; the latter ends at the left or splenic flexure, where the descending colon begins. The descending colon ends at the left iliac crest, where it continues with the sigmoid colon, the end of which is found at the level of the S3. The sigmoid colon is subdivided into iliac and pelvic colons. The iliac colon ends at the medial border of the left psoas muscle, where the pelvic colon begins. The rectum begins at S3 and ends where it is reached by the pelvic diaphragm and where it continues with the anal canal, the end of which is the anus.

The cecum, vermiform appendix, transverse, and sigmoid colons are movable, whereas the ascending and descending colons are fixed (their mesos adhered to the posterior abdominal wall). Both the ascending and descending colons are the medial walls of the right and left parietocolic recesses, respectively.

The vermiform appendix is located in the right iliac fossa, has a mesoappendix and, because of the large

amount of lymphoid tissue, is called the "intestinal tonsil."

The colons contain haustra coli or sacculations, separated by external sulci, which correspond internally with colic semilunar folds. The large intestine shows teniae (mesocolic, omental, and libera or free), which are three condensations of longitudinal musculature that start at the level of the appendiculocecal junction. Adjacent to the teniae the epiploic appendages (fat lobules) enclosed in peritoneal bags) are found.

The tunica mucosa of the large intestine has a simple columnar epithelium with goblet cells, a lamina propria, a muscularis mucosae, and solitary lymph nodules. The tela submucosa is areolar connective tissue, vessels, and nerves (Meissner's submucous plexus). The tunica muscularis has an inner circular and an outer longitudinal (with thickenings or teniae), and an intervening Auerbach's myenteric plexus. The tela subserosa and the tunica serosa are layers of peritoneum, and they form the epiploic appendages.

The rectum* is 15 cm long and has the rectal ampulla; it shows a sacral flexure and, at its junction with the anal canal, the perineal flexure (90°), surrounded by the sling of the puborectal muscle (the medial portion of the levator ani muscle). The rectum is separated from the urinary bladder by the rectovesical pouch (in the male) and by the rectovaginouterine pouch (from the vagina and uterus. The three transverse rectal folds are made up of mucous, submucous, and muscular layers.

The anal canal* is 3 cm long, beginning at the level of the pelvic diaphragm. It is surrounded by the levatore ani and external sphincter muscles. The canal's inner aspect has 5 to 10 anal columns, united by anal valves, each valve limiting an anal sinus. The aboral limit of the anal valves is the pectinate line, followed, toward the anus, by the pecten (a bluish area) and by the anal verge. The external orifice of the anal canal is the anus, which has wrinkles caused by the corrugator cutis ani muscle.

The anal canal mucosa has a simple columnar epithelium and, at the level of the valves, becomes stratified columnar and, subsequently, stratified squamous noncornified epithelium; the skin of the anus is stratified squamous epithelium (epidermis), is pigmented, and has glands and hair. The submucous tela shows a conspicuous venous hemorrhoidal plexus. The muscular layer presents longitudinal and inner circular (sphincteric) coats for the opening and closing of the lumen. The superior fascia of the pelvic diaphragm surrounds the rectum and the rectosacral fascia separates the rectum from the sacrum. The peritoneum partially covers the rectum.

---

* These two organs should be studied topographically with the pelvic viscera, and are included here for the sake of continuity.

Arteries of the cecum and colons: Marginal artery, formed by branches of the superior and inferior mesenteric arteries (ileocecoappendiculocolic or ileocolic artery, right, middle, and left colic arteries; sigmoid arteries) supply the vermiform appendix, cecum, and colons.

Veins: Accompany the arteries and drain the blood to the portal vein through the inferior and superior mesenteric veins.

Lymphatics: Vessels form plexuses and drain into nodes (ileocecocolic; right, middle, and left colic, and inferior mesenteric); from these nodes, the lymph is led to the thoracic duct.

Nerves: autonomic and sensory fibers by way of branches of the celiac, superior, and inferior mesenteric plexuses, which follow homonymous arteries. Parasympathetic fibers (from the pelvic splanchnic nerves and inferior hypogastric plexus) reach the aboral half of the descending and the sigmoid colon.

Arteries of the rectum and anal canal: Superior, middle, inferior rectal, and median sacral arteries.

Veins: From the submucous venous plexus into the superior rectal veins, then inferior mesenteric vein and portal vein; middle rectal vein into internal iliac veins; inferior rectal veins.

Lymphatics: Along superior rectal and inferior mesenteric vessels into inferior mesenteric nodes; along middle and inferior rectal vessels into internal and common iliac and sacral nodes; below he pectinate line that lymph of the anal canal is drained into the superficial ingui nodes.

Nerves: Superior and middle rectal plexuses, inferior rectal nerves; above the pectinate line parasympathetic, preganglionic, and postganglionic fibers; sympathetic postganglionic (vasomotor) and sensory fibers, below the pectinate line motor (sphincter ani externus), vasomotor, and sensory fibers.

Other abdominal viscera include the kidney, renal pelvis, ureter, and suprarenal glands.

The kidney is a bilateral retroperitoneal (on each side of the vertebral column) organ. Each has anterior and posterior aspects, superior and inferior poles, and lateral and medial margins; the latter indented by the renal hilum and sinus. The kidney weighs 150 g and is 12 cm long, 6 cm wide, and 3 cm thick; it is located in front of the psoas muscle at the level of rib 12, T12, L2, and L3 (the right being lower than the left). The renal pedicle is made up of vessels, nerves, renal pelvis, and ureter surrounded by fat. The fibrous capsule of the kidney is surrounded by the adipose capsule. The kidney and the suprarenal gland are both enveloped by the renal fascia with an intervening septum. Pararenal fat is situated outside the renal fascia and perirenal fat is found within the renal fascia. Each kidney is made up of anatomico-surgical segments, the anatomical basis for partial nephrectomy. A segment is an almost independent vascular territory. In each kidney, there are the superior, inferior, anterosuperior, anteroinferior, and posterior aterial renal segments. The venous segments are not as typical as the arterial, but it is possible to recognize the superior, middle, and inferior.

The relations of the anterior aspect of the kidneys differ. On the right, there is the liver, duodenum, right colic flexure, and the jejunum; on the left, there is the pancreas, spleen, stomach, left colic flexure, and jejunum.

The supracellular morphofunctional unit is the nephron (1,250,000 per kidney), made up of a glomerulus, glomerular capsule, 15 mm long proximal convoluted tubule, 20 mm long straight tubule (Henle's loop), which reaches the renal medulla and returns to the cortex, 5 mm long distal convoluted tubule, and collecting ducts. Each of the 500 collecting ducts receives many tributaries and opens into a minor calyx (at a renal papilla in the apex of a pyramid). The glomerlar capsule has two layers of squamous epithelium and a basement membrane. The proximal tubule shows a simple columnar epithelium having a brush border. The straight tubule (Henle's loop) has descending and ascending arms with an intervening thin segment (squamous cells); the ascending arm contacts the glomerular vascular pole and forms the macula densa (packed elongated cells and no basement membrane). The distal tubule has low cuboidal cells and the collecting ducts have cells with clear boundaries, spherical nuclei, and agranular cytoplasm.

The terminal portions of the collecting ducts join to form 18 papillary ducts in the area cribrosa of the renal papilla.

Most glomeruli occupy the cortex and most tubules the medulla. Medullary pyramids (8–12) contain straight tubules and collecting ducts. Renal columns of cortex separate adjacent pyramids and reach the sinus. One or more pyramids is received in one of nine minor calyces, which join the three major calyces; the confluence of the latter forms the renal pelvis, which continues with the ureter.

Vessels and nerves of the kidney are as follows:

Arteries: Renal, its division into anterior and posterior branches, then the segmental arteries (superior, inferior, anterosuperior, anteroinferior, and posterior); interlobar and arcuate arteries, afferent arteriole (juxtaglomerular cells), capillaries (glomerulus), efferent arteriole.

Veins: Stellate, straight, interlobular, segmental (superior, middle, and inferior) veins. The left renal vein is longer than the right and receives the left gonadal (ovarian or testicular), left suprarenal, diaphragmatic veins and veins of the abdominal wall; the left renal vein is clamped by the mesentericoaortic forceps.

Lymphatics: To lumbar nodes after renal hilar nodes.

Nerves: Celiac (aorticorenal) and intermesenteric plexuses, and thoracic and lumbar splanchnic nerves.

The renal pelvis or pelvis of the ureter is retroperitoneal, small, and made up of long major calyces (ramified type) in brachytypes (endomorphic) and is large and made up of short major calyces (ampullar type) in longitypes (ectomorphic).

The ureter is 25 cm long, retrovascular in the hilum, retroperitoneal, and divided into abdominal, pelvic, and intraparietal portions. The abdominal portion is related to the psoas muscle, the right ureter is crossed by the mesentery, and related to the vermiform appendix, while the left is related to the intersigmoid recess. The pelvic portion has different relations according to the sex, crosses the common iliac artery, and reaches the urinary bladder, in the wall of which is the intraparietal portion. In the female, at the ischial spine, the ureter turns medially, below the uterine vessels, 2 cm from the uterine cervix. Vessels and nerves of the renal pelvis and ureter are as follows:

Arteries: Renal, gonadal, common iliac, and inferior vesical arteries.

Veins: Follow the arteries.

Lymphatics: to lumbar and internal iliac nodes.

Nerves: Gonadal, renal, and hypogastric plexuses.

The urinary bladder* is a viscus that stores and expels urine, changing its continuous ureteral flow into an intermittent or periodical micturition. It contains, when full, .5L of urine, but it can store a larger volume; with 350 ml the urge to empty it is felt. The shape, size, position, and relations of the bladder vary with the functional stage, age, and sex. The bladder has a body, fundus, apex, and neck. Only the superior portion of the bladder is covered by peritoneum; the median umbilical ligament (urachus) extends from the apex to the navel.

The bladder is located superior to the small intestine and the sigmoid colon, anterior to the retropubic space, and posterior to the seminal vesicle, ampulla of the ductus deferens, and rectum (between the two ampullae) or to the vagina and cervix. The pelvic diaphragm is attached to the neck; the medial and lateral puboprostatic ligaments and the lateral ligament of the bladder fix the viscus in the pelvis.

---

* The pelvic ureter and the bladder are pelvic organs and are described here for the purposes of continuity.

The inner aspect of the bladder shows the right and left ureteral and the internal urethral orifice, limiting the smooth vesical trigone. Posterior to the internal urethral orifice is the uvula.

The wall of the calyces is thin and becomes thicker in the renal pelvis, ureter, and bladder. The wall has the same structure, in all these passages. (i.e., mucosa, surrounded by smooth musculature and by an adventitia) The mucosa shows a transitional epithelium, being three cells thick in the calyces, five cells thick in the ureter, and seven cells thick in the empty bladder. When the wall contracts, the epithelial cells appear columnar and the epithelium thickens, the opposite occurring during relaxation. The lamina propria has dense connective tissue with lymph nodules and elastic fibers. The musculature comprises an inner longitudinal, a middle circular, and an outer longitudinal coat in the bladder. The inner longitudinal coat of the minor calyces is attached to the junction between each calyx and the papilla it encircles, where the circular forms a sphincter. Except in the bladder, the urinary passages have an inner muscular longitudinal and an outer circular coat. The intraparietal portion of the ureters passes obliquely through the wall of the bladder, where the circular fibers of the ureter disappear, the lamina propria thins, and the longitudinal coat thickens. The latter (dilator muscle) is responsible for the opening of the orifice.

The outer longitudinal musculature of the bladder is more developed anteriorly and posteriorly, forms the pubovesical muscle and the rectovesical muscle. It is possible to consider the three coats as combined in spiral fibers. As the circular and longitudinal musculatures contract to expel urine, they are also called detrusor urinae muscle. The musculature of the trigone (trigonal muscle) is located between the detrusor and the mucosa, receives fibers from the ureteral muscular coat, and extends to the urethra. There is an opening and closing muscular mechanism in the neck of the bladder, assisted by the circular and spiral elastic tissue and supplemented by the voluntary relaxation of the urogenital and pelvic diaphragms.

Where there is no serous coat, the bladder is invested by a fibrous coat. The vessels and nerves of the urinary bladder are as follows:

Arteries: Two superior vesical (from the umbilical) and inferior vesical arteries.

Veins: into the vesical (or prostatic) venous plexus, then into the internal iliac vein.

Lymphatics: Into the external, internal, common iliac, and sacral nodes.

Nerves: From vesical (or prostatic) and inferior hypogastric plexuses, which give the motor (parasympathetic fibers to the detrusor muscle), vasomotor (sympathetic), and sensory (stimulated by detrusor stretching) groups.

The male urethra,* the passage for semen and urine, from the bladder neck to the external urethral orifice, is 20 cm long and divided into prostatic, membranous, and spongy portions. The prostatic portion is 3 cm long and shows posteriorly the median urethral crest continuous with the uvula and, distally, with the colliculus seminalis, where the prostatic utricle and the paramedian openings of the ejaculatory ducts are seen. The membranous portion (1 cm long) is surrounded by the sphincter urethrae muscle (of the urogenital diaphragm). At the bulb of the penis, the urethra turns forward (90° angle). The spongy portion (15 cm long) is contained in the corpus spongiosum, being wider in the bulb (intrabulbar fossa) and in the glans penis (navicular fossa).

The structure of the urethra is made up of a mucous and a muscular layer. The mucosa is lined by transitional epithelium (prostatic portion) or stratified columnar or pseudostratified (the other portions). The navicular fossa has stratified squamous epithelium. Many lacunae have (some may not) openings of urethral glands. The musculature has extensions from the bladder and from the (striated) sphincter of the membranous urethra.

Vessels and nerves of the male urethra are as follows:

Arteries: Inferior vesical and middle rectal arteries (prostatic portion), artery of the bulb of the penis (membranous portion), urethral artery, deep and dorsal arteries of the penis (spongy portion).

Veins: Into the prostatic venous plexus and internal pudendal veins.

Lymphatics: Into internal and (some) into external iliac nodes; from the spongy portion into deep inguinal and (some) into external iliac nodes.

Nerves: Prostatic plexus (for prostatic portion), cavernous nerves (for membranous portion), and pudendal nerve (for spongy portion).

The female urethra* (4 cm long) serves only as a passage for urine and corresponds only to the male prostatic urethra proximal to the openings of the ejaculatory ducts; its external urethral orifice (5 mm in diameter) is anterior to the vagina, between the labia minora, inferior and posterior to the glans of the clitoris. The urethra presents a posterior longitudinal mucosal fold, the urethral crest, and at the posterior wall of the external urethral orifice is the urethral carina.

The structure of the female urethra shows a mucous and a muscular layer. The proximal portion is lined by transitional epithelium and the distal portion by stratified squamous epithelium. There are urethral lacunae with or without openings of urethral glands. The muscular layer is an extension of the bladder and is not present in the distal urethra. The vessels and nerves of the female urethra are as follows:

Arteries: Inferior vesical artery (proximal part), inferior vesical and uterine (middle part), and internal pudendal artery (distal part).

Veins: Into vesical venous plexus and internal pudendal vein.

Lymphatics: Along the internal pudendal artery into internal and external iliac nodes.

Nerves: Vesical and uterovaginal plexuses (proximal part) and pudendal nerve (distal part of the urethra).

The suprarenal glands (adrenal and epinephrine) are paired abdominal endocrine glands, lying on the medial aspect of the superior pole of each kidney, near the adjoining crus of the diaphragm, at the level of intercostal space XI and rib 12. The right gland is posterior to the liver and close to the inferior vena cava; the left gland is posterior to the stomach, and near the pancreas and the omental bursa.

Each suprarenal gland has a cortex and a medulla. The cortex has thin cords of cells separated by sinusoids and is divided into (1) an outermost glomerular zone (with clusters of cells), having columnar cells, deeply staining nuclei, and some fat; (2) a middle fascicular zone, the thickest layer, with parallel cords of cuboidal cells (its outer cells have much fat, whereas its inner cells have very few lipid droplets); and (3) an innermost reticular zone, a network of cells, which resemble those of the fascicular zone on the outside and those near the medulla appear dark and contain more fat. The medulla is similar to the sympathetic nervous system; its cells are polyhedral with basophilic cytoplasm, large vesicular nuclei, and secretion granules. Ganglion cells are also found.

The vessels and nerves of the suprarenal glands are as follows:

Arteries: Inferior phrenic, suprarenal artery (one from the aorta, the other from the renal artery).

Vein: Single vein to the left renal vein and, on the right, to the inferior vena cava.

Lymphatics: To nodes along the sides of the glands (para-aortic nodes).

Nerves: To cortex: greater and lesser splanchnic nerves. Preganglionic fibers start in the 5th to 11th thoracic segments of the spinal cord, enter a ventral root (a white remus communicans to sympathetic chain), then

---

* Described here for the purpose of continuity.

enter a splanchnic nerve to synapse in the celiac or aorticorenal ganglia. Postganglionic fibers follow the arteries of the suprarenal gland; medulla: directly receives preganglionic fibers.

Accessory cortical tissue is found near the kidney or in the pelvis. Other medullary or chromaffin organs are found along sympathetic ganglia (paraganglia, para-aortic bodies).

Blood vessels of the abdomen are the aorta, which has parietal, visceral, and terminal branches. All parietal branches are bilateral except the unpaired median sacral artery. The parietal branches are (1) inferior phrenic arteries (give the superior suprarenal arteries), lumbar arteries, and the median sacral artery. The visceral branches are middle suprarenal, renal, and gonadal arteries, all paired. The renal arteries give off the inferior suprarenal. The gonadal arteries are testicular or ovarian arteries. The testicular artery reaches the deep inguinal ring, follows the ductus deferens, and supplies the spermatic cord and testis. The ovarian artery joins the suspensory ligament of the ovary, runs in the mesovarium, and supplies the ovary.

The unpaired visceral branches are the celiac trunk and superior and inferior mesenteric arteries. The celiac trunk is the artery of the aboral half of the foregut, the limit of which is the middle of the duodenum; that is, the entrance of the common bile duct and pancreatic duct (hepatopancreatic ampulla or major duodenal papilla). It originates between the diaphragmatic crura, and divides into left gastric, splenic, and common hepatic arteries. The superior mesenteric is the artery of the midgut (i.e., from the major duodenal papilla to the left colic flexure) or left third of the transverse colon). It originates just below the celiac trunk and forms, with the aorta, the mesentericoaortic forceps. The superior mesenteric artery enters the mesentery and gives off branches from its convexity (toward the left) to the small intestine (jejunoileum) and from its concavity to the terminal ileum, vermiform appendix, cecum, ascending and part of the transverse colon. The inferior mesenteric is the artery of the hindgut; it originates just above the aortic bifurcation and gives off the left colic artery, sigmoid arteries, and superior rectal artery.

The terminal branches of the aorta result from its bifurcation at the level of L4 into the right and left common iliac arteries; each of the latter are subdivided into external and internal iliac arteries. The right common iliac artery may compress the terminal portion of the left common iliac vein against the lumbar vertebrae and may be a factor in the development of left sided varicose veins.

The veins of the abdomen are the portal, the inferior vena cava, and the vertebral veins.

The portal vein collects the blood from the abdominal esophagus, stomach, intestines, and spleen. It conveys it to the liver, from which it is drained to the inferior vena cava by the right, intermediate, left, and caudate veins.

Portocaval or cavocaval anastomoses are (1) the inferior mesenteric vein and inferior vena cava, at the level of the rectum (superior and middle rectal veins, tributaries to the inferior mesenteric, and inferior rectal veins, tributaries to the internal iliac vein); (2) the gastric veins (tributaries to the portal vein or of the splenic vein) and the superior vena cava, at the level of the esophagus (esophageal, hemiazygos, azygos, and vertebral veins); (3) the small retroperitoneal veins (retrohepatic, retrogastric, retroduodenal, ascending, and descending retrocolic, renal capsular, inferior phrenic), the azygos system, vertebral veins, and pancreatic, duodenal, and hepatic veins; (4) the paraumbilical veins (along falciform and round ligaments), periumbilical subcutaneous veins (to the epigastric veins and vena cavae), epigastric anastomoses, and the left branch of the portal vein; and (5) tributaries to the internal iliac veins, to the vertebral veins, and the external iliac veins (superior and inferior caval veins).

The inferior vena cava is formed by the confluence of the right and left common iliac veins and ascends at the right of the aorta; its superior abdominal portion is embedded almost completely in the liver. Its tributaries are the inferior phrenic veins, lumbar veins, hepatic veins, renal veins, right suprarenal vein, right ovarian, or right testicular vein.

The vertebral venous plexus comprises veins that drain the organs of the vertebral canal, the vertebrae, and the dorsum (or back). It is anastomosed with intracranial veins, and the portal system, and drains into vertebral, posterior intercostal, lumbar, and lateral sacral veins.

Lymphatics of the abdomen include (1) lumbar vessels, located along the vertebral column, ascending from iliac lymph nodes and reaching the thoracic duct; (2) lumbar (aortic) lymph nodes; (3) lymph nodes along vessels supplying the viscera; and (4) thoracic duct, which begins as the cisterna chyli, lies on the right side of the aorta and reaches the thorax through the aortic orifice of the diaphragm.

The nerves of the abdomen are the 7th to 11th thoracoabdominal, right and left phrenic, anterior, and posterior vagal trunks, thoracic splanchnic (greater), lesser, and lowest splanchnic nerves, right and left sympathetic trunks and ganglia (lumbar splanchnic nerves), autonomic plexuses (prevertebral plexus, celiac plexus and ganglia, aortic plexus, superior mesenteric plexus, inferior mesenteric plexus, intermesenteric plexus), and lumbar plexus (ilioinguinal, iliohypogastric, lateral femoral cutaneous, femoral, genitofemoral, obturator, and accessory obturator nerves).

Pelvis

The pelvis (basin) is the lowest portion of the trunk, separated from the abdomen, with which it is freely continuous, by an arbitrary limit, the terminal line. Inferiorly, the pelvis is limited by the superficial aspect of the perineum and on each side by the girdle or roots of the inferior members. The terminal line (pubic crest, pectineal line, medial margin of ilium or arcuateline, sacral wing on each side of the pelvic promontory) may divide the pelvis in a broad sense into a false, superior, or greater pelvis (between the iliac fossae and below the plane uniting the iliac crests) and the true, inferior, or lesser pelvis. The latter, or pelvis in a narrow sense, will be described here.

The bony pelvis is made up of the hip bone (pubis, ilium, and ischium), sacrum, and coccyx. It has an inlet, an outlet, and a cavity in between.

The pelvic inlet (brim) is the superior aperture, limited by the terminal line; it has the following diameters: Anteroposterior, sagittal or true conjugate (12 cm), between the superior margin of the pubic symphysis and the pelvic promontory, or obstetrical conjugate diameter (11 cm), when it is measured between the posterior aspect of the pubic symphysis and the pelvic promontory, thus corresponding to the shortest distance between the two points. The (maximum) transverse diameter (13.5 cm) is the widest distance and the (left) oblique diameter (12.75 cm) is the distance between the left sacroiliac joint to the right pectineal line. The transverse diameter divides the pelvis into forepelvis and hindpelvis.

The pelvis outlet is the inferior pelvic aperture, limited by the inferior border of the pubic symphysis, pubic arch, ischial rami and tuberosities, sacrotuberous ligaments, and coccyx. It has the following diameters: Anteroposterior or pubococcygeal (9 cm), from the inferior border of the pubic symphysis to the top of the coccyx; and transverse (11 cm), between the ischial tuberosities.

According to their inlet, pelves are classified as gynecoid (round, normal, true female type), android (heart-shaped, male type), platypelloid (flat type, fore- and hindpelvis shortened), and anthropoid (narrow, oval, ape type).

The subpubic angle has its apex at the inferior border of the pubic symphysis.

The female pelvis differs from the male as its bones are thinner and have less accentuated markings, the pelvic promontory is less prominent, the pubic symphysis and the sacrum are shorter, the sacral concavity is deeper, the subpubic angle is less acute, the iliac fossae are larger, and the acetabula are farther apart. The female pelvis is more developed transversely, whereas the male pelvis is more developed vertically.

The joints of the pelvis are the lumbosacral, sacroiliac, sacrococcygeal, and pubic symphysis, and the ligaments are the sacrotuberous, sacrospinous, iliolumbar, obturator membrane, interosseus (in the sacroiliac joint), and the posterior sacroiliac. The sacrotuberous ligament converts the lesser sciatic notch into the lesser ischial foramen and the sacrospinous ligament converts the greater sciatic notch into the greater ischial foramen. The pelvic promontory is the most anterior prominent point of the lumbosacral joint (L5, disk or S1), frequently S1.

The pelvis is divided into parietal regions and cavity. The parietal regions include lateral, posterior, and inferior walls; they comprise superficial muscles (gluteus maximus, medius, and minimus), hip bones, sacrum, coccyx, their joints and ligaments, deep muscles, fascia vessels and nerves, and peritoneum. The lateral wall is lined by the obturator nerve and vessels, branches of the internal iliac artery, ureter, round ligament (female) or deferent duct (male), and ovary. The posterior wall is lined by the piriform, ischiococcygeal, and rectococcygeal muscles, and is related to the lumbosacral trunk, sacral plexus, median sacral artery, and coccygeal body (glomus). The inferior wall or pelvic floor includes the peritoneum and the perineum. The regions of the perineum are anal and urogenital. The perineum consists of the following

> Pelvic diaphragm
> > Levator ani*
> > > Pubococcygeal muscle
> > > Iliococcygeal muscle
> > > Ischiococcygeal muscle
> > > Puborectal muscle
> Urogenital diaphragm
> > Deep transversus perinei muscle
> > Sphincter urethrae muscle

The superficial muscles of the perineum are the external sphincter muscle of the anus (pars subcutanea, pars superficialis, and pars profunda), the superficial transverse muscle of the perineum, the ischiocavernous muscle, and the bulbospongiosus muscle.

The centrum tendineum perinei, or corpus perinealis, corresponds to the perineal body, as used in obstetrics and gynecology.

The vessels and nerves of the pelvis are as follows:

Arteries: Internal iliac artery and its parietal and visceral branches. The parietal branches are the iliolumbar artery, lateral sacral arteries, obturator artery, superior gluteal artery, inferior gluteal artery, and in-

---

* The levator prostatae or pubovaginal, prerectal, and rectococcygeal muscles are sometimes recognized.

ternal pudendal artery. The visceral branches are the umbilical artery, superior vesical arteries, inferior vesical artery, uterine artery or artery of the ductus deferens, vaginal artery and middle rectal artery.

Veins: Internal iliac vein and its tributaries which correspond to the arteries.

Lymphatics: Into nodes adjacent to the iliac arteries and their branches. Inguinal nodes, external genitalia, vagina, and uterine cervix drain into external and common iliac nodes; uterine cervix, prostate, rectum, perineum, and gluteal region drain into internal iliac and sacral nodes, then to common iliac nodes. The latter, the testis, and ovary drain into the lumbar group of aortic nodes. The lymph of the anal canal and external genital organs drain into inguinal nodes.

Nerves: Sacral plexus, coccygeal plexus, and autonomic nervous system. The sacral plexus is made up of the lumbosacral trunk, the ventral rami of S1–S3 and the superior division of S4; the pudendal nerve (S2–S4) innervates the perineum with motor, sensory, and postganglionic sympathetic fibers, gives off the inferior rectal nerve, and splits into the perineal nerve and the dorsal nerve of the penis or clitoris; the perineal nerve divides into a deep branch (to perineal muscles) and a superficial branch (to scrotum or labia majora). The pelvic splanchnic nerves (S2–S4) help to form the inferior hypogastric plexus. the coccygeal plexus (S4, S5, Co1) innervates the skin of the coccygeal region. The pelvic part of the autonomic nervous system includes sympathetic fibers, which are inferior extensions of the sympathetic trunks and of the aortic plexus. The sympathetic trunks join in front of the coccyx and form the unpaired ganglion. The aortic plexus continues as the superior hypogastric plexus (presacral nerve), which is divided into right and left inferior hypogastric nerves; these join the pelvic splanchnic nerves and form the right and left inferior hypogastric plexuses, which supply the rectum, bladder, and uterus.

The pelvic cavity contains viscera and is divided into intestinal (rectal), genital (seminal or uterine), and urinary (vesical) regions.

MALE GENITAL SYSTEM

The male genital system is formed by the testis, epididymis, ductus deferens, seminal vesicles, ejaculatory ducts, prostate, bulbourethral glands, and penis.

The testis produces spermatozoa and is located in the scrotum or testicular pouch; each testis has superior and inferior extremities, medial and lateral aspects, and anterior and posterior margins. The testis processes a connective tissue coat (tunica albuginea), which sends fibrous septa (300) internally; the latter form the

mediastinum testis. The albuginea is covered by the tunica vaginalis (peritoneum). Each testicular lobule has convoluted seminiferous tubules (800 in each testis), which join into 25 straight seminiferous tubules. These pass in the rete testis and from this network 20 efferent tubules enter the head of the epididymis. A fibroelastic connective tissue (tunica propria) surrounds each tubule, being separated from the 4 to 8 cell layers of stratified epithelium by a basement membrane. The epithelial cells are spermatogenic or sustentacular. The spermatogonia are peripheral; the intermediate are primary and secondary spermatocytes; and the most differentiated (spermatids and spermatocytes) limit the lumen. Sustentacular cells extend from the basement membrane to the lumen; they have pale, ovoid, prominent nuclei with an infolded nuclear envelope. Between seminiferous tubules there is loose connective tissue containing two types of interstitial cells among fibroblasts, macrophages, and mast cells. The interstitial cells are immature (basophilic) and mature (eosinophilic).

The epididymis is in contact with the posterior margin of the testis, from which it receives efferent ductules. It has a head, body, and tail. Between the body of the epididymis and the lateral aspect of the testis there is the sinus of the epididymis.

The efferent ductules form lobules in the head of the epididymis. The duct of the epididymis receives tributaries from all lobules and at the tail continues as the ductus deferens. Appendix testis and appendix of the epididymis are remnants of the development of the corresponding organs. The efferent ductules lead to a single ductus epididymidis, which is surrounded by connective tissue and is lined by a pseudostratified epithelium. The latter is made up of basal cells and uniform tall columnar cells. Both contain lipid droplets and the columnar cells show pigment and secretion granules as well as stereocilia. The duct has a basal lamina and smooth myocytes.

Artery: Testicular artery supplies testis and epididymis.

Veins: Pampiniform plexus.

Lymphatics: Follow testicular vessels and lead into lumbar (aortic) nodes.

The ductus (vas) deferens runs toward the inguinal canal, turns around the inferior epigastric artery, enters the pelvis, and presents it ampulla just before joining the duct of the seminal vesicle to form the ejaculatory duct. The ductus deferens has a thick wall and a star-shaped narrow lumen. Its epithelium is pseudostratified and the cells have stereocilia. A basal lamina separates the epithelim from the lamina propria, containing many elastic fibers. The submucosa is surrounded by a spiral muscular coat which, in section, appears made up of an inner and an outer longitudinal layer with a middle circular layer. A fibrous adventitia surrounds the muscular coat.

Vessels and nerves of the ductus deferens are as follows:

Arteries: The artery of the ductus deferens also supplies the seminal vesicle and the ejaculatory duct, aided by the inferior vesical and middle rectal arteries.

Veins: From the ductus deferens, the seminal vesicle, and ejaculatory ducts into prostatic and vesical plexuses.

Lymphatics: From the ductus deferens into external iliac nodes, and from the seminal vesicles into external and internal iliac nodes.

Nerves: The ductus deferens receives autonomic fibers from superior and inferior hypogastric plexuses; seminal vesicle from inferior hypogastric and prostatic plexuses.

The seminal vesicle secretes a fluid that contributes to the semen. It is related posteriorly to the rectum and anteriorly to the urinary bladder. The wall of each vesicle contains mucous and adventitial layers. The adventitia has fibrous and elastic connective tissue; the muscular coat is thin and the mucosal folds are lined by pseudostratified or simple columnar epithelium. The epithelial cells contain secretory granules and a yellow pigment; the secretion is deeply acidophilic.

The ejaculatory ducts penetrate the prostatic gland and their openings are found on the colliculus seminalis; they have simple columnar or pseudostratified epithelium, surrounded by fibrous connective tissue.

The spermatic cord extends from the posterior margin of the testis to the deep inguinal ring. It comprises the ductus deferens, arteries veins (pampinriform plexus), nerves, lymphatics, and the processus vaginalis peritonei or its derivative. The coverings of the spermatic cord are the external spermatic, cremasteric (cremaster muscle and genital branch of the genitofemoral nerve), internal spermatic fasciae, and the tunica vaginalis testis.

The prostate is made up of glands, the secretion of which also contributes to the semen. It is situated in front of the rectum, seminal vesicle, and ampulla of the ductus deferens, behind the pubic symphysis, and below the urinary bladder. The prostate has a base, an apex, and anterior, posterior, and inferolateral aspects. Its glands open by ductules into urethral sinuses. Right and left lobes are united by the prostatic isthmus. The median lobe lies between the ejaculatory ducts and the urethra. The fascia of the prostate is an extension of the superior fascia of the pelvic diaphragm, and is separated from the prostatic capsule by the prostatic venous plexus.

The structure of the prostate shows 40 compound tubuloalveolar glands with 25 excretory ducts. Small mucosal glands are surrounded by submucosal glands that are embedded in a dense myofibroelastic stroma, which is continuous with the capsule. The epithelium is cuboidal to columnar. Its cells contain secretory granules and lipid droplets. The secretion may contain prostatic concretions or corpora amylacea.

Vessels and nerves of the prostate are as follows:

Arteries: Prostatic branches from the inferior vesical artery, superior and middle rectal arteries.

Veins: Into the prostatic plexus, which joins the vesical plexus and both into the internal iliac vein.

Lymphatics: To the internal and external iliac and sacral lymph nodes.

Nerves: Prostatic (sympathetic) plexus.

The bulbourethral glands are paramedian, embedded in the sphincter urethrae muscle (urogenital diaphragm), at the level of the membranous portion of the urethra. They contribute to the semen. The ducts of the glands enter the bulb of the penis and, after 3 cm, they open in the spongy urethra. Each gland is a compound tubuloalveolar gland, surrounded by a connective tissue capsule. Elastic and muscular (skeletal and smooth) fibers are contained in the connective tissue septa that divide the gland into lobules. The epithelium is cuboidal or columnar, the cytoplasm contains secretory granules and inclusions; the secretory ducts are lined by a pseudostratified epithelium, containing mucous cells surrounded by smooth myocytes.

FEMALE GENITAL SYSTEM

The female genital system is formed by the ovaries, uterine tubes, uterus, vagina, and vulva (pudendum). The ovaries, uterine tubes, and uterus are pelvic viscera; the vagina is pelviperineal, and the vulva (external genitalia) is anterior to the pubic region.

Each ovary is located in the ovarian fossa, limited superiorly by the external iliac vessels, and inferiorly by the ureter and uterine vessels. Ovaries are attached to the posterior aspect of the broad ligament by the mesovarium.

The ovary has a lateral and a medial aspect, the free and the mesovarian (ovarian hilum) margins, the tubal, and the uterine ends; it is covered by the tunica albuginea (continuous with the peritoneum) and is divided into cortex and medulla. A single layer of cuboidal cells constitutes the superficial (germinal) epithelium on the albuginea. The stroma of the cortex has more cells than that of the medulla. The suspensory ligament of the ovary (infundibulopelvic ligament) contains the ovarian vessels and nerves, and inserts into fascia of the psoas muscle. The ovarian ligament unites the uterine end of the ovary to the superolateral angle of the uterus.

The ovarian medulla shows loose fibrous connective tissue containing numerous elastic fibers, scattered smooth myocytes, blood and lymphatic vessels, and nerves. The cortex contains the ovarian follicles within a stroma of reticular and elastic fibers and fusiform cells. Primary follicles occur before puberty, after which growing follicles, corpora lutea, and atretic follicles are seen. Each follicle contains an immature ovum surrounded by epithelial cells. In the newborn, there are 500,000 follicles, the number of which gradually decreases until disappearance after menopause.

A primary follicle measures 40 μm in diameter and it has an immature ovum surrounded by one layer of follicular cells. A growing follicle has a larger ovum, proliferated follicular cells, and a connective tissue capsule. The ovum is surrounded by a deeply staining membrane, the pellucid zone; fluid increases and accumulates in the antrum. The ovum and follicular cells form an eccentric mound (cumulus oophorus) in the antral cavity. The follicular cells are radially arranged (corona radiata). In the periphery of the follicle, the stroma forms the theca folliculi (inner vascular theca interna and outer fibrous theca externa) separated from the membrana granulosa by the glossy membrane (basal lamina). A follicle reaches maturity in 10 to 14 days, becomes prominent on the ovarian surface, and opens (ovulation) at a point called the stigma, through which the ovum is transported to the uterine tube (where it may be fertilized), uterus, and vagina. After ovulation, the follicular wall is transformed into a glandular corpus luteum. If fertilization does not occur, it degenerates and becomes the corpus luteum of menstruation, and the scar is called corpus albicans (white); if fertilization takes place, the corpus luteum enlarges (corpus luteum of pregnancy) and slowly degenerates during the second half of pregnancy and rapidly after delivery, forming a large corpus albicans. As only 400 follicles reach maturity, the others undergo degeneration (atresia).

Arteries: Ovarian artery and ovarian branch of uterine artery; the latter anastomoses with the ovarian artery.

Veins: From a plexus anastomosed with the uterine plexus two veins arise and fuse into a right ovarian (tributary of the inferior vein cava) and a left (to the left renal vein).

Lymphatics: Accompany the ovarian blood vessels and drain into lumbar (aortic) nodes.

Nerves: Vasomotor fibers from the ovarian plexus.

The uterine tube (salpinx) is trumpetlike and extends between the tubal end of the ovary and the superolateral angle of the uterus. Each tube is 10 cm long and is located in the superior border of the broad ligament. The portion of the broad ligament above the root of the mesovarium is called the mesosalpinx.

The uterine tube has the infundibulum, ampulla, isthmus, and uterine portions. The infundibulum (funnel) contains the tubal fimbriae (the longest is the fimbria ovarica) around the abdominal orifice (2 mm in diameter) at the bottom of the funnel, where the ovum enters directed toward the lumen of the tube. The thin-walled ampulla (the widest and longest portion) is tortuous and continuous with the narrow and short isthmus. The latter is followed medially by the uterine or intramural portion, which ends with the uterine orifice (1 mm in diameter). The ovum is fertilized in the infundibulum or in the lateral third of the tube.

The uterine tube has a serous layer, a subserous tela, a muscular layer, and a mucous layer. The serosa and subserous tela correspond to the mesothelium and loose connective tissue of the visceral peritoneum. The musculature consists of spiral fibers, appearing in a cross section as an outer longitudinal layer and an inner circular layer. The mucosa shows longitudinal, branched folds, and consists of ciliated simple columnar epithelium and a lamina propria (connective tissue with numerous cells).

The uterus is a median pear-shaped hollow organ about 8 cm long, 5 cm wide, and 2.5 cm thick. It has intestinal (rectal) and vesical surfaces, right and left margins and angles (horns or cornua), and a cavity. The uterus is divided into fundus (above the plane of the uterine orifices of the uterine tubes), body, isthmus (narrowing), and cervix. The uterine cervix or neck is related to the superior end of the vagina as would be a cork to a "vaginal" bottle. It is subdivided by the insertion of the vagina around it into a portio supravaginalis (above the level of insertion) and a portio vaginalis (below the insertion).

The uterine cavity is in communication with the lumen of the tubes and, by means of the orifice of the uterus, with the vagina. The orifice is limited by an anterior and a posterior lip. The cervical canal presents an anterior and a posterior longitudinal fold or main column of the palmate folds.

The angle between the body and the cervix is anteflexion, and the angle between the uterus and the vagina is anteversion (90°). The peritoneum is reflected from the rectum onto the posterior aspect of the superior portion of the vagina, the cervix and body of the uterus, then to the urinary bladder. The uterus separates the rectouterine (rectovaginouterine) pouch from the vesicouterine pouch.

The broad ligament, formed at each margin of the uterus by the periotoneum, extends to the lateral walls of the pelvis. Its posterior later constitutes the rectouterine fold, the lateral limit of the homonymous pouch, and the mesovarium, which contains the epo- and paraoophoron as well as the branches of the ovarian and uterine vessels. Above the mesovarium, the broad ligament is called mesosalpinx, and below it is called mesometrium. The broad ligament contains parametrium (i.e., connective tissue and smooth myocytes). The round ligament is inserted into the superolateral angle of the uterus; it crosses the umbilical artery and external iliac vessels, forms a loop around the inferior epigastric vessels, enters in the inguinal canal, and ends in the subcutaneous tela of the labium majus. A remnant of the fetal peritoneal vaginal process is found in the adult inguinal canal accompanying the round ligament. The thickening of the visceral pelvic fascia that forms the lateral aspect of the cervix and superior portion of the vagina runs laterally to the superior fascia of the pelvic diaphragm, and is the lateral or transverse cervical or cardinal ligament related to the uterine artery. Another portion of this thickening runs in the rectouterine fold to insert into the sacrum, and is called uterosacral ligament.

The uterine wall has perimetrium (serous layer), myometrium, and endometrium (mucosa). The perimetrium is made up of a single layer of mesothelial cells on a connective tissue layer. The myometrium is made up of concentric laminae of musculature, which apper in sections as an outer longitudinal, a middle circular and oblique, and an inner longitudinal muscular coat, also interpreted as spirally arranged fibers. The endometrium has simple columnar epithelium, and has scattered ciliated cells and glands, which appear as simple tubules branched at their base. The glands are separated by stroma, and are made up of connective tissue with stellate and lymphoid cells and granular leukocytes. The glands lie on a network of reticular fibers that forms a basal lamina. The endometrium undergoes periodical changes correlated to secretions of the ovary, leading to mucosal destruction (necrosis and hemorrhage), known as menstruation (4 days each at 28 day intervals). Between menarche and menopause, each cycle is divided into the menstrual, proliferative (estrogenic or follicular, follicular growth), progestational or luteal, and ischemic or premenstrual stages.

During pregnancy, the fertilized ovum is transported through the uterine tube to the uterus, while undergoing segmentation. The resulting cellular mass contains a cavity and is the blastocyst, which is implanted in the endometrium (7 days after ovulation). The blastocyst is made up of trophoblast and a cavity containing an "inner cell mass," which will form the embryo. The trophoblast evolves into a cytotrophoblast and an outer layer of cells, the syncytial trophoblast. From the surface of the latter appear the primary villi (epithelial cords).

Embryonic connective tissue and the trophoblast together form the chorion. Connective tissue and fetal vessels penetrate the villi, and are then known as secondary or chorionic villi. On the embedded aspect of the blastocyst, the chorionic villi form the fetal component of the placenta and constitute the chorium frondosum, attached to the chorionic plate. On the luminal surface, the chorion laeve appears. The endometrium will be shed at parturition and is called the decidua, which has three regions: capsular decidua, overlying the blastocyst, basal decidua, underlying the blastocyst, and parietal decidua, the remaining mucosa.

Arteries: Uterine.

Veins: Venous plexus around the arteries; a portocaval anastomosis is provided by veins below the rectouterine pouch, linking the uterine plexus and the superior rectal vein.

Lymphatics: From the fundus and body to the lumbar (aortic) nodes, from the body to the external iliac nodes, and from the cervix to the external and internal iliac and sacral nodes; from the tubouterine junction, lymphatic vessels follow the round ligament and reach the superficial inguinal nodes.

Nerves: Uterovaginal plexuses (autonomic and sensory fibers).

The vagina extends from the uterine cervix to the vestibule, traversing the pelvic and the urogenital diaphragms. It is related to the urinary bladder and urethra anteriorly, and to the rectum posteriorly. The vaginal cavity continues that of the uterus and in cross section is H shaped; the anterior wall is 7.5 cm long and, because of the 90° angle (open anteriorly) between the uterus and the vagina, the posterior wall is 9 cm long. The lateral walls are inserted superiorly to the lateral cervical ligament and inferiorly to the pelvic diaphragm. Between the cervix and the walls of the vagina, there is the fornix of the vagina (anterior, posterior, right, and left fornices). In virgins, the vestibular opening of the vagina presents the hymen, the remnants of which, after intercourse and parturition, are called carunculae hymenales.

The walls of the vagina have an adventitia, a muscular, and a mucosal coat. The adventitia is an extension of the visceral pelvic fascia, containing a large venous plexus. The superior portion of the posterior vaginal wall is covered by peritoneum (rectovaginouterine pouch). The muscular coat is made up of smooth myocytes; most fibers are longitudinal and some are continuous with those superficial of the uterus. There are also skeletal fibers of the pubovaginal muscle (from the medial portion of the pubococcygeal muscle and of the levator ani muscle). The mucosa present transverse vaginal rugae and a longitudinal anterior column and posterior column of the rugae. The inferior portion of the anterior column has the urethral carina or ridge, formed by the urethra. The mucosa is lined by stratified squamous epithelium (nonkeratinizing); its cells have abundant glycogen. The epithelium is nonglandular and is lubricated by cervical mucus. It lies on a lamina propria, containing dense connective tissue, elastic fibers, and lymphocytes.

Arteries: Branches of the uterine artery; 2 to 3 vaginal arteries (from the internal iliac artery), the anastomoses of which are two longitudinal anterior and posterior azygos arteries of the vagina; branches of the artery of the vestibiular bulb.
Veins: Into vaginal venous plexus, which leads into uterine and vesical plexuses.
Lymphatics: From the superior portion of the vagina into external and internal iliac nodes; from the middle into internal iliac nodes, and from the inferior into sacral and common iliac nodes; from the portion near the hymen into the superficial inguinal nodes.
Nerves: Uterovaginal plexus (autonomic and vasomotor fibers) and pudendal nerve for the inferior portion of the vagina.

The pelvic diaphragm (right and left levator ani muscle and coccygeal muscle), surrounded by the parietal pelvic fascia, separates the pelvic cavity from the perineal region. The parietal pelvic fascia forms the superior and inferior fasciae of the pelvic diaphragm, the obturator fascia (internal muscle obturator), and below the origin of the pelvic diaphragm the lateral wall of the ischiorectal fossa, where it has the pudendal canal (for the internal pudendal vessels and pudendal nerve). The obturator fascia has a line of fusion with the superior and inferior fasciae of the pelvic diaphragm, and the resulting thickening (from the pubis to the ischial spine) is the tendinous arch of the levator ani muscle.

The male urogenital triangle (perforated by the urethra) comprises the following layers and spaces (in superoinferior order):

1. Superior fascia of the urogenital diaphragm
2. Deep perineal space
   Urogenital diaphragm
      Deep transverse perineal muscle
      Sphincter muscle of the membranous urethra
   Bulbourethral glands
   Branches of the internal pudendal vessels
   Pudendal nerves
3. Inferior fascia of the urogenital diaphragm
   Transverse perineal ligament
4. Superficial perineal space
   Root of the penis

Muscles of the root of the penis
   Superficial transverse perineal muscle
   Ischiocavernous muscle
   Bulbospongiosus muscle
Membranous portion of urethra
Branches of the internal pudendal vessels
Pudendal nerves
5. Deep perineal fascia
   suspensory ligament of the penis
6. Superficial perineal fascia
   Tela subcutanea
      Superficial fatty layer
      Deep membranous layer
      Branches of the posterior scrotal or labial vessels and muscles
7. Dermis
8. Epidermis

The female urogenital triangle (perforated by the urethra and the vagina) comprises the following layers and spaces (in superoinferior order):

1. Superior fascia of the urogenital diaphragm
2. Deep perineal space
   Urogenital diaphragm
      Deep transverse perineal muscle
      Sphincter muscle of the urethra
3. Inferior fascia of the urogenital diaphragm
4. Superficial perineal space
   Superficial transverse perineal muscle
   Ischiocaverous muscle
   Bulbospongiosus muscle
5. Deep perineal fascia
6. Superficial perineal fascia
   Tela subcutanea
      Superficial fatty layer
      Deep membranous layer
7. Dermis
8. Epidermis

The male external genital organs are located partially in the urogenital triangle (most in front of it). They consist of the scrotum or testicular pouch and the penis.

The scrotum is situated below the pubic symphysis and is subdivided by the scrotal septum into right and left halves; the external indication of this subdivision is the scrotal raphe. Each compartment contains testis, epididymis, part of the spermatic cord, and its coverings. The scrotum has thin, pigmented skin, with abundant sebaceous and sweat glands and a few hairs. The other component of the scrotum is the tunica dartos, essentially made up of smooth muscle fibers, firmly attached to the skin.

Arteries: External pudendal arteries, scrotal branches of the internal pudendal artery, branches of the testicular artery and cremasteric artery.

Veins: Follow the arteries.

Lymphatics: Drain into superficial inguinal nodes.

Nerves: Ilioinguinal nerve, genital branch of the genitofemoral nerve, medial and lateral scrotal branches of the perineal nerve and perineal branch of the posterior femoral cutaneous nerve.

The penis is the organ of copulation made up of erectile tissue. It is divided into root, body, neck, and glans. The root is in the superficial perineal space, between the inferior fascia of the urogenital diaphragm and the deep perineal fascia below. It has crura and a median bulb of the penis. Each crus is inserted into the ischial ramus and covered by the ischiocavernous muscle. The crura join at the level of the pubic symphysis and are called corpora cavernosa. The bulb of the penis is pierced by the urethra, thus surrounded by the corpus spongiosus, which is in turn surrounded by the bulbospongiosus muscle. The body of the penis begins the free portion of the organ, pendulous when flaccid, covered by skin. The anterior aspect of a flaccid penis is the dorsum and the opposite aspect is the urethral surface, where the median raphe penis is found. The neck is a narrowing that separates the body from the glans penis, which contains the extremities of the corpora cavernosa and the enlarged end of the corpus spongiosum. The corona glandis is the posterior border of the glans. The latter presents a median slit called the external urethral orifice. The prepuce is a double layer of skin that covers the glans; the frenulum of the prepuce is a median fold in the urethral aspect of the penis between the deep layer of the prepuce and the area near the external urethral orifice.

The skin of the penis is thin, pigmented, and elastic. The glans contains preputial glands, the sebaceous secretion of which forms the smegma. The subcutaneous tela (superficial fascia of the penis) has connective tissue, smooth muscle fibers, and no fat. It is continuous with the dartos and with the superficial perineal fascia. The deep fascia of the penis continues the deep perineal fascia and, as one sheath, surrounds the corpora cavernosa and the corpus spongiosum, without extending to the glans. The tunica albuginea of the corpora caverosa is a dense fibrous envelope, made up of outer longitudinal and inner circular fibers. The latter form the median septum of the penis, which is incomplete in its distal portion, allowing communication between the corpora cavernosa. The tunica albuginea is thinner around the corpus sponsiosum. The erectile organs are constituted of cavernous spaces (blood lakes) separated by trabeculae, the wall of which is made up of collagen, elastic, and smooth muscle fibers, arteries, and nerves.

The penis has the fundiform and the suspensory ligament. The fundiform ligament arises from the linea alba and the membranous layer of the subcutaneous tela, and splits into right and left portions, which surround the penis and unite on the urethral surface, where they join the scrotal septum. The suspensory ligament is deep to the preceding ligament, arises from the pubic symphysis, and inserts into the deep fascia on the right and left side of the penis.

Arteries: Artery of the bulb, deep artery of the penis, dorsal artery of the penis, which anastomoses with the preceding arteries; their small branches (helicine arteries) run in the trabeculae and supply the erectile tissue.

Veins: Dorsal vein of the penis (between the two dorsal arteries) divides into left and right veins, which drain into the prostatic plexus. The skin is drained by the superficial dorsal vein, then into the great saphenous vein.

Lymphatics: From prepuce into superficial inguinal nodes, from glans into deep inguinal and external iliac nodes.

Nerves: Dorsal nerves of the penis (branches of pudendal nerves) to skin and glans; deep branches of perineal nerves to bulb, corpus spongiosum, and urethra; ilioinguinal nerve to skin and cavernous nerves of the penis to erectile tissue. Autonomic fibers of cavernous nerves originate from lumbar sympathetic ganglia; there are sensory, sympathetic, and parasympathetic fibers.

The female external organs are collectively called pudendum femininum or vulva and consist of mons pubis, labium (lip) majus and minus, vestibule and bulb of the vagina, clitoris, and the vestibular glands.

The mons pubis is a prominence anterior to the pubic symphysis, owing to adipose tissue, covered by hairy skin (postpuberty). The labia majora correspond to the scrotum; they limit the pudendal cleft and are united by the anterior and posterior commissures. The labia minora are hidden between the labia majora, limit the vestibule of the vagina, and are united posteriorly by the frenulum of the pudendal labia. Anteriorly, each labium minus splits into medial and lateral membranes. The right and left lateral membranes join to form the prepuce above the glans of the clitoris, while the two medial folds join below the clitoris to form its frenulum. The vestibule of the vagina contains the orifices of the vagina, of the urethra, and of the ducts of the vestibular glands. The external urethral orifice is posterior to the clitoris and anterior to the vaginal orifice. The orifice of the vagina is a median cleft, and size and form of which depends on the morphology of the hymen.

The orifices of the ducts of the lesser vestibular glands are spread out in the vestibule of the vagina between the urethral and vaginal openings; the right and left orifices of the greater vestibular glands are found on each side of the opening of the vagina, between the hymen (or the remnants of its insertion) and the labia minora. Between the vaginal orifice and the frenulum, the vestibular fossa is found.

The clitoris (homologous to the penis) is hidden by the anterior extensions of the labia minora and arises by the right and left crus from the ipsilateral ischial ramus. Each crus is covered by the ischiocavernous muscle, and, after the median junction of the crura, the corpora cavernosa (erectile organs) are formed. The latter are included in the body of the clitoris, the end of which is the glans of the clitoris. The clitoris is united to the pubic symphysis by its suspensory ligament.

The bulb of the vestibule (homologous to the bulb of the penis) is made up of erectile tissue and is 2.5 cm long, located on each side of the vaginal orifice, deep to the insertion of the labium minus. Each bulb is surrounded by a bulbospongiosus muscle, and both bulbs unite under the glans and body of the clitoris.

Each of the two greater vestibular glands (homologous to the bulbourethral) is located under the epsilateral vestibular bulb.

Arteries: Anterior labial branches (of external pudendal arteries) and posterior labial branches (of internal pudendal); deep arteries of the clitoris; dorsal arteries of the clitoris (to glans); artery of the vestibular bulb, and anterior vaginal artery.

Veins: Follow arteries, homologous to male.

Lymphatics: Into superficial inguinal nodes.

Nerves: Anterior labial nerve (from ilioinguinal) and posterior labial nerve (from pudendal); uterovaginal plexus; cavernous nerves of the clitoris; and dorsal nerve of the clitoris. These nerves have sensory and autonomic fibers (vasomotor and secretory).

The Back

The back, or dorsum, corresponds to the posterior regions of the neck and trunk, which are the following:

Vertebral
    Nuchal (cervical)
    Thoracic
    Lumbar
    Sacral
Scapular
Infrascapular
    Lumbar trigone

The back includes epidermis, dermis, subcutaneous tela, muscles, bones, joints, meninges, spinal cord, vessels, and nerves.

The skin is thick and may reach 6 mm in thickness in the nuchal region and shoulder. The tela subcutanea has variable thickness and adipose tissue content; the subcutaneous nerves are branches of the dorsal rami of spinal nerves.

The vertebral furrow is found in the posterior midline, beginning at the external occipital protuberance, at the junction between the scalp and the nuchal region, and ending at the top of the sacrum. The spinous process of the C7 is responsible for the vertebra prominens (70 percent of the cases). The erector spinae muscle is prominent on either side of the vertebral furrow and the iliac crest can be followed laterally from the posterior superior iliac spine, marked by a dimple. The supracristal or bicristal plane, uniting the uppermost points of the iliac crests, corresponds to the spinous process of L4 (landmark for lumbar puncture). The acromion, the scapular spine, and the inferior angle of the scapula can be palpated, and, in lean individuals, seen.

The muscles are divided into prevertebral (supplied by ventral rami of spinal nerves) and retrovertebral muscles. The prevertebral muscles are the longus capitis, longus colli (cervicis), rectus capitis anterior, and rectus capitis lateralis. The retrovertebral muscles are located on the posterior aspect of the vertebral column and divided into three groups, as follows:

1. Superficial
    Trapezius muscle
    Latissimus dorsi muscle
    Sternocleidomastoid muscle
2. Middle
    Levator muscle of the scapula
    Greater rhomboid muscle
    Lesser rhomboid muscle
    Serratus posterior superior muscle
    Serratus posterior inferior muscle
3. Deep
    Levatores costarum muscles
    Erector muscle of the spin
    Splenius capitis muscle
    Splenius cervicis muscle
    Transversospinales muscles
    Interspinal muscles
    Intertransverse muscles

The thoracolumbar fascia is the fascia of the back, attached to the spinous process of vertebrae and, laterally, inserted into the costal angles, the iliac crest, and the sacrum. It forms a sheath for the latissimus dorsi muscle.

The trapezius muscle originates from the spinous process of C7 and T1–T12, nuchal ligament, and occipital bone, and inserts into the lateral one-third of the clavicle, acromion, and scapular spine. Nerves: XI, C3, C4.

The latissimus dorsi muscle originates from the spinous process of T7–T12, thoracolumbar fascia, iliac crest, inferior ribs, and inferior scapular angle; it inserts into the intertubercular groove of the humerus. Nerve: Thoracodorsal.

The triangle of auscultation is limited by the lateral margin of the trapezius muscle (which overlies the latissimus dorsi muscle), by the superior margin of the latissimus dorsi muscle, and by the medial margin of the scapula. This is the area where there is the least number of superimposed muscles.

The sternocleidomastoid muscle originates from the manubrium sterni and the medial one-third of the clavicle, and inserts into the mastoid process. Nerves: XI and C2–C4.

The levator muscle of the scapula originates from the transverse tubercle of C1–C4 and inserts in the superior portion of the medial margin of the scapula. Nerves: C3–C4.

The greater rhomboid muscle is frequently fused with the lesser rhomboid muscle; they originate from the spinous process of the C7 and T1–T5 and insert into the medial margin of the scapula. Nerve: Dorsal scapular.

The serratus posterior superior muscle originates from the nuchal ligament and spinous process of C7 and superior thoracic vertebrae and inserts into ribs 2–5. Nerves: C8–T3.

The serratus posterior inferior muscle originates from the spinous process of the inferior thoracic vertebrae to ribs 9–12. Nerves: T9–T11.

The levatores contarum muscles originate from the transverse process of C7–T12 and insert into the external aspect of the subjacent rib (between the costal tubercle and the angle). Nerves: Dorsal rami of C8–T11.

The erector muscle spine (sacrospinalis) is divided into the spinalis (medial), subdivided into thoracis, cervicis, and capitis, longissimus (thoracis, cervicis, and capitis), and iliocostalis (lateral), subdivided into lumborum, thoracis, and cervicis. Nerves: Dorsal rami of spinal nerves (inferior C, T, and inferior L).

The splenius capitis muscle originates from the nuchal ligament and spinous process of C7 and T1–T4, and inserts into the mastoid process and lateral one-third of the superior nuchal line. Nerves: Lateral branches of the dorsal rami of the middle C spinal nerves.

The splenius cervicis muscle originates from the spinous process of T3–T6, and inserts into the posterior tubercle of the transverse process of the C1–C3. Nerves: Lateral branches of the dorsal rami of the inferior C spinal nerves.

The transversospinales muscles consist of the following:

Semispinalis muscle
 Thoracis
 Cervicis
 Capitis
Multifidi muscles
 Cervicis
 Thoracis
 Lumborum

The transversospinales muscles include the rotatores along with the semispinalis and multifidi muscles (Table 2-6).

The interspinal and intertransverse muscles extend

Table 2-6. Origins, Insertions, and Innervations of Transversospinales Muscles

Muscle	Origin	Insertion	Nerve
Semispinalis thoracis	Transverse process of T6–T10	Spinous process of T1–T4 and C6–C7	Dorsal rami C and T spinal nerves
Semispinalis cervicis	Transverse process of T1–T6	Spinous process of C2–C5	Dorsal rami C and T spinal nerves
Semispinalis capitis	Transverse process of T1–T6 and C7, articular process of C4–C6	Area between superior and inferior nuchal lines	Dorsal rami C and T spinal nerves
Multifidi	Sacrum, origin of erector spinae, superior, posterior iliac spine, dorsal sacroiliac ligament, mamillary process, transverse processes, articular process of C4–C7	Spinous process of above vertebra	Dorsal rami of spinal nerves
Rotatores C, T, L	Superior and posterior part of the transverse	Inferior border and lateral aspect of lamina of vertebra above	Dorsal rami of spinal nerves

between spinous processes (the former) and between transverse processes of the vertebrae (the latter). The interspinal are supplied by dorsal rami of the spinal nerves, whereas some of the intertransverse are supplied by the dorsal rami and others by ventral rami of the spinal nerve.

The suboccipital triangle is the area limited by the major posterior rectus capitis muscle, the oblique capitis superior and inferior muscles; its roof is the semispinalis capitis muscle and the longissimus capitis muscle and its floor is the posterior atlanto-occipital membrane and the posterior arch of the atlas. With the triangle are related the vertebral artery, the suboccipital nerve and its branches for the suboccipital muscles, the greater occipital nerve (dorsal ramus of C2), and the occipital artery. The suboccipital muscles are the recti (posterior major and minor of the head) and the oblique (superior and inferior of the head), supplied by the dorsal ramus (suboccipital nerve) of the C1.

The bones of the back include the vertebral column, the posterior portion of the ribs, the scapula, and the posterior portion of the hip bone.

The vertebral column has 33 vertebrae, divided into the following groups:

24 Presacral
   7C, 12T, 5L
5 Sacral
   5S (fused)
4 Coccygeal
   4 Co (fused)

The vertebral column of the adult individual has four sagittal (anteroposterior) curvatures; C and L are concave posteriorly, and T, S, and Co are concave anteriorly. A slight right convexity or lateral curvature (scoliosis when accentuated) is due to right handedness.

Each vertebra has a body, an arch (pedicle and lamina), and a foramen. The vertebral arch has articular, transverse, and spinous processes. The superimposition of vertebral foramina forms the vertebral canal, for the meninges, spinal cord, vessels, and nerves.

The C7 have a transverse foramen (in the superior C6 it contains the vertebral artery); the C1 is the atlas and the C2 is the axis. The anterior tubercle of the transverse process of the C6 is the carotid tubercle (the carotid artery can be compressed against it).

The T have on each side a facet for articulation with the head of a rib.

The L present a mamillary process on the posterior aspect of the superior articular process and an accessory process is found in the inferior aspect of the transverse process.

The S fuse and form the sacrum, which has a base, a lateral mass, a pelvic and a dorsal aspect, and an apex. The base has the sacral wing or ala. In 84 percent of the cases, the median anterior point of the base is the pelvic promontory, the most prominent point of the lumbosacral joint (in 15 percent of the cases it is the disk and in 1 percent it is the inferior border of the L5). The pelvic aspect is concave and has on each side four anterior sacral (pelvic) foramina for the ventral rami of S1–S4 and four transverse ridges. The dorsal aspect presents the median, intermediate, and lateral sacral crests; four bilateral posterior sacral foramina for the dorsal rami of S1–S4; and the right and the left sacral cornu, which limit the sacral hiatus (through which caudal analgesia is performed) and articulate with the coccygeal cornua. The superior portion of the lateral mass is the auricular surface (for the sacroiliac joint) limited posteriorly by the sacral tuberosity. The apex may be fused with the superior aspect of the coccyx. The sacral canal contains the dura mater, cauda equina, and filum terminale.

The Co are partially or totally fused.

Vertebrae develop in mesenchyme and cartilage, and most begin ossification during intrauterine life. They have three ossification centers; one for the body and two for the arch. Secondary centers occur in the chondral ends of the spinous and transverse processes and on the superior and inferior aspects of the vertebral body. All centers are fused into a complete vertebra at the age of 25.

The joints of the vertebral column are the intervertebral symphyses, those between the arches, those between the thoracic vertebrae and the ribs, and those between the atlas and the skull. Their classification is as follows:

1. Atlanto-occipital: Ellipsoid joint
2. Median atlantoaxial: Trochoid or pivot joint
3. Lateral atlantoaxial: Plane joint
4. Between vertebral bodies: Symphyses
5. Between laminae of arches: Syndesmoses
6. Between articular processes: Plane joints
7. Costovertebral: Plane joint
8. Sacroiliac: Plane joint

The right and left atlanto-occipital joints are formed between the articular facets of the atlas and the occipital condyles; the arches of the atlas are connected to the margin of the foramen magnum by the anterior and posterior atlanto-occipital membranes.

The median atlantoaxial joint is formed by the anterior arch, transverse ligament of the atlas, and the dens. The cruciform ligament of the atlas comprises the transverse ligament of the atlas and the longitudinal ligaments between the foramen magnum and the axis.

The lateral atlantoaxial joints take place between the corresponding articular processes. The apical ligament of the dens unites the dens to the foramen magnum, the alar ligaments connect the dens to the occipital condyles, and the membrana tectoria extends from the body of the axis to the occipital bone. The nuchal ligament continues with the supraspinous ligament, which extends between successive spinous processes.

The symphyses between superimposed vertebral bodies are united by anterior and posterior longitudinal ligaments and by fibrocartilaginous intervertebral disks. Each disk contains a central nucleus pulposus, surrounded by an anulus fibrosus, and is limited by a superior and an inferior hyaline cartilage plate.

The laminae of the vertebrae are united by yellow ligaments (ligamenta flava).

The costovertebral joints consist of those connecting the costal heads with the vertebral bodies and the costotransverse, (i.e., those between the costal tubercles) with the transverse processes.

The sacroiliac joint is established between the auricular surfaces of the sacrum and ilia. Iliolumbar ligaments unite the ilium and the transverse process of L5.

The meninges surround the central nervous system; thus, like the brain in the skull, the spinal cord is invested by the dura mater, the arachnoid, and the pia mater. The dura mater extends from the foramen magnum to the coccyx. Epidural, peridural, or extradural space, containing adipose tissue and the inner vertebral venous plexus, separates the periosteum lining the vertebral canal from the external aspect of the dura mater. The dura mater has extensions to invest the roots and dorsal ganglia of spinal nerves, and also extends into the epineurium of these nerves. The spinal arachnoid is the continuation of the encephalic or cerebral arachnoid from the foramen magnum to the S2. Between the arachnoid and the pia mater there is subarachnoid space which contains CSF. Because the subarachnoid space reaches S2, whereas the spinal cord only reaches L2, CSF can be removed and its pressure measured, or an anesthetic introduced, by insertion of a needle between these two levels (lumbar puncture). The pia mater intimately surrounds the spinal cord and its anterior spinal artery, penetrates the anterior median fissure, and extends laterally as 21 denticulate ligaments (longitudinal septum between venral and dorsal roots) fuse with the arachnoid and dura mater.

The spinal cord is 45 cm long, extending from the medulla oblongata (bulb) to the L2. Below L2, the vertebral canal contains the fibrous continuation of the spinal cord (filum terminale), attached to the coccyx, roots of spinal nerves, and meninges. The spinal cord has a cervical and a lumbosacral enlargement, and ends as the conus medullaris. Its surface shows the anterior median fissure, the posterior median sulcus, and the anterolateral, posterolateral, and posterior intermediate sulci,

continuous with those of the medulla oblongata. The anterior fissure contains the anterior spinal artery, and the posterior aspect of the spinal cord presents small arteries and veins, and branches and tributaries, respectively, of the posterior and medullary vessels. The anterolateral sulci correspond to the line of emergence of 31 pairs of anterior or motor roots of spinal nerves, and the posterolateral sulci correspond to the line of entrance of 31 pairs of posterior or sensory roots (each presenting a spinal ganglion). The anterior median fissure and the posterior median sulcus divide the spinal cord into symmetrical halves; the anterolateral and posterolateral sulci divide each half into anterior, lateral, and posterior funiculi. A posterior and an anterior root join laterally to form a spinal nerve, the first being located between the atlas and the skull. The remaining cervical nerves leave the vertebral canal above the corresponding numbered vertebra (except the C8 and the other nerves, which leave below it). There are 8 C , 12 T, 5 L, 5 S, and 1 Co nerves on each side. The roots below the spinal cord located in the vertebral canal resemble a horse's tail and are called cauda equina. Filaments emerging from the lateral aspect of the superior portion of the cervical spinal cord are the spinal part of the nerve XI.

The funiculi of the white matter surround the H-shaped gray matter, where the central canal is found, extending from the fourth ventricle to the filum terminale (just above the filum there is a dilation called terminal or fifth ventricle). The gray matter is divided into an anterior (in cross section, horn or cornu), a lateral, and a posterior column. The anterior column contains perikarya of motor neurons, the lateral column contains perikarya of preganglionic fibers of the autonomic portion of the nervous system, and the posterior column contains the central process of the sensory neurons, the perikaryon of which is in the spinal ganglion.

There are anterior and posterior (to the central canal) gray commissures, and an anterior white commissure.

The columns contain the following structures:

    Anterior column
        Nucleus ventrolateralis
        Nucleus ventromedialis
        Nucleus dorsolateralis
        Nucleus dorsomedialis
        Nucleus centralis
        Nucleus of nerve XI
        Nucleus of phrenic nerve
    Lateral column
        Substantia grisea intermedia centralis
            Nucleus thoracicus (T1, L2)
        Substantia grisea intermedia lateralis
            Columna autonomica (C7, L2)
        Nuclei parasympathici sacrales (S2–S4)

Posterior column
Apex, head, neck, and base of the posterior horn
Gelatinous substance
Secondary visceral substance

The funiculi contain the following fasciculi or tractus

Anteriorfuniculus
Fasciculi proprii anteriores
Fasciculus sulcomarginalis
Tractus corticospinalis anterior (pyramidalis)
Tractus vestibulospinalis
Tractus spinothalamicus anterior
Lateral funiculus
Fasciculi proprii laterales
Tractus corticospinalis lateralis (pyramidalis)
Tractus rubrospinalis
Tractus tectospinalis
Tractus olivospinalis
Tractus spinotectalis
Tractus spinothalamicus lateralis
Tractus spinocerebellaris anterior
Tractus spinocerebellaris posterior
Tractus dorsolateralis
Tractus spinoolivaris
Tractus spinoreticularis
Posterior funiculus
Fasciculi proprii posteriores
Fasciculus septomarginalis
Fasciculus interfascicularis
Fasciculus gracilis
Fasciculus cuneatus

Arteries of the spinal cord are the anterior spinal artery, formed by the two branches of the vertebral artery and two posterior spinal arteries, given off by the vertebral or posterior inferior cerebellar arteries. These three longitudinal arteries are reinforced by transversal medullary arteries, from spinal branches of the ascending and deep cervical, vertebral, posterior intercostal, and lateral sacral arteries. Veins join the vertebral venous plexuses, leading to the intervertebral veins, which lead into segmental veins.

The arteries or their branches of the back are the following:

1. Neck: Occipital, ascending cervical, vertebral, and deep cervical
2. Thorax and abdomen: Posterior intercostal, subcostal, and lumbar
3. Pelvis: Iliolumbar and lateral sacral

The veins are the following:

1. Vertebral venous plexus: External anterior and posterior, internal anterior and posterior. The vertebral venous plexus is anastomosed with the cranial dural sinuses, pelvic, azygos, and caval veins. The internal vertebral or epidural venous plexus surrounds the dura mater, includes the basivertebral, anterior, and posterior spinal veins, and is drained by intervertebral veins. The external vertebral venous plexus surrounds the vertebral bodies and arches, drains the bones and muscles, and leads into intervertebral veins.
2. Suboccipital venous plexus: Located in the homonymous triangle, drains the occipital veins of the scalp, anastomoses by emissary veins with the transverse sinus and with the vertebral veins.
3. Vertebral vein has two roots (from the venous plexus at the level of the foramen magnum), drains the suboccipital venous plexus, enters the transverse foramen of the C1, descends through the subjacent foramina, and ends in the brachiocephalic vein.
4. Deep cervical vein (from the suboccipital region) leads into the vertebral vein.

The lymph from the deep organs of the back is drained by vessels that accompany the veins. The lymph from the skin leads into cervical, axillary, and superficial inguinal nodes.

The nerves of the back are meningeal and dorsal rami of the spinal nerves:

1. Meningeal branch or sinuvertebral nerve is given off by each spinal nerve and supply the dura mater, posterior longitudinal ligament, periosteum, epidural, and intraosseous blood vessels.
2. Each dorsal ramus innervates the skin, muscles, joints, and bones, after dividing into medial and lateral branches. There are cervical, thoracic, lumbar, sacral, and coccygeal dorsal rami. The cervical dorsal rami include the following: (a) anastomoses between successive C4 nerves form the posterior cervical plexus; (b) the dorsal ramus of C1 is the suboccipital nerve; (c) the medial branch of the dorsal ramus of C2 is the greater occipital nerve; (d) the medial branch of the dorsal ramus of C3 gives the third occipital nerve. The thoracic dorsal rami innervate the deep muscles and divide into a medial and a lateral cutaneous branch; (e) the lumbar dorsal rami supply the erector muscle of the spine by means of their medial branches, the lateral branches innervating the gluteal regions or buttocks (superior cluneal nerves); (f) S1–S4 and inferior lumbar nerves form the posterior sacral plexus, which gives off the middle cluneal nerves; and (g) the coccygeal nerves and S5 form a single nerve,

which supplies the skin and ligaments of the corresponding area.

Superior member

The superior member comprises a root and a free extremity. The root is the scapular girdle, at the level of the shoulder, and the free extremity consists of arm, axilla, elbow, forearm, wrist, hand, and fingers.

The regions of the superior member are deltoid, arm (anterior and posterior), cubital or elbow, (anterior, posterior, cubital fossa, the latter including the lateral bicipital and the medial bicipital sulci), forearm (anterior and posterior regions and lateral and medial margins), wrist (anterior and posterior carpal regions), and hand (dorsal and palmar, thenar and hypothenar, metacarpal, fingers, each of the latter including ventral and dorsal digital aspects).

SKELETON OF THE SUPERIOR MEMBER

The scapula is connected to the clavicle and the humerus by means of joints. Its body has a costal and a dorsal surface, the latter divided by its spine into supra- and infraspinous fossae. There are the superior (with scapular notch), medial, and lateral (with infraglenoid tubercle) borders, and the superomedial, inferior, and superolateral (which contains the glenoid cavity for the head of the humerus and the supraglenoid tubercle) angles. The spine of the scapula ends laterally with the acromion, which articulates with the clavicle. The coracoid process is located medially to the glenoid cavity.

The clavicle extends from the sternum (sternoclavicular joint) to the acromion (acromioclavicular joint).

The humerus is the long bone of the arm, articulated by its ends to the scapula and to the radius and ulna, at the shoulder and elbow, respectively. The proximal end presents a head, anatomical and surgical neck, greater and lesser tubercles, and the intertubercular groove. The body or shaft has three aspects (anterolateral, anteromedial, and posterior) and three margins (lateral, anterior, and medial). The distal possesses a condyle (capitulum and trochlea), epicondyles (lateral and medial), and three fossae (radial, coronoid, and olecranon).

The radius and the ulna are the long bones of the forearm. The radius is articulated with the humerus, medially with the ulna, and distally with the carpal bones. The proximal extremity has a head, neck, and tuberosity. The body shows anterior, posterior, and lateral aspects, and anterior, posterior, and interosseous margins. In the distal extremity there are the styloid process, the ulnar notch, and the dorsal tubercle.

The ulna is longer than and medial to the radius. Its proximal end has the olecranon, trochlear notch, coronoid process, tuberosity, and radial notch. The body presents the anterior, posterior, and medial aspects. It also presents the anterior, posterior, and interosseous margins. The distal end shows the styloid process and the head, which is in contact with the articular disk, separating it from the carpus.

The carpus is made up of eight carpal bones; those of the proximal row are the scaphoid, lunate, triquetrum, and pisiform; and those of the distal row are the trapezium, trapezoid, capitate, and hamate. The anterior or palmar concavity of the carpus and the flexor retinaculum form the carpal canal, where the flexor tendons are found. The scaphoid (often fractured) and the trapezium are the floor of the anatomical snuffbox. The first bones to ossify are the capitate and the hamate (sometimes before birth).

The metacarpus is made of five bones or metacarpals numbered from I (thumb) to V (little finger); it connects the carpus and the phalanges. Each metacarpal has a shaft or diaphysis and two epiphyses or ends (proximal or base, and distal or head). An endochondral center and a periosteal collar appear at the third intrauterine month. Epiphysial centers occur during infancy and they unite at puberty.

There are three phalanges for each finger, except the thumb, which has two. A phalanx has a base (proximal), a shaft or diaphysis, and a head (distal). The proximal phalanx articulates with a metacarpal. Ossification starts at the third or fourth intrauterine month. Epiphysial centers appear during pregnancy and they unite by puberty.

Two sesamoids are located anteriorly to the head of metacarpal I. Others may occur in other areas of the hand.

The veins of the superior member are valved and divided into superficial and deep. The former are subcutaneous and the latter are paired satellites of the arteries (accompanying veins). The superficial veins form a dorsal venous network, which drains into deep veins. The cephalic vein, accompanied by the accessory cephalic vein, ascends on the radial side from the dorsal network, reaches the anterior aspect of the elbow, follows the lateral border of the biceps, perforates the clavipectoral fascia, and terminates in the axillary vein (which is not paired). The basilic vein (from the dorsal network) ascends on the ulnar side and reaches the elbow in front of the medial epicondyle, perforates the fascia in the arm, follows the brachial artery, and joins the brachial veins to form the axillary vein. The cephalic and basilic veins are anastomosed by the median cubital vein at the level of the anterior aspect of the elbow, a vein that drains also into the deep veins. The deep veins have the same names as the arteries. They follow and drain into the axillary vein. This vein begins at the inferior border of the major teres muscle and, at the lateral margin of rib 1, continues as the subclavian vein.

The lymph from the fingers drains into dorsal and palmar plexuses, then into ducts that follow the main superficial veins. A few ducts lead into the cibital (supratrochlear) nodes at the level of the medial epicondyle. Other ducts reach the deltopectoral (infraclavicular) nodes and the deep lymphatic canals follow the arteries; all are tributaries of the lateral axillary nodes.

The axillary nodes are divided into five groups: Lateral (for superior member), pectoral (for breast and part of thorax), posterior (for posterior portion of the shoulder), central (for the preceding groups), and apical (for the preceding groups and directly from the breast). They lead into subclavian trunks and into the jugulosubclavian venous junction, or into deep cervical nodes.

REGION OF THE SHOULDER

The region of the shoulder includes the deltopectral triangle, the infraclavicular region, the axillary region, the deltoid region, and the scapular region.

The deltopectral triangle is limited by the deltoid muscle, the major pectoral muscle, and the clavicle; it continues with the homonymous sulcus, and contains the cephalic vein. The clavipectoral fascia is attached to the clavicle, the coracoid process, the minor pectoral muscle, and the subclavius muscle (Table 2-7). It is perforated by the cephalic vein, the thoracoacromial artery, and the lateral pectoral nerve. The clavipectoral fascia divides the triangle into a superficial and a deep compartment.

The superficial compartment contains the cephalic vein just before entering into the axillary vein. The axillary artery sends a branch, the thoracoacromial artery, into the area where it subdivides into clavicular, acromial, pectoral, and deltoid branches. Lymph nodes here drain lymph vessels that follow the cephalic vein. The pectoral nerve or nerves accompany the corresponding arteries.

The deep compartment contains the axillary vein and artery, and three nerve cords. The latter consitute the infraclavicular portion of the brachial plexus and are called lateral, posterior, and medial cords. Superiorly and laterally, the suprascapular artery, vein, and nerve are seen.

The minor teres muscle (above), the major teres (below), and the surgical neck of the humerus (laterally) limit an area that is divided by the long head of the triceps into a medial triangular space and a lateral quadrangular space. The triangular space contains the circumflex scapular vessels, whereas the quadrangular space contains the axillary nerve and the posterior circumflex humeral vessels.

The axilla is a four sided pyramidal area between the thorax and the superior member. Its base is the axillary fascia, the anterior wall is the major and minor pectoral muscles and fasciae, the posterior wall is the scapula and scapular muscles, the medial wall is the serratus anterior muscle and fascia, and the lateral wall is the intertubercular groove. The lateral margin of the pectoral margin forms the anterior axillary fold, whereas the major teres and the latissimus dorsi form the posterior fold. A vertical midaxillary line is between these two folds. The apex is made up of the clavicle, the scapula, and rib I; it is occupied by axillary vessels and lymph nodes, and by the brachial plexus and its branches, arriving from or directed to the neck.

The fasciae of the axillary walls are the pectoral, clavipectoral, the axillary, and the muscular fasciae. The costocoracoid membrane extends between the subclavius and the pectoralis minor, and forms the suspensory ligament of the axilla.

The axillary artery is the continuation of the subclavian artery. It begins at the external margin of rib I and ends at the inferior margin of the major teres muscle, where it becomes the brachial artery. The axillary artery is divided into three portions, based on its relationship with the minor pectoral muscle. I (above the muscle), II (behind), and III (below). The cords of the brachial plexus are named according to their position in relation to the II portion. The number of each portion of the artery also indicates the number of branches, as follows:

Portion I: 1 Branch: Superior thoracic artery
Portion II: 2 Branches: Thoracoacromial artery, lateral thoracic artery
Portion III: 3 Branches: Subscapular artery, anterior circumflex humeral artery, posterior circumflex humeral artery

The superior thoracic artery supplies neighboring muscles. The thoracoacromial artery is subdivided into acromial, deltoid, pectoral, and clavicular branches. The lateral thoracic artery supplies mammary branches. The subscapular artery has two branches, the circumflex scapular artery and the thoracodorsal artery. The anterior and the posterior circumflex humeral arteries anastomose around the surgical neck of the humerus.

In the shoulder, around the scapula, there are many arterial anastomoses, establishing the anatomical base for collateral circulation such as the subscapular, circumflex, scapular, descending scapular, and suprascapular arteries and branches of the intercostal arteries.

Table 2-7. Muscles Related to the Shoulder

Muscle	Origin	Insertion	Nerve
Pectoralis major	Clavicle, sternum, costal cartilages I–IV, aponeurosis of EO muscle	Greater tubercle of humerus	Lateral and medial pectoral nerve
Pectoralis minor	Ribs 2–5	Coracoid process	Medial pectoral
Subclavius	Rib 1	Clavicle	From superior trunk of brachial plexus
Serratus anterior	Ribs 1–8	Scapula	Long thoracic
Trapezius	Spinous process of C8 and T1–T12, supraspinous and nuchal ligaments, superior nuchal line, external occipital	Clavicle, acromion, scapular spine, tubercle of the crest of scapular spine	Nerve XI, C3–C4 nerves (of the cervical plexus)
Latissimus dorsi	Spinous process of T7–T12, posterior layer of thoracolumbar fascia (spinous process of L and S), iliac crest, ribs 9–12, inferior angle of scapula	Intertubercular groove of humerus	Thoracodorsal
Levator scapulae	Transverse process of C1–C4	Medial margin of scapula	Branches of C3–C4 nerves, dorsal scapular nerve
Minor rhomboid	Spinous process of C8 and first thoracic vertebrae, nuchal ligament	Medial margin of scapula at root of its spine	Dorsal scapular
Major rhomboid	Spinous process and supraspinous ligament of T2–T5	Medial margin of scapula below scapular spine	Dorsal scapular
Deltoid	Clavicle, acromion, scapular spine	Deltoid tuberosity of humerus	Axillary
Supraspinatus	Supraspinous fossa of scapula	Greater tubercle of humeras	Suprascapular
Infraspinatus	Infraspinous fossa of scapula	Greater tubercle of humerus	Suprascapular
Teres minor	Dorsal aspect scapula	Greater tubercle of humerus	Axillary
Teres major	Dorsal aspect of inferior angle of scapula	Medial lip of intertubercular groove of humerus	Inferior subscapular
Subscapular	Subscapular fossa	Lesser tubercle of humerus	Subscapular

The brachial veins (or vein) join the basilic vein at the inferior border of the major teres muscle, where the axillary vein is then formed. This vein has tributaries that are satellites of the branches of the axillary artery, under which names they are also known. The axillary vein also receives the thoracoepigastric veins, a source of superficial collateral circulation in case of obstruction of the inferior vena cava. At the level of rib I, the axillary vein becomes the subclavian vein, which is separated from the homonymous artery by the scalenus anterior. The subclavian and the internal jugular veins form the brachiocephalic vein, which unites with the contralateral vein to form the superior vena cava.

The brachial plexus innervates the superior member; it is situated in the neck and in the axilla. This plexus comprises the ventral or anterior rami of the C5–C7 nerves, and most of the T1 nerves, and occupies the posterior triangle of the neck. The plexus follows the axillary artery and is enclosed with the axillary vessels in the same sheath.

The anterior rami of C5, C6 nerves unite and form the superior trunk, the C7 nerve constitutes the middle trunk, and the C8 and the T1 nerves make up the inferior trunk. Each trunk splits into an anterior and a posterior division, directed to the corresponding aspect of the superior member.

The anterior divisions of the superior and middle trunks form the lateral cord (lateral to the II position of the axillary artery); the anterior division of the inferior trunk continues as the medial cord (medial to the artery). The three posterior divisions form the posterior (to the artery) cord. At the inferior margin of the minor pectoral muscle the cords split into terminal branches.

The branches of the anterior rami are the dorsal scapular nerve (root of C5) and the long thoracic nerve (C5, C6, C7).

The branches of the trunks are the following:

From the superior trunk: The nerve to the subclavius muscle (C5) and the suprascapular nerve (C5, C6)

From the inferior trunk: Medial pectoral nerves

From the anterior divisions of the superior and middle trunks: Lateral pectoral nerves

The branches of the cords are the following:

From the lateral cord
Lateral pectoral nerve
Musculocutaneous nerve
Lateral head of median nerve
Lateral head of ulnar nerve
From the posterior cord
Superior subscapular nerve
Inferior subscapular nerve
Thoracodorsal nerve
Radial nerve
Axillary nerve
Articular nerve
From the medial cord
Medial pectoral nerve
Medial brachial cutaneous nerve
Medial antebrachial cutaneous nerve
Ulnar nerve
Medial head of median nerve

The median nerve (C5, C6, C7, C8, T1) originates by lateral and medial components or heads from the lateral and medial cords. The heads unite anteriorly to the axillary artery. The median nerve supplies the skin anterior to the lateral part of the hand, to flexor muscles of the forearm, to short muscles of the thumb, to the elbow and (many) hand joints. The muscles supplied by the median nerves are the following:

1. Just below the elbow
   Pronator teres
   Flexor carpi radialis
   Palmaris longus
   Flexor digitorum superficialis
2. Forearm
   Flexor pollicis longus
   Flexor digitorum profundus (II, III digits)
   Pronator quadratus
3. Hand
   Abductor pollicis brevis
   Opponens pollicis
   Flexor pollicis brevis
   Lumbricales (I, II digits)

The musculocutaneous nerve (C5, C6, C7) arises from the lateral cord and supplies the skin of the lateral side of the forearm and the flexor muscles of the arm (i.e., biceps, brachialis, and coracobrachialis).

The ulnar nerve (C7, C8; T1) arises from the medial cord and supplies the medial aspect of the anterior and posterior aspect of the hand and anterior muscle of the forearm and short muscle of the hand, as follows:

1. Proximal forearm
   Flexor carpi ulnaris
   Flexor digitorum profundus (IV, V digits)
2. Palm
   Palmaris brevis
   Abductor digiti V
   Flexor digiti V brevis
   Lumbricales (III, IV digits)
   Interossei
   Adductor pollicis

The radial nerve (C5 – C8; T1) continues the posterior cord and supplies the skin of the back of the superior member and the extensor muscle, as follows:

1. Arm
   Triceps and anconeus
   Brachioradialis
   Extensor carpi radialis longus
2. Forearm
   Extensor carpi radialis brevis
   Supinator
   Extensor digitorum communis
   Extensor digiti V proprius
   Extensor carpi ulnaris
   Abductor pollicis longus
   Extensor pollicis longus
   Extensor pollicis brevis
   Extensor indicis

The axillary nerve (C5, C6) arises from posterior cord, supplies skin of the deltoid region, the deltoid and minor teres muscles.

The joints of the scapular girdle and shoulder are the following:

1. Coracoclavicular: Syndesmosis
2. Acromioclavicular: Plane joint
3. Sternoclavicular: Spheroid joint (on the basis of movement)
4. Shoulder: Spheroid joint

The costoclavicular ligament reinforces the capsule of the sternoclavicular joint.

The shoulder joint is scapulohumeral or glenohumeral (i.e., between the glenoid cavity and the head of the humerus); its capsule has the coracohumeral, glenohumeral, and transverse humeral ligaments.

The transverse scapular ligament closes the scapular notch into an orifice. The suprascapular artery passes

Table 2-8. Muscles of the Arm

Muscle	Origin	Insertion	Nerve
Biceps brachii			
Long head	Supraglenoid tubercle of scapula and glenoid lip.	Tuberosity of radius, fascia of forearm, bicipital aponeurosis, ulna	Musculocutaneous nerve
Short head	Coracoid process	Same as above (both heads are distally fused)	
Coracobrachialis	Coracoid	Humerus	Musculocutaneous nerve
Brachialis	Humerus	Coronoid process tuberosity of ulna	Musculocutaneous nerve
Triceps			
Long head	Infraglenoid tubercle	Olecranon and fascia of forearm for all heads	Radial
Lateral and median heads	Humerus		

over the ligament and the suprascapular nerve passes under the ligament.

REGIONS OF THE ARM AND ELBOW

The arm (brachium) extends from the shoulder to the elbow, the region of the joint between arm and forearm.

The skin of the arm is thin and has hairs. There are medial and lateral bicipital grooves, indicating the corresponding deep intermuscular septa between muscles of the anterior (preaxial) and posterior (postaxial compartment) groups. The cephalic vein and the basilic vein run in the lateral and medial sulcus, respectively. The medial intermuscular septum has two laminae, the anterior contributing to form the neuromuscular compartment.

In the elbow, the following structures and landmarks are recognized: Lateral and medial epicondyles, olecranon, cubital fossa, biceps tendon (landmark for brachial arteries and median nerve), head of radius, median cubital vein, and ulnar nerve.

The brachial fascia covers the deep parts of the arm and continues with the axillary fascia and the fasciae of adjacent muscles (Table 2-8).

Tapping on the area of the tendon of insertion of the triceps muscle causes extension of the forearm (i.e., the triceps jerk). The spinal cord reflex center being segments C6, C7 (Table 2-9).

At the level of the posterior axillary fold or of the inferior margin of the major teres muscle, the brachial artery continues the axillary artery and at the neck of the radius divides into radial and ulnar arteries; its branches are (1) nutrient (to bones); (2) muscular; (3) deep brachial artery (following the radial nerve) and its branches, such as the deltoid, radial collateral, and middle collateral arteries; (4) superior ulnar collateral artery; and (5) inferior ulnar collateral artery. The elbow collateral circulation is provided by the radial collateral, radial recurrent, middle collateral, interosseus recurrent, inferior ulnar collateral, anterior ulnar collateral, superior ulnar collateral, posterior ulnar collateral, and transverse connections (between profunda brachii and inferior ulnar collateral).

Brachial veins accompany the artery; the basilic vein also follows the brachial artery in the middle of the arm, before it joins the brachial veins.

The nerves are the musculocutaneous, the radial and, passing only, the median and ulnar.

The cubital fossa occurs in front of the elbow. It is limited by the brachioradial and the pronator teres muscles. The floor is represented medially by the brachial muscle and laterally by the supinator muscle. The contents of the fossa comprise the biceps tendon, brachial artery, median nerve, and the radial nerve.

The elbow joint, formed by the humerus, radius, and ulna, is a hinge joint; humeroradial, humeroulnar, and proximal radioulnar (trochoid or pivot) joint. The capsule has radial and ulnar collateral ligaments. The proximal radioulnar joint is surrounded by the anular ligament and also has the quadrate ligament.

The forearm extends from the elbow to the wrist. Its skin is thinner on the anterior aspect than on the posterior aspect. The pulse can be felt by compressing the radial artery against the distal radial epiphysis. The muscles of the forearm are divided into anterior and posterior groups and superficial and deep subgroups (Table 2-10).

Table 2-9. Movements and Muscles of Segments of the Spinal Cord

Segments of Spinal Cord	Movements	Muscles
C5, C6	Flexion	Brachial, biceps, brachioradial
C6	Pronation	Pronator teres, pronator quadratus
C6	Supination	Supinator, biceps
C7, C8	Extension	Triceps

Table 2-10. Muscles of the Forearm

Muscle	Origin	Insertion	Nerve
Anterior Superficial			
Pronator teres	Medial epicondyle coronoid process of ulna	Radius	Median
Flexor carpi radialis	Medial epicondyle	Bases metacarpals II–III	Median
Palmaris longus	Medial epicondyle	Flexor retinaculum, palmar aponeurosis	Median
Flexor carpi ulnaris	Medial epicondyle, olecranon	Pisiform, hamate, metacarpal V	Ulnar
Flexor digitorum superficialis	Medial epicondyle, radius	Middle phalanges II–V	Median
Anterior Deep			
Flexor digitorum profundus	Ulna, interosseous membrane	Distal phalanges II–V	Ulnar, anterior interosseous
Flexor pollicis longus	Radius, interosseous membrane	Distal phalanx I	Anterior interosseous
Pronator quadratus	Ulna	Radius	Anterior interosseous
Posterior Superficial			
Brachioradialis	Lateral supracondylar ridge	Distal radius	Radial
Extensor carpi radialis longus	Lateral supracondylar ridge	Base metacarpal II	Radial
Extensor carpi radialis brevis	Lateral epicondyle	Base metacarpals II–III	Radial
Extensor digitorum	Lateral epicondyle	Middle distal phalanges II–V extensor expansion finger V	Radial
Extensor digiti minimi	Lateral epicondyle		Radial
Extensor carpi ulnaris	Lateral epicondyle, ulna	Base metacarpal V	Radial
Anconeus	Lateral epicondyle	Olecranon	Radial
Posterior Deep			
Supinator	Lateral epicondyle	Radius	Radial
Abductor Pollicis Longus	Interosseous membrane Radius, ulna	Base metacarpal I	Posterior interosseous
Extensor pollicis brevis	Interosseous membrane, radius	Proximal phalanx I	Posterior interosseous
Extensor pollicis longus	Interosseous membrane, ulna	Distal phalanx I	Posterior interosseous
Extensor indicis	Interosseous membrane, ulna	Extensor expansion finger II	Posterior

The radius and the ulna are united by the interosseous membrane, which provides insertion to muscles. Between the oblique cord (from the ulnar tuberosity to the radius) and the interosseous membrane there is a space through which the posterior interosseous artery reaches the posterior compartment of the forearm.

The radial artery, lateral to the tendon of the flexor carpi radialis muscle, gives off a recurrent branch, which joins the elbow anastomoses. Carpal and palmar branches are also given. The ulnar artery gives off a recurrent branch for the elbow anastomosing network and the common interosseous artery (which splits into anterior and posterior interosseous arteries, the anterior giving off the median artery); it continues as the superficial palmar arch after giving off the deep palmar branch.

The veins follow the arteries.

The median nerve and its branches (muscular, anterior interosseous, and palmar), ulnar nerve, between the origins of the flexocarpiulnaris muscle, and its branches (muscular, dorsal, and palmar), radial and its branches (posterior antebrachial cutaenous, muscular and its terminal branches, superficial and deep). The superficial branch is cutaneous and articular, and gives the dorsal digital nerve to fingers I, II, and part of finger III. The deep branch is muscular and articular, and continues as the posterior interosseous nerve.

The wrist or carpus (anterior and posterior carpal region) is described as the proximal portion of the hand.

The fingers or digits are distal to the palm of the hand and numbered from the radial to the ulnar side: I (thumb), II (index), III (middle), IV (ring), and V (little). The prominent portions of the hand related to the thumb and the little finger are called thenar and hypothenar eminences, respectively.

The skin of the palm is thick and hairless, whereas that of the dorsum is thin, hairy (except on distal phalanges), and mobile. Palmar papillary ridges are an individual characteristic, and those of digital pads are recorded as fingerprints for identification purposes. Flexure lines correspond to sulci of skin movements, where the dermis is anchored to the tela subcutanea; the tela contains pads of fibrous and adipose tissue. There is a fascia of the dorsum and a palmar aponeurosis. Superficial transverse metacarpal ligaments connect the four bands of the palmar aponeurosis, in the plane of interdigital ligaments.

The flexor retinaculum converts the carpal arch into a canal, containing flexor tendons and the median nerve. The central compartment of the palm is divided into fascial spaces by septa that begin between the lumbrical muscles and the deep flexor tendons, and limit canals.

There is a fat pad between the anterior interosseous fascia and the synovial sheaths of the flexors.

Of the three synovial sheaths, the one for the flexor carpi radialis is short; the other two are called ulnar and radial bursae. The ulnar bursa is the common flexor synovial sheath (all superficial and deep flexor tendons) and the radial bursa envelops only the flexor pollicis longus tendon.

The synovial sheaths in the fingers have mesotendons (vincula).

The muscles of the hand are divided into the thenar, hypothenar, lumbrical, and interossei regions (Table 2-11).

The radial artery gives off the superficial palmar branch, palmar and dorsal carpal branch, dorsal metacarpal arteries, dorsal digital arteries, princeps pollicis artery, and radialis indicis artery. It anastomoses with the deep branch of the ulnar artery to form the deep palmar arch, from which palmar metacarpal arteries originate. The ulnar artery gives off the palmar and the carpal branches and splits into two terminal branches,

Table 2-11. Origins, Insertions, and Innervations of Muscles of the Hand

Muscle	Origin	Insertion	Nerve
	Thenar Region		
Abductor pollicis brevis	Flexor retinaculum, tubercle of trapezium	Lateral sesamoid, base proximal phalanx	Recurrent branch of median
Flexor pollicis brevis	Flexor retinaculum, tubercle of trapezium	Lateral sesamoid, base proximal phalanx	Recurrent branch of median
Opponens pollicis	Flexor retinaculum, tubercle of trapezium	Lateral sesamoid, base proximal phalanx	Recurrent branch of median
	Hypothenar Region		
Abductor digiti minimi	Pisiform	Medial side of proximal phalanx	Deep branch of ulnar
Flexor digiti minimi brevis	Hook of hamate	Medial side of proximal phalanx	Deep branch of ulnar
Opponens digiti minimi	Hook of hamate	Anterior aspect of proximal phalanx	Deep branch of ulnar
Palmaris brevis	Medial margin palmar aponeurosis	Skin, ulnar aspect of hand	Superficial branch of ulnar
	Lumbrical		
I–II	Lateral two tendons of flexor profundus	Lateral side of extensor expansions of fingers II–V	Median (digital branch)
III–IV	Medial three tendons of flexor profundus	Lateral side of extensor expansions of fingers II–V	Median (digital branches) and deep branch of ulnar
	Interossei		
I–IV Palmar	Diaphysis of metacarpals I, II, IV, V	Extensor expansions of fingers I, II, IV, V	Deep branch of ulnar
dorsal	Sides of metacarpals I–V	Extensor expansions, proximal of fingers II–V	Deep branch of ulnar phalanges

the superficial palmar arch (which gives the common palmar digital arteries) and the deep branch to form, with the radial artery, the deep palmar arch.

The veins follow the arteries.

The nerves of the hand are the median, ulnar, radial, lateral, and posterior antebrachial cutaneous. The intrinsic muscles of the hand, supplied by the median and ulnar nerves, depend upon segment T1 of the spinal cord.

The median nerve gives a recurrent branch to the abductor, the flexor pollicis brevis and the opponens muscles; and palmar digital nerves to $3\frac{1}{2}$ fingers, I, II, and III lumbricals and the dorsum of the distal portion of the fingers and matrix of fingernails (fingers II, III, and radial side of finger IV). In cases of carpal tunnel syndrome, caused by compression of the median nerve, there is weakness of the thenar muscles and sensory loss in the cutaneous distribution of the digital branches.

The ulnar nerve gives off a dorsal branch (in the forearm), muscular branches, dorsal digital nerves, a superficial and a deep branch. The superficial branch gives the common palmar digital nerves and the proper palmar digital nerves. Fine movements of the fingers depend upon the ulnar nerve.

The radial nerve provides a superficial branch, which gives off dorsal digital nerves to $2\frac{1}{2}$ fingers.

The joints of the wrist and hand are (1) the distal radioulnar joint (trochoid or pivot); (2) the radiocarpal joint (ellipsoidal), the capsule of which has palmar, dorsal, radial, and ulnar collaeral ligaments; (3) intercarpal joints, among which are the midcarpal and the pisotriquetral; (4) carpometacarpal joints (saddle); (5) metacarpophalangeal joints (ellipsoidal); and (6) interphalangeal joints (hinge), each having a medial and a lateral collateral ligament.

Inferior Member

The inferior member comprises a root and a free extremity. The root is the pelvic girdle, at the level of the hips, and the free extremity consists of the gluteal region, thigh, knee, leg, ankle, and foot.

The regions of the inferior member are gluteal (gluteal sulcus), femoral (posterior, anterior, and femoral trigone), knee (anterior, posterior, and popliteal fossa), leg or crural (anterior, posterior, sural, anterior, and posterior talocrural), and foot (calcaneal, dorsal, and plantar regions, lateral and medial margins, tarsal and metatarsal regions, and fingers).

SKELETON OF THE INFERIOR MEMBER

The hip bone or pelvic bone (coxae) joins the sacrum to form the bony pelvis; each establishes the connection between the inferior portion of the trunk and the free extremity. Each hip bone is made up of the pubis (which joins the contralateral bone at the pubic symphysis), the ilium, and the ischium. The fusion of these three portions occurs at the acetabulum in the adult. The acetabulum has a fossa, a notch, a margin, and an articular (lunate) surface. The obturator foramen is limited by the ischium, pubis, and their rami; it is almost totally closed by the obturator membrane (except at the obturator groove).

The ilium has a body and a wing (ala). The iliac crest is the superior margin, and its extremities are the anterior and posterior superior iliac spines, the former above the level of the anterior inferior iliac spine (just above the acetabulum) and the latter above the posterior inferior iliac spine. Between the external and internal lips of the crest is the intermediate line.

The wing has a gluteal and a sacropelvic aspect. The gluteal aspect contains the iliac fossa and three gluteal lines (anterior, posterior, and inferior). The sacropelvic aspect has the articular surface, the preauricular sulcus, and the iliac tuberosity. The iliopubic eminence corresponds to the fusion between the ilium and the pubis. Below the posterior inferior iliac spine is the greater sciatic notch. The arcuate line is found between the articular surface and the iliopublic eminence at the pelvic brim (medial border of the wing).

The ischium (sciatic bone) has a body and a ramus; it presents the tuber of the ischium or ischial tuberosity, and the sciatic spine, which separates the greater and lesser sciatic notches.

The pubis has a body and superior and inferior rami. In the body are found the pubic tubercle and crest as well as the symphyseal surface. The anterior border of the superior ramus is the pecten or pectineal line, and the inferior border is the obturator crest.

The femur has a long diaphysis and two epiphyses. The superior epiphysis consists of a head, neck, and greater and lesser trochanters, whereas the inferior consists of the medial and lateral condyles. The head has a fovea, where the ligament of the femoral head is inserted. The neck is separated from the diaphysis by the intertrochanteric line. The medial aspect of the greater trochanter shows the trochanteric fossa. The quadrate tubercle is an elevation of the intertrochanteric crest. The diaphysis or shaft has anterior, medial, and lateral aspects and medial, lateral, and posterior (linea aspera) borders. The medial lip of the linea aspera continues with the spiral line and the lateral lip continues with the gluteal tuberosity. The linea aspera is united to the lesser trochanter by the pectineal line. The intercondylar fossa separates the condyles posteriorly; anteriorly, these form the patellar surface. Each condyle presents an epicondyle, medial and lateral, respectively. The adductor tubercle is above the medial condyle.

The patella is the knee cap, the largest sesamoid bone

embedded in the quadriceps tendon. The portion of the tendon between the apex of the patella and the tuberosity of the tibia is the patellar ligament.

The tibia has a diaphysis and two epiphyses, superior or proximal and inferior or distal. The superior epiphysis comprises a medial and a lateral condyle, an anterior and posterior intercondylar area, and an intercondylar eminence. This eminence is surmounted on each side by the medial and lateral intercondylar tubercles. The lateral condyle has an articular surface for the fibula. The diaphysis has medial, lateral, and posterior surfaces, and anterior, medial, and interosseous borders. The shaft anteriorly contains the tibial tuberosity, and the apex of the triangular area that begins between the condyles. The superior portion of the posterior surface has a nutrient foramen and the soleal line. The anterior border is the shin and the interosseous membrane is inserted into the interosseous border. The distal end of the tibia has the medial malleolus and anterior, posterior, medial, lateral, and inferior surfaces. The posterior surface presents the malleolar groove, and the lateral aspect of the distal end has the fibular notch; the inferior articular surface articulates with the talus and so does the articular surface of the malleolus.

The fibula has a diaphysis, a proximal, and a distal epiphysis. The proximal epiphysis or head has an articular surface to articulate with the lateral condyle of the tibia. The common fibular nerve can be palpated laterally to the neck of the fibula. The shaft has an interosseous margin for the insertion of the interosseous membrane. The distal end is the lateral malleolus, which articulates with the lateral surface of the talus.

The tarsus has one bone less than the carpus. Of the seven tarsals the talus articulates with both the tibia and the fibula. The tarsals are the talus, calcaneus, navicular, cuboid, medial, intermediate, and lateral cuneiform.

The talus has a head, neck, and body. The head presents the navicular, anterior calcaneal, and middle calcaneal articular surfaces. Inferior to the talus is the sulcus tali, the roof of the tarsal sinus, occupied by the interosseous talocalcaneal ligament. The body has the trochlea tali, which presents the lateral malleolar surface (with the lateral process of the talus), the medial malleolar surface, the posterior calcaneal articular surface, the posterior process of the talus (related to the flexor hallucis longus muscle), and the medial and the lateral tubercles for insertion of ligaments.

Posteriorly, the calcaneus has the tuber calcanei, which present the lateral and medial processes and in which the calcaneal (Achilles) tendon is inserted. Anteriorly, the articular surface for the cuboid is found. The three articular surfaces on the superior aspect are the anterior, middle, and posterior talar. The calcaneal sulcus, which faces the talar sulcus and forms the tarsal

sinus, is between the middle and the posterior talar articular surfaces. Medially, the sustentaculum tali has the middle talar articular surface. Inferiorly, there is the groove for the tendon of the flexor hallucis longus muscle, and laterally the fibular trochlea is seen. Under this trochlea is the groove for the tendon of the fibularis longus muscle.

The navicular is situated between the talus and the three cuneiforms; it articulates with these four bones. It has a tuberosity for the insertion of the tibial posterior muscle.

The cuboid lies between the calcaneus and metatarsal bones IV and V. It has articular surfaces for these bones, the lateral cuneiform, and the naviciular. Inferiorly, it has a tuberosity and a groove (for the fibularis longus muscle). The calcaneal process is the posterior projection of the plantar aspect, supporting the anterior end of the calcaneus.

The medial, intermediate, and lateral cuneiforms articulate with each other, with the navicular, and with the metatarsals. The medial with metatarsals I and II, the intermediate with metatarsal II, and the lateral with metatarsals II, III, and IV.

Each of the five metatarsals has a proximal epiphysis (base), a diaphysis (shaft), and a distal epiphysis (head). The bases of metatarsals I and V have a tuberosity. The head of metatarsal I has two sesamoids.

The phalanges of the toes are 14 bones, as in the fingers. Toes II, III, IV, and V have three phalanges each, while toe I (hallux), similar to the thumb (pollex), has only two. The proximal phalanges have a proximal base (articulated with a metatarsal), a body, and a head (articulated with the middle phalanx). The middle phalanges are shorter and the distal phalanges are the shortest. The latter present distal phalangeal tuberosities (for the nail and pulp).

Ossification centers appear in each bone, as follows:

Hipbone
    Ilium: Third intrauterine month
    Ischium: Fourth intrauterine month
    Pubis: Fifth intrauterine month
    Synostosis of the three bones: Age 6
    Synostosis of the acetabulum: Age 16
Femur
    Shaft: Seventh intrauterine week
    Distal epiphysis: Tenth intrauterine month
    Head: Age 1
    Greater trochanter: Age 3
    Lesser trochanter: Age 13
Patella: Age 3
Tibia
    Shaft: Seventh intrauterine week
    Proximal epiphysis: Age 1
    Distal epiphysis: Age 2

Fibula
   Shaft: Second intrauterine month
   Malleolus: Age 2
   Head: Age 4
Talus: Seventh intrauterine month
Calcaneus: Fifth intrauterine month
Navicular: Age 3
Cuboid: Tenth intrauterine month
Cuneiforms
   Medial: Age 2
   Intermediate: Age 3
   Lateral: Age 2
Metatarsals
   Shaft: Second intrauterine month
   Epiphysis: Age 2
Phalanges
   Shaft: Second to eighth intrauterine month
   Proximal epiphysis: Ages 1 to 5
Sesamoids: Before birth

The superficial veins of the inferior member begin as two dorsal digital veins that fuse to form dorsal metatarsal veins, then the dorsal venous network. The medial end of this arch continues as the great saphenous vein, which runs anteriorly to the medial malleolus, then posteriorly to the medial condyles, to reach the femoral triangle, where it pierces the cribriform fascia (saphenous orifice) and the femoral sheath to empty in the femoral vein. Its tributaries are several (e.g., superficial epigastric vein). The small saphenous vein is formed on the lateral end of the dorsal venous network, runs posteriorly to the lateral malleolus, then between the heads of the gastrocnemius muscle, pierces the popliteal fascia, and empties into the popliteal or great saphenous vein. The deep veins begin as plantar digital veins, accompany the arteries, and ultimately drain into the popliteal and femoral veins. They are valved and anastomosed. Perforating veins establish communication between superficial and deep veins.

The lymph is drained by superficial and deep lymphatic vessels. The superficial vessels drain ultimately into the inguinal nodes (3–14), while the deep vessels follow blood vessels and drain into the popliteal nodes (1–5). The efferent vessels from the popliteal nodes follow the femoral vessels and end in the deep inguinal nodes. The efferent vessels from the inguinal nodes drain into the external iliac nodes, then into the lumbar (aortic) nodes.

The arteries for the inferior member are the external iliac, femoral, and popliteal arteries as well as their branches. The popliteal artery splits into the anterior tibial artery and common tibiofibular trunk, which divides into posterior tibial and fibular arteries. The anterior tibial artery continues as the dorsal artery of the foot while the posterior tibial splits into the medial and lateral plantar arteries.

The nerves of the inferior member are mostly branches of the lumbar and sacral plexuses.

GLUTEAL REGION

The skin of the gluteal region is innervated by T12 to S3 nerves, as follows:

Cluneal nerves: Superior, middle, inferior
Lateral cutaneous branches
   of subcostal nerves
   of iliohypogastric nerve
Perforating cutaneous nerves

A subcutaneous bursa is located on the greater trochanter.

The fascia of the gluteal region invests the greatest gluteal muscle and continues as the iliotibial tract of the fascia lata (Table 2-12). It is bound inferiorly to the skin at the level of the gluteal fold.

HIP JOINT

The hip joint is a spheroidal joint (ball-and-socket joint), in which the head of the femur articulates with the acetabulum, completed by the acetabular lip and by the transverse ligament. The capsule is reinforced by the iliofemoral, pubofemoral, and ischiofemoral ligaments. The ligament of the head of the femus arises from the ischium, pubis, and transverse ligaments, and inserts into the head of the femur. Nerves are the femoral, obturator, superior gluteal, and the nerve to the quadratus femoris muscle.

Vessels and nerves of the gluteal region are as follows:

Arteries: Superior and inferior gluteal arteries (both from internal iliac artery); the superior gluteal divides into superficial branch (to gluteus muscle) and deep branch, which is subdivided into superior and inferior branch (to supply adjacent muscles). The inferior gluteal artery supplies the gluteal and hamstring muscles, the hip joint, and anastomoses with the first perforating artery and with the transverse branches of the lateral and medial circumflex arteries (cruciate anastomosis). It gives the companion artery of the sciatic nerve.

Veins: Two superior and two inferior gluteal veins accompany the corresponding arteries and drain into the internal iliac veins.

Nerves: Superior gluteal nerve (L4, L5, S1), inferior gluteal nerve (L5, S1, S2), posterior femoral cutaneous nerve (S1, S2, S3) and branches (inferior cluneal, peri-

Table 2-12. Origins, Insertions, and Innervations of Muscles of the Gluteal Region

Muscle	Origin	Insertion	Nerve
Gluteus maximus	Ilium, sacrum, coccyx, sacrotuberous ligament, aponeurosis of erector spinae, gluteal aponeurosis	Gluteal tuberosity of femur, iliotibial tract	Inferior gluteal
Gluteus medius	Ilium, gluteal aponeurosis	Greater trochanter (bursa)	Superior gluteal
Gluteus minimus	Ilium	Greater trochanter	Superior gluteal
Tensor fasciae latae	External lip of iliac crest, anterior superior iliac spine	Iliotibial tract	Superior gluteal
Lateral Rotators			
Piriformis	S2–S4, sacrotuberous ligament, ilium	Greater trochanter	S1–S2 nerves
Obturator internus	Obturator membrane, hip bone	Greater trochanter	From S plexus
Superior gemellus	Ischial spine	Tendon of obturator internus	Nerve to obturator internus
Inferior gemellus	Ischial tuberosity	Tendon of obturator internus	Nerve to quadratus femoris
Quadratus femoris	Ischial tuberosity	Intertrochanteric crest	From S plexus
Obturator externus	Obturator membrane, pubis, ischium	Trochanteric fossa	Obturator

neal, femoral, and sural), sciatic nerve (L4 to S3), and pudendal nerve (pelvis).

THIGH

The thigh is the proximal region of the free portion of the inferior member, interposed between the gluteal region and the knee. For topographical reasons, the thigh and the knee are described together.

The skin of the thigh is innervated by branches of the following:

Femoral nerve
Obturator nerve
Lateral femoral cutaneous nerve
Posterior femoral cutaneous nerve
Ilioinguinal nerve
Genitofemoral nerve (femoral branch)
Subcostal nerve (lateral cutaneous branch)
Iliohypogastric nerve (lateral cutaneous branch)

The subcutaneous tela contains the great saphenous vein and inguinal lymph nodes.

The fascia lata (of the thigh) forms, with tendinous extensions of the vastus medialis and lateralis muscles, the medial and lateral retinacula of the patella. Over the vastus lateralis, the fascia makes up the iliotibial tract. The fascia lata sends toward the linea aspera two septa: (1) The lateral intermuscular septum inserts into the lateral lip of the linea aspera and separates the extensors

from the flexors; (2) the medial intermuscular septum inserts into the medial lip of the linea aspera and separates the vastus medialis from the adductors. The fascia lata has an opening for the great saphenous vein, the saphenous orifice or oval fossa, 4 cm below to the pubic tubercle. The fascia lata is fused with the inguinal ligament and the lacunar ligament (i.e., the pectineal line), and forms the falciform margin (superior and inferior cornua) of the saphenous opening.

The iliopectineal septum separates a vascular (medial) and a muscular (lateral) compartment. The vascular compartment contains the femoral artery and vein. These vessels and the femoral canal (medial to them) are surrounded by the femoral sheath (posterior to the inguinal ligament, between the iliopsoas and the pectineal muscles). The muscular compartment contains the iliopsoas muscle and the femoral nerve. The femoral canal (anterior to the pectineus) contains adipose tissue and lymph nodes; its superior base is closed by the femoral septum and has a lymph node.

The femoral triangle contains the femoral artery, vein, and nerve, and is limited by the sartorius, long adductor, and inguinal ligament. Its floor has the iliopsoas, pectineal, and long adductor muscles, and its ceiling the fascia lata and cribriform fascia. Lateral to the artery are the femoral nerve, saphenous nerve, and the nerve to the vastus medialis. Medial to the artery is the vein.

The adductor canal is limited by the vastus medialis (laterally), the long adductor, and the magnus (medially), and is covered by the sartorius, then the synonym "subsartorial canal"; the canal contains the femoral vessels, saphenous nerve, and nerve of the vastus medialis muscle.

The muscles of the thigh are classified into the posterior, medial, and anterior regions (Table 2-13).

Tapping the patellar ligament causes a reflex sudden extension of the ligament, the center of which is the L3 segment.

The bursae related to the patella are the subtendinous, subfascial, subcutaneous prepatellar, and subcutaneous infrapatellar.

Vessels and nerves of the thigh are the following:

Arteries: The femoral artery and its branches (superficial epigastric, superficial circumflex iliac, and superficial and deep external pudendal, including inguinal branches and anterior scrotal or labial branches), lateral and medial circumflex, descending genicular, and deep femoral arteries. The profunda femoris gives off muscular and three perforating arteries (pierce the insertions of the adductor brevis and magnus); the lat-

Table 2-13. Origins, Insertions, and Innervations of the Muscles of the Thigh

Muscle	Origin	Insertion	Nerve
Posterior (Hamstring Muscles)			
Biceps femoris			
Long head	Ischial tuberosity, sacrotuberous ligament	Head of the fibula lateral condyle of the tibia	Tibial portion of sciatic nerve
Short head	Lateral lip of linea aspera, lateral supracondylar line, lateral intermuscular septum	Head of the fibula lateral condyle of the tibia	Fibular portion of sciatic nerve
Semitendinosus	Ischial tuberosity	Tibia (medial)	Tibial portion of sciatic nerve
Semimembranosus	Ischial tuberosity	Tibial, medial condyle, medial margin, soleal line	Tibial portion of sciatic nerve
Adductor magnus	Ischial tuberosity, ischiopubic ramus	Linea aspera, adductor tubercle	Tibial portion of sciatic nerve
Medial			
Pectineus (anterior muscle)	Pubic pectineal line	Femoral pectineal line	Femoral obturator
Adductor longus	Pubis	Linea aspera (medial lip)	Obturator
Adductor brevis (anterior muscle)	Pubis	Pectineal line, linea aspera	Obturator
Adductor magnus	Ischial tuberosity, ischiopubic ramus	Linea aspera, adductor tubercle	Tibial portion of sciatic nerve
Gracilis	Pubis	Tibia (medial)	Obturator
Obturator externus (gluteal muscle)	Obturator membrane, pubis, ischium	Trochanteric fossa	Obturator
Anterior			
Iliopsoas			
Iliacus	Iliac fossa	Psoas major tendon	Femoral
Psoas major	Lumbar vertebrae	Lesser trochanter	Lumbar plexus (L1, L2, L3, L4)
Psoas minor	T12, L1	Arcuate line, iliopectineal eminence	Lumbar plexus (L1, L2, L3, L4)
Quadriceps femoris			
Rectus femoris	Anterior inferior iliac spine, acetabulum	Patella, tibial tuberosity	Femoral
Vastus lateralis	Linea aspera (lateral lip)	Patella, tibial lateral condyle	Femoral
Vastus medialis	Intertrochanteric and spiral lines	Patella, tibial medial condyle	Femoral
Vastus intermedius	Femur (anterior, lateral)	Tendon of rectus and vasti	Femoral
Articularis genus	Femur (distal fifth)	Knee joint capsule (bursa suprapatellaris)	Femoral
Sartorius	Anterior superior iliac spine	Tibia (medial)	Femoral

ter provide muscular and nutrient branches and the continuation of the profunda femoris is the fourth perforating artery. The lateral circumflex has descending, ascending, and transverse branches. The medial circumflex artery has an acetabular branch, an ascending, and a transverse branch. The descending genicular artery splits into saphenous and articular branches (knee joint).

Veins: The femoral vein is formed by the popliteal veins and continues at the inguinal ligament as external iliac vein. It receives the deep femoral vein, medial and lateral circumflex veins, and the great saphenous vein.

Nerves: Femoral nerve (LN2, L3, L4) nerves and branches (lateral femoral cutaneous, nerve to pectineus and to hip joint, anterior cutaneous, branches to sartorius, muscular branches and saphenous nerve). The anterior cutaneous branches are the medial and the intermediate cutaneous nerves. The muscular branches supply the rectus femoris muscle (and hip joint), the vastus lateralis (and knee joint), intermedius (and articular muscle of the knee and knee joint), medialis (and knee joint). The saphenous nerve is the termination of the femoral and supplies the skin of the medial side of the leg and foot.

The lateral femoral cutaneous nerve (L2, L3) arises from the L plexus or from the femoral and splits into anterior and posterior branches to innervate the anterior and lateral aspects of the skin of the thigh.

The popliteal fossa is the posterior region of the knee, limited by the biceps (laterally), semitendinous and semimembranous (medially), and distally, plantaris and lateral head of the gastrocnemius (laterally), and medial head of the gastrocnemius (medially). Its floor is made up of the femur, the oblique popliteal ligament, and the fascia of the popliteal muscle. The contents of the fossa are common fibular and tibial nerves, popliteal vessels, posterior femoral cutaneous nerve, genicular branch of the obturator nerve, small saphenous vein, lymph nodes, bursae, and adipose tissue.

The vessels and nerves of the popliteal fossa are the following:

Arteries: Popliteal artery, continuation of the femoral artery at the level of the hiatus in the tendon of the adductor magnus muscle, and its branches, including the superficial sural artery, sural arteries (gastrocnemius muscle), genicular arteries (medial and lateral superior genicular arteries, middle genicular artery and medial and lateral inferior genicular arteries), and terminal (anterior and posterior tibial arteries).

Veins: Two popliteal veins, formed by the accompanying veins of the anterior and posterior tibial arteries; their tributaries correspond to the branches of the pop-

liteal artery and include the small saphenous vein. The popliteal veins form the femoral vein at the hiatus of the tendon of the adductor magnus muscle.

Nerves: The common fibular or lateral popliteal nerve (L4, L5; S1, S2), from the sciatic nerve and its branches: Nerve to short head of biceps and knee joint; (2) lateral sural cutaneous nerve; (3) fibular communicating branch; (4) recurrent nerve; (5) terminal, comprised of deep fibular nerve and superficial fibular nerve. The tibial or medial popliteal nerve (L4, L5; S1, S2, S3), from the sciatic nerve, and its branches: (1) to hamstring muscles; (2) to the knee joint; (3) muscular branches to gastrocnemius, soleus, plantaris, popliteus, and tibialis posterior; the nerve to the popliteus gives off the interosseous nerve of the leg; (4) medial sural cutaneous nerve, which is joined by the fibular communicating branch and forms the sural nerve, reaching the foot; and (5) the sural nerve gives off the lateral calcaneal branches and its continuation to toe V is connected with the superficial fibular and is called the lateral dorsal cutaneous nerve.

The knee joint is classified as a condylar or a hinge joint. It involves the femur, the tibia, and the patella. The patella and the patellar ligament correspond to the anterior portion of the capsule. The tibial collateral ligament is medial to the capsule, and the short lateral ligament is covered by the fibular collateral ligament on the lateral aspect. A posterior extension is called the arcuate popliteal ligament. The capsule is reinforced by the medial and lateral retinacula of the patella, and posteriorly by the oblique popliteal ligament. The intra-articular ligaments are the cruciate ligaments and the menisci. The anterior and posterior cruciate ligaments connect the tibia and the femur, anteriorly and posteriorly to the intercondylar eminence; their names correspond to the tibial insertion. The medial and lateral menisci are semilunar cartilages, actually, the medial is like the letter C and the lateral like the letter O; they are connected by the transverse ligament.

LEG

The skin of the leg is innervated by the saphenous nerve, posterior femoral cutaneous nerve, medial and lateral sural cutaneous nerves, sural nerve, superficial fibular nerve, and obturator nerve.

The fascia of the leg continues the fascia lata and receives expansions from other muscular fasciae of the thigh; it forms the anterior and posterior intermuscular septa inserted into the anterior and posterior borders of the fibula, respectively. These septa determine the division of the leg into the anterior (for the extensors), lateral (for the fibular muscles), and posterior (subdivided by

Table 2-14A. Origins, Insertions, and Innervations of the Muscles of the Leg: Anterior Compartment

Muscle	Origin	Innervation	Nerve
Tibialis anterior	Tibial lateral condyle	Medial cuneiform, metatarsal base I	Deep and common fibular
Extensor hallucis longus	Fibula (anterior)	Hallux (distal phalanx)	Deep fibular
Extensor digitorum longus	Tibial lateral condyle, fibula (anterior)	Toes II–V (middle, distal phalanges)	Deep and common fibular
Fibularis tertius	Fibula (anterior)	Metatarsal base V	Deep fibular

the deep transverse fascia of the leg) compartments. The posterior compartment contains the triceps surae muscle behind the deep transverse fascia, the deep flexor muscles in front of it, and, anteriorly to these muscles, the posterior tibial muscle (next to the interosseous membrane) (Table 2-14).

The vessels and nerves of the anterior compartment of the leg are the following:

Arteries: Anterior tibial artery and its branches to supply the skin and the anterior muscles of the leg: (1) Circumflex fibular branch; (2) posterior tibial recurrent artery; (3) anterior tibial recurrent artery; (4) medial anterior malleolar artery; (5) lateral anterior malleolar artery; and (6) terminal, which continues as dorsal artery of the foot.

Veins: Two veins accompany each artery

Nerves: Deep fibular nerve (terminal branch of the common fibular nerve) and its branches: (1) Muscular branches (tibialis anterior, extensor hallucis longus, extensor digitorum longus, and fibularis tertius); (2) articular branch to the ankle joint; (3) terminal, including the medial branch (subdivided into dorsal digital nerves for toes I and II and articular branches), and the lateral branch distributed to the extensor digitorum brevis, interosseous muscles I, II, and III, and joints.

Vessels and nerves of the lateral compartment of the leg are the following:

Arteries: Anterior tibial artery, fibular artery, and its branches.

Veins: Two veins accompany each artery.

Nerves: Superficial fibular and its branches. The superficial fibular nerve is musculocutaneous and is

one of the terminal branches of the common fibular nerve. Its branches are (1) muscular to both fibular muscles and to extensor digitorum brevis; (2) articular branches; (3) terminal, including the medial dorsal cutaneous nerve and the intermediate dorsal cutaneous nerve. The medial dorsal cutaneous nerve supplies the medial side of the hallux, and gives off a branch to join the deep fibular nerve, and a branch that subdivides into dorsal digital branches to adjacent aspects of toes II and III. The intermediate dorsal cutaneous branch splits into two branches, each subdivided into dorsal digital nerves for adjacent aspects of toes III, IV, and V.

Vessels and nerves of the posterior compartment of the leg are the following:

Arteries: Posterior tibial and branches. The posterior tibial artery is one of the divisions of the popliteal artery and its branches are (1) circumflex fibular; (2) fibular artery and its branches (muscular, nutrient to the fibula, communicating with posterior tibial, perforating, lateral malleolar, and calcaneal branches); (3) medial malleolar branch (and calcaneal branch); and (4) terminal, including medial and lateral plantar arteries.

Veins: Two posterior tibial veins accompanying veins for each artery; the posterior tibial vein is formed by both medial and plantar veins.

Nerves: The tibial nerve and its branches, which are (1) muscular (soleus, tibialis posterior, flexor hallucis longus, and digitorum longus); (2) cutaneous (medial calcaneal branches); (3) articular (ankle joint); and (4) terminal (medial and lateral plantar nerves).

The proximal tibiofibular joint is a plane joint. Its capsule is reinforced by the anterior and posterior ligaments of the head of the fibula.

The interosseus membrane connects the diaphysis of the tibia and of the fibula.

The distal tibiofibular joint is a syndesmosis.

Extensor retinacula are fascial reinforcements and are divided into superior and inferior retinacula. The superior retinaculum is located above the ankle and the infe-

Table 2-14B. Origins, Insertions, and Innervations of the Muscles of the Leg: Lateral Compartment

Muscle	Origin	Insertion	Nerve
Fibularis longus	Tibial lateral condyle, fibular head	Medial cuneiform, metatarsal base I	Superficial, common fibular
Fibularis brevis	Fibula (lateral)	Metatarsal V tuberosity	Superficial fibular

Table 2-14C. Origins, Insertions, and Innervations of the Muscles of the Leg:
Superficial and Deep Posterior Compartments

Muscle	Origin	Insertion	Nerve
Triceps surae			
Gastrocnemius	Femoral lateral and medial, condyles, popliteal surface of femur	Calcaneus	Tibial
Soleus	Fibular head, soleal line of tibia	Calcaneus	Tibial
Plantaris	Popliteal surface of femur	Calcaneal tendon	Tibial
Popliteus	Femoral lateral condyle, lateral meniscus	Tibia	Tibial
Tibialis posterior	Fibula (posterior) soleal line of tibia	Navicular tuberosity, tarsals except talus	Tibial
Flexor digitorum longus	Tibia (posterior)	Toes II – V (distal phalanges)	Tibial
Flexor hallucis longus	Tibia (posterior)	Toe I (distal phalanx)	Tibial

rior is located on the dorsum of the foot and is subdivided into proximal and distal bands to keep the tendons in place.

The superior fibular retinaculum binds the tendons of the fibular muscles posteriorly to the lateral malleolus, and the inferior fibular retinaculum keeps the tendons next to the lateral aspect of the calcaneus.

The flexor retinaculum, between the medial aspect of the calcaneus and the medial malleolus, sends septa that limit four compartments: (1) Tibialis posterior tendon; (2) flexor digitorum longus tendon; (3) posterior tibial vessels and tibial nerve; and (4) flexor hallucis longus tendon.

ANKLE AND FOOT

The ankle is the junction between the leg and its most distal portion, the foot. The toes are numbered from the hallux (I) to the little toe (V).

The skin of the dorsum of the foot is thin, whereas that of the plant is thick and hairless. Epidermal lines or papillary ridges are an individual characteristic of the sole (footprints for identification).

The fascia of the foot continues that of the leg and, at each side of the foot, continues the plantar aponeurosis. This aponeurosis is divided into a central, medial, and lateral part. The central part is inserted into the tuber calcanei and extends forward into each of the five toes. The medial part covers the abductor hallucis, and the lateral part extends from the tuber calcanei to the tuberosity of metatarsal V and covers the abductor digiti minimi.

A subcutaneous and a subaponeurotic space are found on the dorsum of the foot. The central compartment in the plantar region has four spaces: (1) Inferior (between the plantar aponeurosis and the short flexor digitorum muscle); (2) between the short flexor digitorum muscle and the quadratus plantae muscle; (3) between the quadratus and tarsal bones; and (4) superior (above the adductor hallucis) (Table 2-15).

In the ankle, there are three synovial tendon sheaths: (1) For the tibialis anterior; (2) for the extensor hallucis longus; and (3) for the extensor digitorum longus and fibularis tertius. As the extensor digitorum longus extends into the foot, its tendons have synovial sheaths as does the extensor digitorum brevis. Both fibularis longus and brevis are invested by one synovial sheath. There is a synovial sheath (1) for the tibialis posterior; (2) for the flexor digitorum longus; and (3) for the flexor hallucis longus, posterior to the medial malleolus.

Stroking the sole causes flexion of the toes (i.e., the plantar skin reflex).

Arteries: (1) Medial and (2) lateral plantar artery, and (3) dorsal artery of the foot. The posterior tibial artery splits into medial and lateral plantar arteries. The medial plantar artery gives off cutaneous, muscular, and articular branches. Its superficial branch supplies the medial aspect of the hallux, and its deep branch provides three superficial digital branches, which anastomose with plantar metatarsal arteries I, II, and III. The lateral plantar artery gives off calcaneal, cutaneous, muscular branches and contributes to the formation of the arterial plantar arch. The dorsal artery of the foot continues the anterior tibial and gives off the following branches: (1) Lateral tarsal artery; (2) medial tarsal arteries; (3) arcuate artery, which provides dorsal metatarsal arteries II, III, and IV, each subdivided into two doral digital arteries for adjacent aspects of two toes; perforating branches anastomose the dorsal metatarsal with the plantar arch and plantar metatarsal arteries. Dorsal metatarsal artery I supplies dorsal digital arteries

Table 2-15. Origins, Insertions, and Innervations of the Muscles of the Foot

Muscle	Origin	Insertion	Nerve
Dorsum			
Extensor digitorum brevis	Tarsal sinus	Long extensor tendons of toes I–IV	Deep fibular
Extensor hallucis brevis	Tarsal sinus (medial)	Base of proximal phalanx of toe I	Deep fibular
Plant (Layers I, II, III, IV)			
(I) Abductor hallucis	Tuber calcanei	Medial sesamoid, proximal phalanx of toe I	Medial plantar
(I) Flexor digitorum brevis	Tuber calcanei	Middle phalanges toes II–V	Medial plantar
(I) Abductor digiti minimi	Tuber calcanei	Proximal phalanx, metatarsal V	Lateral plantar
(II) Quadratus plantae	Tuber calcanei	Tendon of flexor digitorum longus	Lateral plantar
(II) Lumbricals	Long flexor tendons	Medial sides of proximal phalanges of toes II–V	Lateral plantar (I), medial plantar (II–IV)
(III) Flexor hallucis brevis	Tendon tibialis posterior	Sesamoids, proximal phalanx toe I	Medial plantar
(III) Adductor hallucis Oblique head	Sheath of fibularis longus	Lateral sesamoid, proximal phalanx toe I	Lateral plantar
Transverse head	Deep transverse metatarsal ligament		
(III) Flexor digiti minimi brevis	Sheath of fibularis longus	Proximal phalanx of toe V, metatarsal V	Lateral plantar
(III) Plantar interossei (3)	Medial side of the metatarsal bases III, IV, V and sheath of fibularis longus	Medial side of proximal phalanx of toes III, IV, V	Lateral plantar
(III) Dorsal interossei (4)	Shafts of all metatarsals	Bases of proximal phalanges of toes II–IV	Lateral plantar

to the medial aspect of the hallux and adjacent aspects of toes I and II. The plantar arterial arch is the continuation of the lateral plantar and gives off four plantar metatarsal arteries, each of which gives off two plantar digital arteries.

Veins: Are superficial and deep. The deep veins include the plantar digital veins, the plantar venous network, four plantar metatarsal veins, the plantar venous arch, and medial and lateral plantar veins.

Nerves: (1) Sural; (2) deep fibular; (3) superficial fibular; (4) medial plantar; and (5) lateral plantar nerves. The medial plantar nerve has the following branches: (a) Muscular (to abductor hallucis and flexor digitorum brevis); (b) cutaneous; and (c) terminal, including four plantar digital nerves to nailbeds, tips of toes, skin of toes I–IV, joints, and muscles (flexor hallucis brevis, lumbrical I). The lateral plantar nerve gives off (a) muscular branches to quadratus plantae and abductor digiti minimi; (b) cutaneous; (c) terminal, in-

cluding superficial and deep branches. The superficial branch (lateral part) supplies the flexor digiti minimi brevis, and has cutaneous and articular branches; its medial part subdivides into plantar digital nerves for the adjacent aspects of toes IV and V and their joints. The deep branch gives articular and muscular branches to interosseous muscles, to lumbricals II, III, and IV, and to the adductor hallucis muscle.

The joint of the ankle is the talocrural, classified as a hinge joint, involving tibia, fibula, and the trochlea of the talus. Its capsule is reinforced by ligaments (medial or deltoid), having an anterior tibiotalar part, a superficial tibionavicular part, a posterior tibiotalar part, and a tibiocalcaneal part; the lateral ligament is divided into anterior talofibular ligament, posterior talofibular ligament, and an intervening calcaneofibular ligament. The joint is supplied by the tibial and deep fibular nerves.

The subtalar is the talocalcaneal joint, classified as an ellipsoidal joint.

The talocalcaneonavicular is part of the transverse tarsal joint, classified as a spheroidal joint. The socket, formed by the calcaneus and navicular, is completed by the plantar calcaneonavicular ligament (spring ligament).

The calceneocuboid is part of the transverse tarsal joint, classified as a saddle joint. Its ligaments are the bifurcate ligament, the long plantar ligament, and the calcaneocuboid ligament.

The cuneocuboid, the intercuneiform, and the cuneonavicular joints are all plane joints.

The tarsal canal is formed by the inferior aspect of the talus and the superior aspect of the calcaneus. Its anterolateral expansion is the tarsal sinus, which contains blood vessels, ligaments (ligament of the tarsal canal and part of the extensor retinaculum), and adipose tissue. The floor of the sinus has the bifurcate ligament, the origin of the extensor digitorum brevis, the cervical ligament (to the neck of the talus). The intertarsal joints are innervated by the deep fibular, the medial plantar, and lateral plantar, sural, and superficial fibular nerves.

The tarsometatarsal are plane joints; the ligaments of their capsules are plantar, dorsal, and interosseous.

The intermetatarsal are plane joints (there is no joint between the bases of metatarsals I and II). The ligaments are plantar, dorsal, and interosseous.

The metatarsophalangeal are ellipsoidal joints and the interphalangeal are hinge joints. Each articular capsule has two collateral ligaments and a plantar ligament. The plantar ligaments of the metatarsophalangeal joints are united by the deep transverse metatarsal ligament.

Metatarsophalangeal I or joint of the hallux includes the joint of the head of metatarsal I with two sesamoids (embedded in the plantar ligament).

The foot has longitudinal and transverse arches. The medial longitudinal arch is made up of the calcaneus, talus, navicular, cuneiforms, and metatarsals I, II, and III; the lateral longitudinal arch is made up of the calcaneus, cuboid, and metatarsals IV and V. The transverse or metatarsal arch is formed by the five metatarsals, navicular, cuneiforms, and cuboid.

REFERENCES

Allen DJ, Motta PM, DiDio LJA: Three Dimensional Microanatomy of Cells and Tissues. Elsevier-North Holland, New York, 1981

Arey LB: Developmental Anatomy. 7th Ed. WB Saunders Co., Philadelphia, 1966

Bacon RL, Niles NR: Medical Histology. Springer Verlag, New York, 1983

Basmajian JV: Grant's Method of Anatomy. 10th Ed. Williams and Wilkins Co., Baltimore, 1980

Bloom W, Fawcett DW: A Textbook of Histology. 10th Ed. WB Saunders Co., Philadelphia, 1975

Carpenter MB, Sutin J: Human Neuroanatomy. 8th Ed. Williams and Wilkins Co., Baltimore, 1983

Clemente CD: Anatomy: A Regional Atlas of the Human Body. 2nd Ed. Urban and Schwartzenberg, Baltimore, 1981

Crafts RC: A Textbook of Human Anatomy. 2nd Ed. John Wiley and Sons, New York, 1979

DiDio LJA: Synopsis of Anatomy. CV Mosby Co., Saint Louis, 1970

DiDio LJA, Anderson MC: The "Sphincters" of the Digestive System. The Williams and Wilkins Co., Baltimore, 1965

DiDio LJA, Stacchini A: Principles of construction of the human body: Form and beauty. Quad Anat Pratica 37:1, 1981

DiFiore MSH, Mancini RE, DeRobertis EDP: New Atlas of Histology. Lea and Febiger, Philadelphia, 1977

Fawcett DW: The Cell. 2nd Ed. WB Saunders Co., Philadelphia, 1981

Gardner E, Gray DJ, O'Rahilly R: Anatomy. 4th Ed. WB Saunders Co., Philadelphia, 1975

Ham AW, Cormack DH: Histology. JB Lippincott Co., Philadelphia, 1979

Hamilton WJ, Simon A, Hamilton SGI: Surface and Radiological Anatomy. 5th Ed. Heffer, Cambridge, 1971

Han SS, Holmstedt JO: Human Microscopic Anatomy. McGraw-Hill Book Co., New York, 1981

Hollinshead WH: Anatomy for Surgeons. 2nd Ed. Hoeber-Harper, New York, 1971

International Anatomical Nomenclature Committee: Nomina Anatomica, Histologica, Embryologica. 5th Ed. The Williams and Wilkins Co., Baltimore, 1983

Joseph J: A Textbook of Regional Anatomy. University Park Press, Baltimore, 1982

Lachman E: Case Studies in Anatomy. 2nd Ed. Oxford University Press, New York, 1971

McMinn RMH, Hutchings RT: Color Atlas of Human Anatomy. Year Book Medical Publisher, Chicago, 1981

Moore KL: The Developing Human. 3rd Ed. WB Saunders Co., Philadelphia, 1982

Motta PM: Anatomia Microscopica. Casa Editr. Vallardi, Milano, 1972

Motta PM, DiDio LJA: Basic and Clinical Hepatology. Martinus Nijhoff Publ. Co., The Hague, 1982

Pansky B, Allen DJ: Review of Neuroscience. Macmillan Publ. Co., New York, 1980

Romanes GJ: Cunningham's Textbook of Anatomy. 11th Ed. Oxford University Press, London, 1972

Skinner HA: The Origin of Medical Terms. 2nd Ed. Williams and Wilkins Co., Baltimore, 1961

Snell RS: Clinical Anatomy for Medical Students. Little, Brown and Co., Boston, 1973

Snell RS: Clinical Embryology for Medical Students. 2nd Ed. Little, Brown and Co., Boston, 1975

Snell RS: Atlas of Clinical Anatomy. Little, Brown and Co., Boston, 1978

Warwick R, William PS: Gray's Anatomy. 35th British Ed. WB Saunders Co., Philadelphia, 1973

Weir J, Abrahams P: An Atlas of Radiological Anatomy. Year Book Medical Publ., Chicago, 1978

Williams PL, Warwick R: Functional Neuroanatomy of Man. WB Saunders Co., Philadelphia, 1975

Woodburne RT: Essentials of Human Anatomy. 5th Ed. Oxford University Press, New York, 1973

Yokochi C: Photographic Anatomy of the Human Body. Igaku Shoin, Ltd., Tokyo, 1969

Zuckerman S: A New System of Anatomy. 2nd Ed. Oxford University Press, Oxford, 1981

MULTIPLE CHOICE QUESTIONS

Circle the correct statement.

1. A. The trachea is aboral to the main bronchi.
   B. The uterine tube is aboral to the uterus.
   C. The jejunum is aboral to the duodenum.
   D. The rectum is distal to the anal canal.

2. A. Preaxial means corresponding to the thumb or hallux.
   B. Fibular is opposite to peroneal.
   C. Plantar and rostral are synonymous.
   D. Distal is the same as oral.

3. A. Variation is a severe deviation from the normal structure.
   B. Anomaly is a congenital variation incompatible with life.
   C. Teratology is the study of acquired diseases.
   D. In medicine, a normal individual or organ is defined as healthy.

4. A. Newborns are miniatures of human adults.
   B. The prominentia laryngea is better seen in females than in males.
   C. Brachitypes frequently have a long hook-shaped stomach.
   D. Members are relatively more developed than the trunk in longitypes.

5. A. Glycocalyx is a cellular coat made up of glycoprotein and polysaccharides.
   B. Nuclear microvilli are commonly seen in renal tubules.
   C. Nexus or gap junction establishes the communication between cytoplasm and nucleus.
   D. Plasmalemma is the nuclear envelope rich in nuclear pores.

6. A. Mesothelium of the myocardium contains medium-sized granules.
   B. The urinary bladder is lined by squamous keratinized epithelium.
   C. The skin presents various types of epithelium, the transitional being the most frequent.
   D. Ciliated and nonciliated pseudostratified epithelium lines respiratory passages.

7. A. Exocrine glands, such as the salivary glands, are ductless.
   B. Endocrine glands have cells that expel their apexes with the secretion.
   C. Apocrine glands expel hormones without structural loss.
   D. Holocrine glands have cells that disintegrate and become part of the secretion.

8. A. Intercellular substance invests basal lamina and subsarcolemmal mitochondria.
   B. Ground substance contains polysaccharides and nonesterified mucopolysaccharides.
   C. Chondroblasts and epiblasts constitute the primordia of the hematoietic tissue.
   D. Collagenous, elastic, reticular, and hyaluronic fibers are elements of neuronic connections.

9. A. The red color of erythrocytes is due to agglutination.
   B. Hemoglobin is a lipoid, mainly carbamino-esterase and minerals.
   C. Leukocytes may have a myeloid, a lymphoid, or a monocytic line of evolution.
   D. Eosinophils decrease in number in cases of allergy and parasitic infestations.

10. A. Motor endings are terminations of afferent or recurrent fibers.
    B. Glyocytes protect and support neurons and connect them with blood vessels.
    C. Myon is a combination of axon and sarcoplasmic reticulum.
    D. Neuron is the functional unit of the neuromusculoskeletal system.

11. A. The amniotic cavity appears between the ectoderm and the cytotrophoblast.
    B. The trophoblast divides into blastomeres, morula, and blastula.
    C. Chorionic villi form the somatopleure and the splanchnopleure.
    D. Syncytiotrophoblast transforms neurulation into gastrulation.

12. A. Ectoderm originates connective tissue and lymphatic vessels.

B. Epidermis and cutaneous glands are derived from mesoderm.

C. Hypophysis and suprarenal medulla are derived from endoderm.

D. The thyroid and parathyroids are included among endodermic structures.

13. A. Diploë is the layer of spongy substance between the layers of compact substance of a cranial flat bone.

B. The galea aponeurotica connects the vertex and the meninges.

C. Interparietal is the portion of the coronal suture posterior to the obeliac area.

D. Leptorrhine comprises the glabella, the asterion, and the nasal septum.

14. A. The sphenoethmoidal recess contains the opening of the nasolacrimal duct.

B. The middle meatus contains the openings of the frontal and maxillary sinuses, and anterior ethmoidal cells.

C. The inferior meatus contains the opening of the lumen nasi.

D. The superior meatus contains the opening of the sphenoidal sinus.

15. A. The inferior orbital fissure transmits the infraorbital nerve and artery and the zygomatic nerve.

B. The superior orbital fissure transmits the cavernous sinus and the recurrent meningeal branch.

C. The oculomotor nerve supplies all muscles of the eyeball except the medial rectus.

D. The ciliary ganglion is medial to the optic nerve and has two roots from the nasociliary nerve and from the external carotid plexus.

16. A. Choroid and cornea form the ocular fibrous tunica.

B. The sclera comprises iris and ciliary body.

C. The inner tunica contains the bulbar fascia (Tenon's capsule), dividing the eyeball into anterior and posterior chambers.

D. The lens is anchored by the suspensory ligament to the ciliary body.

17. A. The tympanic cavity is situated under the jugular fossa and above the middle cranial fossa.

B. The promontory of the middle ear is formed by the cochlea basal turn.

C. The auditory ossicles are articulated at the malleo-stapedial joints.

D. The spiral organ lies on the secondary tympanic membrane at the fenestra vestibuli.

18. A. Subcortical cerebellar nuclei are the molecular, piriform, and granular.

B. The cerebellar cortex has three layers: dentate, globose, and fastigial.

C. Vestibular (flocculonodular lobe) or archeocerebellum is one of the cerebellar functional areas.

D. The dorsal aspect of the mesencephalon has four colliculi and the rootlets of cranial nerve III.

19. A. The lateral sulcus of the brain separates the sphenoidal from the temporal lobes.

B. The central sulcus separates the parietal from the temporal lobes.

C. The precentral gyrus is Brodmann's area 4.

D. The visual cortex is Brodmann's area 41.

20. A. The olfactory, optic, and oculomotor nerves are sensory.

B. The trochlear and the trigeminal nerves are mixed.

C. The facial and the vesticulocochlear nerves are sensory.

D. The hypoglossal and the abducent nerves are motor.

21. A. The major supraclavicular fossa is located in the carotid triangle of the suprahyoid region.

B. The minor supraclavicular fossa is found in the lateral cervical region, next to the subclavius muscle.

C. The cutaneous branches of the cervical plexus are the lesser occipital, the greater auricular, the transverse cervical, and the supraclavicular.

D. The fascia cervicalis is divided into superficial, deep, pre- and retrotracheal, pre- and retrovertebral, and carotid sheaths.

22. A. The subclavian vein runs in front of the scalenus anterior muscle and joins the external jugular to form the brachiocephalic vein.

B. The roof of the pharynx has the tubal tonsil, the pharyngeal bursa, the torus tubarius, and the pharyngeal recess.

C. The posterior cricoarytenoid muscle is the extrinsic sphincter muscle of the rima glottidis.

D. The blood from the esophagus is drained by the thyroid, azygos, and left gastric veins.

23. A. The superior lobe of the right lung comprises the

apicoposterior, the anterior, the superior, and inferior lingular segments.

B. The lateral and medial segments of the left lung split the middle lobe into halves.

C. The pericardial transverse sinus is a canal between the aorta and the pulmonary trunk.

D. The oblique sinus of the pericardium is located between the inferior vena cava and the pulmonary veins.

24. A. The atrioventricular node is divided into anterior, middle, and posterior internodal tracts, bundle, and right and left branches.

B. The cardiac fibrous skeleton comprises the anuli fibrosi, the right and the left trigonus fibrosus, the conus tendon, and the septal pars membranacea.

C. The right pulmonary artery is connected to the aortic arch by the fibrous, obliterated remains of the ductus arteriosus, the ligamentum arteriosum.

D. The root of the aorta has five sinuses, ordinarily three orifices, and appears in radiograms as the aortic knuckle.

25. A. The inguinal ligament is the inferior margin of the internal oblique muscle, extending from the anterior iliac spine to the iliac crest.

B. The lumbar triangle is limited by the external oblique muscle, the internal oblique muscle, and the latissimus dorsi.

C. The linea semilunaris is the line along which the aponeuroses of the internal and external oblique muscles meet at the lateral margin of the rectus abdominis muscle.

D. The posterior abdominal is made up of serratus posterior superior, rhomboids, and inferior intercostal muscles.

26. A. The lesser omentum originates from the dorsal mesogastrium.

B. The coronary ligament derives from the dorsal common mesentery.

C. The mesoappendix originates from the ventral mesentery.

D. The medial umbilical ligament corresponds to the obliterated umbilical artery.

27. A. The vertex of the intersigmoid recess is related posteriorly to the right ureter.

B. The broad ligament includes the mesovarium, the mesometrium, and the myometrium.

C. The stomach is supplied by the right, left, poste-

rior, right gastroepiploic, left gastroepiploic, and short gastric arteries.

D. The duodenal lymph is drained by collecting vessels into inferior mesenteric, internal iliac, and common iliac nodes.

28. A. The hepatopancreatic ampulla comprises the common hepatic duct and the main pancreatic duct.

B. The mesentericoaortic forceps contains the left renal vein, the duodenum, and the tip of the uncinate process.

C. The pancreas is supplied by the anterior pancreatic and the short gastrosplenic arteries.

D. The lymph of the spleen is drained into gastric, mesenteric, hepatic, and celiac nodes.

29. A. The gonadal and suprarenal arteries are unpaired, whereas the renal arteries are paired.

B. All parietal arteries of the abdomen are bilateral except the median sacral artery.

C. The testicular artery reaches the superficial inguinal canal and supplies the scrotum.

D. The ovarian artery runs in the perimetrion, anastomoses with the middle rectal artery and the inferior vesicular artery, and supplies the ovaries.

30. The triangle of auscultation is limited by the:
A. Sternocleidomastoid, sternal, and subclavian muscles.

B. Sternal muscle, lateral margin of clavicle, and subclavius muscle.

C. Major and minor rhomboid and serratus posterior muscles.

D. Trapezius muscle, latissimus dorsi muscle, and medial margin of scapula.

31. A. The axillary artery becomes the brachial artery at the level of the inferior margin of the pectoralis major muscle.

B. The axillary vein receives the thoracoepigastric veins, a source of collateral circulation when there is obstruction of the inferior vena cava.

C. The branches of the posterior cord of the brachial plexus are the lateral and the medial pectoral nerves.

D. The m. pronator teres and the flexor ulnar muscle are supplied by the radial nerve.

32. A. The femoral triangle contains the adductor canal, vessels, and nerves.

B. The popliteus muscle and the tibial posterior

muscle are supplied by the superficial branch of the fibular nerve.

C. The metatarsophalangeal are plane joints connected by the transverse and longitudinal arches.

D. The ileopectineal septum separates a medial vascular and a lateral muscular compartment in the thigh.

Answers to Multiple Choice Questions

1 C	2 A	3 D	4 D	5 A
6 D	7 D	8 B	9 C	10 B
11 A	12 D	13 A	14 B	15 A
16 D	17 B	18 C	19 C	20 D
21 C	22 D	23 D	24 B	25 C
26 D	27 C	28 B	29 B	30 D
31 B	32 D			

3

Behavioral Sciences

Evan G. Pattishall, jr.

The medical behavioral sciences are an integration of a number of social sciences and biological sciences concerned with the study of human behavior. These include the disciplines of psychology, sociology, anthropology, biology, behavioral genetics, neuroscience, psychophysiology, psychopharmocology, neurochemistry, economics, political science, and psycho-neuroendocrinology. Thus, the medical behavioral sciences represent a true integration of the major sciences and disciplines as they relate to, influence, and are influenced by human behavior.

A number of clinical studies have estimated that at least 50 to 60 percent of all visits to physicians are behaviorally related and that to ignore the biopsychosocial components of any illness seriously handicaps both the physician and the patient. One must also understand that the study of human behavior has now achieved the prominance of a basic medical science in its own right, along with anatomy, biochemistry, microbiology, pathology, pharmacology, and physiology. While the behavioral sciences are basic to psychiatry, just as anatomy is basic to surgery, or physiology to internal medicine, the behavioral sciences are basic in their own right to all clinical specialties of medicine.

The various components of the medical behavioral sciences are summarized here beginning with the more biologically related correlates of behavior, progressing to development and behavior as expressed by the individual, then as the individual interacts with others, singularly and in various groups, followed by the impact of cultural and societal factors, on the individual and the specific applications to behavioral medicine.

An important dimension that should be kept in mind at all times is the interaction and impact of each of these behavioral factors on the health and disease of individual patients. Every fact, concept, and relationship should be examined and applied to current medical diseases and problems in terms of how this behavioral factor would influence the etiology of a specific disease; how it might be used as a diagnostic aid; how it would influence or be influenced by the treatment regimen; how it would impact attempts at rehabilitation; and how these biobehavioral factors might be applied to prevent a specific disease or help to maintain or improve health.

The behavioral sciences cover such an extensive number of disciplines that there is no possibility that one can summarize all of the relevant principles and applications. Thus, the following represents a sample and summary of some of the more important principles, facts, and applications which should help guide one's learning of the medical behavioral sciences and stimulate one's investigation of other relevant behavioral actions and interactions.

BIOLOGICAL BASES OF BEHAVIOR

Genetic Determinants of Behavior

In order to understand human behavior it is important to begin with a better understanding of the crucial role played by genetics. While most social scientists have been concerned with the influence of environmental factors on human behavior, behavior geneticists have been rapidly accumulating evidence to demonstrate the crucial role of genetic factors, especially in such areas as intelligence, mental retardation, schizophrenia, behavioral development, traits, aging, alcoholism, biological defects, and affective diseases such as manic depressive psychosis. This in no way discounts the role of the environment, but does mandate the need to account for both genetic and environmental factors as individual and interactive determinants of behavior. Determining whether a genetic factor is expressed, the time it is expressed, and the conditions under which it is expressed most often involve interactions between environmental and biological factors.

Family studies, twin studies, and adopted child studies are common methods in the study of behavioral genetics, but selective breeding using animal models has also produced significant behavioral differences in such areas as alcohol preference or avoidance, susceptibility to convulsions, and certain parenting behaviors as well as certain aggressive behaviors.

Medical and behavioral disorders caused by genetic aberrations or influences

DOWN'S SYNDROME ("MONGOLISM")

Down's syndrome occurs in about 1 per 700 live births. At an early childbearing age the risk is about 1 per 2,000 live births, increasing dramatically with maternal age, at the age of 35 the risk is 1 per 400, and at the age 40 the risk is about 1 per 100. Down's syndrome is most often due to trisomy 21, but can also be due to translocation of chromosomes 21 and 15. It can be detected through amniocentesis. It is estimated that about 30 percent of all retarded children are victims of Down's syndrome. IQ can be relatively normal in some individuals with Down's syndrome, but most IQ's are between 40 and 60. While individuals with Down's syndrome previously died at a relatively early age, many of the advances in medical science have now extended the average life expectancy to age 40.

PHENYLKETONURIA (PKU)

Phenylketonuria, a genetic disorder from a single gene defect, results from the inheritance of a double recessive gene (autosomal recessive transmission). Serious mental deficiency can result from the inability to metabolize phenylalanine, due to the absence or insufficient amount of the enzyme phenylalanine hydroxylase. If the condition is undetected in time for treatment, there is a build-up of unmetabolized phenylalanine or other alternate pathway metabolites, which alter brain metabolism, producing mental retardation after about 6 months. The incidence is about 1 per 16,000 births, but

it is estimated that about 1 percent of institutionalized retarded persons are retarded because of their inheritance of PKU. Just as genes affect phenotypes, the gene disorder in PKU affects behavior. This is also a good example of how a genetic problem can be bypassed, and retardation prevented through an environmental (behavioral) intervention i.e., dietary control, providing the infant with food of low phenylalanine).

TAY-SACHS DISEASE

Tay-Sachs disease is also an autosomal recessive transmission disorder involving a specific enzymatic deficiency and resulting in progressive mental and physical deterioration. Symptoms occur at about 4 to 8 months of age and affected individuals usually live only 3 to 5 years. It is very rare in the general population, but more prevalent in Jewish groups from eastern Europe. Infants with Tay-Sachs disease have slow development, are hypotonic, and appear weak and apathetic.

TURNER'S SYNDROME

Turner's syndrome is a genetic disorder of women with 45 chromosomes, but with a sex chromosome configuration of XO. It occurs in about 1 per 4,000 female births, and often results in some intellectual impairment, but usually not severe. The women generally have underdeveloped female genitalia and ovaries, a short stature, and webbed neck.

KLINEFELTER'S SYNDROME (XXY)

Klinefelter's syndrome is a genetic disorder of men and is attributed to an extra X chromosome in a person's genotype (XXY). These men exhibit a variety of male morphologic and behavioral characteristics, in that they generally have small testes, low levels of the male hormone (testosterone), are generally sterile, and about 25 percent have varying degrees of mental retardation. About 1 percent of males who are institutionalized for retardation, mental illness, or epilepsy, have Klinefelter's syndrome. XXY genotype is mentioned here for completeness. The so-called supermale is controversial and is alleged to be predisposed to overaggressiveness and violent behavior, but research results are inconclusive at present. The genotype was first noticed among very tall males who had been institutionalized for violent criminal behavior. The incidence is about 1 in 1,000 births.

SICKLE CELL ANEMIA

Sickle cell anemia is the result of homozygous abnormal hemoglobin (SS) in which the red blood cells have a sickle shape that promotes "clumping" and results in a lifetime of recurrent crises, pain, and fever. It is an autosomal recessive disorder and is present in about 0.2 percent of blacks in the U.S. with about 8 percent of blacks being carriers with only one abnormal hemoglobin gene (AS). Carriers are often susceptible to hypoxia in high altitudes. Sickle cell anemia can also occur in persons of mediterranean ancestry. The psychosocial concomitants of the disease are sometimes multiple and severe.

HEMOPHILIA

A recessive sex-linked genetic disorder transmitted by the female (recessive gene on the X chromosome) to the male, hemophilia is characterized by a tendency to bleed or hemorrhage, generally after bruises, tooth extractions, or scratches. It represents a chronic disorder that afflicts much stress on the victim and most family members, with very little normal family activity, requires frequent visits to the doctor or hospital, and often leads to the expression of behavioral factors, such as anxiety, guilt, rejection, alienation, resentment, self-blame, and bitterness.

INTELLIGENCE

Although intelligence is affected by the interaction of hereditary and environmental factors, indeed, heredity accounts for approximately 50 percent of the individual differences found in IQ scores within families. Thus, a major part of the development of individual differences in IQ is due to inheritance. The IQ scores of monozygotic (identical) twins show the highest correlation, compared with the IQs of dizygotic (fraternal) twins which have similar but not identical genes. When identical twins are reared together, their IQs have a correlation coefficient of 0.92, but reared apart, have a correlation coefficient of 0.86. These high correlations may be assumed to be a result of hereditary and environmental factors. Since even monozygotic twins reared together do not have completely identical experiences, one would not expect a perfect positive correlation.

Comparing the correlation between IQs of siblings reared together (0.50) to IQs of siblings reared apart (0.42) suggests that environmental factors affect IQ scores considerably. It also demonstrates a contribution of hereditary factors to intelligence. When siblings are reared apart, the correlation between IQs is lower, however, it is significantly higher than for unrelated persons reared together, who have a correlation factor of 0.25. Thus, hereditary factors are considered to be more potent determinants of IQ than either environmental or experiential factors.

SCHIZOPHRENIA

A complex behavioral and genetic disorder, schizophrenia is considered to be related to more than one gene locus. It exists in about 1 percent of the general population, and the risk for relatives of schizophrenics is considerably higher. Siblings of schizophrenics have about eight times the risk of developing schizophrenia than persons chosen randomly from the general population. If those siblings have an affected parent as well as an affected sibling, that rate is doubled, and if both parents are schizophrenic, the risk is quadrupled again. Such studies have established the importance of behavioral genetic and family history influences. Grandchildren of schizophrenics have about twice the risk as the general population.

MANIC-DEPRESSIVE ILLNESS

Manic-depressive illness also appears to have a major genetic component. An overall heterogenity in the heredity of manic depression seems to be the predominant conclusion. A 100 percent concordance rate in monozygotic twins has been suggested by some investigators who also find evidence for an X-linked dominant transmission.

As more diseases and developmental elements are linked to genetic factors, the interaction and interrelatedness between heredity and environment becomes more evident.

Ethology

Ethology is an outgrowth of biology and psychology, involving comparative studies of animal behavior in relation to natural habitat. While human behavior may be more related to a form of predisposition to learn and respond in a certain way, lower animals are found to display fixed sequences of motor activity which is genetically established and triggered by a sign-stimulus that releases the fixed action pattern of behavior. Sign-stimulus and fixed action patterns appear to exist in humans but are weaker and are more variable because human learning, experience, and cognition are able to override the sign-stimulus and fixed action patterns. *Imprinting* is the phenomenon of a very young animal becoming "fixed" on a member of their own species during an early period of development, usually the result of following their mother, but often another object or another animal may be substituted. The period of maximum receptivity to these critical cues or sign-stimuli is known as the *critical period*. Imprinting is thought to relate to the bond formation between infants and adults in both lower animals and humans.

BRAIN BEHAVIOR

The brain has a direct or indirect neural control of hormone glands and secretion via the hypothalamus. Examples are the thyroid secretion, the pituitary gland, the adrenal glands, and even insulin secretion subject to adrenergic influence from the autonomic nervous system, whereas the parathyroid gland which regulates calcium metabolism is controlled by blood levels of calcium.

It is important to recognize that sexual behavior is influenced by certain hormones. Examples of these are testosterone, estradiol, androsterone, and luteinizing hormone releasing factor. The gonadal steroids and hormones are important for the stimulation and control of appropriate reproductive, parental, and agnostic behavior patterns in many mammals. Testosterone is also the hormone best known for its role in aggression.

The association cortex is the part of the brain that is neither sensory nor motor in function. It mediates a number of higher cognitive functions associated with intelligence. The size and weight of mammal and human brains is not a predictor of intelligence, nor is the ratio of brain to body weight. The relative size of the association cortex is the best morphologic predictor of intelligence differences between species.

In humans, the left hemisphere of the brain generally appears to be particularly involved in language acquisition and mathematical reasoning. Appreciation of music and art, and spatioperceptual abilities are related to the right hemisphere.

The "gate control" theory of pain reception states that the impulse from the primary afferent neurons which carry pain information to the spinal cord is blocked in the substantia gelatinosa by depolarizing impulses from the brain. This is believed to be the mechanism whereby cognitive and emotional factors are able to influence the perceived intensity of pain.

Psychogenic or psychosomatic illnesses are real medical disorders and often involve discomfort and real somatic pain. There are a number of explanations and mechanisms that have been documented such as that the presence of sufficient psychological conflict will cause an organ or body system to become dysfunctional, especially if the organ or body system is predisposed to dysfunction; conditioning or learning processes assume that the physical symptom or dysfunction produces a reinforcement by reducing conflict; and a psychoanalytic view speculates that the physical symptom symbolizes the psychic conflict. While this symbolization has not been able to be verified scientifically, it has provided a number of conceptual ideas that have led to other discoveries.

Sleep

The most recent classification divides sleep into two distinct states of sleep based on their respective EEG activity patterns; D-sleep (desynchronized EEG pattern sleep) and S-sleep (synchronized EEG pattern sleep). D-sleep and S-sleep alternate with each other during the complete sleep session. D-sleep is also known as REM sleep (rapid eye movement sleep and dreaming sleep) and S-sleep as NREM sleep (nonrapid eye movement sleep, also orthodox sleep and quiet sleep). D and REM sleep are used interchangeably, as are S and NREM sleep.

S-sleep (NREM sleep) is divided into stages 1, 2, 3, and 4. Stage 1 is the lightest stage of sleep and stage 4 is the deepest stage of sleep. It is during the deepest stage 3 or stage 4 that enuresis, somnambulism, nightmares, or night-terrors are more apt to occur. D-sleep (REM sleep) is a light sleep but is qualitatively different from S-sleep, and is a time during which vivid dreaming occurs. S-sleep (NREM sleep) typically lasts from 60 to 100 minutes and is followed by 20 to 40 minutes of D-sleep (REM sleep); the cycle is continued throughout the night. About 80 percent of adults' sleep time is spent in NREM sleep and about 20 percent in REM sleep, with REM sleep increasing during the second half of the night and NREM sleep decreasing. In contrast an infant spends about 50 percent of sleep time in REM sleep.

REM sleep was originally termed "paradoxical sleep" because it was a pattern characteristic of the alert waking state even though the muscles were even more relaxed and immobile than during NREM sleep, combined with a relatively high arousal threshold.

Dream deprivation does not appear to produce any major decrement in psychological functions, but it does appear to produce retardation of memory formation, especially impairing the recall of emotionally toned words. Dream sleep appears to assist in the integration of emotional material with memories of other experiences. A deficiency of dream sleep appears to produce a rebound phenomenon of increased dreaming during subsequent uninterrupted sleep.

BIOCHEMICAL CORRELATES

Acetylcholine can be considered to be the ultimate mediator of all behavior since it is the transmitter agent at neuromuscular junctions. Muscular contractions are the substrate of all behavior patterns.

It is thought that the brains of schizophrenic persons may be deficient in dopamine β hydroxylase (an enzyme that catalyzes the conversion of dopamine to norepinephrine which are both capable of functioning as neurotransmitters) as they appear to have either an accumulation of dopamine or a lack of norepinephrine.

The presence of 6-hydroxydopamine in the brain is also implicated in schizophrenia, since 6-hydroxydopamine destroys noradrenergic terminals. A genetic metabolic error could produce a high cerebral concentration of 6-hydroxydopamine.

While more chemicals are expected to be found, acetylocholine, norepinephrine, dopamine, serotonin, epinephrine, and γ-aminobutyric acid are most involved as neurotransmitters in the nervous system.

Barbiturates are sedative hypnotics. In moderate doses, they act as central nervous system depressants, while in higher doses they act as anesthetics. Barbiturates are addicting and are among the most widely abused drugs in our culture. Their effects are potentiated by alcohol, and the difference between a minimum effective dose and a lethal dose is very small.

Cocaine was discovered as a local anesthetic in 1864. It produces reversible nerve block at the site of application, but it is now most frequently used for its central nervous system stimulation characteristics. It is an increasingly popular "street drug," but is regarded as addictive and potentially dangerous.

Amphetamines increase the activity of the biogenic amine norepinephrine by inhibiting monoamine oxidase. They are sometimes used for appetite control. Amphetamines indirectly achieve elevation of norepinephrine levels and are a major drug of abuse.

Meprobamate is a mild tranquilizer, relieves routine tension and free-floating anxiety, and produces a pleasant, drowsy state without marked sedative effects. It is a commonly administered psychotherapeutic agent.

Endorphins are naturally occurring morphinelike peptides. Techniques for pain relief which are thought to operate through the release of endorphins include acupuncture, hypnosis, transcutaneous electrical stimulation, and placebo.

A number of factors interact to control or influence food intake. They are the arteriovenous differences in blood glucose levels which reflect central utilization of glucose, the amount of fat deposited in the body, and the amino acid content of the blood. The absolute level of blood glucose does not appear to be a major factor.

Immune System

Injury to the immune system can be the direct pathologic consequence of an increase in stress-induced plasma cortisone. The neuroendocrine pathways involving the cerebral cortex, the hypothalamus, the pituitary, and the adrenal cortex are the mechanisms whereby psychosocial stress can produce increased levels of adrenal corticoids, which affect the immune system, resulting in increased vulnerability. This is considered to be a possible mechanism for the subsequent action of latent oncogenic viruses or newly mutated cancer cells, which would ordinarily be attacked by the immunologic surveillance and defense mechanisms. It is also known that lymphocytes and lymphatic tissues such as the thymus, nodes, and spleen, are destroyed or weakened by an increase of glucocorticoids in the blood levels over an extended period of time. It has been suggested that such mechanisms can enhance certain pathologic processes, including the development of cancer.

LEARNING

Even though there are different conceptualizations about all of the variables that are actually involved in learning, there is general agreement about the empirical components of learning. Building on a definition offered by Kimble (1961), we can say that learning is a relatively permanent change in behavior potentiality which occurs as a result of reinforced practice, excluding changes due to maturation, fatigue, and/or injury to the nervous system. Learning is relatively permanent because it tends to remain as a new part of the person's behavioral repertoire (even when one thinks it has been forgot, it can be relearned more easily); a change because the behavioral repertoire is altered; behavior potentiality referring to the learning-performance distinction (we observe performance changes and infer that learning has occurred); the result of reinforced practice (not just practice) because the reinforcement (reward) itself becomes a stimulus that makes the reoccurrance of a behavior more probable (a major contribution of B. F. Skinner was to demonstrate that a reinforcing stimulus is a stimulus that increases the probability of a behavior); and the exclusion of maturation, fatigue, and/or injury to the nervous system because changes in behavior can occur as a result of maturation, fatigue, or injury that do not necessarily involve learning. The types of learning are classical, operant conditioning, and observational learning.

Classical Conditioning

In classical conditioning, a reinforcing stimulus elicits a response. This is the classical conditioning known as Pavlovian conditioning, in which meat, an unconditioned stimulus (US) produces salivation, an unconditioned response (UR), meat with bell, a conditioned stimulus (CS) producing salivation (UR), followed by bell alone, a stimulus substitution producing salivation (UR). This is the result of stimulus generalization. A more clinical example would be a cancer patient coming to the clinic for chemotherapy, an US which usually makes him nauseated, an UCR. After one or more associations (pairing) of the anticipated nausea with the clinic, the patient becomes nauseous upon entering the clinic, even before the chemotherapy, an US begins. Entering the clinic becomes the CS and elicits the original UR of nausea. Thus, a previously neutral stimulus (clinic) precedes a US (chemotherapy), and after repeated pairings of the CS and US, the (clinic) elicits the UR (nausea).

Another example might be the experiencing of fright and a pounding heart upon seeing or hearing a stimulus or stimuli previously associated with a frightening experience. Fear of a white coated individual in a hospital may represent another example of classical conditioning.

Classical conditioning is associated with the sympathetic and parasympathetic nervous systems of the autonomic nervous system. While the autonomic nervous system has been regarded historically as independent and not under cognitive control, more recent evidence points to much more connection, interaction, and control by the cortex and CNS than previously realized.

Operant Conditioning

Operant conditioning (also referred to as instrumental conditioning) is the production of a given response by reinforcing that response with an appropriate reward (reinforcer). This principle which was formulated by Edward Thorndike and B. F. Skinner has been one of the major scientific and philosophic advances.

A positive reinforcer increases the probability that the preceding response will occur again and the probability is decreased when the reward (positive reinforcer) is taken away. A negative reinforcer (usually some form of punishment) lowers the probability of the preceding response reoccurring, and when the negative reinforcer is removed, the preceding behavior will tend to reoccur.

There are also two types of reinforcers; primary reinforcers which meet a primary need of the person (e.g., food, water, love, etc.) and secondary reinforcers that are learned (e.g., money, promotion, praise, smile, etc.).

As a general principle, the events that follow a particular stimulus or behavior, control or determine future behavior. Thus, a class of behavior that is controlled by stimulus consequences is known as operant behavior. This significant relationship between behavior and the consequences is the basis for the therapeutic strategies involved in behavior modification. When behavior occurs that is close to or approximates the ideal or desired complex behavior, reinforcing those approximations is called *shaping*. Thus, only those behaviors are reinforced which more closely approximate the desired behavior (successive approximations) until the desired behavior is learned and can be predicted and produced. It is a fundamental educational tool whether teaching physical skills, polite behavior, and even problem solving.

In addition to the positive and negative dimensions of reinforcement, the following patterns or schedules of reinforcement influence the probability of the reoccurrence of the behavior.

Continuous: Reinforcement occurs every time the behavior occurs. New learning will occur most efficiently if rewarded each time. The response reinforcement ratio can then be stretched gradually over time.

Intermittent: Behavior is maintained and more resistant to extinction than with continuous reinforcement. The response-reinforcement varies along two dimensions (fixed or variable), and whether it is controlled by time or the number of responses.

Fixed interval: Schedules reinforce the correct response after a fixed time period has elapsed. Usually the individual learns to wait until just before the time for reinforcement, then produce a burst of behavior until reinforcement, and then the output will fall off again. Cramming for an exam is an example. This schedule produces the fewest responses per unit of time.

Fixed ratio: Reinforcement occurs after a fixed number of responses. It is the piece-work method, where reward occurs only after a certain amount of production (e.g., being reimbursed two dollars for each exam graded). This schedule improves production over the fixed interval schedule.

Variable interval: Reinforcement for response after an unpredictable (variable) time period; better response rate than fixed interval schedule; the surprise visit or pop quiz or irregular bonuses are examples.

Variable ratio: The number of responses needed to gain reinforcement is varied; produces highest and most consistent response rate; gambling with a slot machine is an example, in that a person keeps trying, hoping that the next ratio will be smaller; responses are resistant to extinction; negative behavior, such as whining or throwing tantrums, is reinforced by this schedule since an occasional victory encourages continuing the behavior. This is also the basis of superstitious behavior when, for example, a reinforcement may occur in association with a good luck charm, so that the charm is credited with having averted some danger or unpleasant event.

In general, learning is acquired more easily and retention is greater if it occurs over a series of distributed practice periods rather than the same amount of learning time combined into a mass practice period.

In instrumental conditioning, reinforcement occurs only if the individual responds with the desired behavior. Thus, learning or behavior change occurs through the reinforcement. In one sense, the learner can control the desired response, and hence the occurrence of the reinforcement. Since operant conditioning affects the activity of the autonomic nervous system, the principle of biofeedback was a natural outgrowth and has many applications to modern medicine. If one is attempting to modify a bodily function such as heart rate, hypertension, skin temperature, etc., the technology of *biofeedback* is very appropriate. The process involves providing the person with feedback of physiologic information on the bodily function one is attempting to modify. For example, if one is attempting to lower heart rate, one's heart rate is visible (feedback to the person) on a graph or dial, and the person generates positive reinforcement for themselves (success) each time the heart rate graph or dial turns downward. Biofeedback has also been successfully applied to tension and migraine headaches, hypertension, and peripheral circulatory disorders. Much optimism has been developed by the early work of Neil Miller and his colleagues working with biofeedback.

Observational Learning

Observational learning is a type of learning that does not fall clearly into either a classical conditioning or an operant conditioning process. It is also frequently referred to as *social learning.*

This type of learning is accomplished through the exposure to the behaviors of others, whether in-person or symbolically in television, movies, literature, or the press. In effect, the observer (learner) attempts to produce behaviors by imitating someone who becomes a model. Observational learning is also labeled *imitative learning.* Albert Bandura is probably the most currently identified individual in explorations of observational learning or social learning theory.

Most skills, whether learning to catch a football, sew on a button, bake a pie, or change a spark plug are learned through observation, demonstration, or reading instructions, and are followed by periods of practice, observing a model, practice, observing a model, practice, etc. The learner can observe the model then practice, attempting to observe and analyze his or her own performance, or the model can interact with the learner as a teacher with demonstrations and analyses of performance. Observational learning also operates in nonmotor behaviors, such as values and attitudes, which are often learned by imitating someone else. Nonverbal behavior can also be acquired through the process of observational learning.

Three important factors that have been found to affect imitative performance are the following:

1. Vicarious reinforcement of the observer in terms of perceived consequences to the model of the behavior being observed. If a person sees another person rewarded for a particular behavior, the observing person may attempt to produce the same behavior, perhaps to get the same reward or come to the conclusion that it must be acceptable behavior and therefore worth imitating.
2. Another determinant is the expected and actual consequences to the observer of the first imitative performance, such as expecting a reward, praise, or just being able to hit the ball.
3. It is important that the characteristics of the model be salient to the observer, thus, the imitation will be greater if the model is seen by the observer as having desirable attributes such as power or prestige or "good looking," and if the model is similar to the observer in some important way. Observational learning or socialization is thus facilitated when there is identification with the model by the observer.

As can be seen by the factors that affect imitative performance, cognitive processes play a major role in observational learning. Observational or social learning in infancy and childhood must be considered within the context of the significant developmental changes in cognition which occur throughout infancy and childhood. It is also important to recognize that the process of observational and social learning is very active in terms of the influence of media on various antisocial or undesirable behaviors of children (e.g., aggression, violence, sexuality, etc.) observed on television and movies. Observational or social learning is also actively involved in peer and adult influence in substance abuse. Therefore, the major question is not whether, but how and how much these activities influence children's and adolescent's behavior.

Even though observational and social learning does not appear to rely primarily on reinforcement, it is important to recognize that primary and secondary reinforcement can play an important role in all learning, whether cognitive social learning, operant conditioning, or classical conditioning. If some form of primary or secondary reinforcement does not occur, the newly acquired behavior will tend to extinguish.

Modeling, direct reinforcement, denying the rewards that maintain a particular attitude, and desensitization to establish neutral or positive responses are all based on social learning principles.

Spontaneous recovery, which exists in all three types of learning, was first described by Pavlov. It represents the return of an original response that had been extinguished or forgotten. Most extinguishing occurs due to the lack of reinforcement. In many instances, spontaneous recovery can occur following a single reinforcement which reestablishes the original response, generally, at full strength. If a response is not reinforced for a long enough period of time, it will presumably become extinct.

Overlearning helps stabilize and prolong a learned response. It usually involves continuing practice beyond the point of achieving the optimal criterion for performance. The overlearning increases the time period over which the behavior or skill will be retained without reinforcement. In general, learned responses must be continuously rehearsed or practiced if they are going to be retained.

The phenomenon of proactive interference occurs when older or earlier learned material begins to interfere with the retention of more recently learned material. Retroactive interference occurs when subsequent learning begins to interfere with the retention of earlier learned material or skills.

MARRIAGE AND FAMILY

Even though the American family has lost some of its previous functions, such as educating offspring and providing recreational activity, there are two major functions that are still active and valid; these are socialization of offspring and stabilization of adult personalities. Studies show a powerful socialization influence of parents during a child's early years, even though schools and other agencies have assumed a part of this task. Stabilization of adult personalities is still the major function of the American family and is accomplished when men and women are able to adjust themselves to roles of parental responsibility and sharing of nurture and security. There is no other place in our society where this function can be as powerfully performed.

Marital Status

In comparing marital status with health status, it has been found that married persons have a significant longer life expectancy; married men have a less higher admission rate to state and county psychiatric hospitals than separated or divorced men. Divorced white males have death rates for heart disease and lung cancer twice that of married white males; widowed women have a higher admission rate to state and county psychiatric hospitals than separated or divorced women or never married women; and widowed women have a lower admission rate to state and county psychiatric hospitals than widowed men.

Married persons also have less chronic illness, especially mental illness than formerly married persons, and make fewer visits for health care services. Children raised in single parent families have more illnesses and make more visits to health care services.

Persons tend to marry individuals who are similar to themselves rather than different from themselves, especially with regard to the social characteristics of age, nationality, race, family background, education, intelligence, previous marital status, and religion. Despite the tendency to homogamy, many marriages among persons of dissimilar social backgrounds are quite successful. The most important factors appear to be each individual's personal qualities and total adjustment, even though elements of similarity or difference are important.

Marital adjustment and stability is positively related to the higher the educational level of the married couple. The higher the social class of the couple, the older the couple when they marry, and the more similar the levels of intelligence of the couple, the high the rate of marital adjustment and stability. Divorce is twice as likely to occur if the woman marries in her teens and the man marries under the age of 22. The possibility of higher financial resources may positively affect the persons with upper class backgrounds having better adjusted marriages. Higher educational level is also associated with a later age at marriage and a higher income. If the educational level of the woman is higher than the man, the marital stability appears to be less. One of the major dangers of significant differences in intelligence is that the partners often grow apart with little intellectual stimulation and exchange of ideas.

The birth order of partners in marriage seems to bear some relationship to marital success. The findings are that high marital success is associated with the male being first born and the female being later-born; next, later-born male and first-born female; and middle-born male or female and in any birth order. The birth order of partners with moderate or medium marital success is most often associated with the only child (male or female), and with the first born. The lowest marital success is associated with the first-born male and first-born female; youngest male and youngest female; only male child and only female child.

These findings are not to oversimplify the more important requirements of adjustment to adulthood and marriage, but do serve to illustrate that even children from the same family have different personal and social learning experiences, are treated differently, and have certain behavior patterns reinforced differently, all of which when combined with other factors help to develop independence, leadership, dependence, and other interpersonal skills.

Studies of marital satisfaction find that marital satisfaction is highest during the first few childless years of marriage. It then declines during the rearing of children, during which marital satisfaction reaches a low point. Marital satisfaction slowly recovers to its original level after all children have left home. The lowest satisfaction with family life appears to take place when the children are in adolescence. Satisfaction with spouse companionship appears to be the highest during the first few years of marriage, and then declines rapidly and appears to remain at a relatively low level of satisfaction for the duration of the marriage.

While the current divorce rate is 5 times that for 1910 and double the rate for 1966, it is important to recognize that most people marry and remain married. Sixty-three percent of first marriage partners remain together and 41 percent of second marriages remain intact.

It is also significant that the percentage of individuals who do not marry has shown little variation in this century. For example, in 1910 10.3 per 1,000 population did not marry; 10.4 in 1953; 10.4 in 1968; and 9.9 in 1976.

Family

Absence of the father from the home in situations of separation, desertion, divorce, or death have been demonstrated to show a more detrimental influence on a child's personality in early development than after 5 years of age; absence due to death is not as detrimental for male children as absence due to divorce, separation, or desertion. The earlier the absence of the father, the more the mothers are apt to display overprotection toward their female children; when the father is absent due to divorce, adolescent girls are more active and aggressive in seeking the attention of men; in absence of the father due to death, adolescent girls engage in more active avoidance of male peers and prefer other girls as companions. The absence of the father due to death

seems to provide more interference with overall adjustment for females; absence of fathers due either to divorce or death results in girls expressing more insecurity about their ability to relate to males; absent fathers produces a tendency for conflict and uncertainty as to appropriate masculine orientations, sometimes leading to overcompensation (i.e., "super macho" role), or a more feminine orientation.

Cohabitation (an unmarried male and an unmarried female living together) has become more frequently practiced in recent years. The most common reason given for cohabitation is as a temporary matter of convenience or choice without the commitment to marriage. Trial marriage is the second most frequent reason given to test compatibility or await more favorable circumstances for marriage. The third most frequent reason for cohabitation is as a permanent alternative to marriage. Cohabitation most frequently involves persons in their late teens or 20s, but an increasing number of persons in their 30s, 40s, and 50s are cohabitating, particularly after divorce or separation.

Fertility and attitudes toward child bearing appear to change significantly over a period of time. In 1960, about 1 percent of all couples stated that they did not expect to have children, compared with 1.3 percent in 1967 and 4 percent in 1973. Also, in 1968 41 percent of the public stated that the ideal number of children would be 4 or more, but by 1974, only 19 percent stated the ideal to be 4 or more children. Women, because the mother role is more basic to their sense of self, seem to be more seriously affected personally about fertility problems and not having children than men. Historically, it was generally assumed that the women were at "fault" in infertility, however, more recent studies have indicated that about $\frac{1}{3}$ to $\frac{1}{2}$ of infertility is due to sterility or other problems of the man. Fertility rate is also related to age. Women have the highest potential fertility from age 18 to age 25, followed by a gradual decline until age 35 and a sharper decline to age 49. Fertility also declines in the male, but not as rapidly.

Employment

From 1900 to 1978 the percentage of adult women (age 20 to 64) who were employed rose from 20 to 58 percent. During the same time period, the percentage of married women who were employed rose from 5.5 percent to 48 percent. Black women are more likely to be employed outside of the home than white women, regardless of the educational levels. Despite the increase in the proportion of women in professional graduate schools and in other dimensions of the work force, the vocational role orientations of females and males remain more traditional than one would expect. This is changing, however, as the proportion of women increases in the work force.

Working mothers appear to have a positive effect on the career orientation and feminine roles of their daughters if maternal employment is during childhood or adolescence. The daughters of such mothers generally aspire to a career outside the home, seek more advanced education, get better grades in college, and have less stereotyped views of female roles. They are also more apt to select a traditionally masculine occupation, more apt to emulate their mothers or state that their mother is the person they aspire to be like, and have a broader definition of the female role. It has also been found that daughters of working mothers appear to develop more independence than daughters of nonworking mothers.

Working mothers establish a different family interaction pattern in their homes than nonworking mothers. There is a strong modeling influence toward working and toward the development of an orientation of achievement, often with nontraditional vocational aspirations. Fathers who have achieved a high occupational status are more apt to influence their daughters toward nontraditional vocational achievement. It is hypothesized that the interaction found in such family settings plays a major role in developing nontraditional vocational role orientations and behaviors. Nonworking mothers are more apt to influence their daughters in the direction of the traditional model of the nonworking mother and the daughter is more apt to develop traditional female roles and achievement orientations.

CHILD REARING PRACTICES

Parenting

Some authorities have characterized parental behavior between the following four extremes: Warmth-acceptance, cold-rejectance, autonomy-permissiveness, and control-restrictiveness.

Warm-accepting parents provide understanding and emotional support, express physical affection, and provide a reasonable explanation for their disciplinary reactions, while cold-rejecting parents demonstrate the opposite behaviors. Control-restricting parents impose a system of rigidly enforced rules, obedience, no back talk, and no aggression toward almost every aspect of a child's behavior, while autonomy-permissive parents demonstrate the opposite. It is possible to characterize most parental behavior as a combination of these more extreme descriptions, and each combination results in different reactions and behaviors of their children.

Most authorities stress the importance of an atmosphere of warm-acceptance combined with moderate autonomy-permissiveness, which have been shown to more often lead to traits of responsibility, self-initiative, achievement, goal direction, and independence. It is also generally agreed that inconsistency of parental discipline is very detrimental in the development of a child's personality and general social development.

Independence training in American culture begins early, is prolonged, and is characterized by parents gradually shifting to more permissive attitudes as their child matures. This shift appears to be more pronounced in mothers than in fathers. In societies where the economy is more dependent on male physical strength and motor skills (e.g., hunting and herding v food-gathering cultures) there is greater differentiation between sex and age at which independence occurs.

In general, adolescents view an authoritarian parental attitude as being more appropriate for their fathers than for their mothers. Parental attitudes that encourage autonomy and independence yet express an interest in the adolescent's behavior and opinions contribute significantly to the development of confidence and self-esteem in the adolescent.

The best principles of parental discipline are those which help children become self-actualized, self-directed, socialized adolescents and adults. It is important that parental expectations be maintained consistently through time. Another principle of follow-through requires that parents pay attention to the child's response, and if a disciplinary punishment is stated (unfortunately sometimes threatened), then it must be carried through. The principle of immediate feedback is important so that the quicker the feedback or consequences are experienced, the greater the learning that takes place. In general, delayed consequences are not effective in changing behavior.

The maturational level of the child must be considered and discipline should be consistent with the child's level of maturation and comprehension. Since normal growth and development require mutual trust, adults must be truthful with their children. While children want to feel that their parents are superhuman and infallible, it is important for children to know that parents can make mistakes and admit to them.

The most important principle of parental discipline is to feel, learn, demonstrate, and seek genuine love. This has been described by some specialists as unconditional love; to know that whether you are right or wrong or good or bad, you will still be loved.

In general, parents with a lower socioeconomic status are more strict in enforcing sharply defined sex-typed behavior, and appear to maintain relatively strong sex-role stereotypes among children and adults. Both the father and the mother are important in producing appropriate sex identities in both boys and girls, and not just fathers being important for boys and mothers being important for girls.

While cognitive development is important in the development of an awareness of moral values, standards, and learning to abide by them, parental love and warmth, which provide for positive identification modeling, is also of major significance. It is also important that the parent's conscious and moral standards be mature and reasonable, and not deficient, overly strict, harsh, or inflexible.

Maternal Deprivation

Institutionalization and inadequate care during infancy increases the risk of deficiencies of emotional responsivity, general intellectual functioning, conceptual reasoning, abnormal behavioral and emotional patterns, and impairment of motor skills. Motor skills development is not irreversible, but there is some evidence that there are other deficits of early deprivation that are irreversible. Spitz and Bowlby are renowned for their studies and writing in this area.

Infants deprived of their mother or an adequate mother surrogate have an increased risk of developing anaclitic depression during childhood. In general, there are two stages in the development of such anaclitic depression: During the first stage of separation the infant protests vigorously, and during the second stage the infant enters into what is known as a phase of despair and ceases protesting and withdraws from any interaction, sometimes engaging in self-stimulation or refusing to eat.

Child Abuse

Inconsistency in discipline is the most frequent parental behavior found in most incidences of child abuse. Harsh physical punishment is also more frequently used by abusive parents. Abusive parents also tend to have been abused by their own parents, establishing a generational effect where the practices of one generation serve as a model for the next. Thus, physicians have an opportunity to help break the cycle of parental behaviors. While many child abusive parents may be rejecting and cold toward their children, they are more apt to be overcontrolling than permissive.

The findings of child abuse research show that child abusing parents are found to be more often abused by their own parents, abused children are frequently born prematurely and developed more slowly than their siblings, child abuse occurs more frequently among children below the age of 3, mothers abuse their children more often than fathers (attributed to the fact that mothers have more contact with their children), and parents are more apt to select one child as a scapegoat rather than abuse all their children.

The characteristics of parents who abuse their children include identifying with adult abusing models from their own childhood, maintaining a facade as "good parents" by use of projection and externalization, scapegoating of the child as "bad" to relieve the parents of their own conflicts over aggression and inadequacy, and mothers who abuse their children tend to turn to their children for gratification of personal dependency needs.

LIFE SPAN DEVELOPMENT

It is important to recognize that human development occurs at all points along the life span from conception to death. More traditional views of human development focus on maturation and growth during different stages, such as infancy, childhood, adolescence, etc., while the life span view of human development stresses that human life is multidimensional, must be studied and understood in a multivariate framework, and attempts to identify, describe, explain, and optimize intraindividual and interindividual changes and differences in growth and behavior across the life span from conception to death. As such, any portion of life must be viewed as just one part of the entire life span, and it requires that many academic disciplines, such as biology, psychology, sociology, anthropology, law, medicine, etc., be used to study development.

The Study of Human Development

There are several dimensions of development which are useful in studying and understanding the biological and behavioral components of development.

Chronological age is the most traditional. It is one that is useful in looking for variations that can or should occur in relationship to the chronological age of an individual. We, therefore, speak of certain developmental skills, tasks, concepts, or biological changes as occurring within a certain range of chronological age.

Cohort is also a useful dimension in that an individual born in 1920 or 1960, for example, becomes a member of the 1920 or 1960 birth cohort, so that an individual born within a given range of time may be understood in terms of the history of that particular period, and within the context of all other individuals born at that time and perhaps influenced by parental practices, nutrition, health status, education, and family structure existing during and subsequent to that particular time period.

This projects a longitudinal dimension between and within different birth cohorts.

Life transitions are also useful dimensions to describe normative life events, such as entering an occupation, marrying, the birth of children, retiring, etc. These kinds of transitions are important dimensions to learn more about in order to understand and predict behaviors that are more apt to affect or be effected by such transitions. As previously stated, developmental changes continue to occur throughout adulthood, but there are no general development stages as one finds in childhood or adolescence. One of the reasons is that the range of differences between individuals increases over the life span, therefore, the variability of differences between individuals becomes greater as chronological age increases. While society expects children and adolescents to demonstrate positive growth and change, it does not have the same expectation and encouragement for adults. Thus, the full potential for adult development has never been recognized, demonstrated, or promoted.

Developmental Research

Human growth and development are most often studied utilizing the following methods: Longitudinal design, cross-sectional design, time-lag design, and sequential design.

In longitudinal design the same individuals or group are observed more than one time (i.e., over a period of time). In cross-sectional design a group of individuals are measured at only one point in time. Time-lag design attempts to measure only age level at different times (e.g., in 1960, 1970, and 1980), thus, studying differences in behavior associated with a particular age group at various times in history. In sequential design, repeated measures are secured from each of the different cohort groups that were included in the initial cross-sectional sample, allowing the researcher to assess changes by retesting the initial study group and retesting the control group (i.e., allowing the remeasurement of a cross-sectional sample after a fixed interval of time). John Nesselroade, Warner Schaie, and Paul Baltes are important methodologists in developmental research.

Models and Theories of Human Development

The historical roots of the study of human development extend back into philosophy of more than 2,000 years ago, perhaps beginning with Plato, and progress through all of the major philosophers since that time, including the nature-nurture issue argued for years. The biological roots extend back at least to Charles Darwin's theory of evolution which emphasizes the impact of the physical and psychosocial environment on the biological organism. Other important historical contributors to our knowledge of human development include G. Stanley Hall (theory that ontogeny recapitulates phylogeny), Lewis Terman (measuring intellectual ability), Arnold Gesell (maturational readiness/nature-based), John B. Watson (behaviorism/the laws of classical and operant conditioning), Sigmund Freud (psychosexual stages of development), Jean Binet (measurement of intelligence), Erik Erikson (stages of psychosocial development), Jean Piaget (cognitive development), Konrad Lorenz (instinctive behavior and imprinting), Boyd McCandless (drive arousal and drive reduction), and many modern development theorists (e.g., Alexander Thomas and Richard Lerner individuality/temperment).

Freud's Theory of Development

Psychoanalytic-psychosexual stages of development were proposed by Sigmund Freud. Freud attempted to identify a series of psychosexual stages that children pass through. He believed that these stages could be identified by determining the erogenous zone that gives the child the greatest pleasure during that particular age.

Freud believed that the *oral stage* occurred during the first year because of the oral activities of feeding and biting. The *anal stage,* during the second and third years, was related to supposed gratification occurring during bowel movements. The *phallic stage,* during the fourth and fifth years, when the genital area is identified as providing a source of pleasure. The phallic stage spans the third through the fifth years and involves the libido moving to the genital area. In the male phallic stage, the libido moves to the boy's genital area and gratification is obtained through manipulation and stimulation of the genitals. Freud believed that there was an initial identification with the mother (oedipus complex), and anxiety about the power of the father (castration anxiety), with final identification with the father.

The female phallic stage again resulted in gratification through manipulation and stimulation of the genitals, with an identification with her father and an awareness that she does not have a penis (penis envy). The *latency stage* occurs at the end of the phallic stage (about 5 years of age) and lasts until puberty occurs at about 12 years of age. Freud believed that the libido is latent and not localized in any bodily zone. The *genital stage* was seen as occurring during adolescence, paralleling the maturation of the genitals and the formation of love objects. Freud asserted that if emotional experiences were associated with any given zone or stage, that children could develop a "fixation" at that particular stage of development.

A major factor in Freud's theory of neuroses was that sexual disturbances were the major cause of neurotic development. Freud recognized the existence of sexual feelings and curiosity in children and insisted that as a result of socialization many sexual feelings were repressed, and when repression becomes excessive, enormous amounts of psychic energy are consumed to maintain the repression. Freud reasoned that under various conditions of stress, sexual impulses could emerge or escape and appear in the form of neurotic symptoms.

Free association is one of the most important techniques in psychoanalytic treatment. In free association, a patient is encouraged to say whatever comes to mind. When the patient's flow of thoughts is blocked or lost, the therapist can assume that some resistence has occurred as a defensive maneuver to prevent repressed material from emerging into consciousness.

Transference is the process whereby the patient transfers emotional attachments to the therapist as a substitute for the parental figure. Transference may be either positive or negative, resulting in expressed feelings of love and emotional attachment, or feelings of unfairness and rejection. Thus, the patient seeks the therapist's love and emotional satisfaction that was desired from the parent, or may reject the parental figure as unloving and unjust, and the patient begins to recognize and deal with these feelings and emotions as related to their own parental figures, reflecting previous emotional entanglements.

A major problem and source of error in Freud's psychoanalytic and psychosexual theories was that he attempted to infer and extrapolate normal growth, development, and behavior on the basis of his own neurotic adult Victorian patients' behavioral pathology and their attempts to reconstruct their memories of childhood and of growing up. This has led to much criticism of his concepts of early development, normal behavior and even the origin of behavioral pathology. Nevertheless, one must view Freud's ideas as important historical formulations that had a tremendous impact on the conceptualization and study of human behavior and development. For example, Freud's dividing the mind into the *id* (unconscious instinctual drives, needs, and impulses), the *ego* (the part of the mind that interfaces the internal needs with the external reality), and the *super-ego* (the conscience or value system) has been useful in the conceptualization of how the mind might work. In fact, the term ego has become a household term in popular psychology.

One of the most important contributions of Freud's theories has been the concept of the unconscious, the preconscious, and the conscious. The unconscious portion of the mind refers to material that is not in a person's awareness and generally requires special techniques or situations for it to emerge into consciousness. Freud postulated that material in the unconscious can have a direct and an indirect influence on thinking, emotion, and behavior in everyday situations. The preconscious refers to material that is not in consciousness, but that can be readily brought into consciousness (e.g., names of individuals or places). Consciousness is material that is in a person's present awareness.

Psychosocial Model

Erik Erikson constructed a stage theory of development but, unlike Freud, he focused on the role of the ego in psychosocial development with particular attention to the expectations of society and the adaptations that must be made by the ego to meet those expectations. He proposed that each stage is fixed by a maturational "ground plan" and that development must proceed through each critical stage. Erikson identified the following eight psychosocial stages and tasks that must be accomplished during each stage:

1. Basic trust *v* mistrust (ages 0 to $1\frac{1}{2}$ years). If the basic needs of food and affection are met during this period, the infant develops a sense of basic trust, feeling that the world is intrinsically safe and that people can be trusted to respond to its needs.
2. Autonomy *v* shame and doubt ($1\frac{1}{2}$ to 3 years). The crisis is whether one is able to develop a sense of autonomy (i.e., gaining confidence of being able to use one's own muscles, feed one's self, and being able to operate somewhat independent of one's own parents or others). It is during this period that the 2-year old tests, announces, and practices the responses of "no." It is also the time that the 2-year old becomes toilet trained. Erikson believed that not being able to do these things during this period resulted in a feeling of shame and doubt.
3. Initiative *v* guilt (4 to 6 years). It is during this period that the child learns and practices even more independence, being able to explore and carry out more independent activities without being tied to the parent's "apron strings." Not being able to develop and practice these new initiatives can then lead to a feeling of fear and guilt of inappropriate dependency or inadequacies.
4. Industry *v* inferiority (6 to 13 years). The child focuses much more on accomplishing certain goals of parents, society, and self (e.g., learning to read, write, and compete). Performing well in comparison with one's peers can lead to more industry, confidence, and competitiveness, while lack of success can lead to feelings of inferiority and inadequacies. This time period conforms with Freud's latency period.
5. Identity *v* role confusion (13 to 18 years). This is the period of adolescence. It is also the period of puberty, with rapid changes in physical growth and endocrine

activity. The particular crisis is developing a sense of personal identity (e.g., identifying a role in society and with peers, and believing you can handle adulthood). Inadequate resolution of this crisis can result in role confusion and identity diffusion (e.g., not knowing what one can do in society or with one's talents).

6. Intimacy *v* isolation (18 to 25 years). This is young adulthood and the major development task is to learn to establish an intimate and love relationship with at least one person. If there is not adequate resolution of this task, one is apt to develop a feeling of isolation, being alone, and perhaps being unable to be close to or share their life with anyone.

7. Generativity *v* stagnation (25 to 40 years). According to Erikson, this period of adulthood includes the tasks of generating and raising children and of generating occupational accomplishments, both of which provide meaning to life. If neither of these tasks is accomplished or resolved by age 40, the person is apt to feel a predominate sense of stagnation and without meaning in life. It is expected that during this stage one will take an active responsibility for one's own life and related decisions. It can be a sign of inadequate resolution and inadequate ability to adapt if one continues to blame one's parents or others for this responsibility.

8. Integrity *v* despair (age 40 to death). This psychosocial stage is called maturity. A person begins to examine one's life and to evaluate one's accomplishments, relationships, and status in the sense of self-approval and meaningfulness. A sense of emotional and personal integration occurs; a feeling of personal integrity and that one has led a full, rich life. On the other hand if one looks at the past, present, or future with disapproval (e.g., unhappy and always regretting the lack of a second chance), the result can be despair.

Erikson's psychosocial stages of development provide a useful description of personality development that is consistent with a life span perspective. It provides a more adequate integration of psychological and social factors in normal and abnormal development than does Freud with his psychoanalytic theories. It has also served as a basis for much research about human personality. One limitation is that it does not adequately integrate biological factors. Also, stage-development concepts are useful in identifying major tasks to be accomplished, and when the resolution occurs, but does not often emphasize that even though the developmental tasks (e.g., trust, autonomy, identity, or integrity) may reach their peak at certain ages, in fact, they may begin and continue during all stages or periods of one's life span.

One can also get the impression that the resolution of stages is bimodal, in the sense that one either does or doesn't develop trust or identity or integrity, while in reality the resolutions may represent more of a normal curve distribution at each stage of development, and display much interaction within and between stages throughout one's life span.

Jean Piaget made a major contribution to understanding human development, describing the sequential changes that occur in cognitive ability with special focus on how a child thinks and learns. Piaget viewed children as constantly trying to make some sense of their world and their interactions with people by dealing actively with objects, relationships, and people. He regarded the abstract or mental representation of the significant components of an event and their relation to each other as schema. Through new experiences and ideas the child selectively incorporates those ideas and objects into the schema that the child has already developed.

By studying the cognitive abilities of children, Piaget was able to describe the sequences and levels of thinking through which all children progress, and how the thinking process at one stage differs from another at each of four stages of cognitive development. He considered the developmental stages to be an unfolding response to the interaction of both biological and environmental forces.

1. Sensory motor stage (birth to 2 years). The infant interfaces and coordinates with the environment. He or she relies on real or natural senses and apparently believes that if something is out of sight it no longer exists. Therefore, the game of "peek-a-boo" or "now you see it, now you don't" becomes a fascinating and surprising experience for infants and adults. The interaction with the environment becomes more systematic, and independent motor activities become purposely coordinated in the exploration of the outside world. Eventually, there is a realization that external objects continue to exist, even when not sensed, and that one can intentionally seek an object.

2. Preoperational stage (2 to 7 years). The child is able to mentally and symbolically represent objects and use perception and intuition to comprehend the world. A traditional test is to take two equal sized pieces of clay and make one longer than the other. The child will report the shorter piece to be the smaller and the longer piece to be the larger.

3. Concrete operational stage (7 to 11 years). Internalized actions which are reversible now exist, but cognition is limited since the child can think only about objects which have a concrete and real existence. The child cannot deal adequately with counterfactual or hypothetical phenomena. The child can also add and subtract various elements from each other and yet still converse the essence of the separate elements.

4. Formal operational stage (11 years to adolescence or adulthood). The person now has the ability to think ab-

stractly, think of all possible combinations of elements of a problem in order to find a real or imaginary solution. Tangible objects are not necessary to engage in abstract thought and the person can think in terms of abstract relationships and reversibility.

The three developmental theories that have been described should be viewed as complimentary, with Freud emphasizing the psychosocial/psychoanalytic internal processes, Erikson integrating the psychosocial, interpersonal, and societal issues, and Piaget focusing on analyzing the development of the cognitive aspects of the mind. Today it is most useful to use a pluralism of theories emphasizing nature (biological), nurture (environment and behavior), and various types of interaction between and within each element.

There is now strong evidence of the interaction between nature and nurture. In fact, the same genetic inheritance will lead to different developments or outcomes when expressed in different environments. Likewise, the same environment will have different effects on behavior and growth when it acts on, or reacts with, genetically different organisms. It was once thought that the major influence on growth and/or aging was from the biological changes influencing the behavioral changes, but we now know that behavioral and social changes do indeed also influence, modify, and sometimes cause the biological changes in growth and/or aging.

Cognitive and Intellectual Development

Most children develop cognitive skills in a chronological and predictable pattern. At the age of 18 months, a child can be expected to begin many questions with "what," try to imitate almost everything in his environment, conceptualize space primarily from his own space and activity as he moves through it, can follow simple one-part directions, and can begin to infer causes by observing effects. The two-year old learns more about time sequences (e.g., "in a minute" or "when daddy comes home"), can use several words to form two or three word sentences, can match simple shapes and colors, and can begin to participate and cooperate in toilet training.

A three-year old child asks many "why" questions, uses four or more words in a sentence, can anticipate fears, can remember his first and last name, likes to explore the environment outside of the home, and can sleep through the night and wake up dry. The four-year old child frequently begins questions with "where," often talks to imaginary playmates, can even threaten to run away from home, and is able to give opposites of

hot-cold, up-down, here-there, etc. The five-year old asks questions with "how," can follow a three-step direction, identifies coins, knows the days of the week, asks the meaning of words, talks more continuously, and is often so strongly focused or attending to external objects or activities that he may need to be reminded to eat or go to the bathroom. Monitoring cognitive skills development can help physicians determine normal or typical growth and development of individual children.

A number of programs have been attempted over the past two decades to provide educational stimulation and improved school performance for disadvantaged children. The factors which have contributed most to the success of such programs are providing educational stimulation at as early an age as possible, designing programs to focus directly on cognitive, language, and arithmetic skills, maintaining the program over a long period of time (years), providing stimulation daily, rather than periodically, recognizing powerful influences of the values of the family, community, and the media, and recognizing social class and ethnic group values and motivations.

Learning Disability in Childhood

Failure in academic learning does not necessarily imply impairment in intellectual capacity. Individuals with learning disabilities are more apt to show a selective deficit despite normal schooling exposure, normal family settings, appropriate motivation, normal sense organs, adequate physical status, and normal intelligence. Inspite of these apparently normal dimensions, they still fail to learn with normal proficiency. Most often, the failure to learn to read is the most frequently associated learning disability. Dyslexia is a learning disability involving the failure to learn to read and is a major problem, especially during adolescence.

During the early years, an individual's IQ is somewhat variable, but becomes increasingly stable during adolescence, and reasonably stable by age 18. Early cross-sectional studies of intelligence showed a decrease in IQ scores between adolescence and adulthood, with adulthood showing a general decline throughout life. However, longitudinal research of the same individuals over periods of 10–40 years, showed considerable stability of IQ score, with some individuals decreasing, some remaining fairly constant, and others actually increasing in IQ.

Of the four measures included in the IQ scores (visual-motor flexibility, verbal comprehension, number skills, and ability to organize and process visual information), visual-motor flexibility was the only measure that tended to decline with age, while the others showed a systematic increase in scores.

Many of the levels and types of ability developed during the schooling years can be expected to be maintained or even enhanced into adult and aged years, most often depending on such factors as whether the individual has continued to learn new things, had multiple new experiences, and continued to exercise their cognitive abilities.

Language and Speech

It is important to recognize that the number of sounds needed to produce the world's natural languages are fewer than 100 in number. While these sounds may seem meaningless when considered individually, they can be compounded to produce literally hundreds of thousands of meaningful morphemes.

Speech development is important in assessing the normal development of a child. During the first 6 months, infants invent and experiment with new noises, with cooing beginning at about 2 months of age. Babbling appears by 4 to 5 months of age, and is an important skill to develop so that the child can learn to repeat sounds of other humans, which occurs between 6 and 9 months of age, the infant will attempt to imitate all sounds that they hear, and select those sounds which will help them communicate. By 24 to 36 months of age, they will have 200–300 words in their vocabulary. By 48 months of age, they should have a vocabulary of about 1,500 words.

PERSONALITY DEVELOPMENT

Development of Personality

Personality is a term used to describe consistent predispositions of a person to behave in one distinctive way rather than another. While there has been much speculation and conflict as to how an individual's personality develops, it is an area of particular fascination since we recognize others by their distinctive personality and often use it to predict their behavior. There are many so-called theories of personality and each has helped us to learn more about the etiology of personality. A few will be mentioned here as examples.

The psychodynamic (psychoanalysis) theory developed by Freud has had a profound influence upon Western culture, medicine, and the behavioral sciences. It is an attempt to describe the psychic structure in terms of the id (unconscious source of all energy expressed through biological sex drives and seeking pleasure), the ego (the self which is rational and mediates between the id and the reality and demands of society), and the super-ego (the conscience or moral values, which is partly conscious and unconscious, and generally strives for perfection). One's personality becomes a reflection of how an individual resolves the natural conflicts of the three elements of personality. The ego develops various coping mechanisms and defense mechanisms to control anxiety and impulses. The failure or exaggeration of these mechanisms is described as maladaptive behavior.

The social learning theory maintains that personality develops through the process of reinforcers which shape behavior, which may be vicarious or self-administered. As one matures and gains ability to perceive and process more complex and abstract information, one learns to deal with the consequences of different behaviors. This socialization leads to habits, values, and attitudes which accumulate and become more persistent, resulting in a socially learned personality. By analyzing the antecedents and consequences of the behaviors, one is able to understand the origin of one's personality or behavioral pathology. The development of illness behavior and how it influences health is described in a later section.

HUMANISTIC APPROACH TO PERSONALITY

The humanistic approach to personality is more concerned with the behavioral characteristics which separate humans from animals. A number of personality theorists have described personality development in more experiential and perceptual terms. Abraham Maslow coined the term *self-actualization* as a means of describing the ability of some adults to accomplish their full potential development. By studying individuals who had developed their full potential such as Abraham Lincoln, Eleanor Roosevelt, and Albert Schweitzer, he found that they shared the following characteristics: Spontaneity, unaffectedness, independence, autonomy, creativity, and a fresh appreciation of people and the world. He also found them to be highly selective in their friendships and with only a few truly intimate friends.

Carl Rogers conceptualized two main structural concepts (i.e., the self and the ideal self). When the self and the ideal-self are not in congruence with each other, the individual is more apt to be maladjusted. Self-actualization is accomplished by increasing the alignment of the self and the concept of the ideal-self.

Neil Miller and John Dollard developed a theory of social learning whereby social skills and personality characteristics are acquired by imitative behaviors. Matched-dependent behavior occurs when positive reinforcement is received for emulating the behavior of a model or ideal.

Hans Eysenck used learning and conditioning principles to develop a descriptive theory of personality. He also related personality development to genetic factors and was instrumental in the origin and growth of behavior therapy. He also provided arguments and data to show that traditional psychotherapy and psychoanalysis are without efficacy.

Kurt Lewin developed the concept of field theory as an outgrowth of Gestalt psychology. He postulated psychological field forces existing in all situations and encounters; forces which influenced resulting behavior. He regarded individuals as living within a life space. Personality developed as the total field configurations became more and more differentiated, also allowing for considerable permeability and interaction between the various units of the personality and the life space. Dynamic and interactive concepts, such as need, psychic energy, tension, force or vector, and valence, played a major role in Lewin's field theory.

More recent theories have combined the behavioral/social learning and the humanistic theories into a more cognitive behaviorism which deals with perception of reality and applications of the principles of learning to the interaction between thoughts, feelings, and behaviors.

When an individual's cognitive elements (attitudes, perceived behaviors, etc.) are inconsistent with each other, tension is produced and the individual attempts to reduce this tension or incongruence by adding consonant elements. Thus, the individual attempts to change one of the dissonant elements so that it is either no longer inconsistent with the other, or attempts to reduce importance of the dissonant elements. Thus, dissonance theory allows one to predict attitude change when persons are in a situation that is contrary to their previously expressed beliefs.

Achievement Motivation

The old adage that success breeds success expectations and failure breeds failure expectations is especially true in young childhood. The success or failure expectations are strongly influenced by the expectations and reactions of significant others, particularly parents and other adults. Such encouragement, reward, and expectations can help children develop the traits of achievement motivation, mastery motivation, level of aspiration, frustration, tolerance, and feelings of competence. Such efforts to encourage and reward a child's achievement also develop persistence to set and accomplish higher, but realistic, goals.

Children who are discouraged, expected to fail, ridiculed, or ashamed are more likely to develop fear of failure or feelings of insecurity, inadequacy, or incompetence. They are also more apt to set low goals which can be reached easily, or unrealistically high goals which they can never reach or never try.

David C. McClelland is known for his theory of achievement motivation (nAch) in which the achieve-

ment motive is expressed in terms of a disposition or tendency to seek success in achievement-related situations. Achievement motivation is usually measured by a projective test and appears to be relatively stable from middle childhood through the rest of one's life. A person high in achievement motivation will set goals that involve moderate risks, especially in a task that involves skill. Also, students who are high in achievement motivation are likely to strive for a good grade in a course, whether or not the course is related to career plans. The achievement motive does not appear to be manifest in a situation where success is governed by chance.

Aggression and Development

The expression of aggression in early childhood actually increases the frequency of subsequent aggressive behavior. It has also been found that aggressive behavior appears to occur in children of all classes, cultures, and ethnic groups between 2 and 5 years of age; that physical punishment by parents may actually increase a child's aggression; that even though girls are usually less aggressive than boys, the sex differences often disappear in situations where aggression is allowed without fear of detection; and hyperactivity is frequently associated with aggression.

The "cathartic" approach to aggression therapy has been discredited, and there is considerable evidence that overpermissiveness toward childhood aggression actually increases subsequent aggression. Many children actually want to be helped to control aggressive feelings and behavior.

PRENATAL INFLUENCES

It is becoming increasingly well documented that the mothers' behaviors (activity, consumption, and emotions) have a direct and indirect effect on the developing infant before birth. The consequences of certain chemicals passing through the placental membrane can affect development. Events and phenomena in the environment outside the amniotic sac can also affect development. The major factors that have been associated with physical malformation and behavioral disorders are maternal nutrition, alcohol and tobacco consumption, drug use, maternal age, and teratogens acting through the male.

Undernutrition and malnutrition are most often associated with poor maternal health, miscarriage, premature birth, still birth, long labor, increased death rate in infancy, birth complications, and problems with nervous system development.

Alcohol and tobacco consumption are major behavior

problems and influence fetal development prenatally and postnatally. Both alcohol and tobacco consumption are associated with premature birth, aborted pregnancies, and low birth weight. Furthermore, to engage in both drinking and smoking results in a potential of the effect.

Chronic drinking by a pregnant woman can produce a syndrome of malformations termed the fetal alcohol syndrome. Frequent sequelae of fetal alcohol syndrome are retardation of intrauterine growth, premature birth, microcephaly, congenital eye and ear problems, heart anomalies, extra fingers or toes, patterns of disturbed sleep, face defects, mental retardation, excessive irritability, and hyperactivity. It is estimated that 2 to 4 ounces of hard liquor consumed daily by a pregnant woman can result in a 10 percent risk of this syndrome. The number of infants involved in this syndrome is estimated to be about 6,000 infants per year.

Drug ingestion can have several detrimental effects on the fetus and infant. Thalidomide, a good example of a drug not harmful to mothers, produces gross anatomical defects in the limbs of the fetus. Diethylstilbestrol (DES), which was taken to prevent miscarriage, is now affecting the daughters of the women who took the drug with a higher probability of developing cancer of the cervix. Mothers addicted to heroin, morphine, or psychoactive drugs deliver infants who are also addicted, and who are more often of low birth weight, premature, excitable, and irritable. Physicians now recognize that even well-known drugs can affect the fetus and that drugs should be taken only when absolutely necessary. Many pregnant women have changed their own drug-taking behavior and will take no drugs or medicines while they are pregnant or if they suspect they are pregnant. Central nervous system depressant drugs and even anesthetics used to assist in delivery are now being critically examined. Reed and Lamaze have promoted labor and birth without medication, with fathers present, and with an active support system provided to help both mother and father.

Virus-caused diseases can produce severe defects in the fetus. The contraction of rubella (German measles) in the first trimester can result in heart defects, deafness, cataracts, blindness, or mental retardation. Toxemia greatly increases the infant mortality, and also increases the risk of maternal mortality and the likelihood of infant mental retardation. Rh factor incompatibility can result in miscarriage, anemia, mental retardation, or death (while the Rh factor can be successfully treated today it is not always done). Other diseases of a pregnant woman which can affect the fetus are toxoplasmosis, hepatitis, cytomegalovirus (CMV), chicken pox, mumps, Asian flu, polio, typhoid fever, tuberculosis, cancer, malaria, diabetes, syphilis, and herpes simplex.

Even though there is no direct neural connection be-

tween the mother and the fetus, the mother's emotional state can influence the infants prenatal environment and development. A number of studies have reported emotional disturbances during pregnancy associated with prematurity, abortion, prolonged labor, delivery complications, infant hyperactivity, irritability, sleep problems, and irregular eating behaviors. It is reported that ACTH, epinephrine, and other hormonal products of anxiety, stress, and emotional tension not only affect the mother's physiology, but also cross the placental membrane and affect the fetus, especially with regard to irritability and hyperactivity.

Maternal age (either too young and too old) has a dramatic genetic effect on the fetus as well as on infant and maternal mortality, prematurity, and delivery complications.

There is some evidence that males who are exposed to certain teratogens, before conception, result in a greater incidence of birth defects in the offspring. Implicated are certain anesthetic gases, thalidomide, methadone, and other known teratogens.

Premature versus full-term children often show developmental differences up to school age. The premature infant shows decrements of height, weight, motor skills, and cognitive skills. Prematurity is also more frequent among adolescent pregnancies, and women from lower socioeconomic groups. Such premature babies also recover less rapidly from development deficits.

Adolescent pregnancies most often result in the growth of infants with lower birth weight, higher rate of infant mortality, higher rate of mental retardation, and higher rate of birth defects. Pregnant adolescents are also more likely to have had inadequate prenatal care, more apt to suffer from medical complications of toxemia or anemia, and more likely to have poor nutrition.

PHYSICAL DEVELOPMENT

Infant Reflexes

Reflexes are relatively consistent motor (muscular) movements which occur in response to particular sensory stimulation. Even though there is considerable interindividual variability associated with norms for each reflex, the appearance, existence, or disappearance of certain reflexes are useful behavioral markers to distinguish between normal and abnormal development, especially in the newborn infant. An alphabetical listing of the main primative reflexes follows:

1. Blink: A flash of light or touching of the eyelashes is responded to by a closing of both eyelids. This is a per-

manent reflex and protects the eyes from foreign or strong stimuli.

2. Biceps reflex: A tap on the tendon of the biceps produces a short contraction of the biceps. It is more brisk the first few days than later. It is absent in depressed infants and in congenital muscular disease.

3. Babinski: A stroking or scratching on the lateral side of the foot from heel to toes produces a dorsal flexion of the big toe and extension or fanning of other toes. Disappears after first year and is replaced by plantar flexion of big toe as found in adults. It is absent in defects of the lower spine.

4. Knee jerk (patellar tendon): A tap on the tendon below the patella produces a quick extension or kick of the knee. It is quicker during the first 2 days than later. It is absent or diminished in depressed infants or in certain muscular diseases. It becomes exaggerated in hyperexcitable infants.

5. Moro reflex: Produced by a sudden loud sound, a jarring, sudden movement of infant's head and neck. The moro reflex is also caused by holding the infant horizontally and the examiner lowering his or her hands rapidly about 6 inches with abrupt stop. The infant's arms are thrown out in extension and then brought toward each other in a quick convulsive manner. Hands are fanned out at first and then clenched. It begins to disappear at 3 or 4 months and fully disappears by 5 to 7 months. When the moro reflex is absent or constantly weak, it indicates a diffuse central nervous system depression or disturbance, or other brain stem disorder.

6. Plantar-hand or toe grasp: When a finger is pressed against the infant's palm or ball of the feet it produces a grasp with the fingers or a plantar flexion of all toes. The finger grasp increases during the first month, then gradually declines and disappears in 4 or 5 months and is replaced by voluntary grasp. It is absent or weak in depressed infants. The toe grasp disappears in 8 to 12 months and is absent in defects of the lower spinal cord.

7. Rooting response: When the infant's cheek is stimulated by light pressure of the finger it turns its head toward the finger and opens its mouth to suck the finger. It disappears in about 3 or 4 months and is absent in depressed infants.

8. Sucking response: Inserting tip of finger into mouth of infant produces rhythmical sucking. Sucking may be less in first 3 or 4 days. Poor sucking reflex is found in apathetic infants or due to maternal medication.

9. Other tendon reflexes: Sudden stretching of a tendon by a tap produces a quick contraction. It is absent or diminished in depressed infants and exaggerated in hyperexcitable infants. In addition to the patellar tendon (which relates primarily to L2–L4), others include jaw jerk (C5), biceps (C5–C6), triceps (C6–C8), and ankle (S1–S2).

Infant Motor Development

Motor development and muscular control skills are helpful behavioral guidelines for tracking normal development. There is considerable variability between individuals, and within the same individual, but the normative behavioral data are also helpful in anticipating existing and future developmental problems. Since parents usually follow behavioral development so carefully, a knowledge of such normative data and its variability can help the physician assess development and reassure parents.

The following is presented as a general guide.

1 Month: Raises head and chin briefly while lying on stomach.

2 Months: Raises chest while lying on stomach.

3 Months: Lifts head above body plane; makes stepping motions when held vertically; can retain a hold on objects.

4 Months: Sits with support; looks around; grasps hands together; plays with hands; can use a unilateral openhanded approach to objects.

5 Months: Can sit alone briefly; grasps objects in one hand.

6 Months: Knee push and swimmer movements; gets up on hands.

7 Months: Sits without support; rolls over unassisted.

8 Months: Stands with help.

9 Months: Stands by pulling up and holding on to furniture; sits alone unassisted; makes some crawling progress on stomach.

10 Months: Creeps; scoots backward and is able to crawl.

11 Months: Can walk when led; can grasp object in each hand and clap them together; can use thumb and forefinger to pick up small objects.

12 Months: Pulls self up to stand; takes and releases small objects placing them in a container.

13 Months: Climbs stairs.

14 Months: Stands alone.

15 Months: Can stand up alone and walk alone.

18 Months: Can go up and down stairs without help; can run; walks forward and backward; throws ball; feeds self and uses a cup; turns several pages of a book; builds tower of 4–5 blocks.

24 Months: Can jump and walk backwards; can hold a pencil and draw with it; drinks from small cup using one hand; turns doorknobs; builds tower of 6–7 blocks; turns pages one at a time.

3 Years: The child should be able to pedal a tricycle, use blunt scissors, wash hands, brush teeth, make a bridge of 3 blocks, jump from a low step, and copy a circle with a pencil.

4 Years: A child should be able to hop forward on one foot, walk backwards, copy a square with a pencil, button side buttons, cut around pictures with scissors, and bath himself with some assistance.

5 Years: A child should be able to jump rope, print own name, dress without assistance, put toys away, copy a triangle, and eat with a fork.

Gender Development

A sex role is a set of prescriptions for behavior, defined by society, and expected for a particular sex group. Sex-role behavior is the behavior exhibited in accordance with these prescriptions. Sex-role stereotypes are particular behaviors that are generalized and expected as characteristics of one sex group, usually as opposed to another. Thus, we have "typical" masculine or feminine behaviors.

Biology does play a major role in such psychosocial development, however, it does not occur independently of cultural demands and historical milieu. Gender identity is most strongly influenced by assignment by parents, rather than chromosomal sex, gonadal sex, or morphologic sex. The feeling of being male or female is generally learned by the age of 3 years.

The development of an atypical gender role in boys is most often associated with lack of male playmates, lack of an older male role model, parental encouragement of more feminine behavior, maternal overprotection, unusual physical attractiveness, and paternal rejection.

Children are more apt to develop an identification with a parent through the imitation or modeling of parental mannerisms, the perception of physical and behavioral similarities between themselves and a parent, the perception of desirable attributes, the receipt of communications from others identifying their similarities, and the attractiveness of the parent.

ADOLESCENCE

Richard Lerner has defined adolescent development as that period within the life span when most of the person's processes are in a state of transition from what typically is considered childhood to what typically is considered adulthood. While all developmental stages involve biologic, psychologic, sociologic, cultural, and historical dimensions of stability and change, adolescence appears to have more varying rates of change than any other development period. Society also has recognized and labeled adolescence as a most difficult and trying period of development. The problem of coordinating and adapting to these changes constitutes an enduring and often crisis situation for the individual. The

search for identity is considered to be the major and sometimes overpowering task for the adolescent.

The physical changes of puberty and its associated hormonal and endocrine factors represent a complicated but exciting realm of new behavioral possibilities. From the standpoint of cognitive development, the adolescent is entering the stage of formal operations where intellectual analysis, detachment, and systematic search for ideal answers to both real and hypothetical questions become a major activity and challenge. Adolescence also becomes prolonged (roughly 12–18 years) in our society which leads to the ambiguous status of being neither child nor adult, leading to additional stress.

Prepubescence is the first period of significant bodily change beginning with sexual maturation and ending with the appearance of pubic hair. In males there is a progressive enlargement of the testicles, increase in size of the penis, and toward the end of pubescence, usually a lowering of the pitch of the voice. In females, there is a rounding of the hips and the first visible indications of breast and nipple ("bud") development.

In pubescence, pubic hair and height and weight growth spurts occur for both sexes, however, these changes occur about 2 years earlier in females. The growth spurt for girls usually reaches its peak at about age 12, while for boys, the peak usually occurs at 14 years of age. The growth spurt for girls usually begins at about $10\frac{1}{2}$ ending at age 14, but can begin as early as age $9\frac{1}{2}$ and can continue to age 15. Menarche is usually a late event in puberty, beginning between the ages of 10 and $16\frac{1}{2}$. While the growth spurt for boys peaks at 14 years of age, it can begin as early as age $10\frac{1}{2}$ or as late as age 16, and can end anytime between age $13\frac{1}{2}$ and age $17\frac{1}{2}$. The growth spurt for the testes can begin between the ages of $9\frac{1}{2}$ and $13\frac{1}{2}$ and can end between the ages of $13\frac{1}{2}$ and 17.

In males, there is continued growth of the penis and testes, axillary hair starts after pubic hair, and the voice changes as the larynx enlarges during pubescence. For females, the first menstruation (menarche) occurs at about $12\frac{1}{2}$ years, but the range is between $10\frac{1}{2}$ to 15 years. There is evidence that the onset of mences has been occurring at an earlier age over the past 100 years. The period of postpubescence begins when pubic hair growth is complete and extends until all primary and secondary sexual characteristics are complete.

The major developmental tasks of adolescence are peer and sexual relationships, economic independence, and identity. It is important for the adolescent to be socially acceptable to peers. This often provokes differences between the adolescent and parents. Developing one's own mode of dress, speech, and entertainment is a part of this. The so-called generation gap is often publicized for commercial interests, but is less evident in healthy family environments. Even though peer group influence is strong, the family is still the most important determinant of adolescent attitudes, values, and political and religious beliefs. Economic independence from parents is an increasing need and is also related to emotional independence. Vocational and occupational choice and the training and educational programs to acquire the necessary qualifications assume increasing importance and serve as a source of stress during adolescence.

The achievement of personal identity is related to feeling one is unique, worthy, and an integrated whole. As defined by Erikson, the crisis of adolescence is between identity at one extreme and role confusion (identity diffusion) at the other. Failure to develop this sense of identity makes it more difficult for one to proceed with the subsequent attainment of intimacy and productivity which is later expressed through marriage, occupational achievement, and parenthood. Extended periods of education and dependence sometimes results in delay of the resolution of identity, particularly in terms of occupational choice, affiliation, economic independence, and occupational achievement. Some adolescents resolve occupational identity issues by adopting the identities of their parents with little or no questioning or challenging of those identities. Sexual and moral values, occupational commitments, and social and political attitudes are all considered to be components of the final stage of adolescence.

The development of sexual and affiliative relationships consumes much adolescent thought and energy. Society is also concerned, since the social problems of venereal disease, illegitimacy, and early marriage are all related to adolescent sexuality. Although there has been an increase in sexual behavior, it is argued that there has been a sexual evolution, rather than a sexual revolution. While sexual intercourse may begin in early adolescence for a small number, by late adolescence about half of white females and 5/6 of black females (a higher proportion for males) have become sexually active, with half of them involving only one partner. Not being contraceptively protected results in hundreds of thousands of premarital pregnancies each year. Abortion is the most common alternative, but other options include marriage, single parenthood, or birth with adoption.

Masturbation during adolescence is practiced more frequently by boys; also practiced by girls; varies widely in frequency from individual to individual; and is a prominent source of guilt and anxiety.

The single most predictive factor of male adolescent juvenile delinquency is the nature of the relationship with his parents. The better an adolescent boy gets along with his parents, the less likely he will engage in delinquent behavior. Delinquency is also related to overly severe and overly lax home discipline, and to an atmosphere of mutual hostility and rejection between parents and children. There is little evidence that most delinquents come from broken homes; rather, the incidence of delinquency is increased among boys of unhappy intact homes.

The major reason for the first offense imprisonment of male juveniles is conviction of robbery and burglary (33 percent), not sex and narcotic offenses (11 percent) as many believe. Since the mid-1960s, the percent of first offense imprisonment of male juveniles involved in crimes of violence has increased from 5 percent to over 34 percent. Girls are less likely to be imprisoned for a first offense violent crime than for drug or sex related offenses.

YOUNG ADULTHOOD AND ADULTHOOD

Erikson labeled the young adult as involved in the crisis (process) of developing a sense of intimacy or a sense of isolation. Adulthood was characterized as a period of generativity v stagnation. In real life, young adulthood and adulthood often become fused or overlapping, since the beginnings of occupation, marriage, and producing (children and occupational success) occur at different ages and not always in the same sequence. In fact, development in each of these tasks or activities is most often interwoven and reoccurs over a 15 to 30 year period. With the increasing frequency of second marriages, second families, and second or third occupations, the developmental stages have been interwoven and extended through adulthood and into old age. Perhaps this is one of the main reasons why so little is known about the psychosocial dimensions of these stages, crises, and tasks.

To understand the place of young adulthood and adulthood in the life cycle, one must identify the individual components and recognize: (1) That development is more than an individual process; (2) it involves a dynamic interaction between individuals and society; (3) individuals change over the life span; and (4) that various age cohorts form a series of age strata which vary and interact over time and create a changing demographic profile within the society. It is within this total context that each individual develops, acts, and interacts.

The social processes within society use age as a criterion for allocating various roles and for evaluating one's performance in these roles. Thus, age is used as a criterion for entry into and exit from the roles of society. Age norms have evolved to a normative social and personal clock for the timing and development of the major events in life and also for judging the appropriateness, value, and tolerance of these behaviors. Even though some of these age norms may be weakening, age-related roles are still an important determiner of an individual's participation in different types of roles and role changes over the life cycle. Thus, society has developed many age-related roles and normative expectations associated with definite positions, attributes, responsibilities, and privileges (e.g., men, women, professions, parents, religions, honors, unemployed, elderly, heroes, nonroles, socially unstructured roles, etc).

Tasks of Young Adulthood and Adulthood

Marriage is a major task of young adulthood and adulthood. In spite of its personal, social, and biological fulfillment properties, it is still a stressful event, and provides many opportunities for continuing stress, especially if the partners have misperceived each other's needs and capacity for enduring intimacy. Fortunately, while second marriages are also vulnerable, they tend to succeed as well as the first marriages which endure. (*See* Marriage section.)

Parenthood (*see also* Parenting section) generates even higher levels of stress than marriage. Even though there are many fulfilling rewards of parenthood, there are great physical, emotional, and economic demands placed on young adults, and adults because of the responsibilities involved with parenthood. The potential for and reality of certain failures in the parent role can be devastating to the ego, conscience, and sense of worth of either or both parents. Frustration and depression is a frequent result. Also, not having the economic and family resources to help with the success and failures of parenthood, can exacerbate and potentiate the sense of helplessness and hopelessness. The long-term developmental effects of such deficits of resources are incalculable. Opposingly, infertility is also a source of stress and distress during this period of young adult or adult life.

The postparental stage includes the period when children leave home and when parents become grandparents. This stage can encompass many years. The period and stress of children leaving home is often referred to as "the empty nest syndrome." Stability of the marriage is particularly vulnerable at this time, if the marriage relationship has not been satisfactory, if the parents have been resigned to the marriage for the sake of the children, if either parent has developed an unusual dependency on the children, or if the parents have a disproportionate investment in their children rather than in their marriage. The beginning of menopause can also signal the end of reproductive capacity and precipitate a midlife crisis for women who may have based their identity on motherhood. The late 40s and early 50s are also ages when men are apt to become aware that they will never achieve their youthful aspirations, and in some instances will begin to feel the threat of competition from younger

men and women. This will also become more prevalent among employed women as they enter this stage of their development.

The awareness of mortality usually begins to rise in the late 50s when many adults develop cardiovascular diseases and chronic problems associated with obesity, hypertension, arthritis, fatigue, etc. One's friends, parents, and other significant individuals usually begin to die during this period, further emphasizing an individual's mortality concerns. Many adults rethink their priorities and frequently establish new interests and lifestyles. During this transition from middle age to old age, previously inhibited aspects of the personality are more freely expressed. Men find freer expression of nurturant and affiliative feelings and women are able to express aggressive and egocentric feelings. In general, the middle years represent a turning point with introspection and self-evaluation increasing, a reorientation of time in terms of time left to live rather than time since birth, and the reformulation of new perceptions of self, time, and death. It is important to recognize that we know much more about the psychopathology and adjustment failures of this stage of adulthood than we do about the normative and individual coping skills and successes of this period of development. While there are many adjustive failures at this age, there are many more individuals who find this period a successful and fulfilling experience. It often results in rejuvination of individuality, self-confidence, and self-directedness. It is most often a period of re-allocation of concerns, energies, and commitments. It is a stage during which most of Erikson's integrity work and accomplishment takes place.

The elderly and old age period can begin with retirement, widowhood, or perhaps facing one's own death. Society has designated the age of 65 years as the beginning of old age, but it can occur as early as the middle 50s or as late as 70 years of age. It is generally accompanied by a gradual or fairly sudden decrease in financial resources, social contacts and status, authority, responsibility, and opportunity to continue one's youthful aspirations. It is regarded primarily as a period of disengagement; a gradual reduction in total range of activities, commitments, and social interaction. Disengagement also involves a withdrawal of emotional commitment and involvement from the environment. As aging progresses, the individual is apt to become more concerned with their immediate needs and wishes, and less concerned with the demands of society.

On the other hand, some older persons regard the period as an opportunity to exercise personal, social, and recreational options that have not been possible in the past. Some studies show that sex-role and race stereotypes weaken, women become less submissive and more assertive, men more nurturant, and there are increased opportunities for continued personal growth and a more satisfying life. Contrary to conventional wisdom, individual differences are exaggerated, not diminished, in old age. With continued personal growth, Erikson's concept of integrated acceptance of one's own life and its meaning becomes a reality. Without this development, Erikson postulated the development of despair and depression.

Some of the common, but untrue, stereotypes of the elderly are that most old people feel miserable most of the time, the aged are unhappy, the aged are rarely as happy as when they were younger, a high percentage of the aged live in institutions, most aged are dependent and give up social, physical, and cognitive independence, older drivers have a higher automobile accident rate when compared with middle-aged drivers, and most older drivers have a higher accident rate than drivers under age 30.

These stereotypes are a major problem in attempting to provide health care for the elderly. In general, the five senses do tend to decline with age, but most of the elderly see themselves as being as happy as when they were younger. Boredom and lack of meaningful activity are major factors for the aged and for the individuals providing health care to the elderly. Minorities often suffer from and have to cope with a situation of double jeopardy (i.e., age and race discrimination).

Five percent of persons 65 years of age and over are in long-term institutions and only about 10 percent of persons age 75 and over are in long-term institutions. The aged place a high priority on retaining one's social, physical, and cognitive independence.

As to automobile accident rate, the elderly have about the same accident rate as middle-aged drivers, and have an even lower accident rate than drivers under age 30.

In studies of stress and mortality among elderly persons in nursing homes, who have been transferred from one nursing home to another, it was found that those patients who had adjusted satisfactorily to their initial nursing home have the lowest mortality rates following the move; patients whose attitudes were angry and hostile had much higher mortality rates. Other studies have found depressed patients to have high mortality rates after stress of movement. While patients who were well adjusted had the lowest mortality rates, even negative or hostile attitudes appeared to enhance to some extent the chances of adapting to a new situation, perhaps at least representing some active mode of coping as being preferable to depression.

Most recommendations concerning preparation for old age emphasize the more positive aspects of continued growth and development. Some may prefer to disengage, and others to remain active until they die. Some will need and prefer the companionship of their peers,

but others will seek younger persons and grandchildren. In most, a feeling of helplessness, isolation, and lack of control will be damaging. Much has been written and even more should be known about nutrition and the elderly as undernutrition and malnutrition are very common among the elderly, particularly if they disengage or begin to lose certain cognitive or social skills. The fact that only a minority of the elderly are in nursing homes is a positive indicator for potential health maintenance. Retaining some measure of autonomy and self-sufficiency is very important.

As one can prepare oneself for retirement and old age, so can one prepare oneself for their own death. Reaching the developmental stage of meaningfulness and integrity, and acceptance of the process and reality of dying will do much to accomplish this preparation. The physician's role should be one of facilitating this developmental stage and providing information and counsel that is needed about the particular disease, the patient's condition, or the approachment of death. The physician should also provide the same information and support to the family to help them adjust and cope.

In addition, physicians can best handle other professional responsibilities to dying patients and their families by recognizing the requirements for effective mourning by the patients' relatives and medical personnel who know the patients, developing procedures for the psychologic and organizational aspects of terminal care in the hospital, planning for continuing care of the patients if they leave the hospital, and keeping discussions about death open among relatives and medical personnel.

In attempting to inform a patient or a patient's relative about the patient's serious illness, the following is a summary of factors that have been found to be of major importance: Find out what the patient or patient's relative thinks, knows, or wants to know about the illness; give honest answers that will provide some degree of realistic hope; determine each one's understanding of what you have discussed; always leave the communication channel open for further discussion or questions; recognize that most patients and families have a series of rational and irrational ideas about the illness, its cause, and its prognosis, which should be explored by the physician; and be supportive of the patient or relative regardless of what he or she may be going through. A natural pitfall is for physicians to avoid giving information or discussing the illness until they have all of the facts, tests, etc.; lest the patient's fear or anxiety be increased, or the physician appear not to know the nature of the illness, or risking the possibility of looking bad in the patient's eyes.

The process of grieving places a person at an increased risk for the onset of death from cardiovascular disease, minor somatic complaints, drug and alcohol abuse, and accidents. A study of grieving found mortality to be 40 percent higher than expected in the first 6 months of widowhood.

In the death of a loved person, one is apt to find unconscious anger toward the deceased person, which is often repressed anger that leads to a sense of guilt, which then exacerbates the normal depression that might be associated with mourning. This tends to prolong and intensify the mourning process, frequently leading to pathologic grief reactions. It has also been shown that if a mourner has a history of emotional problems, the grief reaction is more apt to become pathologic.

Other studies have shown that in the treatment of terminally ill patients the number of medical staff contacts with terminally ill patients declines preciptiously when the label "terminal" or "hopeless" is applied to the patients; denial of death is a characteristic defense mechanism used by terminally ill patients and should be respected; expressions of anger and rage by terminally ill patients are frequently directed toward the medical personnel treating them; and the acceptance of death by terminally ill patients and their family members does not preclude the expression of grief.

Kubler-Ross has proposed that the five stages of dying are the following:

1. Denial: A sense of disbelief.
2. Anger: Feelings of distress, hostility, resentment, and "why me?"
3. Bargaining: Favors are asked to extend life or delay death, "I promise to be a better person if I can live a little longer."
4. Depression: Realization that death can't be avoided.
5. Acceptance: Resolved about death, though not happy, the struggle being over.

All people don't go through the sequence, nor do they complete one stage before going to the next (e.g., a person might exhibit denial from time to time throughout the dying process). Other studies have analyzed the dying process as a series of phases such as an acute phase, a chronic living-dying phase, and terminal phase.

COMMUNICATION

Interviewing

In interviewing, the opening statement is important in setting the tone and direction of the interview. It is most important for the physician to learn from the patient why he or she has come, relate in a frank and honest manner what you know about the problem, recognize the information that the patient has given and refrain from duplicating questions already gathered in the chart, and encourage a forthright and open relationship.

Attempting to play the authority role is likely to decrease the exchange of information and increase the dependency role. It has been established that open-ended questions, rather than yes-or-no questions, are most effective in encouraging patients to speak more freely and provide more information. Some examples of types of questions physicians ask are the following:

"Tell me about your problem," an open-ended question.
"Do you have pain in your stomach?" a yes-or-no question.
"Show me where you have the pain," an open-ended question.
"What do you do to relieve the pain?" an open-ended question.
"Do you realize that almost everyone feels this way after it happens?" a reassurance question.
"Are you sure it really hurts?" a confrontation question.
"Since he did that to you, I assume you are still angry?" an interpretive question.
"You say you've never gotten along with her?" a reflective question.
"Some patients report nauseau with this medication; how do you feel?" a leading question.
Silence, with expression of interest, a tell me more question (open-ended).

It is important to recognize that physicians most often focus on symptoms or degree of tissue damage that are apt to have serious implications for the patient's future health status, while patients are more apt to focus on symptoms that interfere with usual activities or routines or the degree of discomfort.

The most typical problems that arise from physician-patient interactions are that "matter-of-fact" statements by the physician often have an emotional impact and generate a high level of anxiety, patients are often presented excessive amounts of information resulting in "data overload," often because of certain time constraints or compulsive physician behavior, technical jargon is most often not understood by the patient and results in ambiguity and uncertainty in the patient's mind, and the social distance between the physician and the patient influences the interaction, so that decreasing the social distance facilitates the therapeutic alliance.

Nonverbal Communication

In general, all forms of communication other than words spoken are considered to be nonverbal communication. These include gesture, posture, touch, facial expression, dress and grooming, physical distance, skin color (blushing, pale, dehydrated, etc.), voice inflection, voice tone, voice volume, body hygiene, and silence. Nonverbal communications communicate much about one's emotions and feelings, and place verbal communication into a context. Intensity, complexity, and subtlety can all be communicated through nonverbal behavioral patterns, and with great accuracy. There is some evidence that women are superior to men in both the reading and transmission of nonverbal facial communications. By attending to nonverbal communication, physicians can secure maximum communication, information, feelings, and context. Different cultural, ethnic, educational, and socioeconomic status backgrounds often learn to express different nonverbal communication patterns.

Physicians must be able to read and interpret nonverbal expressions. Most often these expressions reveal intentional and unintentional feelings. There are a number of terms used to describe nonverbal communication.

Illustrators: Any movement that amplifies or emphasizes an individual's words. These can be hand movements (e.g., flowing v jerky) or facial movements called speech illustrators (e.g., wrinkling brow or moving eyelids to accent or provide emotional context). Outgoing and sociable individuals use many more illustrators than a depressed patient. Many illustrators are learned as a characteristic of different ethnic and cultural groups. As a depression lifts, a person increases the use of illustrators, and a person trying to conceal his or her feelings will decrease the use of illustrators. The voice pitch generally increases as illustrators decrease.

Self-manipulators: An individual doing something with or manipulating another part of the body (e.g., scratching one's head, wringing one's hands). Individuals are often not aware of these movements. The more anxious or uncomfortable the patient, the greater the number of self-manipulators. They may also serve as illustrators by amplifying a verbal description (e.g., licking one's lips while describing a desirable food).

Facial expressions: A fairly universal means of communicating such emotions as happiness, sadness, surprise, fear, disgust, or anger. There are also cultural and ethnic learned variations (e.g., stoicism or increased intensity of emotional response).

Emblem: A movement or gesture used to communicate a special message or meaning in a given culture. For example, indicating "stop" by raising one's hand upright with palm outward and moving the hand toward another person; indicating protest or anger by clenching one's fist, raising it to shoulder level, and moving the hand back and forth toward another person; indicating a sign of hope, or that one is telling a small lie by crossing one's index and middle fingers; indicate "OK" by joining the end of the thumb and the index finger in clear view of another person; indicating "yes" or "no" by a nod of the head; indicating "I don't know" by a shrug of the

shoulders; and indicating approval or disapproval by thumbs up or down.

Eye contact between individuals varies according to the degree of familiarity between the individuals and can communicate threat, anger, or fear. It has been found that listeners maintain eye contact more than talkers.

An often ignored aspect of nonverbal communication is personal space. It is the immediate area surrounding a person, an envelope if you will, which a person carries around as a sort of "portable territory." It varies considerably from person to person and from situation to situation, and generally produces discomfort in the individual when the personal space is invaded or occupied by another individual. Sitting in an audience, standing in an elevator, conversing intimately, and arguing violently will all involve or allow different degrees of intrusion before discomfort is experienced.

Doctor-Patient Relationship

Patients most often judge professional competence on the basis of a physician's behavior and positive interpersonal relationship rather than on an evaluation of the physician's abilities and knowledge. Showing an interest in their patients and a willingness to give of their time are the major criteria used in evaluating a physician's competence. Self-confidence, a willingness to socialize, and the ease with which diagnosis and treatment plan are developed are also important factors that patients use in judging professional competence.

Hospitalized patients pose a special problem as they see themselves being unable to exercise control, yet they fear that exerting control may diminish quality or quantity of care. Furthermore patients want to cooperate, but they have little knowledge of what they should expect or demand as they are unable to evaluate the competence of nurses and physicians. These difficulties often cause the patient to see the hospital as a crisis institution.

A positive physician-patient relationship presents the physician as a strong, stable, nurturant person on whom the patient can depend. An unequal relationship can result between the patient and physician as the patient can express fears and feelings that might be unacceptable under different circumstances, yet that does not allow for emotional reciprocity on the part of the physician. Since most risk factors require that patients make significant changes in their health behavior or life-style, it is crucial that physicians learn the specific educational skills required to accomplish such behavior changes.

Patients often have strong opinions about the nature, cause, and treatment of their illness, and may even insist that the physician give medical care that is consistent with their beliefs. Physicians must be willing to listen to the patient, but cannot necessarily grant a patient's wishes. Such beliefs and convictions can generate physician-patient conflict.

Physicians often have contradictory expectations of their patients. Physicians like to expect their patients to be well informed about their illness so that the patients do not have to call their doctors with minor complaints or during off hours, yet the physician often expects the patient to defer entirely to their professional advice and opinion. Thus, a "double bind" is established for the patient. A double bind is a situation in which an individual (sender) gives another individual (receiver) a mixed message (e.g., an explicit communication may be disqualified or countered by a second, usually somewhat subtle, communication). One may be verbal and the other nonverbal. The receiver is said to be in a double bind, finding it impossible to respond, recognizing that whichever response is chosen, the receiver "loses" (a no-win situation).

Physicians often profess that the physician-patient relationship should be one of reciprocity and cooperation, yet the physician's behavior or expectation may insist that the patient obey instructions and defer to the physician's knowledge. Also, the physician-patient relationship can be put in conflict if the patient seeks a second opinion or if the second opinion conflicts with the original diagnosis or treatment.

Sometimes, illness makes it almost impossible for patients to maintain a normal relationship with their physician, especially when one is the parent or employee. The doctor's special knowledge and skills, when combined with the patient's dependence by being ill, leads to a situation of great power and authority in the treatment situation, further encouraging passive or dependent behavior on the part of the patient. Thus, some patients may even assume a childlike state and surrender responsibility. This poses a significant interpersonal problem, especially as physicians attempt to encourage patients to take more responsibility for their own health and rehabilitation.

GROUP PROCESSES

Attitude and Behavior Change

Attitude and behavior change can be influenced by a group because individuals are social beings and develop considerable dependence on other individuals. It has been found that the most effective means of changing attitudes in a group are by satisfying various personal and social needs, reducing unpleasant motivational states, and comparing one's own attitudes and beliefs with the attitudes and beliefs of others. The credibility of the communicator, the various communication patterns

existing in the group, and other attributes of the communicator and the situation in the group can also cause changing attitudes in groups. Persuasive facts and information are not very effective in changing attitudes and behaviors in groups.

Attitude change is more likely to occur in individuals when they are strongly attracted to a group and are more likely to be maintained under sustained attractiveness. Attitude change is also more likely to occur if an individual participates in the group discussion, opposed to being passive or only listening to a lecture. Soloman Asch research on conformity demonstrated that a majority opinion is more apt to cause an individual to change or give an erroneous response. He also showed that the power of a majority opinion can be weakened by an individual who openly disagrees with the majority. Members who are strongly attracted to the group are less likely to be influenced by communications that are inconsistent with the norms of the group.

A classic experiment demonstrating group influence is the following: In the presence of a group of judges, a person was asked to estimate the relative lengths of two lines. Before making his own estimate, he was told the result of the group's estimate. His tendency to conform to the overall group judgment increased with the number in the group, with the difficulty of the judgment, and with the status of the group members.

Group Interaction

Members of a group are more alike in their group norms, such as what they say they ought to do or be like, than in what they actually do. Social and physical environment may affect the resulting behavior, however, the norm of behavior is generally not affected. Thus, a group may show some variation in attire or the type of clothing worn, but they will still profess a strong belief or acceptance of a group norm.

Members of a group who find that group membership is especially rewarding are more likely to conform to the group's norms and values. Also, if membership in a group is particularly rewarding, individual members are less likely to seek membership in other groups.

Contrary to folk beliefs that opposites attract, it has been well validated that similarity leads to liking. In the development of friendships and liking, the following similarities appear to be of more importance than others: Physical characteristics, social status, attitudes, beliefs, and values; introverts and extraverts both prefer extraverts; similarity of ability; when disagreement is followed by agreement, more liking is produced than agreement followed by disagreement; high ability and high self-esteem individuals dislike a high ability person who blunders, but low ability and low self-esteem individuals tend to like a high ability blunderer.

The Hawthorne Effect is a term used to illustrate that research participation has been found to have a greater influence on behavior than experimental manipulations which may be involved in an investigation. It involves individuals feeling that they have been selected for special attention, which acts as a motivator in itself.

The term originated from a study done at the Hawthorne plant of the General Electric Company which demonstrated that employees involved in a special research project increased their work output more than those who did not participate, and every time a new variation was introduced and studied, production continued to increase. The investigator was unable to demonstrate that pay scales, rest periods, or working conditions had more effect on production than other changes, but did demonstrate the universality of individuals feeling that they were selected for special attention.

In groups where others are present, a psychological phenomenon of deindividuation occurs through a weakening of restraints or individual norms, and sometimes results in impulsive behavior, vandalism, violence, etc. Self-awareness is reduced and one has a decreasing ability to monitor one's own behavior. Anonymity also contributes to less self-awareness and deindividuation and thus, feelings of close group unity, high arousal, or focusing on an external event, can all contribute to deindividuation, which leads to weakened restraint or ability to regulate one's own behavior, less concern for what others may think, less rational planning and other cognitive processes, and weakened restraint against impulse behavior.

A number of studies have demonstrated that during such occasions, individuals do not block out or decrease their sensitivity to other cues in their surrounding, but actually experience an increase in sensitivity to other cues as well as their own emotional state. This is contrary to the folk belief that such group behavior blots out sensitivity and concern for one's environment or emotional condition.

The likelihood of conflict between groups in a community is increased when a minority group's position is rapidly improving, there is a rapid change in intergroup relations, there is a rapid deterioration following a period of improvement, and a minority group's position is rapidly deteriorating.

The degree of social discrimination directed by one group toward a second group increases as the retaliatory capabilities of the second group increase, is related to a history of discrimination by the first group against the second group, and is increased by the extent to which the members of the second group are easily identified.

Leadership and Performance

Group members appear to derive exceptional satisfaction from a leader who demonstrates conformance and competence in a group's major activity or responsibility.

The major responsibilities and activities of a leader are to help the group concentrate on the important goals, focus on the task to be accomplished, maintain interpersonal relations among group members, and demonstrate a commitment and motivation to the task or responsibility. Often, if a leader's motivation is perceived as being strong, he or she will frequently be permitted to vary from certain group standards or expectations.

Individuals are more effective as communicators if they are perceived as having both high expertise and credibility. In general, the more intelligent the audience, the more the audience should be encouraged to draw their own conclusions, rather than the communicator stating them explicitly.

Communicators can be more persuasive, especially when presenting a one-sided argument, when the audience starts out agreeing with the communicator, is generally friendly, or when it is important to achieve an immediate (even though temporary) opinion change.

Exercising influence on the basis of being an expert or authority may assist the task of the group, but often increases the social distance between the individual and the group members. Likewise, coercive power and authority may achieve compliance, but runs the risk of rejection of the group. A phenomenon called *referent power* appeals to the shared elements among group members and promotes closer relationships between the leader and the members of the group.

In general, the more actively an individual participates in a group, the more that individual will be perceived as a group leader. In this case, quality does not seem to be as important as quantity of participation. Quantity becomes an index of motivation in individuals who are highly motivated toward the group and are more likely to be perceived as leaders.

There is considerable literature on the effect of group size as it relates to leadership and group performance. The optimal informal group size for most effective functioning appears to be five to seven persons, however, the effect is also related to the atmosphere of the group, the satisfaction of its members, the task to be accomplished, and the amount of active work that must be done by the leader. While it is true that larger groups have more individuals who are able to contribute, they also increase the potential conflicts and social obstacles and make more demands on the leader. The important and reoccurring factor is related to the extent that the size or other factors enhance an individual gaining a sense of membership in the group.

In considering models of leadership, there is the transactional view of leadership, the situational theory, and the contingency model.

The transactional view regards leadership as a reciprocal process of social influence with leaders and followers influencing and being influenced by each other, whether the leader is regarded as legitimate or illegitimate, and whether each perceives the other in a positive or negative manner.

The situational model regards the task and the general situation or conditions as most important, rather than the personality or dynamics of the leader or the members of the group. In the situational model, the power of the leader over the group members is important.

The contingency model incorporates the leader's personal traits and certain features in the situation that influence the leadership process. It identifies task oriented authoritarian leaders and contrasts them with less authoritarian, less directive, and more relaxed leaders.

Social facilitation refers to the effect of the presence of certain individuals on the group process, sometimes facilitating or impairing the interactions or performance of the group.

Collective behavior is often used to refer to the action of individuals who happen to be at the same place at the same time and who respond to the same stimulus (e.g., persons at the scene of an accident, persons waiting for a bus or a train, persons at a sports event, etc.). Group behavior and leadership may be quite different under these conditions when compared with organized or task oriented gatherings.

Kurt Lewin worked with different styles of group leaders and found that democratic leaders performed best on task goals and maintained very high morale; authoritarian leaders were able to accomplish the task goals, but the groups had low morale; and laissez-faire leaders were least effective in accomplishing the task goals and with variable morale.

George Bavelas identified the function of the leader as planning, giving information, evaluating, arbitrating, controlling, rewarding, and punishing. He postulated that it is more important how these functions are distributed within a particular group than which person may be designated as the leader.

Howard Leavitt studied the effects of group structure on the problem solving ability and morale of groups. He found that groups with a firm hierarchical structure solved more problems more efficiently, but with less morale than democratically structured groups. In a hierarchically structured group, the members who are at the center of the communication network expressed much more satisfaction with the problem solving task, while those who were not a part of the central communication network expressed very little satisfaction.

Robert F. Baltes differentiated between the task leader (concern with getting the job done) and the sociomotive leader (concern with how people are feeling about being in the group).

Fred Fiedler developed a contingency theory of leadership effectiveness, based largely on an individual's preference for a particular leadership style or stated characteristics of the person with whom they like working with most or least. He found leader-group relations to be the most important leadership factor. He further included the type of task structure (also whether the task requirements are clear or ambiguous), and the power that is available for the leader as the three situational factors considered most important in predicting leadership effectiveness.

HEALTH CARE BEHAVIOR

Models of Health

In general, there are three basic models of health. One view of health is a dichotomy; either being present or absent. A second is the more utopian view of health (being more than the presence or absence of disease) as an ideal level of functioning, even though it may not be obtainable. The world health organization has defined health in this manner. A third model involves statistical norms so that extreme values are defined as abnormal and being healthy is to remain within a normal range. These models are contingent upon the values and social structure of a particular culture or social system.

The medical model somewhat narrowly defines health as the absence of disease, as generally identified by physical or behavioral signs or symptoms. Criteria used to determine a pathologic condition are if the problem is undesirable, if it can be treated, if it has a statistical prevalence, if it is associated with pain or discomfort, if it has a related disability, if it conflicts with environmental adaptation, and if it disrupts homeostasis. Unfortunately, most of these criteria have been interpreted as relating primarily to biological or physical signs and symptoms, often, ignoring the important behavioral dimensions that related to the specific pathology. These criteria have also resulted in more interest in pathology than in health, and a search for one cause and effect relationship. The focus of these criteria is on the pathology within the individual rather than external factors, it results in a continual search for biological causes and it assumes that one successful intervention can be applied universally.

The statistical model assumes that behavioral and biological attributes of human beings are normally distributed in any population, so that society or the health care professional can postulate how many standard deviations from the mean will be considered normal and the limits of normality at both extremes. Major problems with the statistical model are that pathology may be labeled as sick rather than unusual, the norms may not come from a representative sample of the population, all attributes may not be normally distributed in certain cultures, races, or sexes, and it forces a label of abnormality that must exist in all populations.

The social system model does not view health as an absolute, but as a relative concept which is identified and labeled according to various cultural values and social norms. In this way, health is defined as a part of a social status as well as biological status, and health is viewed according to an individual's capacities and according to group attributes. This allows for a wide range of responses to the same sign or symptom. Problems with this model relate to differentiating between a person as being sick and another as being eccentric or sinful. The ability of the larger social system to establish a health deviation, the effects of individual beliefs or subcultural norms, and inability to perform everyday roles may result in labeling (e.g., problem drinkers may not be regarded as ill or needing help until they become an alcoholic).

Studies of public beliefs about health show health to be a multidimensional concept. Many people have a view of health that is quite different from the traditional medical model, in that conceptions of health are an admixture of folk beliefs, mass media assertions, spiritual beliefs, and lay understandings and misunderstandings of scientific medicine. Very often, the physician and the patient do not share basic assumptions about disease, the meaning of symptoms, what is necessary to reach a diagnosis, or the reasonableness of treatment.

Andrew Twaddle developed a three dimension taxonomy of health and nonhealth. First, one must consider the disease or the biological state of the person; second, illness or the person's subjective feeling state must be considered; and third, sickness as a behavioral status or social role may be involved. Changes in health do not occur simultaneously across these dimensions (e.g., a person can be hypertensive but not feel ill or act sick; a person may have a common cold, may feel ill but not act sick; or if attempting to avoid a situation, a person may act sick without feeling ill). While this might seem a bit complicated, all three facets must be considered in understanding health because they all have a direct affect on behavior.

An interactionist orientation attempts to deal with two sets of forces impinging upon behavior (i.e., "inside" forces such as personality, cognition, attitudes, beliefs, and motives, and "outside" influences arising from situational, environmental, and group involvements).

Personal attitudes and behavior have at least three components: Cognitions or beliefs and ideas that a person thinks are attributes of an object, person, behavior, or idea (e.g., thinking or believing that smoking is related to the onset of lung cancer, is expensive, offends nonsmokers, etc.); the affective or evaluative component of the attitude whereby feelings, emotions, value, or importance, accompany the cognitions attributed to the object (e.g., having negative feelings toward smoking because of the link between the habit and the disease); and the cognitive component linked to the affect, whereby behavioral tendencies are linked to the affect or feeling involved (e.g., one may have strong feelings about unhealthy, expensive, or socially offensive acts, therefore, they do not smoke). While the affective component is considered to be the most important, it is also the most difficult to change. Many studies now associate cognitions with beliefs and affect with attitudes. All individuals are constantly processing information and actively seeking to construct a comprehensive view of a predictable world. By studying beliefs, values, and attitudes, scientists have attempted to link an individual's view of the world to the way he behaves.

Personal beliefs and attitudes are acquired from our perceptions of common sense or cultural truisms in our everyday experience, by observing our own behavior as well as the behavior of others, from social norms transmitted during a socialization process, from feedback from other people about beliefs and attitudes, from our experience in formal education, and through the mass media. Our membership in groups or association with peers seems to exert the most pressure, whereby other individuals provide us with a frame of reference to compare and evaluate our own reactions to objects, persons, behaviors, ideas, etc. Behavioral scientists have established that the relationships between beliefs, attitudes, and behavior are much less predictable than would be expected. In summary, beliefs and attitudes are hypothetical constructs that represent what a person believes about something and his or her feelings toward it, and one must look at the effects of social relationships and external pressures as well as the situational context in which the behavior occurs.

Inconsistencies between attitudes people express and their actual behavior can be accounted for on the basis that behavior may be more related to norms, expectations, and situational demands rather than attitudes, attitudes are frequently measured unprecisely or they often measure an orientation toward a general category, while behavioral assessments most often involve only one facet of that category, and some individuals measure more inconsistently than others as a matter of personal belief or style.

Historically, it has been known that attitudes do affect behavior, but most recently it has been demonstrated that behavior also affects attitudes. Indeed, it has been postulated that the best way to change an attitude is to induce a behavioral change. Daryl Bem developed a "self-perception" theory. He stated that one does not eat chocolate because one likes it, but one eats chocolate; therefore, one infers one's attitudes from one's own behavior.

Leon Festinger developed a theory of cognitive dissonance (described earlier) which stated that when two or more "cognitive elements" (beliefs, opinions, knowledge, etc.) conflict, the inconsistency sets up a dissonance which is unpleasant and motivates the individual to attempt to resolve or reduce the dissonance. This often results in the individual emphasizing the positive aspects of a chosen alternative and the negative aspects of the unchosen alternative. Cognitive dissonance can also be reduced by attempting to downgrade the importance of a decision or action.

Clark Hull and Kenneth Spence were responsible for several theories of attitude change. In general, they postulated that the strength of any response (attitude) depended on the interaction of habit, strength, drive, incentive motivation (rewards), and inhibitory potential (fatigue).

Illness Behavior

Historically, illness has been regarded as constituting a relatively infrequent, unusual, or abnormal experience. However, more recent studies have documented, through the use of health diaries in populations considered to be healthy, the presence of clinically serious problems is the norm. For example, the frequency of 12 annoying symptoms (headache, upset stomach, sore muscles, chest pains, nasal congestion, watering eyes, ringing in ears, racing heart, dizziness, flushed face, sweating hands, and shortness of breath) was 80 percent at any one time. Thus, illness should be regarded as an every day typical experience. This also raises the possibility that the treated cases are actually only the tip of a clinical iceberg, considering that only a small number of health problems ever result in seeking professional care. Physicians must understand the dynamics involved in the patient's recognition of the presence of symptoms (i.e., the bodily changes and interpretation that patients place on their likely significance). The presence of symptoms alone does not result in the seeking of medical care, even though patients may be aware that the delay of reporting certain symptoms could be quite serious.

The illness behavior that occurs before an individual becomes a patient is just as important to recognize and understand, as is the behavior associated with various illnesses. Thus, it is important to identify the psychological and social factors that influence how individuals per-

ceive and evaluate the significance of their physical and behavioral symptoms.

Psychological and Sociological Perspectives

A major psychological model is called attribution theory. The purpose is to explain how people use such basis as their own information, feelings, and beliefs to make causal inferences or attributions about various types of personal or interpersonal events (signs, symptoms, etc.) they observe. Thus, we attribute certain explanations to the perceived changes and these attributions influence our behavior. Each of us has developed an extensive repertoire of information and beliefs about cause and effect relationships, and we apply these explanations, or search for new explanations, when there are unexpected changes. We also have a tendency to link a cause with an effect whenever the two appear together. It is important to determine why people react so differently to the same type of illness, change, or symptom, and to recognize that individual characteristics must also take into account group and situational influences.

Sociological research has tended to focus more on differences between population subgroups than individual differences. Historically, much emphasis has been placed on social differences found in social class, ethnicity, religion, age, geographic residence, and sex. However, it is important to recognize that social factors such as sex roles, cultural conditioning, etc., do change over time (e.g., the growth of the woman's movement may be narrowing traditional sex role differences). The influence of cultural conditioning with the same type of medical problems has been well documented (e.g., patients raised in an Irish culture tend to exhibit more denial of pain and its personal effects, while patients raised in an Italian culture tend to be more expressive and expansive in their description of their condition and how it affects their daily activities).

Studies of lower social class individuals show them to be more concerned about their health, but also to appear to exhibit greater tolerance of symptoms. However, one must bear in mind that the types of every day pressures and lack of financial resources of lower income persons may mean that such tolerance may not be volitional. This is illustrated by the following report of a poor woman:

I wish I really knew what you mean about being sick. . . . sometimes I've felt so bad I could curl up and die, but had to go on because the kids had to be taken care of, and, besides, we didn't have the money to spend for the doctor. . . . How could I be sick? How do you know when you're sick anyway? Some people can go to bed most any time with anything, but most of us can't be sick . . . even when we need to be. (David Mechanic)

The group based social norms of sex, ethnicity, religion, and social class are learned behaviors, primarily through the socialization process, and are socio-cultural factors which influence how people react to health changes or to the onset of symptoms. It is important to keep in mind that the variation within such groups is often much greater than it is between groups.

A third dimension in explaining illness beliefs and behavior is to recognize that transient and personal and situational factors often have a powerful and sometimes overriding effect on behavior or interpretation of symptoms. For example, psychological distress or anxiety can increase one's concern about health, perceived susceptibility, and the possible consequences of specific symptoms or disease. Also, intense participation in some activity or crisis often deters attention to symptoms.

The coping model of David Mechanic focuses on 10 "contingencies" or dimensions of an illness experience that influence subsequent behavior and interpretation of physiological and behavioral changes. Michael Counte summarizes the 10 criteria as: (1) Symptom salience (how apparent and dramatic is the change); (2) perceived seriousness (how familiar is the symptom); (3) behavioral interference (role disruption); (4) symptom frequency and persistence (does it go away?); (5) tolerance threshold of the person and obervers; (6) cognitive appraisal (information known about the symptom); (7) denial needs (often resulting from psychological anxiety); (8) competing needs (health needs and other goals); (9) alternative interpretations (other attributions available other than disease); and (10) perception of treatment accessibility (personal and social costs, effort required, and cultural barriers). An important aspect of this model is that it entertains the possibility that numerous explanations (other people, and social, psychological, and situational factors) could explain the symptoms rather than those believed by health care professionals.

Another dimension that should be considered in understanding illness behavior is to determine the possible benefits a person can derive from being defined as ill. This is known as secondary gain and is often used by an individual to obtain various benefits, most often in a manipulative fashion. Examples might be fabricating or exaggerating symptoms to collect a claim from an insurance company or workman's compensation, make claims on another person's time or attention, or developing an acceptable reason for social, personal, or occupational failure or inadequate performance.

In summary, many individuals respond quite differently to the same physiological stimulus or health deviation, and the basis of this response is more complex than considered in the past. We also know that many annoying symptoms of illness are quite prevalent even within the general population considered to be healthy. One

must then understand the conditions under which various symptoms are defined as serious enough to seek assistance from others. The physician must be able to determine the psychological framework used by patients to attribute various causes to unexpected physiological changes and their underlying beliefs concerning cause-and-effect relations regarding their health. We also know that sociocultural factors such as sex, ethnicity, religion, and social class shape socialization experiences, resulting in a tendency to exhibit responses that are typical of the group in general; recognizing that these differences sometimes change over time; that various coping strategies relate directly to symptom attributes, psychological states (e.g., anxiety), and situational and social influences. Thus, the physician must determine the patients current psychological state and the context within which the symptoms are experienced.

A person's response to the onset of an illness may be a function of attributes of the symptom (e.g., visibility, pain, incapacitating), a person's current psychological state (e.g., level of anxiety, depression, etc.), the interpersonal responsibilities and pressures (e.g., occupational, family, etc.), and the interaction between each of these three factors. The physician must assess each of these factors to understand an individual patient's reaction to illness, that these reactions eminate from social roles and expectations, and that how an individual reacts to symptoms can have a significant impact upon the ultimate course of the condition or disease, the type of health care or assistance selected, and the specific role behaviors of the patient during treatment. These factors can be considered as prepatient role behavior or how people behave before being defined as sick.

The Sick Role

Talcott Parsons described the sick role and the role expectations that must exist for the American society to accept an individual as sick as the following: (1) The sick person should not be able to be blamed for his or her problems, but is the victim of forces beyond their control; (2) the sick person is excused or not expected to fulfill the usual obligations that accompany their "well roles" in the family, school, or job; (3) the sick person is expected to obtain professional assistance if the illness is defined as a serious problem; and (4) the sick person is expected to participate and cooperate in the treatment process. This translates into two rights (i.e., not being blamed and exemption from well roles) and into two responsibilities (i.e., seeking aid and participating in the treatment).

In order to understand health care seeking behavior and health care utilization, it is useful to consider five interrelated stages of behavior that occur when one develops a health problem: (1) Recognition of symptoms or physical changes, with accompanying emotional effects and cognitive interpretations; (2) the person begins to obtain the advice of others, sometimes referred to as the "lay referral structure" so as to decide what to do, and usually begins to make behavioral adjustments in order to assume the sick role; (3) the individual then seeks assistance from the health care system; (4) the treatment stage consists of the person occupying a dependent-patient role; and (5) the recovery or rehabilitation phase in which the person returns to the "well role" or, occasionally, the "role of the chronic invalid." Very often what happens at one stage is likely to influence the other stages. Models to describe health care utilization are designated as sociocultural, demographic, psychological distress, and the health belief model.

A major dimension of the sociocultural factors in the use of medical services is the lay referral structure whereby a person acquires the support and reassurance of others in the family or group before recognizing or accepting illness, relinquishing social responsibilities, and seeking medical care. Thus, the decision to seek medical care is both personal and consensual within the family or valued referents. The decision to seek medical care is also shaped by social preferences which have their origin in cultural values and norms that one learns through the socialization process. The degree of cultural similarity between the person and the prospective health care professional is an important factor in determining whether health care help will be sought.

Among demographic variables in the utilization of health services is social class. There is a chronically low utilization rate of lower income persons for at least three major reasons (i.e., inadequate financial resources, more alienation from society and its institutions, and systematic barriers encountered by the poor when they attempt to utilize the medical care system, such as greater distance from medical facilities, long waits, depersonalization of health care providers, fragmented services, and lack of understanding as to how to use the system). Even when financial barriers are removed, certain social and psychological dimensions continue to impede utilization of health care facilities. Thus, changing the health beliefs and attitudes of the poor have become important goals for health care planners.

The psychological distress model places emphasis on certain characteristics of the individual and the interaction of the social and the psychological processes, such as stress, distress, anxiety, etc. The development of models of primary care must examine more than the patient's complaint. It must also consider why the patient has sought care at this particular time, what is expected from the consultation, and what does he believe to be the cause of the symptoms. The physician must know the

events that preceded the psychological distress and explore a person's capacities to cope with such problems.

The health belief model asserts that there are basically six important factors that influence health behavior: (1) The person's level of health motivation of value of health; (2) the person's perceived vulnerability or susceptibility to health problems; (3) the person's evaluation of the consequences or of the severity of the health problem; (4) the person's evaluation of the benefits likely to be achieved by seeking aid; (5) the economic, social, physical, and/or psychological costs of seeking health care; and (6) the cues or critical incidents in one's life, such as the occurrence of symptoms, mass media appeals, death or sickness of family members or friends, or advice of family members or friends. These health beliefs moderate other social, demographic, cultural, and individual factors. The health belief model has been recently expanded to include more general system models which include additional dimensions, such as constraints on utilization ranging from individual health beliefs and attitudes to social, structural, and organizational factors of supply and accessibility.

Patient Compliance

Compliance can be defined as patient behavior in which the patient adheres to a program of treatment as prescribed by a medical authority. Compliance is also referred to as cooperation, therapeutic alliance, or adherence. Many health professionals do not like to use the word compliance because of its authoritarian or regimented inferences, but it has become a term of common usage both in practice, teaching, and research settings.

It is estimated that about 50 percent of patients comply with scheduled follow-up appointments and with taking prescribed medicines. Studies of rates of noncompliance range from 30–50 percent depending upon the types of actions being assessed and who is being asked (e.g., doctors have a tendency to overestimate compliance). The impacts of noncompliance are great. A direct impact of noncompliance is the detrimental effect it has on the treatment program which may lead to the need for additional treatment and increased costs. Indirect impacts of low rates of compliance may include a disruptive effect on the patient/doctor relationship and may interfere with evaluation of clinical trials in health research, distorting the results.

The major approaches to the study of compliance/noncompliance are related to the social and psychological bases of compliance behavior. In studying noncompliance, investigators have applied these bases to the characteristics of the patient, special aspects of the treatment, characteristics of the disease, interaction of patients and clinicians, and characteristics of the health care system.

Social bases of compliance have found group values, pressures for conformity, normative behavior, and situational factors to be especially relevant. For example, a medication resulting in a side effect of occasional impotence will affect compliance differently for elderly widowers, compared with young bachelors. Likewise, individuals who rely on folk healers may feel a conflict between their usual reliance on folk remedies and the medicines prescribed by a doctor. Lower adherence is commonly found among young adults and the elderly. Unfortunately, attempting to explain conformance or noncomformance on the basis of individuals belonging to certain social groups is not always of great help for the single physician attempting to explain the behavior of a single patient. While such studies help determine much about the process, they most frequently describe intergroup differences rather than individuals, and there is often as much variation within social groups as there is between them. Therefore, if one looks hard enough compliars and noncompliars can be found in almost any subgroup of age, education, race, ethnicity, etc. in the population.

In general, there are five types of psychological explanations which can be involved in understanding individual compliance behavior: (1) A personality trait in which an individual may be reticent to go along with any recommendation from another person (a sort of obstinacy or a noncooperative "way of life"), (2) a psychodynamic approach asserting that compliance or noncompliance behavior is influenced by underlying unconscious processes, (3) a social reinforcement explanation in which a person does not comply because they do not receive consistent positive reinforcement to establish and continue the new pattern of behavior, (4) a cognitive approach in which an individual patient may attribute certain side effects or other problems to the medication, and (5) a coping approach which may invoke personal denial when a person is told that a disease is present, but the patient is not willing to accept the diagnosis.

Any understanding of compliance/noncompliance must not only incorporate the traditional bases of individual and social factors, but must also focus on the relationships and interactions between patients and health care providers.

Health care providers are often unaware of the emotional impact of many of their "matter of fact" statements which can produce a high level of anxiety and even block the patient's subsequent learning. The phenomenon of data overload can take place when a patient receives an excessive amount of information at one time without any checking for comprehension. Communication obstacles can be produced by the use of technical jargon and lack of specificity. At least five types of social power are often present in the doctor-patient interaction: (1) reward power where the physician may reward a patient and decrease negative sanctions in order to gain cooperation; (2) coercive power where the physician attempts to gain cooperation by using negative sanctions such as disapproval; (3) expert power where physicians may emphasize professional status and knowledge, also creating greater social distance between the doctor and the patient; (4) legitimate power focusing on the patient's obligation to cooperate with the treatment recommendations; and (5) referent power in which the physician may develop a more supportive relationship based on a feeling of friendship. Physicians often use one or more of these different types of interpersonal influence or power to obtain cooperation from their patients. Unfortunately, many physicians develop an excessive dependence on the first four more impersonal types of social power. When the social distance is decreased between the physician and the patient, the therapeutic alliance is facilitated.

Studies have been reported that the greater the amount of information provided by a physician, the higher the level of satisfaction and compliance. Also, the more explicit a physician is in the communication, the greater the compliance and satisfaction. Blue-collar workers and lower socioeconomic status patients often receive less information than upper socioeconomic status patients because they tend to be more passive, do not ask questions, and physicians often underestimate their desire and ability to handle medical information.

Three major recommendations have emerged from compliance/noncompliance studies. One is the importance of having physician knowledge of a patient's lifestyle, belief, attitudes, and behaviors, to anticipate the likelihood of certain compliance problems (e.g., a child may be given an antibiotic intramuscularly when compliance will be low). Second, by understanding a patient's capacities and frame of reference, one can anticipate certain communication barriers, including the expectations of outcome held by the patient and the physician. Third, the physician should make every attempt to ensure that the patient comprehends the information presented during the doctor-patient interaction.

An important enabling variable has been identified as the person's "locus of control" which is an indication of the extent to which a patient may believe that he or she can control events and consequences, as opposed to the control being delegated to chance or fate.

Another summary suggests five ways a physician can improve adherence to a treatment program are the following: (1) Social support to the patient while in treatment, including questions and concerns about the treatment, and assisting in a continuous not fragmented manner; (2) recognize that patients often have motives that compete with the treatment regimen and that the motives must be taken into account (i.e., physicians must get into the frame of reference of their patient); (3) the treatment regimen should be simplified as much as possible, perhaps starting off with a more simplified regimen and gradually adding more steps; (4) making certain that the patient fully comprehends the instructions, procedures, and likely side effects; and (5) physicians should measure their own personal success in securing compliance by periodically monitoring patient compliance using the best methods at their disposal to validate individual compliance.

Changing Health Beliefs and Attitudes

Social norms and personal attitudes are powerful influences on people's life-style, health status, and interaction with the health care providers and the health care system. In attempting to change health behavior it has been assumed that the most powerful force to effect the change, would be to change the attitudes of greatest relevance to the behavior in question. It is also recognized that there are a number of normal processes which activate resistance to change. Specific techniques for attitude change that have been tested include the cognitive consistency model, functional model, persuasive communications model, and group influence model.

The cognitive consistency model recognizes that attitudes are comprised of cognitive, evaluative, and behavioral components. Thus, attitudes, beliefs, and behavior tend to fit together, so that if a person has a fear of contracting cancer, and they believe that birth control pills cause cancer, then they will not use birth control pills. The cognitive consistency explanation is that the attitude change process is one of rationalization and that people are motivated to be and to appear consistent. If the attitude change strategy can arouse a state of inconsistency or dissonance, the individual will tend to try to resolve the inconsistency by developing a rationalization or a change of behavior. New attitudes and beliefs often emerge in order to rationalize new behaviors that people engage in. When a person tries a new behavior and they are not forced to do so, an attitude or belief change often follows in order to reestablish a state of consistency. Role playing is frequently used as a technique of constructing a natural setting for attitude change.

Functional models of attitude change tend to focus on the function that an attitude may provide for an individual, so that when the usefulness of an attitude no longer exists, the individual concludes that a change of attitude may be more useful. Examples are that when an attitude maximizes rewards and minimizes punishment, or when an attitude helps protect an individual from an unpleasant truth about themselves (e.g., prejudice or projection), or provide new information which can sometimes bring about change or sometimes help an individual express their basic values by proclaiming to the world what kind of a person they are.

Persuasive communications is another model for attitude change that attempts to modify attitudes through mass media and other communication techniques. The acceptance of the new opinion or attitude is contingent upon the incentives or rewards that are being suggested by the communication. Persuasive communication is perhaps one of the most frequently employed methods of changing attitudes through written, visual, and audio media. Some conclusions from the use of the persuasive communications model to change attitude are that the similarity of the communicator (e.g., race, sex, age) enhances attitude change; the higher the perceived credibility of the source, the greater the attitude change; a one-sided argument appears to be more effective when an audience lacks knowledge whereas a two-sided message is more effective for knowledgeable audiences; when fear is incorporated into the message (e.g., fear of cancer, alcoholism, venereal disease, or being crushed on a steering wheel), it can produce a "boomerang effect," since attempts to control fear may override attempts to cope with an attitude change; face-to-face attempts are more successful than other approaches with written appeals being one of the lowest persuasive in changing attitudes; the higher the self-esteem of the receiver, the more difficult to change attitudes; and the more that a person is personally involved in an issue, the more difficult it is to modify their attitudes.

Group influence on attitude change is especially powerful, since people tend to compare their attitudes and beliefs to those of other members of their group. High status in a group may result in increased filtering or blocking of messages or information that is dissonant with group values and facilitate messages or information that are consonant. Thus, a leader of Alcoholics Anonymous may not allow a lecture on the use of self-control in moderation drinking, because the message does not fit the values of the group, or social pressures may be exerted in groups to ensure uniformity through self-imposed rules or ethics to force individuals to conform to the norms or values of a reference group.

The changing of health related beliefs and attitudes can be illustrated through two different studies attempting to modify health beliefs and health behavior. One study involved aiming persuasive communication at different levels of perceived vulnerability to cervical cancer among ghetto women. The experimental group exposed to a health education program consisted of stressing the danger of the health problem and the value of seeking professional check-ups on a regular basis.

They found that communication actually served as a trigger or cue to action for those who felt vulnerable and that check-up behavior was more apt to follow if there were situational conveniences such as free taxi and a free babysitter. Another study attempted to change beliefs about the dangers of heart disease, cancer, and tuberclerosis with a group of primarily female university employees, using a health education program stressing the danger of the health problem and the value of seeking professional exams on a regular basis. The researchers were able to change perceived susceptibility and perceived benefits of action and persuaded a greater number of individuals to obtain a check-up, but they were still not successful in changing personal health habits. This is consistent with other research where health beliefs and attitudes, but not health habits, may be altered. Thus, life-style, which is a group of personal behavior habits, is not easily modifiable, even though the health beliefs and the consequences are clearly visible.

A classic three-year community health education study was conducted by Stanford University to determine if a "total push" multiple factor health education campaign could reduce cardiovascular risk factors (i.e., reduce weight, increase exercise, stop smoking, and change to salt-free, fat-free, etc. diets). One community was exposed to a large-scale mass media campaign, another community received the mass media campaign coupled with behavioral modification training of individuals who were identified with high risk of cancer, and a third community served as a control. In both experimental communities cigarette smoking was significantly decreased, including decreases in egg consumption and levels of cholesterol, however, the community receiving the mass media campaign plus the behavioral modification training achieved the most impressive changes. It was concluded that health behavior can be changed in natural settings. They were also able to document the power of significant countervailing pressures in American society; pressures that promote smoking and eating nonnutritional foods. Also, the countervailing force of our high automotive society producing a sedentary state. New knowledge of health values, beliefs, and behaviors and the new technology that is being created to change those health related behaviors and life-styles may allow physicians to help individual patients to change.

Ethnomedicine

Ethnocentrism is the tendency for one to consider one's own group, or way of life (usually national or ethnic) to be superior to other groups and judging other groups against the frame of reference of one's own group. Since American families live in relative isolation from persons of different cultures, they are often considered ethnocentric. This can also cause Americans to have a rather narrow view of marriage and family life.

In determining ethnic differences in response to pain, it has been demonstrated that there are no ethnic differences in the threshold for the sensation of pain, however, there are highly variable differences in ethnic response to pain, which are conditioned by cultural factors. The major factors accounting for these differences in response to pain are the significance and traditions of emotionalism or stoicism regarding pain.

Symptoms, notably pain, are differentially experienced and communicated by people of various cultural backgrounds; and physician's diagnoses and treatments have been shown to be affected by the socioeconomic class and the cultural background of the patient.

People from the upper socioeconomic classes are faster in recognizing symptoms and in seeking professional care than those from the lower socioeconomic classes. Also, willingness to pay for medical services increases with the level of socioeconomic class.

There have been a number of pain response studies among different American ethnic groups. When comparing pain response for disorders of equivalent objective severity, they have established that American Italians and Jews are more likely to be open and vocal about their discomfort than Americans of Irish or "old American" descent (several generations born in the United States); Italians appear to focus more on the pain itself, while the Jews worried more about what the pain meant or might mean for the future; Irish tended to deny the existence of the pain, while "old Americans" tended to provide a detailed description of the pain in a somewhat detached or scientific manner.

As compared to middle and upper socioeconomic classes, conditions seen more commonly in lower socioeconomic classes include behavior disorders, schizophrenia, and alcoholism. Manic-depressive illness is not seen more commonly in lower socioeconomic classes.

Chinese-American medicine postulates the basic symbols of yin and yang. Each person is considered to have a vital life force, within which there is a conflict between the cold forces of yin and the hot of yang through foods and herbals as the basis of many medical treatments in Chinese-American medicine.

Curanderismo is a Mexican-American conception of disease that attempts to identify certain imbalances of heat and cold within the body and relates these imbalances through the cause of specific diseases or illnesses. Cold illnesses, such as measles or an ear infection, are cured with hot foods, such as rice, pork, beans, onions, etc. Hot illnesses, such as bleeding or skin disorders use cold foods, such as lamb, corn, tortillas, cow's milk, and oatmeal as cures. Foods and herbs are categorized as hot or cold on the basis of their relationship to hot and cold forces believed to be within the body.

Curanderos carry on their solo practice, and they are respected and valued by their patients because they reflect and reinforce the culture of the barrio, which is the community. The healer is literally one of the people with the same value system, norms, and belief in certain symbols. Thus, a close healer-patient relationship is developed; one that is all too rare in western scientific medicine.

PERSONALITY

Attempts to characterize certain personalities as typical of individuals with certain diseases, such as asthma, ulcers, hypertension, etc., have received much attention historically, but have been generally invalid. Nevertheless, psychological factors are important and have been documented in most diseases. For example, boys with bronchial asthma have most frequently demonstrated a high level of dependency, where they look to others, particularly their mothers, for protection and on whom they are dependent. Thereby, an attack of bronchial asthma can be precipitated in some individual on whom they are dependent. Studies have demonstrated that about 50 percent of all asthmatic attacks are triggered or precipitated by anticipated or actual separation from an individual on whom he or she is dependent.

In another example, persons with urticaria, or hives tend to perceive themselves as being helpless or powerless. Also, psychogenic hyperthyroidism, which is more common in women than in men, is frequently precipitated by an individual's concern over loss of individuals dependent on them, such as familial dependents, especially children. Therefore, an overdependency on being needed can be a precipitating factor. There are also a number of studies showing that rheumatoid arthritis involves various psychogenic components. For example, the profile of such an individual is more apt to reflect someone who is more righteous, rigid, moral, conforming, and conscientous. Studies of their parents tend to reflect a more domineering and rigid management of conflict.

While there is no migraine personality, empirical research on personality traits clearly associates migraine headaches with a so-called driving personality and compulsiveness along with a tendency to be ambitious, a perfectionist, efficient, orderly, somewhat inflexible, and cautious.

Theodore Adorno and his co-workers developed a measure of authoritarian personality which they called the F-scale (for facism). They found a number of personality characteristics to conform with individuals scoring high on the F-scale. These characteristics included rigidity in thinking, focusing on status differences between themselves and others, strict with subordinates, but differential to superiors, and demonstrating considerable prejudice toward ethnic and minority groups. High scores on the F-scale measuring authoritarian personality have been linked to prejudice behavior. Thomas Pettigrew conducted a classic study demonstrating that prejudice behavior cannot be explained or predicted by the authoritarian personality measures alone because social norms and expectations appear to be even more important than attitudes or personality. Again, it is insufficient to attempt to change attitudes as a means of changing, understanding, or predicting behavior. While the F-scale is rarely used today, it did represent a classic study that began to explore the personality of prejudiced individuals.

David McClelland and others have reported a behavioral cluster for adult men with high power motives (achievement motivation), to include driving highly maneuverable cars, heavy drinking of alcohol, and engaging in exploitative sexual relationships. They also postulate that these behaviors become more severe when attainment of power is blocked. They also differentiate between personal power v social power, so that individuals with a high need for personal power are more concerned with obtaining obedience from others and exhibit more aggressive behavior while persons with a high need for social power tend to facilitate socially constructive behavior in other people and are less competitive.

Type A Behavioral Pattern

There are many behavioral factors related to the incidence and risk of cardiovascular disease, especially diet, smoking, obesity, exercise, stress, and life-style. Raymond Rosenman and Milton Friedman have described and linked a behavior pattern associated with high coronary risk. They labeled it Type A behavior pattern and contrasted it with Type B behavior pattern which is associated with a low coronary risk. A Type A person or personality exhibits the following behaviors: (1) Speaks with explosive accent on key words and tends to speed up toward the end of sentences; (2) moves, talks, and eats rapidly; (3) is impatient with how slowly people, cars, and events move; (4) feels a sense of urgency, particularly time urgency; (5) often does or thinks about two or more things at once; (6) is highly competitive; (7) feels hostile and sometimes threatened by other Type A's; (8) prefers to talk rather than listen; (9) has difficulty or feels some guilt when attempting to relax; (10) is preoccupied with getting v being; (11) has difficulty seeing the most important or most interesting or beautiful things that should be enjoyed; (12) has habitual gestures or tics (e.g., clenching fist, teeth grinding); and (13) is afraid to stop hurrying; believing that hurrying leads to success.

Type B persons are generally free of Type A habits and traits, not generally hostile or competitive, able to play and relax without guilt, and work calmly. While these behavior patterns are more a matter of degree rather than true typology, studies have shown Type A men to be almost three times as likely to develop coronary heart disease as Type B men. When one combines the Type A behavior patterns with other behavioral risk factors, such as smoking, diet, obesity, stress, or a sedentary life-style, the risk of coronary heart disease becomes even greater.

There are also a number of physiological correlates of persons with Type A behavior patterns, for example, elevated serum cholesterol and triglycerides, higher ratios of low density lipoproteins, accelerated blood co-agulation, increased daytime excretion of catechol-amines, and increased blood pressure. These changes usually occur prior to the onset of clinical signs of coro-nary heart disease.

If one lists the 10 major causes of death in the United States (heart disease, malignant neoplasms, cerebrovas-cular diseases, accidents, influenza and pneumonia, dia-betes, liver cirrhosis, arteriosclerosis, suicide, and var-ious causes of infant mortality), behavior is implicated as playing a major role in half of them (heart disease, acci-dents, cirrhosis, arteriosclerosis and suicide) and often a major or minor role in the other half. Thus, individual behavior and life-style (long-term patterns of behavior) are related to over 50 percent of the major causes of death. These behaviors are now recognized as behavioral risk factors and include cigarette smoking, dietary habits, reckless driving, nonadherence to medication, excessive consumption of alcohol, maladaptive re-sponses to social pressures, and use of illicit drugs.

Each year in the United States, almost two million deaths are caused by cardiovascular diseases, cancers, accidents, violence, diabetes, cirrhosis, and respiratory diseases. Seventy-five percent of all deaths are caused by three categories of disease or conditions; heart disease and stroke account for 42 percent, cancer accounts for 22 percent, and accidents and violence account for 11 percent.

If one calculates the average number of years of life lost for each person who died of the top three "killers," it has been determined that almost 12 years of life were lost for each person who died of cardiovascular disease, almost 27 years lost for each person who died of cancer, and almost 36 years for each person who died by acci-dent, poisoning, or violence. Automobile accident deaths have been designated as being of epidemic pro-portions among adolescents and young adults.

All of these diseases or conditions have a significant

life-style component both in terms of causes and preven-tion. Intervention through behavior change is assuming increased importance; however, it is also known that individuals often find it very difficult to change their life-styles, even when they clearly know the risks of not changing. Physicians must become more sensitive to and aware of which behavioral changes are potentially bene-ficial and how such behavioral changes can be accom-plished. In terms of expensive hospitalization costs, a recent hospital study showed that 31 to 69 percent of high-cost patients had at least one high-risk habit of alcohol abuse, smoking, nonadherence to treatment, or overeating to obesity, while only 20 to 45 percent of lower-cost patients had one or more of these high-risk habits.

It has been estimated that the one change that would do more than any other to improve the health of the nation would be to eliminate cigarette smoking. Both mortality and morbidity rates are considerably greater for smokers than for nonsmokers. Furthermore, the risk is consistently increased for both men and women with increasing daily doses of cigarettes. Smoking during pregnancy doubles the risk of low birth weight, and we also know that mortality in the first year of life is 20 times as great for low birth weight infants. Other hazards during the prenatal period have been discussed in other sections of this chapter.

Most smokers begin smoking during adolescence or as young adults. Even though smoking is a difficult behav-ior to change, most successful prevention programs in-clude the active involvement of young people in devel-oping strategies to help each other to avoid the pressures to smoke as found in peers, media, and adults. About 60 percent of regular smokers say that they have tried to quit (but failed) and another 30 percent say that they want to quit. Since smoking is a powerful addiction, the physician must consider the social, psychological, cul-tural, and behavioral factors as well as the pharmacologi-cal, physiological, and neurochemical factors involved (e.g., while nicotine appears to be a prominent pharma-cologic reinforcer, behavioral factors are prominently involved in the initiation of the smoking habit and in the day-to-day fluctuations in smoking).

Unhealthy dietary habits can seriously damage health. The adverse consequences of excess consumption are reflected in the finding that if an individual is 20 to 30 percent overweight, their mortality is 20 to 40 percent greater than for individuals of average weight, and if an individual is 50 to 60 percent overweight, the mortality is 150 to 250 percent greater. In general, obesity increases the risk of most disease, but particularly the risk of hy-pertension, diabetes, hyperlipidemia, heart disease, and cardiovascular disease. Even though much attention has been given to the overconsumption of calories and the resulting obesity, there is an equal concern for the consumption of the type of foods, for example, fats (especially saturated fats), cholesterol, salt, food preservatives, sugar, and pollutants.

It has been estimated that 10 million adult men and women in the United States are heavy drinkers, consuming an average of four drinks per day. For teenagers, the estimate is 3.5 million heavy drinkers, consuming five or more drinks per drinking occasion. Teenager consumption of alcohol appears to be increasing. It is also known that mortality is 2.5 times greater for heavy drinkers, with the greatest increase in mortality among younger alcoholics. Sixty to 80 percent of alcohol-related deaths are due to cirrhosis of the liver. The consumption of alcohol is also directly related to accidents, suicides, and homicides. Alcohol is also associated with cancer, particularly of the esophagus and mouth, with primary liver cancer almost exclusively attributed to alcohol consumption. People who drink and smoke have even greater increases in esophageal cancer rates. About 80 percent of 12 to 17 year olds report having had a drink, more than half drink at least once a month, and nearly 3 percent drink daily. Nearly 80 percent of male high school seniors drink at least once a month and more than 6 percent drink daily.

Reactions to Stress

Stress research has included research on physiological systems through which stress affects bodily function, and research on how individuals cope with stress. Some of the more exciting research involves understanding the nervous system. There is a rapidly expanding number of neuroregulators being identified as well as studies on the coordinated responses of the nervous and endocrine systems to stressors. The links between being exposed to a stressor and developing a disease are being demonstrated.

The other dimension of stress research involves identifying successful and unsuccessful coping patterns, and attempting to apply this knowledge to the prevention of disease and promotion of health by helping people to improve their coping strategies. This involves the application of basic learning principles, such as operant conditioning, social learning, and cognitive problem solving. Coping mechanisms attempt to resolve conflicts in socially or personally effective ways, for example, by confronting the problem, generating possible solutions, securing more information, getting help, and allowing oneself or others to take action to eliminate the undesirable behavior or condition causing the conflict. Coping generally attempts to change either the condition or behavior or both. Defense mechanisms *v* coping mechanisms generally do as the word implies; they "defend"

the individual and do not generally change behavior or resolve conflict.

Life change events of predictable and unpredictable nature are a normal part of human existence. However, these events may produce life stress that exceeds an individual's coping ability. This stress can then become a major factor in the onset of a wide variety of physical and mental illnesses and can also increase the severity of existing symptoms. Therefore, physicians must be alert to life changes in the lives of their patients.

Stress conditions can induce significant increases in blood pressure, plasma potassium, plasma sodium, plasma aldosterone, ACTH, and renin-angiotensin. The secretion of aldosterone can be increased through behaviorally induced changes in potassium, ACTH, and renin-angiotensin. It is thought that the development of chronic elevation of blood pressure can result from the interactions between these behaviorally induced physiological factors. Stress also increases systolic blood pressure, heart rate, plasma norepinephrine, plasma epinephrine, cortisol, serum cholesterol, serum triglycerides, platelet aggregation, serum corticotropin, and causes a decrease in occipital alpha activity, and clotting time.

Many neuroregulator systems are involved in stress reactions. The catecholamines (adrelines found in the adrenal gland and in several parts of the brain) have long been linked to stress. The endorphins, which are recently discovered morphinelike peptides in the brain, pituitary gland, and adrenals are involved in perception of and response to pain, with the ability to ease pain and induce a feeling of euphoria. The release of endorphins in response to stress appears to have an adaptive value in that they appear to counter adrenal-triggered overreactions by slowing respiration, lowering blood pressure, and calming motor activity throughout the body. It is known that chicken pox and herpes simplex viruses can be latent for years, but when the individual is under stress they begin to multiply and cause disease. When viruses invade the body and begin to grow within certain cells, their growth is impeded due to chemical processes in the cell. These chemical processes can be significantly reduced under conditions of stress, thus, resulting in vulnerability to disease.

Thomas Holmes and Richard Rahe conducted a classic study on the relationship between environmental events and disease by assessing recent life change events, ranking them according to severity of life change, and arriving at an individual score compiled from the various weights given to each life change event. Receiving a traffic ticket or taking a vacation might be given a low score, while the death of a spouse, or divorce would be given a high score.

Individuals with a high score of stressful life change

events were demonstrated to be more susceptible to disease. Richard Lazarus put more emphasis on the individual's perceptual appraisal of the stressful event as being more important than the experimenter's or society's ratings of relative stressfulness of life change events. He also postulated that "daily hassles" may generate even more stress than a life change event.

Hypertension affects one in six Americans, often beginning early in life and becoming progressively more severe. It is the most important risk factor for stroke and one of the most important risk factors for a coronary heart disease. Hypertension is more frequent in men up to age 55, but more frequent for women after age 55. Blacks are twice as likely to have hypertension as whites, and it is more frequent in lower socioeconomic groups and in lower education levels. Only 10 percent of people with hypertension can account for the hypertension with known causes, such as kidney disease or toxemia of pregnancy, while 90 percent of the patients with hypertension have no known organic cause. Many people do not take required medications, because hypertension does not usually produce symptoms, patients fail to understand the significance of the disease and its control, and they often experience adverse reactions to the medications.

Risk of hypertension has been associated with age, sex, race, obesity, emotional problems and stress (particularly during prehypertension), and other stress-related factors, such as time pressure, anxiety, noxious stimulation, and stressful events. High levels of epinephrine and norepinephrine can elevate blood pressure. Blacks living in low stress areas of a city will exhibit fewer cases of hypertension than those living in high stress areas. Highly stressful occupations have been shown to contribute to hypertension; for example, air traffic controllers have a greater increase in blood pressure when stress is high than when they are in less stressful settings. The relationship between blood pressure, onset of hypertension, and stress has also been demonstrated when patients attach a highly emotional meaning to specific stressful events, when compared with stressful events without the attachment of highly emotional meaning. The ability of biofeedback and relaxation treatments to lower blood pressure in patients with hypertension also supports a psychosocial link with the disease. Likewise, there are a number of successful programs which help patients learn how to deal with social pressures and reduce stress, resulting in the reducing of blood pressure. Nutrition is also a factor, in that a reduction in obesity can lower blood pressure and a reduction of salt consumption is effective in reducing blood pressure, probably linked in part to a genetic predisposition. Hypertension control involves using resources and services from a variety of sectors, dealing with different kinds of individ-

ual motivation, life-style changes, and long-term intervention.

MEASUREMENT AND RESEARCH METHODS

Intelligence

Intelligence quotient (IQ) is calculated by dividing the mental age (calculated from a test score) by the chronological age, times 100, producing a quantitative representation of the intelligence quotient. The Stanford-Binet and the Wexler Intelligence tests produce a test score from which a mental age is calculated, based on the average performance of an individual at a particular chronological age. Therefore, a mental age of 12 would indicate a test performance of the average 12 year old person, and a chronological age of 12 times 100 would produce an IQ of 100. If the mental age is greater than the chronological age, then the IQ will be above 100.

Projective Tests

In projective tests, the stimuli are usually relatively ambiguous, the task is unstructured, and the subjects are less aware of what the tester is looking for and hence the patient is better able to provide a more free and less inhibited response. It is also possible that projective techniques are less apt to activate defensive reactions, and encourage fantasy that can lead to a disclosure of unconscious material, attitudes, and motivations.

Projective techniques are considered to have serious limitations due to the lack of adequate normative data, thus relying too heavily on an individual clinician's interpretations. Also, the reliability and validity of projective techniques are difficult to assess.

A number of projective tests have been developed in an attempt to assess personality, or to determine an individual's attitudes, motivations, defensive maneuvers, or characteristic ways of responding to a situation. The projective technique involves asking an individual to respond to unstructured and ambiguous stimuli, and for which there are no correct answers. An analysis of these responses is assumed to reflect an individual's personality characteristics, more so than structured tests, where the responses of the individual are more apt to be determined by the nature of the test and the specific items and choices than by the nature of the individual.

Examples of projective tests are the Thematic Apperception Test, Draw-A-Person Test, Sentence Completion Test, and Rorschach Test. The Minnesota Multiphasic Personality Inventory (MMPI) is a personality inventory of 550 items, but it is a structured test in that the subject must answer "true," "false," or "cannot say."

The Thematic Appreception Test (TAT) is a projective test consisting of 30 rather ambiguous pictures with the subject being asked to make up a story for each picture, describing what has led up to the depicted scene, what is occurring in the picture at the present time, describing the feelings of the characters involved, and what the outcome will be. The stories are recorded verbatim and it provides a case-study exploration of an individual's motivational variables and personality. It does not provide an adequate assessment of intellectual level. It can be followed by an interview to obtain more in-depth information about specific stories so as to aid the diagnostic process.

Validity

The four types of validity involved in psychologic assessment are content, construct, predictive, and incremental. Content validity exists when the content of the test is demonstrated to be representative of the behaviors to be measured. Construct validity exists when the tests relates, at least theoretically, to other relevant tests and measures. Predictive validity exists when the test allows the tester to predict a future behavior or test score. Incremental validity exists when a test, or specific items in the test add to information that has been secured from prior tests or test items.

Measurements

There are a number of methods for rating attitudes or feelings.

The Likert method involves a 5-point scale on which subjects indicate the extent of their agreement or disagreement (i.e., strongly agree, agree, don't know, disagree, strongly disagree). The ratings are then added to yield a total attitude or agreement score.

The Thurstone technique requires that a group of judges sort the various statements into 11 equally-spaced categories, with subjects indicating whether they agree with each of the series of attitude statements, which are equally spaced along a continuum of attitude.

The Guttman scalogram involves arranging a series of items in the order of "difficulty of acceptance," so that the subjects check all acceptable items in the series of statements. Since the items are assumed to be cumulative, the acceptance of one statement implies acceptance of all other less extreme statements.

C. E. Osgood approach is a multidimensional approach, using a series of 7-point bipolar scales (e.g., strong-weak, active-passive, good-bad), with the subject rating a single word or concept along a 7-point scale between (e.g., good or bad, etc.).

"Significant at the 5 percent level of confidence" means that the results will occur by chance only 5 percent of the time, and that the probability that the samples were drawn from the same universe is less than 5 percent.

The normal frequency distribution as derived mathematically has an identical mean, median, and mode; the curve is perfectly symmetrical around the mean; the proportion of observations that will lie in the interval between the mean itself and the mean plus any multiple of the standard deviation can be calculated theoretically; and the dispersion of the distribution is measured by its standard deviation.

Aspects of the distribution are the following:

An unsymmetrical distribution is called skewness.
The center of the distribution is the mean.
Kurtosis is the degree of peaked or flattened distribution.
A standardized statistic is a Z statistic.

The double-blind aspect of an experimental design is introduced in an attempt to control bias because of the experimenter, and the subject. It will not compensate for poorly matched experimental groups, nor errors in sample size.

REFERENCES

Carr JE, Dengerink HA (Eds): Behavioral Science in the Practice of Medicine. Elsevier Science Publishing Co., New York, 1983
    An excellent review and application of the behavioral sciences to clinical medical problems, including health care delivery, behavioral medicine, pain hypertension, depression, and aging.
Counte MA, Christman LP: Interpersonal Behavior and Health Care. Westview Press, Boulder, 1981
    An excellent review and discussion of the behavioral sciences as related to illness behavior, health care services, patient/clinician interaction, and health beliefs and attitudes. This is one of a series of other good reviews of biological bases of human emotion and cognition, stress, development, health care delivery, behavioral intervention, and social epidemiology.
Department of Health, Education, and Welfare: Healthy People: The Surgeon General's Report on Health Promotion and Disease Prevention. U.S. Government Printing Office, Washington, DC, 1979
    An excellent summary and review of major health problems in the United States with many behavioral implications and supporting data.
Gatchel RJ, Baum A: An Introduction to Health Psychology. Addison-Wesley Publishing Co., Reading, 1983
    An excellent overview of health psychology with good supporting data of major behavioral science applications to medicine and health, such as physiological bases, stress, psychological assessment, cognitive behavioral treatment, and pain.

Lerner RM, Hultsch DF: Human Development: A Life Span Perspective. McGraw Hill Book Co., New York, 1983
An excellent comprehensive integration of biological, psychological, social, and cultural dimensions of life span development with excellent applications to medical and health problems. Also presents helpful tables and graphs to further explain concepts of facts.

Norton JC: Introduction to Medical Psychology. The Free Press, New York, 1982
A good review and discussion of the behavioral sciences as applied to various medical specialties, including preventive medicine.

Weiss SM, Herd JA, Fox BH: Perspectives on Behavioral Medicine. Academic Press, Inc., New York, 1981
A good detailed, comprehensive, and scholarly presentation of data and discussion of topics in behavioral medicine with special reference to cardiovascular and neoplastic diseases, with discussion of life events, stress, and animal models.

Winefield HR, Peay MY: Behavioral Science in Medicine. George Allen and Unwin, London, 1980
A good comprehensive review of the behavioral sciences as applied to medicine, including predisposition in behavior, perception, learning individual differences, life span development, groups in society, and cross-cultural perspectives.

MULTIPLE CHOICE QUESTIONS

Circle the correct statement.

1. The Type A behavior pattern is characterized by all of the following except:
   A. Talks, moves, and eats rapidly
   B. Impatient with how slowly people move
   C. Feels a sense of time urgency
   D. Difficulty concentrating on more than one thing at a time
   E. Hostility

2. Suicide is more prevalent among the:
   A. Adolescent
   B. Young adult
   C. Elderly
   D. Middle Aged
   E. Preadolescent

3. The most important contributions of Sigmund Freud to understanding human behavior was the concept of:
   A. Retroactive inhibition
   B. Autonomy versus shame
   C. Preoperational stage
   D. The unconscious
   E. Cognitive dissonance

4. Females aged 15 to 19 facing a premarital pregnancy most frequently:
   A. Marry
   B. Have an abortion
   C. Have a spontaneous abortion (miscarriage)
   D. Give birth to the child and keep it
   E. Give birth to the child and give it up for adoption

5. The elimination of which behavioral factor would do the most to improve the health of the nation?
   A. Alcohol consumption
   B. Cigarette smoking
   C. Illicit drugs
   D. Compliance with medication
   E. Malnutrition

6. Mental retardation is apt to be more severe and more frequent in:
   A. Klinefelter's syndrome
   B. Tay-Sachs disease
   C. Turner's syndrome
   D. Down's syndrome
   E. Phenylketonuria

7. Erik Erikson's psychosocial developmental task of accomplishing integrity occurs during which stage of development?
   A. Young adult
   B. Age 40 to death
   C. Middle age
   D. Adolescence
   E. Age 25 to 40

8. In learning, the pattern or schedule of reinforcement which produces the highest and most consistent response rate is:
   A. Continuous reinforcement
   B. Fixed ratio
   C. Fixed interval
   D. Variable interval
   E. Variable ratio

9. The admission rate to state and county psychiatric hospitals is highest for:
   A. Married women
   B. Separated women
   C. Divorced women
   D. Widowed women
   E. Never married women

10. In the measurement of marital success when considering the birth order of partner in marriage, which of the following has been found to achieve the highest marital success?
    A. Male only child/female only child
    B. Firstborn male/firstborn female

C. Youngest male/youngest female
D. Male firstborn/female later-born
E. Only male child/only female child

11. All of the following statements are true about changing attitudes, except
    A. People are motivated to be consistent
    B. Changing behavior is also effective in changing attitudes
    C. Role playing is effective in changing attitudes
    D. An individual tends to modify their attitudes when they are no longer functional
    E. Mass media presentations are generally ineffective in changing attitudes

Each question below contains four suggested answers of which one or more is correct. Choose the answer:

A	if 1, 2, and 3 are correct
B	if 1 and 3 are correct
C	if 2 and 4 are correct
D	if 4 is correct
E	if 1, 2, 3, and 4 are correct

12. Methods most often used to study human growth and development include:
    1. Cross-sectional design
    2. Time-lag design
    3. Longitudinal design
    4. Cross-psychosocial design

13. Observational learning usually involves which of the following:
    1. Imitation
    2. Practice
    3. Modeling
    4. Biofeedback

14. The medical model tends to define disease as:
    1. The presence of physical signs and symptoms
    2. Having a statistical prevalence
    3. Associated with pain or discomfort
    4. Normally distributed in the population

15. Basic models of health include the:
    1. Medical model
    2. Social system model
    3. Statistical model
    4. Secondary gain model

16. Which of the following are true of patient compliance?
    1. Doctors have a tendency to underestimate compliance
    2. About 50 percent of patients comply with taking medicine
    3. About 25 percent of patients comply with follow-up appointments
    4. Lower compliance is commonly found among young adults and the elderly

17. Producing a given response by reinforcing that response with an appropriate reward is the mechanism used in which of the following?
    1. Classical conditioning
    2. Instrumental conditioning
    3. Observational learning
    4. Operant conditioning

18. Talcott Parsons has described the sick role as requiring which of the following?
    1. Person is not responsible for their illness
    2. Person is excused from usual obligations
    3. Person is expected to seek professional help
    4. Person is expected to cooperate with treatment

19. Patients most often evaluate professional competence on which of the following physician abilities?
    1. Establishing a positive interpersonal relationship
    2. Giving of their time
    3. Showing an interest in the patient
    4. Demonstrating extensive knowledge

20. The health belief model asserts which of the following factors as influencing health behavior?
    1. Level of health motivation
    2. Perceived vulnerability
    3. Evaluation of the consequences
    4. The costs of seeking care

Answers to Multiple Choice Questions

1 D	2 C	3 D	4 B	5 B
6 D	7 B	8 E	9 C	10 D
11 D	12 A	13 A	14 A	15 A
16 C	17 C	18 E	19 A	20 E

Biochemistry

Cara-Lynne Schengrund

MOLECULAR CONSTITUENTS OF CELLS

Water

The major molecular component of cells is water. Within this aqueous environment are four main classes of organic compounds: Proteins, carbohydrates, lipids, and nucleic acids, plus small quantities of inorganic ions.

Water serves as the solvent in which cellular chemical reactions occur; it plays a role both in maintaining the structure and aggregation of macromolecules, and in temperature control. The ability of water molecules to form noncovalent hydrogen bonds, in a tetrahedral array, with four adjacent water molecules contributes to its unique properties. As a result of hydrogen bonding the melting point of water at $0°C$ and boiling point at $100°C$ are much higher than those of other compounds which appear to have similar electronic structures (e.g., NH_3). The high specific heat, heat of vaporization, and heat of fusion of water minimize fluid loss during large temperature changes, aid in maintenance of body temperature, and, through the oceans, minimizes fluctuations in atmospheric temperatures as the seasons change. The high dielectric constant of water accounts for the solubility of electrolytes in water as well as for the tendency of nonpolar hydrocarbon groups, present in lipids and proteins, to aggregate, thereby, minimizing their interactions with water.

Water exists in equilibrium with hydroxyl (OH^-) and hydronium (H_3O^+) ions: $2H_2O \rightleftharpoons H_3O^+ + OH^-$ and the equilibrium constant for this reaction is:

$$K_{eq} = \frac{[H_3O^+][OH^-]}{[H_2O]^2}$$

$K_{eq}\ H_2O \sim 3 \times 10^{-18}$ which means that at equilibrium the $[H_3O^+]$ and $[OH^-]$ are about 10^{-7} mol/L. The ion product for water is defined as:

$$K_{H_2O} = [H_2O]^2\ K_{eq} = [H_3O^+][OH^-] = 10^{-14}\ \text{at}\ 25°C$$

If there is an alteration in the amount of either ion caused by the addition of an acid or a base, there will be an alteration in the concentration of the counter ion, so that the K_{H_2O} remains constant.

In the aqueous environment of the cell there are many compounds which act as weak acids (ones not completely dissociated). In solution they exist in an equilibrium: $HA \rightleftharpoons H^+ + A^-$ and their dissociation (ionization) constant is:

$$K_a = \frac{[H^+][A^-]}{[HA]}$$

For ease of manipulation $[H^+]$ and K_a values are usually expressed as pH and pKa which are the negative logs of the values obtained. The expression of $[H^+]$ values in this way is the basis of the pH scale. pH and pKa of a weak acid are related:

$$[H^+] = \frac{K_a[HA]}{[A^-]}$$

$$pH = pK_a + \log\frac{[A^-]}{[HA]} = pK_a + \log\frac{[salt]}{[acid]}$$

The final form is known as the Henderson-Hasselbalch equation. It can be used to calculate the ratio of salt to acid present in, or needed for, a buffer of known pH since pKa values are available for biologically important compounds.

Proteins

The protein components of cells play a variety of roles in their function. Enzymes are proteins; carriers for molecules as diverse as oxygen and vitamin B_{12} are proteins, as are hormones such as insulin and glucagon; proteins serve as receptors for homones and neurotransmitters; they are components of the immune system; and proteins serve as structural and motile components. The characteristic properties of a protein depend upon the sequence of the 20 different α-amino acids which can be used in its synthesis. Amino acids have a carboxyl group and, on the α-carbon, an amino group, a hydrogen atom, and a side chain or R group. This introduces an asymmetric center into all of the amino acids except glycine (R = H). All of the amino acids have the same absolute configuration as L-alanine which is similar to that of L-glyceraldehyde. The R group determines the properties of a particular amino acid and permits their classification as either ionic, polar, nonpolar, or aromatic.

Amino acids with nonpolar aliphatic side chains have the R groups shown below:

Glycine
(Gly,G)

R = H—

Alanine
(Ala,A)

R = H_3C—

Leucine
(Leu,L)

$R = H - \overset{CH_3}{\underset{CH_3}{C}} - CH_2 -$

Valine
(Val,V)

$R = H - \overset{H_3C}{\underset{H_3C}{C}} -$

Isoleucine
(Ile,I)

$R = H - \overset{H_3C-CH_2}{\underset{H_3C}{C}} -$

Proline
(Pro,P)

(imino acid)

Amino acids with aromatic side chains and their R groups are as follows:

Phenylalanine
(Phe,F)

R = ⟨phenyl⟩—CH_2—

Tyrosine
(Tyr,Y)

R = HO—⟨phenyl⟩—CH_2—

Tryptophan
(Trp,W)

R = ⟨indole⟩—CH_2—

Amino acids with polar side chains and their R groups are as follows:

Serine
(Ser,S)

R = HO-CH_2—

Asparagine
(Asn,N)

$R = H_2N - \overset{O}{\overset{\|}{C}} - CH_2 -$

Threonine
(Thr,T)

$R = H_3C - \overset{H}{\underset{OH}{C}} -$

Glutamine
(Gln,Q)

$R = H_2N - \overset{O}{\overset{\|}{C}} - (CH_2)_2 -$

The R groups of amino acids with ionic side chains are as follows:

Aspartic acid
(Asp,D)

R = ^-OOC-CH_2—

Glutamic acid
(Glu,E)

R = ^-OOC-$(CH_2)_2$—

Lysine
(Lys,K)

R = H_3N^+-$(CH_2)_4$—

Arginine
(Arg,R)

$R = H_2N - \overset{H_2N^+}{\overset{\|}{C}} - \overset{H}{\underset{}{N}} - (CH_2)_3 -$

Histidine
(His,H)

R = ⟨imidazole HN$^+$...NH⟩—CH_2—

Sulfur containing amino acids have the R groups indicated below:

Cysteine   Methionine
(Cys,C)   (Met,M)

R = HS-CH$_2$—   R = H$_3$C-S-(CH$_2$)$_2$—

Three of the 20 amino acids are sometimes modified after incorporation into peptide chains. Serine can be phosphorylated to phosphoserine, an alteration which can serve to activate (e.g., skeletal muscle phosphorylase) or inactivate (e.g., glycogen synthetase) an enzyme. In collagen, proline can be converted to hydroxyproline, and in prothrombin, glutamate can be converted to γ-carboxyglutamate.

The charge of an amino acid varies with the pH. An amino acid at a low pH bears a positive charge due to the presence of a charged ammonium ion. As the pH is raised the number of charged carboxylate ions increases until at the isoelectric point there are equivalent numbers of ammonium and carboxylate ions. The result is that the molecule bears no net charge. A further increase in the pH results in loss of protons with the charge of the amino acid becoming negative due to the loss of the ammonium ion and the formation of a carboxylate ion.

$$R-\underset{\underset{H}{|}}{\overset{\overset{NH_3^+}{|}}{C}}-COOH \overset{K_1}{\rightleftharpoons} H^+ + R-\underset{\underset{H}{|}}{\overset{\overset{NH_3^+}{|}}{C}}-COO^- \qquad K_1 = \frac{[H^+]\,[-COO^-]}{[-COOH]}$$

$$R-\underset{\underset{H}{|}}{\overset{\overset{NH_3^+}{|}}{C}}-COO- \overset{K_2}{\rightleftharpoons} H^+ + R-\underset{\underset{H}{|}}{\overset{\overset{NH_2}{|}}{C}}-COO^- \qquad K_2 = \frac{[H^+][-\overset{\overset{NH_2}{|}}{C}H-COO^-]}{[-\underset{\underset{[-CH-COO^-]}{}}{\overset{\overset{NH_3+}{|}}{}}]}$$

At the pH at which there is no net charge (pI) it can be determined that: $pH = pI = \frac{1}{2}(pK_1 + pK_2)$. For a diamino, monocarboxylic acid the pI will be the pH halfway between the pK values for the two ammonium groups, since at that pH the net charge will be zero. Conversely, a dicarboxylic, monoamino acid will have a pI at the pH halfway between the pK values for the two carboxylic acid groups.

In proteins, the amino acids are linked together by peptide bonds (i.e., amide bonds formed between the carboxyl and α-amino groups of two amino acids).

$$R-\underset{\underset{}{|}}{\overset{\overset{NH_3^+}{|}}{C}}H-\overset{\overset{O}{||}}{C}-NH-\underset{}{\overset{\overset{R}{|}}{C}}H-COO^-$$

Di-, tri-, tetra- etc. peptides result from two, three, four, or more amino acids forming polymers via the formation of peptide bonds. Polypeptides contain many amino acid residues (i.e., >10) and proteins are longer polypeptide chains. The primary structure of a protein is defined by the amino acid sequence. With 20 different amino acids many different proteins can be synthesized. The overall amino acid composition of a protein is determined by ion-exchange chromatography of its hydrolysate. There are standard enzymatic or chemical hydrolytic methods, which give rise to polypeptide fragments which can be separated by electrophoretic and chromatographic procedures and sequenced by end group analysis, for determining the actual sequence. It is essential to have pure material and a single polypeptide. Sulfhydryl bonds present in cystine moieties formed between cysteine residues on two different polypeptides can be broken by reducing with mercaptoethanol and protected by blocking with iodoacetic acid as shown:

$$R_1-S-S-R_2 + 2HSCH_2CH_2OH \rightleftharpoons$$
$$R_1SH + R_2SH + HOCH_2CH_2-S-S-CH_2CH_2OH$$
$$RSH + ICH_2COO^- \longrightarrow R-S-CH_2COO^- + HI$$

where R refers to the peptide chains.

The secondary structure of a protein describes the folding of the polypeptide chain. While rotation about the peptide bond (—NH—CO—) is limited due to its having partial double bond characteristics, there is a large degree of rotational freedom around the bonds between the α-carbons and the carbonyl carbon and nitrogen atom. Two main types of polypeptide secondary structures result, the right-handed (clockwise) α-helix and the β pleated sheet. In the α-helix there are 3.6 amino acid residues per turn and the amino acid side chains all point away from the helix. Hydrogen bonds formed between amide hydrogens and the cabonyl oxygens stabilize the helix. The amide group is on an amino acid four residues removed from the carbonyl oxygen with which it hydrogen bonds. In contrast, in a β pleated sheet the polypeptide chain is almost fully extended rather than coiled and it is stabilized by hydrogen bonds between the amide hydrogen and carbonyl oxygen groups in different polypeptide strands. When adjacent polypeptide strands in a β pleated sheet run in the same direction it is a parallel pleated sheet, when they are in opposite directions it is an antiparallel sheet. β bends or turns permit the peptide chain to fold back upon itself. In these turns, formed by four consecutive amino acid residues in the peptide, the carbonyl oxygen of the first residue is hydrogen bonded to the amide hydrogen of the fourth residue. Some proteins contain much secondary structure, as defined by α-helices, β pleated sheets, and β bends, while others have little. Even though the amino acid sequence determines a protein's three-dimensional structure, it alone is insufficient for predicting protein conformation, although it is known that some amino acids are found more often in an α-helix and others in β pleated sheets.

Tertiary structure, the three-dimensional structure of the protein, reflects the noncovalent interactions between side chains and between helixes and β-structures as well as backbone interactions. Hydrophobic residues tend to be buried in water soluble globular proteins thereby minimizing their interactions with water. VanderWaal's interactions help stabilize the structure. Ionic groups tend to be exposed to the aqueous environment. The disulfide bridges, formed when cysteine residues are positioned appropriately, add to the stability of the tertiary structure. When a protein contains subunits, the quaternary structure is defined by the subunits' interactions with each other to give rise to the active protein. Disruption of protein conformation by a reagent such as 6 M guanidine hydrochloride or by heat results in loss of protein function.

ENZYMES

Within a cell a wide variety of chemical reactions occur, which under normal conditions would take place very slowly or not at all, but in the presence of the appropriate catalyst are accelerated by a factor of a million or more. In the cell these catalysts are proteins which exhibit specificity for the substrates with which they interact and for the type of reaction which they catalyze. In fact, enzymes are classified according to the type of reaction they catalyze. The International Union of Biochemistry has developed a system of nomenclature based on six main categories of reactions. Within each category there are further subdivisions permitting complete identification of the enzyme. The six main classifications for enzymes are the following:

1. Oxidoreductases: Catalyze oxidation-reduction reactions.
2. Transferases: Catalyze transfer of a group containing C, N, P, or S from one substrate to another.
3. Hydrolases: Catalyze a hydrolytic cleavage or its reversal.
4. Lyases: Catalyze the breakage of C—C, C—O, C—N, and other bonds by elimination or addition of groups to double bonds but not by hydrolysis or oxidation-reduction.
5. Isomerases: Catalyze an intramolecular rearrangement.
6. Ligases: Catalyze formation of bonds between two substrate molecules with the concommitant hydrolysis of a high energy bond (e.g., ATP).

The specificity of an enzyme results from its having a conformation which allows formation of an active site, the structure of which determines what compounds can fit as well as the subsequent reactions. Once the substrate is associated with the active site it is located so that certain bonds can be destabilized (making them more reactive) through interactions with specific groups on the enzyme. For example, some of the amino acid side chains can act as general acid (donate a proton) or general base (accept a proton) catalysts. As a result of the interaction of a substrate and enzyme the energy of activation (ΔG) for the reaction is lowered. The equilibrium of the reaction is unaffected by the enzyme, although it is attained more rapidly.

Many enzymes contain a prosthetic group known as a cofactor. The protein plus cofactor is known as the holoenzyme, and the protein moiety alone as the apoenzyme. The cofactor can be a metal ion or an organic molecule. Some organic cofactors are derived from molecules which mammalian cells cannot synthesize. They are essential nutrients known as vitamins. A specific cofactor can be required by several different enzymes.

Knowledge of the kinetics of an enzyme catalyzed reaction can help to define the mechanism of action of the enzyme. It also provides a basis for understanding what factors may influence the reaction rate as well as how they affect it. For any enzyme catalyzed reaction, the rate of reaction is dependent upon the concentration of both a substrate and enzyme if all other conditions are constant. If the enzyme concentration is fixed and the substrate concentration gradually increased, the velocity will increase hyperbolically (Fig. 4-1A). At maximum velocity, all of the active sites of the enzyme are occupied by substrate, the enzyme is saturated, and additional substrate will not enhance the rate. The enzyme catalyzed reaction in which one substrate (S) reacts with the enzyme (E) can be written as:

$$E + S \underset{k_2}{\overset{k_1}{\rightleftharpoons}} ES \underset{k_4}{\overset{k_3}{\rightleftharpoons}} P + E$$

The Michaelis-Menten equation describes the velocity of this type of reaction when (1) it occurs under conditions in which the rate of ES formation equals its rate of breakdown, and (2) the initial velocity is measured, which means that only a very small amount of product is present, therefore $P + E \rightarrow ES$ can be ignored. These assumptions permit derivation of the Michaelis-Menten equation:

$$V = \frac{V_{max} + S}{K_M + S}$$

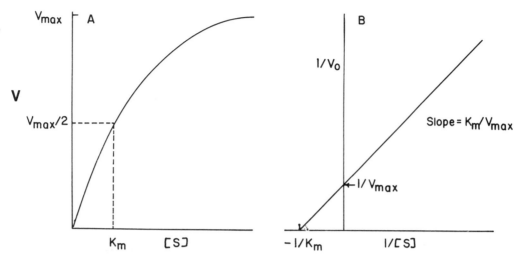

Fig. 4-1. (A) Plot of velocity versus substrate concentration for an enzyme catalyzed reaction. V_{max} is obtained when all of the active sites on the enzyme are occupied by substrate. $V_{max}/2$ occurs when $\frac{1}{2}$ of the active sites are occupied; the substrate concentration needed to obtain $V_{max}/2$ is equal to K_M, the Michaelis constant. (B) Plot of the reciprocal of the initial velocity v the reciprocal of the substrate concentration. The Lineweaver-Burk equation permits identification of the slope as K_M/V_{max}, the Y-intercept as $1/V_{max}$ and the X-intercept as $-1/K_M$.

In this equation V is the velocity, S the substrate concentration, V_{max} the maximum velocity and K_M the Michaelis constant (substrate concentration in moles per liter at which $V = \frac{1}{2}V_{max}$). A low value for K_M indicates a high degree of interaction between enzyme and substrate. V_{max} and K_M can be obtained by measuring the velocity at different substrate concentrations, under conditions in which the rate of the reverse reaction is negligible. The reciprocal of the Michaelis-Menten equation gives a linear relationship, the Lineweaver-Burk equation:

$$1/V = (K_M/V_{max})\,(1/[S]) + 1/V_{max}$$

in which K_M/V_{max} defines the slope, $1/V_{max}$ the Y-intercept and $-1/K_M$ the X-intercept (Fig. 4-1B).

A reaction catalyzed by an enzyme may involve more than one reactant (e.g., $A + B \rightleftharpoons C + D$). The kinetics of such a reaction are much more complex. There are several mechanisms possible for this type of reaction. Substrates may be bound prior to release of products giving a sequential mechanism. The reaction may be ordered, with substrates added and products leaving in a defined way. A random mechanism is one in which either substrate may bind to the enzyme first. The term ping-pong describes the mechanism in which a substrate reacts with the enzyme with release of a product and the retention of a functional group by the enzyme. A second substrate is then bound, the functional group is transferred to it and the final product released. As the number of substrates increases the possible mechanisms for the reaction become more complex.

Obviously, enzymatic reactions must be regulated in order to maintain the proper metabolic balance within the cell. The rate of a reaction can be affected by altering the substrate, product, or enzyme concentration and by the interaction with molecules which affect the catalytic activity of the enzyme. Knowledge of enzyme regulation can provide information about a metabolic pathway and/or about the type of molecule (e.g., a drug) which could serve as a more effective substrate or inhibitor.

Product inhibition reflects the ability of an enzyme to catalyze both the forward and reverse reactions while not altering the final equilibrium. This implies that as the product concentration increases, it will compete with the substrate for binding sites thus slowing the rate of the forward reaction. Many metabolic pathways involve several enzymatically catalyzed reactions prior to formation of the product (e.g., cholesterol biosynthesis). Feedback inhibition is an important regulatory mechanism in many pathways. In feedback inhibition the pathway end product inhibits an enzyme that catalyzes a step earlier in the pathway (e.g., cholesterol inhibits 3-hydroxyl-3-methylglutaryl-CoA-reductase), blocking production of a substrate needed for continued synthesis of the accumulated product. As the concentration of the final product decreases, its inhibition of the prior step decreases.

The three types of inhibition that can be recognized by kinetic analysis are competitive, noncompetitive, and uncompetitive (Fig. 4-2). In competitive inhibition the inhibitor binds at the substrate binding site; the substrate must compete with the inhibitor for access to the active site. As the substrate concentration increases the inhibition decreases. In a Lineweaver-Burk plot the intercept

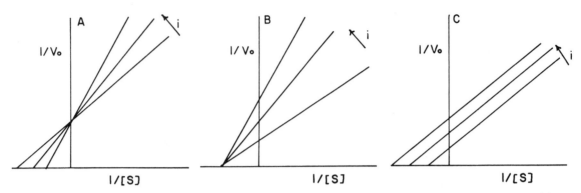

Fig. 4-2. Lineweaver-Burk plots illustrating the effects of (A) competitive, (B) noncompetitive, or (C) uncompetitive inhibitors on reaction velocity and K_M.

$(1/V_{max})$ remains constant and the slope varies when the rate of reaction is measured in the presence of different amounts of inhibitors. In noncompetitive inhibition, inhibition is only dependent upon the concentration of the inhibitor. It binds at a site distinct from the substrate and alters the enzyme so that conversion of substrate to product cannot occur. Lineweaver-Burk plots of this type of inhibition show that as the inhibitor concentration increases the value for V_{max} decreases ($1/V_{max}$ increases), but the value for K_M remains constant. Uncompetitive inhibition occurs when the inhibitor binds to the ES complex blocking product formation. In this instance, Lineweaver-Burk plots of the values for $1/V$ v $1/[S]$, obtained in the presence of increasing inhibitor, result in parallel lines which differ in both V_{max} and K_M.

Enzyme activity can be regulated by the binding of compounds (effectors) at specific sites other than the substrate binding site (allosteric sites). If the reaction rate is enhanced, it is allosteric activation, if it is reduced, it is allosteric inhibition. Enzymes with allosteric sites contain two or more subunits. The interaction of an effector with a subunit alters the subunit's conformation which in turn may influence the conformation of the second subunit, modifying its catalytic activity. A plot of V v [S] for this type of enzyme is often sigmoidal. The Hill equation

$$-\log\,(V_{max} - V)/V = n_H \log\,[S] - \log K,$$

is used in studies of enzymes with allosteric sites. A plot of log $V/(V_{max} - V)$ v log[S] gives a straight line the slope of which is n_H, the Hill coefficient. An n_H value greater than one indicates positive cooperativity (binding of first ligand enhances binding of second), a value less than one, negative cooperativity. The value of n_H cannot be greater than the maximum number of substrate residues that can bind to the protein. Examples of this type of control are seen in the kinetics of the binding of oxygen to hemoglobin and in the action of phosphofructokinase.

Alteration of an enzyme by covalent modification of an amino acid residue can result in either activation or inactivation of an enzyme. A common covalent modification is the phosphorylation of the hydroxyl groups of serine, threonine, or tyrosine residues. This occurs via the action of a protein kinase which catalyzes the transfer of the phosphate group from ATP to the enzyme. The phosphate group can be removed via the action of a phosphoprotein phosphatase. Glycogen phosphorylase is an example of an enzyme activated by phosphorylation. This type of regulation provides more control than the others since the enzymes involved in the phosphorylation and dephosphorylation provide additional opportunities for modulation.

Carbohydrates

Carbohydrates have the general formula $(CH_2O)_n$ indicating that they are hydrates of carbon. They are either polyhydroxyaldehydes or polyhydroxyketones, depending upon whether they carry an aldehyde or ketone function. The value of n for naturally occurring carbohydrates ranges from three to nine. Simple carbohydrates are referred to as sugars (e.g., glucose, sucrose) and are mono- or disaccharides. Cells can contain polysaccharides which are composed of many monosaccharide residues and may have molecular weights ranging up to a million (e.g., glycogen). Carbohydrate residues can also be found linked to lipid moieties (glycolipids) and to proteins (glycoproteins). In addition to serving the cell as a source of energy and as precursors for other components, carbohydrates as glycoconjugates (compounds in which sugar moieties are covalently bound to proteins or lipids) have been implicated in cell-cell and cell-substratum recognition, contact inhibition, and as receptors and antigenic determinants.

Glyceraldehyde and dihydroxyacetone are the only sugars containing three carbon atoms in a molecule (trioses), and they serve as the basis for sugars containing more carbon atoms. D-glyceraldehyde is the precursor for the aldoses and dihydroxy-acetone is the precursor for the ketoses.

```
   CH2OH            CHO              CHO
   |                |                |
   C = O           HOCH             HCOH
   |                |                |
   CH2OH           H2COH            H2COH

dihydroxyacetone  L-glyceraldehyde  D-glyceraldehyde
```

The D and L designate configuration about the asymmetric carbon furthest from the carbonyl group. In the Fischer projection, when the hydroxyl group at the two position is to the right, the configuration is D; when it is to the left, the configuration is L. Sugars found in glyco-conjugates are usually of the D-form, however fucose and iduronic acid have the L-configuration.

Sugar solutions can rotate the plane of polarized light to the right (dextrorotatory) or to the left (levorotatory) indicated by a (+) and a (−) respectively. The optical rotation of freshly prepared sugars such as glucose or fructose changes with time due to mutarotation. This results from the ability of the sugars to form a hemiacetal or hemiketal (condensation product of the carbonyl function with an alcohol group). This introduces another asymmetric center at the former aldehydic or ketosidic carbon atom. The α- and β-anomers thus formed reach equilibrium through the open chain aldose or ketose. It is this attainment of equilibrium that alters the optical rotation of the freshly prepared sugars.

```
  HCOH              HCO              HOCH
  |                 |                |
  HCOH              HCOH             HCOH
  |                 |                |
  HOCH  O  ⇌   HOCH  ⇌   HOCH  O
  |                 |                |
  HCOH              HCOH             HCOH
  |                 |                |
  HC ─              HCOH             HC ─
  |                 |                |
  CH2OH             CH2OH            CH2OH

α-D-glucopyranose  D-glucose  β-D-glucopyranose
```

Formation of the hemiacetal or hemiketal gives rise to a sugar containing a five- or six-membered ring. Sugars containing five-membered rings are called furanoses and those with six-membered rings are called pyranoses.

In oligosaccharides and glycoconjugates, only a limited number of different monosaccharide residues are found in nature. Glucose, galactose (4-epimer of glucose), and mannose are the neutral hexoses found. The

amino sugars are glucosamine, galactosamine, and sialic acid. Derivatives of glucose containing a carboxy group at C_6 are glucuronic and iduronic acid. Two other neutral sugars found are L-fucose, a 6-deoxy sugar, and xylose, a pentose. Nucleic acids contain either ribose or deoxyribose.

```
  CHO          CHO          CHO          CHO
  |            |            |            |
  HCOH        HOCH         HCOH         HCOH
  |            |            |            |
  HOCH        HOCH         HOCH         HOCH
  |            |            |            |
  HOCH        HCOH         HCOH         HCOH
  |            |            |            |
  HCOH        HCOH         HCOH         HOCH
  |            |            |            |
  CH2OH       CH2OH        COOH         COOH

D-galactose   D-mannose  D-glucuronic acid  L-iduronic acid
```

N-acetyl glucosamine and galactosamine have an acetylated amino group (—HN—CO—CH$_3$) at the two position.

```
        COOH
        |
        C = O
        |
        CH2
        |
        HCOH
        |                      CHO              CHO
H3C-CO—HN—CH                  |                |
        |                     HCOH            HOCH
        HOCH                  |                |
        |                     HOCH            HCOH
        HCOH                  |                |
        |                     HCOH            HCOH
        HCOH                  |                |
        |                     CH2OH           HOCH
        CH2OH                                  |
                                               CH3

N-acetylneuraminic acid      D-xylose         L-fucose
    (a sialic acid)
```

```
   CHO             CHO
   |               |
   HCOH            CH2
   |               |
   HCOH            HCOH
   |               |
   HCOH            HCOH
   |               |
   CH2OH           CH2OH

 D-ribose      2-deoxy-D-ribose
```

Under appropriate conditions, these sugars can react with each other to form poly- or oligosaccharides via formation of acetals or ketals. Maltose, isomaltose (derived upon glycogen hydrolysis), and cellobiose (derived from cellulose) are disaccharides of glucose residues linked α1,4, α1,6, and β1,4, respectively. In each instance the anomeric carbon of one glucose residue is unsubstituted and is free to act as a reducing agent. The ability of sugars to act as reducing agents provides a convenient method for the measurement of blood glucose levels. The reduction of Cu^{+2} to Cu^{+1} is monitored. In contrast, sucrose (glc αl-2 fru) is a nonreducing sugar; both anomeric carbons are substituted. When oligosaccharides are found covalently bonded to protein it is by one of four types of linkages: N-acetylglucosamine can be N-glycosidically linked to the β-amide nitrogen of an asparagine residue, N-acetylgalactosamine can be O-glycosidically linked to the β-hydroxyl of either serine or threonine, galactose through an O-glycosidic linkage to the hydroxyl group of 5-hydroxylysine, or xylose through an O-glycosidic linkage to the hydroxyl group of serine. The latter two are found primarily in glycoconjugates of connective tissue.

Lipids

Lipids are the third major class of organic compounds found in cells. They are generally soluble in solvents such as methanol, chloroform, ether, or mixtures thereof. Lipids serve the cell as a source of potential energy and as the basic building blocks for cell membranes. They can also function as receptors, vitamins, and hormones. The simplest lipid is a fatty acid. Neutral acylglycerols and phosphoglycerides are complex lipids containing glycerol. Complex lipids lacking glycerol include glycosphingolipids, terpenes, steroids, and waxes.

Fatty acids are aliphatic monocarboxylic acids, often containing an even number of carbon atoms; the chain can be saturated or unsaturated. Chain length and degree of unsaturation affect the physical characteristics of fatty acids. For example, as the chain length decreases, the melting point decreases. The double bonds in unsaturated fatty acids are generally in the cis configuration and, if there is more than one double bond, they are methylene interrupted. The cis double bond introduces a kink in the chain and as a result increases the fluidity or lowers the melting point of the fatty acid. Fatty acids have both hydrophobic (aliphatic chain) and hydrophilic (carboxyl) regions. They are weak acids and in an aqueous environment they dissociate, $RCOOH \rightleftharpoons RCOO^- + H^+$. The dissociation constant (pK) for all fatty acids, with the exception of formic acid (pK = 3.75), is about 4.8. Free fatty acids are only found in small quantities. Usually they are found in ester or amide linkages in the more complex lipids. It should be noted that mammalian cells cannot synthesize fatty acids in which the double bond is within the terminal seven carbon atoms (carboxyl carbon is number one,

ω-carbon is the terminal methyl carbon). Essential fatty acids, those with a double bond within the terminal seven carbons, serve as the precursors for the eicosanoids (biologically active compounds derived from C_{20} unsaturated fatty acids).

Fatty acids are named for the parent hydrocarbon. For example $CH_3(CH_2)_{14}COOH$ is called hexadecanoic acid. The parent hydrocarbon is hexadecane; in naming the corresponding acid the e is removed and oic is added. Insertion of one double bond results in substitution of anoic with enoic, while two or three double bonds results in substitution of noic with dienoic or trienoic, respectively. Fatty acids may be represented by a numerical symbol, for example, 18:3 (9,12,15) is the designation for octadecatrienoic acid in which the double bonds are between carbons 9 and 10, 12 and 13, and 15 and 16. Common or trivial names are also used for many fatty acids.

Fatty acids which serve as an energy source are stored as triacylglycerols (glycerol esterified with fatty acids at all three positions). Mono- and diacylglycerols are also present in cells but in much lesser amounts. Hydrolysis of triacylglycerols catalyzed by acid or enzymes (lipases) gives three free fatty acids and one glycerol molecule. Base catalyzed hydrolysis is known as saponification. The released carboxylate ions react with the cations present to give soaps. The solubility of the neutral fats is determined primarily by the hydrophobic hydrocarbon chains. The free hydroxyl groups, found in mono- and diacylglycerols, and ester linkages, are nonionic and weakly polar. Therefore, when triacylglycerols are stored in adipose tissue cells they are found in droplets which exclude water molecules from the interior. This stored reservoir of triacylglycerol is a much more compact storage form of potential energy than the hydrated carbohydrates which proportionately occupy more space. Because the fatty acids are reduced, a higher caloric yield is obtained when they are fully oxidized than is obtained from the oxidation of a comparable amount of carbohydrate.

The second group of lipids containing a glycerol backbone is the phosphoglycerides. These lipids are derivatives of L-glycerol-3-phosphate (sn-glycerol-3-phosphate):

$$
\begin{array}{l}
H_2COH \\
| \\
HO\text{-}C\text{-}H \\
| \quad\quad O \\
| \quad\quad || \\
H_2C\text{-}O\text{-}P\text{-}O\text{---} \\
\quad\quad | \\
\quad\quad O\text{-}
\end{array}
$$

Further classification is based on the polar groups, other than phosphate, that are present and the type of linkage between the hydrocarbon moiety and the glycerol. These molecules are more amphipathic than triacylglycerols and interact more with water. Phospholipids are essential structural components of cell-membranes and also help to "solubilize" fat droplets (e.g., chylomicra).

Phosphatidyl compounds are derived from L-phosphatidic acid (1,2-0-diacyl-L-glycerol-3-phosphate). As the proper name indicates, there is a fatty acid residue esterified at the one and two positions and a phosphate group at position three. In phosphatidylcholine, phosphatidylethanolamine, and phosphatidylserine there is a nitrogenous base, choline [$HO-CH_2-CH_2-N^+(CH_3)_3$], ethanolamine ($HO-CH_2-CH_2-{}^+NH_3$), or serine ($HO-CH_2-CH-{}^+NH_3$), respectively, in
$$COO^-$$
ester linkage to the phosphate residue. Phosphatidylcholines are sometimes referred to as lecithins.

Plasmalogens are 1-alkenyl-2-acyl derivatives of L-glycerol-3-phosphate. The fatty acyl residue found at position one of phosphatidyl compounds is replaced by an α-unsaturated alcohol in an ether linkage. These phosphatidal compounds contain the same bases as those of phosphatidyl compounds. Although plasmalogens are found in a variety of cells, they account for only a small percentage of the phosphoglycerides.

Mammalian cells also contain phosphatidylinositols and diphosphatidylglycerols (nitrogen-free phosphatidyl compounds). Phosphatidylinositol usually has myoinositol esterified to the phosphate residue. The myoinositol can be phosphorylated at the four, or four and five positions. Diphosphatidylglycerol consists of two moles of L-phosphatidic acid and one mole of glycerol. The common name for this lipid is cardiolipin. Note that all phospholipids bear either no net charge or a negative charge at physiological pH.

Sphingolipids are complex lipids whose core structure is provided by the long-chain aminoalcohol, sphingosine (*trans*-1,3-dihydroxy-2-amino-4-octadecene), or a derivative thereof. C_{18} sphingosines are the most prevalent, however, C_{16}, C_{17}, C_{19}, and C_{20} derivatives are also found. The simplest sphingolipid is ceramide, in which a fatty acid is linked via an amide bond to sphingosine.

ponents but are present at lower concentrations than are phospholipids. Sphingomyelins are derived from ceramides by the introduction of a phosphorylcholine moiety at the one position of the sphingosine base.

$$CH_3(CH)_{12}-CH=\text{-}CH\text{-}CH\text{-}CH\text{-}CH_2\text{-}O\text{-}R$$

HO   NH-CO-(CH_2)_n-CH_3

R = H in ceramides

$$R = -P-O-CH_2-CH_2-N^+(CH_3)_3$$
in sphingomyelins

R = one or more sugar residues in glycosphingolipids

Glycosphingolipids contain ceramide with one or more sugar residues. Cerebrosides have either D-galactose (more common) or D-glucose at position one of the sphingosine moiety. The galactosyl residue can be sulfated. Most common is the presence of sulfate in an ester linkage with the three hydroxyl of the galactose; these lipids are referred to as sulfatides. Ceramides which contain more than one sugar residue are termed ceramide disaccharide, ceramide trisaccharide, etc. Ceramide oligosaccharides define the ABO and Lewis blood group antigens. Gangliosides, found in enriched concentrations in nervous tissue, are ceramide oligosaccharides which contain at least one sialic acid residue in addition to the other sugars.

Fatty acids can be esterified to long chain alcohols (excluding glycerol) giving a product commonly known as a wax. Cetyl palmitate is a major component of spermaceti found in the head oil of the sperm whale. It results from the esterification of palmitic acid by cetyl alcohol.

Some of the vitamins (A, E, and K), dolichol, coenzyme Q, and the steroids have carbon skeletons which can be considered polymers of isoprene (e.g., 2-methylbutadiene):

$$CH_2{=}\overset{\displaystyle CH_3}{\underset{\displaystyle |}{C}}{-}CH{=}CH_2$$

Compounds with open chains or with simple rings are referred to as terpenes (e.g., dolichol):

$$H(CH_2{-}\overset{\displaystyle CH_3}{\underset{\displaystyle |}{C}}{=}CH{-}CH_2)_{18-20}{-}CH_2{-}\overset{\displaystyle CH_3}{\underset{\displaystyle |}{CH}}{-}CH_2{-}CH_2{-}OH$$

The more complex sphingolipids have ionic and/or polar groups at the one position of the sphingosine moiety. These molecules are found as membrane com-

The steroids contain a fused ring system comprised of three fused cyclohexane rings in a phenanthrene-type structure and a fourth, terminal, cyclopentane ring. An example is cholesterol:

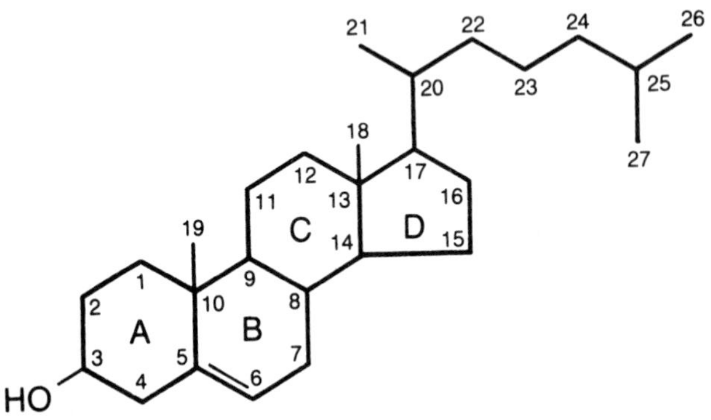

Steroid molecules are fairly planar and rigid with low water solubility. The A ring in some instances is aromatic in which case the methyl group shown at position 10 is deleted. The length of the hydrocarbon chain at C_{17} can vary and serves in part as a basis for classifying different types of steroids (i.e., corticoids have two carbons, and androgens none, while estrogens also have none and in addition have an aromatic ring A). In addition to functioning as hormones, steroids are important membrane components.

Nucleic Acids

The expression of the different protein, carbohydrate, and lipid moieties found in a cell is under the control of the nucleic acids, the cellular components that carry genetic information. Nucleic acids are polymers of nucleotides. Nucleotides consist of a pyrimidine or purine base linked to a sugar, either D-ribose or D-2-deoxyribose, and a phosphate residue esterified to the five position of the sugar. Nucleic acids synthesized from nucleotides containing deoxyribose are known as deoxyribonucleic acid (DNA), while those from nucleotides containing ribose are called ribonucleic acid (RNA). Nucleoside refers to the base-sugar moiety alone. The pyrimidine bases found in DNA are cytosine and thymine; in RNA uracil replaces thymine:

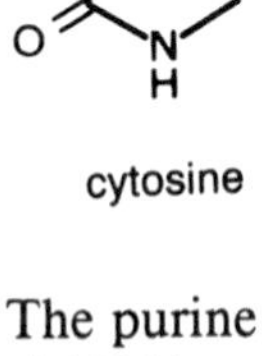

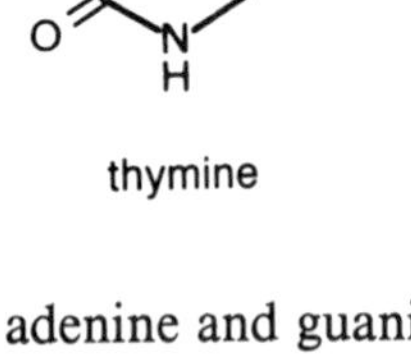

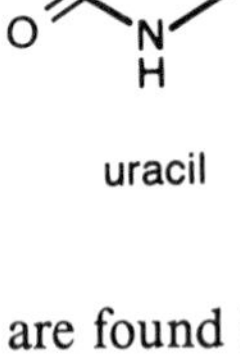

The purine bases adenine and guanine are found in both DNA and RNA.

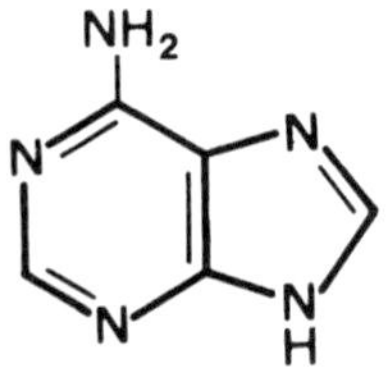

The addition of ribose to the base is indicated by altering the names to adenosine, guanosine, cytidine, thymidine, and uridine. If the sugar is deoxyribose, deoxy is used prior to the name (e.g., deoxyadenosine). The exception is thymidine which does not carry the prefix since it is found in DNA but not RNA. In the nucleotides the position of the phosphate residue on the sugar is indicated by the carbon number followed by a prime (e.g., adenosine-5'-phosphate).

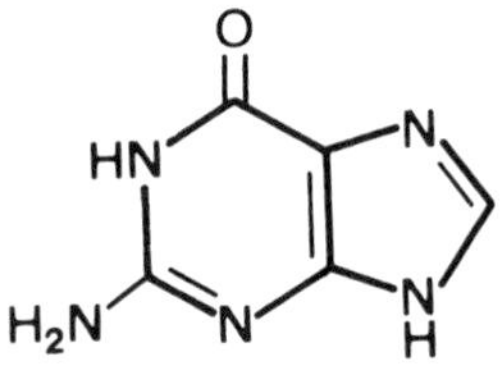

BIOCHEMICAL ASPECTS OF MOLECULAR BIOLOGY

DNA

DNA contains equal amounts of purines and pyrimidines; this reflects the structure of DNA. It is composed of two polynucleotide strands that run in opposite (antiparallel) directions and twist into a right-handed double helix. This results in exposure of the sugar-phosphodiester backbones on the surface of the helix and brings the bases together in the center. The phosphodiester bridges occur between the 5'-phosphate of one nucleotide and the 3'-hydroxyl of the adjacent one. Hydrogen bonds are formed between complementary base pairs: adenine with thymine, and guanine with cytosine. In each instance one purine and one pyrimidine base make up the pair, and the hydrogen bonds are formed between an amino and keto group or between an amino group and a ring nitrogen. Two hydrogen-bonds are formed between adenine and thymine and three hydrogen-bonds between guanine and cytosine. Double-stranded DNA can be represented as:

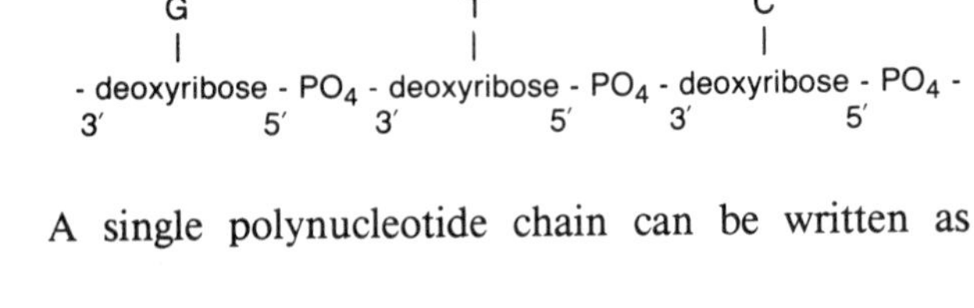

A single polynucleotide chain can be written as

pdCpdApdG, where a p to the left represents esterification by phosphate at C-5' and a p to the right esterification at C-3'. The sequence is written in the 5' → 3' direction (CAG).

Methods have been developed for determining the nucleotide sequence of DNA. The DNA chain can be cleaved by one or more restriction endonucleases (catalyze the cleavage of internucleotide linkages at specific base sequences), and the fragments can be separated by electrophoresis. The DNA fragments can be labelled with ^{32}P at their 5'-hydroxyl termini in a reaction catalyzed by polynucleotide kinase. Chemical methods can then be used to cleave at a specific purine or pyrimidine base with the conditions set so that there is an average of one break per chain. This yields a set of radioactive products extending from the ^{32}P-terminus to each of the positions of the base. These fragments can be separated by polyacrylamide gel electrophoresis and located by autoradiography. By running the cleavage products obtained for each base in parallel a complete map can be obtained. The sequence is determined by starting with the shortest polynucleotide (migrated furthest) and reading up the gel.

Double-stranded DNA can be denatured by heat, acid, alkali (although DNA is insensitive to alkali hydrolysis), and low ionic strength. The conversion of DNA from a double- to a single-stranded structure results in decreased viscosity, optical rotation, and an increased ultraviolet absorption (absorption maximum ~ 260 nm). Heating a DNA sample results in disruption of the hydrogen bonds between base pairs; this disruption can be monitored by measuring the increase in ultraviolet absorption that occurs. The more guanine and cytosine that is present the narrower and higher is the temperature range over which "melting" takes place. T_m refers to the temperature at which 50 percent of the DNA is denatured. Cooling of the denatured solution permits the complementary DNA strands to anneal. This requires that the two strands reassociate correctly after which hydrogen bonds reform between the aligned complementary bases. The initial part of the annealing (reassociation of the two strands) follows second-order kinetics. It can be expressed as $C/C_o = 1/(1 + K_2C_ot)$, where C_o is the initial concentration of denatured DNA; C is the concentration of denatured DNA at time t; and K_2 is the second order rate constant. Algebraically it can be seen that when half the DNA is renatured, $K_2 = 1/C_ot_{1/2}$. K_2 decreases as the time required for renaturation increases. The time required reflects the number of base pairs in the DNA when there are no repeated sequences. Hence $C_ot_{1/2}$ is directly proportional to the number of base pairs in the DNA.

In eukaryotes, DNA is complexed with histones, a group of basic proteins which neutralize the negative charges of the phosphate groups in DNA. There are five major classes of histones, which can be differentiated in part by their arginine and lysine content. DNA can wrap around histone octamers giving a supercoiled structure resulting in a condensation of the DNA in eukaryotic chromosomes. The condensed structured is called a nucleosome. These are packed, possibly around a nonhistone protein structure, to give a further condensation of the DNA. At certain times during the cell cycle, modifications (phosphorylation, acetylation, and polyadenosinediphosphate ribosylation of specific classes of histones occur; these alterations may mediate changes in chromatin structure necessary for transcription.

Replication of DNA occurs by a semiconservative process in which the daughter DNA molecules formed contain one strand from the parent and one new strand. In eukaryotic cells, instead of having one origin of replication as in *Escherichia coli,* there are multiple origins, each of which forms two replication forks which move in opposite directions, permitting rapid replication. DNA polymerase α catalyzes the 5' to 3'-directed addition of mononucleotides from the deoxyribonucleoside-5'-triphosphate to the 3'-hydroxyl terminus of the growing DNA chain. The directionality of polymerase α permits continuous replication of the 3' → 5' parent (leading strand). Replication of the 5' → 3' parent (lagging strand) however, occurs in a discontinuous manner. Short complementary sections of the 5' → 3' parent (Okazaki fragments) are synthesized in the 5' → 3' direction using a short RNA primer. Subsequently the sections are linked together in reactions catalyzed by DNA ligase. After synthesis, DNA bases can undergo modification which may play a role in regulating transcription in eukaryotes. Also, after DNA is synthesized, cells are able to repair it if it becomes damaged. In the inborn error, xeroderma pigmentosum, cells have a reduced ability to excise thymidine dimers formed between adjacent thymidine residues in response to the ultraviolet component of sunlight. Such individuals are extremely sensitive to sunlight and have a high incidence of skin cancer.

RNA

Although DNA is found in the nucleus with a small amount present in the mitochondria in eukaryotic cells, translation of genetic information carried by nuclear DNA occurs in the cytoplasm. This requires three types of RNA, transfer (tRNA), messenger (mRNA), and ribosomal (rRNA). In contrast to DNA, RNAs are single-stranded molecules. The backbone consists of ribose residues linked 5'→3' by phosphodiester bridges. The bases extend outward. After formation of the RNA, modification of the purines and pyrimidines can occur. Secondary order is induced in the RNA strand by base stacking and by hydrogen bonding between complementary base sequences within the molecule. The latter introduces folds in the chain which can have unpaired loops at the end. Transfer RNA, for example, has four loops of different sizes; one of these loops (the anticodon loop) functions as the tRNA's anticodon during protein synthesis. In addition RNAs are associated with proteins which tend to stabilize them.

Transcription, transfer of genetic information from DNA to RNA molecules, is mediated by DNA-dependent RNA polymerases. There are three different RNA polymerases which catalyze the transfer of nucleotides from nucleoside triphosphates to the RNA chain with the release of pyrophosphate. RNA polymerase I, in the nucleolus, catalyzes the synthesis of rRNAs; RNA polymerase II, in the nucleoplasm, catalyzes the synthesis of mRNAs; and RNA polymerase III, also in the nucleoplasm, catalyzes the synthesis of 5S rRNA and tRNAs. Mitochondria contain an RNA polymerase which is different from the three nuclear enzymes.

Transcription starts with the binding of the polymerase to a defined sequence on the DNA known as a promoter. Synthesis of RNA starts with the 5'-terminus ($3' \rightarrow 5'$ direction on the DNA template) with either ATP or GTP as the initial nucleotide. Additional nucleotides are added in stepwise fashion, until a temination sequence is reached, at which point the polymerase is released. In some instances binding of a termination protein to the polymerase DNA complex facilitates release of the RNA.

Several modifications of the transcribed RNAs take place in eukaryotic cells. Ribosomal RNA is transcribed as a large 45S precursor RNA. It is cleaved by endonucleases to give an 18S fragment which is associated with the 40S ribosomal subunit, and a 28S plus hydrogen bonded 5.8S fragment which is associated with the 60S ribosomal subunit. Messenger RNAs have a "cap" at their 5'-terminus which aids in initiation of transcription and may stabilize the molecule. The cap consists of 7-methyl-G (5') ppp (5')-initial nucleotide transcribed. The initial nucleotide and less frequently the second nucleotide can be methylated at the 2'-O-position. After transcription, a poly(A) tail is added to most mRNAs, possibly by the action of a poly(A) polymerase. At this stage the mRNA often contains nonfunctional intervening sequences termed "introns" between sequences termed "exons." Endonucleases catalyze loss of the introns. The exons are ligated together to give functional mRNA. Transfer RNA is synthesized as a large precursor which is then cleaved at the appropriate 5' and 3' termini to give tRNA of the correct size. Transfer RNAs contain many modified nucleosides and at their 3' terminus contain the sequence —pCpCpA$_{OH}$.

TRANSLATION

Translation of the information transcribed in RNA molecules into proteins occurs on polyribosomes and involves three steps (i.e., chain initiation, elongation, and termination). Synthesis of the aminoacyl-tRNAs, amino acids bound to specific tRNA carriers, utilizes a molecule of ATP. To initiate peptide synthesis, Met-tRNA$_i^{Met}$ (unlike prokaryotes the eukaryote met-tRNA$_i^{Met}$ is not formylated) is bound to a specific initiation factor, which also binds GTP, and this complex then binds to the 40S ribosomal subunit. At this stage mRNA associates with the 40S subunit, forming an initiation complex, in a step requiring ATP and several initiation factors. The 60S subunit then associates with the 40S initiation complex, with release of initiation factors and hydrolysis of GTP. The Met-tRNA$_i^{Met}$ then associates with the peptidyl (P) site of the ribosome, leaving the aminoacyl (A) site of the complex free for the next aminoacyl-tRNA. In elongation, the aminoacyl-tRNA specified by the next codon complexes with GTP and an elongation factor. It is bound at the A site releasing GDP and phosphate. The amino group on the amino acid residue of the new aminoacyl-tRNA reacts with the carbonyl carbon of the methionine (Met-tRNA$_i^{Met}$) in a reaction catalyzed by peptidyltransferase. The result is that tRNA$_i^{Met}$ remains associated with the P site with a dipeptidyl-tRNA moiety at the A site. As the next aminoacyl-tRNA unit is added to the ribosome, the dipeptidyl-tRNA anticodon-mRNA-codon-complex moves to the P site in a translocase and elongation factor-mediated step. At the same time, the tRNA$_i^{Met}$ is released and a molecule of GTP is hydrolyzed. The addition of each amino acid requires the expenditure of one ATP molecule (formation of the aminoacyl-tRNA) and two GTP. Repetition of these steps results in synthesis of a polypeptide which always occurs from the amino terminus toward the carboxy end. Chain termination occurs at a specific termination codon present on the mRNA. It is recognized by a protein release factor which requires GTP in order to bind to ribosomes. This factor binds at the A site in place of an aminoacyl-tRNA. The result is that the peptidyl-tRNA linkage at the P site is hydrolyzed, giving the free carboxyl terminus of the peptide. The peptide, tRNA, mRNA and ribosomal subunits are released and synthesis is terminated.

From the above it can be seen that information for the primary structure of a protein is carried in the mRNA base sequence. The nucleotide sequence (codon) defining a specific amino acid is a triplet. The anticodon present in tRNA consists of the three complementary bases. There are 64 possible codons comprising the genetic code. Three of the codons code for termination of the peptide chain, and one codes for methionine, needed for chain initiation as well as for protein synthesis *per se.* Changes in even one base (point mutation) in the sequence of DNA being transcribed will be reflected in the RNA synthesized. A single base change in mRNA might result in the replacement of one amino acid by another, as in sickle cell disease; in premature chain termination, as in β°-thalassemia; or in failure to terminate with resultant chain elongation, as in hemoglobin McKees Rocks. A frameshift mutation, caused by the addition or deletion of a single base, can result in an altered amino acid sequence or in the addition or deletion of a stop codon. In addition to mutations which result from errors in replication or repair, chemicals can induce mutations by converting one base to another (e.g., nitrous acid deaminates cytosine, converting it to uracil). Analogs of nucleotides may be incorporated into the DNA resulting in point mutations; others can induce deletions during transcription. Sometimes these mutations are corrected by changing the altered codon back to the original, or by the occurrence of a second mutation, at a different site, which suppresses the first mutation.

Often, newly synthesized protein must undergo post-translational modification in order to become functional. Proteins composed of subunits can result either from aggregation of subunits synthesized separately or from cleavage of a larger precursor. In the first instance, controls have evolved so that appropriate amounts of the different subunits are synthesized, as in the synthesis of the α- and β-globins needed for hemoglobin. Insulin illustrates activation of a protein by cleavage of the precursor. Finally, amino acids can undergo modification to give the active protein.

Regulation of gene expression in eukaryotes can occur at a number of points. It is apparent that regulation occurs because even though all nucleated cells in an animal carry the same genetic information, different cell types express different phenotypes. Mechanisms for regulating the expression of genetic information include amplification or rearrangement of the genes to be expressed, alteration of the rate of production of functional mRNA, and alteration of the rate of translation or post-translational processing of the polypeptide synthesized.

CLONING

Of special interest is the development of a methodology for cloning mammalian genes in *E. coli.* Two major clinical goals of research in this area are (1) the production of proteins needed for clinical use (e.g., factors needed for blood clotting) and (2) to be able to use the appropriate cloned human gene to replace that which is defective in an individual patient with a genetic disease. The following outlines the general procedure developed for cloning mammalian genes in *E. coli.*

An antibiotic resistant plasmid (small extrachromosomal DNA present in bacteria) and the strand of mammalian DNA to be inserted are cleaved using a restriction endonuclease in order to obtain complementary ends on the separate DNA fragments. The plasmid and mammalian DNA are allowed to anneal and the breaks in the nucleotide sequence are ligated in a reaction catalyzed by DNA ligase. The plasmids are inserted into the *E. coli* and the transformed *E. coli* are selected by their plasmid-induced resistance to a specific antibiotic. The plasmid-mammalian-DNA complex is transcribed and translated into its gene products, which can then be isolated, purified and used. Methods have been developed for isolating or for synthesizing (if the base sequence is known) the gene to be incorporated into the plasmid.

Several mammalian gene products have been produced using this type of procedure; including, for examples, somatostatin and insulin.

ENERGY METABOLISM

A source of energy is needed for cells to carry out such diverse functions as muscle contraction and the synthesis of macromolecules needed for cell maintenance. The required energy is obtained from the catabolism of lipid, carbohydrate, and protein. To understand the metabolic conversions involved in the formation of chemical compounds which serve as a source of chemical energy (e.g., ATP) it is necessary to review some thermodynamic relationships. The first law of thermodynamics states that energy can neither be created nor destroyed; the second law states that all processes tend toward maximum disorder or randomness. At equilibrium, disorder of the system is maximum. Entropy (S) is the term used to indicate the degree of disorder in the system. If a reaction does not result in an increase in entropy it cannot be spontaneous, and will require external energy to occur. Entropy and free energy for a reaction at constant temperature and pressure are related in the equation $\Delta G = \Delta H - T\Delta S$, in which ΔG is the change in free energy, ΔH the change in enthalpy (heat content), T the absolute temperature, and ΔS the change in entropy. At equilibrium, $\Delta G = O$. If ΔG is negative, the process occurs spontaneously; energy is given off and the reaction is exergonic. If ΔG is positive the reaction is not spontaneous because energy is required. For a chemical reaction, the change in free energy (ΔG) is related to the equilibrium constant for that reaction. For example, in the reaction $A + B \rightleftharpoons C + D$,

$$\Delta G = \Delta G^\circ + RT \ln \frac{[C][D]}{[A][B]}$$

Here, ΔG is the free energy change; ΔG° the standard free energy change for the chemical reaction when the reactants and products are present at concentrations of 1.0 M, R is the gas constant (1.987 cal/mol°K) and T the absolute temperature. [C][D]/[A][B] is the equilibrium constant, K_{eq}. At equilibrium $\Delta G = 0$. Therefore the equation can be written as $\Delta G° = -RT \ln K_{eq}$. In a multistep system the $\Delta G°$ for the initial reactants giving rise to the final products is equal to the sum of the standard free energy changes of the individual reactions. If that sum is negative the pathway will proceed spontaneously even though some of the individual reactions have positive standard free energy values.

Tricarboxylic Acid Cycle

The breakdown of glycogen to glucose and further catabolism of glucose (glycolysis), the β-oxidation of free fatty acids obtained from triacylglycerols and the deamination and oxidation of most amino acids obtained from proteins, provide precursors for the formation of acetyl coenzyme A (acetyl CoA). When energy is required by the cell, acetyl CoA is completely oxidized in a series of reactions known as the tricarboxylic acid (TCA) cycle, the citric acid cycle, or the Krebs cycle. These reactions occur in the mitochondrial matrix, which is also the site of action of pyruvate dehydrogenase (catalyzes the conversion of pyruvate to acetyl CoA and CO_2) and the locus for β-oxidation of fatty acids, two direct precursors for production of acetyl CoA. The oxidation of acetyl CoA produces two molecules of CO_2, free coenzyme A and four pairs of electrons. These reducing equivalents (electrons) are then passed down the electron transport chain in a process which is coupled to oxidative phosphorylation (ATP production).

In the initial step of the TCA cycle citrate synthase catalyzes the condensation of the acetyl moiety of acetyl CoA with oxaloacetate to produce an enzyme-citroyl-SCoA intermediate; this intermediate is then hydrolyzed to produce citrate and CoASH ($\Delta G° \sim -9$ kcal/mol). Citrate is converted to *cis*-aconitate and then to isocitrate in a reaction catalyzed by aconitase (equilibrium favors reactants). Isocitrate is then oxidized to α-ketoglutarate ($\Delta G° \sim -5$ kcal/mol). Isocitrate dehydrogenase catalyzes this reaction with NAD^+ (nicotinamide adenine dinucleotide) as a coenzyme. The conversion of α-ketoglutarate to succinyl CoA is catalyzed by the α-ketoglutarate dehydrogenase multienzyme complex in which thiamine pyrophosphate, lipoic acid, CoASH, FAD (flavin adenine dinucleotide), and NAD^+ serve as coenzymes; NAD^+ is reduced to NADH and H^+, and CO_2 is released ($\Delta G° = -8$ kcal/mol). Succinyl CoA synthetase catalyzes the conversion of succinyl CoA to succinate and CoASH with the concomitant conversion of GDP plus P_i to GTP ($\Delta G° = -0.7$ kcal/mol). (GTP can be used to convert ADP to ATP via a nucleoside diphos-

phokinase catalyzed reaction.) Succinate is oxidized to fumarate in a reaction catalyzed by the iron containing succinate dehydrogenase (associated with the mitochondrial inner membrane) utilizing FAD as an electron acceptor. In a freely reversible reaction, fumarase catalyzes the addition of water to fumarate to produce L-malate, which in the final step of the cycle is oxidized to oxaloacetate with the concomitant reduction of NAD^+. This step is catalyzed by malate dehydrogenase. The final reaction has a $\Delta G° = +7$ kcal/mol, but the conversion of oxaloacetate to citrate and the subsequent reactions in the cycle pull the reaction toward the production of oxaloacetate. The net effect of the passage of one acetyl CoA molecule through the cycle is the production of $2CO_2$, $3NADH + 3H^+$, $1FADH_2$ and 1GTP (Fig. 4-3).

Regulation of the TCA cycle is needed so that a continuous supply of ATP is available to meet the cell's energy requirements. When ATP, NADH or succinyl CoA levels are high relative to ADP, NAD^+ or succinate they exhibit inhibitory effects on the cycle. Conversion of isocitrate to α-ketoglutarate appears to be the rate-limiting reaction of the cycle; ATP, NADH, and NADPH (nicotinamide adenine dinucleotide phosphate-reduced) are inhibitory while ADP enhances activity. The NADP-specific protein, present in both the mitochondria and cytoplasm, is of importance because it serves as a source of reducing equivalents. α-Ketoglutarate dehydrogenase activity is inhibited by NADH but the main control appears to be exerted by succinyl CoA. GTP may also act as an inhibitor of this step. Succinyl CoA may inhibit the citrate synthase catalyzed reaction and oxaloacetate may inhibit conversion of succinate to fumarate.

The conditions which result in inhibition of the TCA cycle are those which occur when acetyl CoA is being produced and is available for the cycle (i.e., well fed state). Reduction in the rate of reactions in the TCA cycle coupled with the positive effect this has on other processes (e.g., increased citrate stimulates fatty acid synthesis) permits utilization of TCA cycle components for other cell functions. Acetyl CoA moieties can leave the mitochondria as citrate and in the cytosol serve as the two carbon precursors needed for fatty acid and sterol biosynthesis.

α-Ketoglutarate can be reductively aminated to yield glutamate which can serve as an amino donor in transamination reactions (e.g., oxaloacetate → aspartate). Succinyl CoA can react with glycine to give δ-aminolevulinic acid, a precursor in porphyrin synthesis. Succinyl CoA is added to the cycle by the methylmalonyl CoA mutase-catalyzed conversion of methylmalonyl CoA ($^-OOC—CH—COSCoA$) which is produced during

$\quad\quad\quad |$

$\quad\quad\quad CH_3$

the metabolism of both fatty acids of odd chain length

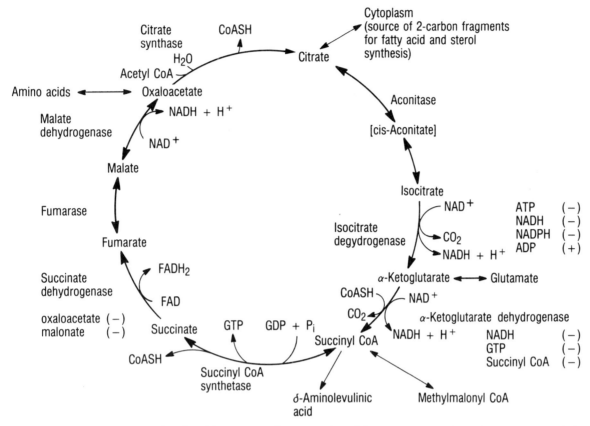

Fig. 4-3. The tricarboxylic acid cycle. Inhibitors (—) and activators (+) of the enzymes are indicated as are sites at which intermediates may be added or removed from the cycle.

and the branched chain amino acids (valine and isoleucine).

Electron Transport/Oxidative Phosphorylation

The mitochondria, site for the TCA cycle described above, are subcellular organelles which function in the production of energy via the oxidation of NADH and $FADH_2$ and conserve it by synthesizing ATP. Concentration of mitochondria within a cell reflects its function; tissue very dependent on aerobic metabolism (e.g., cardiac muscle) contains a large number of mitochondria per cell. Mitochondria are made up of two membranes separated by an intramembrane space. Within the inner membrane is the matrix. The outer membrane is composed of approximately equal amounts of protein and lipid. It is readily permeable to molecules up to 10,000 daltons (dalton refers to the mass of a molecule expressed in atomic units based on ^{12}C, for example, one atom of ^{12}C has a mass of 12 daltons). The inner membrane is characterized by invaginations toward the matrix (cristae). It is very hydrophobic and more dense than the outer membrane reflecting that it is composed of

approximately 75 percent protein and 25 percent lipid. About two-thirds of the lipid associated fatty acid residues are unsaturated, and it is this membrane that contains almost all of the cardiolipin of the cell. Protruding from the inner surface of the cristae are small structures called elementary particles which consist of spherical head pieces connected to the cristae by narrow stalks. These particles contain the components of the electron transport chain and enzymes for oxidative phosphorylation. The inner membrane also has several selective transport systems.

One important function of these transport systems is to shuttle reducing equivalents from NADH produced in the cytoplasm into the mitochondrial inner membrane, where they can subsequently be reoxidized by the electron transport chain. The α-glycerol phosphate shuttle is an example. In glycolysis, glyceraldehyde-3-phosphate is converted to 1, 3-bisphosphoglycerate with the reduction of NAD^+. The NADH is oxidized in the cystoplasmic, glycerol 3-phosphate dehydrogenase-catalyzed conversion of dihydroxyacetone phosphate to glycerol-3-phosphate. The shuttle is completed by the action of a glycerol-3-phosphate dehydrogenase, associated with the outer surface of the inner mitochondrial membrane, catalyzing the conversion of the glycerol 3-phosphate back to dihydroxyacetone phosphate. However, the coenzyme is FAD which is reduced to $FADH_2$. A somewhat more complex system is the malate-aspartate shuttle. Briefly, the reduction of oxaloacetate to malate regenerates cytoplasmic NAD^+; the malate crosses the inner mitochondrial membrane in exchange with α-ketoglutarate. Malate dehydrogenase catalyzes the oxidation of malate to oxaloacetate producing matrix NADH and H^+. Aspartate aminotransferase (also known as glutamic-oxaloacetate transaminase) catalyzes the transamination of oxaloacetate by glutamate producing aspartate and α-ketoglutarate. The aspartate can cross the inner membrane in exchange with cytoplasmic glutamate. In the cytoplasm the aspartate is deaminated (cytoplasmic aspartate aminotransferase) to give oxaloacetic acid and glutamate completing the cycle.

The oxidation of NADH and H^+ by oxygen can be written as:

$$NADH + H^+ + \tfrac{1}{2}O_2 \longrightarrow NAD^+ + H_2O$$

Similarly the oxidation of $FADH_2$ can be described as:

$$FADH_2 + \tfrac{1}{2}O_2 \longrightarrow FAD + H_2O$$

In each of these reactions the oxygen is reduced and the coenzyme is oxidized. The standard free energy of this type of reaction can be calculated providing the redox potential (E_o' defined as the midpoint potential that would be measured by a potentiometer inserted between a standard hydrogen electrode and an inert electrode in a solution containing equimolar amounts of the oxidized and reduced components under defined conditions) of the reactants is known. The standard free energy and standard reduction potential are related by the equation:

$$-\Delta G^\circ = nF\Delta E_o'$$

in which ΔG° is the standard free energy of the reaction, $\Delta E_o'$ the difference between redox potentials (E_o') for the two systems, n the number of electrons transferred per mol, and F is the Faraday (96,500 coulombs). The units for $F\Delta E_o'$ are coulomb-volts, or joules, and can be converted to calories using the relationship 4.18 J equal one calorie. Therefore, when NADH is oxidized in electron transport, the net redox reaction (sum of the oxidation and reduction half reactions) is:

$NADH \longrightarrow NAD^+ + H^+ + 2e^-$	$E = E_o' = +0.320V$
$\tfrac{1}{2}O_2 + 2H^+ + 2e^- \longrightarrow H_2O$	$E = E_o' = +0.816V$
$NADH + \tfrac{1}{2}O_2 + H^+ \longrightarrow NAD^+ + H_2O$	$\Delta E_o' = 1.14V$

$\Delta G^\circ = -nF\Delta E_o' = -(2)(23.1 \text{ kcal/V})(1.14 \text{ V}) = -52$ kcal/mol. The oxidation of NADH results in the formation of three ATPs, that of $FADH_2$ in the formation of two ATPs. Hydrolysis of ATP to produce ADP and P_i yields 7.3 kcal/mol, so hydrolysis of three moles of ATP would produce 21.9 kcal. Therefore, the efficiency of ATP synthesis via oxidative phosphorylation of NADH is 21.9 kcal/mol/52 kcal/mol or about 40 percent.

The electron-transferring components of the electron transport chain are organized in a sequential arrangement in the inner mitochondrial membrane. The sequence of electron carriers and the sites of ATP formation are as shown:

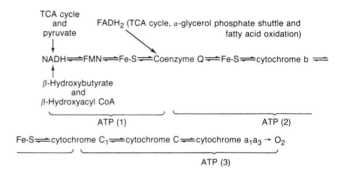

The system is set up so that as one member is oxidized the next component is reduced. In the final step oxygen is reduced to water with the reoxidation of cytochrome a_1a_3. It has been shown that one molecule of ATP is produced as the electrons move down the components of the chain in such a way that a drop in redox potential of about 0.3 V occurs. The change in potential when electrons are transferred from $FADH_2$ to coenzyme Q is too low to permit ATP synthesis, hence oxidation of $FADH_2$ results in production of two ATP while oxidation of NADH results in production of 3 ATP. Therefore, the oxidation of acetyl CoA to produce CO_2 and water results in the production of a total of 12 ATP molecules (1GTP, 3NADH + $3H^+$ and $1FADH_2$).

Currently, the chemiosmotic hypothesis provides an explanation for how the production of protons during electron transport results in ATP synthesis. This hypothesis proposes that the components of the electron transport chain are situated so that as they are oxidized the protons are released on the outer side of the membrane, thereby establishing an electrochemical gradient. Subsequent reduction of this gradient is coupled to synthesis of ATP in a reaction catalyzed by a $Ca^{2+} - Mg^{2+}$ dependent ATPase associated with the inner surface of the inner mitochondrial membrane. The ATPase consists of a water soluble component, F_1 and a hydrophobic portion, F_o. The active site of the enzyme is in the F_1 unit. The F_o portion may provide the channel through which protons can pass to the active site and in some manner drive ATP formation. The tight coupling of electron transport with ATP formation provides a coarse control for the rate at which potential energy sources are completely oxidized. If no ADP and P_i are available for ATP synthesis, the chemiosmotic hypothesis also explains the shut down of electron transport (i.e., the ATPase will not permit protons to pass from the intermembrane space to the matrix). With the increase in proton concentration, the oxidative process is inhibited and electron transport is blocked.

Glycolysis

In glycolysis, glucose is converted to pyruvate (aerobic) or lactate (anaerobic):

$$\text{Glucose} + 2\text{ADP} + 2P_i + 2\text{NAD}^+ \longrightarrow$$
$$2 \text{ pyruvate} + 2\text{ATP} + 2\text{NADH} + 2\text{H}^+$$

In the formation of lactate from pyruvate, NADH is oxidized to NAD^+, which can then be used again in the pathway. The first step in the cellular metabolism of glucose is its essentially irreversible reaction with ATP to form glucose-6-phosphate ($\Delta G° = -5$ kcal/mol) in a phosphorylation catalyzed by hexokinase or glucokinase. There are three isoenzymes of hexokinase (I, II, and III) present in cells. Type I is the major form found in brain; type II is enriched in skeletal muscle. All have low K_m values for glucose, can use other monosaccharides as substrates albeit less efficiently, and are inhibited by glucose-6-phosphate. Type II is more sensitive to inhibition by glucose-6-phosphate than Type I and the presence of P_i does not lessen the glucose-6-phosphate inhibition of type II as it does for type I. These properties reflect the needs of the cells (i.e., muscle hexokinase (type II) responds to changes in glucose levels, while brain, which normally has a steady supply of glucose, has a hexokinase (type I) which responds primarily to P_i levels). Glucokinase (also called hexokinase IV) associated primarily with liver cells, has a much higher K_m for glucose and is not inhibited by glucose-6-phosphate. Liver cells are freely permeable to glucose and in the hyperglycemic state, as occurs after eating, glucokinase converts excess blood glucose to glucose-6-phosphate without product inhibition. The glucose-6-phosphate can then be used in glycolysis or stored as glycogen.

Phosphoglucose isomerase catalyzes the reversible conversion of glucose-6-phosphate to fructose-6-phosphate, which, in an essentially irreversible reaction requiring ATP, is converted to fructose-1,6-bisphosphate ($\Delta G° = -4.5$ kcal/mol). The enzyme responsible for catalyzing this *committing step* in glycolysis is phosphofructokinase. In muscle, low ATP concentration results in the phosphofructokinase exhibiting hyperbolic ki-

netics (V v S plot) while high ATP concentrations result in sigmoidal kinetics with an increased K_m. The liver enzyme is activated by fructose-2,6-bisphosphate which also inhibits fructosebisphosphatase the enzyme which catalyzes the conversion of fructose-1,6-bisphosphate to fructose-6-phosphate in gluconeogenesis. Glucagon, a hormone released by the pancreas in response to low blood glucose levels, stimulates release of glucose by liver cells. It functions by inhibiting fructose-2,6-bisphosphate kinase, the enzyme which catalyzes the conversion of fructose-6-phosphate to fructose-2,6-bisphosphate, via a cascade series of reactions starting with activation of adenylate cyclase and terminating with phosphorylation of the kinase. This results in reduction of the phosphofructokinase activity (increases the K_m) and activation of the phosphofructophosphatase thereby stopping glycolysis and enhancing gluconeogenesis (synthesis of glucose).

Aldolase catalyzes the formation of two-three carbon moieties from fructose-1,6-bisphosphate:

$$\text{Fructose-1,6-diP} \rightleftharpoons$$
$$\text{dihydroxyacetone-P} + \text{D-glyceraldehyde-3-P}$$

where P indicates phosphate. $\Delta G° = 5.7$ kcal/mol for this reaction. Triose phosphate isomerase catalyzes the conversion of dihydroxyacetone phosphate, which cannot be used in subsequent glycolytic reactions, to glyceraldehyde-3-phosphate ($\Delta G° = 1.8$ kcal/mol). Alternatively, dihydroxyacetone phosphate can be reduced to glycerol-3-phosphate (precursor for complex lipid synthesis) in a reaction catalyzed by glycerol-3-phosphate dehydrogenase and requiring NADH and H^+ as a cofactor.

The two glyceraldehyde-3-phosphate molecules undergo a series of alterations resulting in production of two lactate molecules and four ATP molecules. The conversion of glyceraldehyde-3-phosphate to 3-phosphoglycerate results in formation of ATP:

$$2 \text{ D-glyceraldehyde-3-P} + 2 \text{ NAD}^+ + 2 P_i \xrightarrow{\text{glyceraldehyde-3-P dehydrogenase}}$$
$$2 \text{ 1,3-bisphosphoglycerate} + 2 \text{ NADH} + 2 \text{ H}^+ \ (\Delta G° = 1.5 \text{ kcal/mol})$$

$$2 \text{ 1,3-bisphosphoglycerate} + 2\text{ADP} \xrightarrow{\text{phosphoglycerate kinase}}$$
$$2 \text{ 3-phosphoglycerate} + 2 \text{ ATP} \ (\Delta G° = -4.5 \text{ kcal/mol})$$

The formation of 3-phosphoglycerate pulls the unfavored aldolase and isomerase catalyzed reactions toward the products needed for glycolysis. Phosphoglucomutase catalyzes the reversible conversion of 3-phosphoglycerate to 2-phosphoglycerate ($\Delta G° = 1$ kcal/mol) which is then dehydrated to phosphoenolpyruvate in an enolase catalyzed reaction ($\Delta G° = 0.4$ kcal/mol). Pyruvate kinase catalyzes the essentially irreversible conversion of phosphoenolpyruvate to pyruvate with formation of ATP ($\Delta G° = -7.5$ kcal/mol). The liver kinase is inhibited by ATP and alanine (feedback inhibition) and activated by fructose-1,6-bisphosphate (feed forward regulation). Diet also affects kinase activity; fasting and glucagon decrease kinase activity, thereby enhancing gluconeogenesis, while insulin and a carbohydrate-rich diet increase liver kinase activity. Finally, pyruvate is reduced to give lactate ($\Delta G° = -6$ kcal/mol) with oxidation of an amount of NADH and H^+ equivalent to that produced in formation of 1,3-bisphosphoglycerate. This step, catalyzed by lactate dehydrogenase, provides for the reoxidation of NADH and H^+ in an anaerobic environment, maintaining the supply of NAD^+ required for glycolysis. Lactate cannot be further catabolized but it can diffuse from the cell and be carried to the liver where it can be oxidized to pyruvate. A pyruvate carrier facilitates transport of pyruvate across the inner mitochondrial membrane (in exchange for OH^-) where the pyruvate dehydrogenase complex catalyzes its conversion to acetyl CoA and CO_2:

$$\text{Pyruvate} + NAD^+ + \text{CoASH} \xrightarrow{\overset{\text{Pyruvate}}{\text{dehydrogenase}}}$$
$$\text{acetyl CoA} + CO_2 + NADH + H^+ \quad \Delta G° = -8 \text{ kcal/mol}$$

The pyruvate dehydrogenase complex contains three catalytic subunits (pyruvate dehydrogenase, dihydrolipoyl transacylase, and dihydrolipoyl dehydrogenase) and five coenzymes (thiamine pyrophosphate, lipoic acid, coenzyme A, FAD, and NAD^+). Initially, pyruvate reacts with pyruvate dehydrogenase-bound thiamine pyrophosphate, losing CO_2 and forming α-hydroxyethyl thiamine pyrophosphate. The hydroxyethyl moiety reacts with the disulfide of lipoic acid bound to the dihydrolipoyl transacetylase, reducing the disulfide and forming acetyllipoamide. The acetyl group is transferred to the sulfhydryl group of CoA and FAD bound to dihydrolipoyl dehydrogenase is reduced in the reoxidation of the lipoyl residue. The $FADH_2$ is then oxidized in a reaction in which NAD^+ in the matrix is reduced to NADH and H^+. Several factors help regulate the activity of the pyruvate dehydrogenase complex. The complex is inactive when phosphorylated; an ATP-Mg-dependent protein kinase catalyzes its phosphorylation while phosphoprotein phosphatase *a* catalyzes loss of the phosphate residue. Acetyl CoA and NADH (products of the reaction) inhibit the active form of the complex and also

activate the protein kinase, resulting in inactivation of the complex by phosphorylation. NAD^+ and coenzyme A inhibit the kinase as does pyruvate. Insulin activates the complex in adipose tissue (in the fed state, acetyl CoA produced can be used for fatty acid synthesis), and epinephrine can activate it in cardiac tissue (oxidation of acetyl CoA to give ATP).

In summary, glycolysis results in the *net* production of 2 ATP, 2 NADH and 2 H^+ when pyruvate is the product. Conversion of two pyruvate to two acetyl CoA produces 2 NADH and 2 H^+. Oxidation of the two acetyl CoA molecules yields 6 NADH and 6 H^+, 2 $FADH_2$ and 2 ATP. Oxidation of the reduced coenzymes produces 34 ATP which gives a total of 38 ATP molecules produced per glucose molecule oxidized:

$$\text{Glucose} + 6 O_2 + 38 \text{ ADP} + 38 \text{ P}_i \longrightarrow$$
$$6 CO_2 + 6 H_2O + 38 \text{ ATP}$$

Gluconeogenesis

Pyruvate or other glucogenic precursors can be produced in the metabolism of all of the amino acids except leucine and lysine. Pyruvate can be converted to oxaloacetate and serve to replace depleted intermediates in the TCA cycle plus it serves as an initial reactant in gluconeogenesis (glucose synthesis). Gluconeogenesis cannot occur by a reversal of glycolysis, since some of the glycolytic reactions are essentially irreversible. For example, the conversion of pyruvate to phosphoenolypyruvate, the first step of gluconeogenesis, requires an alternative pathway. Two steps are involved. The first, catalyzed by the biotin-containing enzyme pyruvate carboxylase, results in the production of oxaloacetate:

$$\text{Pyruvate} + CO_2 + \text{ATP} \longrightarrow \text{oxaloacetate} + \text{ADP} + \text{P}_i$$

pyruvate carboxykinase then converts oxaloacetate to phosphoenolpyruvate:

$$\text{Oxaloacetate} + \text{GTP} \longrightarrow$$
$$\text{phosphoenolpyruvate} + \text{GDP} + CO_2$$

Pyruvate carboxylase is in the mitochondria and the carboxykinase is associated with the cytoplasm. Since oxaloacetate cannot cross the inner mitochondrial membrane, it is transaminated to give aspartate (glutamate $\rightarrow$ α-ketoglutarate) or reduced to malate ($NADH + H^+ \rightarrow NAD^+$). Both can cross the mitochondrial membrane via shuttle mechanisms. In the cytoplasm, aspartate and malate are converted back to oxaloacetate. If lactate is the pyruvate precursor, its conversion to pyruvate produces NADH which can be reoxidized during conversion of the phosphoenolpyruvate to glucose. When pyruvate is produced from other sources, the malate shuttle results in production of cytosolic NADH. In glycolysis, conversion of phosphoenolpyruvate to pyruvate produces one ATP while the reverse step in gluconeogenesis requires the equivalent of two ATP (GTP can reversibly phosphorylate ADP in a nucleoside diphosphate kinase catalyzed reaction).

Reversal of glycolysis converts phosphoenolpyruvate to fructose-1,6-bisphosphate. This cannot be converted to fructose-6-phosphate by reversing the step catalyzed by 6-phosphofructokinase. Instead, the enzyme fructose bisphosphatase catalyzes the irreversible hydrolysis of fructose-1,6-bisphosphate to fructose-6-phosphate. It is then converted to glucose-6-phosphate in the reaction catalyzed by phosphoglucoisomerase. The glucose-6-

phosphate is converted to glucose in a reaction catalyzed by glucose-6-phosphatase (unique to kidney, liver and intestinal mucosa) since the glucokinase which catalyzes the first step of glycolysis cannot catalyze the reverse reaction. While lactate production from glucose results in the net production of two ATP, the synthesis of glucose from lactate requires the utilization of six ATP (four ATP in the synthesis of two phosphoenolpyruvate, and two ATP in the conversion of two molecules of 3-phosphoglycerate to two 1,3-bisphosphoglycerate).

The points of regulation for glycolysis, the reactions catalyzed by hexokinase, phosphofructokinase, and pyruvate kinase, are the steps that are not reversed in gluconeogenesis. Similarly, the enzymes regulated in gluconeogenesis are pyruvate carboxylase and fructose-1,6-bisphosphatase. Conditions which inhibit glycolysis tend to enhance gluconeogenesis (Fig. 4-4). Immediately

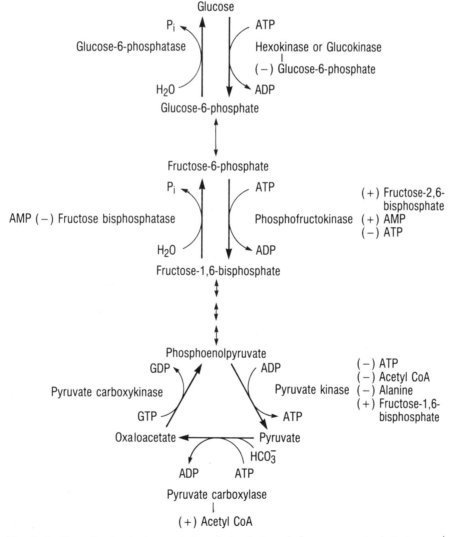

Fig. 4-4. Control points in the regulation of glycolysis and gluconeogenesis. Activators and inhibitors of the enzymes are indicated by a (+) and (−), respectively.

after eating (blood glucose and insulin levels are relatively high) gluconeogenesis is depressed. However, a few hours after eating insulin levels have fallen and glucagon concentration has increased and liver glycogen will be utilized to keep blood sugar levels stable. This is essential because brain is dependent upon glucose as its main source of energy. Pyruvate kinase and 6-phosphofructokinase are inactivated by phosphorylation which is regulated in a positive manner by glucagon. An increase in glucagon activates adenylate cyclase producing cAMP which in turn activates a protein kinase that catalyzes phosphorylation of both the pyruvate and phosphofructokinases. Glucagon also stimulates mobilization of fatty acids from adipose tissue to the liver, where they can undergo β-oxidation in the mitochondria to produce acetyl CoA. Acetyl CoA serves as a positive effector of pyruvate carboxylase, while the ATP generated by β-oxidation can be used to drive gluconeogenesis and serves as a negative effector of both phosphofructokinase and pyruvate kinase. The later enzyme is also inhibited by acetyl CoA.

Glycogen

Glycogen, which accounts for not more than 10 percent of the energy stored in the body (lipids account for greater than 90 percent), is a glucose polymer in which the residues are linked in an $\alpha 1,4$ linear linkage except at branch points, which are introduced by $\alpha 1,6$ linkages. While glycogen occurs in most tissues, skeletal muscle (which stores glycogen at $1-2$ percent of its wet weight) contains about two-thirds of total body glycogen, while liver contains most of the remainder (as much as 10 percent of its wet weight). Liver glycogen serves as a source of glucose for maintenance of blood glucose concentrations ($70-90$ mg per 100 ml blood). In contrast "white" muscle uses its glycogen stores as a source of energy in times of stress. The production of glucose-1-phosphate in the first step of glycogenolysis only requires P_i whereas the first step of glycolysis (glucose $\rightarrow$ glucose-6-phosphate) requires ATP. This means that a net of three ATP molecules are produced during conversion of a glycogen glucose residue to lactate. During times of rest the muscle cells replenish their glycogen stores.

Glycogen synthesis starts with glucose-6-phosphate produced by the initial step in glycolysis. Glucose-6-phosphate can be reversibly isomerized to glucose-1-phosphate in a reaction catalyzed by phosphoglucomutase. Glucose-1-phosphate reacts with UTP to produce an activated glucosyl residue, UDP-glucose, and pyrophosphate which is hydrolyzed to produce inorganic phosphate, making the reaction essentially irreversible. Glycogen synthase specifically catalyzes the transfer of the activated glucosyl moiety to the four position of the growing glycogen chain forming an $\alpha 1,4$ linkage and liberating UDP:

$$(\text{Glucose})_n + \text{UDP-glu} \longrightarrow (\text{glucose})_{n+1} + \text{UDP}$$

The UDP can react with ATP producing UTP and ADP. The addition of one glucose to glycogen requires the equivalent of two ATP, one for the phosphorylation of glucose and one for its activation. Glycogen synthase requires preformed glycogen; the initiation steps in the *de novo* synthesis of glycogen are not known. The branches are introduced by the action of a branching enzyme, amylo $(\alpha 1,4 \rightarrow \alpha 1,6)$ transglucosylase. It cleaves a block of six or seven glucosyl residues and transfers it to form an $\alpha 1,6$-linkage with a glucose residue at least four glucosyl residues from the last branch point. In Type IV (Anderson's) glycogen storage disease the branching enzyme is defective and glycogen with long branches is synthesized.

Glycogen phosphorylase catalyzes glycogen phosphorolysis at the $\alpha 1,4$ bonds:

$$(\text{Glucose})_n + P_i \longrightarrow \text{glucose-1-phosphate} + (\text{glucose})_{n-1}$$

Phosphoglucomutase catalyzes the conversion of glucose-1-phosphate to glucose-6-phosphate which can be used in glycolysis. Liver, kidney, and intestinal mucosal cells contain glucose-6-phosphatase which catalyzes the conversion of glucose-6-phosphate to glucose. These are the cells which can release glucose to the blood and help maintain blood glucose levels. In Type Ia (von Gierke's) glycogen storage disease, this enzyme is inactive with the result, severe hypoglycemia. In Type Ib the glucose-6-phosphate translocase is defective and the substrate fails to enter the lumen of the endoplasmic reticulum which is the site of action for the glucose-6-phosphatase. Glycogen phosphorylase functions until only four residues remain from a branch point. Continued glycogen degradation depends on the activities associated with the "debranching" enzyme. The first reaction it catalyzes is the transfer of the triglucoside attached to the $\alpha 1,6$-linked glucose to a different chain in an $\alpha 1,4$-linkage. Its second action is as an $\alpha 1,6$-glucosidase which catalyzes cleavage of the $\alpha 1,6$-linked glucose. The resulting $\alpha 1,4$-linked glucose polymer can then be further degraded by the glycogen phosphorylase. The "debranching" enzyme is defective in Type III (Cori's) glycogen storage disease. Note that the "debranching" enzyme produces free glucose when it acts as a glucosidase.

Multiple controls exist which affect the activities of glycogen synthase and phosphorylase, the key enzymes in glycogen metabolism. Both enzymes are affected by metabolites; glucose-6-phosphate activates the D or inactive form (now designated b) of glycogen synthase, while AMP activates the inactive "b" form of glycogen phosphorylase. The major control for both enzymes is covalent modification by phosphorylation. Glycogen phosphorylase is converted to the active "a" form by phosphorylation while the synthase is converted from the active "a" form to the inactive form when phosphorylated. The letter "a" designates the active form and "b" the inactive form regardless of the effect of phosphorylation.

Several interrelated reactions occur in the covalent modification (phosphorylation) of phosphorylase "b" to give phosphorylase "a" (Fig. 4-5). The first of the series of reactions can be initiated by the interaction of epinephrine or glucagon with the appropriate membrane receptor. This results in cAMP formation. The cAMP activates a cAMP-dependent protein kinase (insulin inhibits) which catalyzes the phosphorylation of phosphorylase kinase "b" producing phosphorylase kinase "a". The phosphorylase kinase "a" catalyzes the phosphoryl-

ation of glycogen phosphorylase "b" to give phosphorylase "a" which will catalyze the degradation of glycogen. While AMP does not activate the a form of phosphorylase to any extent, it does bind to it to prevent it from being dephosphorylated (inactivated) by phosphoprotein phosphatase. Other controls include the positive effect of Ca^{2+} on phosphorylase kinase activity. Phosphorylase kinase activity is lacking in Type VIII glycogen storage disease which usually presents with mild clinical symptoms. There is also an inhibitory protein which inhibits phosphoprotein phosphatase. The inhibitor is also covalently modified by phosphorylation in a reaction catalyzed by cAMP-dependent protein kinase. In contrast to the phosphorylase kinase and the phosphorylase which are phosphorylated on serine residues, the inhibitory protein is converted to the "a" form by phosphorylation of a threonine residue. The inhibitor is converted to its "b" form by the phosphoprotein phosphatase that it inhibits.

While the steps involved in glycogenolysis and its regulation appear to be similar in liver and muscle, the

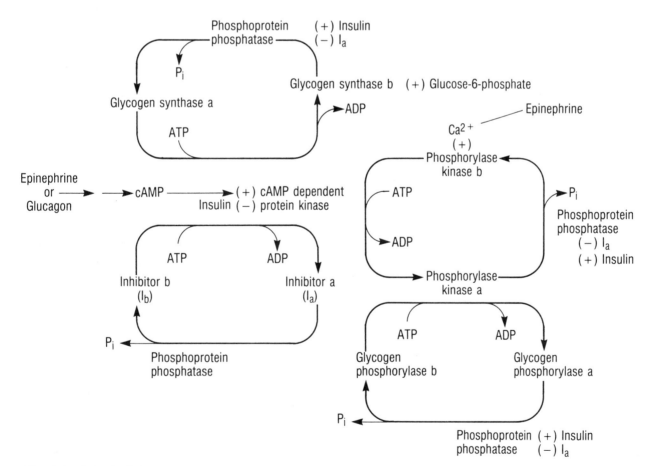

Fig. 4-5. Controls of glycogen metabolism. An "a" indicates the active form of the enzyme, a "b" the inactive form. The cAMP dependent protein kinase is central in the regulation of glycogen metabolism in that it affects the activity of glycogen synthase, phosphorylase kinase, and the inhibitory protein. Activators of individual enzymes are indicated by a (+) and inhibitors by a (−).

phosphorylases isolated from these cells show poor immunocross-reactivity. This difference is consistent with the fact that there are two different glycogen storage diseases in which phosphorylase activity is defective. In Type V (McArdle's disease) the defect is associated with muscle glycogen phosphorylase; in Type VI (Hers' disease) liver glycogen phosphorylase is inactive. Skeletal muscle is affected by the former; liver and leukocytes by the latter.

Unlike glycogen phosphorylase, glycogen synthase can be phosphorylated in a reaction catalyzed by cAMP-dependent protein kinase. Phosphorylation converts the synthase to the inactive form. Insulin enhances glycogen synthesis by inhibiting cAMP-dependent protein kinase and by enhancing phosphoprotein phosphatase activity. Phosphorylase kinase can also catalyze phosphorylation of the synthase. The kinase is affected positively by Ca^{2+}, which can be increased by the action of epinephrine and also made available by the nervous stimulation of muscle contraction. Neural stimulation of muscle cells results in membrane depolarization and release of Ca^{2+} from the sarcoplasmic reticulum into the sarcoplasm of the muscle cells. It can be seen that glycogen synthesis and breakdown are regulated by a cascade system which in response to glucagon and epinephrine slows down glycogen synthesis and accelerates glycogenolysis while insulin exerts opposing effects.

Pentose-phosphate Pathway

An alternative pathway to glycolysis for glucose oxidation is the pentose-phosphate pathway (also known as the 6-phosphogluconate pathway or the hexose monophosphate shunt). While glucose is oxidized to CO_2 and H_2O, no ATP is generated. This pathway functions to produce NADPH which provides reducing equivalents for many biosynthetic reactions (e.g., fatty acid synthesis) and it results in the synthesis of five-carbon sugars needed for nucleotide and nucleic acid synthesis. This pathway can be considered in two parts. The initial reactions:

Glucose-6-phosphate → glucose-6-phosphate dehydrogenase → 6-phosphoglucono-lactone → lactonase → 6-phosphogluconate → 6-phosphogluconate dehydrogenase → Ribulose-5-phosphate + CO_2 → isomerase → Ribose-5-phosphate

result in formation of two NADPH and one CO_2. The second series of reactions in this pathway can be visualized as converting three ribulose-5-phosphate moieties

to glyceraldehyde-3-phosphate and two fructose-6-phosphate:

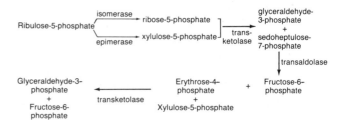

Glyceraldehyde-3-phosphate and fructose-6-phosphate are intermediates of the glycolytic pathway.

The way in which glucose is used by different types of cells reflects their specialized needs. Red blood cells lack organelles (e.g., mitochondria) and use glucose as an energy source (glycolysis) and for the production of NADPH (phosphate-pentose shunt). The lactate produced in glycolysis is released to the blood stream. The NADPH reduces oxidized glutathione making it available to block free radical reactions by reducing organic peroxides. This protects cellular proteins from inactivation by oxidation and is particularly important in red blood cells which lack the machinery necessary for protein synthesis. In brain, glucose enters (as it does red blood cells) via an insulin-independent facilitated diffusion. Glycolysis produces pyruvate which in brain is oxidized completely to CO_2 and H_2O. Glucose also provides NADPH, needed for reductive synthesis as well as for maintenance of protein integrity. Muscle, heart, and adipose cells have *insulin-dependent* facilitated transport systems for glucose. Muscle and heart use glucose for energy production forming lactate when conditions are essentially anaerobic and pyruvate, which is completely oxidized, under conditions in which oxygen is available. Again the pentose-phosphate pathway is utilized for NADPH production. Muscle and heart cells are able to synthesize glycogen which they will use in times of stress. Adipose tissue metabolizes glucose to produce pyruvate which is converted to acetyl CoA by pyruvate dehydrogenase. However, the primary use of acetyl CoA is for fatty acid synthesis rather than energy production. NADPH synthesis is of particular importance to these cells which need the NADPH for the reductive steps in fatty acid biosynthesis. While adipose tissue can synthesize glycogen, it is not as quantitatively significant as it is in muscle. Liver cells have an *insulin-independent* glucose transport system and metabolize glucose to produce a variety of products reflecting the diverse processes its cells carry out. Glycolysis produces pyruvate which can serve as a source of acetyl CoA for fatty acid synthesis or be completely oxidized to produce ATP. The pentose-phosphate pathway produces essential NADPH plus ribose phosphate needed for liver nucleotide synthesis. Glucose is also used for glycogen synthesis and liver cells can convert three-carbon precursors to glucose by gluconeogenesis, thus the liver serves as a source of glucose for maintenance of blood sugar levels. Finally, liver cells can convert glucose to glucuronic acid which can form conjugates with the amino, carboxy, hydroxyl, or sulfhydryl groups of drugs as part of a detoxification system.

Glucose can be metabolized to produce other monosaccharides found in cells. UDP-glucose can epimerize producing UDP-galactose. Utilization of dietary galactose requires its conversion to the UDP-derivative. This occurs via formation of galactose-1-phosphate which reacts with UDP-glucose to produce UDP-galactose and glucose-1-phosphate. Galactosemia results if either the galactokinase (catalyzes phosphorylation of galactose) or the uridyltransferase is inactive. A clinical symptom of these metabolic errors is cataract formation. The high galactose concentration results in formation of galactitol which accumulates in the lens. Fructose-6-phosphate (glycolysis intermediate) can be aminated (glutamine serves as the amino group donor) in an essentially irreversible reaction to form glucosamine-6-phosphate. It serves as the precursor for UDP-*N*-acetylglucosamine and UDP-*N*-acetylgalactosamine. UDP-*N*-acetylglucosamine can epimerize at the two or four position to form *N*-acetylmannosamine or UDP-*N*-acetylgalactosamine, respectively. *N*-acetylmannosamine can be phosphorylated producing *N*-acetylmannosamine-1-phosphate. This can be converted to *N*-acetylmannosamine-6-phosphate which condenses with phosphoenolpyruvate to form *N*-acetylneuraminic acid-9-phosphate; hydrolysis yields *N*-acetyl-neuraminic acid (sialic acid). Fructose-6-phosphate can also be converted to mannose-6-phosphate in a mutase catalyzed reaction. The mannose-6-phosphate undergoes a series of reactions resulting in GDP-fucose formation. Ingested fucose must likewise be activated to GDP-fucose, which can then be utilized for oligosaccharide synthesis.

Lipids

The major source of potential energy for tissue utilization is stored in adipose tissue in the form of triacylglycerols, which can be synthesized from nonlipid precursors. The only required lipid nutrients are the essential fatty acids (linoleic and linolenic) and the lipid-soluble vitamins (A,D,E, and K). Triacylglycerols can be synthesized by most tissues but the primary sites are liver and adipose tissue. The triacylglycerols synthesized in adipose tissue can be stored there as lipid droplets in the cytoplasm; those synthesized in the liver are used primarily in lipoprotein formation. The precursors for triacylglycerol synthesis are glycerol-3-phosphate (produced by an NADH-dependent reduction of dihydroxyacetone phosphate formed in glycolysis) or dihydroxyacetone phosphate and three fatty acyl CoA residues.

Fatty Acid Biosynthesis

The synthesis of fatty acids is a cytoplasmic process, and can be considered to be the result of the condensation of two-carbon, acetyl CoA, fragments which are a product of carbohydrate, amino acid, and lipid catabolism. The committing step in fatty acid synthesis is the carboxylation of acetyl CoA to produce malonyl CoA. This reaction utilizes ATP, requires bicarbonate as the CO_2 source, and is catalyzed by the enzyme acetyl CoA carboxylase:

$$AcetylCoA + ATP + HCO_3 \longrightarrow malonylCoA + ADP + P_i$$

The enzyme from rat liver is composed of two subunits, each of which contains a molecule of biotin (serves as the CO_2 carrier) as its prosthetic group. The protomeric form of acetyl CoA carboxylase is inactive; the active form is polymerized in a citrate activated conversion. Citrate causes a shift in equilibrium to the active, filamentous form of the enzyme. Palmitoyl CoA shifts the acetyl CoA carboxylase equilibrium back to the inactive promoter. Carboxylase activity is also regulated by a cAMP-dependent phosphorylation, with the phosphorylated enzyme less active than the dephosphorylated form. Glucagon is believed to promote phosphorylation and insulin to promote the presence of the dephosphorylated, active carboxylase. When blood levels of insulin are high, blood sugar levels are elevated, and glucose is available as an energy source. This results in increased glycolysis, producing acetyl CoA which can be oxidized with concomitant formation of ATP. As the ATP level increases it inhibits isocitrate dehydrogenase, resulting in citrate accumulation. This can be shuttled from the mitochondria to the cytoplasm. There, the citrate can be cleaved in an ATP-dependent reaction catalyzed by citrate lyase, to produce oxaloacetate and the acetyl CoA needed for fatty acid synthesis. Citrate also serves as a positive effector of the carboxylase. A diet high in carbohydrate results in an increase in the synthesis of enzymes needed for fatty acid biosynthesis (ATP-citrate lyase, acetyl CoA carboxylase, and fatty acid synthetase) providing a long-term control.

Fatty acid synthetase and palmitate synthetase are the common names given the multifunctional enzyme which catalyzes the subsequent reactions necessary for fatty acid biosynthesis. There are seven catalytic functions associated with the enzyme. The first step in fatty acid synthesis catalyzed by the acetyl transferase activity of the enzyme is the transfer of the acetyl group from CoA to first the phosphopantetheine residue of the acyl-carrier protein (ACP) unit of the enzyme and then to a sulfhydryl group. The transfer of malonate from malonyl CoA to the ACP phosphopantetheine sulfhydryl reflects the malonyl transferase activity of the enzyme. β-ketoacyl-ACP synthetase catalyzes the condensation of the acetyl moiety with the malonate producing acetoacetyl-ACP and CO_2. In an NADPH-dependent reaction catalyzed by β-hydroxyacyl-ACP reductase acetoacetyl-ACP is reduced to β-hydroxybutyryl-ACP, which can be dehydrated to yield crotonyl-ACP in a reaction catalyzed by β-hydroxyacyl-ACP dehydratase. The carbonyl moiety can be reduced in a second NADPH-dependent reaction catalyzed by 2,3-*trans*-enoylacyl reductase. Transacylase catalyzes the transfer of the butyryl moiety from the phosphopantetheine sulfhydryl to the sulfhydryl group of the synthetase, preparing the enzyme for the addition of another malonyl residue to the ACP phosphopantetheine residue. If the cycle is repeated seven times, palmitoyl-S-enzyme will be produced. At this point a deacylase specific for palmitate catalyzes the hydrolysis of palmitate from the synthetase. In summary, the synthesis of palmitate can be considered the result of the condensation of eight two-carbon fragments, seven of which are introduced as malonyl moieties. Each addition of a malonyl unit requires two NADPH and two H^+. Therefore, the reaction can be written as:

$$\text{AcetylCoA} + 7 \text{ malonylCoA} + 14 \text{ NADPH} + 14 \text{ H}^+ \longrightarrow$$
$$\text{palmitate} + 7CO_2 + 14 \text{ NADP}^+ + 8 \text{ CoASH} + 6 \text{ H}_2\text{O}$$

However, the synthesis of malonyl CoA requires ATP:

$$7 \text{ AcetylCoA} + 7 \text{ CO}_2 + 7 \text{ ATP} \longrightarrow$$
$$7 \text{ malonylCoA} + 7 \text{ ADP} + 7 \text{ P}_i$$

Hence the stoichiometry for the synthesis of palmitate from acetate is:

$$8 \text{ AcetylCoA} + 7 \text{ ATP} + 14 \text{ NADPH} + 14 \text{ H}^+ \longrightarrow$$
$$\text{palmitate} + 8 \text{ CoASH} + 7 \text{ ADP}$$
$$+ 7 \text{ P}_i + 6 \text{ H}_2\text{O} + 14 \text{ NADP}^+$$

The synthetase is inhibited by long chain fatty acyl CoAs and activated by NADPH.

Fatty Acid Modification

Elongation of palmitate or dietary fatty acids can occur in the endoplasmic reticulum and in the mitochondria. The sequence of reactions in the endoplasmic reticulum is similar to those catalyzed by the cytoplasmic fatty acid synthetase, with malonyl CoA serving as the source of two-carbon fragments; the difference is that the intermediates are linked to coenzyme A instead of the ACP. Palmitoyl CoA is synthesized from palmitate, ATP, and coenzyme A in a reaction catalyzed by a chain-length specific fatty acid CoA ligase. ATP is hydrolyzed to AMP and PP_i during the reaction. Stearic acid is the primary product of this pathway in most tissues. In brain, however, there appears to be at least one, and possibly more, additional endoplasmic reticulum-associated elongation systems; one for C_{16} and C_{18} and one for C_{20}-CoA and above derivatives. This may reflect the need for the longer chain fatty acids found in the lipids present in myelin membranes. The mitochondrial elongation system differs in that acetyl CoA serves as the source of two-carbon units. Acetyl CoA acyltransferase catalyzes transfer of the fatty acyl chain to acetyl CoA producing a β-ketoacyl CoA derivative. An NADH-dependent dehydrogenase catalyzes formation of the 3-hydroxyacyl CoA derivative. This is then dehydrated (enoyl CoA hydratase catalyzed reaction) and subsequently reduced in a reaction catalyzed by an NADPH-dependent acyl CoA dehydrogenase.

Other systems which can modify fatty acids include α-oxidation and ω-oxidation. α-Oxidation results in formation of the 2-hydroxy fatty acid or, if the reaction continues, in a fatty acid of one carbon less than the original. ω-Oxidation initially forms an ω-hydroxy fatty acid which can be further oxidized to an α,ω-dicarboxylic acid. Fatty acids can be converted to unsaturated fatty acids in a reaction catalyzed by a desaturase complex consisting of cytochrome b_5, NADH-cytochrome b_5 reductase and a desaturase. Molecular O_2 is required. Palmitoleoyl CoA is formed from palmitoyl CoA and oleoyl CoA from stearoyl CoA. The introduction of the double bond permits subsequent synthesis of triacylglycerols which are not solids at body temperature. Triacylglycerols with high melting points are not incorporated into transport lipoproteins as well as those with lower melting points, nor do they make as good substrates for lipases (enzymes which catalyze the degradation of complex lipids). Formation of desaturase is induced by diets high in carbohydrate or saturated fatty acids.

Triacylglycerol Synthesis

Fatty acids can be converted to their coenzyme A derivatives in an ATP requiring reaction catalyzed by a chain length-dependent microsomal fatty acyl CoA ligase. Acyl CoA reacts with L-glycerol-3-phosphate to form 1-acylglycerol-3-phosphate (lysophosphatidic acid). This reaction is catalyzed by glycerol-3-phosphate acyltransferase. A second fatty acid moiety is added at the two position forming phosphatidic acid in a reaction catalyzed by lysophosphatidic acid acyltransferase. Phosphatidic acid phosphatase catalyzes hydrolysis of the phosphate residue. Diacylglycerol acyltransferase, the only enzyme unique to triacylglycerol synthesis, catalyzes the formation of triacylglycerol. When dihydroxyacetone phosphate is the precursor, dihydroxyacetone phosphate acyltransferase catalyzes esterification of the one position and the acyl-dihydroxyacetone phosphate formed is reduced to lysophosphatidic acid in an NADPH-dependent reaction catalyzed by an oxidoreductase. Subsequent reactions to form TAGs are the same.

Triacylglycerol Mobilization

As a person goes from the well fed to the fasted state, the rate of fat mobilization increases gradually rising to a maximal rate seen only during prolonged periods of fasting. During the transition from the fed to the fasted state, insulin and blood glucose levels decrease, glucagon levels increase, and sympathetic nerve activity to the adipose tissue increases. These changes result in formation of the phosphorylated (inactive) form of acetyl CoA carboxylase and an increase in mitochondrial isocitrate dehydrogenase activity, which reduces the amount of citrate available for transport to the cytoplasm. Since citrate activates the conversion of acetyl CoA carboxylase to the active form, lower citrate levels have a negative effect on fatty acid synthesis. Under conditions of prolonged fasting, the amounts of citrate lyase, acetyl CoA carboxylase, and palmitate synthetase decrease. Specific catecholamine receptors are present on adipocytes. When they are occupied by the appropriate transmitter (norepinephrine is released by the sympathetic neurons innervating adipose tissue) the result is an increase in the activity of adenylate cyclase which in turn increases cAMP concentration. The elevated cAMP levels result in activation via phosphorylation of an adipose tissue hormone-sensitive lipoprotein lipase necessary for hydrolysis of triacylglycerols. The free fatty acids are released to the blood, where they associate with serum albumin, and are transported in the circulation to various tissues. The fatty acids are taken up by the cells and activated to the coenzyme A derivative in an ATP-de-

pendent acyl CoA synthetase catalyzed reaction:

$$RCOOH + HSCoA + ATP \xrightarrow{Mg^{2+}, K^+} RCOSCoA + AMP + PP_i$$

Acyl CoA synthetases (differ in chain length specificity) are associated with the endoplasmic reticulum and the outer mitochondrial membrane. In order for the acyl CoA to be oxidized it must enter the mitochondrial matrix, the site of β-oxidation. The inner mitochondrial membrane is impermeable to coenzyme A and derivatives thereof. This is circumvented by transferring the acyl moiety from coenzyme A to carnitine, which is carried across the inner mitochondrial membrane by a translocase that exchanges it for matrix carnitine. On the inside surface of the inner membrane, the acyl residue is transferred back to coenzyme A and the free carnitine can cross back through the membrane in exchange with another acylcarnitine moiety. Substrate availability for β-oxidation can be controlled by regulating activity of the palmitoyl CoA carnitine palmitoyl transferase, which catalyzes the transfer of palmitate from coenzyme A to carnitine. Malonyl CoA inhibits this reaction, suggesting that when malonyl CoA levels are high (fatty acid synthesis) β-oxidation is reduced due to a decrease in the amount of substrate available.

β-Oxidation of Fatty Acids

β-Oxidation of fatty acyl CoA derivatives results in a shortening of the acyl chain by two carbon atoms, and occurs in a series of four reactions. Initially, an FAD-dependent acyl CoA dehydrogenase catalyzes the formation of a trans double bond between carbons two and three:

$$R-CH_2-CH_2-CO-SCoA + FAD \longrightarrow R-CH=CH-CO-SCoA + FADH_2$$

The double bond is then hydrated (enoyl CoA hydratase) to give L-3-hydroxyacyl CoA,

$$R-CH=CH-CO-SCoA + H_2O \rightleftharpoons RCHOH-CH_2-CO-SCoA$$

NAD$^+$-dependent L-β-hydroxyacyl CoA dehydrogenase catalyzes the oxidation of the C$_3$-hydroxy group yielding the 3-keto derivative:

$$RCHOH-CH_2-CO-SCoA + NAD^+ \rightleftharpoons RCO-CH_2-CO-SCoA + NADH + H^+$$

In the final step, the β-ketoacyl CoA reacts with free coenzyme A (thiolase catalyzed reaction) to form acetyl CoA and a fatty acyl derivative two carbon atoms shorter:

$$RCO-CH_2-CO-SCoA + HSCoA \rightleftharpoons$$
$$RCOSCoA + CH_3COSCoA$$

Each set of reactions results in reduction of one FAD and one NAD^+, which when oxidized produce a total of five ATPs. The complete oxidation of an acetyl residue through the TCA cycle produces 12 ATPs. To completely oxidize palmitate the cycle must be repeated seven times. This yields seven NADH, seven reduced flavoproteins and eight acetyl CoAs which when oxidized produce 131 ATPs. The equivalent of two ATPs are required to activate the palmitate to palmitoyl CoA, therefore, a net of 129 ATPs are produced during the complete oxidation of palmitate.

Unsaturated (monoenoic or polyenoic) fatty acids can undergo β-oxidation as described until the double bond is at the 2-or 3-position. When it is at the two position, the enoyl CoA hydratase can catalyze the addition of water to the cis-double bond, but the D-3-hydroxy CoA derivative is formed. This can not be acted upon by the L-β-hydroxyacyl CoA dehydrogenase. There is, however, a 3-hydroxyacyl CoA epimerase which catalyzes the conversion of the D- to the L-isomer, making it available for the rest of the cycle. If the cis-double bond is at the three position, enoyl CoA isomerase can catalyze the isomerization of the double bond from the cis, C_3 position to the trans, C_2 position. Note that in each instance the presence of the double bond eliminates the need for the initial dehydrogenase reaction in which FAD is reduced to $FADH_2$; therefore, the energy yield obtained upon oxidation of an unsaturated fatty acid is reduced. β-Oxidation of odd chain fatty acids yields propionyl CoA which undergoes a series of reactions (carboxylation, racemization, and an intramolecular transfer of the thioester group) to produce succinyl CoA, an intermediate of the TCA cycle. The methylmalonyl CoA mutase which catalyzes the formation of succinyl CoA from methylmalonyl CoA requires vitamin B_{12} as a coenzyme. Lack of mutase activity causes methylmalonic acidemia resulting in mental retardation and failure of the affected individual to grow. Retardation appears to be the result of progressive demyelination, possibly reflecting the accumulation of methylmalonyl CoA. In one type of mutase deficiency the enzyme protein is defective and in another it is due to a vitamin B_{12} dependency.

Ketone Body Formation

Not all of the acetyl CoA is oxidized via the TCA cycle. In the liver, much of the mitochondrial acetyl CoA is converted to acetoacetate and D-β-hydroxybutyrate, referred to as "ketone bodies." Acetyl CoA acetyl transferase catalyzes the head-to-tail condensation of two acetyl CoA residues to produce acetoacetyl CoA and free coenzyme A. The acetoacetyl CoA reacts with another molecule of acetyl CoA to form 3-hydroxy-3-methylglutaryl CoA (HMGCoA, which in the cytoplasm is a precursor for synthesis of isoprenoid-derived lipids). HMGCoA is cleaved in a HMGCoA lyase-catalyzed reaction to produce acetoacetate and acetyl CoA. Reduction of the acetoacetate yields β-hydroxybutyrate. The ketone bodies are released from the liver to the circulation. They are cleared rapidly from the blood—especially by muscle cells. In the fasting state, even though the brain still requires glucose, it can use acetoacetate and β-hydroxybutyrate to meet much of its energy needs. The β-hydroxybutyrate is oxidized to acetoacetate. Mitochondrial succinyl CoA-acetoacetyl CoA transferase (not present in the liver) catalyzes the transfer of CoA from succinyl CoA to the acetoacetate to form acetoacetyl CoA and succinate. The acetoacetyl CoA is then cleaved, in a thiolase catalyzed reaction, to give two molecules of acetyl CoA which can enter the TCA cycle. In starvation, where glycogen stores are depleted and energy is derived primarily from fatty acids obtained through mobilization of depot fat, there is an increase in ketone body formation. A similar increase is seen in diabetes mellitus. Even though glucose in the blood is elevated the lack of insulin prevents its utilization at a normal rate. The insulin deficiency results in sustained activation of the horomone-sensitive triacylglycerol lipase, causing continued mobilization of adipose triacylglycerol fatty acids, with results similar to those seen in starvation. An uncontrolled diabetic, with severe ketosis, can have a blood concentration of ketone bodies over 30-times greater than normal (< 3 mg/dl) and secrete as much as 5000 mg/day in urine (~20 mg/day is normal).

Amino Acid Catabolism

Unlike excess carbohydrates and lipids which can be stored until needed, excess amino acids (those not needed for protein or other synthetic reactions) cannot be stored; they are degraded to pyruvate, TCA cycle intermediates, or acetyl CoA, compounds formed in the metabolism of carbohydrates and fatty acids. Amino acids which yield products that can result in net glucose formation are referred to as glycogenic, those producing acetyl CoA as ketogenic.

Alanine, glutamate (glutamine can be converted to glutamate by glutaminase), and aspartate (asparagine can be converted to aspartate by asparaginase) can be transaminated to yield the keto acids, pyruvate, α-ketoglutarate, and oxaloacetate, respectively. All are glycogenic. The enzymes catalyzing the transaminations (transaminases) require pyridoxal phosphate as a coenzyme. Glutamate can also be oxidized to form α-ketoglutarate and ammonia in a reaction catalyzed by glutamate dehydrogenase (NAD^+ or $NADP^+$ serves as a coenzyme).

Threonine can be catabolized via three different pathways. It can be converted to α-ketobutyrate in a threonine dehydratase catalyzed reaction. The α-ketobutyrate can then undergo a series of reactions (propionyl CoA and methylmalonyl CoA intermediates) to form succinyl CoA. Threonine can be cleaved (threonine aldolase) producing glycine and acetaldehyde. The acetaldehyde can be oxidized to acetate, a precursor of acetyl CoA. If the glycine is not used for protein synthesis or for formation of other more complex molecules, it can either be decarboxylated to CO_2 and NH_3 in a reversal of the 5,10-methylene tetrahydrofolate requiring glycine synthase catalyzed reaction; converted to serine by reversal of the serine transhydroxymethylase reaction; or oxidized to glyoxylic acid (D-amino acid oxidase). The two carbon glyoxylate can be oxidized to oxalate or react with α-ketoglutarate forming α-hydroxy-β-ketoadipate which can undergo successive loss of two CO_2 to yield α-ketoglutarate. Finally, threonine can be decarboxylated and dehydrogenated to form aminoacetone which can be converted to 2-ketopropanol. This can be oxidized to pyruvate or converted to methylglyoxal and then to lactate.

Arginine, proline, and histidine can be degraded to α-ketoglutarate. Arginine can be cleaved (arginase) to urea and ornithine. The ornithine is transaminated to glutamic acid semialdehyde which is then oxidized to glutamate and transaminated to α-ketoglutarate. Proline is oxidized to give the intermediate Δ^1-pyrroline-5-carboxylic acid which undergoes spontaneous hydrolysis to glutamic semialdehyde. While hydroxyproline does not produce α-ketoglutarate, it undergoes initial reactions similar to those of proline. It is oxidized to Δ^1-pyrroline-3-hydroxy-5-carboxylic acid which hydrolyses to erythro-L-γ-hydroxyglutamate. α-keto-γ-hydroxyglutarate is formed by transamination and is cleaved to glyoxylic acid and pyruvate. In brain, hydroxy-glutamate is converted to malate. Histidine undergoes deamination followed by hydration to yield 4-imidazolone-5-propionic acid, which undergoes ring cleavage to form N-formiminoglutamic acid. The formi-

mino group is transferred to the N^5 position of tetrahydrofolate and glutamate is produced.

The branched chain, aliphatic amino acids, valine, leucine, and isoleucine provide important sources of energy for extrahepatic tissues. The initial step in their catabolism, transamination with α-ketoglutarate as the aceptor, produces the corresponding α-keto acid. One aminotransferase catalyzes the transamination of valine (hypervalinemia occurred in a child, while transamination of leucine and isoleucine was normal) and another catalyzes the transamination of both leucine and isoleucine. A branched chain α-ketoacid dehydrogenase complex catalyzes the oxidative decarboxylation of each forming the acyl CoA derivatives with one less carbon atom. The dehydrogenase catalyzed reaction uses coenzyme A and NAD^+. It is inhibited by the end-products of the reaction, the branched chain acyl CoA derivatives, and NADH. If the enzyme is defective the three branched-chain α-keto acids are found in urine and are the cause of the characteristic odor associated with the autosomal recessively transmitted, maple syrup urine disease, which results from this defect. Elevated levels of the corresponding amino acids also accumulate in the blood and urine of affected children. These children show severe mental retardation and failure to myelinate nerves; they usually survive for only a few years. Subsequent catabolism of valine leads to formation of succinyl CoA (glycogenic product); of leucine, to formation of acetoacetate and acetyl CoA (ketogenic products); and of isoleucine, to formation of acetyl CoA and propionyl CoA, ketogenic and glycogenic products, respectively.

Cysteine is catabolized to pyruvate upon loss of the amino and sulfur moieties. Transamination of cysteine gives β-mercaptopyruvate which loses sulfur in a β-mercaptopyruvate transulfurase catalyzed reaction in the presence of an appropriate acceptor such as CN^- or RSH. Cysteine can also be converted to cysteine sulfinic acid in a reaction catalyzed by an Fe^{2+} containing dioxygenase. The sulfinic acid undergoes transamination and then loss of sulfite to give pyruvate. The sulfite is oxidized to sulfate by sulfite oxidase. Lack of sulfite oxidase activity results in accumulation of thiosulfate and sulfite in the urine. Children with this defect present with neurological problems at birth, undergo progressive deterioration, and die at an early age. Methionine can undergo a series of reactions (formation of S-adenosylmethionine, loss of a methyl group followed by loss of the adenosine moiety, and condensation with serine) to form cystathionine. This can be cleaved to yield homoserine and cysteine. Homoserine can undergo deamination giving α-ketobutyrate, a propionyl CoA precursor.

Phenylalanine not utilized for protein synthesis is converted to tyrosine in a reaction catalyzed by phenylalanine hydroxylase, a mixed function oxygenase requiring NADPH and tetrahydrobiopterin. Lack of phenylalanine hydroxylase activity results in the clinical symptoms seen in phenylketonuria, and in minor pathways for phenylalanine metabolism becoming prominent (e.g., transamination of phenylalanine to phenylpyruvate). Children with this inborn error exhibit severe mental retardation. Restriction of dietary phenylalanine reduces blood levels of phenylalanine and phenylpyruvate as well as the clinical symptoms. Tyrosine undergoes transamination and oxidation to form homogentisic acid which undergoes ring scission and subsequent cleavage to produce both fumarate and acetoacetate. Therefore, these amino acids are both glycogenic and ketogenic.

Tryptophan undergoes catabolism via two major pathways. It serves as a precursor for serotonin (5-hydroxytryptamine) or it can be oxidized to N-formylkynurenine in a reaction catalyzed by tryptophan-2,3-dioxygenase. The N-formylkynurenine loses its formyl group to yield kynurenine. This can be cleaved producing alanine and anthranilic acid, or it can lose alanine and undergo a series of reactions which result in ring cleavage and formation of two acetyl CoA moieties. 3-Hydroxyanthranilic acid, one of the intermediates of tryptophan catabolism, is a precursor for niacin (nicotinic acid) which is necessary for $NAD^+/NADP^+$ synthesis. In Hartnup's disease the renal and intestinal absorption mechanism for neutral amino acids are defective and they are excreted in the urine. Affected individuals develop rashes and neurological symptoms similar to those of pellagra (niacin deficiency). These symptoms can be alleviated by oral feeding of nicotinamide, thereby eliminating the need for tryptophan conversion to nicotinic acid. The clinical symptoms seen in niacin deficiency have not yet been correlated with the metabolic functions of NAD^+ and $NADP^+$.

The primary pathway for lysine catabolism is initiated by its condensation with α-ketoglutarate to form saccharopine which is converted to α-aminoadipic-ϵ-semialdehyde by loss of glutamate. The semialdehyde undergoes a series of reactions (oxidation, transamination, and oxidative decarboxylation) to form glutaryl CoA. The glutaryl CoA is then oxidized in an FAD-dependent acyl CoA dehydrogenase catalyzed reaction, loses CO_2 and is then hydrated to form β-hydroxybutyryl CoA. Conversion of the β-hydroxy to a keto group results in formation of acetoacetyl CoA.

In summary, pyruvate is produced by the catabolism of alanine, cysteine, glycine, hydroxyproline, serine, threonine, and tryptophan; α-ketoglutarate by arginine, glutamate, glutamine, histidine, and proline; succinyl CoA by isoleucine, methionine, and valine; fumarate by phenylalanine and tyrosine; malate by hydroxyproline;

and oxaloacetate by aspartate and asparagine. In addition to forming glycogenic precursors, catabolism of isoleucine, tryptophan, phenylalanine, and tyrosine produce acetyl CoA or acetoacetate, ketogenic products. Catabolism of leucine and lysine results only in production of acetoacetyl CoA and/or acetyl CoA. These are the only amino acids which yield exclusively ketogenic products. All of the catabolic products can be oxidized to provide ATP or converted to carbohydrate or fatty acids and stored as potential energy reserves. Pyruvate can be transaminated to produce alanine. This is believed to play an important role in muscle metabolism. Alanine comprises not more than 10 percent of muscle protein. However, it accounts for more than 30 percent of the α-amino nitrogen transported from muscle to liver. It has been suggested that alanine, synthesized in muscle by transamination of pyruvate, is transported to the liver. There the amino group is used in urea formation and the pyruvate is converted to glucose. The glucose is then transported to the muscle and the cycle can be repeated.

METABOLIC PATHWAYS OF SMALL MOLECULES

Urea Cycle

The ammonia produced in amino acid catabolism is detoxified in the liver by conversion to urea (quantitatively the liver is the most important organ for urea production). The urea is transported in the blood to the kidneys. It is excreted in urine where it accounts for up to 90 percent of urinary nitrogen, or up to 17 g of urea nitrogen per day (corresponds to about 100 g of protein). Ammonia is produced by the action of FMN-dependent amino acid oxidase and pyridoxal phosphate-dependent dehydratases. The ammonia can react with glutamate and ATP in a glutamine synthetase catalyzed reaction to form glutamine, ADP, and P_i. Glutamine thus serves as a nontoxic carrier of ammonia. In the mitochondria, glutamate dehydrogenase catalyzes the formation of α-ketoglutarate with release of ammonia.

Urea synthesis is carried out in a series of reactions known as the urea cycle or the Krebs-Henseleit cycle. The formation of carbamoyl phosphate, which supplies the carbamoyl group to the cycle, is catalyzed by mitochondrial carbamoyl phosphate synthetase I and uses ammonium ion, bicarbonate, and ATP:

$$HCO_3^- + NH_4^+ + 2ATP \longrightarrow$$
$$H_2N-CO-OPO_3 + 2ADP + P_i$$

N-acetylglutamic acid (synthesized from glutamate and acetyl CoA) is required as a positive allosteric effector by the enzyme. A cytoplasmic carbamoyl phosphate synthetase II requires glutamine as the nitrogen donor and catalyzes the reaction:

Glutamine + HCO_3 + H_2O + 2ATP $\longrightarrow$
        carbamoyl phosphate + 2ADP + P_i + L-glutamate

which supplies carbamoyl phosphate for pyrimidine biosynthesis. Ornithine transcarbamoylse activity is associated with the carbamoyl phosphate synthetase I. The transcarbamoylase catalyzes the formation of citrulline, which can passively diffuse from the mitochondrial matrix to the cytoplasm where it condenses with aspartate producing argininosuccinic acid. This is cleaved to yield arginine and fumarate in a reaction catalyzed by argininosuccinate lyase. Arginase catalyzes the hydrolysis of arginine to yield urea and ornithine. Ornithine can be transported back into the mitochondria, thus, completing the cycle.

N-acetylglutamate serves as a control of the urea cycle. In the well-fed state, the level of *N*-acetylglutamate increases and activity of the carbamoyl phosphate synthetase I increases in a parallel fashion. Diet affects the level of urea cycle enzyme activity. A carbohydrate-rich diet results in decreased levels of enzyme activity, while increasing dietary protein above the normal results in increased enzyme activity. In starvation, the body catabolizes tissue proteins to obtain amino acids which can be oxidized for ATP production, and there is an even greater increase in enzyme activity than seen for a protein-enriched diet. The increased activity is necessary to remove the excess nitrogen generated during the catabolism of the amino acids. In errors of metabolism which result in loss of activity of a urea cycle enzyme, mental retardation generally is seen and many of the individuals die within the first few weeks of life.

Amino Acids

The essential amino acids, those whose carbon chains cannot be synthesized *de novo* by the body at a rate able to meet metabolic needs, include arginine and histidine in infants, and isoleucine, leucine, lysine, methionine, phenylalanine, threonine, tryptophan, and valine throughout life. The nonessential amino acids, those which can be synthesized in adequate amounts, include alanine, asparagine, aspartate, cysteine, glutamate, glutamine, glycine, proline (hydroxyproline), serine, and tyrosine. Tyrosine is derived from phenylalanine and cysteine derives its sulfur from methionine, so they are both dependent upon adequate ingestion of essential amino acids. The liver and to a lesser degree the kidney are principal sites of amino acid synthesis.

Alanine, aspartate and glutamate are synthesized by the transamination of pyruvate, oxaloacetate, and α-ketoglutarate, respectively. The enzymes catalyzing these reversible reactions are aminotransferases which require pyridoxal phosphate as a coenzyme. While most amino acids participate in transamination reactions (lysine and threonine are exceptions) glutamate is the most common donor of amino groups. Asparagine and glutamine also serve as amino group donors and as a result are converted to the ω-amides of the corresponding α-keto acids. These are converted to the keto acid by loss of ammonia in reactions catalyzed by ω-amidases. Glutamate and ammonia are converted to glutamine in a reaction requiring ATP and catalyzed by glutamine synthetase. This reaction provides a mechanism for the removal of the potentially toxic ammonia. Glutamic acid also serves as the precursor for the synthesis of ornithine and proline. Glutamate is converted to γ-glutamylphosphate and then reduced to glutamic semialdehyde; transamination gives ornithine, ring closure forms Δ^1-pyrroline-5-carboxylic acid which can be reduced to give proline.

3-Phosphoglycerate, a glycolytic intermediate, provides the carbon skeleton of serine. The 3-phosphoglycerate is oxidized in an NAD^+-dependent reaction to 3-phosphopyruvate which undergoes transamination producing 3-phosphoserine. Hydrolysis of the phosphate moiety completes the synthesis of serine. Serine serves as a precursor of cysteine and can also be converted to glycine, in a reversible reaction catalyzed by serine hydroxy-methyltransferase. Conversion of serine to glycine results in transfer of the β-carbon atom of serine to tetrahydrofolate forming the 5,10-methylene derivative, which is a source of 1-carbon units. Glycine can also be synthesized from ammonia and CO_2 in an NADH-dependent reaction catalyzed by glycine synthase.

Cysteine synthesis is more complex. When *S*-adenosylmethionine serves as a methyl donor it is converted to *S*-adenosylhomocysteine. Adenosylhomocysteinase catalyzes release of homocysteine which can condense with serine forming cystathionine (cystathionine β-synthase). This is cleaved (cystathionine γ-lyase) giving cysteine and α-ketobutyric acid. Cysteine inhibits cystathionine γ-lyase and suppresses synthesis of the cystathionine β-synthase thereby preventing unnecessary utilization of methionine for this pathway.

Purine and Pyrimidine Synthesis

Amino acids play an important role in the synthesis of purines and pyrimidines, donating most of the ring carbons and all of the nitrogen atoms. The purine moiety:

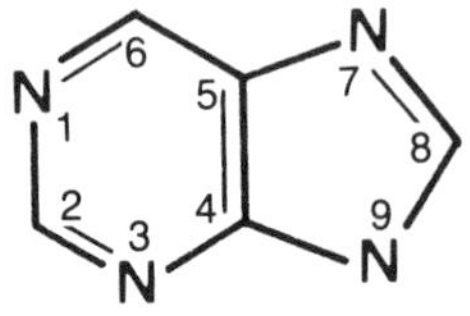

obtains the N_1 from aspartate, and N_3 and N_9 from the amide nitrogen of glutamine. C_2 and C_8 are derived from formate, C_6 from CO_2 and C_4, and C_5 and N_7 from glycine.

5-Phosphoribosyl-1-pyrophosphate (PRPP) is the starting material for purine biosynthesis. It is synthesized from ribose-5-phosphate (product of the pentose-phosphate pathway) and ATP in a reaction catalyzed by PRPP synthetase. PRPP amidotransferase catalyzes the reaction which results in the transfer of the amide of glutamine to PRPP forming 5-phosphoribosyl-1-amine, glutamate, and pyrophosphate. This is the committing step of purine synthesis. PRPP is a positive effector of the PRPP amidotransferase while purine nucleotides are negative effectors (feedback inhibition). GMP and AMP have synergistic inhibitory effects on the enzyme suggesting that there are different binding sites for the two nucleotides.

The following reactions result in the synthesis of the purine inosine-5′-monophosphate from 5-phosphoribosyl-1-amine. Glycine is added to the amino group in a reaction catalyzed by phosphoribosyl glycineamide synthetase, which is dependent upon hydrolysis of ATP to ADP and P_i for energy. N^{10}-formyltetrahydrofolate serves as the donor of the formyl group added to the amino group of the phosphoribosyl glycineamide. Next, the keto-oxygen is replaced with an amino group; this is followed by ring closure, forming 5′-phosphoribosyl-5-aminoimidazole. Two ATP are hydrolyzed to ADP and P_i to provide energy for the synthesis and ring closure. CO_2 is then added at the four position of the imidazole ring. This is followed by an ATP-requiring reaction in which aspartate serves as the amino donor to form 5′-phosphoribosyl-5-aminoimidazole-4-carboxamide. A formyl group from N^{10}-formyltetrahydrofolate is added to the amino group at the five position. Ring closure with loss of a water molecule gives rise to inosine-5′-monophosphate (IMP):

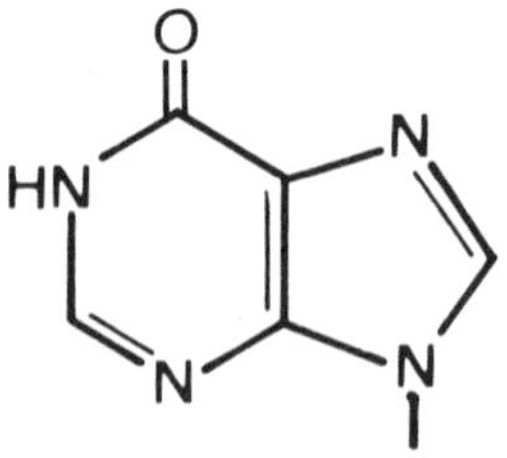

Ribose – 5′ – phosphate

The conversion of IMP to AMP requires aspartate and GTP, which react to form adenylosuccinate, GDP, and P_i. Adenylosuccinase catalyzed cleavage of the adenylosuccinate releases fumarate and AMP. Formation of GMP from IMP is initiated by oxidation of IMP to xanthosine-5′-monophosphate (XMP) in an NAD^+-dependent reaction catalyzed by IMP dehydrogenase. XMP can then react with glutamine in an ATP-requiring reaction to form GMP and AMP and pyrophosphate. Note that *de novo* synthesis of AMP requires GTP while formation of GMP requires ATP as the energy source. GMP inhibits formation of XMP while AMP inhibits synthesis of adenylosuccinate. GMP cannot be converted directly to AMP, but both purine nucleotides can be converted to IMP, the precursor for each. GMP reductase catalyzes conversion of GMP to IMP and is inhibited by XMP and activated by GTP. AMP is converted to IMP in an AMP-deaminase catalyzed reaction activated by ATP and inhibited by GDP and GTP (Fig. 4-6).

The *de novo* synthesis of purine nucleotides requires a high energy input in the form of ATP. To circumvent the energy drain, salvage pathways exist which permit synthesis of purine nucleotides from free purines and purine nucleosides. Guanine and hypoxanthine (lacks amino group found at the two position of guanine) can react with PRPP to form the corresponding nucleotide in a reaction catalyzed by hypoxanthine-guanine phosphoribosyltransferase (HGPRT). GMP and IMP are competitive inhibitors of HGPRT in this reaction. Patients expressing the Lesch-Nyhan syndrome (elevated blood uric acid and neurological problems such as mental retardation and self-mutilation) are defective in hypoxanthine-guanine phosphoribosyltransferase activity. The corresponding reaction for adenine is catalyzed by adenine phosphoribosyltransferase which is inhibited by AMP. Red blood cells cannot synthesize 5-phosphoribosyl-1-amine and therefore cannot synthesize purines *de novo*; they are dependent upon these salvage pathways for necessary nucleotides and for formation of nucleotide coenzymes.

Uric acid is the end product of purine catabolism in man. GMP is converted to guanosine by loss of P_i. The ribose moiety can then be cleaved in a reaction catalyzed by the P_i-requiring purine nucleoside phosphorylase to produce guanine and ribose-1-phosphate. The reaction is readily reversible and the enzyme can act on the deoxyribose sugar nucleoside as well. Replacement of the amino group with a keto function at C_2 results in formation of xanthine which is oxidized to uric acid in a reaction catalyzed by xanthine oxidase.

AMP can undergo one of two initial catabolic reactions. It can lose P_i forming adenosine or be deaminated to form IMP. Adenosine is deaminated to form inosine which is also produced by loss of P_i from IMP. Purine

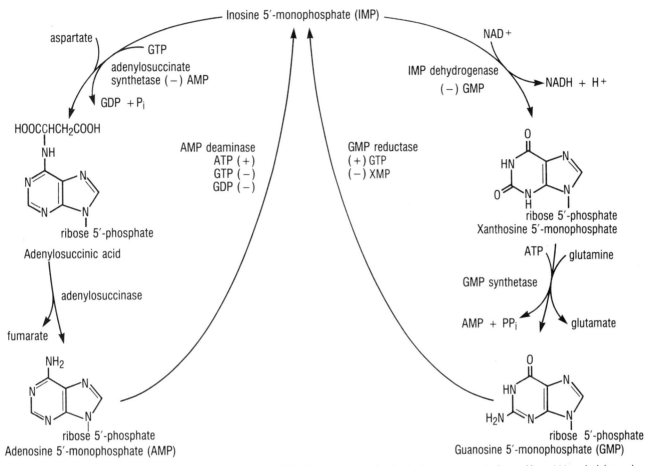

Fig. 4-6. Pathways for the interconversion of IMP, AMP, and GMP. Activators of individual enzymes are indicated by a (+) and inhibitors by a (−).

nucleoside phosphorylase (probably a different enzyme from that which acts on guanosine) catalyzes the removal of the ribosyl moiety as ribose-1-phosphate with formation of hypoxanthine. Hypoxanthine can undergo two successive oxidations (catalyzed by xanthine oxidase) to form first xanthine and then uric acid.

crystals (tophi) are found in the joints of the extremities. Crystalline deposits can also result in renal damage or urinary obstruction. Gout is not necessarily due to an enzymatic problem since it can be caused by an impaired renal clearance of urate. It is commonly treated with the drug, allopurinol, a hypoxanthine analog. Allopurinol

Hypoxanthine → (xanthine oxidase, O_2, H_2O_2) → Xanthine → (xanthine oxidase, O_2, H_2O_2) → Uric Acid

The normal concentration of uric acid in plasma ranges from 2-7.5 mg/dl. Females average somewhat less than males (4.1 mg/dl as compared to 5.0 mg/dl). Above a concentration of 6.4 mg/dl, monosodium urate is no longer soluble and crystals can form. In gout there is an increase in uric acid concentration and deposits of urate

inhibits xanthine oxidase resulting in decreased uric acid synthesis. This results in decreased *de novo* synthesis of purines because of increased reutilization of hypoxanthine for purine nucleotide synthesis.

In the *de novo* synthesis of the pyrimidine ring, N_1, C_4, C_5, and C_6 are from aspartate, C_2 from CO_2, and N_3 from the amide nitrogen of glutamine. In contrast to purine nucleotides, the synthesis of pyrimidine nucleotides is initiated by pyrimidine ring synthesis:

which is followed by attachment to ribose phosphate. The six enzymatic activities required for UMP synthesis are found in association with three different proteins in animals. The first three reactions are catalyzed by a multifunctional complex enzyme which contains carbamoyl phosphate synthetase II, aspartate transcarbamoylase, and dihydroorotase. Carbamoylphosphate reacts with aspartate producing P_i and N-carbamoyl aspartate which upon loss of water forms dihydroorotate. The second protein contains the dihydroorotate dehydrogenase activity which in the presence of NAD^+ catalyzes the oxidation of dihydroorotate to orotate. The third protein contains the final two activities, orotate phosphoribosyltransferase and orotidylate decarboxylase. The transferase catalyzes the addition of ribose-5-phosphate from PRPP to orotate (uracil and thymine can also serve as substrates) forming orotidine-5'-monophosphate (OMP). Loss of CO_2 from OMP yields uridine-5'-monophosphate (UMP).

The formation of cytidine nucleotide requires UTP as the starting reactant. UMP is converted to UTP by two successive ATP-dependent phosphorylations. In the presence of ATP, UTP can be aminated by glutamine to produce CTP, ADP, P_i, water, and glutamate.

Formation of the deoxyribonucleotides occurs by reduction of the ribosyl moiety of the corresponding ribonucleotides, catalyzed by ribonucleoside diphosphate reductase. It can reduce ADP, GDP, CDP, and UDP to their deoxy (d) derivatives. dATP inhibits the reduction of all four nucleoside diphosphate substrates; dGTP inhibits reduction of CDP and UDP; dTTP also inhibits reduction of CDP; and ATP inhibits reduction of ADP. The deoxynucleotide dTMP is synthesized by methylation of dUMP with N^5, N^{10}-methylenetetrahydrofolate as the methyl donor. Deamination of dCMP to form dUMP provides a source of dUMP for the reaction.

Catabolism of the pyrimidine nucleotides is accomplished by their conversion to first the nucleoside and then to the free base, either uracil or thymine. dUTP is converted to dUMP and pyrophosphate in a reaction catalyzed by dUTPase, whose high activity prevents the cell from having a pool of dUTP available to serve as a substrate for DNA polymerase. The free bases uracil and

thymine are then further degraded; uracil yields the products CO_2, NH_3, and β-alanine; thymine yields CO_2, NH_3, and β-aminoisobutyric acid.

Nucleotide Coenzyme Metabolism

NAD^+, FAD, and coenzyme A are synthesized by mammalian cells when the appropriate vitamin (niacin, riboflavin, and pantothenic acid, respectively)

HO—CH_2—$C(CH_3)_2$—CHOH—CO—NH—$(CH_2)_2$—COO^-
Pantothenic acid

or precursor is available. In the synthesis of NAD^+, nicotinate, nicotinamide, or quinolate (derived from tryptophan) can react with PRPP to form either nicotinate- or nicotinamide mononucleotide in reactions catalyzed by nicotinate- or nicotinamide phosphoribosyltransferase, respectively. The latter enzyme is inhibited by NMN, NAD^+, $NADP^+$, and NADPH, while ATP enhances its activity. NAD^+-pyrophosphorylase catalyzes the reaction of ATP with the mononucleotide to form either nicotinate- or nicotinamide adenine dinucleotide and pyrophosphate. In an ATP-requiring reaction, NAD^+ synthase catalyzes the reaction of nicotinate adenine dinucleotide with glutamine to form nicotinamide adenine dinucleotide (NAD^+). NAD^+ is converted to $NADP^+$ in an ATP-requiring reaction catalyzed by NAD^+-kinase. NAD^+ and $NADP^+$ serve as coenzymes in oxidation-reduction (electron transfer) reactions. For example, NAD^+ serves as a coenzyme for pyruvate dehydrogenase while NADPH serves as a coenzyme for fatty acid synthetase. In general NAD^+ is utilized in reactions in which the transferred electrons will be subsequently used for ATP synthesis, while NADP is used for synthesis of cellular metabolites. NAD^+-glycohydrolase catalyzes the degradation of NAD^+ to nicotinamide and adenosine diphosphoribose. The latter is further broken down to adenosine-5'-phosphate and ribose-5-phosphate. The effect of the glycohydrolase catalyzed reaction is to permit the net conversion of niacin (nicotinate) to nicotinamide which can then be methylated with S-adenosylmethionine serving as the methyl-donor. Both nicotinamide and the methyl derivatives are excreted in the urine.

FAD is synthesized from riboflavin in a two-step reaction with the utilization of ATP for each step. First, riboflavin is phosphorylated to form riboflavin phosphate which is often, inappropriately, termed "flavin mononucleotide." Riboflavin phosphate reacts with a second ATP molecule in a FAD-pyrophosphorylase catalyzed reaction to form FAD and pyrophosphate. The flavins also serve as coenzymes in electron transport reactions (e.g., FAD is a coenzyme for fatty acyl CoA dehydrogenase and succinate dehydrogenase) in which the electrons are used for subsequent ATP synthesis.

Coenzyme A is synthesized from pantothenic acid. Pantothenate is phosphorylated by ATP to form 4-phosphopantothenate which can react with cysteine in the presence of ATP to give 4-phosphopantothenoylcysteine. This can lose CO_2 (phosphopantothenoylcysteine decarboxylase) to form 4-phosphopantotheine, which serves as a feedback inhibitor of the reaction. 4-Phosphopantotheine can react with ATP in a dephosphocoenzyme A pyrophosphorylase catalyzed reaction to form dephosphocoenzyme A and pyrophosphate. Dephosphocoenzyme A kinase catalyzes the formation of coenzyme A in the presence of ATP. Coenzyme A serves as a carrier of activated fatty acyl residues.

Phospholipids

The synthesis of phosphatidic acid, which can serve as an intermediate in triacylglycerol synthesis, has been described. Phosphatidic acid is a key intermediate in the synthesis of phospholipids. It can react with CTP to form CDP-diacylglycerol and pyrophosphate or it can lose its phosphate moiety to form diacylglycerol. CDP-diacylglycerol is the precursor for the phosphatidylinositols and phosphatidylglycerols. It can react with inositol to give CMP and phosphatidylinositol or it can react with glycerol-3-phosphate to form 3-phosphatidyl-1'-glycerol. Two molecules of phosphatidylglycerol can react to form cardiolipin (diphosphatidylglycerol) and glycerol, provided CDP-diacylglycerol is present as a cofactor.

In contrast to the phosphatidylinositols and phosphatidylglycerols, the phospholipids containing the nitrogenous bases, serine, ethanolamine, and choline, are synthesized in reactions in which 1,2-diacylglycerol reacts with the activated nitrogen-containing moiety. In the synthesis of phosphatidylethanolamine, the ethanolamine is converted to phosphoethanolamine in an ATP-requiring reaction catalyzed by ethanolamine kinase. Phosphoethanolamine is then converted to CDP-ethanolamine in a CTP-dependent reaction catalyzed by phosphorylethanolamine cytidyltransferase. CDP-etha-

nolamine can then react with 1,2-diacylglycerol to form phosphatidylethanolamine and CMP in an ethanolamine phosphotransferase catalyzed reaction. Phosphatidylethanolamine can be converted to phosphatidylcholine by the successive addition of three methyl residues from S- adenosylmethionine. The methylations are catalyzed by N-methyltransferases. This series of reactions provides the only endogenous pathway for the *de novo* synthesis of choline.

When dietary choline is used for the synthesis of phosphatidylcholine it is activated to form CDP-choline in reactions analogous to the formation of CDP-ethanolamine. The CDP-choline reacts with 1,2-diacylglycerol in a choline phosphotransferase catalyzed reaction to form phosphatidylcholine and CMP. In mammals the mechanism for phosphatidylserine synthesis is via a phosphatidylethanolamine (i.e., serine transferase catalyzed exchange between phosphatidylethanolamine and serine, with phosphatidyl serine and ethanolamine as the products).

Plasmalogens are synthesized from monoacyl dihydroxyacetone phosphate. The acyl residue is exchanged for a fatty alcohol to form O-alkyl dihydroxyacetone phosphate which is reduced to O-alkylglycerol phosphate. Fatty acyl CoA provides the acyl moiety for the synthesis of 1-alkyl-2-acylglycerol phosphate. This is converted to the appropriate phospholipid via reactions analogous to those described for the phosphatidyl compounds. The final step involves the introduction of the double bond, which is catalyzed by a specific desaturase in an O_2-requiring, NADH or NADPH-dependent reaction.

Phospholipases catalyze the breakdown of phospholipids. Phospholipases A_1 and A_2 catalyze the hydrolysis of acyl residues esterified at C_1 and C_2, respectively. Phospholipase C catalyzes hydrolysis of the phosphoryl moiety esterified to the glycerol backbone while phospholipase D catalyzes hydrolysis of the terminal diester bond. The enzymes catalyzing the reactions for *de novo* synthesis of phospholipids do not appear to exhibit much specificity for the type of fatty acids incorporated. Evidence suggests that phospholipase A_2 can function in the formation of phospholipids containing specific fatty acyl residues at the two position. Phospholipase A_2 cleaves the fatty acyl group at position two to form the lysophosphatidyl compound. Remodeling can then occur via reacylation by a fatty acyl residue (fatty acyl CoA) specified by the acyl CoA transacylase. It can also occur for lysophosphatidylcholine via an exchange reaction in which a fatty acyl group from a phospholipid is transferred to the two position of the lysophosphatidylcholine producing phosphatidylcholine and a lysophosphatidyl compound. Lysophospholipids can also serve as the fatty acid source in remodeling reactions; in which case the products are the phosphatidyl compound and the glycerol phosphoryl base.

Sphingolipids

Synthesis of sphingolipids starts with the long-chain base sphingosine or a derivative thereof. The synthesis of sphingosine results from the reaction of palmitoyl CoA with serine. The carboxyl group of serine is lost as CO_2 during formation of 3-dehydrosphinganine which can be reduced in an NADPH-dependent reaction to D-sphinganine. The D-sphinganine can be oxidized to D-sphingenine (*trans* 1,3-dihydroxy-2-amino-4-octadecene, termed, "sphingosine") in an FAD-dependent reaction. In the initial reaction with serine, fatty acyl groups of chain length C_{14}–C_{18} can be used as substrates by the enzyme resulting in a family of sphingosines which may or may not contain the *trans* double bond at C_4. Free sphingosine is not normally found in cells. Ceramide-*N*-acyltransferase catalyzes the addition, through an amide linkage, of a fatty acyl group from CoA to the sphingosine base forming ceramide. The physical properties of ceramide are somewhat analogous to those of diacylglycerol in that each contain two hydrocarbon tails and a polar hydroxyl group. Sphingomyelin, both a sphingolipid and a phospholipid since it is comprised of ceramide to which a phosphorylcholine group has been esterified at the one position, has CDP-choline as the major source of the phosphorylcholine moiety although phosphatidylcholine can also serve as a donor.

Glycosphingolipids (sphingolipids containing one or more sugar moieties) are synthesized by the sequential action of glycosyltransferases which catalyze the transfer of the appropriate monosaccharide from its nucleotide carrier to either the C_1-hydroxyl of the ceramide or to the growing saccharide chain. In general, glycosyltransferases are specific for the nucleotide sugar donor and catalyze the synthesis of specific sugar linkages. Specificity for the acceptor molecule is not always observed. Within the broad classification of glycosphingolipids there are subclasses characterized by the sugar moiety present. In addition to serving as membrane components, glycosphingolipids serve as antigenic determinants, as receptors for toxins, function in transmitter recognition, and are believed to play a role in cell-cell interactions.

The simplest glycosphingolipids are the cerebrosides (ceramide monohexosides) which are either glucosyl- or galactosylceramides. They are synthesized from the activated sugars UDP-glucose or UDP-galactose and ceramide. Glucosylceramide (glucocerebroside) functions primarily as an intermediate in the metabolism of the more complex glycosphingolipids. Galactosylceramide is found in highest quantities in the brain. Galactosylceramide can be converted to sulfatide (sulfuric acid esters of galactosylceramide) in a reaction catalyzed by a sulfotransferase which uses 3′-phosphoadenosine-5′-phosphosulfate as the sulfate donor. Galactosylceramide-3-sulfate is the major cerebroside sulfatide found in brain. Addition of more sugars to glucosylceramide gives rise to ceramide oligosaccharides. The ABO and Lewis blood group antigens are defined by the carbohydrate moieties of the neutral ceramide oligosaccharides.

Gangliosides form the fourth (in addition to cerebrosides, sulfatides, and ceramide oligosaccharides) subgroup of glycosphingolipids. They differ from the others in that they contain sialic acid. Sialyltransferases catalyze the transfer of the sialyl moiety from CMP, its nucleotide carrier, to the oligosaccharide portion of the molecule. Gangliosides are often indicated by the letter G followed by a subscript M, D, T, or Q to indicate whether there are 1, 2, 3, or 4 (mono-, di-, tri-, or quatra-) sialyl residues. The numerical subscript which follows the letter indicates the number of sugar residues present in the oligosaccharide portion of the molecule (e.g., cer-glc-gal-galNAc-gal is designated by a 1 while cer-glc-gal-galNAc is indicated by a 2). Removal of a sugar residue results in increasing the value of the subscript by one.

Sphingolipids are catabolized by hydrolytic enzymes present in the liposomes. Their degradation takes place in a sequential fashion with specific exoglycosidases catalyzing each step. The glycosidases purified so far are glycoproteins which have an absolute specificity toward the anomeric linkage but not necessarily absolute epimeric specificity. Often multiple forms of the same enzyme exist which exhibit different specificities for the glycoconjugate substrate (not for the anomeric linkage). The structures of some glycosphingolipids and the enzymes which catalyze their degradation are shown in Figure 4-7. The free monosaccharides can cross the lysosomal membrane and be reutilized by the cell. Inborn errors which result in the inactivation (or reduced activity) of specific hydrolases are referred to as the sphingolipidoses.

Inborn errors of metabolism result from the presence of a mutant gene which translates into synthesis of a functionally defective protein. The protein affected may be an enzyme, a cofactor, or a transport protein. The result is an interruption of a normal biochemical pathway; this can result in disruption of normal systemic metabolism as expressed in an accumulation of metabolites proximal to the affected step and a depletion of metabolites distal to the defect. The errors often result in a progressive expression of the effects of the error. Some errors of carbohydrate and amino acid metabolism have been indicated and have contributed to an understanding of those metabolic pathways. Errors affecting the activity of a lysosomal hydrolase result in the accumulation of the undegraded substance within the lysosome. In

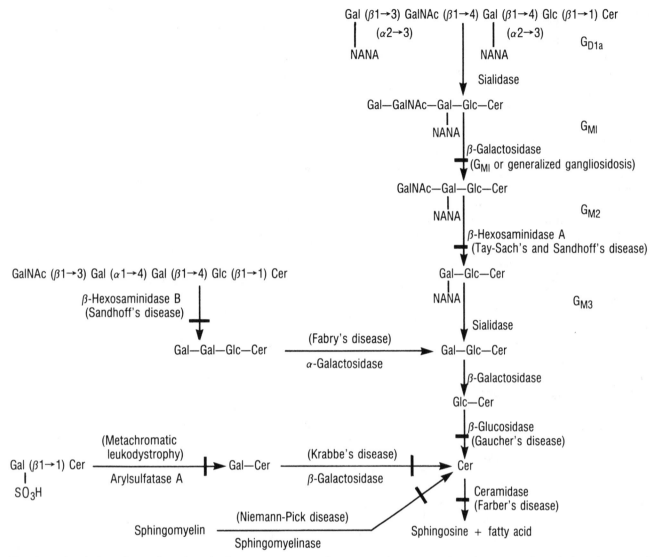

Fig. 4-7. Catabolic pathways for sphingolipids. Cross bars across the arrows indicate a site of an inborn error of metabolism; the name of the resultant disease is given in parentheses.

the sphingolipidoses, as in other errors affecting lysosomal hydrolases, the severity of the clinical symptoms reflects in part the cellular distribution of the affected lipid. The diagnosis of these errors as for many other known errors of metabolism can be made via assay of enzymatic activity against the specific substrate. Unlike some of the errors of carbohydrate and amino acid metabolism in which the symptoms can be ameliorated by diet; thus far there is no therapy for the sphingolipidoses, although enzyme replacement is being investigated.

Cholesterol

Cholesterol is found in essentially all cell membranes and is especially abundant in the myelinated structures of the brain and the central nervous system. It also serves

as a precursor of steroid hormones and the bile acids (catabolic products). Cholesterol is also a primary component of the plaques found in the walls of arteries in atherosclerosis.

All of the carbons in cholesterol are derived from the acetyl group of acetyl CoA. The acetyl CoA is obtained from citrate through the action of ATP-citrate lyase. In discussing the synthesis of ketone bodies, the synthesis of HMGCoA within the mitochondria was described. A similar series of reactions generates HMGCoA in the cytoplasm where it serves as a precursor for cholesterol synthesis. Enzymes for cholesterol synthesis are associated with the cytoplasm and the endoplasmic reticulum. HMGCoA is reduced to form mevalonic acid in an NADPH-requiring reaction catalyzed by 3-hydroxy-3-methylglutaryl CoA reductase (HMGCoA reductase). Formation of mevalonic acid is the committing step in the synthesis of polyisoprenoid lipids. Cholesterol inhibits HMGCoA reductase through a feedback mechanism which results in reduction of both the activity and rate of synthesis of the enzyme. Fasting and cholesterol feeding result in inhibition of the reductase while refeeding increases its activity. HMGCoA reductase activity is also hormonally regulated, primarily by glucagon and insulin. Glucagon binding stimulates cAMP production which results in activation by phosphorylation of HMGCoA reductase kinase; it catalyzes the phosphorylation of the HMGCoA reductase which results in reduced HMGCoA reductase activity. The result is reduced cholesterol synthesis. Insulin activates a protein phosphatase which acts to dephosphorylate both the reductase kinase (inactivates it) and the HMGCoA reductase (activates it). The effects of these hormones on cholesterol synthesis are similar to their effects on glycogen formation and lipogenesis [i.e., insulin enhances synthesis (glycogen, triacylglycerols, and cholesterol) while glucagon enhances glycogen catabolism, fatty acid mobilization, and retards cholesterol synthesis].

Mevalonate undergoes two consecutive phosphorylations by ATP to form 5-pyrophosphomevalonic acid. Loss of the carboxyl as CO_2 and of the hydroxyl group in an ATP utilizing reaction (probably involving formation of the intermediate 3-phospho-5-pyrophosphomevalonate) produces isopentenyl pyrophosphate. This can undergo isomerization to form 3,3-dimethylallyl pyrophosphate. Dimethylallyl pyrophosphate can be transferred to the N_6 position of certain adenosines on preformed t-RNA molecules. Dimethylallyl pyrophosphate and isopentenyl pyrophosphate undergo head-to-tail condensation forming geranyl pyrophosphate which reacts with an isopentenyl pyrophosphate to form farnesyl pyrophosphate. Both condensations are catalyzed by a prenyltransferase (catalyze transfer of units which can be considered derivatives of isoprene) specifically named geranyltransferase.

Farnesyl pyrophosphate serves as a major branch point in polyisoprene synthesis. It serves as a precursor for the formation of the side chain of coenzyme Q, for dolichols, carriers of oligosaccharide chains prior to their use in synthesizing *N*-glycosidically linked glycopeptides, and for cholesterol. In the isoprenoid side chain of coenzyme Q all of the double bonds are *trans* and the enzyme which catalyzes the head-to-tail condensations of 6 to 10 isopentenyl pyrophosphates is a transprenyltransferase. Dolichols, composed of 16 to 22 isoprene residues, are synthesized from farnesyl pyrophosphate through repeated additions of isopentenyl residues in reactions catalyzed by *cis* prenyltransferase. In dolichols the double bonds from the farnesyl moiety are *trans* and the rest are *cis*. Squalene synthetase, in an NADPH-

requiring reaction, catalyzes the condensation of two molecules of farnesyl pyrophosphate to form squalene plus two pyrophosphates. This is the committing step for cholesterol synthesis. Squalene then undergoes a series of reactions to form cholesterol.

ROLE OF LIPOPROTEINS IN LIPID METABOLISM

Lipids are not very soluble in an aqueous environment; their transport in blood requires that they be associated with protein. Both triacylglycerols and cholesterol are carried from either the mucosal cells of the intestine or the liver (major synthetic site) to their sites of utilization in the form of lipoproteins. There are four main classes of lipoproteins defined by their sedimentation properties which are indicative of their composition. Chylomicra are the least dense, remain at the origin upon paper electrophoresis, and are composed of ~85 percent triacylglycerol, ~2 percent protein, ~8 percent phospholipid, and low levels of cholesterol esters and free cholesterol. They are synthesized in the intestinal mucosal cells and function as carriers of triacylglycerols. Very low density lipoproteins (VLDL) are synthesized by the liver. They are more dense and on paper electrophoresis migrate towards the anode and are termed "pre-B." VLDLs contain more protein, phospholipid, and cholesterol (both esters and free), and a lesser quantity of triacylglycerols (50–65 percent) than do chylomicra. Of increasing density are the low density lipoproteins (LDL) and high density lipoproteins (HDL). LDLs are composed of up to 50 percent cholesterol with most of it esterified and ~20 percent phospholipid and ~20 percent protein. They contain low levels of triacylglycerols. HDLs are the most dense, move furthest toward the anode on paper electrophoresis (α), and have been subdivided into HDLs and VHDLs. HDLs contain more than 30 percent protein, while VHDLs have more than 50 percent protein. The protein constituents of lipoproteins, referred to as apoproteins when not associated with lipid, have properties which appear to contribute to the function of the lipoproteins with which they are associated.

A major apoprotein component associated with the chylomicra and VLDL is apoprotein C_{II}. This protein is a potent activator of lipoprotein lipase. The lipase synthesized by the tissue is secreted by the cells and becomes associated with the surface of the endothelial cells of capillaries. In the well fed animal, lipoprotein lipase activity is increased in adipose tissue; in the fasted state the lipoprotein lipase activity associated with heart increases. The lipase catalyzes hydrolysis of triacylglycerols to form free fatty acids and 2-monoacylglycerol which can be taken up by the cells. When the concentration of triacylglycerols in the lipoprotein decreases so that the concentration of apoprotein C_{II} is greater than 2 percent of their concentration, the apoprotein becomes inhibitory to the lipoprotein lipase. VLDL is converted to an intermediate density lipoprotein (IDL) which is converted to an LDL upon loss of more triacylglycerol and of essentially all apoproteins but B. IDL can be removed by the liver or may be converted to LDL at the cell surface since hepatic lipoprotein lipase is not activated by C_{II}.

The LDL and HDL are the lipoproteins believed to have primary roles in maintenance of cholesterol levels. LDLs carry cholesterol to the cells and HDLs carry cholesterol from the tissue to the liver where it can be further metabolized. HDLs are synthesized in the liver and the intestine. In the circulation they contain apoprotein A_I (added in intestine) which activates plasma lecithin: cholesterol acyltransferase (LCAT) and apoprotein E (added in the liver) which is recognized by receptors on liver cells. It is probable that HDLs can take up unesterified cholesterol from the surface of membranes of peripheral cells. The apoprotein A_I activates LCAT which catalyzes the esterification of cholesterol. The cholesterol or cholesterol esters are then transported as part of the HDL or may be transferred to VLDL. Approximately two-thirds of cholesterol in the circulation is esterified, while that in membranes is not. In this manner the cholesterol is transported to those tissues which can further metabolize it (i.e., to the liver, the primary site for synthesis of bile salts, or to the adrenal cortex for conversion to steroid hormones).

The pathway for LDL utilization has been elucidated through studies of their metabolism by fibroblasts derived from normal subjects and from patients with genetic disorders of cholesterol metabolism. The general sequence is (A) binding of LDL through its apoprotein B moiety to high affinity receptor sites on the cell surface; (B) endocytosis of the LDL and subsequent uptake by cellular lysosomes; and (C) degradation of the LDL component by lysosomal enzymes. The last step results in hydrolysis of the cholesterol esters making free cholesterol available to the cell. The cholesterol represses both the synthesis and activity of cellular HMGCoA reductase as well as the synthesis of LDL receptors. Acyl CoA, cholesterol acyltransferase (catalyzes esterification of cholesterol) activity is enhanced under these conditions. When circulating LDL levels are low, the number of cellular LDL receptors increases as does HMGCoA reductase activity and, hence, cellular cholesterol synthesis.

Several mutations exist which affect the normal LDL pathway; five have been identified at the cellular level and one which affects the synthesis of plasma LDL itself. In abetalipoproteinemia, apoprotein B is lacking and

individuals with this error do not synthesize LDLs. The cholesterol associated with other plasma lipoproteins cannot be taken up by cells so there is no suppression of HMGCoA reductase activity and cellular cholesterol synthesis is elevated. Familial hypercholesterolemia is a genetically dominant error in which the cells fail either to bind or to take up circulating LDLs. The symptoms associated with this error (elevated LDL levels, clinical signs of atherosclerosis at an early age, and excessive cholesterol synthesis) reflect either (1) a lack of LDL receptors on the surface, (2) a reduction in the number of LDL receptors, or (3) failure to internalize the LDL after binding. Both Wolman's disease and cholesterol ester storage disease result from a reduction in lysosomal acid lipase activity to less than 2 percent of normal in the former and to 5 percent in the latter. Failure to hydrolyze the cholesterol esters in the lysosomes results in their accumulation in the lysosomes and continued HMGCoA reductase activity. These errors result in cholesterol ester accumulation in the arterial wall and advanced atherosclerosis.

Atherosclerosis is believed to be initiated by leakage of blood components, including LDLs, through a damaged endothelium into the artery wall. Smooth muscle cells of the middle (medial layer) of the artery wall proliferate and migrate into the inner (intima) layer where they phagocytose the foreign components. LDLs phagocytosed by the muscle cells are degraded in the lysosomes. The cholesterol released cannot leave the muscle cell and enter the plasma unless it has a carrier molecule to solubilize it. Therefore, it accumulates in the muscle cell where some will be esterified and stored as the cholesterol ester. With time, the accumulation of cholesterol esters gives rise to overt clinical symptoms. To minimize this problem it is desirable to keep sufficient LDL levels to supply cholesterol to the cells but not in excess. In vitro, a LDL concentration of 15 μg protein/ml (equivalent to 25 μg LDL-cholesterol/ml) results in suppression of HMG-CoA reductase activity. Evidence suggests that the concentration of LDL-cholesterol in the interstitial fluid is about 10 percent of that in plasma. In order to maintain LDL-cholesterol levels of 25 μg/ml in the interstitial fluid, the LDL-cholesterol level in the plasma would have to be 250 μg/ml (25 mg LDL-cholesterol/dl). Normal newborn humans have ~30 mg/dl of LDL-cholesterol while a normal adult western man has ~150 mg/dl, a level five times greater than may be needed.

BILE ACIDS

Cholesterol can be metabolized in the liver to form bile acids, the major form in which cholesterol is excreted. The bile acids, referred to as bile salts since their carboxyl group is ionized at pH 7, are secreted into bile canaliculi, move to the bile ducts, and then into the gallbladder. In bile, the bile acids are found with phospholipids in mixed micelles. The micelles can contain cholesterol in up to a 1:1 ratio with the phospholipid. Excess cholesterol has a tendency to crystallize out from the micelles, forming stones. This occurs most often in the gallbladder because the bile is there for a relatively long time; until it is secreted into the intestine. The tendency to secrete bile supersaturated with cholesterol is inherited, found more often in females than males, and is often associated with obesity.

Conversion of cholesterol of bile acids involves (1) the loss of three carbons from the side chain with the terminal carbon of the chain oxidized to a carboxyl, (2) the insertion of hydroxyl groups, (3) reduction of the C_5 double bond, and (4) epimerization of the C_3 hydroxyl. The insertion of hydroxyl groups at C_7 and C_{12} is catalyzed by a 7 α-hydroxylase and a 12 α-hydroxylase, respectively. The bile acid formed, cholic acid, can be conjugated via an amide bond to either glycine or taurine to form glycocholic or taurocholic acid:

cytochrome P_{450}s which catalyze scission of the side chain of cholesterol and β-hydroxylations at C_{11} and C_{18}. The cytochrome P_{450}s associated with the endoplasmic reticulum catalyze β-hydroxylations at C_{17}, C_{19}, and C_{21}. In the liver, cytochrome P_{450}s that catalyze hydroxylations at C_2, C_7 and C_{16}, are associated with the endoplasmic reticulum.

Conversion of cholesterol to pregnenolone results from the insertion of hydroxyl residues on C_{20} and C_{22}, followed by cleavage between C_{20} and C_{22}. The product, pregnenolone, contains only 21 carbons and has a ketone group at position 20. Pregnenolone serves as a feedback inhibitor of this step, which appears to be rate-limiting for steroid hormone formation. Synthesis is stimulated by adrenocorticotrophin hormone (ACTH) in the adrenal cortex and luteinizing hormone (LH) in the testes and ovaries. Both hormones are secreted by the pituitary. ACTH and LH bind at specific cellular receptors, activating adenylate cyclase which results in elevated cAMP levels; this activates a protein kinase which catalyzes the phosphorylation of cholesterol esterase.

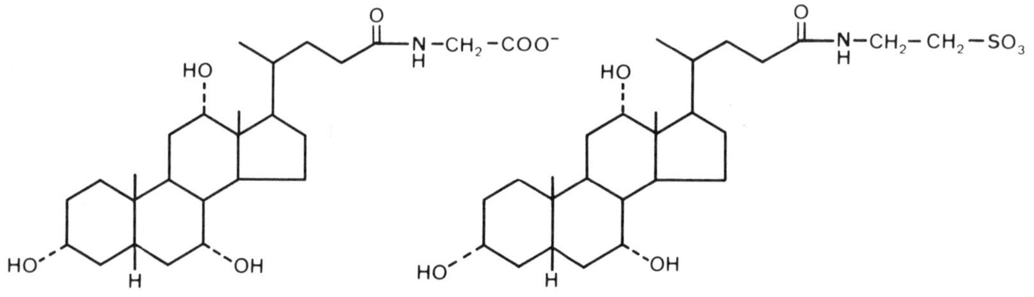

Glycocholic acid

Taurocholic acid

In the intestine the bile acids can either be reabsorbed after removal of the glycine or taurine residue or converted by action of bacteria (remove the C_7 or C_7 and C_{12} hydroxyl groups) to deoxycholate or lithocholate.

Steroid Hormone Synthesis

Synthesis of steroid hormones involves an initial oxidative shortening of the side chain which is often followed by additional hydroxylations, reactions catalyzed by enzymes referred to as hydroxylases in earlier literature or currently as cytochrome P_{450} enzymes. The term "cytochrome P_{450}" designates a group of heme-containing proteins which in the reduced state form a complex with carbon monoxide that has a major absorption band at 450 nm. Their function is to catalyze the monooxygenation of lipophilic substrates. They are found in association with the mitochondria and endoplasmic reticulum. In the adrenal cortex, the mitochondria contain

The esterase catalyzes the hydrolysis of cholesterol esters providing free cholesterol. There is also an enhanced uptake of cholesterol from the circulation and an increase in HMGCoA reductase activity. Metabolism of the cell is altered so that cholesterol is made available for pregnenolone synthesis.

Pregnenolone can be oxidized to give progesterone or 17 α-hydroxypregnenolone. Both products can be oxidized to form 17 α-hydroxyprogesterone. Progesterone can be oxidized to yield corticosterone and aldosterone:

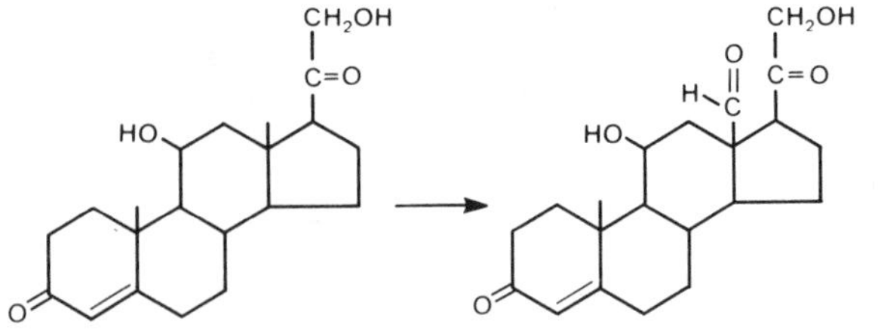

Corticosterone

Aldesterone

while 17 α-hydroxyprogesterone is the precursor for cortisol and cortisone.

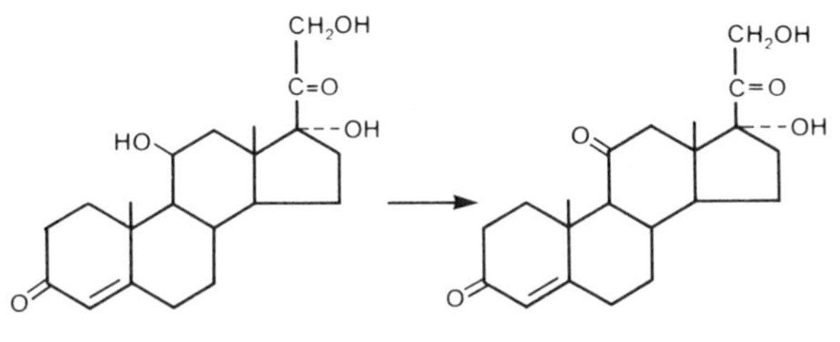

Cortisol   Cortisone

17 α-hydroxypregnenolone can be oxidized to dehydroepiandrosterone which can be further oxidized to form androstenedione.

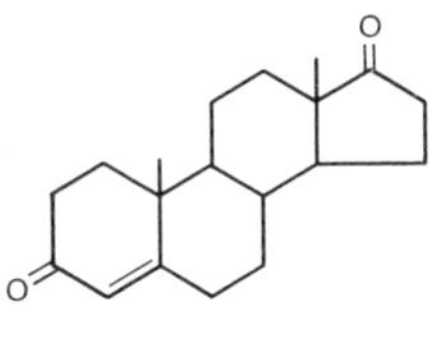

Androstenedione

Reduction of the 17-ketone of androstenedione to a hydroxyl group produces testosterone, which in turn serves as a precursor for synthesis of the estrogens, estradiol, and estrone.

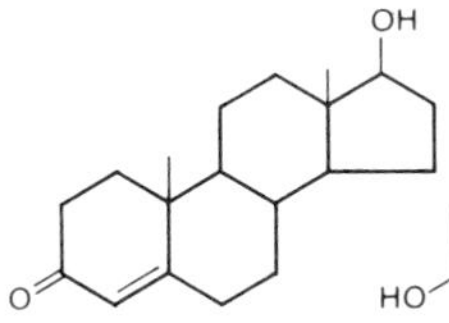

Testosterone 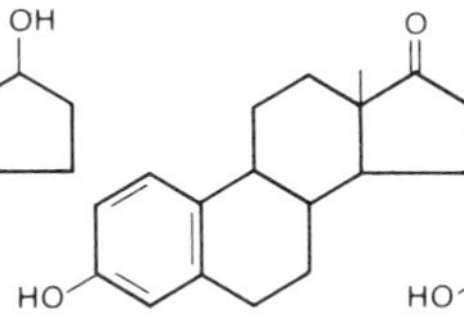   Estrone 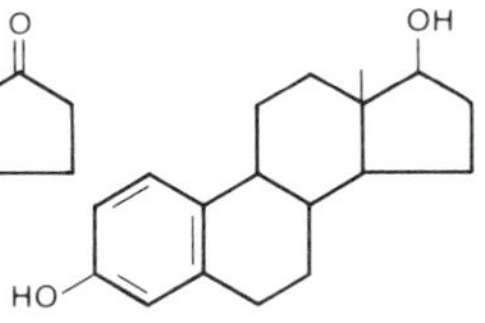   Estradiol

Androstenedione also serves as a precursor for estrone. The final steroid hormone formed from pregnenolone via reactions catalyzed by hydroxylases and dehydrogenases depends upon which enzymes are present and active in the endocrine tissue.

The steroids are secreted into the blood stream where

they can bind to different blood proteins with varying affinities. In this manner they are transported from their sites of synthesis to their sites of utilization. Then, they diffuse across the plasma membrane and are bound by specific cytoplasmic receptors; this induces changes which result in translocation of the hormone receptor complex to the nucleus. The complex binds to the chromatin activating the synthesis of certain mRNAs resulting in increased synthesis of specific proteins.

Eicosanoids

Eicosanoids are derived from C_{20} unsaturated fatty acids and include the prostaglandins, thromboxanes, some hydroperoxy and hydroxy fatty acids, and the leukotrienes. In contrast to steroid hormones, eicosanoids tend to act locally rather than circulating to a distant site. Also, eicosanoids rarely act on their own, instead they enhance or antagonize an ongoing cellular process or sensitize tissue to the effects of other hormones.

The C_{20} fatty acid precursor for eicosanoid synthesis is provided by phospholipase A_2 catalyzed hydrolysis of the fatty acid residue at position two of certain phospholipids. Arachidonic acid (5,8,11,14-eicosatetraenoic acid) is the major precursor for eicosanoid synthesis although 8,11,14-eicosatrienoic and 5,8,11,14,17-eicosapentaenoic acids are also used. Two different enzymes catalyze the initial steps in eicosanoid synthesis. Cyclooxygenase, also known as prostaglandin endoperoxide synthetase, catalyzes the formation of an unstable endoperoxide which serves as the precursor for prostaglandins, prostacyclin, and thromboxanes. These compounds have been implicated in a wide variety of effects. The basis of these effects probably involves the utilization of messengers such as cAMP, cGMP, and Ca^{2+}. Lipoxygenases catalyze the initial step in the formation of hydroperoxy and hydroxy eicosanoids and the leukotrienes. Cyclooxygenase is found in a variety of tissues while lipoxygenase activity is associated with the leukocytes, mast cells, platelets, and lung. The positional specificity of the lipoxygenase differs in different tissues.

Prostaglandins are considered derivatives of the C_{20} compound, prostanoic acid, which contains a five-membered ring formed by a bond between C_8 and C_{12}, with the C_8 hydrogen above the plane (β) and the C_{12}-hydrogen below the plane (α).

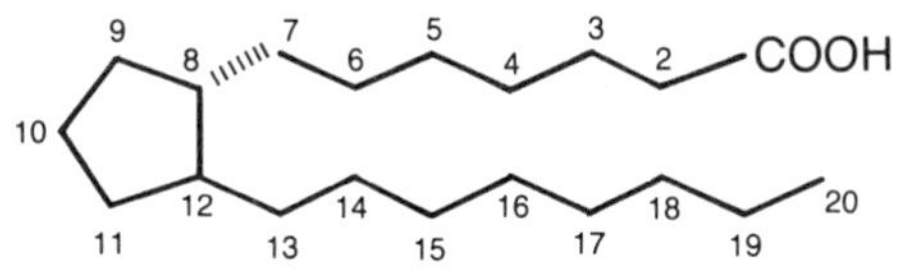

Prostanoic acid

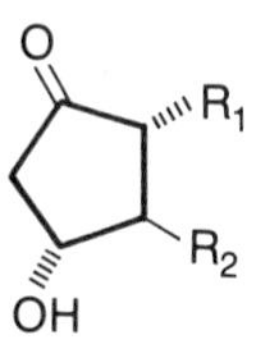

PGE 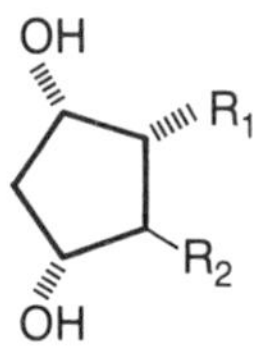   PGFα 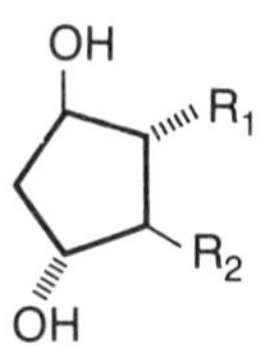   PGFβ

There are two main classes of prostaglandins identified as PGE and PGF. The E and F refer to the ring substituents. In the E series there is a keto group at C_9 and an α-hydroxy at C_{11}; the PGF_α series has an α-hydroxy at C_9 and C_{11} while PGF_β has a β-hydroxy at C_9. Other series exist which are designated as A (keto group at C_9, double bond at C_{10}), C (which is similar to A except the double bond is at C_{11}), B (also similar to A but with the double bond between C_8 and C_{12}), and D (α-hydroxy at C_9 and a keto group at C_{11}). Subscripts in the prostaglandin abbreviations refer to the number of double bonds in the R_1 and R_2 side chains. Those with a subscript of 1 have a saturated R_1 while the 2 and 3 series have a *cis* double bond at C_5 of R_1. In the 1 and 2 series R_2 has an α-hydroxy at C_{15} and a *trans* double bond at C_{13}, while in the 3 series R_2 has an additional *cis* double bond at C_{17}. The 3-series is derived from eicosapentaenoic acid, the 2-series from arachidonic acid, and the 1-series from eicosatrienoic acid. Prostacyclin (PGI) contains the 5-membered ring formed between C_8 and C_{12} plus an additional 5-membered ring formed by an oxygen atom bridging carbon atoms C_9 and C_6. Thromboxanes differ from prostaglandins in that they contain a 6-membered oxane ring formed between C_8 and C_{12} with the oxygen atom inserted between C_{11} and C_{12}. Prostacyclin and the thromboxanes have very short half-lives. The endoperoxide PGH_2, formed by the action of fatty acid cyclooxygenase on arachidonate, is converted to thromboxane by action of thromboxane synthetase, to PGI_2 by prostacyclin synthetase, and to PGE_2 by endoperoxide isomerase. Cyclooxygenase catalyzes the rate-limiting reaction once substrate is available. Corticosteroids have an antiinflammatory activity which is related to their ability to block release of arachidonate via induction of the synthesis of a protein inhibitor of phospholipase activity. Cyclooxygenase is inactivated by the free radical generated during the conversion of arachidonate to an endoperoxide. New protein must be synthesized to continue the reaction. Catecholamines can augment cyclooxygenase activity, while drugs such as aspirin and indomethacin can block it. Oxidation at C_{15}, reduction of the double bond at C_{13}, and β and ω-oxidations give rise to the C_{16}-dicarboxylic acid products of prostaglandin catabolism.

Lipoxygenase products may function as mediators of allergic and inflammatory reactions. The products formed by action of the 11-, 12-, or 15-lipoxygenases on arachidonate are the corresponding 11-, 12-, or 15-hydroperoxyeicosatetraenoic acids which can be converted to the corresponding hydroxy compounds. 5-Lipoxygenase catalyzes the synthesis of 5-hydroperoxyeicosatetraenoic acid which can form 5-hydroxyeicosatetraenoic acid or, in the presence of glutathione, can be converted to leukotriene A_4 (LTA_4) in a reaction catalyzed by LTA

synthetase. LTA_4 has an oxygen atom bridging C_5 and C_6, *trans* double bonds at C_7 and C_9, and *cis* double bonds at C_{11} and C_{14}. The glutathione residue is found at C_6. LTA_4 serves as a precursor of LTC_4 which has a β-hydroxy at C_5. Loss of the glutamyl residue of glutathione converts LTC_4 to LTD_4. LTD_4 is degraded to LTE_4 by loss of the glycine residue. Subscript numerals refer to the precursor fatty acid which determines the number of double bonds in the product; eicosatrienoic acid is the precursor of the 3 series and arachidonate for the 4 series. Eicosapentaenoic acid is a poor substrate for the lipoxygenases so the 5 series is rare. The B series differs from C,D, and E in that it has two hydroxy residues, one at C_5 and one at C_{12}, a *cis* double bond at C_6, *trans* double at C_8 and C_{10}, and no amino acids. Leukotrienes C_4 and D_4 are of particular interest because they are the slow reacting substances of anaphylaxis.

Vitamins

In addition to the nucleotide coenzymes several other coenzymes have been mentioned which are derived from water soluble vitamins. These include pyridoxine (vitamin B_6), thiamine (vitamin B_1), biotin, folic acid, cobalamine (vitamin B_{12}), and ascorbic acid (vitamin C). The water-soluble vitamins are not stored in the body to a significant degree and therefore must be ingested on a frequent basis.

Pyridoxol, pyridoxal, or pyridoxamine are the three natural forms of vitamin B_6. Pyridoxol is phosphorylated to form pyridoxol phosphate in a kinase catalyzed reaction and then oxidized to form pyridoxal phosphate.

Pyridoxal phosphate   4-Pyridoxic acid

Pyridoxal phosphate serves as a coenzyme in transaminations, forming a Schiff's base (arrow indicates the active site) as an intermediate. It is also required for synthesis of the transmitters serotonin and norepinephrine, and for the synthesis of the heme precursor, δ-aminolevulinic acid. A mild pyridoxal deficiency results in irritability and nervousness; severe deficiency can result in convulsions. Pyridoxal phosphate can be oxidized to 4-pyridoxic acid, the form in which it is excreted.

Thiamine is converted to thiamine pyrophosphate, the coenzyme form, by reacting with ATP.

Thiamine pyrophosphate

It is required by the pyruvate and α-ketoglutarate dehydrogenases, in the oxidative decarboxylation of the α-keto acids derived from the branched chain amino acids and by the transketolase of the pentose-phosphate pathway. A deficiency of thiamine results in the symptoms of beriberi (loss of weight, muscle wasting, and muscle weakness). Thiamine can be excreted as thiamine or it can be converted to 4-amino-5-hydroxymethyl-2-methylpyrimidine by the action of thiaminase present in intestinal microorganisms.

Enzymes requiring biotin to function contain the compound in an amide linkage to the ϵ-amino group of a lysine residue. Formation of the amide bond requires the ATP-dependent activation of biotin to biotinyl-5'-adenylate prior to its reaction with the enzyme.

Biotinyl-enzyme

Biotin serves as a prosthetic group for enzymes that catalyze the fixation of CO_2 (e.g., pyruvate and acetyl CoA carboxylases). Proteolysis of the holoenzyme releases biotinyllysine which can be cleaved to biotin and lysine. The side chain of biotin can then undergo β-oxidation. Biotin is synthesized by intestinal bacteria; therefore, a deficiency does not occur normally. Raw egg white is rich in avidin, a glycoprotein that binds biotin tightly, and if ingested in sufficient quantity can induce a biotin-deficiency.

Folic acid serves as a precursor for 1-carbon tetrahydrofolate derivatives used in amino acid metabolism and for the synthesis of purines and the pyrimidine, thymine.

Folic acid consists of 2-amino-4-hydroxy-6-methylpteridine, p-aminobenzoic acid, and glutamic acid.

Folic Acid

Folic acid usually has two to seven glutamic acid residues which are removed during digestion by a conjugase present in the lysosomes of intestinal mucosal cells. The folic acid is reduced to tetrahydrofolate and circulates as the N^5-methylderivative of tetrahydrofolate. In cells it is found as the polyglutamate formed by tetrahydrofolate undergoing successive reactions with glutamate in the presence of ATP. The reactions are catalyzed by folylpolyglutamate synthetase. The ATP is hydrolyzed to ADP and P_i. A deficiency in folic acid results in growth failure and a macrocytic anemia. The latter results from decreased DNA synthesis which among other changes results in a slowed maturation of erythrocytes producing abnormally large red blood cells. The cells also have fragile membranes which undergo hemolysis.

Cobalamin in food is usually found bound to protein in the methyl or 5'-deoxyadenosyl form, while in supplements it is found as hydoxy- or cyanocobalamin. Cobalamin has cobalt coordinated in four positions to the nitrogens of a corrin ring, in one position to a benzimidazole nitrogen, and in the sixth position to a methyl, deoxyadenosyl, cyano, or hydroxyl group. During digestion it is hydrolyzed to give hydroxycobalamin which binds to an intestinal glycoprotein, intrinsic factor, which carries it to the mucosal cells of the ileum. There a specific receptor binds the complex which dissociates with release of the cobalamin inside the cell. Deoxyadenosylcobalamin is synthesized intramitochondrially; after reduction of the cobalamin the adenosyl group is transferred from ATP in a reaction catalyzed by an adenosyltransferase. Methylcobalamin is synthesized in the cytosol; after reduction of the cobalt, a methyl group is transferred to it from N^5-methyltetrahydrofolate. Deoxyadenosylcobalamin is essential for the methylmalonyl CoA mutase catalyzed conversion of methylmalonyl CoA to succinyl CoA, while methylcobalamin is needed for the conversion of homocysteine and N^5-methyltetrahydrofolate to methionine and tetrahydrofolate. Pernicious anemia and neurological impairment are the symptoms associated with a cellular vitamin B_{12} deficiency. The deficiency is usually caused by a lack of functional intrinsic factor.

Ascorbic acid is used as a reducing agent in hydroxylation reactions in which molecular oxygen is a substrate.

O C
|
HO C
‖
HO C   O
|
HC
|
HO CH
|
CH$_2$OH

L-Ascorbic acid

Examples include the conversion of tryptamine to 5-hydroxytryptamine (serotonin), and the hydroxylation of proline and lysine residues in the synthesis of collagen. It also aids in the absorption of iron and in the utilization of folic acid. A lack of vitamin C results in symptoms of scurvy such as capillary fragility, anemia, and bone disease.

A variety of inborn errors have been identified which result in a vitamin dependency, the need for an increased quantity of the vitamin, or for its administration via a different route. Errors can occur which affect (1) intestinal absorption, (2) transport of the vitamin in the plasma and/or into the cell, (3) conversion of the vitamin to the coenzyme, and (4) formation of the holoenzyme. Juvenile pernicious anemia (described above), resulting from a lack of intrinsic factor for the transport of vitamin B_{12}, is an example of the first type of error. Transcobalamin I and II carry vitamin B_{12} in the circulation. Transcobalamin II-associated cobalamin is cleared from plasma rapidly; when there is a lack of functional transcobalamin II, symptoms similar to those associated with a lack of intrinsic factor appear. Failure to convert B_{12} to deoxyadenosyl cobalamin results in changes in peripheral and central myelin. This error is accompanied by the urinary excretion of elevated amounts of methylmalonate due to lack of conversion of methylamalonyl CoA to succinyl CoA. Vitamin B_6 responsive disorders have been observed in which the mutation affects the apoenzyme. Inborn errors which can be classified as vitamin dependencies can usually be treated by altering the route of administration of the vitamin and/or giving pharmacological (*not* physiological) doses of a specific vitamin.

Cytochrome P$_{450}$s, Oxygenases, Hydroxylases, and Oxidases

In amino acid and steroid metabolism, oxidations occur in which molecular oxygen is a substrate. Hydroxylations of the steroid nucleus or its side chain are catalyzed by hydroxylases referred to as cytochrome P$_{450}$s; enzymes which catalyze the general reaction:

$$RH + O_2 + NADPH + H^+ \longrightarrow ROH + H_2O + NADP^+$$

The active site of a cytochrome P$_{450}$ contains an iron-protoporphyrin IX moiety in a relatively open hydrophobic depression in the surface of the apoprotein. The iron binds to four pyrrole nitrogen atoms and to a cysteine in the protein. The sixth is open in the ferrous form and occupied by water in the ferric form. During a reaction, Fe^{3+} is reduced to Fe^{2+} by one electron from NADPH; the oxygen then binds to the iron. A series of changes occur which culminate in release of a water molecule and the insertion of a hydroxyl group into the substrate. In liver the cytochrome P$_{450}$s are associated with the endoplasmic reticulum; in the adrenal cortex they are associated with the mitochondria.

One of the most important functions of the liver is to protect the body against drugs (e.g., smoke, particles, dyes, preservatives, and therapeutic agents) which might interfere with essential cellular biochemical reactions. Lipid soluble drugs are excreted slowly by the kidney and would accumulate, possibly at toxic levels, if they could not be converted into more water-soluble compounds which are often less toxic and more readily excreted. The liver uses the cytochrome P$_{450}$ system to convert drugs to more water-soluble metabolites. Induction of this system in response to a drug is accompanied by the proliferation of the smooth endoplasmic reticulum, the site of cytochrome P$_{450}$ activity. The problem with this method of detoxification is that formation of a more polar (water-soluble) drug may result in one that is more toxic.

Oxygenases are divided into monooxygenases which catalyze reactions in which one atom of molecular oxygen is found in the product and one in water; and dioxygenases which catalyze reactions in which both atoms of molecular oxygen are found in the product. The cytochrome P$_{450}$ enzymes are a special group of monooxygenases. Dopamine-β-monooxygenase (dopamine-β-hydroxylase) is a Cu^{2+}-containing enzyme, which requires ascorbate to reduce the inactive Cu^{2+}-enzyme to the active Cu^{+1} form, that catalyzes the synthesis of norepinephrine from dopamine. Lipoxygenases act as dioxygenases catalyzing formation of hydroperoxy derivatives of eicosatetraenoic acid (both atoms of oxygen are incorporated in the product). Tryptophan-2,3-dioxygenase catalyzes the insertion of both atoms of molecular oxygen into tryptophan to produce N-formyl-kynurenine.

Oxidases catalyze the oxidation of a substrate in such a manner that hydrogen peroxide is produced. Glucose oxidase, in the presence of molecular oxygen, catalyzes the oxidation of glucose to gluconic acid with the concomitant reduction of oxygen to hydrogen peroxide.

SUPEROXIDE AND PEROXIDE METABOLISM

During evolution enzymes developed which enabled aerobic organisms to metabolize hydrogen peroxide (H_2O_2) and the superoxide ions (O_2^-) produced during the reduction of molecular oxygen by the spontaneous oxidation of reduced coenzymes such as NAD(P)H and flavoproteins or the iron of compounds such as cytochrome b and hemoglobin. Superoxide dismutases catalyze the reaction:

$$2O_2^- + 2H^+ \longrightarrow O_2 + H_2O_2$$

There are two dismutases in mammalian cells, one associated with the cytoplasm and one with the mitochondria. Catalase and peroxidases catalyze reactions to prevent the accumulation of H_2O_2. Catalase acts to convert $2 H_2O_2$ to $2 H_2O$ and O_2. Peroxidases, less widely distributed in animal tissues than catalase, catalyze the reaction of hydrogen peroxide with two molecules of the substrate to be oxidized (e.g., glutathione or a halide) to form $2 H_2O$ and the oxidized substrate (e.g., oxidized glutathione or halogen).

CELLULAR BIOLOGY

Membranes

Membranes serve to delineate cells (plasma membrane) and to form compartments within the cell (organelles) thereby permitting a variety of reactions to occur simultaneously, under quite different conditions. They function as very selective permeability barriers, contain receptors for external stimuli, participate in intercellular communication, and play a role in many metabolic reactions. When viewed under the electron microscope, membranes appear to have a trilaminar composition comprised of two dark bands separated by a lighter band.

Membranes consist of two main components, lipid and protein. The relative amounts of each can vary from one membrane to another. For example, the erythrocyte plasma membrane has a lipid to protein ratio of about one to one, while in myelin it is greater than three to one and in the inner mitochondrial membrane it is less than one to three. The carbohydrate associated with membranes is found as glycoprotein and glycolipid. Currently, the accepted general explanation of membrane structure is that given by the fluid mosaic model in which membranes are described as being composed of a lipid bilayer with both peripheral and integral membrane components.

The actual lipid composition varies in different membranes, but phospholipids generally comprise 50 percent or more of the total lipid with cholesterol and glycolipids accounting for the rest. Phospholipids will spontaneously aggregate in an aqueous environment to form a bimolecular bilayer in which their polar groups interact with the water and their hydrocarbon chains interact with each other. The hydrophobic interactions between the fatty acyl chains and the hydrophilic interactions of the polar groups with water stabilize the lipid bilayer. The lipid composition determines the fluidity of the bilayer. When a phospholipid is heated there is a transition point at which a pronounced endothermic change occurs and the fatty acyl chains are said to "melt." Phospholipids composed of shorter fatty acyl chains or chains with a higher degree of unsaturation (cis double bonds introduce kinks in the fatty acyl chains preventing their close packing) have a lower transition phase temperature than phospholipids with longer chain, saturated fatty acyl groups. Cell membrane functions require that the bilayer be fluid. Cholesterol helps to maintain membrane fluidity. It interacts with the membrane so that its polar hydroxyl group is on the surface of the bilayer while its planar steroid rings interact with the hydrocarbon chains nearest the polar head groups. This prevents the close packing required for the phospholipids to crystallize when cooled. By decreasing the mobility of the fatty acyl chains, cholesterol increases the viscosity at the middle of the bilayer.

The distribution of lipids within a membrane is asymmetric. An example of this is seen in the erythrocyte plasma membrane in which the total phospholipids are distributed evenly on both sides. However, the aminophospholipids, phosphatidylethanolamine and phosphatidylserine, are found predominantly on the cytoplasmic side while phosphatidylcholine and sphingomyelin are enriched on the outer surface. Glycolipids are associated with the outer surface of plasma membranes.

Peripheral and integral membrane proteins are differentiated by the ease with which they can be dissociated from the membrane. Peripheral proteins are dissociated by mild treatments such as changing the ionic strength. Upon dissociation they are free of lipids, and they are relatively soluble in aqueous solvents. Integral membrane protein components require harsher methods such as treatment with detergents for dissociation. Upon dissociation they often remain associated with lipids and they usually are not very soluble in neutral aqueous buffers. The integral protein can span the width of the bilayer, with parts exposed at both the inner and outer surface. The distribution of integral proteins within a membrane has been found to be essentially random. Proteins can move laterally within the membrane and are distributed asymmetrically in the membrane.

Glycosylation of nascent proteins, which will be the glycoprotein constituents of membranes, is catalyzed by enzymes found on the luminal side of the rough endoplasmic reticulum and Golgi apparatus. It is this asymmetric glycosylation which accounts for the observation that glycoproteins are found on the outer surface of the plasma membrane and the noncytoplasmic surfaces of intracellular membranes. Synthesis of oligosaccharides linked glycosidically to the hydroxyl group of a serine or threonine residue occurs through the sequential addition of sugars in reactions catalyzed by specific glycosyltransferases. Biosynthesis of the asparagine-linked (N-linked) oligosaccharides is much more complex. First, glycosyl transferases catalyze the sequential addition of specific monosaccharides to dolichol phosphate which is bound to the endoplasmic reticulum. N-Acetylglucosamine is the first sugar added; it is transferred as the sugar-phosphate from its UDP-carrier to dolichol phosphate forming N-acetylglucosaminyldiphosphoryldolichol. A second N-acetylglucosamine and five mannose residues are then added in a similar fashion. The last four mannose and three glucose residues are added in reactions catalyzed by glycosyl transferases which use the monosaccharide monophosphoryldolichol as the sugar donor instead of the sugar nucleotide. The complete oligosaccharide is then transferred to the appropriate asparagine which is found in the sequence asparagine-x-threonine (serine) and is present at the surface of the protein. Addition of the oligosaccharide to the protein can occur as the peptide emerges on the luminal side of the rough endoplasmic reticulum. The oligosaccharide is then processed as the glycoprotein moves to the smooth endoplasmic reticulum and subsequently to the Golgi. Initially, the three glucose residues are removed by the action of α-glucosidases (endoplasmic reticulum) and then the four mannose residues are cleaved by α-mannosidases (Golgi). N-acetylglucosaminyltransferase catalyzes the addition of N-acetylglucosamine prior to re-

lease of two more mannose residues forming:

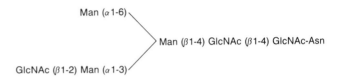

which can then be converted to the finished glycoprotein by the sequential addition of the appropriate sugars.

Since a major function of membranes is to serve as permeability barriers, it is necessary to understand how small molecules and macromolecules are transported across them. Small, nonpolar molecules such as oxygen and nitrogen can readily diffuse across a lipid membrane as can small uncharged polar molecules such as ethanol, carbon dioxide, and water. Larger, uncharged polar molecules such as monosaccharides and charged molecules of all sizes cannot diffuse across the membrane. Membrane transport proteins transport a specific class of compounds or an individual member of that class across the membrane. Some transport proteins function in passive transport (concentration gradient determines the direction of flow) while others function in active transport (requires a source of energy). Passive transport can occur by simple diffusion, via channel proteins which form aqueous channels allowing molecules of certain size and charge to pass through, or by facilitated diffusion in which the molecule to be transported binds to a carrier protein which transfers it across the membrane. Facilitated diffusion can be differentiated from channel diffusion in that the rate of passage of the molecule being transported reaches a maximum when the carrier protein is saturated; addition of more of the molecule to be transported does not increase the rate. In channel mediated diffusion increasing the concentration of the molecule to be transported results in a continuing increase in the rate of transport. Proteins which transport only one molecule across the membrane are called uniports while those for which transport of one molecule requires simultaneous or sequential transport of a second are called cotransport systems. Cotransport can be in the same direction (symport) or in the opposite direction (antiport).

In active transport there is a net movement of the solute against its concentration gradient (from lower to higher concentration). An illustration of active transport is the $Na^+ - K^+$ pump which maintains the Na^+ and K^+ concentration gradient across the plasma membrane of a cell. Hydrolysis of ATP to ADP and phosphate provides the energy required to keep the concentration of K^+ higher inside the cell and that of Na^+ higher outside. The

$K^+ - Na^+$ gradient maintains the cell's membrane potential, helps control cell volume (prevents an influx of Na^+ and Cl^- down a concentration gradient which would upset the osmotic balance causing the cell to swell), and provides energy in the form of the ion gradient for the active transport of some sugars and amino acids into cells.

Macromolecules are transported across membranes by endocytosis and exocytosis. In endocytosis the material being ingested is enclosed by a portion of the cell's plasma membrane which then pinches off to form an intracellular vesicle containing the ingested substance. In pinocytosis small vesicles are ingested while in phagocytosis large particles are taken up. Pinocytosis and endocytosis can be used interchangeably for most cells, however, macrophages and polymorphonuclear leucocytes tend to be phagocytic. Most mammalian cells can remove specific macromolecules from the extracellular mileu via receptor-mediated endocytosis. The substance to be taken up binds to its receptor which is associated with cell surface coated pits (identified by electron microscopy). The material thus bound is then internalized as part of a vesicle. This provides a mechanism for the uptake of specific macromolecules in a concentrated fashion. An example of this is the receptor-mediated uptake of LDLs previously described. Cell surface receptors can also be distributed across the cell surface, and become associated in coated pits only after binding the substrate as seen in the binding and uptake of insulin by fibroblasts.

Exocytosis can be considered the reverse of endocytosis. Vesicles that pinch off from the Golgi can fuse with the plasma membrane releasing their contents to the extracellular environment. Small molecules that are to be secreted can be actively transported into secretory vesicles, where they may bind to macromolecules. This permits their storage at high concentrations without an appreciable alteration in cell osmolarity. Material in secretory vesicles is usually released in response to an extracellular signal, such as Ca^{2+}, as in the release of acetylcholine by neurons. In both endocytosis and exocytosis the molecules ingested or secreted are localized in vesicles and do not mix with the other cellular components, except for those associated with the specific membrane with which the vesicle fuses.

Cellular Organelles

Membrane bound cellular organelles found in most eucaryotic cells include the nucleus, mitochondria, lysosomes, peroxisomes, Golgi, and the endoplasmic reticulum. The plasma membrane can also be separated for study using standard cell fractionation procedures. In addition some cells contain secretory vesicles. The membranes delineating these organelles are the sites of many biological processes, many of which have been indicated.

The nucleus is the site of DNA replication and synthesis. It is bordered by a double membrane, the nuclear envelope. The outer membrane of the envelope and the perinuclear space between it and the inner membrane are continuous with the endoplasmic reticulum and its lumen, respectively. Nuclear pores which are surrounded by a discoid structure, the nuclear pore complex, provide channels for the transport of water-soluble molecules between the nucleus and cytoplasm. Edges of the pores appear to be formed by fusion of the inner and outer membranes, which could allow the lateral flow of lipid soluble components from their site of synthesis in the endoplasmic reticulum to the inner nuclear membrane. The structure of the pores is probably maintained by a fibrous protein network that lines the inner nuclear membrane and is referred to as the nuclear lamina. Within the nucleus there is often a large, diffuse, non-membrane bound structure, the nucleolus. It is the site of rRNA synthesis and of its packaging into the large and small ribosomal subunits; the final steps occur as the subunits are transferred to the cytoplasm.

The endoplasmic reticulum (ER) whose membrane often accounts for over half of the total cellular membrane, is the site of synthesis of the protein and lipid components found in cell membranes; it separates cytoplasmic molecules from noncytoplasmic ones. The ER consists of two functionally distinct areas: the smooth ER, not involved in protein biosynthesis, and the rough ER which has ribosomes associated with it and is involved in protein synthesis. Smooth ER is the site of synthesis of the lipid components of lipoproteins, the site of steroid hormone biosynthesis, and the site of the detoxification reactions catalyzed by cytochrome P_{450}s. It is also the area from which vesicles carrying newly synthesized lipid and protein for intracellular transport are pinched off. Proteins synthesized on the rough ER are those which will be secreted or incorporated into other intracellular organelles. The ribosomes associated with the rough ER are held there in part by the growing peptide chain and by specific binding proteins present in the ER membrane. Proteins synthesized on the ER contain an extra leader peptide of ~20 amino acid residues which is not found in the finished product. This leader sequence is believed to act as a "signal" which directs the ribosome to the ER. This sequence is cleaved on the luminal side of the rough ER. Phospholipid and cholesterol synthesis associated with the smooth ER require metabolites found in the cytoplasm. This suggests that lipid synthesis occurs on the outer membrane of the ER. It is not yet known how newly synthesized lipids are transferred to the inner membrane. The synthetic activity results in the formation of additional ER which contains the carbohydrate moieties of glycoproteins on the luminal side as are the amino termini of transmembrane proteins. Vesicles which pinch off and become associated with the other cellular organelles maintain this sidedness; fusion of an ER vesicle with the plasma membrane results in the luminal side of the ER membrane being on the outer surface of the plasma membrane.

After synthesis in the ER, many molecules pass to the Golgi apparatus which consists of stacks of flattened disk-shaped vesicles. Small membrane bound vesicles are found near the Golgi. The Golgi is the site for final modification of the asparagine-linked oligosaccharide chains of glycoproteins, and of protein alteration by glycosylation of select serine and/or threonine residues, by proteolysis, and by sulfation. Macromolecules destined for specific cellular organelles appear to become enriched in localized areas of the *trans* side (plasma membrane side) of the *trans* most Golgi, suggesting that vesicles carrying these components are packaged in defined regions. These areas are probably delineated by receptors specific for the macromolecules to be transported. Proteins which will be secreted are packaged in secretory vesicles. Initially, condensing vacuoles are synthesized on the *trans* side of the Golgi stack. With time, the material to be secreted becomes more concentrated in the condensing vacuoles resulting in formation of mature secretory vesicles. These are stored in the apical portion of the cell and are released to the extracellular environment in response to a certain stimulus.

LYSOSOMES

Lysosomes serve as the digestive component of the cell. The hydrolases they sequester have acidic pH optima which permit them to be active in the acidic ($\sim$pH5) environment of the lysosome. Primary lysosomes, delineated by a single membrane, are formed by budding from the Golgi. Specific receptors exist in the ER and Golgi which recognize the hydrolases destined to become lysosomal constituents. In studies of the inborn error, I-cell disease (characterized biochemically by the very low hydrolase activity associated with lysosomes) it was found that a mannose-6-phosphate containing oligosaccharide was the marker recognized. It is lost once the hydrolase is packaged in the lysosome. Material to be digested is made available to the lysosome through its fusion with a phagocytic, endocytotic, or autophagic vesicle. Lysosomes which have been exposed to substrate for digestion are known as secondary lysosomes.

PEROXISOMES

Peroxisomes contain enzymes which catalyze catabolic reactions that utilize molecular oxygen. This membrane bound organelle is formed by budding from the smooth ER, although many never break completely free. Catalase is sequestered in peroxisomes where it catalyzes the conversion of hydrogen peroxide, produced in other reactions, to water and molecular oxygen.

MITOCHONDRIA

Mitochondria are the organelles which convert energy to forms usable by mammalian cells. Like the nucleus, mitochondria are bound by a double membrane. They can be divided into the outer and inner membranes, the intramembrane space, and the lumen or matrix. Fatty acid oxidation and the tricarboxylic acid cycle occur in the mitochondria and the reducing equivalents produced are carried down the electron transport chain and are finally used to reduce molecular oxygen to water. Electron transport is linked to production of ATP, a high-energy phosphate compound which upon hydrolysis provides energy for a variety of metabolic processes.

CYTOSKELETON

The cytoskeleton of eukaryotic cells maintains cell shape, cell movement, and the arrangement of cell organelles. It is formed by actin filaments and microtubules. Microtubules form the mitotic spindle needed for cell division. Evidence suggests that cell organelles are associated with the cytoskeleton and that they move along the cytoskeleton via an energy dependent process.

Biochemistry of the Cell Cycle

During embryogenesis cells proliferate at a rapid rate while in mature individuals the rate of cell replication is normally reduced to a rate sufficient to replace those cells which die. For a cell to divide, it has to reproduce its DNA and double its cell contents. Then it can undergo nuclear division (mitosis) and cytoplasmic division (cytokinesis). The cell cycle consists of four successive phases. The M phase which consists of mitosis and cytokinesis; the G_1 phase in which new cells exhibit a high rate of biosynthetic activity; the S phase which starts with DNA replication and ends when each chromosome has been replicated; and the G_2 phase which occurs between DNA replication and mitosis. In a rapidly dividing cell system the M phase is relatively brief (1 to 2 hrs); the G_1 and S phases occupy the majority of the time involved in one cycle. The length of G_1 is the principal determinant of how rapidly cells divide. If the division of cells grown in vitro is reduced (due to a lack of essential nutrients or overcrowding, etc.) the cell cycle is arrested in the G_1 phase. Cells in this stable, resting state are often said to be in the G_0 phase of the cell cycle. Once cells pass a restriction point in G_1 they are committed to complete the cycle.

The event which causes the actual initiation of DNA replication that occurs in S phase is not known. In an analogy with yeast where spindle pole body duplication is necessary for DNA replication, it may be that a particular point in the replication of the centriole stimulates DNA replication. As described previously, the DNA winds around a histone octameric protein core forming a nucleosome. These pack together to form a chromatin fiber which folds into looped domains. Each loop is believed to contain a single origin of replication. During replication different units are activated at different times, in an order believed to be determined in part by the degree of compactness of the chromatin. The bulk of histone synthesis also occurs during the S phase. During replication the histones appear to remain associated with the DNA and are found in association with one daughter strand (that synthesized on the leading side of the replication fork). Newly synthesized histones become associated with the lagging strand within minutes of its replication.

Protein synthesis which occurs during G_2 is essential for mitosis. One of the essential proteins synthesized is a kinase, believed to catalyze the phosphorylation of histone H1 present in nucleosomes. This may initiate chromosome condensation which defines the initiation of the prophase stage of mitosis. There are six stages in the M phase (i.e., prophase, prometaphase, metaphase, anaphase, and telophase in mitosis; and cytokinesis). In prophase, defined chromosomes are formed which consist of two sister chromatids (synthesized during S phase) that are joined at the centromere. During this time the nucleolus disappears and the microtubules of the cytoskeleton come apart. The tubulin molecules are then used in formation of the extranuclear mitotic spindle. Each of the two pairs of centrioles (the original pair was replicated in S phase) become the focal points for a radial arrangement of microtubules, termed asters. By late prophase, bundles of polar microtubules extend between the asters. Prometaphase sees the breakdown of the nuclear envelope and the spindle enters the nuclear area. Kinetochores, specialized structures which form on either side of the centromeres, become attached to microtubules forming kinetochore fibers. These radiate in opposite directions and interact with fibers of the spindle. During metaphase the chromosomes become aligned so that their centromeres are in a single plane. Anaphase involves the separation of the paired kinetochores which

results in movement of each chromatid to a spindle pole. During telophase the separated chromatids arrive at the poles, the kinetochore fibers disappear and a nuclear envelope forms around each group of daughter chromatids. The condensed chromatin expands, the nucleolus reforms, and mitosis is completed. Cytokinesis, which starts during late anaphase or telophase, is initiated by a perpendicular drawing of the cell membrane toward the spindle axis between the two daughter nuclei. This cleavage furrow deepens and eventually reaches the narrow mitotic spindle where it breaks forming two separate daughter cells.

During development, different cell types become associated with each other. The question is how does this recognition and aggregation occur. In the simplest case of tissue formation, newly synthesized cells are held in the extracellular matrix and therefore remain associated with each other. The problem arises when cells are synthesized in one area and migrate to another. Mixing experiments have shown that single cells are able to recognize and aggregate preferentially with cells isolated from the same tissue rather than with those from other tissues. Studies have shown that cell interactions can be moderated by specific molecules mediating cell-cell adhesion (e.g., neuronal-cell adhesion molecule) and substrate adhesion (e.g., fibronectin). A third mechanism for cell communication is the contacts cells form with each other (e.g., gap and tight junctions).

SPECIAL BIOCHEMISTRY OF TISSUES

Digestion and Absorption of Nutrients

The process of digestion (enzymatic hydrolysis of large molecules) provides the substrates which can be absorbed and used for the normal metabolic functions of cells. Digestion occurs in the lumen of the gastrointestinal tract. The mucosal cells lining the gastrointestinal tract are coated by mucins, glycoproteins containing a high percentage (60–85) of carbohydrate in O-glycosidic linkage to serine or threonine. These molecules form very viscous solutions and serve as lubricants and as protective agents for the mucosal cells.

Ingestion of food stimulates secretion of saliva by the parotid and submaxillary and sublingual glands. Salivary enzymes include a phosphatase, a lipase, α-amylase, carbonic anhydrase, and kallikrein (a serine protease). Mucin is also secreted in saliva. The secreted saliva serves to lubricate the food and initiates digestion. As the food passes down the gastrointestinal tract it enters the stomach, where four components active in the digestive process are secreted by cells of the gastric mucosa. Specifically, intrinsic factor (vitamin B_{12} transport) and HCl are secreted by the parietal cells, pepsinogen (converted to pepsin by the acidic environment) by the peptic cells, and mucins by the surface epithelial cells. Pepsin initiates protein hydrolysis yielding a mixture of polypeptides. It catalyzes hydrolysis of peptide bonds involving the carboxyl group of an aromatic amino acid.

The bulk of the digestive process occurs in the small intestine. The epithelial cells lining the intestine contain numerous microvilli which provide a large surface area for absorption. The microvilli are covered by a brush border membrane which is protected on the luminal side by a carbohydrate-rich glycocalyx. Associated with the luminal side of the brush border membrane are di- and oligosaccharidases, esterases, and peptidases. In response to hormonal stimuli induced by the flow of gastric chyme into the duodenum, the pancreas secretes large amounts of the enzymes needed for digestion (trypsinogen, chymotrypsinogen, procarboxypeptidases, proelastase, a triacylglycerol lipase, a phospholipase, α-amylase, ribonuclease, and deoxyribonuclease) into the descending portion of the duodenum. The gallbladder is also stimulated and secretes bile acids into the same area. Pancreatic fluid is more alkaline and neutralizes the acidic chyme from the stomach. In the lumen, enteropeptidase (produced by duodenal epithelial cells) catalyzes the essential conversion of trypsinogen to trypsin, which in turn catalyzes the conversion of inactive zymogens and proenzymes to their active form. There is a trypsin inhibitor present in pancreatic juice which prevents premature digestion by any trypsin which might be formed within the pancreas.

Each of the proteolytic enzymes have different substrate specificities. Trypsin, chymotrypsin, and elastase are referred to as "serine" proteases because each has a serine residue that is essential for activity. Trypsin catalyzes hydrolysis of peptide linkages involving the carboxyl bonds of arginine and lysine; chymotrypsin hydrolyzes those involving carboxyl bonds of the aromatic amino acids; and elastase cleaves peptide bonds of neutral aliphatic amino acids. Carboxypeptidases A and B require Zn^{2+} for their activity. In contrast to the aforementioned endopeptidases, the carboxypeptidases are exopeptidases; carboxypeptidase A catalyzes hydrolysis of carboxyl-terminal amino acids possessing aromatic or aliphatic side chains, while carboxypeptidase B acts only on terminal arginine or lysine residues. Aminopeptidases present on the surface of the intestinal mucosal cells catalyze hydrolysis of peptide bonds adjacent to amino acids with a free α-amino group. Small peptides are hydrolyzed by peptidases. Prolidase, present in the cytoplasm of the mucosal cells, hydrolyzes proline containing dipeptides.

Four carrier-mediated active transport systems for amino acids have been identified in the epithelial cells of the intestinal mucosa. They are also present in the renal tubules. All four are Na^+ symport systems which transport the amino acids against their concentration gradient while transporting Na^+ down its concentration gradient. $Na^+ - K^+$ ATPase provides the necessary energy. The groups of amino acids transported by each system are neutral amino acids (monoamino, monocarboxylic), dibasic amino acids, dicarboxylic amino acids, and glycine and imino acids. Specific inborn errors have been identified which affect each of the transport systems. Hartnup disease, cystinuria (dibasic aminoaciduria), dicarboxylic aminoaciduria, and Joseph's syndrome (iminoglycinuria) result from defective absorption of each of the aforementioned classes, respectively. Oligopeptides can also be transported into the epithelial cells of the intestinal mucosa. Di- and tripeptides are transported via a system which is believed to be a Na^+ symport. Within the cells they are hydrolyzed by cytoplasmic peptidases. Larger peptides are hydrolyzed at the cell surface and the amino acids and peptides are then absorbed. After uptake by the mucosal cells, the amino acids diffuse into the portal blood and are carried to the liver. A few peptides resistant to hydrolysis are absorbed intact and can also enter the portal circulation. This explains why the tripeptide, thyrotropin releasing hormone, can be taken orally.

Carbohydrates, ingested in the form of glycogen, amylase or amylopectin, or disaccharides, must be hydrolyzed to monosaccharides prior to absorption. Salivary α-amylase, an endosaccharidase which catalyzes hydrolysis of internal α1,4-glucosidic bonds, initiates digestion of the plant starches amylose (linear chain of glucose molecules linked α1,4), amylopectin (branched chain glucose polymer with α1,6 linkages introducing branch points), and of the animal polysaccharide, glycogen, which is similar to amylopectin except that it has more branch points. Amylases are not present in gastric juice and the low pH therein precludes continued action of the salivary enzyme. The major site of carbohydrate digestion is the small intestine. Pancreatic α-amylase continues the degradation of ingested starch. However it cannot hydrolyze the α1,4 bonds adjacent to α1,6 branch points. Therefore α-limit dextrins are produced in addition to maltose and maltotriose. These di-, tri-, and oligosaccharides plus ingested disaccharides (sucrose and lactose) are hydrolyzed to yield monosaccharides in reactions catalyzed by glycosidases associated with the luminal surface of the membranes of epithelial cells in the small intestine. Maltase (hydrolyzes glucose from the nonreducing ends of α1,4-linked glucose chains) and isomaltase (hydrolyzes α1,6 bonds present in dextrins) catalyze the hydrolysis of the α-dextrins to give glucose monomers.

Fructose, glucose, and galactose are the three principal

monosaccharides produced during digestion of carbohydrates. Sucrose (glc α1-2 fru) and lactose (gal β1-4 glc) are the major sources of fructose and galactose, respectively. Fructose is absorbed from the lumen by epithelial cells via facilitated diffusion (it is carried down its concentration gradient). Glucose and galactose are transported by the same carrier, which has separate binding sites for both the sugar and Na^+. Sodium ions are transported across the membrane with the sugar. Immediately after eating, glucose and galactose are transported down a concentration gradient; with time the sugar concentration gradient shifts and the sugar is transported against its concentration gradient. Energy for this is provided by $Na^+ - K^+$ ATPase which pumps the Na^+ out of the cell, thereby maintaining the Na^+ gradient. Phlorizin can block the sugar binding site of the Na^+-dependent transport molecule. After entering the epithelial cell, some of the glucose can diffuse out of the cell at the contraluminal side but the majority is transported out via a Na^+-independent mechanism. This glucose transport system is blocked by phloretin and cytochalasin B.

Di- and oligosaccharides not hydrolyzed by α-amylase or one of the glycosidases associated with the small intestine are not absorbed from the lumen. They pass to the lower portion of the intestine where bacterial saccharidases act on the sugars to release monosaccharides which can be further metabolized by bacteria present in the lower portion of the intestine. The products formed which include methane, hydrogen, CO_2, and lactate can cause fluid secretion resulting in diarrhea. Inborn errors in which a disaccharidase is affected have been characterized. Lactase deficiency in infants necessitates their being fed a lactose-free formula; human and cow's milk are not suitable since they contain lactose. Sucrase and sucrase-isomaltase deficiencies have been observed. As as result of these errors, the affected individual develops diarrhea if they eat foods containing the particular disaccharides which they cannot properly digest.

The bulk (~90 percent) of dietary lipid is in the form of apolar triacylglycerols. Cholesterol, cholesterol esters, phospholipids, and free fatty acids comprise the difference. By definition these molecules are not very soluble in an aqueous environment; this results in formation of lipid droplets in which lipid-water interactions are minimized. A lipase is secreted in saliva but under normal conditions digestion of lipid at this point is minimal due to the limited exposure of the triacylglycerols to the aqueous environment of the enzyme. The stomach has an acid stable lipase which catalyzes the hydrolysis of some of the surface triacylglycerols to 2-monoacylglycerols and free fatty acids. The products of lipase action have both polar and nonpolar portions and can act as surfactants. This results in an increase of the surface area

of the lipid phase in contact with the water, resulting in the availability of more triacylglycerol for lipase action. The major site of lipid digestion is the same as that for carbohydrates and proteins, the small intestine. Pancreatic lipase continues the degradation of triacylglycerols with fatty acyl residues of 12 carbons or more. The amphipathic bile salts, released by the gallbladder into the duodenum, act as emulsifying agents and, in conjunction with the churning effect of the small intestine, cause formation of smaller lipid-bile acid droplets. This increases the availability of triacylglycerols to lipase action. Bile salts inactivate pure pancreatic lipase. However, a colipase is secreted in the pancreatic juice and this protein stabilizes the lipase. At least two different classes of esterases are also present in the pancreatic juice; one catalyzes the hydrolysis of short-chain (C_{10} or less) fatty acyl residues from triacylglycerols and the other acts on cholesterol esters, monoacylglycerols, and other lipid esters (e.g., vitamin A). Phospholipids are degraded via the action of phospholipases.

The products of lipid digestion, monoacylglycerols, fat soluble vitamins, cholesterol, and the longer-chain free fatty acids ($>C_{12}$) are incorporated into mixed micelles formed with the bile salts. The micelles carry the products to the surface of the epithelial cells of the intestinal mucosa. There the free fatty acid, monoacylglycerols, fat soluble vitamins, and cholesterol leave the micelles and passively diffuse across the epithelial cell membrane. This process is essentially completed in the upper jejunum. However, reabsorption of the bile salts occurs primarily in the ileum via an active transport mechanism. From there the bile salts enter the enterohepatic circulation and are recycled. Within the epithelial cells the longer-chain free fatty acids ($>C_{10}$) can react with coenzyme A in the presence of ATP, in an acyl CoA synthetase catalyzed reaction, to form fatty acyl CoA. In a reaction believed unique to the intestinal mucosa, monoacylglycerol can react with two fatty acyl CoA moieties to form triacylglycerol. The triacylglycerol molecules are incorporated into chylomicra, which are secreted into the lymph and enter the blood via the thoracic duct. Short chain fatty acids (C_{10} or less) are soluble in water and are directly absorbed by epithelial cells; from there they directly enter the portal circulation.

Blood

Blood serves to circulate gases as well as nutrients and waste products to and from the cells of the body. Removal of cells by centrifugation leaves a yellowish supernatant, the plasma. Removal of the cells by allowing them to clot also removes fibrinogen from the blood leaving what is known as serum. Erythrocytes are the specialized cells of blood which serve to transport oxygen and carbon dioxide and to maintain its pH. The erythrocyte lacks a nucleus, mitochondria, Golgi apparatus, lysosomes, ribosomes, and endoplasmic reticulum. These cells derive their metabolic fuel from glucose via glycolysis and reducing equivalents from the phosphogluconate pathway. Nucleotides are synthesized from preformed purines. The average life span for an erythrocyte in the circulation is 120 days. Its major cytoplasmic constituent is hemoglobin, the blood component which actually transports oxygen to and carbon dioxide away from cells.

An oxygen carrier is needed because not enough oxygen is soluble in blood (~0.3 ml O_2/dl blood) to meet the body's requirements. Each g of hemoglobin can combine with 1.34 ml of oxygen and there are ~15 g of hemoglobin/dl blood. Therefore, the hemoglobin in one dl of blood can carry 20.1 ml of oxygen (an almost 70-fold increase). The amount of gas present in solution can be calculated using the equation $C = kP$. C is defined as the mls of gas dissolved per ml of solvent, P is the partial pressure (mm Hg) of the gas in the vapor phase, and k, the Bunsen absorption coefficient, is a constant for the gas in a specific solvent at a given temperature. The tension of a gas in solution, given in mm Hg, is defined as the partial pressure of the gas in the total gas mixture with which the solution is in equilibrium.

Hemoglobin is made up of four protein subunits, two α and two β. A wide variety of abnormal human hemoglobins have been identified and are the result of point, deletion, extended, frameshift, insertion or fusion mutations. Each normal subunit contains one heme molecule which can bind a single oxygen molecule via the iron atom it contains. Therefore, each hemoglobin molecule, when fully oxygenated, can bind four molecules of oxygen. The oxygen binding curve of hemoglobin is sigmoidal indicating a cooperative interaction in binding of oxygen. The Hill coefficient for human hemoglobin is ~2.7. Since it is positive, it indicates that binding of the first oxygen to hemoglobin increases its affinity for binding additional oxygen molecules. Physiologically the cooperative effect seen in oxygen binding is very important. The steepest portion of the binding curve occurs at partial pressures of oxygen between 20 and 50 mm Hg which is in the range of oxygen tension in extrapulmonary tissues. This means that small changes in oxygen tension will result in relatively large changes in oxygen release. Hemoglobin is fully oxygenated at a partial pressure of oxygen of approximately 80 mm Hg. When blood leaves the lungs it is saturated with oxygen (~100 mm Hg); when it reaches extrapulmonary tissues such as the capillary bed of active muscle the oxygen

tension drops (~20 mm Hg) and oxygen is released from the hemoglobin. It diffuses from the erythrocyte through the plasma to the interstitial fluid and into the cells of the tissue. In contrast, carbon dioxide is present at a pressure of approximately 40 mm Hg in arterial blood, and at higher levels in the interstitial fluid surrounding extrapulmonary tissue. Therefore, the carbon dioxide diffuses from the interstitial fluid into the erythrocyte. There carbonic anhydrase catalyzes its reaction with water to form carbonic acid which at pH ~ 7.4 dissociates:

$$CO_2 + H_2O \rightleftharpoons H_2CO_3 \rightleftharpoons H^+ + HCO_3$$

When oxygen binds to hemoglobin, it results in release of protons from His β146, val α1 and His α122 due to an apparent change in pKa. This can be written as:

$$H^+Hb + O_2 \rightleftharpoons HbO_2 + H^+$$

Therefore when arterial blood enters the tissues and takes up carbon dioxide the H^+ concentration increases and this results in a decrease in the affinity of hemoglobin for oxygen, a phenomenon known as the Bohr effect. 2,3-Diphosphoglycerate, which is a major form of erythrocyte phosphate, also affects the binding of oxygen by tetrameric hemoglobin. It can bind to hemoglobin and reduce its affinity for oxygen. Therefore an increase in diphosphoglycerate results in dissociation of oxygen from hemoglobin. The concentration of diphosphoglycerate increases at high altitudes and aids in the release of oxygen to peripheral tissues.

δ-Aminolevulinic acid serves as the precursor for heme synthesis. It is formed when glycine reacts with succinyl CoA in a δ-aminolevulinic acid synthetase catalyzed reaction which occurs in the outer membrane of the mitochondria:

$$H_2N-CH_2-COOH + HOOC-(CH_2)_2-CO-SCoA$$
$$\text{glycine} \qquad\qquad\qquad \text{succinly CoA}$$
$$\longrightarrow CO_2 + HOOC-(CH_2)_2-CO-CH_2-NH_2$$
$$\text{δ-aminolevulinic acid}$$

This step is the rate-limiting step of heme synthesis. The enzyme is coded for by nuclear DNA, synthesized in the cytoplasm and then translocated to the mitochondria. Controls are exerted at the levels of synthesis and translocation. The δ-aminolevulinic acid enters the cytoplasm where δ-aminolevulinic acid dehydrase catalyzes the condensation of two molecules of δ-aminolevulinic acid to form porphobilinogen:

2 HOOC—(CH$_2$)$_2$—CO—CH$_2$—NH$_2$ ⟶
δ-aminolevulinic acid

porphobilinogen

Uroporphyrinogen I synthetase and uroporphyrinogen III cosynthetase catalyze the reaction of four porphobilinogen molecules to form uroporphyrinogen III. The acetate groups on each of the four pyrrole rings are then decarboxylated in a uroporphyrinogen decarboxylase catalyzed reaction to form coproporphyrinogen III. The final three steps of heme synthesis occur back in the mitochondria with conversion of the propionic acid groups on two pyrrole rings to vinyl groups, formation of the four methene bridges that link the pyrrole rings, and insertion of Fe^{2+} to form heme.

Heme

As red blood cells age, changes occur within the cell membranes and approximately 120 days after their release from bone marrow the cells are removed from the circulation by cells of the reticuloendothelial system. Most red blood cell components are reutilized, including the iron associated with heme. However, the protoporphyrin ring of heme is not. It is oxidized at the α-meth-

ene bridge (see heme structure, above) releasing carbon monoxide and Fe^{2+} and forming biliverdin. The reaction is catalyzed by a microsomal heme oxygenase which acts in conjunction with NADPH-cytochrome C reductase. The carbon monoxide reacts with hemoglobin and is released in expired air in the lung. Biliverdin is oxidized to bilirubin which is then carried (usually as an albumin complex) to the liver where it is converted to bilirubin mono- or diglucuronoside. These soluble bilirubin derivatives enter the bile and are subsequently excreted.

Plasma contains proteins which serve to transport other molecules than gases. (Some examples follow.) In addition to transporting bilirubin (above), albumin also transports fatty acids and aldosterone. Transcortin binds and transports corticosterone and cortisol; thyroxine binding globulin carries thyroxine as does transthyretin which also transports the retinol binding protein that transports retinol. Cerruloplasmin and transferrin function as carriers for copper and iron respectively.

Plasma also contains the proteins and other factors needed for blood coagulation. The circulating factors are inactive until activated by an event which stimulates clotting (e.g., a cut in which a blood vessel is severed). Activation of the coagulation pathway requires the systematic conversion of proenzymes to their active form. In the extrinsic system (involves a tissue factor in addition to blood components) factor VII is activated by a tissue factor or thrombin. Factor VII then activates factor X (Stuart factor) which in turn converts prothrombin to thrombin. The thrombin acts to convert fibrinogen to fibrin which polymerizes to form the fibrin clot. In the intrinsic system (involves factors present in the circulation) factor XII (Hageman factor) is activated upon contact with the acidic phospholipids of membranes of disrupted platelets or the action of kallikrein. Activated factor XII activates factor XI which in turn activates factor IX (Christmas factor). Factor X is activated by factor IX and catalyzes the conversion of prothrombin (factor II) to thrombin. The rest of this pathway is the same as the extrinsic pathway and both are shown below:

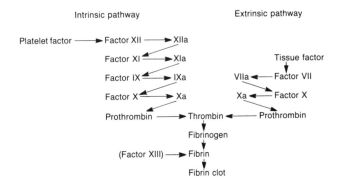

Factor XIII (activated by thrombin) acts to crosslink] fibrin to form a hard clot. Many of these steps were identified in studies of hemophilias in which one of the reactions was found to be defective.

Vitamin K is essential for the normal synthesis of prothrombin and factors VII, IX, and X. The structure of vitamin K_1

is that of the vitamin found in liver. Although other side chains may be associated with the ring, they are removed and the C_{20} side chain added. Vitamin K is an essential cofactor in a reaction catalyzed by a carboxylase (associated with the lumen of the endoplasmic reticulum) in which glutamic acid residues in prothrombin and factors VII, IX, and X are carboxylated to form γ-carboxyglutamate. This is believed to play a role in the binding of Ca^{2+} (factor IV) by these proteins. Vitamin K deficient animals produce γ-carboxyglutamate deficient proteins which do not bind Ca^{2+} as well. Dicumarol is an antimetabolite of vitamin K and inhibits the correct synthesis of the above factors. It is used to reduce the possibility of clot formation in individuals who are at risk for thrombosis, and as a rodent poison.

Fibrinolysis (dissolution of fibrin in a blood clot) occurs upon activation of plasminogen to plasmin. Plasminogen is synthesized in the kidney and is activated by a serine protease. Plasmin catalyzes the hydrolysis of fibrin. Fibrinogen has plasminogen and plasminogen activators associated with it, however, little activation of plasminogen occurs until clotting is initiated. α_2-Antiplasmin present in the plasma inactivates any plasmin that might dissociate from the clot.

Immunoglobulins

Immunoglobulins are plasma proteins which serve as antibodies. The three main classes of antibodies are IgG, IgM, and IgA; IgD and IgE are minor classes. Each class of immunoglobulins consists of two light (L) and two heavy (H) chains or multiples thereof. There are two types of L chains each consisting of about 220 amino acids and designated as κ or λ. Each class of immunoglobulin has a different H chain, consisting of about 440 amino acids and designated as α in IgA, δ in IgD, ϵ in IgE,

γ in IgG, and μ in IgM. There are two parts to each protein chain, the N terminal variable region (V) and the C terminal constant region (C). The L chain has only one C region (CL) while the heavy chain has three C regions (CH1, CH2, and CH3). In the heavy chain there is a hinge region (H) between CH1 and CH2. It is to the CH2 region that the C1 component of complement binds. The amino acid sequences of the V regions are quite variable while those of the C region show much more homology. It is the V region which contains the antigen-binding site. Within the V region there are some sections which show more variation in amino acid sequence than others and these are termed hypervariable (HV) regions. The other areas in the V region are called framework (FR) regions. The amino acid sequence of the HV regions of the light and heavy chains are different. Limited proteolysis of IgG with papain results in cleavage of amide bonds in the hinge region of the H chain. This results in formation of two identical Fab fragments, each consisting of one L chain and the amino-terminal half of the H chain linked by a disulfide bond, and of one Fc fragment, which consists of the two carboxy-terminal halves of the H chains linked together via disulfide bonds. Pepsin also catalyzes proteolysis in the hinge region but produces Fab' fragments. They differ from the Fab fragments in that the two Fab fragments remain linked to each other (Fig. 4-8).

Each B cell usually produces only a single antibody. Upon exposure to an antigen, the B cell producing an antibody to the antigen will be stimulated to divide producing more B lymphocytes which will secrete the antibody. The antibody-producing cells stimulated by the antigen are somatic cells. The question is, how are the wide variety of antibodies (10^6 or more) produced synthesized by the different B cells. The λ chain of mice immunoglobulins is coded in four DNA segments referred to as V, J, and C, after the portions of the chain and the L for leader sequence. The L exon is separated by a single intron from the V segment as is the J segment from the C exon. The V region is quite distant from the C region. The portion coded for by the J segment is the joining region (framework region 4) and contains the last few amino acids of the V region. The V–J segment of the intact gene is necessary for synthesis of the complete V region of the polypeptide. In mice there are only two $V\lambda$ genes, $V_{\lambda 1}$ which can be linked to either J-$C_{\lambda 3}$ or J-$C_{\lambda 1}$, and $V_{\lambda 2}$ which is linked to J-$C_{\lambda 2}$. In humans there are many V_λ regions and at least six C_λ genes allowing for more diversity. In mice λ chains account for about 5 percent of the L chains while in humans they account for about 40 percent. Kappa genes are assembled in a manner analogous to λ; they have a leader sequence, multiple (up to 300) V_κ genes, five different J_κ genes (one of which is inactive in the mouse), and one C_κ region. Since each

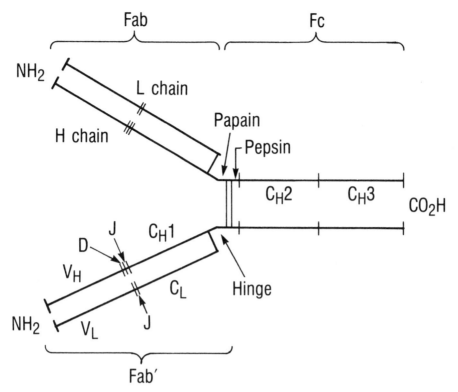

Fig. 4-8. Schematic representation of an immunoglobulin molecule. V refers to the variable region, D the diversity region, J the joining region, and C the constant portion of the chain. Fab fragments are produced by limited proteolysis with papain and Fab' fragments by limited digestion with pepsin. The Fc fragment contains the constant portions, CH2 and CH3, of the heavy chain.

V_κ region can combine with each J region this provides for about 1,200 different κ chains.

In heavy chains the VH genes only code for the amino acid sequence through framework 3. Hypervariable region 3 is coded for by the D (diversity) region and framework 4 by the J region as in κ and λ chains. There are ~300 LH–VH segments, ~12 D segments, and 4 J segments. This permits a possible 12,000 combinations. The product of each can combine with any of the 1,000 light chains to form about 10^7 different antibodies. In man there are a variety of CH genes, μ and δ, γ genes 1-4, three ϵ genes plus two α genes. Only one CH gene is usually expressed in any given cell.

The formation of genes which code for specific antibodies occurs at various points in the maturation of a B lymphocyte. In stem cells, no DNA rearrangements have occurred. The stem cell differentiates to a pre-B lymphocyte which has rearranged genes for heavy chains and can synthesize the μ heavy chain (Fig. 4-9). Formation of immature B lymphocytes is accompanied by the expression of light chain genes and the presence of IgM monomers in the cell membrane. Production of IgM monomers means that introns were removed from precursor-mRNA. Kappa and λ light chain precursor-mRNA had introns between the L and V region and between the J and C regions. The heavy chain precursor-mRNA also had to have the introns between the various C domains deleted. Upon interaction of the membrane IgM with the appropriate antigen, the B lymphocyte is signaled to differentiate into a mature antibody-secreting plasma cell. At this stage the cells may switch from producing one class of heavy chain to another.

Connective Tissue

Connective tissue is found throughout the body. It is present in bone, cartilage, ligaments, tendons, underlying skin, and in the intracellular matrix. The major protein in connective tissue is collagen, which constitutes about 30 percent of total body protein. Collagen provides a framework for the maintenance of the shape and structural integrity of tissue. It is an asymmetric fibrous protein composed of three polypeptide chains (each about 1,000 amino acids in length) which form tropocollagen which associates to form collagen. There are five types of collgen categorized by their three polypeptide chain components; some have three identical subunits, some have two different subunits, and one has three different subunits. The polypeptides differ in

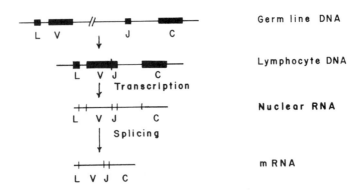

A λ Light chain

Germ line DNA

Lymphocyte DNA

Nuclear RNA

mRNA

B κ Light chain

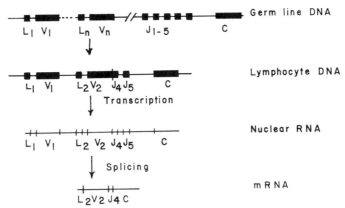

Germ line DNA

Lymphocyte DNA

Nuclear RNA

mRNA

C H Heavy chain

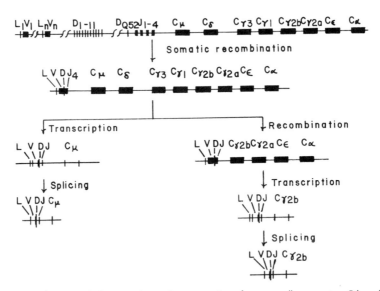

Fig. 4-9. Genetic changes which occur during the maturation of a stem cell to a mature B lymphocyte capable of synthesizing immunoglobulins. Steps in formation of λ and κ light chain and heavy chain mRNA are shown in parts A, B, and C, respectively. L refers to the portion of DNA or RNA that codes for the leader sequence, V, D, J, and C for those portions coding for the variable, diversity, joining, and constant portions, respectively, in the immunoglobulin chains. Unidentified spaces on the molecules are introns which are lost during the course of mRNA formation. During somatic recombination introns separating the V and J or V, D, and J regions are lost. After transcription the introns between the L and V sequences and the J and C regions are spliced out. Initially the Cμ portion is transcribed for the heavy chain, however, when the B lymphocyte differentiates into a mature antibody-secreting cell further recombination of the DNA can occur resulting in production of another class of heavy chain such as the IgG shown.

amino acid composition. However, about 33 percent of the amino acid residues of each are glycine, 10 percent proline, 10 percent hydroxyproline, and 1 percent hydroxylysine. Glycine is present as every third amino acid in the bulk of the chains so the amino acid sequence is (gly-X-Y)n. There are many sequences of gly-X-pro or gly-X-hyp and this results in the polypeptides having a helical secondary structure with three amino acid residues per turn. In the formation of tropocollagen, three of the helical polypeptide chains wind around each other. In collagen there are four evenly spaced areas at which there are regions of polar amino acids. The space between these clusters of polar amino acids is referred to as the "D" period. In collagen fibrils each tropocollagen has associated so that its amino acid terminus is one D period down from the amino end of the adjacent tropocollagen molecule. This results in thicker, overlap zones, and thinner, hole zones.

The synthesis of collagen is of interest because of the many posttranslational events which occur prior to formation of the mature product. The immediate translation product is the preprocollagen polypeptide chain. The gene which codes for the preprocollagen m-RNA has about 50 introns which means that about 50 splicing events have to occur during formation of the mRNA. After cleavage of the signal sequence from the preprocollagen, the following posttranslational modifications occur: (1) Conversion of proline and lysine to the corresponding hydroxy compounds; (2) glycosylation of certain hydroxylysine residues; (3) helix fomation; (4) cleavage of the amino- and carboxy-terminal propeptides by extracellular peptidases to form tropocollagen; and (5) spontaneous self-association of tropocollagen molecules to form collagen fibrils which are stabilized by intermolecular cross links.

The hydroxylases which catalyze the hydroxylations of proline and lysine act on amino acids in the Y position of (X-Y-Gly)n. Both require ascorbate for activity. Reduction of hydroxyproline synthesis due to a lack of ascorbate (as in scurvy) results in collagen which is less stable than normal at body temperature. A deficiency in lysylhydroxylase activity results in a reduction in δ-hydroxylysine residues and subsequent crosslinking of the collagen fibrils is reduced; the clinical manifestation of this is referred to as type VI Ehlers-Danlos syndrome. Lysine and hydroxylysine residues can be converted to the ϵ-aldehydes by oxidative deamination. The aldehydes form Schiffs bases with the ϵ-amino groups of lysine and hydroxylysine residues in adjacent chains. These undergo an Amadori rearrangement to form stable cross-linkages. The cross-links formed by the aldehydes of hydroxylysine are most stable. Studies of inborn errors affecting collagen biosynthesis have helped elucidate the steps involved.

Collagen hydrolysis is initiated by collagenases which catalyze the cleavage of each of the polypeptide chains at a site about $\frac{3}{4}$ of the distance from their amino ends. The secreted form of collagenase is activated by proteolysis. After collagenase action, the polypeptides are more susceptible to the action of other proteases and can also be cleaved by lysosomal proteases.

In addition to collagen, the protein elastin is also found in connective tissue. Glycine accounts for about 33 percent of the amino acid residues in elastin as it does in collagen. However, the total proline plus hydroxyproline content is lower in elastin while alanine and valine content is increased. The initial translation product in the synthesis of elastin is proelastin; proteolysis yields tropoelastin. Association of several tropoelastin molecules gives rise to elastin. The association of tropoelastin monomers is stabilized by cross-linkages formed by allysine residues (ϵ-aldehyde of lysine described for collagen synthesis). However, in elastin the majority of crosslinks are formed by three allysine residues reacting with a lysine residue to form desmosine or isodesmosine bridges. Elastase (produced by trypsin acting on proelastase) catalyzes the hydrolysis of elastin.

In contrast to the proteins of connective tissue, proteoglycans or glycosaminoglycans (previously termed mucopolysaccharides) are polyanionic macromolecules which can contain more than 95 percent carbohydrate. The carbohydrate moieties of the various classes are made up of repeating disaccharide units; in hyaluronic acid it is GlcUA $\beta 1 \rightarrow 3$ GlcNAc $\beta 1 \rightarrow 4$; in chondroitin sulfate, GlcUA $\beta 1 \rightarrow 3$ GalNAc6S $\beta 1 \rightarrow 4$ and GalNAc4S $\beta 1 \rightarrow 4$ GlcUA $\beta 1 \rightarrow 3$; in dermatan sulfate, IdUA $\alpha 1 \rightarrow 3$ GalNAc $\beta 1 \rightarrow 4$ and GlcUA $\beta 1 \rightarrow 3$ GalNAc $\beta 1 \rightarrow 4$; and in keratan sulfate, Gal $\beta 1 \rightarrow 4$ GlcNAc6S $\beta 1 \rightarrow 3$. In heparin and heparan sulfate the repeating unit is GlcNAc $\alpha 1 \rightarrow 4$ UA $\alpha/\beta 1 \rightarrow 4$. Iduronic acid is the major one in heparin while glucuronate is in heparan sulfate. In heparin, the majority of glucosamine residues are N-sulfated with a few N-acetylated; the opposite is found for heparan sulfate. In heparin, the 6-hydroxy group of glucosamine and the 2-hydroxy residues of iduronate tend to be O-sulfated; in heparan sulfate O-sulfation is lower. To summarize, glucosamine or galactosamine is present in each repeating unit; all of the glycosaminoglycans except keratan sulfate have a uronic acid in the repeating unit; and hyaluronic acid is the only one lacking ester sulfate groups while heparin and heparan sulfate are the only proteoglycans containing N-sulfated groups.

The addition of the sugars to the polypeptide chains probably occurs in the Golgi and is via their sequential addition in reactions catalyzed by specific glycosyl transferases. 3'-phosphoadenosine-5'-phosphosulfate serves as the donor of the sulfate groups. The repeating units of chondroitin sulfate, dermatan sulfate, heparin, and heparan sulfate are covalently linked to a polypeptide backbone via glycosidic linkage to the trisaccharide Gal-Gal-Xyl, which is linked through the xylose to a serine residue. Type I keratan sulfate saccharide units are linked through N-acetyl-glucosamine to an asparagine (synthesis of this proteoglycan may involve dolichol-phosphate dependent transferases) while in type II the saccharides are in an O-glycosidic linkage through N-acetylgalactosamine to serine or threonine. Both types contain additional monosaccharides not found in the repeating unit. Hyaluronic acid contains little if any protein.

While the different classes of glycosaminoglycans are found in association with different tissues, all are polyanionic and form viscous solutions (the result of their absorbing large volumes of water). Hyaluronic acid, which is very viscous, is believed to lubricate joints. Glycosaminoglycans can reduce the flow of water caused by concussion, can restrict the movement of cations, and can serve as molecular sieves.

Degradation of proteoglycans is initiated by proteolysis catalyzed by cathepsin D. The partially degraded material can then be broken down to its monomeric components via the action of lysosomal glycosidases and proteases. The mucopolysaccharidoses (MP) are a series of inborn errors affecting proteoglycan catabolism. Hydrolysis of the sugar residues occurs in a stepwise manner and if one of the enzymes is not active the partially degraded material accumulates within the lysosome. The errors are designated as MPI → MPVII or by the

names of the people who first described them (Fig. 4-10). The symptoms which accompany these errors include skeletal abnormalities, distinct facial features, corneal opacities, hepatosplenomegaly, and cardiac problems.

Neurochemistry

The nervous system consists primarily of neurons and glia. Neurons consist of a cell body (soma), an axon (carries impulses away from the cell body), and dendrites (carry impulses to the cell body). In the central nervous system oligodendroglia form the myelin sheath which surrounds the axon of myelinated nerves while in the peripheral nervous system Schwann cells are the myelin precursors. Between the myelinated sections of an axon are unmyelinated areas called the nodes of Ranvier. At a certain point during development the oligodendroglia or Schwann cell is stimulated to elaborate myelin. The Schwann cell myelinates the internodal area of only one axon while a single oligodendroglial cell can myelinate an internodal area on several different axons. As the cell wraps around the axon the multiple layers become compressed and a cross-sectional view (electron microscopy) shows concentric layers of cell membrane. In fact it was from early studies of myelin that initial membrane models were constructed. During the peak period of myelination an oligodendroglial cell can synthesize about three times its own weight of myelin per day.

Myelin serves to insulate the axon with the result that transmission (via membrane depolarization) down the

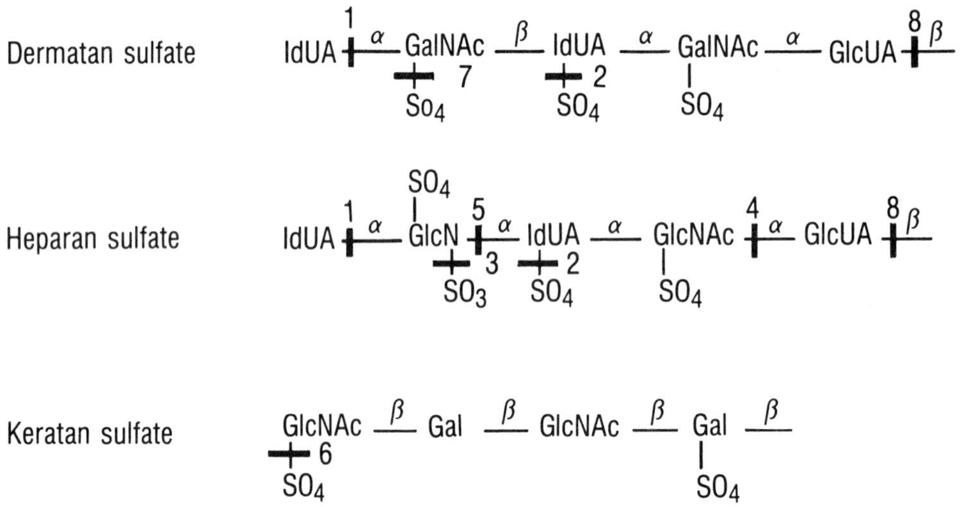

Fig. 4-10. Sites of defined inborn errors of glycosaminoglycan catabolism. 1, Mucopolysaccharidosis (MPS) IH (Hurler) and MPS IS (Scheie) result from deficiencies in α-L-iduronidase activity. 2, MPS II (Hunter) in which L-iduronosulfate sulfatase activity is reduced. 3, MPS IIIA (Sanfilippo A), 4, MPS IIIB (sanfilippo B) and 5, MPS IIIC (Sanfilippo C) in which the activities of sulfamidase, α-N-acetylglucosaminidase and α-glucosaminidase, respectively, are reduced. 6, MPS IV (Morquio) in which N-acetylhexosamidase-6-SO₄ sulfatase activity is reduced. 7, MPS VI (Maroteaux-Lamy) is the result of reduced arylsulfatase B (N-acetylhexosaminidase-4-SO₄ sulfatase) activity. 8, MPS VII results from a deficit in B-glucuronidase activity.

axon "jumps" from node to node and is markedly more rapid down axons that were greater than one micron in diameter prior to myelination than in unmyelinated axons of similar size. The lipid composition of myelin contributes to its stability and ability to insulate the axon. Lipids account for approximately 70 percent of the dry weight of myelin and protein for 30 percent. The lipid content of myelin is greater than that for any other normal tissue or subcellular fraction except for adipose tissue. It consists of about 28 percent cholesterol, about 28 percent galactolipid (galactosylcerebrosides and sulfatides), and about 43 percent phosphoglycerides by weight. The average chain length of galactolipid fatty acids is C_{24}. Myelin contains about 10-fold more long-chain fatty acids ($C_{19}-C_{26}$) and fewer unsaturated fatty acids (1 in 17 compared to 1 in 5) than gray matter does. The longer chain length and high degree of saturation of myelin lipid fatty acid moieties allows them to form a relatively compact bilayer. The compactness is enhanced by the large amount of cholesterol present in the membranes. The three major proteins in myelin are a proteolipid protein, an acidic proteolipid protein (Wolfgram protein), and a basic protein. Injection of an animal with myelin basic protein induces antibody production and produces an autoimmune disease termed experimental allergic encephalomyelitis; demyelination occurs in a manner that resembles multiple sclerosis.

Under normal physiological conditions the brain uses glucose as its main source of energy. The energy requirement of neurons is high and while the brain accounts for only about 2 percent of body weight, it accounts for about 20 percent of the oxygen utilized in the resting state. Glucose transport across the blood brain barrier is accomplished by a carrier specific for D-glucose, is not energy dependent, and the amount transported usually varies directly with blood glucose concentration. In addition to glucose the brain can also use ketone bodies and under conditions of starvation or in the newborn where there are elevated levels of acetoacetate and β-hydroxybutyrate they can account for 25 percent of the oxygen consumed.

Pathways of carbohydrate metabolism are the same in the brain as in other tissues but they have been adapted to meet the high energy requirements of the brain. In glycolysis, hexokinase type I (primary form in the brain) catalyzes the essentially irreversible conversion of glucose to glucose-6-phosphate. Hexokinase type I has the lowest K_M of the hexokinases for ATP and is most active when associated with mitochondria. The amount bound to mitochondria is inversely related to the ATP/ADP ratio, resulting in lower activity when ATP levels are elevated. The responsiveness to ATP as both a substrate and an inhibitor permits close regulation of the activity of brain hexokinase. Enzymes which catalyze the phosphorylation steps of glycolysis (hexokinase,

phosphofructokinase, phosphoglycerate kinase, and pyruvate kinase) are present in higher amounts in the brain than the liver. Most of the glucose which undergoes glycolysis is broken down to CO_2 and H_2O via the tricarboxylic acid cycle. However, about 10 percent of it is utilized for the production of amino acids. The intermediates removed from the cycle for biosynthetic processes are primarily replaced by the formation of oxaloacetate via the pyruvate carboxylase catalyzed carboxylation of pyruvate. The capacity of the liver to fix CO_2 in this reaction is much greater than that of brain. Enzymes necessary for glycogen synthesis and degradation (phosphoglucomutase, glycogen synthase, and glucose-6-phosphatase) are present in much lower levels in the brain than the liver, in agreement with the fact that glycogen stores in the brain are less than 1 percent of those in the liver. The pentose-phosphate shunt probably uses 5–8 percent of the glucose taken up by an adult brain. During active myelination this pathway probably utilizes a much greater percentage of glucose to meet the need for NADPH for the reductive reactions of lipid synthesis.

In addition to using ATP as a source of energy, the brain as well as muscle utilizes creatine phosphate as a storage form of energy. Creatine kinase catalyzes formation of phosphocreatine from creatine and ATP.

Creatine synthesis involves two steps. Initially arginine and glycine react in an arginine-glycine amidinotransferase catalyzed reaction to form ornithine and guanidinoacetic acid. S-adenosylmethionine-guanidinoacetate-N-methyltransferase catalyzes the methylation of the guanidinoacetate to form creatine and S-adenosylhomocysteine. These reactions occur in the liver and pancreas and the creatine produced is released to the blood; brain and muscle cells convert it to creatine phosphate. The brain has high levels of creatine phosphokinase and the level of phosphocreatine in the brain is greater than that of ATP. The phosphocreatine provides high energy phosphate for ADP phosphorylation thereby maintaining ATP levels.

Much of the energy generated by the oxidation of glucose is used by neurons for the transmission of nerve impulses. In chemical transmission, an impulse travels down the axon to the presynaptic terminal at which point the transmitter is released into the synapse (space between the presynaptic terminal and the postsynaptic cell). The transmitter diffuses across the synapse, is recognized by its receptor, and through its interaction with the receptor induces changes within the cell. The signal is terminated by either cellular uptake of the transmitter or by its degradation.

Upon stimulation a neuron transmits an electrical signal down its axon. When a nerve cell is at rest there is a potential difference across its plasma membrane of about -70 mV. This results from the following: (1) The concentration of K^+ is much higher inside the axon than outside, (2) the extracellular concentration of Na^+ is much greater than that of K^+, (3) Na^+ cannot cross the neuronal membrane as readily as K^+ does, and (4) anions inside the cell (nucleic acids and protein) cannot leave and the Cl^- outside the cell crosses the membrane slowly. Since the membrane is essentially only permeable to K^+, it tends to diffuse out down its concentration gradient resulting in polarization of the cell. Some Na^+ does leak into the resting cell and to maintain the membrane potential Na^+ is exchanged for K^+ by Na^+, K^+-ATPase in the membrane. In response to a stimulus, the local transmembrane potential drops below -50 mV and a local change in membrane permeability to Na^+ occurs. Na^+ channels open and Na^+ flows in, down its concentration gradient. Initially more Na^+ flows in than K^+ out and this results in a transmembrane potential of about $+30$ mV. The resting potential is restored by the Na^+, K^+-ATPase transporting Na^+ out and K^+ in. The Na^+, K^+-ATPase pump is driven by the hydrolysis of ATP.

The Na^+ channels (formed by an integral membrane protein) are distributed throughout the plasma membrane of an unmyelinated nerve and the effect of depolarization in one area can affect the next channel. In a myelinated nerve many Na^+ channels are tightly packed in the unmyelinated areas at the nodes of Ranvier. The result is that the depolarization which occurs at one node creates a potential gradient between nodes. The positive current flows through the axoplasm to the next node, the transmembrane potential is reduced, and the process is repeated. This results in very rapid conduction down myelinated axons.

When the impulse reaches the presynaptic terminal, internal Ca^{2+} concentration increases as a result of the membrane depolarization. The increased Ca^{2+} concentration is necessary for release of transmitter from synaptic vesicles (contain transmitter molecules) associated with the presynaptic membrane. The transmitter diffuses across the synapse ($\sim 200A$) and binds to its receptor. Transmitter binding at its postsynaptic site causes membrane alterations which can result in altered membrane polarization and/or formation of a second messenger (e.g., c-AMP).

A variety of putative transmitters have been identified. The criteria used to define a molecule as a transmitter include (1) localization of the transmitter as well as

the enzymes required for its metabolism within the neuron; (2) the substance is released in physiologically significant amounts in response to stimulation of a specific neuronal pathway; and (3) exogenous application of the molecule induces a response identical to that of the specific neuron acting on the target cell. Additional criteria include the presence of specific receptors for the transmitter in close association to the presynaptic terminal, and the presence of mechanisms for rapid inactivation of the transmitter.

Synaptosomes, pinched off nerve endings which include the nerve terminal, synapse, and a piece of the postsynaptic membrane, and are an artifact of subcellular fractionation, have been used in many studies designed to elucidate synaptic events. Much of the information concerning the action of acetylcholine,

$$(CH_3)_3N^+ - CH_2 - CH_2 - O - \underset{\underset{O}{\|}}{C} - CH_3,$$

the transmitter of motor neurons innervating skeletal muscle, some regions of the central nervous system, and preganglionic and some postganglionic neurons of the autonomic system has been obtained in studies using synaptosomal preparations. Acetylcholine plus the enzymes involved in its metabolism, choline acetyl transferase (catalyzes synthesis of acetylcholine from choline and acetyl CoA), and acetylcholine esterase (catalyzes hydrolysis of acetylcholine to form choline and acetate) are enriched in synaptosomes prepared from cholinergic neurons. Coated vesicles present within the cholinergic synaptosomes contain thousands of acetylcholine molecules and ATP. Morphologically it has been shown that some of these vesicles are present on the inside of the presynaptic membrane with their coats apparently fused to the membrane itself. Alterations induced by the action potential result in release of vesicle contents to the synapse. Two different types of acetylcholine receptors have been identified. Muscarinic receptors mediate slow (seconds) responses, can be inhibitory (decrease the rate of neuronal discharge by lowering the resting potential) or excitatory (increase the rate of neuronal discharge), can use the drug muscarine to induce a similar response, and are blocked by atropine. Nicotinic receptors mediate quick (msec) responses, are excitatory, can use the drug nicotine to induce the same response, and are blocked by curare type drugs. Injection of an animal with the nicotinic receptor results in the production of antibodies to the receptor. These can also react with nicotinic receptors normally present in cells with the visible result, myasthenia gravis type symptoms.

Acetylcholine esterase, present in the basal lamina between the pre- and postsynaptic membranes, catalyzes hydrolysis of the acetylcholine. Liberated choline is rapidly taken up by the presynaptic cell by a high affinity transport system; the activity of which is inversely related to the acetylcholine content of the synaptic bouton. Neurons cannot synthesize choline *de novo;* they are dependent upon uptake of choline from plasma and on the recycling of choline released upon acetylcholine hydrolysis.

Catecholamines are transmitters derived from tyrosine and include dopamine, norepinephrine, and epinephrine. Tyrosine hydroxylase present in the nerve terminals catalyzes the rate-limiting step in catecholamine biosynthesis, the conversion of tyrosine to dihydroxyphenylalanine (DOPA). Catecholamines inhibit tyrosine hydroxylase; release of catecholamines during transmission (reduces their concentration in the nerve terminal) results in increased DOPA synthesis. DOPA is converted to dopamine in a reaction catalyzed by DOPA decarboxylase. Dopamine β-hydroxylase (Cu^{2+} containing enzyme requiring ascorbate or other reducing agent as a cofactor) catalyzes the conversion of dopamine to norepinephrine which can undergo *N*-methylation to yield epinephrine,

DOPA   Dopamine   Norepinephrine   Epinephrine

the main catecholamine of the adrenals. It has also been found as a transmitter in nerves in the brain stem. Dopamine is associated with neurons in the substantia nigra which innervate areas of the corpus striatum involved in the control of movement. A reduction of dopamine due to degeneration of the nigrostriatal tract is responsible for the symptoms associated with Parkinson's disease. L-DOPA can cross the blood brain barrier, and its administration has been found to alleviate the symptoms of some Parkinson's disease patients. Norepinephrine producing neurons are present in various areas of the brain and in postganglionic fibers of the sympathetic nervous system.

There are two classes (α and β) of receptors for norepinephrine. Binding of norepinephrine to the β receptors results in synthesis of cAMP which subsequently activates a kinase. Phosphorylation of a postsynaptic protein in a kinase dependent reaction results in hyperpolarization and a decline in the rate of transmission of the cell. Dopamine exerts similar effects on its target cells. Re-

ceptors for norepinephrine appear to be associated with the presynaptic membrane. Binding of norepinephrine to the α_2-receptors terminates its release into the synapse. Action of norepinephrine is terminated by its uptake back across the presynaptic membrane via a high affinity, energy dependent mechanism. A similar uptake mechanism exists for dopamine. The receptor on norepinephrine secreting neurons can take up dopamine and vice versa. Catecholamines not taken up by cells can be methylated at their 3 position in a reaction catalyzed by catechol-*O*-methyltransferase present in the synapse. Monoamine oxidase associated with the outer mitochondrial membrane catalyzes the oxidative deamination of excess catecholamine present within the neuron to its corresponding aldehyde.

The indoleamine transmitter, serotonin (5-hydroxytryptamine), is synthesized from tryptophan. Tryptophan hydroxylase catalyzes the rate-determining reaction, the formation of 5-hydroxytryptophan; this undergoes decarboxylation to form 5-hydroxytryptamine which has been identified as a transmitter in the raphe nuclei which function in the control of sleep patterns. Destruction of the serotoninergic neurons in that area results in insomnia. Similar results can be induced by inhibiting tryptophan hydroxylase. After release of serotonin from synaptic vesicles into the synapse, serotonin can bind to pre- and postsynaptic receptors; its binding to presynaptic receptors, which differ from the postsynaptic receptors, inhibits its further release. *d*-Lysergic acid diethylamide (LSD) binds to the presynaptic receptors thereby decreasing the release of serotonin. LSD also reduces the rate of conversion of tryptophan to serotonin. Serotonin transmission, like that of the catecholamines, is terminated by reuptake by the serotoninergic neurons. Monoamine oxidase converts cytoplasmic serotonin to the corresponding aldehyde which undergoes further oxidation to yield 5-hydroxyindole acetic acid. This can be excreted in the urine.

Of interest is the fact that the concentration of serotonin is much greater in the pineal gland than in any other area. Levels of serotonin in the pineal gland show diurnal variations; they are much higher during the day than at night. In addition, the pineal gland has two unique metabolic pathways for serotonin which result in its conversion to melatonin or 5-methoxytryptophol, inhibitors of gonadal activity.

In addition to the monoamines described, at least three amino acids, *γ-aminobutyric acid* (GABA), glycine, and glutamate, have been implicated as transmitters. GABA found in the brain and spinal cord acts as an inhibitory transmitter. It acts by increasing membrane permeability to Cl^-, resulting in hyperpolarization of the postsynaptic membrane. GABA is synthesized from L-glutamate in a one step reaction catalyzed by glutamic acid decarboxylase which requires pyridoxal phosphate

as a coenzyme. The activity of the decarboxylase, enriched in presynaptic nerve endings, is believed to regulate GABA levels. Transmission is terminated by active
uptake of GABA by the postsynaptic and glial cells and
to a lesser extent by the presynaptic neuron. GABA-
transminase, primarily associated with the mitochondria of the glial cells and neuronal cell soma (rather than
the nerve terminals), catalyzes the conversion of GABA
to succinic semialdehyde which can be oxidized to succinate, a tricarboxylic acid cycle intermediate.

Glycine also appears to serve as an inhibitory transmitter and is found in the brain stem and spinal cord.
The primary pathway in the central nervous system for
glycine synthesis is via 3-phosphoglycerate produced
during glycolysis. The 3-phosphoglycerate is hydrolyzed
to form D-glycerate. The subsequent conversion of
D-glycerate to hydroxy pyruvate, catalyzed by D-glycerate dehydrogenase, may be the rate-limiting step in glycine synthesis. Glycine acts as a feedback inhibitor at this
step. The hydroxypyruvate is transaminated to form serine; this is converted to glycine in a tetrahydrofolate
dependent reaction catalyzed by serine hydroxymethyl
transferase. Glycine released into the synapse binds to
postsynaptic receptors resulting in increased permeability of the membrane to Cl^-. Its action is terminated by its
active transport into pre- and postsynaptic cells and glia.
There, the glycine can be converted back to serine or
undergo transamination to form glyoxylate.

While L-glutamate is present throughout the nervous
system, its uneven distribution in the spinal cord suggested that it might function as a transmitter. It has also
been found in the granule cells of the cerebellum. Addition of glutamate to neurons results in their depolarization; it serves as an excitatory transmitter by increasing
membrane permeability to sodium ions. The action of
glutamate is terminated by its uptake via a high affinity
system present in glial cells. There it is converted to
glutamine which can be transferred to neurons where it
is converted back to glutamate.

A variety of peptides are believed to be neurotransmitters in that they can induce changes in the postsynaptic
cell that are identical to those produced by stimulating
the presynaptic cell. Some of the peptides identified include β-endorphin, substance P, met- and leu-enkephalin, vasoactive intestinal peptide (VIP), luteinizing
hormone-releasing hormone, and adrenocorticotropin
(ACTH). While some of these peptides were first found
in brain (e.g., the enkephalins) others were first identified
as hormones (e.g., VIP and ACTH). In contrast to the
transmitters described above, the peptides are synthesized on ribosomes found in the cell body and carried
down the axon to the terminal. They are synthesized as
large essentially inactive precursor molecules which
undergo posttranslational proteolysis (probably in the
Golgi) which releases the active peptide. The function of
many of the peptides is not known but those studied
appear to help regulate behavioral systems.

The biochemistry of vision (conversion of light energy
into a signal transmitted to the brain) is still being elucidated for the light-sensitive cells (rods and cones) found
in the retina of the eye. These cells form synapses, at the
terminals of their inner segments, with nerve cells
present in the retina. Nerve impulses travel from these
cells along the optic nerve to the brain. The central portion of the retina contains primarily cones which function in bright light and are responsible for color vision.
Rods are found in the peripheral portion and account for
vision in dim light (night vision). The outer membrane
segments of rods and cones which contain the visual
pigment have a resting potential of about −30 to −40
mV with the inside of the cell more negative. Photo-
bleaching of the visual pigment results in hyperpolarization of the cell, the extent of which is dependent upon the
wavelength and intensity of the irradiating light. Studies
of the outer segments of rod cells have provided much of
the information concerning the chemistry of the hyperpolarization process.

Rhodopsin is an integral membrane protein present in
the lipid bilayer of the disks of the rod outer segments.
The ε-amino group of a lysine residue of opsin forms a
Schiff's base with the aldehyde group of 11-*cis*-retinal;
the latter is derived from vitamin A (*trans*-retinol):

Night blindness results from a deficiency of vitamin A; there is less rhodopsin than normal. Liver is a good dietary source of vitamin A because it is the organ in which retinol is stored, usually at *trans*-retinylpalmitate. An esterase catalyzes release of the retinol; it enters the plasma where it is carried by retinol-binding protein (RBP). The retinol-RBP complex in turn is bound by transthyretin which transports the complex to the eye. The pigment epithelium (single layer of cells next to the outer segments) cells specifically bind the retinol-RBP. The RBP is released and the retinol enters the cells where it is converted to 11-*cis*-retinal. When there is more retinal than visual pigment proteins to which it binds, it can be stored in the pigment epithelial cells.

The initial event triggered by light results in a series of reactions resulting in conversion of the 11-*cis*-retinal of rhodopsin to *trans*-retinal which dissociates from the protein yielding free opsin. Light is required only for the first reaction in which rhodopsin is converted to bathorhodopsin. It is believed that the primary photochemical step is the conversion of the 11-*cis*-retinal to the *trans*-isomer; if a retinal analog is used in which the 11-*cis* bond cannot undergo isomerization the visual pigment is stable to light. Bathorhodopsin then undergoes thermal decay through the intermediates lumirhodopsin, metarhodopsin-I, and metarhodopsin-II to yield opsin and *trans*-retinal. The question is how does this series of reactions result in a change in the electrical properties of the plasma membrane of the cell so that the information is transmitted from the outer segment of the cell to the synapse.

In the dark, sodium ions flow down a concentration gradient into the outer segment of a rod cell. They diffuse to the inner segment where they are pumped out via a $Na^+ - K^+$-ATPase system. In response to interaction with light the dark current is shut down and the rod cell hyperpolarizes. The following model has been proposed to explain the observed membrane changes. (1) The light-induced conversion of a single rhodopsin molecule to opsin results in hydrolysis of thousands of c-GMP. Light-activated rhodopsin (R^*) is believed to bind a G-protein (can exist in two forms, one binds GDP the other GTP) to which GDP is bound (G_{GDP}). R^*G_{GDP} exchanges its GDP for GTP forming R^*G_{GTP}. The G_{GTP} dissociates from the R^* (R^* can reenter the cycle) and interacts with a phosphodiesterase (PDE), activating it. $PDE-G_{GTP}$ catalyzes the hydrolysis of c-GMP to GMP and H^+. Hydrolysis of the GTP present in the $PDE-G_{GTP}$ inactivates the PDE. The $PDE-G_{GDP}$ dissociates giving G_{GDP} and PDE which can subsequently reenter the cycle. The cycle is probably terminated by the phosphorylation of opsin in an ATP-requiring reaction catalyzed by opsin kinase. The cycle is completed by recombination of opsin with regenerated 11-*cis*-retinal (accompanied by loss of phosphate groups from the protein) to give rho-

dopsin. (2) The protons released upon hydrolysis of c-GMP exchange for calcium ions stored within the disks. (3) Released Ca^{2+} diffuses to the plasma membrane and blocks the Na^+ channels shutting down the dark current. This model explains the observed membrane changes and how the signal might be amplified. The hyperpolarization of the cell which is observed affects synaptic transmitter release and therefore the information transmitted.

Cone cells differ from rods in structure and function, an aspect of which is seen in the presence of pigments which permit color vision. There are three different visual pigments; each cone cell has one of the visual pigments present in its plasma membrane (cone cells do not have separate disk membranes as rods do). The protein component of the pigments differs but each combines with 11-*cis*-retinal. The absorption maximum of the different pigments are 430 nm (blue), 540 nm (green), and 575 nm (red). In hereditary color blindness, one or more of the three visual pigments is missing or present in reduced amounts. The protein portions of the green and red pigments are coded for by genes on the X chromosome and the gene for the blue pigment is on an autosome. Thus far little is known of the chemistry of cone function.

Muscle

Knowledge of the chemistry of skeletal muscle contraction has contributed to our understanding of locomotion in general because the mechanism of function of contractile proteins appears to be similar in other types of muscle and even in cilia. The movement produced by muscle is the result of active contraction. Myofibrils are the contractile units of muscle fibers. When viewed under a light microscope, skeletal muscle myofibrils have a striated appearance generated by repeating units termed "sarcomeres." These are composed of two sets of parallel and partially overlapping thick and thin filaments; myosin is the protein which forms the thick filaments and actin the major protein component of thin filaments (Fig. 4-11).

Myosin contains six polypeptide chains. Two identical heavy chains which associate to give a fibrous, predominantly α-helical structure which ends in a globular domain at each amino terminus (referred to as the "head" of the protein). Associated with each globular domain are two light chains. One of the light chains associated with each globular domain is the same; they can undergo reversible phosphorylation of a serine residue and are believed to function in the interaction of myosin and actin. The other two light chains, designated A_1 and A_2, are necessary for myosin ATPase activity and for myosin binding to actin. In solution, myosin molecules aggregate to form filaments. They associate so that

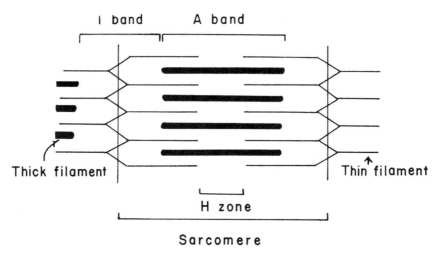

Fig. 4-11. *Schematic representation of a sarcomere (length of myofibril bounded by two adjacent Z bands). The heavy filaments represent myosin and the thin filaments actin. α-Actinin and desmin are found in the region of the Z bands at the ends of the sarcomere. α-Actinin is believed to anchor the actin filaments and desmin is believed to help keep the myofibrils in register.*

their heads are spaced at fixed distances (14.3 nm) from each other, and each is rotated by 120°. The fibers formed in this way meet tail-to-tail giving a bipolar structure, a heavy filament of a sarcomere. The central region, where the two tails come together, is devoid of the heads of the myosin molecules.

Actin consists of a single polypeptide which has a globular conformation and is referred to as G actin. A noncovalently bound ATP and one Ca^{2+} are associated with each actin molecule. In solution in the presence of Mg^{2+}, actin polymerizes to form actin filaments (helical double strand of polymerized actin monomers) designated as F actin. The hydrolysis of the ATP, associated with G actin, to ADP and P_i accelerates but is not essential for polymerization. Troponin and tropomyosin are associated with the actin filaments. Tropomyosin is composed of two nonidentical, α-helical polypeptide chains which twist around each other forming a rod-shaped protein that is found in the grooves formed by the two strands of actin filaments. Troponin consists of three polypeptides designated as troponins T, I, and C. Troponin T binds the complex to tropomyosin, troponin I inhibits the interaction of actin and myosin (probably by holding tropomyosin in a position that blocks the actin binding sites), and troponin C binds up to four Ca^{2+}. When troponin C has bound Ca^{2+} it can reverse the troponin I inhibition of the interaction of actin with myosin. It is these proteins which form the thin filaments of the sarcomere.

Muscle contraction occurs in response to stimulation of the muscle by a motor neuron. The action potential induced in muscle cells by the action of acetylcholine on its receptors present in muscle membrane travels along the sarcolemma to the transverse tubules to the sarcoplasmic reticulum, where it induces release of Ca^{2+}. The released Ca^{2+} raises the concentration to a level sufficient to have Ca^{2+} bound by all the troponin C binding sites. This permits the binding of actin to myosin. Actin binding stimulates the activity of the myosin associated ATPase by increasing the rate of release of ADP and P_i from the myosin. It is the hydrolysis of ATP which provides the energy for muscle contraction. The following series of events is believed to best describe muscle contraction. The myosin head in association with ADP and P_i binds to an actin filament; this results in a change in conformation which enhances the release of the ADP and P_i. Loss of the ADP and P_i causes the myosin head to pull against the actin filament moving it in toward the H region of the sarcomere (*see* Figure 4-11). ATP then binds to the myosin head causing its release from the thin filament. Hydrolysis of the ATP reinitiates the cycle. A second role for Ca^{2+} is in the phosphorylation of the light chain protein associated with each myosin head. This is catalyzed by a Ca^{2+}-calmodulin activated kinase. The phosphorylated form of the protein is believed to modulate the force of the contraction. The cycle is terminated by reuptake of the released Ca^{2+} by the sarcoplasmic reticulum. When the stimulus is removed, a Mg^{2+}, Ca^{2+}-ATPase exchanges Mg^{2+} for Ca^{2+} and pumps the Ca^{2+} against its concentration gradient back into the sarcoplasmic reticulum.

During muscle contraction the utilization of ATP can increase by several hundred-fold. While the oxidative catabolism of sugars, ketone bodies, and some amino acids provides more than enough ATP for the needs of resting muscle, it is not always sufficient for active muscle. ATP levels are maintained by transfer of an active phosphate from phosphocreatine to ADP to form ATP and creatine.

ACKNOWLEDGMENTS

The author would like to acknowledge and thank FJ Cramer for typing this manuscript and Dr. EA Davidson and medical students HM Grasmeder and GS Gerhard for their assistance in proofreading it.

REFERENCES

Alberts B, Bray D, Lewis J, et al: Molecular Biology of the Cell. Garland Publishing, Inc., New York, 1983

Brown MS, Goldstein JL: Receptor-mediated control of cholesterol metabolism. Science 191:150, 1976

Brown MS, Goldstein JL: Multivalent feedback regulation of HMG CoA reductase, a control mechanism coordinating isoprenoid synthesis and cell growth. J Lipid Res 21:505, 1980

Devlin TM (ed): Textbook of Biochemistry with Clinical Correlations. John Wiley and Sons, Inc., New York, 1982

Dorfman A, Matalon R: The mucopolysaccharidoses (a review). Proc Natl Acad Sci USA 73:630, 1976

Edelman GM: Cell adhesion molecules. Science 219:450, 1983

Hammarstrom S: Leukotrienes. Annu Rev Biochem 52:355, 1983

Hers HG, Hue L: Gluconeogenesis and related aspects of glycolysis. Annu Rev Biochem 52:617, 1983

Krieger DT: Brain peptides: what, where, and why? Science 222:975, 1983

Lewin B: Genes. John Wiley and Sons, Inc., New York, 1983

McGilvery RW: Biochemistry. 3rd Ed. WB Saunders Co., Philadelphia, 1983

O'Brien DF: The chemistry of vision. Science 218:961, 1982

Richardson JJ: The anatomy and taxonomy of protein structure. Adv Protein Chem 34:168, 1981

Rosenberg LE: Vitamin-responsive inherited metabolic disorders. Adv Hum Genet 6:1, 1976

Sandhoff K, Christomanou H: Biochemistry and genetics of gangliosidoses. Hum Genet 50:107, 1979

Singer SJ, Nicholson GL: The fluid mosaic model of the structure of cell membranes. Science 175:720, 1972

Smith EL, Hill RL, Lehman IR, et al: Principles of Biochemistry: General Aspects. McGraw-Hill Book Co., New York, 1983

Smith EL, Hill RL, Lehman IR, et al: Principles of Biochemistry: Mammalian Biochemistry. McGraw-Hill Book Co., New York, 1983

Svennerholm L: Gangliosides. p. 425. In Lajtha A (ed): Handbook of Neurochemistry. Vol. 3. Plenum Press, New York, 1970

Tonegawa S: Somatic generation of antibody diversity. Nature 302:575, 1983

Yamada KM: Cell surface interactions with extracellular materials. Annu Rev Biochem 52:761, 1983

MULTIPLE CHOICE QUESTIONS

For each numbered statement, select the one lettered heading that is most closely related to it. Each lettered heading may be selected once, more than once, or not at all.

1. Site of fatty acid biosynthesis
2. Location of enzymes needed for oxidative-phosphorylation
3. Primary location of cardiolipin

A Mitochondrial cristae
B Mitochondrial matrix
C Inner mitochondrial membrane
D Outer mitochondrial membrane
E Cytoplasm

4. Glucose-6-phosphatase deficiency
5. Inactive glycogen "debranching" enzyme
6. Phosphorylation converts this enzyme to the active "a" form

A Type IV glycogen storage disease
B Type Ia glycogen storage disease
C Glycogen phosphorylase
D Type III glycogen storage disease
E Glycogen synthetase

7. A deficiency in this compound can result in pellagra
8. Niacin is derived from this molecule
9. Maple syrup urine disease

A Histidine
B Phenylalanine
C Branched chain α-keto acid dehydrogenase
D Tryptophan
E Phenylalanine hydroxylase

10. Lesch-Nyhan syndrome
11. GMP reductase catalyzes the reduction of GMP forming _____.
12. AMP deaminase catalyzes the deamination of AMP forming _____.

A Allopurinol
B Hypoxanthine-guanine phosphoribosyl transferase deficiency
C Gout
D IMP
E IMP dehydrogenase deficiency

13. is associated with a β-hexosaminidase A deficiency
14. is associated with an arylsulfatase A deficiency

15. is associated with an α-galactosidase deficiency
 - A Tay-Sach's disease
 - B Metachromatic leukodystrophy
 - C Gaucher's disease
 - D Niemann-Pick disease
 - E Fabry's disease

16. Lipoprotein lipase activator
17. Mediates LDL uptake by binding to cell surface receptor sites
18. Plasma lecithin: cholesterol acyltransferase activator
 - A Apoprotein C_{II}
 - B Apoprotein A_I
 - C Apoprotein B
 - D Apoprotein E
 - E Apoprotein C_I

19. Prosthetic group for enzymes that catalyze the fixation of CO_2
20. Functions by forming a Schiff's base in transamination reactions
21. A deficiency of this vitamin can result in a person expressing the symptoms of pernicious anemia
 - A Thiamine pyrophosphate
 - B Pyridoxal phosphate
 - C Biotin
 - D Folic acid
 - E Cobalamin

22. The phase in which cytokinesis occurs
23. The phase in which DNA replication occurs
24. Lack of an essential nutrient will probably arrest the cell cycle in which phase
 - A G_1 phase
 - B S phase
 - C G_2 phase
 - D M phase
 - E G_0 phase

For each of the incomplete statements below, one or more of the completions is correct. Answer

        A   if only 1, 2, and 3 are correct
        B   if only 1 and 3 are correct
        C   if only 2 and 4 are correct
        D   if only 4 is correct
        E   if all are correct

25. An enzyme is a protein which
 1. Alters the equilibrium of the reaction it catalyzes.
 2. Exhibits specificity for substrate and type of reaction catalyzed.
 3. Acts by raising the energy of activation for the reaction.
 4. Contains an active site, the structure of which determines the substrate it acts upon.

26. Carbohydrates
 1. Have the general formula $(CH_2O)_n$.
 2. Can be polyhydroxyaldehydes or polyhydroxyketones.
 3. Can be associated with lipids or proteins.
 4. Can serve as a source of energy for the cell.

27. Water can function in the maintenance of structure and aggregation of macromolecules as well as in temperature control due to
 1. Its ability to form hydrogen bonds.
 2. Its heat of vaporization.
 3. Its heat of fusion.
 4. Its low dielectric constant.

28. Triacylglycerols
 1. Serve as an energy source.
 2. Are hydrophilic.
 3. Give a higher caloric yield when fully oxidized than does the oxidation of a comparable amount of carbohydrate.
 4. Contain two hydrocarbon chains per molecule.

29. Complex lipids
 1. Include phospholipids and sphingolipids
 2. Are essential structural components of cell membranes.
 3. Bear a neutral or net negative charge.
 4. Are less hydrophilic than triacylglycerols.

30. DNA replication in eukaryotes
 1. Is catalyzed by DNA polymerase α which directs the addition of mononucleotides in the 3′ to 5′ direction.
 2. Involves multiple origins of replication.
 3. Is catalyzed by DNA polymerase β which directs the addition of mononucleotides in the 3′ to 5′ direction forming Okazaki fragments.
 4. Requires the linking together of Okazaki fragments in reactions catalyzed by DNA ligase.

31. Transcription
 1. Is the transfer of genetic information from DNA to RNA molecules.
 2. Is catalyzed by DNA-dependent RNA polymerases.
 3. Results in synthesis of m-RNA which may contain introns which must be removed prior to the m-RNA being functional.
 4. Results in synthesis of RNAs which do not undergo modification after transcription.

32. The change in free energy (ΔG) of a reaction
 1. Equals 0 at equilibrium.
 2. Is directly proportional to $\ln K_{eq}$.

3. Is negative for a spontaneous reaction.

4. Is positive if energy is not required.

33. Acetyl CoA is produced by the catabolism of
    1. Lysine
    2. Glycogen
    3. Leucine
    4. Triacylglycerol

34. In fatty acid biosynthesis
    1. The committing step is the synthesis of malonly CoA from acetyl CoA.
    2. Palmitoyl CoA inhibits the acetyl CoA carboxylase.
    3. Insulin activates the acetyl CoA carboxylase by converting it to the active dephosphorylated form.
    4. Increased ATP levels inhibit isocitrate dehydrogenase resulting in increased citrate concentration which activates the acetyl CoA carboxylase.

35. Ketone bodies
    1. Are elevated in the blood of a person with uncontrolled diabetes mellitus.
    2. Are elevated in the starving individual.
    3. Are formed by the condensation of acetyl CoA molecules.
    4. Can be utilized by the brain as a source of energy (as long as some glucose is present).

36. The urea cycle
    1. Occurs in the cytoplasm.
    2. Enzymes are more active during starvation than during times of normal food intake.
    3. Enzymes are activated by a carbohydrate rich diet.
    4. Serves to detoxify the ammonia produced by the catabolism of amino acids.

37. In purine biosynthesis
    1. 5-Phosphoribosyl-1-pyrophosphate is the starting material.
    2. Acetyl CoA serves as the source of two of the ring carbons.
    3. Phosphoribosyl pyrophosphate amidotransferase catalyzes the committing step.
    4. Purine nucleotides are positive effectors.

38. In isoprenoid metabolism
    1. Formation of mevalonic acid is the committing step in isoprenoid synthesis.
    2. Farnesyl pyrophosphate serves as a major branch point in the synthesis of isoprenoid compounds.
    3. Squalene synthetase catalyzes the committing step of cholesterol biosynthesis.
    4. Isopentyl pyrophosphate can be transferred to the N_6 position of certain adenosines in t-RNA.

39. Steroid hormone synthesis
    1. Is initiated by the synthesis of pregnenolone, a C_{25} compound.
    2. Involves reactions catalyzed by cytochrome P_{450} enzymes.
    3. Is inhibited by ACTH.
    4. Is dependent upon the availability of free cholesterol for synthesis of pregnenolene.

40. Hemoglobin
    1. Consists of 3 subunits, 2 α and 1 β.
    2. Increases the amount of oxygen that can be carried per dl of blood.
    3. Binds oxygen more strongly as the H^+ concentration increases.
    4. Has a sigmoidal oxygen binding curve.

41. In heme metabolism
    1. The synthesis of δ-aminolevulinic acid from glycine and succinyl CoA is the rate-limiting step.
    2. Two porphobilinogen molecules react to form uroporphyrinogen.
    3. Some of the synthetic steps occur in the cytoplasm, others in the mitochondria.
    4. The protoporphyrin ring of heme can be reutilized by the red blood cell.

42. In cell membranes
    1. Cholesterol serves to enhance the ability of phospholipids to crystallize when cooled.
    2. Glycolipids are found on the cytoplasmic side.
    3. The lipids are symmetrically distributed.
    4. Proteins are categorized as either peripheral or integral depending on the ease with which they can be dissociated from the membrane.

43. The endoplasmic reticulum (ER)
    1. Consists of two functionally distinct areas, the smooth and rough ER.
    2. Can form vesicles which pinch off and if they fuse with the plasma membrane do so in such a way that the luminal side of the ER membrane is on the outer surface of the plasma membrane.
    3. Is the site of synthesis of the lipid and protein components of cell membranes.
    4. May account for over half of the total cellular membrane.

44. In blood coagulation
    1. Vitamin K is essential for the normal synthesis of prothrombin and factors VII, IX, and X.
    2. γ-carboxyglutamate is believed to play a role in the binding of Ca^{2+}.
    3. The polymerization of fibrin is the final step in clot formation.
    4. Dicumarol enhances the possibility of clot formation.

45. Scurvy
    1. Is accompanied by an increase of δ-hydroxylysine residues present in collagen.
    2. Is caused by a lack of ascorbate.
    3. Is accompanied by an increase in stability of the triple helix.
    4. Is accompanied by a reduction in the conversion of collagen proline to hydroxyproline.
46. Myelin
    1. Of the peripheral nervous system is elaborated by oligodendroglial cells.
    2. Contains a higher proportion of lipids containing short chain or unsaturated fatty acids than is found in neurons.
    3. Contains a wide variety of proteins, all of which are present in about equal amounts.
    4. Contains a high proportion of lipid (~70 percent) with galactolipids and cholesterol accounting for over 50 percent of the lipid components.

Select the one best answer for the question or incomplete statement.

47. In a Lineweaver-Burk plot, the slope varied while the intercept $(1/V_{max})$ remained constant, the rate of reaction was measured in the presence of varying amounts of an inhibitor indicating
    1. Competitive inhibition.
    2. Noncompetitive inhibition.
    3. Uncompetitive inhibition.
    4. Feedback inhibition.
    5. Allosteric inhibition.
48. A weak acid in solution
    1. Has a $pH = pKa + \log \dfrac{[acid]}{[salt]}$.
    2. Has a dissociation constant equal to $\dfrac{[HA]}{[H^+][A^-]}$.
    3. Exists in an equilibrium $HA \rightleftharpoons H^+ + A^-$.
    4. Has an anion concentration equal to $\dfrac{[H^+]}{K_a[HA]}$.
    5. Has a hydrogen ion concentration equal to 10^{-7}.
49. The tricarboxylic acid cycle
    1. Provides ATP to meet the cell's energy requirements.
    2. Results in complete oxidation of the acetyl moiety of acetyl CoA.
    3. Provides intermediates for purine and pyrimidine synthesis.
    4. Is influenced by diet.
    5. Provides NADH for biosynthetic reactions.
50. Secondary structure of a protein can best be described as:
    1. An α-helix.

2. The amino acid sequence.
3. The interactions of polypeptide subunits with each other.
4. The folding of the polypeptide chain.
5. A β pleated sheet.
51. $NADH + \frac{1}{2}O_2 + H^+ \rightarrow NAD^+ + H_2O$
$$\Delta G^\circ = -52 \text{ Kcal/mol}$$
$ATP \rightarrow ADP + P_i$
$$\Delta G^\circ = -7.3 \text{ Kcal/mol}$$
ΔG° for these two reactions indicate that the efficiency of the storage as ATP of enery released by the oxidation of NADH is about
    1. 10 percent.
    2. 20 percent.
    3. 40 percent.
    4. 60 percent.
    5. 75 percent.
52. In glycolysis
    1. Formation of glucose-6-phosphate is the committing step.
    2. Glucose is converted to lactate (aerobic).
    3. The formation of glucose-6-phosphate catalyzed by glucokinase (hexokinase IV) is readily reversible.
    4. Brain hexokinase (type I) responds to changes in glucose levels.
    5. Phosphofructokinase catalyzes the committing step.
53. The β-oxidation of fatty acyl CoA derivatives
    1. Is carried out by enzymes that are associated with the outer mitochondrial membrane.
    2. Requires NADPH as a cofactor.
    3. Occurs via a reversal of the synthetic pathway.
    4. Results in a shortening of the acyl chain by two carbons.
    5. Is stimulated by insulin.
54. In the metabolism of phospholipids
    1. CMP-ethanolamine reacts with 1,2-diacylglycerol to form phosphatidyl ethanolamine.
    2. Phosphatidyl ethanolamine can be converted to phosphatidylcholine by the successive addition of methyl residues from methylene tetrahydrofolate.
    3. Phospholipase D catalyzes the hydrolysis of the phosphoryl moiety esterified to the glycerol backbone.
    4. Phosphatidylserine is formed via the reaction of phosphatidic acid with serine.
    5. Remodeling can occur at position two via the successive actions of phospholipase A_2 and an acyl CoA transacylase.
55. During digestion of ingested food
    1. Cells of the gastric mucosa secrete α-amylase and proenzymes such as trypsinogen.

2. Pepsinogen initiates protein hydrolysis.
3. The pancreas secretes trypsin and chymotrypsin in response to hormonal stimuli.
4. Free amino acids are transported into the epithelial cells of the intestinal mucosa via a carrier mediated active transport system.
5. The stomach serves as the site of the bulk of the digestive process.

56. In carbohydrate digestion
    1. The exosaccharidase α-amylase, which is found in saliva, catalyzes the initial degradation.
    2. Amylases present in gastric juice continue the digestion initiated by salivary α-amylase.
    3. Di- and oligosaccharides must be hydrolyzed to free monosaccharides prior to their absorption from the lumen of the small intestine.
    4. Monosaccharides are able to diffuse freely across the epithelial cells of the lumen.
    5. Maltase catalyzes the hydrolysis of $\alpha 1,6$ bonds present in dextrins.

57. Cytochrome P_{450} enzymes
    1. Catalyze the general reaction: $RH + O_2 + FADH_2 \rightarrow ROH + FAD + H_2O$.
    2. Catalyze reactions which convert lipid soluble drugs to more water-soluble metabolites.
    3. Are dioxygenases.
    4. Are always associated with liver mitochondria.
    5. Contain a copper moiety as part of their active site.

58. Lysosomes
    1. Contain hydrolases which exhibit basic pH optima.
    2. Have membranes that are freely permeable to tri- and tetrapeptides.
    3. Are delineated by a double membrane.
    4. Serve as the digestive component of the cell.
    5. Acquire material for synthesis via fusion with a phagocytic, endocytotic or autophagic vesicles.

59. Immunoglobulins
    1. Can have one of three different types of light (L) chains.
    2. Are synthesized by T cells.
    3. Contain the antigen-binding site in their variable (V) region.
    4. Bind the C1 component of complement to their L chain constant region.
    5. Are separated into classes such as IgG on the basis of their type of L chain.

60. Proteoglycans
    1. Can contain as much as 50 percent carbohydrate.
    2. Generally bear no net charge.
    3. Are separated into different classes on the basis of their repeating disaccharide units.
    4. Always have their carbohydrate moieties in an

N-linkage to asparagine residues present in the peptide chains.
    5. Form solutions of low viscosity.

61. Phosphocreatine
    1. Is found in relatively high levels in the liver.
    2. Serves as a source of high energy phosphate for the maintenance of ATP levels in brain and muscle.
    3. Is used to meet the energy needs of resting muscle.
    4. Is derived from the amino acids lysine and alanine.
    5. Serves as a general source of high energy phosphate for the maintenance of ATP levels in all cells.

62. In vision
    1. Rod cells are responsible for color vision.
    2. Cone cells are responsible for vision in dim light (night vision).
    3. The light induced conversion of rhodopsin to opsin results in hydrolysis of thousands of c-AMP molecules.
    4. The visual pigments which permit color vision have absorption maximum at the wavelengths associated with red, indigo and blue.
    5. The primary photochemical step is the conversion of 11-*cis*-retinal to the trans-isomer.

Each set of lettered headings is followed by a list of numbered words or phrases. Answer

A if the item is associated with (A) only,
B if the item is associated with (B) only,
C if the item is associated with both (A) and (B),
D if the item is associated with neither (A) nor (B).

63. Found in DNA
64. Found in RNA
65. Purine base
    A Adenine
    B Uracil
    C Both
    D Neither

66. Catalyzes an ATP requiring reaction
67. Is a biotin containing enzyme
68. Is activated by citrate
    A Pyruvate carboxylase
    B Acetyl CoA carboxylase
    C Both
    D Neither

69. Play a role in the synthesis of triacylglycerols
70. Unique to phospholipid synthesis
71. Unique to triacylglycerol synthesis
    A Diacylglycerol acyltransferase
    B Phosphatidic acid
    C Both
    D Neither

72. Nucleotide coenzyme
73. When oxidized supplies energy for the synthesis of only 2 ATP
74. Is a carrier for fatty acyl residues
    A Nicotinamide adenine dinucleotide (NAD$^+$)
    B Coenzyme A
    C Both
    D Neither

75. Involves a net movement of the solute against its concentration gradient.
76. The material is taken up by the cell enclosing it with a portion of the plasma membrane.
77. The direction of transport of the solute is dependent upon its concentration gradient.
    A Passive transport
    B Active transport
    C Both
    D Neither

78. Is derived from arachidonic acid.
79. May contain an amino acid residue.
80. Contains a 5-membered ring, formed between C_8 and C_{12}.
    A Prostaglandins
    B Leukotrienes
    C Both
    D Neither

81. Is a putative neurotransmitter.
82. Its synthesis requires loss of a carboxyl group from the immediate precursor.
83. A reduction in the level of this transmitter due to degeneration of the nigrostriatal tract results in the symptoms associated with Parkinson's disease.
    A Dopamine
    B Serotonin
    C Both
    D Neither

Answers to Questions

1 E	2 A	3 C	4 B	5 D
6 C	7 D	8 D	9 C	10 B
11 D	12 D	13 A	14 B	15 E
16 A	17 C	18 B	19 C	20 B
21 E	22 D	23 B	24 A	25 C
26 E	27 A	28 B	29 A	30 C
31 A	32 A	33 E	34 E	35 E
36 C	37 B	38 A	39 C	40 C
41 B	42 D	43 E	44 A	45 C
46 D	47 1	48 3	49 2	50 4
51 3	52 5	53 4	54 5	55 4
56 3	57 2	58 4	59 3	60 3
61 2	62 5	63 A	64 C	65 A
66 C	67 C	68 B	69 C	70 D
71 A	72 C	73 D	74 B	75 B
76 D	77 A	78 C	79 B	80 A
81 C	82 C	83 A		

5

Microbiology and Immunology

Thomas D. Flanagan

BACTERIAL MORPHOLOGY AND PHYSIOLOGY

Cell Structure

The prokaryotic cells of bacteria occur in three basic shapes (i.e., spheres or cocci, rods or bacilli, and spirals or spirilla). The sizes of these cells vary considerably. Bacilli occur over a range $1\,\mu m \times 2\,\mu m$ to $2\,\mu m \times 8\,\mu m$. Cocci range from $1\,\mu m$ in diameter of $1.5\,\mu m$. Spirilla are $0.4\,\mu m$ to $0.8\,\mu m$ wide by $10\,\mu m$ to $50\,\mu m$ long. The shape of a cell is a stable characteristic of a bacterial species and, within considerable limits, so is its size. Cell size is affected by the physiologic state and the environment of the organism.

CELL WALL

Bacteria occur in three groups depending on the characteristics of their outer cell boundary. There are bacteria which lack a rigid cell wall. These organisms belong to the class *Mollicutes* (*Mycoplasma*). The other two groups have rigid cell walls and differ from each other by the composition of the wall and by their reaction to the Gram stain. Gram-positive bacteria have a cell wall consisting of a single thick layer of peptidoglycan. The organisms retain the crystal violet dye after treatment with iodine when decolorized with alcohol or acetone in the Gram procedure.

In contrast, gram-negative organisms have cell walls consisting of two distinct layers. One of the layers, the outer membrane, is a typical unit membrane. It contains phospholipids, proteins, and lipopolysaccharides (LPS). The inner layer is a thin structure of peptidoglycan. The two layers are linked by lipoprotein molecules that are covalently bound at the carboxy termini to diaminopimelate residues in the peptidoglycan and bear fatty acid residues covalently bound to glycerylsterine at the amino termini. This distal terminus is thus highly hydrophobic. In contrast to gram-positive cells, gram-negative organisms do not retain crystal violet after treatment with iodine when decolorized with alcohol or acetone. The decolorized cells must be counterstained in order to be visible in the microscope (Fig. 5-1).

CONSTITUENTS OF CELL WALLS

The bipolymer peptidoglycan is a constituent of the cell wall both gram-positive (40–90 percent of total cell wall mass) and gram-negative (5–20 percent) bacteria. This substance forms a three-dimensional mesh which encloses the cell. The basic structure of the molecule is an alternating sequence of *N*-acetylglucosamine and *N*-acetylmuramic acid. Parallel polysaccharide strands of these residues are cross-linked by two tetrapeptide chains attached to the *N*-acetylmuramic acid residues on each polysaccharide. The tetrapeptide bridges are covalently bound to each other by a peptide between the terminal D-alanine residue and the penultimate diaminopimelic acid or lysine on the tetrapeptide (Fig. 5-2). Thus the peptidoglycan forms a single giant covalently bound mesh-like structure. Variations in the cross-link-

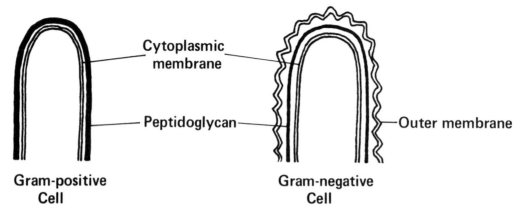

Fig. 5-1. Schematic representation of the cell wall of a gram-positive and a gram-negative cell. (Milgrom F, Flanagan TD: Medical Microbiology. Churchill Livingstone, New York, 1982.)

ing occur among bacterial species. The structure described occurs in the cell wall of *Escherichia coli* but variations of this general theme occur in other bacteria. For example, the cross-linking in *Staphylococcus aureus* is done by a pentaglycine unit bound to the terminal D-alanine of one tetrapeptide and the penultimate L-lysine of the other.

Biosynthesis of peptidoglycan begins in the cytoplasm of the cell with the precursors of the molecule, uri-

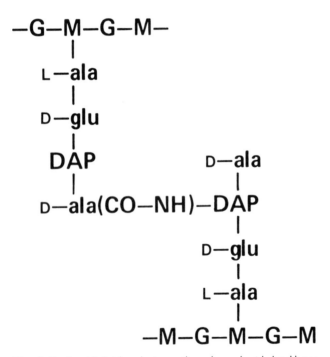

Fig. 5-2. Peptide bridges between the polysaccharide backbone *E. coli* are cross linked. G, N-acetylglucosamine; M, N-acetylmuramic acid; L-ala, L-alanine; D-ala, D-alanine; DAP, mesodiaminopimelic acid; D-glu, D-glutamic acid. (Milgrom F, Flanagan TD: Medical Microbiology. Churchill Livingstone New York, 1982.)

dine diphosphate (UDP)-*N*-acetylmuramic acid, and UDP-*N*-acetylglucosamine (Fig. 5-3). A pentapeptide residue is attached to the *N*-acetylmuramic acid. This unit is then attached to a membrane lipid carrier (i.e., bactoprenol or undecaprenyl phosphate). The *N*-acetylglucosamine is added from the UDP-*N*-acetylglucosamine to form a disaccharide-(pentapeptide)-bactoprenol molecule. Subsequently the disaccharide-(pentapeptide) is added to the growing peptidoglycan with release of bactoprenol pyrophosphate. After dephosphorylation the bactoprenol can again accept *N*-acetylmuramic acid-(pentapeptide). This process mediates the transport across the cytoplasmic membrane as well as the synthesis of the polymer. The final step in synthesis of peptidoglycan is the cross-linking by a transpeptidation reaction. The terminal D-alanine of the pentapeptide is removed by D-alanine carboxypeptidase yielding the characteristic tetrapeptide bridge.

Teichoic acids are major constituents (up to 50 percent of cell weight) of the cell walls of gram-positive bacteria. These substances are composed of ribitol or glycerol residues linked by phosphodiester bonds. They are attached to the peptidoglycan by phosphodiester bonds to *N*-acetylmuramic acid residues. In some organisms teichoic acids are linked to glycolipids in membranes (lipoteichoic acids).

Lipopolysaccharides (LPS) are important constituents of the outer membrane of gram-negative bacteria (Fig. 5-4). They carry the major antigenic determinants referred to as O or somatic antigens and possess potent toxic properties. In the latter case, they are called endotoxins. LPS are complex molecules with three major domains. Lipid A forms the hydrophobic region of the molecule. It is made up of a phosphorylated glucosamine disaccharide linked by ester and amide bonds to long chain fatty acids. This part of the LPS molecule is responsible for toxicity. Lipid A is linked to a polysaccha-

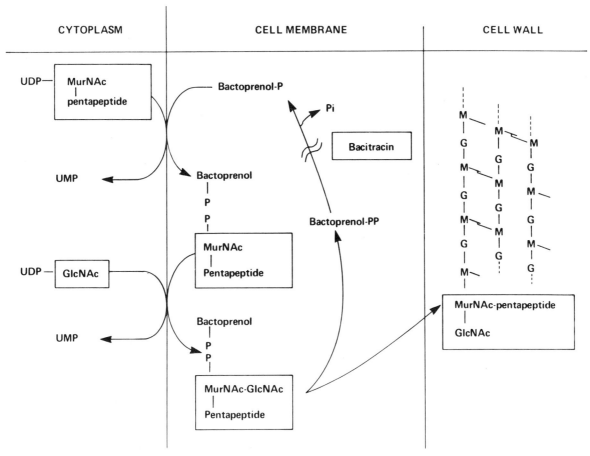

Fig. 5-3. The synthesis of a linear peptidoglycan. GlcNAc or G, N-acetyl-glucosamine; MurNAc or M, N-acetylmuramic acid. (Milgrom F, Flanagan TD: Medical Microbiology, Churchill Livingstone, New York 1982.)

ride core containing three residues of an unusual eight carbon sugar, ketodeoxy-octonoate (KDO), through a glycosidic bond with a glucosamine molecule. The core consists of KDO, heptose, glucose, galactose, and N-acetylglucosamine. The third domain of the LPS molecule consists of the O-specific side chains. These are made up of repeating tri-, tetra-, or pentasaccharide units attached to the core. The O-specific side chains are responsible for the strain- or species-specific serologic characteristics of the bacteria. The variety of sugars, bonds, and modifications such as acetylation confer almost unlimited possibility for antigenic uniqueness. The core structure of different genera differ from one another (e.g., *Salmonella, Shigella,* etc.) but within a genus the structure is relatively constant.

In nature most strains of gram-negative bacteria bear O-specific side chains, however, mutants which lack them do occur (R-strains) and some of these mutants also lack much of the core structure. Bacteria without lipid A and the three KDO residues have not been isolated, suggesting these elements are essential for survival.

CYTOPLASMIC MEMBRANE

The cytoplasmic membrane of a bacterium is a typical unit membrane approximately 10 nm wide and accounts for 10 percent of the dry weight of the cell. It is composed of 20–30 percent lipid, mostly phospholipid, and 60–70 percent protein. The phospholipid molecules are in a double layer with the polar head groups oriented outward toward the aqueous environment and fatty acid chains oriented inward, creating a hydrophobic milieu. Integral proteins of the membrane penetrate through or into the bilayer while peripheral proteins are associated with the hydrophilic head groups and are easily removed.

Many important functions are carried out by or are associated with the cytoplasmic membrane. The membrane functions as an osmotic barrier which is impermeable to most organic and inorganic molecules. It functions in the active transport of many substances from the environment to the interior of the cell as well as the reverse. It is the site of ATP generation for cellular me-

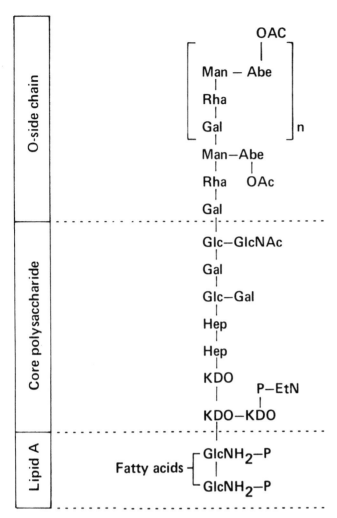

Fig. 5-4. Structure of the *Salmonella typhimurium* lipopolysaccharide. Abe, abequose; EtN, ehtanolamine; Gal, D-glactose; Glc, D-glucose; GlcNH₂, glucosamine; GlcNAc, N-acetylglucosamine; Hep, L-glycero-D-mannoheptose; KDO, ketodeoxyoctononate; Man, D-mannose; OAc, O-acetyl; P, phosphate; PP, pyrophosphate, Rha, L-rhamnose. (Milgrom F, Flanagan TD: Medical Microbiology. Churchill Livingstone, New York, 1982.)

NUCLEUS

Although prokaryotic cells do not have a membrane-bound nucleus, the bacteria do have an area composed of closely packed DNA fibrils; this area is devoid of any other structures. The chromosome of a typical bacterium such as *E coli* is a single circular molecule of DNA with a molecular weight of 3×10^9 daltons. It is composed of 5×10^6 base pairs and is about 1 mm in length.

CYTOPLASM

The cytoplasm of the prokaryotic cell lacks the membraneous structures which serve to organize much of the metabolism of eukaryotic cells. In contrast, the processes of the bacterial cell go on in the cytosol. The bacterial ribosomes, sites of protein synthesis, appear as fine granular structures in electron micrographs. Their abundance varies with the physiologic state of the cell. They are composed of a 30 S subunit and a 50 S subunit. The whole ribosome has a 70 S sedimentation constant. Other structures found in the cytoplasm include poly β-hydroxybutyrate granules, glycogen-like polysaccharide granules, sulfur granules, and polyphosphate deposits called volutin or metachromatic granules and sulfur granules.

CELL SURFACE STRUCTURES

Many bacteria secrete substances which remain adherent to the surface of the cell. These substances are biopolymers, usually polysaccharides, but other substances occur as well. Large accumulations of these substances are called capsules. Bacterial capsules are important factors in determining the pathogenicity of some species. Encapsulated strains of *Streptococcus pneumoniae* are virulent, whereas, mutants which do not form capsules are avirulent.

Motile bacteria have long fibrillar structures called flagella which are organelles of locomotion. Flagella are composed of a type of protein called flagellin. The structures are anchored within the cytoplasmic membrane of the cell and protrude through the cell wall and outer membrane into the environment. They are frequently two to three times the cell length. They impart linear movement to the cell by means of a rotatory motion. The arrangement of flagella on a cell is usually constant for a species. Thus, cells which have a single flagellum at a polar position are monotrichous, those with a tuft of several flagella at a pole are lophotrichous, and those which have many flagella emerging all over the cell are peritrichous.

Fimbriae are short filamentous appendages on the

tabolism. The enzymes involved in the synthesis of membrane and cell wall are located in the cytoplasmic membrane. Attachment sites for the bacterial chromosome and plasmids are on the membrane and it plays a role in replication and segregation of these structures. It is the site of synthesis and secretion of many extracellular enzymes which function to breakdown macromolecules in the environment for subsequent use by the bacterial cell. There are structures called mesosomes made up of folded or rolled membranes which are attached to the cytoplasmic membrane that appear to play a role in transverse septum formation and/or DNA attachment.

surface of gram-negative bacteria. They are composed of a particular type of protein, pilin, and are thought to play a role in adherence of bacteria to tissues. A special type of fimbria, called the sex pilus, is found among bacteria which engage in conjugation. This structure plays a role in the transfer of DNA from one bacterial cell to another.

BACTERIAL ENDOSPORES

The genera *Bacillus* and *Clostridium* contain medically important species. Vegetative cells of both of these genera are characterized by the ability to differentiate into another cell form called an endospore. The endospore is a small cell formed within the vegetative cell from which it later is released. It is highly resistant to heat, drying, and toxic chemicals. Endospores retain viability for long periods (over 50 years). They germinate to form a vegetative cell after the period of dormancy. Because of their ability to withstand highly unfavorable conditions, endospores are used to test the efficacy of various procedures of sterilization. The heat resistance of endospores is related to their highly dehydrated state and to their content of calcium dipicolinate.

Growth of Bacteria

There are two aspects of bacterial growth to be considered, the increase in size of an individual bacterial cell, and the increase in number of cells, growth of the bacterial population. The growth of individual cells is of course the basis of population growth. Under appropriate conditions, a bacterium increases in size by synthesizing more of all its components. This process continues, accompanied by duplication of its DNA, until a critical size is reached when a transverse septum divides the cell and binary fission takes place yielding two daughter cells. Thus a linear increase in bacterial mass and a geometric increase in number occurs in relation to time.

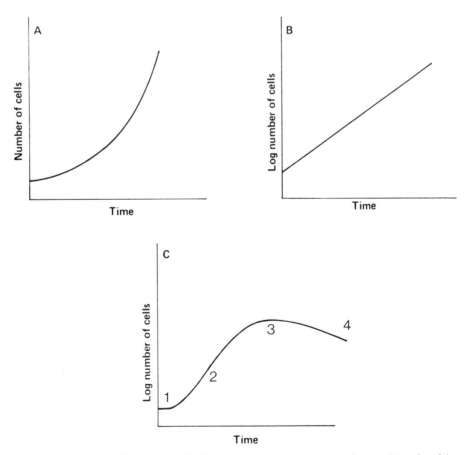

Fig. 5-5. (A) A plot of the number of cells v time results in an exponential curve. (B) A plot of the logarithm of cell number v time gives rise to a straight line. (C) Growth curve showing various phases of growth: (1) lag phase; (2) exponential phase; (3) stationary phase; and (4) death phase. (Milgrom F, Flanagan TD: Medical Microbiology. Churchill Livingstone, New York 1982.)

BACTERIAL GROWTH CURVE

The plot of the number of bacterial cells in a culture in relation to the time after inoculation of the culture is known as the bacterial growth curve. Theoretically, there should be an exponential increase in cell numbers. However, the internal changes occurring within the culture (nutrient depletion, toxic product accumulation) dramatically alter the outcome of population growth (Fig. 5-5). Plots of the actual numbers of bacterial cells in a culture are distinguished by four characteristic phases. An initial phase, called the lag phase, is observed when inoculum is obtained from an older stationary culture or from a culture grown on another carbon or nitrogen source. This phase is characterized by a lack of increase in cell number although there is an increase in average cell size. During this lag the cells are accumulating the enzymes and other metabolites necessary for optimal growth. The lag phase is followed by entry into a period of rapid cell proliferation, the exponential or logarithmic phase. This phase is characterized by an exponential increase in cell numbers. The average period of time between cell divisions is the shortest of all phases. The time between divisions is called the generation time

and is characteristic for a bacterial species under defined conditions. Cells in a culture growing at the exponential rate achieve the largest size for the species. They also have the greatest RNA content in relation to cell mass during this phase. When cells from logarithmic phase cultures are used to initiate new cultures on the same growth medium, growth of the new cultures begins immediately without a lag phase and maintains the characteristics of exponential growth.

Since logarithmic phase cells are growing in an environment with limited nutrients and space with consequent accumulation of toxic products, the conditions for continued exponential growth are rapidly lost and the culture enters into a stationary phase. In this stage, cell replication is offset by cell death, resulting in a steady state in which no increase in numbers of viable cells is observed. The stationary phase cells are the smallest for the species; they contain little RNA in relation to the cell mass. Use of theses cells to initiate a new culture results in a lag phase before exponential growth occurs.

After variable lengths of time (for various species), the death rate exceeds the rate of division and the culture enters the death phase. Cells from cultures in this stage are frequently atypical in size, shape, and even reactivity

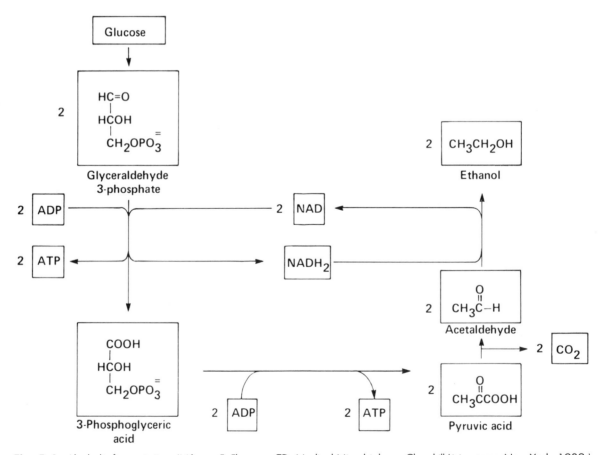

Fig. 5-6. Alcoholic fermentation. (Milgrom F, Flanagan TD: Medical Microbiology. Churchill Livingstone, New York, 1982.)

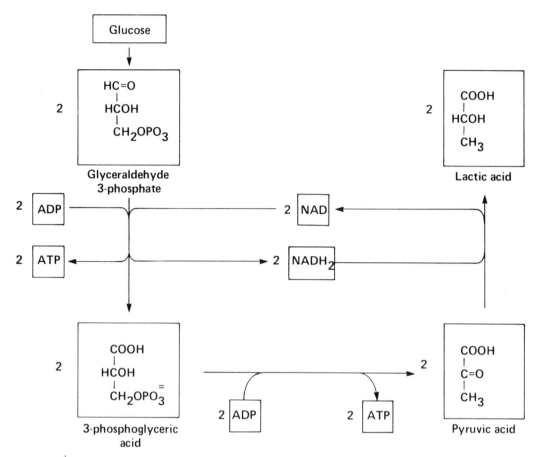

Fig. 5-7. Homolactic acid fermentation. (Milgrom F, Flanagan TD: Medical Microbiology. Churchill Livingstone, New York 1982.)

to the Gram stain. Some species of bacteria (e.g., *Streptococcus pneumoniae* and *Haemophilis influenzae*) release enzymes which bring about autolysis thus accelerating the death rate of cells in culture.

It is important to realize that for many species of bacteria the entire cultural cycle is completed within 24 to 36 hours. Therefore it should be kept in mind that examination of cultures after overnight incubation will result in observation of cells in the stationary or even death phase of the culture. This may result in misleading or difficult to interpret findings in procedures such as the Gram stain.

Energy Metabolism and Nutrition

Bacteria derive energy through a variety of mechanisms basically involving the production of adensosine triphosphate (ATP). Heterotrophic organisms utilize or-

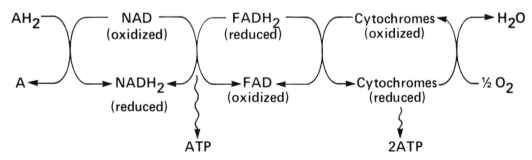

Fig. 5-8. The electron transport system. (Milgrom F, Flanagan TD: Medical Microbiology. Churchill Livingstone, New York 1982.)

ganic carbon sources transformed by the processes of fermentation and respiration to produce ATP as well as for the basic substances for cell structure. Autotrophs utilize light (photoautotrophs) for oxidation of inorganic substances (chemoautotrophs) to derive energy and use carbon dioxide as the basic carbon source for cell structure.

Since all pathogens and other bacteria which directly affect human health are heterotrophic, we will discuss only fermentation and respiration.

FERMENTATION

Fermentation is an energy releasing process in which organic compounds serve as electron donors (oxidation) and as electron acceptors (reduction). A basic process of fermentation occurring in many bacteria involves glycolysis of glucose to two molecules of pyruvic acid with the generation of two molecules of ATP and two molecules of $NADH_2$. Subsequently, the $NADH_2$ is reoxidized to NAD with the pyruvate acting as electron acceptor to generate two lactic acid molecules. Generation of ATP by this process is known as substrate level phosphorylation. In alcoholic fermentation pyruvic acid is enzymatically split to yield carbon dioxide and acetaldehyde (Fig. 5-6). The acetaldehyde acts as the final electron acceptor from $NADH_2$ to produce ethanol and NAD. When the end product of fermentation is a single compound the process is called homolactic (Fig. 5-7). When more than one product results it is called heterolactic fermentation. Many substances are fermented by bacteria including amino acids, purines, pyrimidines, and carbohydrates.

RESPIRATION

Respiration is an energy yielding process in which inorganic molecules act as electron acceptors. If the final acceptor is oxygen, the process is aerobic respiration; if the final acceptor is carbonate, nitrate, or sulfate, the process is anaerobic respiration.

During respiration, electrons are passed from the substrate to NAD to yield $NADH_2$. The $NADH_2$ is reoxidized by passage of the electrons to other acceptors which in chainlike relationships are alternately oxidized and reduced until the electrons are passed to the final acceptor (oxygen or other). As this process called oxidative phosphorylation progresses, energy is trapped at ATP molecules (Fig. 5-8). Respiration is more efficient in deriving energy (ATP) than fermentation. The tricarboxylic acid cycle is a respiratory cycle in which pyruvate is oxidized to carbon dioxide and water and ATP is generated through oxidative phosphorylation. Organisms which require oxygen as a terminal electron acceptor are

termed "obligate aerobes." Some organisms can use fermentation as an energy source in the absence of oxygen but will use aerobic respiration when oxygen is present. They are called facultative anaerobes. Obligate anaerobes are organisms which cannot grow in the presence of oxygen; indeed these organisms are killed as a result of their inability to remove toxic by-products of oxygen consumption such as H_2O_2 or the superoxide radical. Obligate anaerobes lack the enzyme superoxide dismutase which catalyzes superoxide to hydrogen peroxide and the enzyme catalase which converts hydrogen peroxide to oxygen and water.

BACTERIAL GENETICS

Inheritance in Bacteria

Bacterial characteristics are governed by genes present in the DNA chromosome of the cell and in extra chromosomal pieces of DNA called plasmids. Both of these structures duplicate and segregate to daughter cells during binary fission of a cell.

CHROMOSOMAL REPLICATION AND SEGREGATION

The circular DNA molecule of *E coli* has proved to be an important model for understanding the events of replication and segregation of the bacterial chromosome. The molecule is a covalently closed circle with a molecular weight of 3×10^9. Replication initiates at a single locus on the molecule, the replicator site, and proceeds bidirectionally around the circle. DNA synthesis takes place at two replication forks which move away from each other. The strands of DNA separate and short segments of complementary RNA are synthesized on the strands by an RNA polymerase. These sequences serve as primers for DNA polymerase III which synthesizes a complementary DNA sequence in the 5′ to 3′ direction. The antiparallel template strand is copied in short sequences, referred to as Okazaki fragments which are segments of about 1,000 bases connected to an RNA primer. The segments are processed by ribonuclease H which removes the primer and DNA polymerase I which replaces the removed RNA with DNA. The fragments are finally completed into a continuous strand by DNA ligase which joins the 5′ phosphoryl and 3′ -OH ends of the segments (Fig. 5-9).

The replication requires an unwinding of the supercoiled DNA strand which creates strains within the molecule. This is relived by a swivelase enzyme that causes breaks in a strand for a short period that are resealed immediately after unwinding.

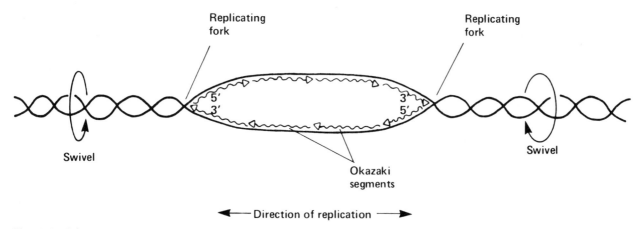

Fig. 5-9. Schematic representation of chromosome replication. (Milgrom F, Flanagan TD: Medical Microbiology. Churchill Livingstone, New York 1982.)

Replication takes place while the chromosome is attached to the cytoplasmic membrane of the cell. The daughter molecules are also attached at close but different sites. As replication ensues, membrane synthesis takes place between the sites of DNA attachment moving the molecules apart. This serves to separate the chromosomes toward opposite poles of the cell prior to cytokinesis (Fig. 5-10).

PLASMIDS

Many important bacterial characteristics such as drug resistance, the ability to transfer DNA between bacterial cells, toxigenicity, bacteriocin production, and metabolic activities are conferred by DNA in extrachromosomal segments called plasmids. Plasmids are circular, double stranded DNA molecules ranging from 5 to 140 megadaltons in size (7 to 200 genes). They attach to specific sites on the cytoplasmic membrane of the bacterial cell and undergo replication independently but often in synchrony with the bacterial chromosome.

Some plasmids have sequences of homology with the bacterial cell chromosome and are able to become integrated into the chromosome forming a single replicon. The same plasmid in one bacterial species may integrate readily into the host chromosome whereas in another species it may be separate.

Plasmids which carry information for a process of cell to cell transfer called conjugation are referred to as conjugative plasmids. Other plasmids may be transferred by temperate bacteriophages in the process of transduction.

BACTERIAL VARIATION

The complement of genes, chromosomal and plasmid, that are carried by a bacterium constitute the genotype of the cell while the expressed products of the genes constitute the phenotype.

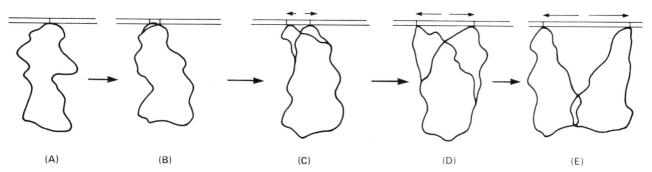

(A)   (B)   (C)   (D)   (E)

Fig. 5-10. Segregation of membrane-attached bacterial chromosomes during replication. (A) The chromosome is attached at or near the replication site. (B) After replication of this region, both daughter chromosomes are attached to the membrane. (C,D, and E) As replication ensues, the attachment sites are separated by biosynthesis of membrane between the sites. (Milgrom F, Flanagan TD: Medical Microbiology. Churchill Livingstone, New York 1982.)

PHENOTYPIC VARIATION

Among bacteria the phenotype is highly variable since the expression of various genes is stringently regulated and frequently affected by the physiologic state and environment of the cell.

Genetic regulation is usually achieved by induction, the initiation of synthesis of a gene product, or by repression, the shutting down of synthesis. In inducible systems, the inducer, usually a low molecular weight molecule and often the substrate of an induced enzyme, binds to the protein product of a regulator gene. The function of this regulator gene product is to bind to the operator locus of the inducible gene, thereby inhibiting transcription of that gene (Fig. 5-11). When the inducer binds to the regulator protein, it inhibits its function. Consequently, transcription of the inducible gene ensues and the protein is synthesized.

In repressible systems, regulator gene products are inactive (i.e., they fail to bind to operator loci). The system is activated when a low molecular weight molecule, often an end-product of metabolism, binds to the inactive regulator protein. This complex of regulatory protein and corepressor binds to the operator site and shuts off transcription of the gene in question.

GENETIC VARIATION

Variation in the genotype of an organism can occur by changes in the nucleotide bases of their DNA or by acquisition of new genetic material from exogenous sources. Change in the intrinsic DNA is mutation. It can occur spontaneously or result from the action of specific mutagenic agents. Mutant genes at a single locus are called mutant alleles in contrast to the wild-type allele found in organisms when first isolated from nature. Mutations which bring about changes in proteins compatible with continued replication will survive; whereas, those causing incompatible changes are lost. Several types of changes can occur in DNA to generate a mutant organism. Among the most frequent is base pair substitution, or point mutation, a change of a single base pair (e.g., thymidine-adenine may be replaced by guanine-cytosine). Such a mutation results in a change in the coding specificity of one codon which in turn may result

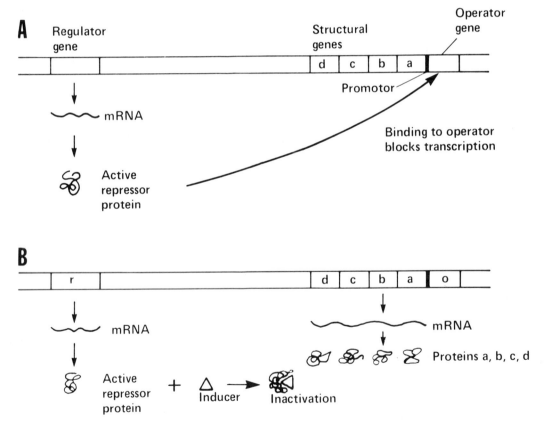

Fig. 5-11. The operon model for the regulation of inducible enzyme synthesis. (A) In the absence of inducer, the regulation gene product (repressor protein) binds to the operator gene and block transcription of genes a through d. (B) Inducer molecules react with the repressor protein, inactivating it and allowing transcription of genes a through d. (Milgrom F, Flanagan TD: Medical Microbiology. Churchill Livingstone, New York 1982.)

in an amino acid change in the primary structure of the polypeptide. Mutations of this type frequently are non-lethal or only conditionally lethal. Another frequently encountered mutation is the frame-shift mutation which results from the insertion or deletion of one or two base pairs in a sequence as a result of breakage of the sugar backbone of the DNA molecule. This changes the entire downstream reading sequence generating an entirely new set of codons. The other type of mutation is the deletion of long sequences from the DNA.

Spontaneous mutations occur in bacterial populations at a rate of 1 per 10^6 to 10^8 cell divisions. In any population, therefore, there is a small number of mutant cells. Most of these cells do not survive since mutation usually results in some impairment of function. However, the mutant may have some survival advantage under unusual environmental conditions and may proliferate at a greater rate than the wild-type bacterium. This process is referred to as selection and the environmental factor as the selecting agent. Many factors may act as selecting agents; some of the most significant in medical settings are antimicrobic drugs. Antimicrobic resistant mutants are selected in the presence of the drugs. This has important implications in the use and misuse of antimicrobics.

Genetic recombination is the other way in which variation of genotype occurs. DNA from exogenous sources can be transferred to bacterial cells wherein the DNA may become functional and confer new attributes on the recipient cells. Transfer of whole bacterial chromosomes in nature probably never occurs to any significant degree. However, fragments of bacterial DNA are transferred and often with significant frequency. The fragment of donated DNA is called the exogenote while the resident DNA of the recipient is called the endogenote. The recipient cell after acquisition of the exogenote is referred to as a merozygote as it is partially diploid. The capacity of an exogenote to survive in a recipient cell is dependent upon the DNA restriction-modification system of the donor and recipient strains of bacteria. Bacterial cells contain endonuclease enzymes (restricting enzymes) which cleave DNA molecules at specific sites. Endogenotes are protected from the activity of these enzymes by modification, usually methylation, of the bases at sites cleaved by the endonuclease. Exogenotes which do not have the same protected sites are degraded by the restricting endonucleases before methylation can occur. There exist complex patterns of restriction-modification compatibilities among genera, species, and strains of bacteria.

Recombination, the insertion of the exogenote into the endogenote, takes place by one of three mechanisms. Generalized recombination requires extensive homology of base sequences between the exogenote and endogenote. The process requires hydrogen bonding between bases, cleavage and crossing over of parental DNA strands, synthesis of a complementary sequence, and finally ligation of the strands. In *E coli* these activities are controlled by three chromosomal genes (i.e., *rec A*, *rec B*, and *rec C*). The process may produce an asymmetric recombinant molecule or a symmetrical molecule when the exogenote is double stranded.

Site-specific recombination is a special case which does not require sequence homology and is independent of the *rec* gene system. The circular DNA of lambda bacteriophage is inserted into the *E. coli* chromosome by this process. The two double stranded DNA molecules possess identical short (15 base) sequences at which integration occurs. A viral gene product, lambda integrase, mediates the breaking and rejoining of the strands at the site. Another viral gene product, excisionase, mediates the excision of the viral DNA (prophage) from the chromosome.

The third mechanism is called illegitimate recombination. This process does not exhibit site specificity and is independent of the *rec*-system. It is the way in which DNA sequences are transposed within and among replicons. Bacterial chromosomes and plasmids have sequences of 800–1400 base pairs, insertion sequences (IS), which can be transposed to another region of a DNA molecule. When inserted next to a gene, the IS can influence gene function. IS can carry other DNA sequences when transposed thus effecting transposition of other genes. When flanked by IS these genes are called transposons (Tn). IS and their included Tn elements undergo replication during transposition; one copy remaining in situ, the other integrating at another site.

Exogenotes do not always achieve integration into resident DNA. If the exogenote contains information for its own replication, it can function as an independent replicon. Several viral prophages and plasmids display this kind of autonomous replication. When an exogenote does not have the capacity for directing its own replication, it still may function (i.e., express its genetic information), but since it cannot replicate, it will be diluted out during cell growth. This situation occurs frequently in cases in which exogenotes are transferred by the process of transduction and is called abortive transduction.

TRANSFER OF DNA

Three processes for the transfer of bacterial DNA have been described. Several bacterial genera have been studied for their ability to take up DNA from the environment. The process, called transformation, occurs in *Streptococcus, Haemophilus, Neisseria,* and *Bacillus.* Some species of other genera can be induced to take up DNA by modification of the permeability of their outer membranes. Transformation has been most extensively studied in *Streptococcus pneumoniae* and *Bacillus subtilis.*

Transformation begins with the binding of the exogenous DNA to specific sites on the cytoplasmic membrane of the recipient cells. This is followed by cleavage of the double stranded molecule at the binding site. One strand of the exogenote enters by active transport across the membrane, the other strand is digested by nucleases. The ability of a bacterial cell to take up DNA in this manner is referred to as competence. It is associated with certain stages in the life cycle of cells, specifically during transverse septum formation and is probably a function of a protein responsible for binding, processing, and transporting the DNA molecule. *S pneumoniae* culture supernatants contain a protein, competence factor, which can confer competence on other *S pneumoniae* cells.

Competent cells take up DNA molecules between 3×10^5 to 3×10^6 daltons in size, excluding smaller and processing larger molecules. Bacteria such as *E coli* and *Pseudomonas aeruginosa* which require special treatment to become competent can take up quite large segments, the size of whole plasmids or bacteriophage genomes.

Another mechanism of genetic transfer is bacterial conjugation. This process has been intensively studied only among *Enterobacteriaceae* and some other gram-negative bacteria. Recent reports have also described similar cell-to-cell transfer in *Streptococcus faecalis.* The ability to initiate and carry out the transfer of DNA from one cell to another is dependent upon the presence of a plasmid in the donor cell. The plasmid contains the genetic information for its own transfer and replication. Such plasmids are called conjugative plasmids or fertility factors. Studies of the F1 plasmid in *E. coli* have resulted in elucidation of the conjugative transfer process. Cells containing the F1 plasmid or F factor are designated F^+ or male cells. They possess a surface appendage, the F pilus, which bears structures specific for receptors found in the outer membrane of F^- or female cells. Interaction of the F pilus with the receptor establishes and maintains cell-to-cell contact during DNA transfer. The exact role of the pilus in transfer is unknown. It may act as a bridge through which DNA is passed from the donor cell to recipient or it may function to draw cells together to establish a more intimate surface-to-surface contact. In either case, it is known that after contact is made, the F plasmid breaks at a specific site on the circular DNA molecule. One strand of the plasmid DNA is extruded from the F^+ cell into the F^- cell. The strand remaining in the original donor duplicates; thus maintaining the F^+ characteristic of the cell. The donated strand duplicates in the new cell and converts that cell from F^- to F^+. The

F1 plasmid contains 40 to 60 genes. Although specific gene products are not yet identified, it contains all the information for its own replication and transfer, including the structural elements of the F pilus. There are base sequences in the F1 plasmid homologous to sequences in the *E coli* chromosome. This permits the insertion of the plasmid into the chromosome by a double crossover event. In the integrated condition the plasmid replicates in concert with the chromosome. It retains its function of mediating transfer and, after contact of the sex pilus with an F^- cell, can bring about the transfer of part of the plasmid and some bacterial genes by the conjugative process. Strains bearing the integrated plasmid are designated Hfr. There are two significant differences in the conjugation of Hfr and F^+ bacteria. Hfr conjugation does not usually accomplish the transfer of the entire F1 plasmid because the break point divides the plasmid into two segments separated from each other by the entire bacterial chromosome. The fragile conjugation bridge usually breaks before an entire transfer can be accomplished leaving the recipient cell with part of the F1 plasmid and a variable complement of new bacterial genes. Since the complement of bacterial genes is a function of the time of contact, experimental disruption of conjugation after specified periods of time have enabled the construction of a detailed genetic map of the *E coli* chromosome. If Hfr conjugation the F^- recipient is not converted to F^+ (or Hfr) since in most cases the trailing segment of the F1 plasmid is not transferred.

In nature most strains of *E coli* are F^- because the plasmid replicates asynchronously (when not integrated) and more slowly with the chromosome. Hence the plasmid is diluted out among bacterial progeny. Also several other factors such as temperature and the existence of male-specific bacteriophages tend to give selective advantages to F^- strains.

Integration of F plasmids into the bacterial chromosome is a reversible event. In F^+ strains there are always a few Hfr cells and conversely in Hfr strains there are always a few F^+ cells. This situation arises because the plasmid can be excised by a double strand crossover event similar to that which brings about integration. One important consequence of this incision-excision dynamic is the occasional inclusion of bacterial genes in the excised segment. The entire plasmid with the included bacterial genes can be transferred by conjugation in a relatively efficient manner making recipient cells F^+ and stable diploid cells for those bacterial alleles transferred with the plasmid. Such modified F plasmids are called F′ or F′ genotes and the process of transferring the bacterial genes is called sexduction.

Probably the most common method of gene transfer in nature is transduction. This process involves the incorporation of bacterial genes into a bacteriophage particle and subsequent introduction of the genes into a recipient cell by the phage. All transducing phages are temperate; they enter into a state of lysogeny in the bacteria they infect. (For a description of lysogeny *see* the Medical Virology section.) There are two types of transduction, generalized and specialized or restricted. In generalized transduction, the prophage of the lysogenic bacterial cell becomes derepressed and vegetative phage replication takes place. As part of this replicative process, phage enzymes degrade bacterial DNA into fragments of variable size. During maturation of the phage, condensing factors interact with DNA and mediate the packing of the molecule into the bacteriophage head. For most particles, the head packages viral DNA, however, some particles package bacterial DNA, since the head structure only controls the amount of DNA not the type (bacterial or viral). Phage particles containing bacterial DNA are identical to those with viral DNA and are capable of adsorbing to bacterial cells. They introduce the bacterial DNA into the recipient cell by the same processes that viral DNA is introduced by normal virus particles. The bacterial genes thus introduced are subject to the same factors as any exogenote but if compatible, and recombination occurs, they become part of the genome of the recipient cell. The head capacity of a phage particle is 6×10^7 daltons or about 2 percent of the *E coli* chromosome. The efficiency of generalized transduction is related to the number of transducing particles, usually 1 in 10^5 to 10^6, and the compatibility of the modification-restriction systems of the donor and recipient bacteria. Generalized transduction can occur whether the prophage is integrated or nonintegrated.

Specialized transduction occurs only when a prophage is integrated at a particular site in the bacterial chromosome. When an integrated prophage is derepressed to enter into the vegetative phage of replication, it is excised from the chromosome. In a manner similar to the F′ genote, the prophage acquires some bacterial genes, those immediately adjacent to the integrated viral DNA. The excised prophage carrying the bacterial genes undergoes replication (amplification) and packaging into phage heads. As the head capacity is fixed, some DNA must be deleted, therefore, transducing phages are defective for some viral functions. This defect can be compensated for by infection of a bacterium by more than one phage particle.

RECOMBINANT DNA TECHNOLOGY

In vitro methods of DNA cleavage using restriction endonucleases and ligation with ligase enzymes have enabled the construction of DNA molecules carrying genes from different sources. Most commonly mammalian genes are spliced into plasmid or viral DNA which serves as a vector for insertion of the recombinant molecule into a host bacterial cell by the process of transformation. The presence of the recombinant molecule in the cell and its progeny confers a potential for production of large amounts of the gene product. Insertion of human genes for insulin, interferon, clotting factors, or other biologically important molecules gives promise of more highly enriched sources for human use.

ANTIBIOTICS AND CHEMOTHERAPY

Antimicrobial chemotherapy is based on the principle of selective toxicity. An ideal antimicrobial drug is one which is highly toxic to a defined group of microorganisms at low concentration and nontoxic to the patient. Antimicrobials in current use fall short of the ideal in several respects yet they represent one of the most important and effective tools for controlling human infectious disease. Selective toxicity is achieved by interrupting processes or destroying structures found in the microorganism and absent in the host. Such processes as cell wall synthesis, nucleic acid synthesis, cytoplasmic membrane function, protein synthesis, and intermediary metabolism are targets of antimicrobial action (Table 5-1).

Drugs are often referred to as bacteriostatic or bacteriocidal. "Static" drugs are those that inhibit microbial growth enabling the host defense mechanisms to clear the body of the organism. Removal of the drug allows renewed growth. "Cidal" drugs are those that kill the organisms directly and growth does not occur after its removal. The distinction breaks down when one realizes that drug concentrations can determine static or cidal results or that prolonged maintenance of bacteriostasis brings about bacterial death.

Many antimicrobial drugs are natural products of the metabolism of microorganisms which exercise an inhibitory effect on other microorganisms. Thus the agents of this antibiosis are called antibiotics. Medically useful drugs are often derived from cultures of these microorganisms. Most often they are derived from members of the genera *Bacillus, Streptomyces,* and *Penicillium.* Chemical modification of native antibiotic molecules has allowed production of drugs with different characteristics such as resistance to enzymatic breakdown or enhanced absorption.

In reality, few antimicrobial drugs are ideally selective in their toxicity. Most have some untoward side effects as a result of their pharmacological activity. In addition to direct toxicity of drugs, some have the potential to evoke an allergic response on the part of the host. Drug allergies may manifest with severe detrimental effects such as systemic anaphylaxis.

Table 5-1. Antimicrobic Drugs

Drug	Mode of Action	Spectrum of Activity	Comments
Penicillins	Inhibitors of cell wall synthesis by blocking transpeptidation		
Penicillin G		Gram-positives, *Neisseria*	Unstable in acid
Penicillin V		Gram-positives, *Neisseria*	Stable in acid
Ampicillin		Gram-positives and gram-negatives	
Methicillin		Gram-positives and gram-negatives	Resistant to penicillinase
Cephalosporin	Inhibits cell wall synthesis by blocking transpeptidation	Gram-positives and gram-negatives	Low allergenic potential
Bactitracin	Inhibits cell wall by binding to udecapsglycophosphate	Gram-positives	
Vancomycin	Inhibits cell wall synthesis by complexing with acyl-D-alanyl-D-alanine	Gram-positives	
Polymyxins	Cell membrane, detergent action	Gram-negatives	
Polymyxin B			
Polymyxin E			
Polyenes	Cell membrane, affinity for sterols	Fungi, mycoplasmas	Quite toxic
Nystatin			
Amphotericin B			
Griseofulvin	Inhibition of mitosis	Dermatotrophic fungi	Orally administered for prolonged periods in order to accumulate in keratinized skin
Rifampin	Inhibits transcription of DNA by RNA polymerase II by binding to the subunit of the enzyme	Pyogenic cocci, mycobacteria chlamydiae	Used in combination therapy to avoid emergence of resistant mutants
Aminoglycosides	Inhibit protein synthesis by binding to the 30 S subunit of bacterial ribosome blocking chain elongation and causing misreading of mRNA		
Streptomycin		Gram-positives, gram-negatives and mycobacteria	Chromosome resistance
Kanamycin		Gram-negatives (except pseudomonads and serratiae)	Systemic toxicity is high, used topically
Neomycin		Gram-negatives (except pseudomonads and serratiae)	
Gentamicin		Gram-negatives	
Tobramycin		Gram-negatives	Highly effective against pseudomonads
Amikacin		Gram-negatives	
Spectinomycin	Inhibits protein synthesis by binding to 30 S subunit of bacterial ribosome	Gram-negatives	Used to treat penicillinase-producing gonococci
Tetracyclines	Inhibit protein synthesis by binding to 30 S subunit	Gram-positives, gram-negatives, chlamydia, rickettsia, mycoplasma	Plasmid-mediated resistance
Tetracycline			
Chlortetracycline			
Minocycline			
Oxytetracycline			
Deoxytetracycline			
Chloramphenicol	Inhibits protein synthesis by binding to the 50 S subunit of the bacterial ribosome blocking peptide bond formation	Gram-positives, gram-negatives, chlamydia, rickettsiae, mycoplasma	Chromosomal and resistance, high level of systemic toxicity
Macrolides	Inhibit protein synthesis by binding to 50 S subunit of the bacterial ribosome blocking	Gram-positives, gram-negatives, chlamydiae, rickettsiae, mycoplasma	Chromosomal and plasmid resistance, low toxicity
Erythromycin			
Oleandomycin			

(Continued)

Drug	Mode of Action	Spectrum of Activity	Comments
Carbomycin Spiramycin	peptide bond formation		
Lincomycin Clindamycin	Inhibit protein synthesis by binding to 50 S subunit of the bacterial ribosome blocking peptide bond formation and chain initiation	Gram-negatives including *Bacteroides* spp.	
Sulfonamides Sulfalamide Sulfadiazine Sulfisoxazole Sulfamethazole	Inhibit folic acid synthesis	Gram-positives, gram-negatives, norcadiae, chlamydiae	Differential solubilities of drugs dictate use
P-aminosalicylic acid	Inhibits folic acid synthesis	Mycobacteria	Used in combination therapy
Isoniazid	Not known, possibly competitive inhibition of pyridoxine or nicotinamide metabolism	Mycobacteria	Used in combination therapy
Sulfones	Block folic acid synthesis	*Mycobacterium leprae*	
Ethambutol	Not known, possibly inhibits RNA synthesis	Mycobacteria	Used in combination therapy
Trimethoprin	Blocks DNA synthesis	Gram-positives and gram-negatives	Used in combination with sulfones for enteric fevers, urinary tract infection
Nalidixic acid	Blocks DNA synthesis damages cell membrane	Gram-negatives	Used in chronic urinary tract infections
Nitrofurantoin	Not known	Gram-negatives	Used for urinary tract infections
Flucytosine	Blocks RNA function	Fungi	Used in combination with Amphoterican B

Drug Resistance

Microbial resistance to the action of the various antimicrobial drugs is achieved through two basic mechanisms. Mutation plays a role in resistance mechanisms which are based on altered structure of a microbial binding component such as a ribosomal site or an enzyme. These altered binding sites have reduced or absent affinity for the antimicrobic and therefore the drug is not active on the organism. When a mutation like this occurs in a population of drug-sensitive bacteria in the presence of the drug, the resistant cell and its progeny have a selective advantage and rapidly replace the sensitive bacteria. Mutations of this type occur with a frequency of 1 in 10^7 to 10^{12} cell divisions.

Bacteria can also acquire resistance by gene transfer mechanisms. Chromosomal and plasmid resistance genes may be acquired by transformation, conjugation or transduction. Plasmids may contain several genes conferring resistance to several different antimicrobic drugs. The mechanisms of resistance include synthesizing enzymes which inactivate the drug, altering receptor sites, changing permeability to the drug, and mediating alternative metabolic reactions blocked by the antimicrobic.

Table 5-1 itemizes the major classes of antimicrobic drugs, their mechanisms of action, and their spectrum of use.

STERILIZATION AND DISINFECTION

The ability to inactivate or eliminate microorganisms, through the various physical and chemical agents of sterilization and disinfection, is critical to the control of infection in virtually all aspects of surgery and medicine (Tables 5-2 and 5-3). The methods used to achieve this are based on the problems presented by the most resistant of microbial forms, the bacterial endospore. Also

Table 5-2. Physical Methods of Decontamination

Agent or Process	Conditions		Effective On	Acts On	Remarks
Heat (with water)	5 to 10 min at pH < 3.5	55 to 60°C	Vegatative bacterial cells	Enzymes	Pasteurization
	30 min	62°C			
	1 min	72 to 85°C			
	20 min	121°C	Spores, fungi, vegetative bacterial cells, viruses	Enzymes, membranes, nucleic acids	Sterilization by autoclaving
Heat (without water)	1 to 2 hr	160°C	Spores, fungi, vegetative bacterial cells, viruses	Enzymes, membranes, nucleic acids	
Radiation	Infrared	>7600 Å	Spores, fungi, vegetative bacterial cells, viruses	Enzymes, membranes, nucleic acids	Actually sterilizes by heat
	Visible	3600 to 4500 Å			No antimicrobial activity; photo-reactivation
	Ultraviolet	2600 to 3100 Å	Spores, fungi, vegetative bacterial cells, viruses	Nucleic acids	Dimer formation between adjacent thyidine and uracil bases
	X-rays, gamma rays		Spores, fungi, vegetative bacterial cells, viruses	Enzymes, nucleic acids	Oxidation by free radicals; denaturation of DNA
Filtration Membrane filters	0.8 μm pore diameter	Yeasts, some large bacterial cells			
	0.45 μm pore diameter	Most vegetative cells			
	0.2 μm pore diameter	All bacterial cells and spores, some viruses			
	0.02 μm pore diameter	All microbial forms including viruses			

(Milgrom F, Flanagan TD: Medical Microbiology. Churchill Livingstone, New York, 1982.)

intrinsic to the problem is the role of water in affecting microbial death. Water is an active participant in the denaturative process which is the basis of most methods of sterilization and disinfection. In general, an agent (physical or chemical) which affects denaturation, does so more efficiently in the presence of water.

IMMUNOLOGY

Parenteral introduction of foreign substances (antigens) into the vertebrate host evokes a set of cellular interactions which result in the generation of effector molecules (antibodies) and cells (cytotoxic and other T-

Table 5-3. Action of Chemical Agents on Microorganisms

Agent	Concentration	Effective Against	Acts On	Remarks
Acids				
Mineral (HCl and others)	$0.01N$ to $>1N$	Spores, vegetative cells, viruses	Cell membrane, enzymes	Mycobacteria are relatively resistant
Organic (lactic and others)	1000 ppm	Vegetative cells	Cell membrane, enzymes	Mycobacteria are relatively resistant
Alkalis				
NaOH and others	$0.01N$ to $>1N$	Spores, vegetative cells, viruses	Cell membrane, enzymes	Mycobacteria are relatively resistant
Alkylating agents				
Ethylene oxide and formaldehyde	100 to 1000 ppm in solution	Spores, vegetative cells, viruses	Cell membrane, enzymes, nucleic acids	Can be used as a gas
Detergents				
Anionic	1000 ppm	Vegetative cells		Effect principally due to washing action
Cationic	1 to 1000 ppm	Vegetative cells	Cell membrane, enzymes	Some effect on spores
Dyes				
Crystal violet and others	0.1 to 100 ppm	Vegetative cells	Nucleic acids	Used in selective media, principally active on gram-positive organisms
Organic solvents				
Ethanol and other alcohols	50 to 70%	Spores, vegetative cells, some viruses	Cell membrane, enzymes	Not active against nonenveloped viruses
Oxidants				
Halogens				
I_2	2 to 7%	Spores, vegetative cells, viruses	Cell membrane, enzymes	Spores more resistant to Cl_2, O_3, and $KMnO_4$
Cl_2	200 ppm			
O_3	6 to 7%			
$KMnO_4$	1000 ppm			
Sulfhydryl poisons		Spores, vegetative cells, viruses	Enzymes	Very toxic
Hg and other heavy metals	>1.0 ppm			

(Milgrom F, Flanagan TD: Medical Microbiology. Churchill Livingstone, New York, 1982.)

lymphocytes). The effectors specifically recognize and react with the antigen which stimulated their production. Two unique characteristics of this response are specificity, the ability to recognize the particular antigen which stimulated the response, and immunologic memory, the ability to respond more quickly and with greater magnitude to antigens encountered previously. The mechanisms of the immune response reside in the cells of the immune system, particularly the various subpopulations of lymphocytes. The immune state may be active in that the individual may be stimulated by antigens to produce the effectors, antibodies or cells, or the immunity may be passive in that the effectors are produced by one individual and transferred to another. In the case of humoral immunity, that mediated by an antibody, transfer can be affected with serum. Cell-mediated immunity can only be transferred by cells.

Structure and Function

The immune system consists of collections of lymphocytes and other cells distributed in organs and tissues as well as in the blood and lymph. Lymphocytes are cells with a large nucleus and a thin rim of cytoplasm which vary from 5μm to $15\ \mu$m in diameter. They arise from pluripotent hematopoietic stem cells. During ontogeny, hematopoietic stem cells are found in the fetal liver and later in the bone marrow. The marrow remains the

Table 5-4. Distinguishing Characteristics of Human T and B Lymphocytes

	T-Lymphocytes	B-Lymphocytes
Maturation of precursor cells	Thymus	Fetal liver Gut-associated lymphoid tissue (?) Bone marrow (?)
Location in lymph nodes	Deep cortical region	Germinal centers and medullary cords
Electrophoretic mobility	High	Low
Surface by scanning electron microscopy	Tends to be smooth	Tends to be more hairy
Forms rosettes with sheep erythrocytes	Yes	No
Specific antigens by absorbed heteroimmune sera	Yes, raised against thymus	Yes, raised against chronic lymphatic leukemia or other B-cell sources
Surface receptor for Fc of IgG	No in most; yes for small subpopulation	Yes
Surface receptor for C3b	No	Yes
Presence of surface immunoglobin	No	Yes
Responsiveness to: PHA and Con-A Pokeweed mitogen *E coli* lipopolysaccharide	 High High Low	 Low High, in presence of T-lymphocytes High
Basis of surface specificity and capacity to combine with antigen	V region recepto on cell surface	IgM or IgM and IgD, other immunoglobulins

(Alexander, Good: Fundamentals of Clinical Immunology. WB Saunders, Philadelphia, 1977.)

source of lymphocytes throughout the life of the individual. Further maturation of lymphocytes occurs as the pluripotent stem cell gives rise to a precommitted (pre-B, pre-T) cell which undergoes further maturation in a central lymphoid organ. In mammals, the thymus serves to mediate the antigen-independent maturation of T-cells and bursal-equivalent tissues of the gut serve to mediate the antigen-independent maturation of B-cells. In birds there is a discrete well organized organ, the bursa of Fabricius, that mediates the maturation of B-cells (Table 5-4). Migration of B and T cells to peripheral lymphoid organs (lymph nodes and spleen) are necessary for further maturation which is dependant on the presence of antigen.

The mammalian thymus arises from the third and fourth branchial clefts of the embryo. The organ is organized into a cortex and a medulla. Connective tissue septa, contiguous with the capsule of the organ, form an infrastructure in the cortex around which small lymphocytes are densely packed. The medulla is characterized by epithelial cells organized into discrete aggregates, Hassal's corpuscles, surrounded by loosely packed lym-

phocytes. The microenvironment of the thymus is necessary for maturation of T-lymphocytes. These cells mature in the cortex and pass through the medulla into the blood and lymph principally through the thoracic duct. Many, perhaps most thymic lymphocytes do not leave the thymus but die in that site. The organ also has an endocrine function, producing hormonelike factors which are necessary for extrathymic maturation of T-cells. Among these factors are thymosin, thymic humoral factor, thymopoietin, and serum thymic factor.

Antigen-dependent maturation of T-cells and B-cells takes place in peripheral lymphoid organs, the spleen, and the lymph nodes. In certain pathologic processes peripheral lymphoid tissue functions can take place in the site of the process (e.g., lymphoid follicles in the thyroid in cases of Hashimoto's thyroiditis). The node is divided into three general areas, the outer cortical area made up of distinct germinal centers, the deep cortical area, and the medulla containing the cords (Fig. 5-12). The germinal center is made up of a central core of densely packed B-cells surrounded by a relatively sparsely populated rim containing both B and T-cells.

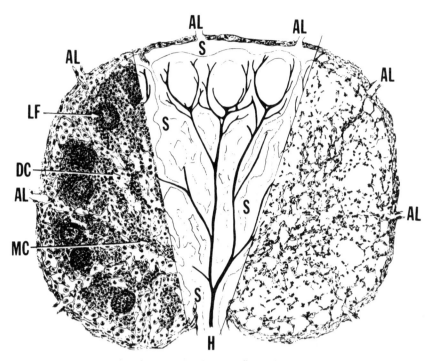

Fig. 5-12. Three views of a lymph node. AL, afferent lymph vessel; DC, deep cortical region; LF, lymphoid follicle; MC, medullary cords; S, sinus; H, hilus. (Weiss L: The Cells and Tissues of the Immune System: Structure, Functions, Interactions © 1972, p. 42. Reprinted by permission of Prentice-Hall, Inc., Englewood Cliffs, N.J.)

The rim is surrounded with a denser population of T-cells. Clinically, patients with Bruton type agammaglobulinemia have depleted B-cells populations in their nodes. In contrast, patients with DiGeorge's syndrome have depleted T-cells. The nodes of patients with severe combined immunodeficiency (Swiss type agammaglobulinemia) lack both types of cells. The spleen has a similar partitioning of B- and T-cells as seen in the lymph node but the areas of concentration are recognized in relation to the brachiating arteriolar system. In general germinal centers are found between bifucating penicilliary arterioles while T-cells are concentrated in periarteriolar sheaths.

Lymphocyte Populations

Reference has been made to the existence of two types of lymphocyte (B-cells and T-cells) differing from one another in the site at which they undergo "education," the bursal equivalent tissue of the gut or the thymus. These two types of lymphocytes are further distinguished by structural and functional characteristics. Table 5-4 lists these characteristics for human B- and T-cells. Analysis of each of these populations has revealed further complexity resulting from developmental and functional attributes. On their surfaces B-cells have immunoglobulins (Ig) which bear the specificity of the

antibody molecules to be secreted. However, the isotype of the heavy chain of the molecules is different during different stages of B-cell maturation. In addition certain other cell surface markers are associated with B-cell differentiation. These include receptors for the Fc portion of IgG molecules. C3b receptors and a class of molecules called class II (Ia in mice) associated with the gene complex governing the immune responses, the major histocompatibility complex (MHC) (Table 5-5).

T-cells bear marker molecules identifiable by allogeneic antisera and monoclonal antibodies. Thus the human T1 marker present on immature and mature thymocytes and all T lymphocytes is analogous to the murine Lyt-1 marker. Similarly, T3 bears resemblance to the Thy-1 marker appearing on mature thymocytes and T lymphocytes. The T4 marker has been associated with Lyt-1, however it is found on about 60 percent of peripherial T-lymphocytes and has been identified with helper/inducer function and delayed type hypersensitivity functions of these cells (Table 5-6). Further, a subpopulation of T4 bearing cells carry another marker, juvenile rheumatoid arthritis (JRA), associated with T-T helper functions. The T5–T8 subset, analogous to Lyt-2, Lyt-3 in the mouse, are associated with suppressor and cytotoxic functions.

An important aspect of lymphocyte biology is their ability to proliferate. Both T- and B-lymphocytes re-

Table 5-5. Isotype and Location of Associated Immunoglobulin and Presence of Class II Molecules on Cells of the B-Lymphocyte Line

	Cell Types				
	Pre-B-cell	Immature B-cell	B-cell	B-memory cell	Plasma cell
Location	Cytoplasm	Membrane	Membrane	Membrane	Secreted
Ig isotype	IgM	IgM	IgM+IgD	IgG, IgA, or IgE	IgM, IgG, IgA, or IgE
Presence of Class II molecules (Ia)	−	±	+	+	−

spond to mitogens by synthesizing DNA and cell division. T-cells are stimulated by conconavalin A (Con A) and phytohemagglutinin (PHA). Both T- and B-cells respond to polkweed mitogen (PWM), however B-cell response requires the presence and participation of T-cells. B-cells respond to bacterial LPS. Both types of lymphocytes exhibit antigen-driven proliferation. Antigen-driven responses are confined in their initiation to subpopulations of lymphocytes capable of binding a particular antigen on their surfaces (thus bearing specific receptors). This is the basis of clonal selection.

The Antibody Response

Humoral immunity is a property of an animal derived from the presence of specific immunoglobulins (Ig) in the serum and secretions which react with antigens. Antigens are defined as substances which, when introduced into the vertebrate body, evoke the production of Ig (and other effectors of response) that specifically react with them. Antigens are usually macromolecules and foreign to the body of the responder. Certain substances, haptens, can combine specifically with Ig but are unable to elicit an Ig response by themselves. Haptens are usually low molecular weight molecules often occurring as antigenic determinents or epitopes attached to or part of

larger molecules (carriers). The word immunogen is often used to specify the stimulatory aspect of antigen activity.

The mechanisms in the Ig response involve interactions among various subpopulations of lymphocytes and accessory cells, usually macrophages. In relation to the requirements for cell-cell interaction, we recognize two classes of antigen, T-dependent and T-independent. T-dependent antigens require the participation of antigen-specific T-helper lymphocytes to engender a response in the B-lymphocyte population leading to B cell clonal proliferation and eventual differentiation of B memory cells and Ig secreting plasmacytes. Removal of T-helper cells results in a lack of response to T-dependent antigens. T-independent antigens do not require T-helper cells, although macrophages normally participate in the stimulation by these antigens. The property of T-independence is apparently related to the molecular structure of an antigen. T-independent antigens are large molecules with repeating units of structure such as polysaccharides; in contrast, T-dependent antigens are often proteins and lack repeating units.

The antigen-dependent differentiation of B-cells begins with the recognition of the antigen by presentation on macrophages or T-lymphocytes. Recognition presumably is a function of the Ig combining site of the

Table 5-6. T-Lymphocyte Cell Surface Markers

Marker		Expression
Human	Murine	
T1	Lyt-1 (?)	Immature and mature thymocytes, A cell T-lymphocytes
T3	Thy-1 (?)	Mature thymocytes, all T-cells
T4	Lyt-1 (?)	Immature and mature thymocytes 60% mature T-cells (T helper)
T5 and T8	Lyt-2, Lyt-3	Immature and mature thymocytes, 30% mature T-cells (cytotoxic T, T suppressor)
T6	TL	Immature and intermediate thymocytes
T10		All thymocytes
T11		All T-cells (sheep erythrocyte receptor)

surface IgM and or IgD molecules on resting immature B-cells. Antigen recognition by surface Ig is necessary but apparently insufficient to stimulate B cells. Another condition must be met; the antigen must be presented in the context of an appropriate class II (Ia) molecule. These molecules are found on macrophages and lymphocytes and are products of genes found in the MHC. Physiologic stimulation occurs when there is a self-self relationship between the Ia molecules of the antigen presenting cell and the responding B-cell. Proliferation of the cells results in giving rise to mature B-cells bearing surface either IgG, or IgA, or IgE or IgM. B-memory cells bearing these isotypes do not undergo further differentiation but cease to proliferate and become resident in peripheral lymphoid organs. Other mature B cells continue proliferation and further differentiate into Ig-secreting plasmacytes. Plasma cells secrete Ig molecules of the identical isotype and specificity as the B-cells from which they arose.

This process is normally under stringent regulation of the immune system itself. The T-suppressor cell population functions to directly or indirectly inhibit lymphocyte proliferation. Other mechanisms which may or may not involve T-suppressors such as the idiotype-anti-idiotype network may also be operative in regulation. Antigen-driven proliferation occurs in T-cell populations as well as B-cell, thus enhancing T-helper and T-suppressor responses.

The classical description of primary and secondary antibody response can now be understood in terms of the cells involved. In the primary response, small numbers of specific IgM- or IgM and IgD-bearing immature B lymphocytes encounter and bind an antigen for the first time. The cells undergo proliferation giving rise to a limited number of clones specific for that antigen. Some cells differentiate into B-memory cells bearing either IgG or IgE or IgA on their surfaces. Others differentiate into IgM or IgG or IgA or IgE plasmacytes which secrete their Ig into the serum or secretions. In the primary response, most secreting cells produce IgM at least early in the response or when confronted with low immunogenic doses of antigen. Upon a second or subsequent exposure to the same antigen, B-memory cells resident in peripheral lymphoid tissues immediately begin differentiation into Ig-secreting cells. Thus the characteristic dramatic increase in antibody titer is detected within hours of antigen administration. The magnitude and rapidity of IgG, IgA, and IgE responses reflect the number of Ig-bearing memory cells with those isotypes.

Antibody Structure

Antibody activity is the property of globulin molecules found in blood serum and various other body fluids and secretions. Because of their common characteristic of being synthesized as a result of antigenic stimulation and of being able to react with (bind to) the antigen, they are called immunoglobulins (Ig) (Table 5-7). The basic structure of all Ig is a four chain molecule, two identical light (L) chains of 23,000 molecular weight (MW) and two identical heavy (H) chains of 53,000 to 71,000 MW depending upon the isotype of the Ig. H chains are bound to each other by disulfide bonds while each L chain is associated with one H chain. In some isotypes disulfide bonds hold the L and H chains together, in others, other forces are operative. Antibody activity (combining site) is associated with the amino termini of both L and H chains while other biological properties (i.e., complement fixation, placenta passage, etc.) are associated with the carboxy termini of the chains, particularly the H chain.

Ig are divided into five classes (or isotypes) which differ from one another in several characteristics. They have different molecular weights, electrophoretic mobilities, and biological properties, and are found predominantly in different body sites. The basic differences such as size, composition (carbohydrate components), and antigenicity reside in the H chain of the molecules. Class or isotypic specificities on H chains determine the five types, μ in IgM molecules, γ in IgG, α in IgA, δ in IgD, and ϵ in IgE. L chains also have two antigenic types, κ and λ, either of which may associate with H-chains of any class. Thus the molecular formula of any Ig molecule may be expressed using the chain composition (i.e., an IgG molecule may be 2 γ-2 κ or 2 γ-2 λ).

The classes of Ig molecules may be further subdivided into subclasses based upon antigenic make-up and other properties. There are four subclasses of IgG in humans, IgGl, IgG2, IgG3, and IgG4 which vary in their ability to participate in complement fixation as well as antigenicity. Similarly there are subclasses of IgM (IgM1, IgM2) and IgA (IgA1, IgA2).

Ig molecules are found associated with B lymphocyte plasma membranes in their basic monomeric form (H_2L_2) whatever their isotype. However, IgM and IgA molecules are found in polymeric form in serum or secretions. IgM occurs as a pentamer held together by another 15,000 MW polypeptide, termed J-chain, thus the formula is $(\mu_2\lambda_2)_5 J$. IgA is found in serum as either a monomer $(\alpha_2\lambda_2)$, a dimer $(\alpha_2\lambda_2)_2 J$ or a trimer $(\alpha_2\lambda_2)_3 J$. In secretions, IgA occurs as a dimer with an addition 74,000 MW polypeptide termed secretory piece or transport ("T") component. One formula for secretory IgA (sIgA) is $(\alpha_2\lambda_2)_2 JT$. Secretion of sIgA across epithelial tissues involves transit through epithelial cells which is apparently mediated by the T component.

The electrophoretic mobilities of Igs in serum have long been used to describe them. The partition of globulins into alpha, beta, and gamma classes was observed in early investigations, thus antibody activity was asso-

Table 5-7. Various Properties of Human Immunoglobins

	IgG	IgA	AgM	IgD	IgE
Normal adult serum concentration (per dl)	1.0–1.4	0.2–0.3	0.4–0.15	0.003	10^{-3}–10^{-4} (average $\approx$ 10^{-4})
Distribution	Intravascular and extracellular fluid	Intravascular and internal secretions	Mainly intravascular	Mainly intravascular	Intravascular and skin, respiratory and GI tracts
Molecular weight	150,000	155,000 (395,000 for sIgA)	900,000	185,000	187,000
Molecular weight of the H chains (MW of the L chains $\approx$ 23,000)	53,000	55,000	65,000	70,000	71,000
Nomenclature of H chains	γ	α	μ	δ	ϵ
Molecular formula	$\gamma_2\kappa_2$, $\gamma_2\lambda_2$	$\alpha_2\kappa_2$, $\alpha_2\lambda_2$	$\mu_{10}\kappa_{10}J$, $\mu_{10}\lambda_{10}J$	$\delta_2\kappa_2$, $\delta_2\lambda_2$	$\epsilon_2\kappa_2$, $\epsilon_2\lambda_2$
Valency	2	2 (monomer)	10	2	2
Normal κ/λ chain ratio	2/1	5/4	3/1	1/6	–
H chain subclasses	IgG1, IgG2, IgG3, IgG4	IgA1, IgA2,	IgM1, IgM2	Ja, La	–
Approximate occurrence of the H chain subclasses (%)	75, 15, 7, 3	93, 7	–	85, 15	–
Number of domains per H chain	4	4	5	5	5
Allotypes (all immunoglobulins wih κL chains have InV = Km allotypes)	Gm	Am	Mm	–	–
Carbohydrate (%)	2.9	5–10	12	13	12
Synthetic rate (g/day/70 kg)	2.3	1.7	0.1	0.03	2×10^{-4}
Half-life (days)	23	6	5	3	
Complement binding (via the classical pathway)	+	–	+	–	–
Involvement in opsonization	+	–	+[a]	–	–
Placental transport	+	–	–	–	–

(Continued)

	IgG	IgA	AgM	IgD	IgE
Other important biological properties	Major Ig in antimicrobial defense; Ig with strongest precipitating capacity	Major Ig (in secretions) in antiviral defense	Major Ig produced in the primary response; Ig with strongest agglutinating capacity	Present on the surface of B lymphocytes of the new born	Involved in atopic allergy; increased in parasitic infections

a In the presence of complement only.

(Reprinted with permission from van Oss CJ: General physical and chemical and biological properties of the human immunoglobulin. In Greenwalt, TJ, Steane EA (Eds): Blood Banking, Vol. II CRC Handbook Series in Clinical Laboratory Science. CRC Press, Cleveland, 1980. Copyright, The Chemical Rubber Co., CRC Press, Inc.)

ciated principally with the slowest moving species, the gamma globulins, although some activity was observed among beta globulins. These terms are now somewhat supplemented by other more precise terms yet the designation gamma globulin as used is roughly equivalent to IgG. (Similarly the terms 7 S and 19 S globulins deriving from sedimentation characteristics in reference to IgG and IgM are sometimes encountered.) The properties of human Ig are summarized in Table 5-7.

Structural studies on Ig molecules have been carried out on preparations of myeloma proteins. These proteins are the products of plasmacytomas and unlike Ig found in normal serum, are structurally identical. Digestion of IgG preparations with the enzyme papain yields

two fragments termed Fab and Fc. Two Fabs are generated for each Fc residue, and contain whole L chains and part of the H chains. The Fc fragment is constituted of parts of the two H chains. When generated from purified antibody molecules, the ability to bind to antigen resides on the Fab fragment.

Further structural analysis of myeloma Igs revealed that certain regions of the molecules were constant in their composition when different myelomas were compared; these regions were called constant (C) regions. These regions were further divided into domains which were globular in structure and tended to aggregate. The C regions were found to reside on both L and H chains, with one domain on an L chain and three or four domains (depending on isotype) on the H chains. IgG and IgA have three H chain C domains while IgM, IgD, and IgE have four. It was also found that each Ig molecule had unique regions that were variable in their amino acid sequences, that is each myeloma Ig had unique and characteristic variable regions (V) as well as constant (C) regions identical to other myeloma proteins of the same isotype. The V regions were found on the Fab portion of the molecule and both the L chain and H chain components of the Fab had one variable region each. Thus each polypeptide chain of the Ig molecule is composed of a V region and C region. The C region further divided into one domain for L chains and three or four domains for H chains (Fig. 5-13).

ANTIBODY SYNTHESIS

One of the classical problems of immunology was to account for the capacity of the immune system to recognize a seemingly unlimited variety of antigens and respond by the production of antibody molecules specific for those antigens. To account for this, two kinds of theories were evolved, instructive theories and selective theories. Instructive theories held that the antigen directly or indirectly influenced the conformation of the Ig molecule conferring the specificity of the antibody com-

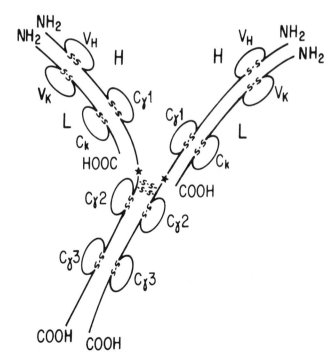

Fig. 5-13. Diagram of the domains of the tetrapolypeptide IgGl. (Milgrom F, Abeyounis CJ, Kano K. Principles of Immunological Diagnosis in Medicine. Lea and Febiger, Philadelphia, 1981.)

bining site. Selective theories held that all specificities are preexisting and that the antigen merely selects the proper Ig molecule. Present understanding of cellular mechanisms and antibody synthesis confirms selection as the basis for the immune response.

The clonal selection theory of Burnet was based on the theory of Jerne which had postulated the existence of natural antibodies of all possible specificities. Jerne held that the antigen selected the proper antibody and thereby evoked an overproduction of that particular molecule. Burnet elaborated the idea of selection by assigning the production of an antibody to particular lymphoid clones and accounting for changes in amounts of antibody of a particular specificity to expansion of a clone. His theory also accounted for several other characteristics of the immune response including self-recognition and immunologic memory.

Modern efforts using the techniques of molecular genetics have produced insights into the mechanisms of antibody formation and provided a basis for understanding antibody diversity. Sequencing studies on purified myeloma proteins had demonstrated the basic structure of immunoglobulins and revealing the existence of variable (V) and constant (C) regions of the polypeptide chains. It was clear that antibody specificity was associated with the variable regions and perhaps more precisely with the hypervariable sequences within them. Since the V regions were part of the same polypeptide chain as the C regions, a new concept in polypeptide synthesis was required; that two genes could give rise to one polypeptide molecule. Initial work on the kappa light chains of the mouse showed that the gene sequences for V-kappa and C-kappa regions were widely separated in embryonic cells. Later in ontogeny the sequences were found in closer proximity separated by several sequences termed J sequences and other interviewing sequences. Eventually in fully mature Ig secreting cells, the V sequence was separated from C by one J sequence. This change in location was acccomplished by a rearrangement of DNA sequences and excision and splicing of RNA transcripts to form the functional mRNA. Amino acid sequence data suggests there are about 30 V-kappa genes and since four to six related V-kappa genes are demonstrable with each V-kappa DNA probe, there are probably 100–200 V-kappa genes in germ line DNA. Similar analyses have demonstrated only one C-kappa gene. Since there are four functional J sequences (of five known), it is clear there is considerable potential for diversity in the structure of mouse kappa light chains.

Analysis of heavy chain structure has proceeded in a similar manner. The problem here is more complicated in that the antibody specificity associated with the V_H region must accompany two or three different isotypes carried on the C_H portion of the chain (i.e., a clone of cells carries surface Ig of a given specificity, V_H, on a mu chain and/or delta chain, later switching to secretion of Ig bearing the V_H associated with gamma-chain). Germ line DNA contains all sequences determining isotype borne on the C domains in the left to right order $C\mu$, $C\delta$, $C\gamma3$, $C\gamma1$, $C\gamma2b$, $C\gamma2a$, $C\epsilon$, and $C\alpha$. During ontogeny, the particular V_H sequence characterizing the specificity of the antibody, associates with two other sequences termed D and J by rearrangement of DNA. In the immature B cell these sequences are expressed by their transcription in tandem with the $C\mu$ or $C\delta$ immediately adjacent. Processing of the transcript gives rise to an mRNA molecule with the VDJ region attached to a $C\mu$ or $C\delta$ sequence. Later in ontogeny, a rearrangement and deletion occurs in the DNA, inserting another C region bearing another isotypic determinant, for example $C\gamma2a$, adjacent to the VDJ sequence. Transcription and processing then gives an mRNA coding for a heavy chain of the $\gamma2a$ isotype bearing the specificity determined by the VDJ sequence which had previously been on μ or δ chains. This rearrangement is called the "heavy chain switch." The recombination of DNA necessary for this process is a property of specific homologous sequences termed S or switching sequences at the 3′ end of each C_H sequence.

The random combination of V_L chains (100–200 κ and 4λ) with 5J chains and C_L chains (1 κ and 2λ) can give rise to 1,004 different chains. When these light chains associate with heavy chains arising from the combination of 200 V_H genes, 10 D sequences and 4 J_H regions there are some 8×10^6 possible different specificities generated. In addition to this potential diversity generated by combination of different DNA sequences, still further diversity is generated by apparent somatic mutation in V_H sequences. The total number of specificities possible has been estimated to be of the order of 10^9.

ANTIBODY-ANTIGEN INTERACTIONS

The capacity of an Ig molecule to recognize and bind to its antigen is its distinguishing characteristic. This reaction in vivo is the basis of protective immunity as it may lead to subsequent lysis of cells or phagocytosis and clearance of the antigen or neutralization of some toxic property or infectivity of the antigen. It is also the basis of a number of harmful reactions such as anaphylaxis, immune complex deposition, and autoimmunity.

Studies of antibody-antigen reactions in vitro are termed "serologic studies" and serology is the source of much of our knowledge concerning these reactions. Serologic procedures are also important tools in the diagnosis and management of many diseases.

The reaction of antibodies with antigens borne on the

surface of particles or cells (as opposed to molecules) results in the agglutination of the particles or cells. The agglutination reaction is a very sensitive procedure for the detection of antibodies. The reaction is relatively rapid, taking place within a few minutes, and visible clumping is readily observed. In the laboratory, agglutination tests are often centrifuged to enhance the reaction. Agglutination reactions, because of their sensitivity, are desirable methods for the detection of antibodies. To exploit this many passive agglutination tests have been developed. In these tests soluble antigens are attached to particulate carriers such as red blood cells or latex particles and reaction with an antibody can then be detected readily by agglutination. Sensitive detection of an antigen can be enhanced by using these tests in an inhibition format.

The reaction of antibodies with soluble antigens can result in precipitation. This results from the cross-linking of bivalent IgG (usually) and a multivalent antigen. The reaction is conceived as a two-step phenomenon. The first step is the reaction of the Ig with individual antigen molecules followed by a second stage in which large cross-linked lattices of antigen-antibody complexes form which ultimtely precipitate from solution. This probably is a simplistic view of the reaction which may well result from other nonspecific aggregating effects such as nonpolar interactions created by the initial antibody-antigen reaction. It is possible to set up a series of dilutions of antigen, varying the concentration over considerable range. Precipitate forming after the addition of antibody can be weighted, thus an accurate quantitative measurement may be made of the reactions. An observation frequently made in such precipitating systems is that there is less precipitate formed in tubes containing higher concentrations of antigens than that formed in tubes with lower concentrations. At still lower concentrations, small amounts of precipitate are formed. This phenomenon is referred to as the prozone phenomenon and has led to the concept of optimal proportions of immune precipitations. This concept holds that under conditions of high antigen concentration (antigen excess) the available antibody molecules are consumed by the many antigen molecules leaving few opportunites for cross-linking. At the other end of the scale, at very low antigen concentration (antibody excess) the opposite conditions exist and antibody molecules saturate all available antigen sites and cross-linking is again reduced. At the optimal concentrations of antigen and antibody the proper stoichiometry exists to promote extensive cross-linking and hence an optimal amount of precipitate. Experimental testing of this concept has shown that precipitates can be dispersed by the addition of antigen to create antigen excess or of antibody to create antibody excess. In general precipitation reactions are not particu-

larly sensitive methods to detect antibody (usually requiring more than 10^{-4} to 10^{-6} g of Ig). However, they can be quite useful for demonstrating antigen in some cases. The precipitation method has proved to be a powerful analytical tool when the reaction has been allowed to take place within a gel matrix. The most familiar of gel techniques is the double-diffusion technique of Ouchterlony. In this method antibody and antigen solutions are placed in wells in a gel. The reactants diffuse radially from the well and at some point between the wells encounter one another. The reaction takes place at that locus and when enough reactants have participated, precipitation takes place. The precipitation takes the form of a line in the gel (actually a plane or surface). The contours of the line may form an arc due to differences in diffusion rates between the reactants. Thus the position of the precipitate and shape of the line are functions of the diffusion rates and these rates are in turn functions of concentration and size of the diffusing molecules (Fig. 5-14). The method can discriminate two or more react-

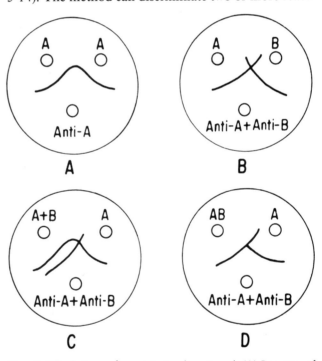

Fig. 5-14. Pattern of precipitation lines in gel. (A) Reaction of identity. The same antigen from the two upper wells diffuses into the gel and precipitates with its antibody diffusing from the lower well. (B) Reaction of nonidentity. Two different antigens diffusing from the upper wells form independent precipitin lines when each antigen reacts with its antibody. (C) Multiple reactions. Mixture of antigens in one well and a single antigen in the other react with a mixure of antibodies. (D) Reaction of ''partial'' identity. Two antigenic determinants on one particle form a spur of precipitate with mixture of antibodies to each determinant. The A-anti A precipitation forms a reaction of identity, the spur results from the B-anti B reaction. (Van Oss CJ: Antigens in Antibodies. p. 21. In Milgrom F, Abeyounis CJ, Kano K (eds): Principles of Immunology Diagnosis of Medicine. Lea & Febiger, Philadelphia, 1981.)

ing systems in any mixture of antigens and multispecific antiserum. Each reacting antibody-antigen system will form its own line of precipitation. The method can be used to examine the antigenic relatedness of antigens by diffusing them from separate wells against a single antiserum.

A widely used modification of the double diffusion gel precipitation technique is immunoelectrophoresis. In this technique a complex antigen mixture such as serum is electrophoresed to separate antigens by differential migration in the electric field. These now separated antigens are allowed to diffuse against an antiserum containing one or more antibodies. Precipitation arcs form showing each antibody-antigen system. Immunoelectrophoresis of human serum is used to detect abnormalities in serum proteins such as in multiple myeloma (Fig. 5-15).

In counterimmunoelectrophoresis the reaction between the antibody and antigen is enhanced by the enforced undirectional migration of the antigen by electrophoresis (antibody moves anodally because of endosmosis). The sensitivity of the reaction can further be enhanced by the addition of an antiglobulin reagent (antibody raised to Ig in another species) to the gel after removal of all soluble (nonprecipitated) reactants.

Other precipitation methods in gels include the radial diffusion technique in which antigen in a well is allowed to diffuse into gel containing its antibody to form a ring of precipitate. Since there is a constant concetration of antibody, different concentrations of antigen will form

rings of different diameters. The diameters of the rings can be used to calculate the concentration of antigen in unknown preparations. This technique is often used to quantify various Igs in serum.

Another important serologic test is complement fixation, a procedure based upon the ability of antigen-antibody complexes to bind a series of normal serum proteins collectively called complement. An important property of complement when fixed by antigen-antibody complexes on the surface of cells is the capacity to lyse the cells. The reaction is called immune lysis or hemolyis when erythrocytes are used. In the classical complement fixation test, as may be used in serodiagnosis of mumps, a known amount of antigen is added to dilutions of a patient's serum and a measured amount of exogenous complement is also added. The normal complement present in the patient's serum must be inactivated by heating prior to the test. After incubation, an indicator system consisting of sheep erythrocytes reacted with rabbit antisheep erythrocyte antibody, is added to the test. If complement has been consumed ("fixed") by reaction of any antibody in the patients' serum with the antigen there will be no lysis of the sheep erythrocytes. On the other hand, hemolysis will take place in any dilution in which there is insufficient antibody.

Labeled antibody techniques have become widely applied techniques. All of these techniques are based on the attachment of a marker to an antibody molecule. Fluorochromes such as fluorescein and rhodamine allow the localization of antibody-antigen reactions in immunofluorescence (IF) procedures. The technique can be used as a direct test in which the fluochrome is conjugated to the antibody which reacts with the antigen in question. For example, the demonstration of herpes simplex virus antigen in biopsy material is often carried out by direct IF. The biopsy tissue is usually fixed to a glass slide and overlaid with a dilution of antiherpes simplex antibody conjugated with fluorescein isothiocyante. After washing, the tissue is examined microscopically with ultraviolet light. The presence of a green flourescence in cells of the biopsy constitutes a positive test. If tests are also conducted using indirect procedures. Indirect tests utilize fluoresceinated antiglobulin antibodies which are applied as a second step after reacting the antigen with an unlabeled antibody. The antiglobulin conjugate may be directed against whole globulin of the species of the antibody or may be more specific, directed against the isotype of reacting Ig. Using known antigen substrates the indirect IF procedure may be used to detect and quantify antibodies in serum.

Radioimmunoassay (RIA) and enzyme immunoassays (EIA) have very wide application. Both techniques are highly sensitive and used for the detecion of antigens as well as antibodies. RIA procedures are based upon the

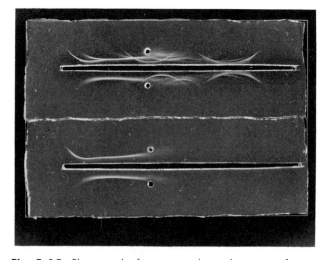

Fig. 5-15. Photograph of an immunoelectropherogram of serum from a patient with a monoclonal gammopathy (upper wells) and a normal subject (lower wells) run against anti human serum (upper trough) and antihuman IgG (lower trough). (Photograph courtesy of Dr. C. J. van Oss and Mr. D. T. Mount.)

radiolabeling of the antibody and subsequent measurement of radioactivity as the method of quantification. In EIA, enzymes such as horse radish peroxidase or alkaline phosphatase are conjugated to the antibody molecule. An enzyme substrate which gives a colored reaction product is added to the system and the color measured.

Complement

Normal serum and plasma contain a series of eleven proteins which when activated react in sequential fashion to produce a number of important effects in immune clearance and inflammation (Table 5-8). This system, the complement system, can be activated in two ways, referred to as the classical pathway and the alternative pathway (Fig. 5-16). The activation of the classical pathway is dependant upon the reaction of the first complement component, C1, with an appropriate Ig molecule or molecules. Reaction of IgM, IgG1, IgG2, or IgG3, but not IgG4, IgA, IgD, or IgE with antigen brings about a conformational change in the Ig which enables a reaction with C1q. The bound C1q in concert with C1r, C1s, and Ca ions forms an active enzyme which cleaves its natural substrates C2 and C4. Binding of the C1 complex requires one IgM or at least two IgG molecules to react

Table 5-8. Proteins of the Complement System

Components	Molecular Weight
C1q	410,000
C1r	168,000
C1s	83,000
C2	117,000
C3	200,000
C4	209,000
C5	205,000
C6	95,000
C7	120,000
C8	163,000
C9	79,000

with antigen. (Definitive studies on the C pathways are conducted in erythrocyte-antierythrocyte systems and therefore hemolysis is the end result of complement activity. It should be kept in mind that C can react with antibody-antigen complexes other than those on cell surfaces.) Control of C1 activity is achieved by the action

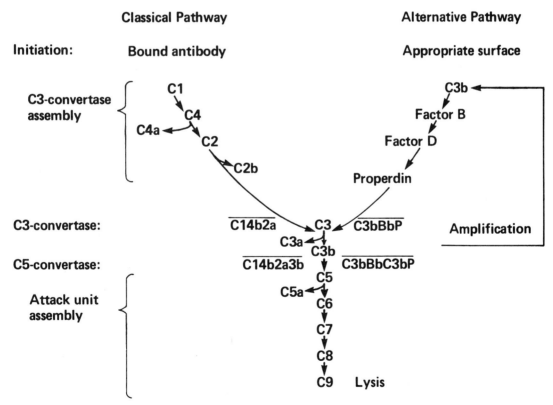

Fig. 5-16. The sequence of events in activation of complement by the classical and alternate pathways. (Milgrom F, Flanagan TD: Medical Microbiology. Churchill Livingstone, New York, 1982.)

of C1 esterase inhibitor (C1 IHN). A genetic defect leading to absent or reduced levels of C1 INH results in hereditary angioedema. The fixed C1 complex, called the recognition unit, cleaves C4 into two fragments, a low molecular weight C4a and a larger C4b which adheres to the antigen surface (of a cell) in proximity to the C1. C1 also cleaves C2 into two fragments, a small C2b and a large C2a. C2a and C4b, in the presence of magnesium ions, form an enzymatically active complex, C3 convertase. C2b and C4a are released into the fluid phase. The C3 convertase (C2aC4b) cleaves its natural substrate C3 to release a small C3a fragment and fix a larger C3b fragment. The C3a is an anaphylotoxin causing histamine release from mast cells or other granulocytes thereby participating in inflammation. The C2aC4b complex can be inactivated by the action of a C4 binding protein found in serum. This affects a regulation of the system at this point. The C2aC4bC3b complex cleaves the C5 protein into the small C5a, another anaphylotoxin, and a larger fragment, C5b. The activity of C2aCrbC3b is the last enzymatic activity in the complement cascade; the subsequent reactions are binding activities. C3b is regulated by two proteins β_1H globulin which binds to it causing inactivation by cleavage by C3b inactivator (C3bINA). The latter also inactivates C4 in the presence of the C4 binding protein.

The C5b fragment has affinity for membranes and immune complexes. The fragment is rather unstable and will become inactive unless stabilized by C6 (either on a membrane or in fluid phase). The complex C5b67 constitutes the initial element in the attack or cytolytic sequence. The complex has affinity for cell membranes and binds to them. The binding is independent of the recognition (C1) and activating complexes (C2aC4bC3b) and may take place on adjacent (bystander) cells. C5b67 further bind the last two components of the system C8 and C9. This final complex C5b6789 forms transmembranal channels in cell membranes allowing influx of water, ions, and small molecules thereby affecting cytolysis.

The alternative pathway of complement activation occurs in the absence of a functional recognition unit (C1) and implements another mechanism to produce C3 convertase activity rather than the C2a4b complex of the classical pathway. The activity is generated by the unique properties of certain surfaces such as those of zymosan, some bacteria, some immune complexes, and those of dialysis membranes. These surfaces are capable of binding C3b in serum. In the normal metabolism of C3, small amounts of C3b are constantly being formed. Most of this material is inactivated by β_1H globulin and C3bINA. However, certain surfaces can bind C3b in a way to protect it against inactivation. Another serum factor, B is cleaved by and binds to C3b to form a com-

plex C3bBb which is analogous to C2aC4b. Cleavage of factor B is dependent upon the presence of another serum factor, D, and magnesium ions. The C3bBb complex is unstable and may be stabilized by yet another serum factor, properdin (P). Thus the stabilized complex C3bBbP acts to generate activated C3b fragments which in concert with it (the C3bBbP) acts as C5 convertase. The analogous C5 convertase complexes are C2aC4bC3b for the classical pathway and C3bBbPC3b for the alternative pathway. The generation of C5a and C5b has the same consequences for the alternative pathway as for the classical.

BIOLOGICAL ACTIVITIES OF COMPLEMENT

The lytic property of the complement cascade is operative in vivo and is a basic mechanism of defense against certain bacteria. Both the classical and alternative pathways undoubtedly participate in bacteriolysis. In addition, the complement may enhance phagocytosis through the mediation of C3b. This factor whether generated by the classical or alternative pathways, fixes to surfaces. Many phagocytic cells have a C3b receptor on their surfaces, thus the presence of the factor on the surface of a cell or particle, may mediate interaction of the receptor-bearing cell and the target surface. Precise data demonstrating this mechanism has not been published, however. There are important in vivo activities ascribed to the C5a and C3a fragments relating to chemotaxis and vascular permeability. In addition C5a seems to augment the adhesiveness of PMN to surfaces and cause aggregation of these cells. The factor also stimulates the oxidative metabolism of the PMNs. All of the C5a stimulated responses of PMNs are related to a specific receptor on the phagocyte's surface. Activities of C5a and C3a are regulated by another serum enzyme, a carboxypeptidase-B like activity.

Major Histocompatibility Complex

The major histocompatibility complex (MHC) is a set of genes found in all vertebrate species (so far examined) which codes for two types of glycoprotein molecules found on the surface of cells. Some of the genes code for class I molecules which are single glycopeptide chains of 43 k MW with three globular domains (similar to domains on Ig) and are anchored in the cell membrane. The chains are associated with β_2 microglobulin. Class II molecules are coded for by other genes of the MHC. These molecules consist of an α chain and a β chain both of which are anchored in the cell membrane. Each chain is glycosylated and has two globular domains. Alpha chains are larger (34 k in humans, 33 k in mice) than β chains (28 k in humans and mice). The two chains are apparently coded for by two very closely linked genes which are never expressed independently of one another. Conceptually, they are treated as a single gene. A third class of molecule, class III, is coded for within the MHC but structurally and functionally these molecules are unrelated to class I and class II.

Class I and class II molecules are distributed widely in the tissues and each tissue varies in amount of the molecules expressed. Lymphocytes and macrophages are rich sources. Functionally class I and class II molecules are critical in the antigen-presenting and recognition steps in the immune response. Class I molecules are concerned with the activities of cytotoxic lymphocytes while class II molecules are concerned with helper and suppressor functions. Present understanding of cell-cell cooperation in immune response and its regulation conceives that antigen presentation under normal physiologic conditions must take place within the context of self-self recognition, a function of the MHC gene products.

The MHC is a highly polymorphic system. In the human system, the human leukocyte antigen (HLA), there are four loci, A, B, C, and D(DR). At the HLA-A locus there are at least 17 serologically defined (SD) alleles. HLA-B has 32 SD alleles and HLA-C has 8 known SD alleles. HLA-A,B, and C code for class I molecules. The HLA-D(DR) locus was originally defined by mixed lymphocyte reactions and therefore is designated lymphocyte defined (LD). Twelve alleles have been demonstrated at this locus. D(DR) genes code for class II molecules. In mice, the best studied species, the MHC is called H-2 and consists of three regions, K, D, and I. Another region, S, is found within H-2, but it codes for class III molecules. The I region of H-2 is divided into five subregions, A, B, J, E, and C. Genes within the H-2K and H-2D regions code for class I molecules while those in the I region code for class II. The H-2 class I genes are extremely polymorphic; there are 29 H-2K alleles and 38 H-2D alleles. The class II genes of the I region were once assumed to be five in number but experimentally only products of two regions have been demonstrated, I-A and I-E. These products, Ia molecules, have been shown to be actually the product of two very closely linked genes in the I-A region A_α and A_β (Ia-1). The I-E region product has also been shown to be a product of two genes, A_e (in the I-A region) and E_α in the I-E (Ia-5). There are 21 known alleles for the I-A (A_α-A_β) loci and 6 known alleles for the I-A and I-E loci. The gene products of H-2 genes are serologically defined with allogeneic antisera although cell-mediated immune responses are also demonstrable.

The gene products of the MHC are alloantigens and evoke strong immune responses in allogeneic hosts. They were first described as blood group antigens and later as transplantation antigens. While we currently recognize their significance in their function of antigen recognition and regulation of immune response, they are also important in the biology of transplantation.

Cell-mediated Immunity

The immune state mediated by Ig is referred to as humoral immunity. In contrast, there are immunologic reactions in which the effectors are cells. These cells recognize and react with antigens in the same way as Ig molecules. The immune state confirmed by these cells is called cell-mediated immunity. While humoral immunity may be transferred by serum, cell-mediated immunity (CMI) can only be transferred from one individual to another by lymphocytes. More specifically CMI resides in the T-cell population. The afferent limb (stimulatory) of the response is similar to humoral immunity as it requires recognition of antigen by T-helper cells within the context of the Ia or Ia-like class II molecule on the surface of a macrophage. T-T interaction ensues through the agency of soluble factors including interleukin-2 and perhaps direct contact.

The effectors of CMI are T-lymphocytes belonging to the subsets identified by the T4 marker (T_{DH}) and by the T5–T8 markers (T_c). The T_{DH} cells are the cells which participate in classical delayed hypersensitivity reactions such as the tuberculin reaction. They are characterized by their proliferative response to antigen and their concomitant release of biologically active soluble factors (lymphokines) during proliferation (Table 5-9).

The T5–T8 subpopulation contains cytotoxic T-lymphocytes (T_c). These cells are able to recognize antigen-bearing cells and kill them by direct contact. The direct interaction of the T_c cell and the target cell requires compatibility at the MHC locus. This phenomenon has been called associative recognition.

Other Types of Cellular Cytotoxicity

Several other types of cellular cytotoxicity have been described. Macrophages can, upon activation, exhibit direct cytotoxic activity on target cells. They do not exhibit immunologic specificity in this reaction although the state of activation results from antigen-triggered T-cell activity. Antibody molecules bound on the surface of macrophages by Fc receptors can confer specificity of antigen recognition for cytotoxic interactions.

Other cell-types also display this form of antibody-mediated cellular cytotoxicity (ADCC), among them are immature monocytes, eosinophils, polymorphonuclear neutrophils, and null cells (lymphoid cells without surface Ig or T-cell markers). Null cells active in ADCC are called killer or K cells.

Natural killer (NK) cells are a population of lymphoid

Table 5-9. Lymphokines

Factor	Active On	Activity
Migration inhibitory factor (MIF)	Macrophages	Inhibits cell migration
Macrophage activation factor (MAF)	Macrophages	Increased cell adherence, phagocytosis pinocytosis, glucose metabolism, bacteriocidal activity
Monocyte chemotactic factor (MCF)	Macrophages, monocytes	Positive chemotaxis
Leukocyte inhibitory factor (LIF)	Granulocytes	Inhibit cell migration
Neutrophil chemotactic factor (NCF)	Granulocytes	Positive chemotaxis
Lymphocyte mitogenic factor (LMF) (Blastogenic factor)	Lymphocytes	Causes lymphocyte proliferation
Lymphotoxin (LT)	Variety of target cells	Cytotoxicity
Osteoclast-activating factor (OAF)	Osteoclasts	Increase osteclastic activity
Interferon (IFN)	Variety of cells	Antiviral, antiproliferative activity, stimulates NK activity
Transfer factor (TF)	Lymphocytes (?)	Transfer of specific reactivity

cells which are directly cytotoxic for a variety of tumor cells and virus-infected cells. They lack surface Ig and T-cell markers but murine NK cells bear a unique alloantigen NK-1. NK cytotoxicity apparently does not require MHC compatibility.

Manifestations of CMI

The in vivo demonstration of CMI is carried out by skin testing. In the classical tuberculin test, purified protein derivative (PPD) of tuberculin is injected into the skin. A positive test is manifested by induration and erythema at the site of injection. The intensity of the response is greatest 24–48 hours after introduction of the antigen. Histologically, the positive reaction is characterized by infiltration with mononuclear cells (both lymphocytes and macrophages). The reaction, as exemplified by the positive tuberculin skin test, is often referred to as a delayed hypersensitivity reaction. Cells found in the sites bear the T4 marker and are capable of elaborating lymphokines as stated above. Various in vitro tests for lymphokine activities have been developed. However, unequivocal demonstration of these activities in vivo has not been reported.

Immediate Hypersensitivity

Hypersensitivity refers to an exaggerated immune response which results in harm to the host. There are four mechanisms of hypersensitivity, three of which are due to the action of antibody molecules. The best studied of these mechanisms is that mediated by IgE. Upon stimu-

lation with antigen, some genetically predisposed individuals respond by elaborating an antibody response, a major part of which is IgE. This class of Ig is homocytotropic and as such adsorbs to the surface of mast cells and basophils. If the cell-bound IgE encounters antigen as a result of reexposure of the individual, cell surface antibody-antigen complexes are formed and the cell releases granules into the environment. Bridging of two or more IgE molecules by the antigen is necessary to effect degranulation of the mast cells or basophils. Chemical mediators released by degranulation are responsible for the symptoms of immediate hypersensitivity. The more important mediators in humans are histamine, serotonin, and the slow reacting substance of anaphylaxis (SRS-A).

Release of large amounts of mediators at disseminated sites can cause anaphylactic shock. The mediators evoke smooth muscle contraction and extravasation of fluids. These responses can precipitate symptoms in humans dependent upon the particular site at which the antigen is introduced (Table 5-10).

Two other forms of antibody-mediated immediate

Table 5-10. Manifestations of Anaphylaxis in Man

I. *Dermal:* Flushing erythema, urticaria, angiodema

II. *Pulmonary:* Laryngeal edema, bronchospasm

III. *Gastrointestinal:* Nausea, vomiting, diarrhea

IV. *Circulatory collapse:* Oppression in chest, apnea, fall in blood pressure

Rose NR, Milgrom F, Van Oss CJ: Principles of Immunology. MacMillan, New York, 1978.

hypersensitivities are ADCC reactions and immune complex-mediated reactions. The clinical significance of ADCC is unknown, on the other hand, immune complex-mediated responses seem to be the basis of a number of disease states. Serum sickness is a well studied model of immune complex disease in which deposition of the complexes in extravascular sites is accompanied by complement activation and inflammation at the site. Most frequently the glomerlus is involved. However, other sites such as the choroid plexus and the lung can be involved.

Immunology of Transfusion and Transplantation

The practice of blood transfusion and the transplantation of solid tissues are based upon the recognition of allogeneic antigens. Alloantigens are antigens present in some individuals of a species and absent in others. Upon introduction into individuals who do not have the antigen as a part of their constitution, an immune response is mounted. The first studied allogenic system was the ABO blood group system. Landsteiner, in 1900, observed the agglutination of human erythrocytes by human sera and deduced from the pattern of reactions that humans belonged to one of four groups. Groups were determined by the presence of two antigens, A and B, on the erythrocyte surface. Cells bearing A alone determined the A blood group, B alone, the B blood group, A and B, the AB blood group. Cells bearing neither antigen determined the O blood group. Landsteiner and his colleagues further determined that antibodies against the A and B antigens occured naturally in the serum of persons whose red cells did not bear an A or B antigen. Thus group A persons have anti-B, group B have anti-A, group O have both anti-A and anti-B and group AB have neither antibody. The source of immunologic stimulation for these antibodies is not known. However, the A and B substances occur widely and their presence on enteric bacteria probably provide antigenic stimulation. The anti-A and anti-B agglutinins are usually IgM but IgG antibodies also occur.

The clinical significance of the ABO bloodgroup system relates to the severe reactions which occur upon the transfusion of incompatible cells into a recipient. Intravascular hemolysis results from the fixation of complement by the reaction of the natural antibody with the incompatible cells. The concept of universal donor, group O and universal recipient, group AB arise from the fact that O cells have neither A nor B antigen and AB individuals have neither antibody.

The inheritance of the ABO blood groups is determined by three alleles A, B, and O. The A allele codes for

α-D-N-acetygalactosamine transferase while the B allele codes for α-D-glalactose transferase. The O allele is apparently amorphic. Expression of the A or B phenotype is dependent upon another independent gene, H, which codes for fucosyl transferase, an enzyme which catalyzes the transfer of α-L fucose to the terminal galactose of erythrocyte glycolipids. This reaction generates H substance, the substrate for the A and B transferase reactions.

A and B are codominant alleles, therefore the presence of either gene results in expression of the antigen. Heterozygous AO and BO persons are phenotypically group A and group B respectively while A and B heterozygotes are group AB. The homozygotic AA and BB individuals are phenotypically indistinguishable from AO and BO. Group O persons are always homozygous OO. The A and B substances as well as H are present on the cells of several organs other than erthrocytes. In addition they can be found in soluble form in secretions from about 80 percent of the population. The ability to secret the substances is controlled by a secretor gene. The dominant allele *Se* codes for a glycosyl transferase whose action permits the activity of fucosyl transferase producing H substance on soluble or cell-bound substrates. The recessive allele *se* inhibits the fucocyl transferase activity except on cell-bound substrates; thus H and consequently A and B are not found in secretions.

The other clinically significant human blood group system is the Rh system. While controversy exists over nomenclature and the precise nature of the antigens, it is agreed that several antigenic specificities are coded for by the genes of this system. Two systems of nomenclature based upon different concepts of the system have arisen and are in common use. The Weiner system, based upon a single locus theory, uses the designations Rh_0, rh, hr, rh', hr', rh," and hr" for specificities detected within the system. The Fisher-Race model holds that there are three very closely linked alleles (such that crossover between them does not occur) which are inherited as a block. The system uses the designations, C, D, E, c, d, and e for the alleles (Table 5-11).

There are two clinical situations of importance involving this system. The first concerns incompatible pregnancy. In this case D/d alleles are most significant. Pregnant women lacking the D allele (Rh_0-) can be immunized by their fetus' D-bearing erythrocytes. Such anti-D (Rh_0) antibodies can cross the placenta and react with the erythrocytes of the fetus causing their removal from the fetal circulation and deposition in various tissues. This can result in death of the fetus in severe cases or in hemolytic disease of the newborn (HDN). The antigenic potency of the Rh antigens is of low order; therefore, the first incompatible pregnancy rarely results

Table 5-11. Most Common Alleles (Haplotypes) of the Rh System and Their Specificities

Allele or Haplotype[a]	Allele (Haplotype) Frequency in Whites	Phenotypic Specificity[b]			
R^1	0.41	rh′	Rh$_0$	hr″	rhi
CDe		C	D	e	Ce
R^2	0.14	hr′	Rh$_0$	rh″	–
cDE		c	D	E	cE
R^0	0.03	hr′	Rh^0	hr″	hr
cDe		c	D	e	ce(f)
R^z	0.002	rh′	Rh$_0$	rh″	–
CDE		C	D	E	CE
r	0.39	hr′	–	hr″	hr
cde		c	–	e	ce(f)

[a] Allele and haplotype correspond to Wiener's concept of a single locus or to Fisher's concept of three loci.
[b] Designations correspond to Wiener's (first line), Fisher's (second line) nomenclatures.
(Modified from Zaleski, Dubiski, Niles, et al: Immunogenitics. Pitman, Marshfield 1983.)

in HDN. The antigenic stimulus provided by the large influx of fetal red cells into the maternal circulation at parturition serves to sensitize the mother. Subsequent incompatible pregnancy will provoke an anemnestic response and the IgG antibodies will cross the placenta. The disease can be avoided by treating mothers who deliver incompatible infants with an anti-D antibody preparation. Apparently this passively acquired antibody serves to remove the incompatible red cells from the maternal circulation without allowing significant antigenic stimulation.

The second clinically significant aspect of the Rh blood group system is related to transfusion. Donor and recipient of blood are matched for the D(Rh$_0$) antigen as well as the ABO blood group. While natural antibodies against the D(Rh$_0$) antigens do not occur, incompatible blood can evoke an antibody response. Such antibodies could cause HDN in fetuses carried by women recipients of incompatible transfusions. Also, the immune response could cause a hemolytic reaction if further transfusions of incompatible blood were done.

In transfusion practice, donor and recipient are matched for the ABO blood group and the D(Rh$_0$) antigen. In addition a major compatibility crossmatch is conducted. This procedure is carried out to detect any antibodies in the recipient serum which will react with antigens on the donor cells.

As stated previously, the products of the MHC are potent alloantigens, and as such are important in transplantation. The human MHC, called HLA, codes for class I, class II, and class III molecules. The alleles at three loci, A, B, and C, code for class I and a single (or two very close loci) D(DR) locus has alleles which code for class II. Class III molecules are irrelevant to transplantation. The class I and class II molecules constitute a major barrier to the transplantation of tissues because they evoke a vigorous immune response in recipients. Thus the name major histocompatibility antigens is applied to them. There are also minor histocompatibility antigens which evoke weak immunologic responses. These minor histocompatibility antigens can be demonstrated in mice when grafts are exchanged among animals that are compatible as the major histocompatibility loci. In humans, these minor antigens seem to have some significance in bone marrow grafting. The major antigens have significance in the clinical practice of transplantation of kidneys and other organs as well as bone marrow.

The modern practices of transplantation have developed through the use of immunosuppressive therapy and the ability to match donor and recipient by tissue typing. The HLA phenotype is determined by complement-mediated cytotoxicity using reagent antisera. The antisera are derived from multiparous women or recipients of many blood transfusions. They are usually monospecific, reacting with class I molecules on lymphocyte surfaces. The alleles at the A and B loci are usually determined in clinical tissue typing procedures by testing the peripheral lymphocytes of a prospective recipient against a panel of reagent sera. The panel consists of one or more antisera against each of the known A and B specificities. Matching of donor and recipients at these loci within nuclear families (since siblings share parental chromosomes) reduces allogeneic differences and may increase the survival of grafts.

MEDICAL BACTERIOLOGY

Bacteria cause disease by the invasion of the tissues of the body and/or by the elaboration of toxins. These two facets of pathogenicity, invasiveness and toxigenicity, are usually both active to some degree in any infection; however, some diseases are principally intoxications (e.g., botulism) whereas others are due almost exclusively to invasiveness (e.g., pneumococcal pneumonia). A third factor contributing to the pathogenesis of any infection is the immune status of the host in regard to the significant antigens of the bacteria. For example, *Corynebacterium diphtheriae* causes diphtheria by elaborating a potent toxin which contributes to the local infection in the throat and to the systemic disease. Humoral antibodies to the toxin in an immunized host neutralize the toxin and protect against the systemic expression of the disease. These antibodies do not prevent the colonization of the nasopharynx with *C diphtheriae* nor the development of localized wound infections with the organism. This example emphasizes a protective role for the immune response and in most cases the response to infections is beneficial to the host. However, immune response itself can contribute to pathology and form an integral component in the pathogenesis of some diseases. For example, the formation of immune complexes and their subsequent deposition in glomeruli are seen in cases of bacterial endocarditis caused by several bacteria.

The following pages present various groups of bacteria with their salient morphologic and cultural characteristics and their disease associations.

The Pyogenic Cocci

Pyogenic cocci are associated with infections characterized by pus formation. The group consists of the gram-positive genera *Staphylococcus* and *Streptococcus* and the gram-negative genus *Neisseria* (Tables 5-12 and 5-13). While they are involved in local infections, there are also many situations in which they participate in generalized disease including intoxications.

THE STAPHYLOCOCCI

The two type species of the genus *Staphyloccus* are the prototypic pathogen, *S aureus* and the prototypic non-pathogen, *S epidermidis.* The pathogenic *S aureus* causes a variety of diseases from abcesses to systemic intoxication. The pathogenicity of the organism is attributed to its ability to elaborate a variety of enzymes and toxins, coupled with its ability to evade the host response. Staphylococci produce four hemolysins (α, β, γ, and δ) and a leukocidin all of which contribute to tissue destruction. The organism further protects itself against host response by the action of coagulase, the leukocidin, and Protein A. These factors are regarded as operative in the hallmark lesion of staphylococcal infection, the abcess. The organisms can also elaborate toxins which have other effects. Exfoliatin, a toxin active in the scalded skin syndrome, brings about the exfoliation of stratum granulosum cells of newborns. Other toxins are apparently active in disease such as toxic shock syndrome and Kawasaki disease. Most strains of *S aureus* produce an enterotoxin which causes food poisoning. The enterotoxin is odorless, tasteless, and relatively resistant to heat and proteolysis. It is often responsible for early onset food poisoning (2–6 hrs after ingestion).

S epidermidis is found on the skin and mucous membranes as is *S aureus.* It is regarded to have low pathogenic potential and has principally been associated with small local lesions of the skin but occasionally with endocarditis and urinary tract infections.

THE STREPTOCOCCI

Streptococci are ubiquitous microorganisms found in many environments. They are regarded as fastidious in their nutritional requirements and are usually associated with animals or their products. The streptococci pathogenic for humans fall into several catagories. The most prominent pathogenic species is *Str pyogenes* (Group A,β-hemolytic). This organism causes infections which are often characterized by extension and spreading through tissues, in contrast to the abcess formation of the staphylococcus. The streptococcal disease process is attributed to a variety of enzymes and toxins which promote spread. Some strains of *Str pyogenes* also produce an exotoxin, erythrogenic toxin which causes scarlet fever. Certain strains are also associated with acute post-streptococcal glomerulonephritis. This is an immunopathologic disease caused by deposition of immune complexes in the kidney. Another immunologic consequence of *Str pyogenes* infection is rheumatic fever. *Str agalactiae* (Group B,β hemolytic) is an important pathogen in the newborn period. It is the leading cause of meningitis in the first few weeks of life. Infections during this period frequently involve the lung as well as the meninges. In adults, Group B infection are much less frequent and similar in nature to Group A disease.

The enterococci are a group of streptococci which are found in the enteron. As a group, they are generally more resistent to environmental conditions then are other streptococci. They are normal inhabitants of the human body and are regarded as opportunistic pathogens. They are most frequently involved in endocarditis (about 4 percent of the cases) and urinary tract infections (16.3 percent of cases). Enterococci are more resistant to the usual antibiotics and therefore etiologic diagnosis is important in cases where they are active.

The viridans group of streptococci are normal inhabitants of the mouth and oropharynx. Certain members are active in caries formation (*Str mutans*) and perhaps peridontal disease. They are also the most frequent organisms associated with endocarditis.

The organism *Str pneumoniae* is an opportunistic pathogen of major significance. While the organism is frequently found in the normal throat, introduction into the lower respiratory tract leads to lobar or bronchial pneumonia. Pneumococci are the most frequent causes of lobar pneumonia with 50 percent of all cases caused by serotypes 1, 2, and 3. In childern type 14 is the most frequent cause. There are 82 serotypes defined by the antigenicity of their capsular polysaccharide. This structure is regarded as the principal pathogenic factor and antibody against the type-specific antigen is responsible for recovery from infection and protection against subsequent infection with the same serotype. Pneumococci

Table 5-12. Gram Positive Cocci

Name	Colonial Morphology	Microscopic Morphology	Clinical Diseases Forms	Toxins and Pathogenicity Factors	Significant Antigens	Significant Biochemical or Serologic Tests
Staphylococcus aureus	1.5 mm, golden pigment on nutrient agar strains cause clear hemolysis on sheeps blood agar	Clusters of gram + cocci	Abses formation in skin and other organs, pneumonia, enterocolitis, food poisoning, associated with scalded skin syndrome, toxic shock syndrome, Kawasaki disease	α-Lysin β-Lysin α-Lysin δ-Lysin Exfoliatin, enterotoxin, leukocidin, protein A	Teichoic acids (ribotal type)	Coagulase test (positive), techoic acid antibodies, strain typing by bacteriophage
S epidermidis	1.5 mm, white pigment on nutrient agar, few strains cause clear hemolysis on sheeps blood agar	Clusters of gram + cocci	"Stitch" abseses		Teichoic acids (glycerol type)	Coagulase test (negative)
Streptoccus pyogenes (Group B, β hemolytic)	0.3–0.5 mm, clear glistening on sheep or human blood agar, clear (β) hemolysis	Gram + cocci in chains, some strains are encapsulated	Acute pharyngitis and extension into middle ear, sinuses and mastoid air cells, skin infections, cellulitis, puerperal sepsis, pneumonia, scarlet fever, poststreptoccal glomerulonephritis, rheumatic fever, poststreptococcal arthritis	Streptolysin O Streptolysin S Hyduronidase Streptokinase Streptodornase Erythrogenic toxin	C substance (determining Lancefield Group A) M protein (60 serologic types) T proteins	Antistreptolysin O (ASO), antistreptococcal enzyme tests, sensitive to bacitracin in vitro
Str agalactiae (Group B, β hemolytic)	0.3–0.5 mm, clear glistening on sheep or human blood agar, β hemolytic	Gram + cocci in chains	Early onset meningitis of newborns (1st week), late onset meningitis of newborns (2–4th week), other infections in adults similar to Group A	Type-specific antigens	Type Ia, Ib, Ic, II, and III antigens	Resistant to bacitracin, cAMP test positive
Str faecalis (Group D enterococcus) variety *faecalis* variety *liquifacieus* variety *zymogenes*	0.3–0.5 mm, clear glistening on sheep or human blood agar, nonhemolytic (*faecalis, liquifacieus*) or β hemolytic (*zymogenes*)	Gram + cocci in chains	Endocarditis, urinary tract infections			Growth in 6.5% NaCl, blackening of bile esculin agar

Name	Colonial Morphology	Morphology	Clinical Disease Forms	Toxins and Pathogenicity Factors	Significant Antigens	Significant Biochemical or Serologic Tests
Str. faecium (Group D enterococcus) variety *faecium* variety *durans*	Colonies as above α hemolysis (*faecium* and *durans*) or β hemolysis (*durans*)	Gram + in chains	Endocarditis, urinary tract infections			As above
Str pneumoniae	0.3–0.5 mm, clear glistening crater-form colonies on sheep or human blood agar, α hemolytic	Gram + lancet-shaped cocci, in pairs with prominent capsule	Lobar pneumonia, bronchopneumonia, meningitis, otitis media, sinusitis, cellulitis, bacteremia	Capsular polysaccharide	Capsular polysaccharides (82 types)	Bile solubility Optochin sensitivity Quellung (swelling) reaction with type-specific antiserum

Table 5-13. Gram Negative Cocci

Name	Colonial Morphology	Morphology	Clinical Disease Forms	Toxins and Pathogenicity Factors	Significant Antigens	Significant Biochemical or Serologic Tests
Neisseria gonorrhoeae	0.5 mm, opaque colonies on chocolate agar	Gram – diplococci	Gonorrhea and complications (prostatitis seminal vesiculitis, epididymitis in males; salpingitis, pelvic inflammatory disease, peritonitis in females), ophthalmic neonatorum	Fimbriae, endotoxin (LPS)	Sixteen serotypes of cell outer membrane proteins	Acid and gas production from glucose
N meningitidis	0.5 mm, opaque colonies on chocolate agar	Gram – diplococci encapsulated	Meningitis, sepsis (meningococcemia)	Capsule endotoxin (LPS)	Group-specific polysaccharide capsule groups A,B,C,D,X,Y,Z,Z¹, and W135	Demonstration of capsular polysaccharide in CSF by counter immunoelectrophoresis acid and gas production from glucose and maltose, Quellung test with group-specific antisera

are also significant causes of other infections; these include meningitis, sinusitis, and otitis media.

THE NEISSERIA

Neisseria has two pathogenic species, *N gonorrhoeae,* the cause of gonorrhea, and *N meningitides,* a principal cause of purulent meningitis. Both organisms are gram-negative diplococci, often seen within PMN in gram-stained smears of exudate. Gonorrhea is a sexually transmitted disease resulting from the implantation and proliferation of *N gonorrhoeae* on mucous membranes of the genitourinary tracts. It occurs principally as a cervicitis in women and as a urethritis in men. The pathogenic potential of the gonococcus is related to its ability to colonize tissues, a function of the surface fimbriae, to endotoxin and perhaps to the presence of a capsule. Complications of gonorrhea in women result from extension of the infection from the primary site, usually the endometrium, to other sites of the genital tract or adjacent tissues. Thus salpingitis, pelvic inflammatory disease, pelvic peritonitis, proctitis, and perihepatitis can result. In men, epididymitis and prostatitis as well as inflammation of the seminal vesicles have been attributed to the gonococcus although solid microbiologic evidence has not been recorded. *N gonorrhoeae* can also cause pharyngitis and ocular infections. Ophthalmia neonatorum is a serious eye infection of newborns that can lead to blindness.

N meningitides is the second most common cause of bacterial meningitis and an important cause of sepsis presenting as meningococcemia. The pathogenic potential is related to its capsule and endotoxin. The capsule antigens are used to classify the organism into eight serogroups. Group A is the most frequently associated with disease followed by B, C, and Y. Immunity results from response to capsular antigens. Vaccines using type A and C polysaccharides are effective in preventing disease due to these serogroups.

Gram-Positive Bacilli

CORYNEBACTERIA

The genus *Corynebacterium* is made up of species of aerobic gram-positive, nonsporulating, tapered club-shaped bacilli. They are nonmotile and stain unevenly. Metachromatic granules in the cytoplasm of older cells cause the irregular staining. The principal pathogen is *C diphtheriae,* the causative agent of diphtheria. Three colonial variants of *C diphtheriae* are differentiated as, *gravis, mitis,* and *intermedius* (Table 5-14). All of these forms can cause disease. The ability to cause diphtheria

is dependent on the presence of a prophage, *tox* which codes for the diphtheria toxin. Nonlysogenic strains do not produce toxin. Diphtheria toxin is a 62 k polypeptide. The polypeptide can be split into two fragments A and B by proteolysis. The B fragment attaches to cell surfaces and the A fragment enters the cytoplasm where it inhibits protein synthesis by inactivating elongation factor 2. The lethal dose for man is 130 ng/kg. The extensive local necrosis and the systemic pathology of diphtheria are due to the toxin. Immunity is a function of antitoxic antibodies. Immune status can be determined by the Shick test. The test is conducted by the injection of minute amounts of toxin into the skin and observation of the response. A positive reaction at the site consisting of necrosis indicates a lack of antibody. The test also includes a control injection of toxoid to better discriminate hypersensitive states. Nonimmune individuals can be immunized by administration of toxoid, a formalin-inactivated preparation of diphtheria toxin.

Nontoxigenic strains (*tox-*) can cause local infections of the oropharynx. Cord factor is recognized as the principal pathogenic factor in these cases. Other members of the genus are animal pathogens and rarely are associated with human disease.

LISTERIA

Listeria monocytogenes and closely related species *L innocua* and *L murraya* are aerobic asporogenic gram-positive to gram variable rods. They are motile by peritrichous flagella. *L monocytogenes* causes a variety of infections in humans and in animals, as illustrated in Table 5-14. It is primarily associated with meningitis and a systemic "grippe-like" syndrome accompanied by sepsis.

Gram-Positive Spogenous Bacilli

The genus *Bacillus* consists of species of aerobic sporeforming bacilli most of which are saprophytic. There is one significant pathogen, *B anthracis* the causative agent of anthrax. This organism is nonmotile and possesses a capsule of poly D-glutamic acid. *B anthracis* elaborates a toxin complex of three factors which act in concert to exert toxic effects. The factors are the edema factor, protective antigen, and lethal factor. *B cereus* is a common saprophyte which is capable of causing food poisoning. The organism elaborates two enterotoxins one of which causes diarrhea and the other emesis (Table 5-15).

The genus *Clostridium* consists of many species of anaerobic sporeforming bacilli (Table 5-16). The organisms are common soil inhabitants and cause disease

Table 5-14. Gram Positive Asporagenous Bacilli

Name	Colonial Morphology	Microscopic Morphology	Clinical Disease Forms	Toxins and Pathogenicity Factors	Significant Antigens	Significant Biochemical or Serologic Tests
Corynebacterium diphtheriae variety *gavis*	Semi-rough colonies on Loeffler's medium 0.5 mm	Pleomorphic short rods, (1.0 μm) club shaped, metachromic granules	Diphtheria, wound infections	Diphtheria toxin (produced by lysogenic *tox*$^+$ strains of *C diphtheriae*) cord factor, neuraminidase	Diphtheria Toxin	Ouchterlony-Elek agar gel diffusion test for toxigenicity
variety *mitis*	Smooth colonies on Loeffler's medium 0.5 mm	Pleomorphic long rods (3.0–6.0) club shaped, metachromatic granules				
variety *intermedius*	Dwarf-smooth colonies on Loeffler's	Pleomorphic rods, club shaped, metachromatic granules				
Listeria monocytogenes	Smooth entire colonies, 0.5 mm on sheeps blood agar, clear hemolysis	Short, gram + rods	Meningitis, meningoencephalitis, septicemia glanular swelling and monocytosis (wide-spread infections in domestic and wild animals)	Monocytosis-producing lipids, hemolysin	Four serogroups based on somatic (O) and flagella (H) antigen	Anton test (development of kerato-conjunctivitis after instillation of broth culture into conjunctival sac of a rabbit)

Table 5-15. Gram Positive Sporogenous Bacilli (Aerobic)

Name	Colonial Morphology	Microscopic Morphology	Clinical Disease Forms	Toxins and Pathogenicity Factors	Significant Antigens	Significant Biochemical or Serologic Tests
Bacillus anthracis	2.4 mm, rough (incubated in air) or smooth to mucoid (in CO_2) on nutrient agar, hemolytic on sheeps blood agar	Large, square ended bacilli in chains (2.5–5 μm) encapsulated (in vivo) centrally located spores when grown aerobically	Cutaneous anthrax inhalation anthrax gastrointestinal anthrax, anthrax septicemia	Polyglutamic acid capsule, anthrax toxins	Protective antigen (component of anthrax toxin)	Fluorescent antibody (presumptive), animal inoculation
B cereus	2.5 mm, rough on nutrient agar hemolytic on sheeps blood agar	Large bacilli (2.0–5 μm) nonencapsulated, spores central in cell	Food poisoning	Enterotoxins, diarrheal, emetic	Nineteen serotypes	Serotyping for confirmation of food poisoning outbreaks

Table 5-16. Gram Positive Sporogenous Bacilli (Anaerobic)

Name	Colonial Morphology	Microscopic Morphology	Clinical Disease Forms	Toxins and Pathogenicity Factors	Significant Antigens	Significant Biochemical or Serologic Tests
Clostridium botulinum	Large, irregular translucent with granular surface, hemolysis on horse blood agar	Large, plump bacilli oval central or subterminal spores	Botulisms, infant botulism	Botulinum toxin 7 serotypes based on neutralization	Serogroups based on cross reaction of toxins A B and F, C D and E G	Serologic indentification of serotype
C tetani	Large, fine filamentous growth, hemolysis on horse blood agar	Slender rods, spherical terminal spores of diameter greater than the negative cell	Tetanus, neonatal tetanus	Tetanospasmin tetanolysin	Ten types of flagellar antigens	
C perfringens	Low, convex semiopaque 1.0–1.5 mm double zone hemolysis on sheep or horse blood agar	Slender, blunt end rods, spores (when present) central and greater diameter than cell	Gas gangrene, food poisoning, enteritis necroticans (Type C)	Twelve exotoxins α-τ and enterotoxin, α-toxin (lecithinase) of type A, β-toxin (necrotizing) of types B and C, ϵ-toxin (necrotizing) of types B and D and ι-toxin of type E are the most significant	Five serotypes A-E (most human disease associated with type A)	Production of opacity on egg yolk agar and its inhibition by antiserum to α-toxin
C novyi	Irregular, semitranslucent colonies with crenated edges	Large gram + bacilli, swollen subterminal spores	Gas gangrene	Eight exotoxins α-toxin (necrotizing), lecithinase C	Four serotypes A-D (human disease associated with A and B)	Opacity on egg yolk agar and inhibition by type-specific antiserum (types A, B and D)
C histolyticum	Small, circular shiny with entire edge; hemolytic on horse blood agar	Gram + rods, swollen subterminal oval spores	Associated with gas gangrene	4 exotoxins (α–δ)	No egg yolk reaction	
C difficile	Low convex, circular whitish matt surface	Large gram + rods, motite, oval subterminal spores	Antibiotic-associated pseudomembranous enterocolitis	Cytotoxin		Tissue culture cytotoxicity and inhibition by antiserum

principally by the elaboration of potent exotoxins. *C botulinum* causes botulism which results from the action of bolutinum toxin. There are seven serologically distinct types of toxin which define the serotypes of the organism. They are identical in their toxic effect in that they act at the neuromuscular junction inhibiting the release of acetylcholine by motor neurons. The lethal dose for a human has been estimated as about 7 ng/kg. Botulism usually results from ingestion of preformed toxin in contaminated food. Infant botulism has been attributed to intestinal colonization with *C botulinum,* often from contaminated honey. *C tetani* is the causative agent of tetanus. This disease results from the elaboration of tetanus toxin (tetanospasmin) by the organism growing in infected sites. The toxin binds to the gangliosides of the motor end-plates and interferes with synaptic inhibition resulting in muscular tetany. *C perfringins* and other clostridia are causes of gas gangrene. These organisms elaborate a number of tissue-destructive toxins which are active in the pathogenesis of the disease. *C difficile* causes antibiotic-associated pseudomembranous enterocolitis. The organism is apparently favored by changes in the enteric flora brought about by antibiotic therapy (Lincomycin and Clindomycin are often involved). Growth is accompanied by elaboration of a cytotoxin which causes the pathology.

Gram-Negative Aerobic Bacilli

ENTEROBACTERIACEAE

The Enterobacteriaceae are a family of five tribes of gram − asporogenous bacilli that ferment glucose and reduce nitrates to nitrites. The normal habitat of many species is the intestine of man and animals and others are found in soil and water. Morphologically the organisms are similar to one another; they are short rods (2 − 3 µm × 0.4 − 0.6 µm), motile by peritrichous flagella (the genus *Shigella* and some other organisms are nonmotile) and often have fimbriae. All members have LPS present in the outer membrane of the cell wall. The organisms are differentiated on the basis of biochemical tests and by serology. Three classes of antigens, flagellar (H), somatic (O), and capsular (K) are used in serologic classification. Complex patterns of antigen sharing reflect close phylogenetic relationships as well as the common occurrence of plasmid-determined characteristics.

The tribe Escherichieae contains five genera, *Escherichia, Edwardsiella, Citrobacter, Salmonella,* and *Shigella.* The organism *E coli* is usually regarded as the prototype of the Enterobacteriaceae because of the accumulated knowledge of its biochemistry and genetics. *E coli* is a normal inhabitant of the human and animal intestine and forms a significant proportion of the microbial population of the site. It is also regarded as an opportunistic pathogen when introduced into other body sites such as the urinary tract or the respiratory tract. Some strains of *E coli* are frankly pathogenic; these strains are significant causes of diarrheal disease. Three kinds of *E coli* intestinal pathogens are distinguished. Enterotoxigenic strains (ETEC) are responsible for "travelers diarrhea" and some cholera-like diseases of developing countries. These strains elaborate enterotoxin, a plasmid encoded gene product. Two types of enterotoxin have been described; a thermostable (ST) toxin which is not immunogenic and a thermolabile (LT) protein toxin which is immunogenic. Both cause diarrhea by water and electrolyte loss due to increase adenyl cyclase activity of epithelial cells. Enteroinvasive strains (EIEC) cause dysentery-like disease by invasion of the epithelial cells in a manner similar to the *Shigella.* These strains are also associated with food poisoning. Enteropathogenic strains (EPEC) are responsible for diarrhea in infants (usually in institutions). The factors which cause pathogenicity are unknown.

The genus *Salmonella* contains more than 1,500 serotypes, all of which are considered pathogenic for humans. The serotypes can be considered as separate species and as such are designated by a binomial (e.g., *S newport, S herschfeldii,* etc.). Another, more favored, approach to classification, holds that there are three species: *S cholerasuis,* the prototype, *S typhi,* the cause of typhoid fever, and *S enteritidis,* containing all other serotypes. Analysis of the salmonellae on the basis of shared antigens (principally O and H) has divided the organisms into six groups A, B, C_1, C_2, D, and E.

The source of *S typhi* is a human patient or carrier of the organism. Ingestion of the bacilli is followed by invasion of the intestinal wall and bacteremia. The bacilli are seeded into many sites including the bone marrow, kidney and gallbladder. During the first 10 days, bacteria are found in the blood, later the organisms can be found in the stool and sometimes in the urine and saliva. Serologic response can be detected 2 to 3 weeks after onset as rising titers of both anti O and anti H antibodies. During this period, intracapillary agglutination of bacilli leads to the characteristic "rose spots" associated with typhoid fever. LPS is apparently the principal pathogenic factor; although the ability to penetrate the small intestine and survive in nonactivated macrophages are certainly important but as yet unelucidated contributors. Infection with this pathogenesis when caused by other salmonellae, is referred to as salmonella or enteric fever. Other diseases caused by these organisms take the form of gastroenteritis (food poisoning or food infection) and extraintestinal infections.

The genus *Shigella* contains four species, *S dysenter-*

iae, S flexneri, S boydii, and *S sonnei,* all of which cause bacillary dysentery. The shigellae differ from other species of Enterobacteriaceae in that they do not have flagella (therefore are nonmotile and do not have H antigens). The pathogenesis of bacillary dysentery involves invasion of the epithelial cells of the colon sparing other regions of the enteron. The bacilli multiply within the cells causing cell death and sloughing. Invasion is accompanied by inflammation and limited to the superficial mucosa. Dysentery is characterized by blood and mucous-containing stools. The pathogenic potential of shigellae is related to the ability to adhere to and invade mucosal cells and apparently to LPS. *S dysenteriae* and some strains of *S flexneri* and *S sonnei* elaborate a potent exotoxin which has cytotoxic and neurotoxic activity. While the role of this toxin is presently undefined, it is assumed to play a role in the pathogenesis of the disease, although cell invasion is clearly a more critical factor.

Citrobacter and *Edwardsiella* are regarded as opportunistic pathogens of low pathogenic potential in normal subjects yet can be of considerable significance in the compromised host.

The tribe Klebsielleae contains the genera *Klebsiella, Enterobacter, Hafnia,* and *Serratia.* Among these genera, the species most frequently associated with human infection is *K pneumoniae.* This organism is responsible for about 25 percent of community-acquired pneumonias due to gram-negative bacilli. It is also significant as a cause of nosocomial gram-negative pneumonias as are many other Enterobacteriaceae. Members of the tribes Proteeae, Yersineae, and Erwineae are, with some notable exceptions, regarded as opportunistic pathogens of variable pathogenic potential. Species of *Proteus* are associated with several infections, notably complicated urinary tract infections, chronic ear infections, and some gram-negative pneumonias.

Yersinia pestis is the cause of plague. The classification of this organism has undergone some revision. It was long classified as *Pasteurella pestis* but moved to the genus *Yersinia* on the basis of glucose fermentation and reduction of nitrates. The other species *Y pseudotuberculosis* and *Y enterocolitica* cause enteritis in humans as well as other diseases in birds and animals. These organisms elaborate an enterotoxin and have LPS. *Y pestis* are small pleomorphic rods, nonmotile, and often show bipolar staining. The pathogenic potential of the organism is related to a capsular antigen (Fraction 1) which is antiphagocytic and two factors V and W which allow intracellular multiplication of the organism. In addition, virulent strains of *Y pestis* elaborate an exotoxin which is lethal for rodents and possess LPS. There is evidence to suggest that there are quantitative considerations also important for the expression of virulence.

VIBRIO, CAMPLYLOBACTER, AND PSEUDOMONAS

Organisms in the genera *Vibrio, Campylobacter,* and *Pseudomonas* are not taxonomically closely related to the Enterobacteriaceae, yet because they are frequently encountered in similar clinical situations, they are often considered together.

Vibrio cholerae is the cause of Asiatic cholera. It is a short, comma-shaped, gram-negative organism, motile by means of a single polar flagellum. The organism has H and O antigens. Three O antigens (A, B, and C) occur in three antigenic combinations determining the Ogawa (AB), Inaba (AC), and Hikojima (ABC) serotypes. A fourth type, A, occurs rarely. *V cholerae* gains entrance by ingestion. Since it is relatively sensitive to many conditions, including low pH, the infecting dose is thought to be large. In the alkaline environment of the small bowel, the vibrios adhere to the mucosa and proliferate. The organism elaborates an enterotoxin similar to *E coli.* Cholera toxin is an 84 k protein composed of six light chain entities and single heavy chain. The light chains apparently interact with ganglioside receptors of cell membranes and the heavy chain acts to stimulate adenyl-cyclase. The levels of cAMP increase in the cells followed by an outpouring of water and electrolyte.

The *Campylobacter* species *C intestinalis* and *C jejuni* cause a variety of human infections, principally of the gastrointestinal tract. The organisms resemble the vibrios and are usually associated with domestic animals.

Pseudomonas aeurginosa is a member of the genus *Pseudomonas,* a group of bacteria widely disseminated in nature. *P aeurginosa* is the most frequently encountered of these organisms in human infections. It is regarded as an opportunistic pathogen. Pseudomonads are aerobic gram-negative motile rods with a single polar flagellum. They are nonfermentative and catalase positive. *P aeurginosa* is an important cause of postburn sepsis and nosocomial infection in compromised patients. Neonates are also vulnerable to the organism. The pathogenic potential of the organism is attributed to LPS, elaboration of proteases and lipases, and an exotoxin A. The activity of exotoxin A is similar to diphtheria toxin. The organism also elaborates other products apparently unrelated to pathogenicity but helpful in identification. Among these is pyocyanin, a blue-green soluble pigment which diffuses into laboratory media and frequently can be seen in pus from *P aeurginosa* infections.

BRUCELLA

The brucellae are short, coccobacillary, gram-negative rods that are nonmotile and not encapsulated. Three species, *Brucella melitensis, B abortus,* and *B suis* cause infection in humans. The organisms cause similar disease in the human host. They are also significant animal pathogens. Brucellae are highly invasive entering the host by direct penetration of the oral and intestinal mucosa or through abrasions in the skin. The source of infection is often animals or animal products including unpasteurized milk. The pathogenic factors appear to be LPS and the ability to remain viable in macrophages. Human brucellosis manifests as an acute febrile disease with chills, sweats, headache, and various influenza-like symptoms. Immune response is humoral and cellular with the cellular component contributing to the pathogenesis. The lesions of the disease are granulomatous and sometimes necrotic foci in the liver, spleen, and lymph nodes. The three species share antigens and differ from one another by the quantity of antigens. The *B abortus* organism has increased quantities of the A antigen in relation to the M antigen, while *B melitensis* has high M and low A. *B suis* has about equal amounts of each antigen.

BORDETELLA AND HAEMOPHILUS

Organisms in the genera *Bordetella* and *Haemophilus* are important pathogens of humans. The bacilli of both are small, coccobacillary, gram-negative forms which are nonmotile (with the exception of *B bronchiseptica*). Humans are susceptible to infection with *B pertussis* and *B parapertussis*. Both organisms cause whooping cough; the former about 95 percent of cases, the latter about 5 percent. Initial cultivation of *B pertussis* on complex medium gives an organism defined as antigenic phase I. Repeated subculturing on simple medium yields an organism defined as phase IV. This phase change is accompanied by loss of a number of antigens, some of which function to evoke protective immunity. The pathogenesis of whooping cough involves the adherence of *B pertussis* to the ciliated epithelium of the upper respiratory tract. The adherence antigen of phase I organisms plays a role in colonization as does the hemagglutinin (fimbriae). In phase I organisms a toxin which paralyzes cilia is elaborated and the LPS of the cell wall is a potent endotoxin. Protective antigen (PA), a protein of the cell wall, is the most important cell component in evoking protective antibody. A number of other biologically active components have been described which may contribute to pathogenicity. Histamine-sensitizing factor and lymphocyte-promoting factor appear to be a single entity showing two biologic activities both of which could contribute to pathology.

Haemophilus influenza, H ducreyi, and *H aegypti* are the three principal human pathogens in the genus *Haemophilus*. The organisms are distinguished by their nutritional requirements for growth in vitro. They are un-

able to synthesize either hematin or NAD or both; therefore these factors must be supplied. Historically, the factors were referred to as X (hematin) and V (NAD) and were recognized as critical constituents for growth. *H influenza* and *H aegypti* require both X and V while *H ducreyi* requires only X. *H influenzae* is encapsulated and the capsular polysaccharide occurs in six serologically distinct types, a–f. Endotoxin is also a constituent of the outer membrane. The organisms in serotype b are responsible for almost all human infections with *H influenzae*. The organism is the leading cause of bacterial meningitis and it also causes epiglottitis, otitis media, suppurative arthritis, osteomylitis, pericarditis, and pneumonia. *H aegypti* is the cause of a contagious purulent conjunctivitis which is endemic in warm climates. *H ducreyi* causes chanchroid, a disease characterized by multiple (usually) vesicular eruptions on the skin or mucosa of the genitalia. It is a sexually transmitted infection which often occurs with other such diseases.

Pasteurella and Francisella

The genus *Pasteurella* contains the animal pathogen *P multicida* which occasionally infects humans. The organism is a pleomorphic gram-negative coccobacillus that is frequently encapsulated. It is asporogenous and nonmotile. The organism is highly pathogenic for several mammalian and avian species but only occasionally causes human infections. Most human infections take the form of local infections by cat scratch or animal bite. Other human infections include respiratory tract infections and systemic infections such as meningitis or bacteremia.

Francisella tularensis is the causative agent of tularemia. It is a very small gram-negative coccobacillus that tends to be pleomorphic. The organism is a facultative intracellular parasite which may persist for many years in an infected host. Infection of humans can occur by direct contact with the carcasses of infected wild animals, by aerosols, through the bite of ticks or deer flies, or by drinking contaminated water.

Legionella

Legionella pneumophilia is a small gram-negative pleomorphic rod that grows aerobically. It is fastidious, nonsporulating, and nonmotile. It is an opportunistic pathogen found in soil and water. It is spread to humans by aerosal; human-to-human spread has not been documented. *L pneumophilia* causes a number of clinical entities ranging from mild respiratory disease to disseminated multiorgan infection. Two distinctive forms have been described: Legionaires disease which is a severe multilobar atypical pneumonia and Pontiac fever which is a mild to moderate pleuritis. The factors that confer pathogenicity are unknown although there is clear evidence of strain differences. The organism has LPS but its role in pathogenicity is unknown.

Acid Fast Bacilli

MYCOBACTERIUM

The genus *Mycobacterium* contains the two human pathogens *M tuberculosis* and *M leprae,* the causes of tuberculosis and leprosy, respectively. In addition, several other species regularly cause human infections including tuberculosis-like pulmonary disease. Mycobacteria are slender rods that fail to stain well in the Gram procedure. The bacilli have a high lipid and wax content that interferes with the usual staining procedures. The organisms can be stained by the Ziehl-Neelsen method with heated carbol fuchsin. Clearing of smears stained in this way with HCl in 95 percent ethanol fails to remove the stain from mycobacteria thus the description, acidfast. This property is apparently related to the wax and lipid content of the cells. The bacilli appear deep red and are often irregularly stained. The organisms are also often stained using fluorchromes and observed using ultraviolet light. In the case of tuberculosis, clinical specimens such as sputum are usually digested with a mucolytic agent and NaOH to reduce the viscosity and kill contaminating bacteria. Then the specimens are centrifuged to concentrate the mycobacteria. The digested and concentrated material is examined microscopically after acid-fast staining and used to inoculate culture media. The media of choice are Löwenstein-Jensen or Middlebrook 7H10. Drug susceptibility tests are also initiated directly on quadrant plates containing the primary antimicrobics, isoniazid, ethambutol, and rifampin. Other frequently used drugs are pyrazinamide and ethionamide. The rapidity of mycobacterial growth on laboratory media is a differential characteristic in identification. In general, saprophytic mycobacteria grow rapidly, while the organisms of more frequent significance as pathogens take longer than 14 days to replicate sufficiently to form colonies.

M tuberculosis has a generation time of 13 to 18 hours. Further differentiation is possible on the basis of pigment production, the lack of it, and whether pigment is produced in the dark. Thus organisms can be classified as photochromogens, scotochromogens, or nonchromogens. *M tuberculosis* forms small, hard, heaped-up, buff colored (nonpigmented) colonies in 3 to 6 weeks after inoculation. Further, the organism is niacin positive. *M bovis* an organism which was responsible for many cases of human tuberculosis and is not now often encountered

in the United States, can be differentiated on its inability to secrete niacin (some *M bovis* strains are positive). The other atypical mycobacteria do frequently cause tuberculosis-like disease and must be differentiated. The pathogenic potential of *M tuberculosis* has been ascribed to the high content of waxes and lipids which are present in the cell wall of the organisms. They survive well as intracellular parasites and are capable of replication within nonactivated macrophages. Infection with mycobacteria evokes a CMI response, and with activation of macrophages by lymphokine activity, replication of bacilli is controlled. In most cases, mycobacterial infections are controlled at this point. Modulation of the immune response can lead to reactivation of replication and extension of infection. Pathologic changes accompanying reactivation and the subsequent response, favor replication of bacilli and cavitation of pulmonary lesions. The classical diagnositic procedure for tuberculosis is of course the tuberculin skin test for delayed hypersensitivity to tuberculoproteins. In this test, five test units of purified protein derivative (PPD) are introduced into the skin. A positive test is signaled by the development of erythema and induration at the site 48 to 72 hours after inoculation. Induration of 1.0 cm is interpreted as a positive reaction due to infection with *M tuberculosis* (or *M bovis*). Other mycobacterial infections usually produce reactions of smaller dimensions.

M leprae is the cause of leprosy or Hansen's disease. The organism has not been cultivated on laboratory media but studies on its biology have been conducted in vivo in the foot pads of mice and the nine-banded armadillo. Studies in these animals indicate a generation time of 13 days. The pathogenicity of the organism apparently derives from its ability to survive and proliferate as an intracellular parasite. Clinically, the extremes of response are tuberculoid leprosy and lepromatous leprosy. The former is characterized by an intact and functional CMI state and comparative rarity of *M leprae* in the tissues. The prognosis is good. Lepromatous leprosy is characterized by an absence of CMI and exaggerated humoral response. The bacilli are numerous in tissue and the prognosis is poor.

NOCARDIA AND ACTINOMYCES

The genera *Nocardia* and *Actinomyces* contain slender filamentous branching bacilli which are grampositive. The *Nocardia* are weakly acid-fast. *Nocardia* are aerobic and *actinomyces* are anaerobic. The organism *N asteroides* is the principal pathogen although *N brasiliensis* and *N caviae* cause human infections. Nocardiae are soil microorganisms and cause disease usually by entry through broken skin. In subcutaneous tissue they form multiple and confluent abcesses characterized by intense suppuration. Pulmonary nocardiosis can be acquired by inhalation. The disease has some similarities of pulmonary tuberculosis including cavitation. *Actinomyces* species are normal inhabitants of the human oral cavity, particularly the gingival sulcus and the tonsilar crypts. They are also present in and contribute to the formation of dental plaque. *A viscosus* and *A naeslundii* have been implicated in peridontitis and gingivitis while *A odontolyticus* and *A naeslundii* have been shown to cause root surface caries. *A israeli* and *A naeslundii* cause actinomycosis in humans. Most cases of actinomycosis are cervicofacial and present as a painless swelling which hardens into a "woody" nodule. Suppuration occurs and sinus tracts open to the external surfaces. Pus is characterized by "sulfur" granules, small pigmented agglomerates of bacteria. Actinomycosis also occurs as pulmonary disease and abdominal abcesses.

Nonsporulating Anaerobes

Various nonsporulating anaerobic bacteria are part of the normal flora of the human body (Table 5-17). They populate the skin, alimentary tract, oral cavity, and urogenital mucosa. They are regarded as opportunistic pathogens, causing disease when they gain access to sites not normally colonized. Anaerobic infections are usually mixed infections involving one or more anaerobes and often an aerobe.

The diagnosis of anaerobic infections is aided by a well prepared Gram stain of lesion material. Distinct pleomorphism of the cells is a hallmark of the infection. Culture and identification of organsims is helpful. Proper precautions to maintain an anaerobic environment are necessary to obtain useful results of culture attempts.

BACTERIODES

Bacteriodes are gram-negative rods of highly variable morphology depending on the medium and gaseous environment. They form convex, white to gray, translucent colonies on blood agar. Some species are hemolytic and one, *B melaningenicus,* produces a black pigment. The principal organisms encountered clinically are *B fragilis* and *B melaninogenicus*. These organisms cause abcess formation in the brain, lung, and peritoneum. They are also involved in infections of the urogenital tract and are the most frequent anaerobic isolates in blood culture. The organisms have LPS; other pathogenic factors have not been identified. *B fragilis* is resistant to the usual levels of penicillin. However, *B melaninogenicus* and other clinically significant anaerobes are sensitive. Clindomycin is often used in anaerobic infec-

tions since *B fragilis* is most frequently a component of the normal intestinal flora.

FUSOBACTERIUM

Fusobacterium nucleatum is the most frequent encountered species of the genus. It is a slender gram-negative rod with delicately pointed ends. It is a normal inhabitant of mouth, upper respiratory tract, gastrointestinal tract, and the urogenital tract. The organism is encountered in pleuropulmonary infections and lung abcesses. It also is frequently isolated in blood cultures. *F nucleatum* produces a neuraminidase that along with LPS may play a role in pathogenicity.

The Spirochetes

TREPONEMA

The genus *Treponema* contains the important human pathogens *T pallidum, T pertenue,* and *T carateum* the causes of syphilis, yaws, and pinta, respectively. *T pallidum* is a slender spiral organism 5 to 20 μm by 0.1 to 0.2 μm. It stains poorly by most conventional methods, but is gram-negative. The Levaditi silver impregnation method allows the visualization of the organism in tissues. Examination of material from lesions uses darkfield microscopy to visualize the living treponemes. *T. pallidum* has not been grown on laboratory media. It is propagated by animal inoculation (intratesticular inoculation of rabbits). The factors which contribute to the pathogenicity of the organism are unknown. Syphilis is sexually acquired. The primary lesion, the chancre, appears 14 to 21 days after exposure on the skin or mucous membranes of the genitalia or other site of entry. The chancre heals spontaneously in 3 to 6 weeks. Disseminated secondary lesions appear on the skin usually within 3 weeks of the appearance of the chancre. There may be several "crops" of secondary lesions. Treponemes are demonstrable in primary and secondary lesions. Serologic response in syphilis occurs as anticardiolipin antibody detected in various tests such as VDRL or RPR and as antitreponemal antibody. The latter may be detected by the FTA, FTA-ABS, or TPI tests. In primary syphilis, about 75 percent of patients are VDRL positive while about 90 percent are FTA-ABS positive. In secondary syphilis almost all patients are positive by both types of test. VDRL reactivity is usually lost within 6 months after adequate treatment. In untreated cases about 50 percent of patients lose VDRL reactivity in late stages of syphilis. Antitreponemal antibodies are not lost after treatment nor in late syphilis. Yaws and pinta produce similar serologic responses as

Table 5-17. Selected Anaerobic Bacteria of Medical Importance

Characteristic	Genus	Species
Sporulating Gram-positive bacilli	*Clostridium*	*C tetani* *C botulinum* *C perfringens* *C septicum* *C. novyi* and many others

Nonsporulating
Gram-negative bacilli
	Bacteroides	*B fragilis*
		B thetaiotaomicron
		B vulgatus
		B distasonis
		B ovatus
		B melaninogenicus
		    Subspecies *melaninogenicus,*
		      intermedius, and *levii*
		B oralis
		B ureolyticus

	Fusobacterium	*F nucleatum* *F necrophorum* and others
Gram-positive bacilli	*Actinomyces* *Bifidobacterium* *Corynebacterium* *Eubacterium* *Propionibacterium*	Many various species
Gram-negative cocci	*Veillonella*	*V parvula*
Gram-positive cocci	*Peptococcus* *Peptostreptococcus*	*P magnus* *P anaerobius* *P intermedius*
	Sarcina	*S ventriculi*

(Milgrom F, Flanagan TD: Medical Microbiology. Churchill Livingstone, New York, 1982.)

does syphilis. In addition, anticardiolipin antibodies sometimes occur in nontreponemal infection, autoimmune disease, and in patients with cirrhosis and malignancy.

LEPTOSPIRA

One species, *Leptospira interrogans,* is currently recognized although it has been suggested that the saprophytic strains be classified in a separate species. Pathogens are found in a group of organisms designated as the "interrogans complex" which is divided into 16 serogroups containing 130 serotypes. The serologic groupings are based on cross reactivity demonstrable by agglutination reactions. Analysis is carried out by cross absorption tests. The organisms are fine spiral cells best observed by darkfield microscopy. They are gram-negative but hardly visible in stained preparations. *L interrogans* is grown aerobically on simple artificial media. Liquid or semisolid media are better than solid. The pathogenicity of the organisms is apparently related to their ability to gain entry and to their endotoxin. Most

human exposure is through the medium of contaminated water. The organisms are shed in the urine of infected rodents and contaminate stagnant water. Entry to the human host can be through abraded skin or mucosa. Incubation is about 14 days followed by the onset of fever and chills. This may be followed (in 10 percent of cases) by icterus. Leptospires can be observed in the blood during the early phase of infection by darkfield examination. Isolation can be accomplished from the blood in the early phase and later from the urine.

BORRELIA

The genus *Borrelia* contains pathogens that cause human relapsing fever. The organisms are classified according their vector. Thus *B recurrentis* is spread by the human body louse, *Pediculus humanus* while *B hermsii* is spread by the tick *Ornithinodoros hermsi.* Several other species of borreliae can cause the disease in humans. Borreliae are anaerobic organisms which are not easily cultivated on artificial media. They are gram-negative and easily visualized in stained preparations. They are also readily observed in blood smears. The louse-borne and tick-borne diseases are clinically similar. Typically, there is sudden onset with elevated fever and chills accompanied by splenomegaly, often jaundice and rash. The symptoms remit suddenly in 3 to 10 days to be followed in 4 to 5 days by a second episode of fever. The second is shorter in duration than the first and remission again occurs. If a third attack takes place it is shorter yet than the second and occurs after a longer period of remission. Borreliae are found in the blood during the symptomatic periods but not during remission.

Mycoplasma and Cell Wall-Less Bacterial Variants

MYCOPLASMA

Members of the genus *Mycoplasma* and the closely related genus *Ureaplasma* as well as the genus *Acholeplasma* are all bacteria that do not have cell walls. They are free-living organisms capable of growth on cell-free media. The smallest unit capable of replication is $0.3\,\mu m$ in diameter. They contain both RNA and DNA. The organisms form small ($50-600\,\mu m$ in diameter) colonies which have a characteristic "fried egg" appearance. Human infection is most frequently associated with *M pneumoniae*. It causes primary atypical pneumonia as well as tracheobronchitis and occasionally hemorrhagic bullous myringitis. *U ureolyticum* is associated with infections of the genitourinary tract including nongonococcal urethritis. *M hominis* has been implicated in septicemia, abcesses, endometritis, and salpingitis.

Under certain conditions bacteria can survive and even replicate without a cell wall. Antibiotics such as penicillin that inhibit cell wall formation affect bacterial death because the bacterial cell undergoes lysis without the cell wall. However, if the osmotic environment is high enough or stabilization of the membrane occurs the cells can survive without a cell wall. Some conditions for stabilization have been demonstrated in vivo and therefore, strains for cells that have no cell walls have been suggested as etiologic agents in some chronic and recurrent infections. Formal proof of these associations has not been offered.

RICKETTSIA

Three genera, *Rickettsia, Coxiella,* and *Rochalimaea* contain species causing human disease. Rickettsiae are intracellular parasites with limited metabolic capacities. They are small coccobacillary to bacillary forms with a typical gram-negative cell wall. They replicate by binary fission. With the exception of *R quintana,* they cannot be grown on lifeless medium; they require a living cell as a host. Members of the genus *Rickettsia* cause human diseases that have been grouped according to their general symptomatology. The typhus fever group include epidemic typhus and Brill-Zinsser disease caused by *R prowazekii* and endemic typhus caused by *R typhi.* Humans acquire *R prowazekii* by being bitten by an infected louse. *Pediculus humanus* is the vector that spreads the agent in the human population. Thus epidemics of typhus fever accompany conditions such as war, famine, and other catastrophes under which normal hygiene breaks down. Brill-Zinsser disease is recrudescent typhus. This form of the disease occurs in a person who has previously been infected with *R prowazekii* and recovered from the infection. Under conditions of stress there can be a recrudescence of the disease. Individuals manifesting the renewed disease can be a source of infection for lice and thus initiate an outbreak of typhus. *R typhi* causes endemic typhus, a disease that is clinically similar to epidemic typhus but considered to be milder by some investigators. The agent is inoculated into the human host by fleas and lice from rodent hosts. The rat flea is the most important vector for humans. Human to human spread of endemic typhus has not been documented. There is cross protective immunity between epidemic and endemic typhus. The infections both engender the production of antibodies against the OX-19 strain of *Proteus vulgaris* resulting in a positive Weil-Felix agglutination reaction. Antibodies are also produced against the antigens of the rickettsiae and are demonstrable by a variety of techniques.

SPOTTED FEVERS

Rickettsiae cause a number of geographically defined diseases in many regions throughout the world designated as spotted fevers. The etiologic agents are serologically related yet each disease is caused by different species of rickettsiae and is disseminated by a different vector. Two spotted fevers occur in the United States, Rocky Mountain spotted fever (RMSF) and Rickettsial pox. RMSF is caused by *R rickettsii* and is spread humans by ticks. In the western states, the wood tick, *Dermacentor andersoni* is the most important source of RMSF while in the east, the dog tick, *D variabilis* is most important. *R rickettsii* infects a variety of wild rodents that serve as a reservoir for the organism. The agent is passaged vertically though the ova in ticks; therefore ticks also serve as a reservoir. Patients with RMSF develop OX-19 agglutinins and agglutinins to another *Proteus* strain OX-2 with variable frequency. Specific antirickettsial serologic tests are more reliable. Rickettsial pox is caused by *R akari* and is spread to humans by mites. The reservoir is the common house mouse. Rickettsial pox is a benign disease occurring in small localized outbreaks throughout the world.

SCRUB TYPHUS

The causative agent of scrub typhus is *R tsutsugamushi* an antigenically diverse species of rickettsia. The infection is spread to humans from wild rodent reservoirs by mites. The infection occurs in regions of Southeast Asia, the Pacific, and Japan.

Q FEVER

Coxiella burnetti is the causative agent of Q fever. The agent differs from the other rickettsiae in some respects. It is more resistant to environmental conditions and can be spread to human and animal hosts without an anthropod vector. Most human infections occur among animal handlers. The infection is acquired by inhalation of aerosols or dust. Human to human spread does occur although the number of secondary cases is few indicating the spread is inefficient. The most frequent presentation of Q fever is pneumonitis but other systemic manifestations such as hepatitis and endocarditis also occur. *C burnetti* does not engender a Weil-Felix response, therefore specific tests must be used.

TRENCH FEVER

R quintana causes a disease, trench fever, spread by the human body louse. The infection is encountered in wartime. It has a low case fatality rate.

Biology of Viruses

Viruses are obligate intracellular parasites at the genetic level. They invade cells and redirect the synthetic capacities of the cell to the production of viral proteins and nucleic acids. Viruses exist as extracellular particles, called virions and as intracellular replicating entities, referred to as vegetative viruses. In addition, some viruses can mediate the insertion of their genomes into host cellular DNA and exist as cellular genes. The latter state is referred to as a proviral state. Virions are small noncellular particles made up of proteins and one type of nucleic acid. The type of nucleic acid, its size (MW), strandedness, configuration (linear of circular), and segmentation are important determinants used in classification. Virions of some viruses also contain lipids in the form of an outer membrane or envelope. The size of virions vary from about 20 nm in diameter to over 300 nm. For different viruses, virion size is quite constant and a useful criterion for classification. The shape of virions is another characteristic useful for classification; virions may appear spherical, ovoid, or rod-shaped. In addition, some bacterial viruses (bacteriophages) have a complex head and tail shape. Analysis of the structure by electron microscopy has revealed regular and symmetrical relationships among the structural subunits (capsomers) of virions. Three types of symmetry have been observed, cubic, helical, and radial. Cubic symmetry is most often seen in the icosahedral capsid of many viruses while helical symmetry is frequently encountered in the nucleocapsids of many enveloped viruses. In viruses that have cubic symmetry the number of capsomers in the capsid is characteristic of a given virus and thus is another criterion for classification. The combination of structural and compositional characteristics of the virion is the basis for the modern taxonomy of viruses. At present only two taxa, family and genus, are used. Another informal taxonomy, virus groups, has served as an interim system during the development of a formal taxonomy. Thus names such as herpesvirus, adenovirus, and picornavirus are frequently used for obviously similar viruses. Many group designations have been adopted into the formal classification, thus Herpetoviridae, Adenoviridae, and Picornoviridae appear as family names.

Bacteriophages

Studies of bacterial viruses have contributed greatly to our understanding of viral replication and viral effects on host cells. Much of this information comes from studies of the T phages and their hosts, *E coli*.

LYTIC CYCLE

The interaction between bacteriophage and host bacterium that leads to replication of the phage and lysis and death of the bacterium is known as the lytic cycle. The structure of T-4 bacteriophage includes the head which is a polyhedral structure composed of protein. It contains the viral genome, a 106×10^6 dalton DNA molecule, and associated polypeptides. The DNA is linear and double stranded. The tail is a complex structure consisting of an inner hollow core surrounded by a contractile sheath. The distal end of the tail has a hexagonal baseplate to which are attached six long (140 nm) fibers and six short pins (Fig. 5-17). The replicative cycle has been elucidated by the analysis of the biochemical and morphological events taking place under one-step growth (Fig. 5-18). Replication is initiated by adsorption of the phage to the surface of the bacterium by the interaction of the tail fibers with specific receptors in the cell wall. The next event is the close approximation of the tail base plate to the surface; the tail of the phage is perpendicular to the surface of the cell. The next event is a contraction

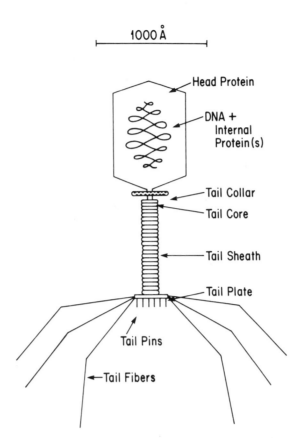

Fig. 5-17. Schematic drawing of bacteriophage T-4. (Milgrom F, Flanagan TD: Medical Microbiology. Churchill Livingstone, New York, 1982.)

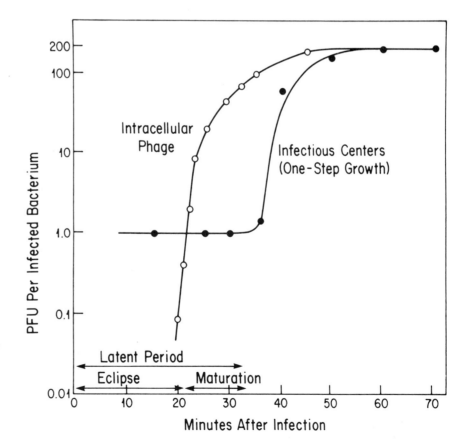

Fig. 5-18. One-step growth curve of bacteriophage T-4 in *E. coli* cells. ●, number of infectious centers per bacterium in cultures inoculated with bacteriophage and sampled at various times after infection. O, number of infectious centers per bacterium in cultures inoculated with bacteriophage and sampled after artificial lysis at various times after infection. (Milgrom F, Flanagan TD: Medical Microbiology. Churchill Livingstone, New York 1982.)

of the sheath thrusting the core through the cell wall and the expulsion of the DNA on to the cell membrane. The DNA crosses into the cytoplasm and begins to function. Immediate early transcription of the viral DNA is accomplished by host RNA polymerase. The mRNA produced is translated into products that shut down host macromolecular synthesis, modify host RNA polymerase, and inhibit host ρ factor. Modified host RNA polymerase transcribes a second set of genes, delayed early genes, producing mRNA which is translated into proteins active in further shutdown of host processes; the mechanism of viral DNA synthesis and initiation of late gene transcription. Late transcription produces mRNA that is translated into structural proteins that function in assembly of progeny virions and that lyse the bacterium. Viral DNA synthesis begins during delayed early synthesis. It is carried out by viral-encoded enzymes and resident host enzymes. Precursors for DNA synthesis come from degraded host DNA and from the medium in which its cells are growing. T-even phage DNA has a unique base, 5-hydroxymethylcytosine. In addition, the base is glucosylated to various extents. These modifications of molecular structure serve to protect viral DNA from destruction by endonucleases of the host. DNA replication takes place at the membrane of the host cell, initially as circular forms. Later, linear forms, concatemers, containing several genome equivalents are found in the cytoplasm of the cell. During maturation, DNA is packaged into the head of the progeny virion. The length of the molecule, hence the amount of genetic information, is governed by the capacity of the head. The maturation of the progeny is accomplished by three independent assembly processes (Fig. 5-19). One process is the assembly of the head and packaging of DNA. The head is made up of a major protein and several minor proteins. The DNA molecule is incorporated by the association of basic polypeptides, removal of a scaffolding protein from the interior of the head and clipping of the concatemeric DNA. The tail is assembled separately and joined to the DNA-filled head. Finally the tail fibers are added. Progeny virions are released from the infected bacterium by lysis of the cell. The lysis is accomplished by the action of viral gene products, lysozymes.

LYSOGENY

An alternative to the lytic cycle is lysogeny (Fig. 5-20). In this state a temperate bacteriophage infects a bacterium. Rather than the production of virions, the viral genome is integrated into the bacterial genome and remains in that site during the growth and replication of the host cell. Thus the viral genome is distributed to all of the progeny of the bacterial cell. The insertion of the viral DNA into the host DNA is carried out by a viral gene

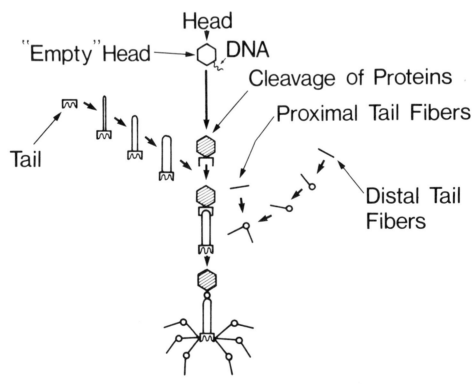

Fig. 5-19. Assembly of bacteriophage T-4. (Reprinted from Wood, Edgar, King, et al: Bacteriophage assembly. Fed Proc 27:1160, 1968.)

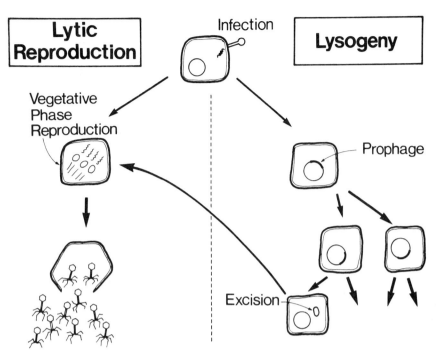

Fig. 5-20. Comparison of lytic reproduction and lysogeny of bacteriophages. (Milgrom F, Flanagan TD: Medical Microbiology. Churchill Livingstone, New York, 1982.)

product and the maintenance of the lysogenic state is also a function of viral genes. A repressor protein acts to inhibit the transcription of viral genes involved in vegetative growth of the virus. The presence of the prophage (the integrated viral genome) has consequences which affect the characteristics of the bacteria. For example, the ability to produce toxins and the presence of surface antigens may be the result of prophage. The acquisition of new characteristics in this manner is called lysogenic conversion. Lysogenic strains of bacteria (those carrying prophages) spontaneously produce bacteriophages at very low frequency. About 1 in 10^6 cells will enter into a vegetative phase of phage replication and produce progeny viruses. This process is initiated by a reduction of the concentration of the repressor allowing excision of the genome from the bacterial chromosome and entry into vegetative viral replication. Simultaneous phage production can be induced in a lysogenic strain of bacteria by exposure to ultraviolet light or other agents. This event results in the lysis of the entire population of bacterial cells.

Animal Viruses

CELL-VIRUS INTERACTION

As do the bacteriophages, animal viruses must recognize and attach to host cells. They must enter the cell and have the capacity to produce mRNA that can be trans-

lated on host ribosomes. They must also be able to replicate their genomes and finally they must have a mechanism to transfer their genomes to other cells. The stages of animal virus replication are similar to the bacteriophage, adsorption, penetration, synthesis, maturation, and release. Among animal viruses however variations on this theme are recognized. Rapidly cytocidal viral growth does occur. For example, poliovirus infection of HeLa cells is completed within 6 to 8 hours resulting in death of the cell and release of progeny poliovirions. Moderate growth is a variation wherein viral release from infected cells occurs over prolonged periods without loss of cell viability or integrity. Release of progeny virions is accomplished by extrusion through the plasma membrane of the cell, a process called budding. The cell membrane is altered by the insertion of viral proteins and the nucleocapsid becomes enveloped in the altered membrane as it buds through to the cell exterior. Moderate growth may continue for a short period (24 to 48 hours) after which the cell may die or, in other cases, the process may continue for rest of the life of the cell. One principal consequence of this process is the antigenic conversion of the cell surface, thus making the cell a target for immune response. Another variation is latent infection. The analogy to bacterial lysogeny seems appropritate in that the viral genome is sequestered in the cell yet it does not express by the production of progeny. Latency is often accompanied by the production of some virus gene products. In many cases these are detected as virus antigens within the cell. Another type of infection is the transforming infection in which the virus confers new properties of growth or behavior on the infected cell.

METHODS OF STUDY

Viruses require living cells for replication. Laboratory hosts for the study of viruses are usually cultures of eukaryotic cells although other hosts are occasionally used. Two types of cell cultures, primary and continuous, are available. Primary cultures are those directly established from animal or embryonic tissues. Under usual conditions, these cultures have a finite life. They can be subcultured once or twice but infrequently more. They retain species markers such as species specific antigens, isoenzymes, and chromosomes. They are euploid. Continuous cell cultures are cultures in which the cells are passaged for extended periods. Some of these cells, called cell strains, remain euploid and carry species antigens and enzymes for 30 to 40 passages in vitro. Other cultures, referred to as cell lines, are capable of unlimited replication in vitro. They are aneuploid and often have characteristics of malignant cells. They retain species characteristics.

Infectivity is a basic property of viruses that must be measured. Three types of assays are used. Quantal assays are methods that give estimates of infectious units based on an all-or-none response of an inoculated host. They are usually carried out by a serial of ten-fold dilutions of the material to be assayed and inoculation of each dilution into an appropriate host. The evidence of viral growth or lack of it (development of cytopathology, appearance of viral antigen) is recorded for each host. The infectivity is usually expressed as doses which infect 50 percent of inoculated hosts (ID_{50}) per unit volume of original preparations. Graded dose assays are those that measure some element of the host response to infection that occurs on a continuous scale. Such measurements as tumor size, time until death, or spleen weight are related to virus dose. Enumerative assays are those that give direct data based on one response for each infectious unit. Plaque assays and focus-forming assays are enumerative. Infectivity titers are usually expressed as plaque-forming units (PFU) or focus-forming units (FFU) per unit volume.

Other properties of viruses may be used to quantify virus studies. Some viruses have surface peplomers that interact with receptors on the surface of erythrocytes, thus they can bring about the agglutination of red cells. This phenomenon is the basis of viral hemagglutination (HA) assays. Since the reaction can be inhibited by antibodies against the viral peplomers, it is the basis of the hemagglutination-inhibition (HI) assay for antiviral antibodies. Other properties such as the ability to cause hemolysis can also be used to quantify virus preparation and measure antibody activity by their inhibition. The enzymatic activities of some virions (i.e., neuraminidase, RNA polymerase) can be used. The antigenic characteristics of viruses can also be used for measurement. These methods bring an exquisite degree of sensitivity and specificity to viral studies. Diagnosis of viral infections rely heavily on serologic methods.

VIRAL GENETICS

Viruses as living organisms retain and transmit their characteristics through their genomes. The genetic message is found in the DNA or RNA in the virions. There is constancy in transmission of properties from generation to generation by faithful reproduction of the base sequence of the nucleic acid. They also have the capacity to change their genetic endowment by mutation or by recombination. Genetic studies on viruses require markers for recognition of genetic variation and methods to isolate differentiated clones. Several types of viral mutants have been used in genetic studies. Plaque-forming mutants, drug resistant mutants, and drug dependent mutants have all been used. The most important type of mutant for studies of viral replication have been the conditionally lethal mutants, temperature-sensitive, and host range mutants. These mutants result from point mutations in the nucleic acid causing changes in single codons. The protein products of such changes often function under certain conditions (temperature, host cell) yet fail to function under other conditions.

INTERACTION OF VIRAL GENES AND GENE PRODUCTS

When more than one virion infects a cell, there is the opportunity for interaction between the infecting viruses. Genetically distinct yet closely related viruses often interact under these circumstances. Several types of interaction have been described. Recombination between different strains of related viruses occurs with variable frequency. Single strand RNA viruses seem rarely to recombine. Double stranded DNA viruses can recombine by conventional crossover quite readily. Viruses with segmented RNA genomes undergo recombination by the process of reassortment very readily. Complementation is another form of interaction in which defective viruses may replicate using a gene function of a coinfecting virus. This may occur when a defective virus coinfects a cell with a nondefective virus or when two defective viruses coinfect. In the latter case the viruses must not be defective in the same function. The replication facilitated by complementation does not repair the genetic lesion as the progeny viruses are still defective.

Phenotypic mixing is an event when two viruses infect a cell and viral progeny bear proteins of both parental strains. For example, if two related viruses, strain 1 and strain 2, coinfect a cell, progeny virions with the genome of strain 1 may bear capsids of strain 2 or mixtures of strain 1 and strain 2 capsomers. The progeny of these mixed virions will "breed true" in that they will only reproduce Strain 1 virions because that is the genetic constitution of the genome. A similar phenomenon can occur with budding viruses in that the nucleocapsid of one type of virus is enveloped in a membrane carrying peplomers of a second type. This is called pseudotype formation.

Another interaction is an interference interaction in which the replication of one virus interfers with the replication of another. One well studied example of interference interaction is that concerning defective interfering (DI) viruses. DI viruses are defective viruses which cannot complete their own replication. They are usually deletion mutants. To be replicated DI viruses must be complemented by a standard nondefective virus; however, the DI interferes with the replication of the standard virus.

PATHOGENESIS AND RESPONSE TO VIRUS INFECTION

Viral replication is a result of virus-cell interaction yet virus disease is a composite of cellular and systemic effects. One aspect of virus infection that affects pathogenesis is the cytotropism of the virus. Cytotropism is the ability of a virus to preferentially infect certain cells while not infecting others. For example, the cytotropism of the influenza virus is the epithelial cells of the respiratory tract while the Epstein-Barr virus infects B-lymphocytes. Cytropisms are often determined by cell surface receptors and occasionally by the presence of essential enzymes (i.e., RNA polymerases). A particularly important cytotropism is the ability of viruses to infect macrophages. Those viruses capable of infecting macrophages are often involved in systemic diseases while those not capable are more often involved in local infections. Infected macrophages can serve as vehicles for the dissemination of viruses and as a source of viremia.

A cellular response to virus infection that is of particular importance is the interferon response. Interferons (IFN) are proteins produced by cells in response to certain stimuli. Among stimuli that evoke IFN production is virus infection. IFN acts to evoke a state of refractoriness to viral infection in cells (other than the cell that produces it usually). A number of agents can stimulate IFN production by cells; among them are ultraviolet-irradiated viruses, natural double standard RNA molecules, synthetic polyribonucleic acids (e.g., polyinosinic

and polycytodylic acid), and polycarbonates. Three types of IFN have been described α, β, and γ. α and β IFN are obtained by stimulation of leukocytes and fibroblasts, respectively. They share common properties of acid stability but are antigenically distinct. γ IFN is produced by antigen stimulated lymphocytes (it is a lymphokine) and is acid labile as well as antigenially distinct from α and β IFN. IFN are species specific, protecting cells of the same species in which they were produced by in large. They do not exhibit any viral specificity, protecitng against many viruses. The mechanisms by which IFN evokes the antiviral state is now know completely. It is known that IFN treated cells must transcribe and process mRNA and that protein synthesis must take place to affect protection. For some viruses the IFN induced activity inhibits viral transcription, whereas others are inhibited at translation.

SYSTEMIC FACTORS

As previously cited the cytotropism of a virus is a factor in the pathogenesis of virus disease. A number of other factors are also important determinants. Among these are route of entry, viral susceptibility to specific and nonspecific mechanisms of protection, temperature preference of the virus, and immunologic status of the host. Reinfection with viruses usually produces a highly modified course of infection; in many cases there is no clinical manifestation of infection at all.

Immune response to virus infection is influenced by the type of infection. Infections of the respiratory tract or alimentary tract stimulate a vigorous local response characterized by secretory IgA and to a variable degree systemic IgM and IgG responses. Immunologic memory of the secretory immune system is not long lived and anemnestic responses are not apparent. Local infections do engender memory in the central immune system and local infections do provoke anemnestic responses in this system. Systemic virus diseases have an initial period in which viruses replicate at some local site at the portal of entry. Virus spreads by the blood vascular system, by the lymphatics, or in some cases by neurons to sites of secondary replication. Primary viremia may be accompanied by clinical signs such as fever but most often no manifestations are apparent. Secondary sites of replication for viremic spread are the spleen and liver. Macrophages become infected in these sites and function as a source of virus for the secondary viremia. This phase is characterized by frank clinical symptoms such as fever. Virus disseminated in this viremia infects cells of the target organ characteristic of the disease. Varicella virus, for example, is disseminated to the epithelium and the rash ensues. In some exanthamata the rash results from immunologic reactions in skin sites. Measles and rubella have this type of rash. IgM and IgG antibodies are engendered by systemic infections. Interactions of these antibodies with virions, in most cases, results in the abolition of viral infectivity. In vivo reactions undoubtedly involve the complement system as well. Neutralization of the infectivity is one of the basic mechanisms of protection attributed to the immune response. Phagocytic removal of aggregates by activated macrophages and PMN plays a role in recovery from infection. CMI is also engendered and is active in recovery. The target of CMI responses is the moderately-infected cell. Cytotoxic interaction by T-cells and other cells (K-cells, NK-cells) eradicate the source of virus. Activation of macrophages is also a critical CMI function as it converts the cell from a source of virus to a cell acting to inactivate virus.

Models of Virus Replications

All viruses must accomplish a common series of events to replicate. They must have their genome transcribed to produce mRNA which can be translated on host cell ribosomes, they must replicate their genomes, and they must generate the virions that are to be released from the cell. Different viruses have different methods of transcription and translation (Table 5-18). Below are examples of some strategies for replication of RNA and DNA viruses.

POLIOVIRUS

Polioviruses belong to the *Enterovirus* genus of the Picornaviridae. They are small (30 nm) positive single stranded RNA-containing viruses. They have four major proteins that make up the icosahedral capsid. There are 32 capsomers. The four proteins are VP1, VP2, VP3, and VP4. The genome is a linear molecule of 2.6×10^6 daltons; it is polyadenylated at the 3′ end and has a small (2,000 daltons) polypeptide, VPg attached to the 5′ end. Infection is initiated by adsorption of the virion to cell surface receptors. The first stage is divalent cation dependent, independent of temperature, and is dissociable. The second stage of the interaction involves a reorientation of capsid proteins, loss of VP4, and is nondissociable. The structural changes in the virion occurring in the second stage are accompanied by changes in antigenic expression. The native virion is an antigenic form referred to as D. Antibody reacting with D forms bring about neutralization. The reoriented virion, without VP4, is referred to as C and antibody reacting with this form does not affect neutralization. (The C antigenic form is also present in the provirion before cleavage of the VPO polypeptide). The reorientation also changes the hydrophilic-hydrophobic character of the virion allowing traverse of the cell plasma membrane. In the cytoplasm, the RNA is released from the capsid, the VPg

Table 5-18. Clinical Syndromes Associated with Coxsackieviruses and Echoviruses

	Coxsackieviruses		Echoviruses
	Group A	Group B	
Aseptic meningitis	+	+	+
Encephalitis	+	+	+
Cerebellar ataxia	+	+	+
Muscle weakness and paralysis	+	+	+
Exanthemata (vesicular, maculopapular)	+	+	+
Epidemic pleurodynia	−	+	−
Pericarditis, myocarditis	−	+	−
Orchitis, parotitis, epididymitis	−	+	−
Generalized disease in early infancy (myocarditis, encephalitis, hepatitis)	−	+	−
Respiratory (acute upper respiratory) disease, summer grippe, pneumonia	+	+	+
Herpangina	+	−	−
Hand, foot, and mouth disease	+	−	−

(Milgrom F, Flanagan TD: Medical Microbiology. Churchill Livingstone, New York 1982.)

residue is cleaved from the molecule, and the entire RNA is translated into a 2.5×10^5 dalton polypeptide that immediately undergoes cleavage into three fragments (Fig. 5-21). The cleavage is carried out by host enzymes. Two fragments, NCVP0 and NCVP1 are cleaved from the polypeptide and are further processed. NCVPO is cut into a smaller fragment NCVP2 which is further cut to NCVP4 and VPg. The NCVP4 fragment may be cut into a polypeptide possessing protease activity as well as one with polymerase activity. The NCVP1 is cleaved by the viral protease into three fragments VP0, VP1, and VP3. These three residues associate during the morphogenesis of progeny virions into aggregates that ultimately form the capsid. A final cleavage of the VP0 peptide occurs after incorporation of the progeny RNA molecule; the cleavage yields a VP2 and a VP4 polypeptide. Replication of the genome occurs by the formation of a replicative intermediate (RI). This entity is a complex formed of the NCVP2 and RNA. The RNA component is made up of one antimessenger (negative) molecule from which several messenger-sense (positive) strands are copied by the NCVP2 polymerase. Attachment of VPg to the 5′ end of progeny ⁺RNA strands is required for the molecule's incorporation into progeny capsids. Morphogenesis of poliovirions takes place in the cytoplasm of the cell. Sixty units, each composed of one VP0, VP1, and VP3 residue, associate to form an entity called the procapsid. Progeny polyadenylated RNA with VPg attached is incorporated and the entity becomes a provirion. Final cleavage of all VP0 residues to VP2 and

VP4 completes the virion. Poliovirus-infected cells undergo rapid shutdown of cellular function soon after infection. The entire replicative cycle is completed in 6 to 8 hours and the cell slowly lyses.

ADENOVIRUS

Human adenoviruses belong to the genus *Mastadenovirus* in the family Adenoviridae. The virions are icosahedral particles without envelopes. They have 252 capsomers, 240 hexons, and 12 pentons. There are 12 penton fibers attached to the pentons on each of the vertices of the icosahedron. Ten different proteins are in the virion. The virion contains a double stranded linear DNA molecule (23×10^6 daltons) that has a 55 K protein attached on each 5′ terminus. Initiation of infection takes place by the interaction of penton fibers and an undefined cell surface receptor. Virions traverse the cell membrane and appear in the cytoplasm minus the pentons and penton fibers. The particles appear larger than the mature virion suggesting some conformational change. Infecting virions migrate to the nucleus of the cell during which time they undergo further change losing hexons and releasing DNA which remains associated with proteins. In the nucleus, early transcription of the viral DNA is carried out by host RNA polymerase. About 15 percent of the genome is transcribed from sequences on each strand. Early mRNA is translated in the cytoplasm yielding products active in DNA synthesis. Five to 6 hours after initiation of infection, viral DNA synthesis begins in the nucleus of the cells. It is carried out by viral enzymes and host enzymes. Semiconservative DNA synthesis takes place by 5′–3′ polymerization of a daughter strand. As polymerization progresses, one parental strand is displaced. The displaced strand forms a "pan handle" due to terminal inverted repeat sequences of bases on the strand. A second daughter strand is then polymerized 5′–3′ using the panhandle strand as template. Late synthesis begins with late transcription of the viral progeny DNA molecules. Late transcription yields 13 species of mRNA that are produced by a process of excision and splicing. Translation of these molecules produces the structural proteins of the progeny virions. Morphogenesis of virions takes place in the nucleus of the cell. Crystalline arrays of complete and incomplete virions along with excess viral DNA and proteins make up the characteristic intranuclear inclusion of adenovirus-infected cells. Infected cells lose their capacity for macromolecular synthesis gradually but remain metabolically active for considerable periods. Virions are very poorly released from the cells, less than 10 percent can be found extracellularly. The replicative cycle is prolonged up to 24 hours before infectious progeny are detected.

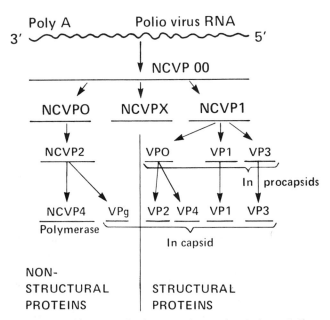

Fig. 5-21. Cleavage of poliovirus polypeptides. (Milgrom F, Flanagan TD: Medical Microbiology. Churchill Livingstone, New York, 1982.)

INFLUENZAVIRUS

Influenzavirus is a genus in the family Orthomyxoviridae. It contains influenza viruses A, B, and C. The viruses are similar in biology and the replication of influenza A will serve as a model for negative strand RNA viruses. The virion is spherical in shape and it is enveloped. There are two types of peplomer in the envelope, a hemagglutinin (HA) and a neuraminidase (NA) peplomer. The genome of the virus occurs in eight fragments within the envelope. Each is encapsidated in a helical nucleocapsid composed of many molecules of a nucleoprotein (NP) and three polymerase (P1, P2, P3) molecules. A matrix protein (M) is found lining the inner face of the envelope. Thus seven different proteins are found in the virions (an eighth, NS, is found in virus-infected cells). The eight RNA segments are in antimessenger configuration. The total mass of the genome is 4.8×10^6 daltons. Infection of host cells is initiated by binding of the HA peplomer to sialic acid residues on the cell surface. Fusion of the viral envelope with the plasma membrane of the cell is affected by the hydrophobic end of the HA2 fragment of the HA molecule. In the cytoplasm of the cell the RNA fragments are transcribed giving eight mRNA species, each of which is translated into a protein. The NS polypeptide modifies the activity of the P1, P2, P3 complex bringing about replication of the gene segment. Progeny nucleocapsids appear in the nucleus of the cell and viral glycoproteins HA and NA appear on the surface of the cell as integral parts of the plasma membrane. Progeny nucleocapsids are transported to cytoplasmic regions beneath the viral modified membrane. The M protein apparently plays some role in recognition of the sites. Virion morphogenesis takes place as the nucleocapsids are enveloped by the modified membrane by budding out of the cell. Release from the surface is a function of the NA peplomer which cleaves *N*-acetylneuraminic acid from surface mucoprotein receptors.

HERPESVIRUS

Herpes viruses are large enveloped viruses, 180 nm in diameter. The envelope encloses a iscosahedral capsid made up of 162 hollow pentagonal capsomers. The virion contains a linear double stranded molecule of DNA that has a mass of 100×10^6 daltons. The herpes virus genome found in the virion has a unique structure. There are two segments of unique sequences, a long sequence and a short sequence, bracketed by repeated sequences. Two regions of repeated sequences are found at the ends of the molecule and two additional inverted repeat sequences separate the unique sequences. This arrangement allows the generation of four isomers of the genome by the rearrangement of the unique sequences relative to each other.

Replication is initiated by adsorption to the plasma membrane of the host cell. Entry is accomplished by fusion or viropexis. Viral DNA takes up a nuclear site in the cell and immediate early transcription, referred to as α transcription, takes place. The transcription is carried out by host RNA polymerase II. After transcription and processing in the nucleus, the mRNA is translated into proteins; the process is α synthesis. Some products of α synthesis function to promote transcription of a second set of viral genes and some function in viral DNA synthesis. The second set of genes produce mRNA called β mRNA that when translated in the cytoplasm gives rise to β proteins. The β products function to modulate the α synthesis, to function in viral DNA synthesis and to initiate γ transcription. The third set of viral genes are transcribed into γ mRNA that is translated into functional and structural proteins. One function is to modulate β synthesis. Viral DNA synthesis takes place in the nucleus of the cell. A variety of circular and circular-linear forms are found along with long linear concatemers of viral DNA. Morphogenesis of the herpesvirions begins in the nucleus of the infected cell. Viral capsids are assembled in that site and DNA is packaged in the progeny virions. Viral glycoproteins appear in all of the membranes of the infected cell. Envelopment of the capsid takes place by budding through the inner lamella of the nuclear membrane. Additional budding events may take place producing virions with more than one envelope. Enveloped virions are found in cisternae in the cytoplasm and eventually are emptied into the extracellular medium. Herpes virus infections are moderate in nature but eventual cell death is the usual end result. Some cell types apparently have the capacity to remain latently infected yet produce infectious virus intermittantly. The nature of these cell-virus relationships is unknown.

Clinical Virology

ORTHOMYXOVIRUSES

Influenza A, influenza B, and influenza C are serotypes of the viruses that cause epidemic and endemic influenza in the human and in animal populations. Serotype is based on the antigenicity of the nucleoproteins (NP) and matrix (M) proteins in the virion. Influenza A and B are responsible for most disease and for the epidemic and pandemic forms of influenza. Influenza C is encountered in endemic or sporatic cases. The replicative cycle of Influenza A is outlined above. The most salient aspect of the structure and replication of this virus is its fragmented genome. Recombination by reassortment of genome fragments is thought to be an important determinant in the epidemiology of the disease. It enables the virus to change its antigenicity so as to evade the herd immunity engendered by exposure to previous strains. The classification of influenza A strains is based upon the antigenicity of the surface peplomers of the virus, the hemagglutinin (H), and the neuraminidase (N). All human and animal strains of influenza A are described by the place of isolation, the number of the particular prototype isolate, the year of isolation, and the antigenic class of its H and N peplomers. Thus the designation A/USSR/90/77(H1N1) describes a strain of influenza A isolated in the USSR, the 90th such isolate in the year 1977 that has H1 hemagglutinin and an N1 neuraminidase. To date, human strains of influenza A have H1, H2, or H3 hemagglutinin and N1 or N2 neuraminidase. A major change in the H antigen (i.e., H1 to H2 in the prevalent strain in a region) is called antigenic shift. It occurs as a result of recombination in which the gene for H2 is substituted for H1. The consequences of this change is opportunity for the new strain to infect individuals whose immunity has been engendered against the H1 peplomer. Changes in antigenicity of a given H or N peplomer also occur by mutation, a process described as antigenic drift. Such changes may give rise to greater or less abilities to survive in an immune host. Changes arising by antigenic shift are thought to be responsible for pandemics and widespread occurrence of influenza. Changes arising from antigenic drift are thought to be responsible for the 1 to 3 year epidemic cycles of the disease experienced in various regions. Influenza B strains are described by the place of isolation, number of prototype, and year. There are no designations of the antigenicity of the peplomers. Antigenic shift has not been observed with influenza B or C viruses although they have a segmented genome similar in structure to influenza A. Influenza B does undergo antigenic drift and these changes are responsible for epidemics of influenza B that occur every 3 to 5 years. Influenza is a respiratory disease. The virus gains entry by inhalation of droplets and implants on the respiratory epithelium. Viral replication in this site leads to local destruction of the epithelium in the trachea and bronchi. Viremia is not a consistant occurrence; however, constitutional symptoms are usually present. The patient suffers fever, chills, and myalgia. Respiratory distress occurs to a variable extent. Diagnosis can be accomplished by isolation of the virus and by serologic means. A four-fold rise in the hemagglutination inhibition (HI) titer of serum antibodies against the prototype A or B strain between the acute phase and the convalescent phase is indicative of infection. Vaccination of high risk populations (elderly, debilitated, etc.) is carried out by parenteral inoculation with a polyvalent (type A and type B) preparation of inactivated virus.

PARAMYXOVIRUSES

The family Paramyoviridae contains three genera, *Paramyxovirus, Morbillivirus,* and *Pneumovirus.* The viruses are large (about 200 nm) RNA-containing enveloped viruses. The RNA of the genomes is a single stranded molecule about $5-6 \times 10^6$ daltons in molecular mass and is in the negative (antimessenger) configuration. The genomes are not segmented and the genetic code is inscribed in sequences that are transcribed into 7 to 10 monocistronic mRNA molecules by a virion transcriptase. The surface of the virions have two types of surface peplomers, a cell recognition peplomer and a fusion peplomer.

The paramyxoviruses have two biologic activities associated with the cell recognition peplomer, hemagglutination and neuraminidase. The structure is made up of a dimer of the HN glycoprotein. The fusion peplomer is also a dimer of the F glycoprotein. Morbilliviruses do not have neuraminidase but do have hemagglutinin; therefore cell recognition is a function of an HA peplomer. These viruses also have F. The Pneumoviruses have neither hemagglutination nor neuraminidase functions associated with the cell recognition peplomer. The structure is made up of a glycoprotein, however. The viruses do have a fusion peplomer made up of F glycoprotein.

The principal human pathogens in the genus *Paramyxovirus* are parainfluenza types 1–4 and mumps virus. The parainfluenza viruses are respiratory pathogens. Types 1–3 are the most frequently encountered. They cause upper and lower respiratory tract infections in children. They cause croup and bronchiolitis in primary infections of children 6 to 18 months. Type 3 is also an important cause of pneumonia in infants. In adults, the viruses cause mild upper respiratory disease. Reinfection with the parainfluenza viruses is common. Diagnosis can be carried out by isolation of the viruses, by demonstration of viral antigen in exfoliated cells from the nasopharynx, and by serology. The HI test is used for antibody testing.

Mumps virus causes a systemic disease in distinction to the local infection of the respiratory tract caused by the parainfluenzas. The mumps virus gains entry through the respiratory tract but there is viremia and systemic dissemination of the virus. The usual symptoms of mumps is parotidis accompanied by fever. Other glands may also be involved. In postpubital males, orchitis occurs in about 20 percent of the cases. Meningoencephalitis is another manifestation of the infection that may occur even in the absence of parotidis. In children less than 2 years, mumps virus infection often takes the form of an upper respiratory infection. Systemic immunity is the result of infection in almost all cases and second episodes are very rare. Diagnosis can be accomplished by viral isolation from throat swabs or urine.

Serodiagnosis is carried out by HI or complement fixation (CF). A four-fold rise in antibody titer between the acute phase serum and the convalescent phase sample is diagnostic. Vaccination against mumps is carried out using a live attentiated strain of mumps virus.

MORBILLIVIRUS

The genus *Morbillivirus* contains measles virus, canine distemper virus, and rhinderpest virus. The virions of these agents resemble the other Paramyxoviridae in that they are large, enveloped, and bear surface peplomers. Unlike the viruses of the *Paramyxovirus* genus, there is no neuraminidase activity associated with the cell-recognition peplomer. There is hemagglutinating activity, however. The F protein is similar in structure and size to that found in the other genus.

Measles virus is the human pathogen of the genus, infecting humans and some other primates. Infection is initiated in the respiratory epithelium where primary viral replication takes place. Virus spreads from the primary site probably by infecting lymphocytes and macrophages. Secondary sites of replication include lymph nodes, spleen, and other aggregates of lymphoid tissues. Primary and secondary replication ensues for about 9 to 10 days when the infection becomes clinically apparent with the onset of the prodrome. This period is characterized by coryza, cough, and fever. The prodrome last from 3 to 5 days. The typical rash is heralded by the appearance of Koplik spots on the buccal mucosa followed quickly by the development of a macular rash. The rash first appears on the forehead later spreading over the face, limbs, and trunk. Concomitant with the appearance of the rash, IgM and IgG antibodies are demonstrable in the serum. Soon after the appearance of the rash, the fever begins to subside. The skin becomes brown over the area of the macules and desquamates. Patients frequently have photophobia. Significant complications of measles are encephalitis and giant cell pneumonia. The diagnosis of measles is usually made on the basis of clinical presentation. In the present postvaccine era, laboratory confirmation may be necessary. The viruses can be isolated from the throat and urine during the prodrome and early period after onset of the rash. Serodiagnosis may be carried out using the HI test to compare acute phase serum antibody titers and convalescent phase titers. Immunity after infection is lifelong. Vaccination is practiced using an attenuated strain of live measles virus.

PNEUMOVIRUS

The human pathogen respiratory syncytial virus is a member of the genus *Pneumovirus*. This virus has neither hemagglutinating nor neuraminidase activity. It is highly fusogenic when growing in cell cultures (and in vivo). Respiratory syncytial virus is the leading cause of viral pneumonia and bronchiolitis in infants less than 6 months of age. In other children and adults, it causes mild upper respiratory disease. Diagnosis of infection is carried out by the demonstration of viral antigen by immunofluorescence in exfoliated cells of the nasopharynx. The virus can also be isolated in cell cultures. There is no effective vaccine for the infection.

PICORNAVIRUSES

The Picornaviridae contains two genera with human pathogens, *Enterovirus* and *Rhinovirus*. The viruses have small (30 nm) virions and are icosahedral in shape with 32 capsomers. They are not enveloped and have four abundant polypeptide species in the virion. The genome is in the form of a single stranded RNA molecule, 2.6×10^6 daltons in mass. The RNA is polyadenylated at the 3′ terminus and has a small polypeptide (about 2,000 daltons) covalently linked to the 5′ terminus. The genomic RNA can be directly translated on host ribosomes after removal of the terminal polypeptide. The replication of these viruses, as exemplified by poliovirus, was previously described.

Rhinoviruses are agents of the common cold. They differ from the enteroviruses in two properties. They are acid labile and they grow preferentially at 33°C. There are currently 89 defined serotypes and another 20 viruses that may be established as serotypes. Rhinoviruses cause the common cold, a mild upper respiratory infection characterized by lack of fever, coryza, and rhinitis. The viruses do not invade the lower respiratory tract. Immunity is serotype specific and principally a function of secretory IgA.

The enteroviruses were divided into four groups, polioviruses, Coxsackie viruses A and B, and echoviruses based upon their pathogenicity in primates, infant mice, and growth in cell cultures. The polioviruses are neurovirulent in monkeys. The Coxsackie A viruses cause a widespread myocitis leading to flaccid paralysis in infant mice while the Coxsackie B viruses cause spastic paralysis with viral growth in brown fat, nerve, and other tissues. The echoviruses do not cause neurologic symptoms in monkeys nor do they grow in infant mice. Echoviruses cause cytopathology in primate cell cultures as do the polioviruses, the Coxsackie B viruses, and some serotypes of Coxsackie A. Serotypes are defined by neutralization tests. There are 3 serotypes of poliovirus, 23 of Coxsackie A, 6 of Coxsackie B, and 31 of echovirus. Recognition that the traditional distinctions among these viruses are not absolute has led to the recent decision not to attempt characterization of new enterovirus isolates according to previous criteria. New isolates are now designated a serotype of enterovirus. There are four serotypes, enterovirus 68–71. A number of serotypes have been reclassified, echovirus 10 is reovirus 1, echovirus 28 is a rhinovirus, and echovirus 34 is a strain of Coxsackie A24. Coxsackie A23 is identical to echovirus 9 and the Coxsackie A designation was never officially sanctioned. The most serious clinical manifestation of infection with the enteroviruses is poliomyelitis. It is caused by poliovirus types 1–3. Occasionally, paralytic disease has been associated with the Coxsackie A viruses. The disease entities associated with the enteroviruses other than poliovirus are shown in Table 5-18.

Diagnosis of enterovirus infection can be accomplished by isolation and identification of the agent. Serodiagnosis is feasible only for the polioviruses and the Coxsackie B viruses. In the United States, active immunization against poliovirus infection is carried out by a polyvalent live virus vaccine (OPV) containing all three serotypes. In some other countries, a formalin-inactivated polyvalent preparation (IPV) is used.

RUBELLA

Rubella virus belongs to the *Rubivirus* genus of the Togaviridae. It differs from other togaviruses in that it does not require an arthropod vector for dissemination. The virion is 42–45 nm in diameter, and enveloped with an icosahedral nucleocapsid containing a positive stranded RNA genome 4×10^6 daltons in mass. The virus causes rubella, a benign disease of childhood, and the congenital rubella syndrome, a serious generalized infection in fetuses that can result in a range of congenital defects. Rubella virus is acquired by airborne droplet and replicates in the respiratory epithelium. Secondary sites of viral replication are established in many organs and tissues including lymphoid tissue. The incubation period averages 18 days. Onset is marked by low grade fever and an ephemeral maculopapular rash. The usual duration of rash is to three days. Prominent cervical lymphadenopathy is a consistant finding even in cases where the rash is not apparent. The diagnosis is usually based on clinical findings but the virus can be isolated from nasopharyngeal secretions and urine during the late incubation period and early onset phase. Serodiagnosis can be done by comparing acute phase antibody titers and convalescent phase titers by HI or ELISA tests. Caution in interpretation must be practiced since the rise in titer occurs very early in relation to the onset of rash. High titers are not unusual seven to 10 days after the rash. Demonstration of IgM antibody is a good positive indicator of recent infection.

Congenital rubella syndrome can result from an in utero infection of the fetus. A primary infection in a nonimmune pregnant woman involves viral replication in the placenta which spreads to the fetus and fetal membranes. Most defects are associated with infection during the first trimester of pregnancy. Stillbirth often occurs as a result of infection in the first month, later infection causes deafness, cataracts, cardiac defects, microcephaly, and motor deficits. Rubella infants are often actively shedding virus at birth and many continued to shed for variable periods up to 12 to 18 months. The fetus mounts an immune to the infection and IgM antibody can be demonstrated in the serum.

Immunity after rubella infection is usually lifelong and second episodes are extremely rare. Immune status can be established by serology. The HI test is used. Titers greater than 20 are indicative of immunity. Vaccination of children and adult susceptibles is carried out using an attenuated strain of live rubella virus.

Rotaviruses and Other Viruses Causing Acute Gastroenteritis

The family Reoviridae contains the genera *Reovirus, Rotavirus,* and *Orbivirus* which contain viruses infecting humans. The viruses are characterized by a double-capsid structure, icosahedral shape, lack of true envelope (orbiviruses are inactivated by ether but not detergents), and a segmented double stranded RNA genome. The molecular mass of the genomes is $10-15 \times 10^6$ daltons. There are 10 segments in the reovirus genome, 11 in the rotavirus, and 8 in the orbivirus genome. Replication of the viruses takes place in the cytoplasm of infected cells. One strand of each segment of the double stranded RNA genome is transcribed by a virion polymerase to produce a messenger RNA molecule. Each segment is a single gene directing the synthesis of a single polypeptide. The virions are assembled and mature in the cytoplasm of the cell. They do not bud from cell membranes, however viral antigens can be detected in the membranes.

Reoviruses types 1, 2, and 3 have been associated with respiratory and with enteric infections of humans. Their role as etiologic agents is not well established. The only human pathogen among the orbiviruses is Colorado tick fever virus. This agent is transmitted to humans by a tick vector from its wild rodent reservoir. The infection in humans is usually mild and self-limiting. There is no human-to-human spread.

Rotaviruses are the principal cause of nonbacterial gastroenteritis in humans. The human viruses are morphologically identical to rotaviruses which infect other species such as cattle, pigs, mice, and monkeys. There is some serologic relationship among the viruses but cross infection among the viruses and other species apparently does not occur. Rotaviral diarrhea occurs in infants and children 6 to 24 months of age. The disease is relatively benign in healthy well nourished children but can be very serious in malnourished children. The virus is spread by the fecal-oral route. It infects the differentiated enterocytes of the intestinal villi, sparing the crypt cells and other elements. Viral cytopathology causes denuding of the villi with subsequent loss of fluid. There appears to be at least two serologically distinct types of human rotavirus. Definitive studies on the serology and epidemiology of the viruses have not been carried out because the viruses cannot be regularly propagated in the laboratory.

Another group of viruses associated with human diarrhea appear to be caliciviruses. The prototype of the human agent is called the Norwalk agent of acute viral gastroenteritis. The virus has not been grown in the laboratory and information on its role in human disease is incomplete.

HEPATITIS VIRUSES

Many viruses such as human cytomegalovirus, Epstein-Barr virus, herpes simplex virus, and yellow fever virus can cause hepatitis. By convention, these agents are not referred to as hepatitis viruses. There are two well defined viruses causing human hepatitis (hepatitis A virus and hepatitis B virus) and a third entity (non A non B) that are designated hepatitis viruses. Non A non B hepatitis virus is also called hepatitis C virus.

Hepatitis A virus causes a clinical disease formerly referred to as infectious hepatitis. The virus is spread by the fecal-oral route. Common source outbreaks are often associated with contaminated food, frequently shellfish. The virus is a typical human enterovirus in morphology and composition. It cannot be propagated well in the laboratory; therefore, definitve studies on its biology are incomplete. There appears to be only one serotype. The virus is usually acquired by ingestion although it may be spread by parental infection in a manner similar to hepatitis B virus as outlined below. The incubation period is 15 to 40 days and onset of the acute phase is sudden with fever and frank evidence of heptatic inflammation. Virus can be demonstrated in the blood during the late incubation and early onset phases. Virus is shed in the feces during this period. Antibody becomes demonstrable soon after onset and increases in titer. Lifelong immunity is conferred by the infection. Diagnosis is frequently established on clinical and epidemiologic grounds although serologic tests for antibody are becoming available. Prophylaxis is affected by adminstration of pooled human IgG.

Hepatitis B virus does not fall into any of the recognized families or genera in the current taxonomy (although the name *Hepadnavirus* has been suggested). The agent occurs as a 42 nm particle containing lipids, proteins, and glycoproteins with a circular interrupted double stranded DNA genome. In addition to the complete virion, several other morphologic forms are found in the serum of patients with hepatitis B. A 22 nm spherical particle and a 22 nm diameter rod-like particle can be seen by electron microscopy. The antigenicity of these three forms are the same and are referred to as HB_sAg. The complete virion, the Dane particle or 42 nm particle, has a central core composed of DNA and protein. The surface of the Dane particle has the same antigenicity of the 22 nm particle, HB_sAg. The core is antigenically distinct and referred to as HB_cAg. Another antigenic specificity, HB_eAg is found on a small particle present in the serum of acutely infected patients. It is a viral gene product but its role in replication is unknown. Finally, there is a DNA polymerase activity associated with the Dane particle core and core structures found in infected cells. All HBV surface antigen preparations (HB_sAg) contain a common antigen, a, and two other antigens each of which is present in one of two allelic forms, d or y and w or r. Thus any HB_sAg preparation is adw or adr or ayw or ayr. The significance of these alleles is unknown; however, they are useful in epidemiologic studies. Immunity is associated with anti HB_s antibodies. The clinical course of hepatitis B is similar to hepatitis A but there are some differences. The virus is acquired (in nonthird world countries) by parenteral inoculation of blood from patients or carriers. This may occur by transfusion or use of blood contaminated needles, syringes, or other instruments. In certain institutional situations and in cases of sexual contact, the virus may be spread directly person-to-person. The incubation period is prolonged, 60 to 160 days and onset is frequently insidious. HB_sAg can be found in the blood late in incubation and during the acute phase. HB_sAg is also present in bile, semen, urine, feces, and nasopharyngeal secretions during the acute phase. Anti-HB_c and HB_eAg are also present in blood during this phase of illness. Their presence is considered the strongest evidence of high potential for infectivity. During convalescence, HB_eAg and anti-HB_c disappear rapidly, while a gradual drop in HB_sAg titer occurs. Eventually rising titers of anit-HB_s can be detected in the serum. In about 10–15 percent of adult patients and 35 percent of children, antigenemia persists longer than 6 months. These patients are classified as chronic carriers and about 50 percent of them have no evidence of liver pathology or dysfunction.

Diagnosis can be carried out by demonstration of HB_sAg in serum, usually by RIA or ELISA. In addition, further documentation for purposes of prognosis may be done by demonstration of anti-HB_c and HB_eAg.

Control of hepatitis B is practiced by vaccination of high risk groups including physicians, dentists, nurses, hemodialysis unit personnel, and others with an inactivated virus preparation derived from pooled antigenemic serum. Prophylaxis with pooled IgG from donors having high titers or anti HB_s has efficacy.

HERPESVIRUS

There are five human herpesviruses, herpes simplex virus–type 1 (HSV-1), herpes simplex virus–type 2 (HSV-2), varicella-zoster virus (VZV), cytomegalovirus (CMV), and Epstein-Barr virus (EBV). Humans are also susceptible to occasional infection with other primate herpes viruses.

One of the important characteristics of herpes viruses is their ability to enter into latency after primary infection. The latent infection has the potential to develop into an episode of active viral replication and recrudescent expression of disease. The factors that stimulate recurrent herpes virus disease are not entirely defined although for each virus certain agents, occurrences, and physiologic states are associated with exacerbation.

Primary infection with HSV-1 usually occurs in early childhood. By age 15, over 90 percent of humans have anti HSV-1 antibodies. Infection is often protean in nature with a clinically nondescript presentation. Gingivostomatitis characterized by vesicle formation is the most frequent recognizable presentation, occuring in 10–15 percent of cases. Other primary infections do occur, with encephalitis the most serious. Newborns and malnourished children suffer more serious infections and encephalitis occurs with greater frequency. Saliva is the usual source of virus but direct inoculation of vesicular material is also an important source.

Subsequent to primary infection, the virus becomes latent. Studies have shown the virus present in greater than 50 percent of trigeminal ganglia cultured on autopsy. The virus can also be recovered from cervical and vagus ganglia. Twenty five percent of the population suffer from recurrent HSV-1 disease, usually as vesicular eruptions around the mucocutaneous junctions of the nose and mouth. A number of inciting factors have been described including emotional stress, ultraviolet irradiation, fever, menses, and x-irradiation. Reactivation can also occur without the development of lesions. About 3 percent of persons can be demonstrated at any given time to shed HSV-1 in the oropharynx.

Immune response to primary HSV-1 infection consists of antibody and cellular responses. The role of antibody in protection is ambiguous. It does not prevent cell-to-cell spread of virus although cell-free virus is neutralized. Reinfection from exogenous sources as well as reactivation of latent infection occurs in spite of demonstrable antibody. CMI is important in the resolution of lesions.

Reinfection from exogenous sources occurs readily under conditions in which the normal skin barrier is compromised. Eczyma and burns make the skin particularly vulnerable to herpes simplex infection. Abraded skin such as that which occurs in high school and that of college wrestlers also is fertile ground for viral growth. Dentists and physicians often acquire infections through small abrasions of the skin around finger nail beds leading to herpetic whitlows.

HSV-2 is serologically related to HSV-1, sharing many common antigens. The genomes of the two viruses share about 50 percent homology. HSV-2 causes infections characterized by vesicular eruptions of the skin and mucosa of the genitalia and adjacent areas. The virus is spread by sexual contact and the infection is the second most frequently occurring of the sexually transmitted disease (STD). Primary infection usually occurs in adolescence in persons who already have been infected with HSV-1. HSV-2 can establish latency in the sacral nerve ganglia. Exacerbation of vesicular eruption usually involves the skin or mucosa of the genitalia, perineum, or perianal area. Infection of newborns is affected at birth by passage of the infant through the birth canal in which HSV-2 is present. Newborns are particularly vulnerable to infection which often presents as generalized vesicular eruptions and/or encephalitis. There is a 70 percent case fatality rate with untreated herpes encephalitis whether caused by HSV-1 or HSV-2. Central nervous system infection of adults with HSV-2 usually manifests as aseptic meningitis rather than encephalitis as seen with HSV-1.

Both HSV-1 and HSV-2 have been associated with neoplasia, HSV-1 with tumors of the mouth and tongue, and HSV-2 with carcinoma of the cervix. While most evidence is epidemiologic in nature, both viruses have the potential to transform cells in vitro and there is evidence of viral DNA in tumor tissues.

Diagnosis of HSV-1 or HSV-2 infections can be affected by isolation of the virus from vesicular fluid or tissue biopsies. In the case of encephalitis in adults the lesion is usually focal in nature and occurs most often in the orbital-frontal and temporal lobes. It is usually unilateral. In neonates the encephalitis is usually diffuse in nature. Demonstration of viral antigen in biopsy tissue can be carried out using immunofluorescence. Serodiagnosis is useful in cases of primary infections. The antibody response in recurrent infection is not a reliable indicator, since many cases of verified infection (viral isolation) have failed to cause a rise in antibody titer.

At present there is no vaccine for the viruses and development of a vaccine will be difficult in that the oncogenic potential of the viruses presents a significant obstacle. Treatment of serious infections (i.e., encephalitis) is carried out with acyclovir and vidarabine. Topical treatment of vesicles with acyclovir reduces the period of eruption. No treatment has been proved effective for preventing the recurrence of disease.

VZV causes varicella (chickenpox) in susceptible individuals. The virus enters by the airborne route in droplets from an infected individual. The virus multiplies locally in the epithelium or lymphoid tissues. There is a 14 to 16 day incubation period before the onset of fever and a papular rash disseminated over the skin and mucous membranes. The papules vesiculate and scab over. Several crops of lesions are present in any given area of skin. CMI is an important factor in recovery. Antibody is important in immunity to subsequent infection. Varicella is a relatively benign disease in children; however, it is quite severe in adults, often causing diffuse pneumonia. Immunocompromized patients such as children with leukemia or those receiving corticosteroids suffer extensive disease. The recurrent form of VZV infections is zoster (shingles). This disease manifests as vesicular eruptions usually confined to the dermatome innervated by a single dorsal root sensory ganglion. Onset of zoster is signaled by pain at the eventual site of eruption. The vesicles may persist for 2 to 4 weeks. Zoster occurs in spite of demonstrable antibody in the serum. There is usually a rise in titer which can help in serodiagnosis. An individual usually experiences only one episode of zoster as opposed to the repeated exacerbation occurring with HSV.

There is an attenuated live virus vaccine available for immunization. It is used for children with leukemia and others particularly vulnerable to VZV. Treatment of severe case with vidarabine has been done and may be efficacious.

CMV is the cause of a variety of clinical syndromes the most important of which is cytomegalic inclusion disease (CID). Primary infections with CMV manifest in adults as a mononucleosis. The disease is somewhat less severe than that caused by EBV and is characterized by the absence of Paul-Bunnell antibodies in the serum. Other manifestations of CMV infections in adults are hepatitis, Guillain-Barré syndrome, and encephalitis.

Acquisition of CMV infection during fetal life leads to CID. This infection presents as a characteristic syndrome seen in the newborn as hepatosplenomegaly with jaundice. There are a variety of defects associated with CID the most serious being microcephaly. Approximately 40 percent of CID infants show evidence of retardation during development. Infection during the newborn period causes symptoms similar to CID but evidence of significant damage to the CNS has not been demonstrated.

CMV is also responsible for disease seen in patients receiving tissue transplants and those receiving immunosuppressive therapy for other reasons. Also patients receiving large volumes of blood show increased incidence of CMV infections. A mononucleosis syndrome is the usual presentation in these cases. In severely immunodeficient patients, CMV can cause pneumonia and serious disseminated disease.

Reactivation of latent infection usually manifests as mild disease. Both primary and reactivated disease can lead to congenital CID in fetuses of pregnant women. Cervical shedding of CMV is common and held to be a source of infection for newborns.

The usual spread of CMV among adults and children is by saliva. Thre is also evidence for sexual transmission of the virus.

Diagnosis of CMV infection can be carried out by demonstration of characteristic giant cells with intranuclear inclusions present in urine sediments or exfoliated from other sites. The cells also carry viral antigens demonstrable by immunofluorescence. Isolation, usually from urine, is possible and serologic diagnosis using ELISA and immunofluorescent techniques is commonly done.

Control of CMV infection is difficult. There is no vaccine and because of the transforming capacity of the virus, the prospects for one are presently remote. Severe cases have been treated with acyclovir and vidarabine but evidence for efficacy is not strong.

EBV causes infectious mononucleosis (IM). IM is a mononucleosis characterized by a triad of findings. Clinically the patient has malaise and a moderately severe pharyngitis. Low grade fever may be present. Hematologically, there is an absolute lymphocytosis with greater than 50 percent lymphocytes of which 10 percent are atypical. Serologically, Paul-Bunnell antibodies are demonstrable in the serum. IM as a clinical entity is seen most frequently in young adults and represents primary infection with EBV. In childhood, typical IM is not seen in EBV infection, although, sensitive tests for Paul-Bunnell antibodies have shown them present.

In Africa, EBV is associated with Burkitt's lymphoma. This tumor, usually occurring on the head or neck of African children, carries EBV antigens and DNA in the neoplastic cells. Cell-free EBV is capable of transforming lymphocytes in vitro and the transformed cells bear EBV antigens and DNA. The virus is also associated with nasopharyngeal carcinoma occurring in southeast Asia. The EBV nuclear antigen, EBNA is found in the epithelial elements of this tumor in contrast to its presence in the lymphoid cells of Burkitt's lymphoma.

Diagnosis of IM rests on the triad of findings described above. Antibodies against EBV antigens, viral capsid antigen (VCA), and early antigen (EA) are usually present during the acute phase of the disease. Therefore, only demonstration of IgM antibodies to VCA is helpful. It is also important to note that anti EBNA antibodies appear late, about 6 months after the acute phase. While the virus cannot be isolated in the usual sense, its presence in oropharyngeal secretions can be demonstrated by its ability to induce EBNA in cord lymphocytes.

There is no vaccine for EBV and at present no effective

regimen for antiviral therapy. Acyclovir is currently being tested.

ADENOVIRUS

Human adenoviruses belong to the genus *Mastadenovirus*. There are 31 serotypes classified by serum neutralization tests. In addition the viruses may be grouped according to their ability to hemagglutinate various species erythrocytes. Subgroup 1 agglutinate rhesus monkey red cells, subgroup 2 agglutinate rat and monkey red cells and subgroup 3 agglutinate rat red cells. The viruses may also be classified on their oncogenic potential. Highly oncogenic (for rodents) serotypes 12, 18, and 31 are differentiated from weakly oncogenic, 8, 9, 10, 13, 15, 17, 19, and 20 and the remaining serotypes that are not oncogenic. Immunologically, the type specific antigenic determinants are found on the hexons and or the penton fibers while family (all human adenoviruses) determinants are present on the hexons and pentons.

Adenoviruses cause a variety of human diseases (Table 5-19). Certain serotypes are associated with certain infections. There is a live virus vaccine used in military populations for the prevention of acute respiratory disease due to types 4 and 7. Diagnosis can be carried out by viral isolation. Serodiagnosis is usually done by CF tests for antibody to the adenovirus family antigen.

POXVIRUSES

Several poxviruses infect humans. Principal agents of interest are variola virus, the cause of smallpox and vaccinia virus, the agent used to vaccinate against smallpox. Other poxviruses that infect humans are cowpox virus, molluscum contagiousum virus, paravaccinia virus which causes milker's nodules, and orf virus which causes contagious pustular dermatitis.

Poxviruses are large ovid particles of complex structure. They have an outer membrane surrounding an inner core and two lateral or elliptical bodies. The virus genome is found in the core as a double stranded linear molecule, 200×10^6 daltons in mass. The strands of the molecule are covalently joined at each terminus. In contrast to other kinds of viruses, poxviruses have a number of enzymes present in the virion. Among these is a DNA-dependent RNA polymerase that functions in producing immediate early mRNA during the replicative cycle. Viral replication occurs in the cytoplasm of infected cells in areas referred to as "factories." In fixed and strained preparations these factories appear as eosinophilic inclusions. Viral maturation including biosynthesis of the membrane occurs in the cytoplasm; the virions do not bud from cell membranes as with conventional enveloped viruses.

Variola virus is the causative agent of smallpox. The last recorded case occurring under natural circumstances was in Somalia in October, 1977. Two other cases were laboratory-acquired infections in England in 1978. The ability to bring about the apparent eradication of smallpox was based upon two factors. First, smallpox was a human disease having no animal reservoir for the virus and second, solid immunity could be evoked by vaccination. The World Health Organization undertook a vigorous progam of case-finding and vaccination that resulted in the present state of freedom from smallpox. Currently in the United States, universal childhood vaccination against smallpox is no longer practiced. The risk of complications of vaccination with vaccinia virus far exceeded the risk of contracting smallpox and therefore the practice was discontinued.

Vaccinia virus is regarded as a laboratory virus. It was maintained by passage in animal hosts for the purpose of immunization. It is virtually identical to variola virus in antigenic constitution. Vaccination is carried out by implantation of live vaccinia into the dermis by scarification. In naive hosts, viral replication takes place in the site and a major reaction takes place. This reaction consists of the appearance of a papule that evolves to a vesicle, a pustule, umbilication of the pustule, and finally scab formation. The sequence begins about 72 hours after inoculation and the scab falls off about 13 to 14 days after inoculation. A major response in partially immune individuals consists of the same sequence of changes but over a shorter time period. A delayed hypersensitivity response to vaccinial antigens sometimes occurs and can be a cause of confusion. This response can be elicited by inactive virus, however, viral replication is necessary to evoke protective immunity.

Currently, vaccinia is being investigated as a possible vehicle for immunization against several diseases by the use of recombinant DNA techniques. Genes coding for various antigens (i.e., HB$_s$Ag or measles HA and F glycoproteins) would be spliced into the vaccinia genome.

Table 5-19. Adenovirus Serotypes and Diseases

Diseases	Serotypes
Acute respiratory disease (recruits)	4,7
Pharyngitis, pharyngoconjunctival fever, conjunctivitis	3,7,14
Keratoconjunctivitis	8
Primary atypical pneumonia	4,7
Primay atypical pneumonia in infants	Several
Hemorrhagic cystitis	11,21
Disseminated disease in immunocompromised patients	Several

Replication of the virus in a host would stimulate immunity against several agents simultaneously.

ARBOVIRUSES AND RABIES VIRUS

The arboviruses are viruses that require an insect or other vector for transmission to new hosts. This classification cuts across the official taxonomy based on structural and compositional criteria. Arboviruses are found in the families Togaviridae, Bunyaviridae, Arenaviridae, and Rhabdoviridae.

Typically, arboviruses infect a particular species of animal or bird producing little or no disease. The infection in the species is characterized by a prolonged period of viremia. The viremic period must be sufficiently long to ensure the passage of the virus to a hematophagus insect or arachnid. Arboviruses usually replicate in the vector and are inoculated into a susceptible host during a subsequent blood meal. Thus the virus is propagated from infected individual to susceptible individual. The species within which the cycle regularly occurs in nature is called the reservoir species. A virus may have more than one reservoir species. Introduction of the virus into other species can occur and the frequency of such introduction is a function of several factors in the ecology of the reservoir species, the vector, and the new host. Some of these factors are the host preference of the vector, the population size of the reservoir, the population size of the vector, and the number of nonreservoir hosts available. In turn, several factors affect these issues, weather, rainfall, presence of predators, etc. For most arbovirus infections, humans are incidental hosts and do not participate in the maintenance of the virus in nature. Two exceptions are the urban form of yellow fever virus infection and dengue fever virus infections.

The togaviruses are small enveloped viruses that have positive single stranded RNA genomes. There are two genera, *Alphavirus* and *Flavivirus*. In older classifications these were referred to as Arbovirus A and B respectively. Alphaviruses replicate in mammalian and insect (mosquito) cell lines. The positive RNA is infectious. After penetration of the host cell, the RNA is translated into a large polyprotein that is cleaved into four nonstructural viral proteins. These proteins function to transcribe a negative strand of RNA and to transcribe from the negative template a 42 S (genomic size) RNA and 26 S messenger RNA. The mRNA is translated into a polyprotein that is cleaved into the structural polypeptides of the virion. Virion assembly and maturation occurs at the plasma membrane of the cell and the mature virion buds through the membrane to be released. Replication of the flaviviruses is similar except virions bud into intracytoplasmic cisternae.

Antigenically, the alphaviruses are all related to each other as shown by overlapping patterns of cross reactivity in HI tests. Flaviviruses show similar patterns of cross reactivity among members of the genus. Alphaviruses and flaviviruses do not cross react with each other.

In North America, the alphaviruses of greatest significance are eastern equine encephalitis (EEE) virus, western equine encephalitis (WEE) virus, and Venezuelan equine encephalitis (VEE) virus. EEE or WEE cause more serious disease in man, contrast to the generally milder, nonencephalitis infection caused by VEE. EEE causes disease marked by a biphasic course. The inoculated virus replicates in local lymph nodes followed by a period of primary viremia producing constitution symptoms of fever and malaise. A second period of viremia results from viral replication in viseral sites such as the spleen. The infection then enters the encephalitic phase in which virus invades the CNS. This phase is marked by fever, headache, and lethargy. This biphasic character of infection is also seen in WEE infections. Outbreaks of EEE have had case fatality rates as high as 25 percent with significant residual damage in survivors. There are about 50 to 100 inapparent human infections with EEE for every case. Disease caused by WEE virus is clinically milder with a lower case fatality rate. The virus is usually more widespread and more inapparent infections occur, perhaps 300 to 500 for each clinically apparent case.

Diagnosis of EEE and WEE is usually conducted serologically using HI tests. Demonstration of an increase in titer indicates infection, however, single serum specimens with high titers are also useful.

Epidemiologically, the viruses are propagated in several species of birds and each can be disseminated by several species of mosquito. EEE is distributed along the East coast of the United States, in the Caribbean, and in Central and South America. WEE has a broad distribution across the United States occurring in the East as well as the West. In the United States VEE occurs principally in Texas and Florida and is widespread in Central and South America.

Flaviviruses found in North America are St. Louis encephalitis (SLE) yellow fever (YE), dengue viruses, and Powassan virus. SLE is the most frequently occurring virus, causing outbreaks of disease every 2 to 3 years in the United States. Clinically, the infection is similar to WEE in severity and incidence of inapparent infection. The reservoir is wild birds, and a number of mosquitos especially *Culex tarsalis* serve as vectors. There is also some evidence for vector transmission from human to human of SLE.

Yellow fever flavivirus infections is characterized by a biphasic clinical course in which the second phase is characterized by hepatitis and hemorrhagic lesions in the skin. There are two epidemiologic forms of yellow fever. One form is an urban form in which the virus is passed from human to human by means of a mosquito vector, usually *Aedes aegypti*. The other form is sylvan yellow fever in which the reservoir consists of several primate species and is disseminated by a number of mosquito species.

Dengue virus occurs in four serotypes, 1–4, that are widespread in tropical and semitropical areas throughout the world. Infections also occur from time to time in temperate areas. Humans and perhaps other primates serve as the reservoir and the virus is passed by a number of mosquito species. Clinically, there is a prodrome of malaise and headache 5 to 8 days after infection followed by an acute onset of fever, severe periorbital headache, and pain in the joints. A hemorrhagic form of the infection leading to shock, that is apparently caused by a more virulent strain, is seen. All four serotypes cause the hemorrhagic shock syndrome but type 2 is the most frequently involved.

Control of togavirus infection is usually directed to control of the vector species. However, vaccines are made for some of the viruses both for human use and veterinary use. The yellow fever vaccine is a highly efficacious live virus preparation.

The Bunyaviridae are a large group of viruses with worldwide distribution. The enveloped virions are 100 nm in diameter and contain a three segmented RNA genome of negative polarity. In the United States, the California encephalitis complex of bunyaviruses causes the most frequently occurring human infections. There are six related viruses in the complex and the LaCross and California serotypes and the most important. Clinically, infection with these viruses can range from mild to moderately severe encephalitis. While fatality is rare, there are reports of sequelae of variable severity. The viruses are maintained in nature in small mammals and spread by mosquitos especially *Aedes triseriatus*. The mosquito passes the virus transovarially, thus can also function as a reservoir. Control of California and LaCross viruses can only be attempted by vector control.

RABIES

Rabies virus is a member of the *Rhabdovirus* genus, a group of viruses characterized by a bullet-shaped, enveloped virion with a single negative strand of RNA as the genome. Rabies virus has a worldwide distribution and is maintained in various wildlife populations. Bats are recognized as a principal reservoir as they can harbor the virus for long periods without clinical manifestations of disease. In all other species the virus causes disease and death. Humans acquire rabies virus by being bitten by a rabid animal. The virus is shed copiously in the saliva of rabid animals and enters through the wound. Various

other routes of entry such as airborne have been documented but these are very rare. There is a prolonged incubation up to a year before the onset of clinical signs. Short incubation periods are associated with severe wounds of the head, neck, and fingers. Onset is signaled by headache, fever, malaise, and frequently paraesthesia or pain at the site of the initiating wound. The encephalitis progresses rapidly to anxiety convulsions, coma, and death. The virus is disseminated throughout the body and viral antigen can be demonstrated in corneal scrapings or exfoliated buccal cells.

Control of rabies in humans is affected by vaccination of domestic animals, dog and cats, which are (or were) the principal sources of human exposure. Vaccination of humans is practiced whenever reasonable expectation of exposure has occurred. The current vaccine is a human diploid cell grown, inactivated virus preparation. In addition, rabies immunoglobulin can be used to rapidly induce passive immunity. Live virus vaccines are available for veterinary use.

Oncogenic Viruses

Four groups of viruses have been recognized as capable of evoking changes in infected cells that result in transformation. Three of the groups, the papovaviruses, adenoviruses, and herpesviruses, contain DNA as their genetic material while the fourth group, the retroviruses, have RNA in the virion and a DNA transcript of the RNA in the infected cell. The oncogenic DNA viruses usually cause a cytolytic, nontransforming infection in cells of the species in which they usually occur. However, in cells of another species or under conditions that inhibit lytic infections (such as damage to the viral genome), they can express their potential to cause transformation. For example, polyoma virus replicates lytically in mice cells yet transforms rat cells. Similarly, HSV-1 normally grows lytically in human cells yet if it is ultraviolet-irradiated, it can transform the cells.

Transformation is the induction of new properties in cells as a result of virus infection (Table 5-20). Transformation in necessary but not sufficient to cause neoplasia in vivo. Therefore, a virus may cause transformation of cells in vitro yet not affect oncogenesis in vivo.

PAPOVAVIRUS

The Papovaviridae has two genera *Polyomavirus* and *Papillomavirus*. The polyomaviruses have nonenveloped icosahedral virions about 45 nm in diameter. They have a circular double stranded DNA genome of 3×10^6 daltons. The best studied viruses in the genus are polyoma virus of mice and SV_{40} virus of monkeys. The human viruses, JC virus associated with progressive

Table 5-20. Properties of Cells Transformed by Viruses

Property	Normal Cell	Transformed Cell
Response to contact with another cell	Inhibition of movement	No inhibition of movement
Requirement for anchorage	Requires solid substrate	Grows in suspension
Growth in agar	Fails to replicate	Replicates to form colonies
Pattern of growth on solid substrate	Ordered monolayer	Disordered, multiple cell layers
Comparative requirement for serum in medium	High	Low
Agglutinability by lectins	Low	High

(Milgrom F, Flanagan TD: Medical Microbiology. Churchill Livingstone, New York, 1982)

multifocal leukencephalopathy (PML) and BK virus isolated from immunosuppressed patients belong to the group.

Lytic replication of polyoma virus takes place in mice cells. Early transcription of the genome gives rise to three mRNA molecules that are translated into three polypeptides having molecular masses of 22 K, 55 K, and 100 K. Collectively, the polypeptides are known as "T antigen" and individually as small T, middle T, and large T. They are detected in the nucleus of the infected cells. In lytic growth, the T polypeptides function in viral DNA replication which is semiconservative in nature. After a period of DNA synthesis, late transcription occurs giving rise to another three mRNA species. The translation products of these molecules are the structural proteins of the capsid. Virions are assembled in the nucleus of the cell which undergoes lysis with release of the progeny virions.

Transforming infection can be illustrated by infected rat cells which are nonpermissive (no lytic growth of virus) with polyoma virus. Early transcription occurs in the cells and T antigen appears. In most cells, evidence of viral infection is lost; such cells are abortively transformed and return to the normal phenotype. However, some cells become permanently transformed and retain the viral antigens and the transformed phenotype. Viral DNA is integrated into the cellular DNA in the transformed cells. Transformation is apparently caused by activity of the middle T polypeptide.

SV_{40} virus carries out very similar events except there are only two polypeptides in early synthesis, small T and large T.

ADENOVIRUS

Various adenoviruses, members of the *Mastadenovirus* genus and of the *Aviadenovirus* genus have been shown to be oncogenic. Among the human adenoviruses, serotypes 12, 18, and 31 are highly oncogenic for rodents and they as well as many other adenoviruses can

transform cells in vitro. The transforming potential of the adenovirus genome had been mapped to one end of the viral DNA molecule. It resides in a segment that constitutes 7 percent of the entire genome. Adenovirus transformed cells have a nuclear antigen analogous to the T antigen.

HERPESVIRUS

In nature, several herpesviruses have been associated with tumors. The Marek's disease virus causes viseral lymphomytosis of chickens. A significant finding in regard to this disease is that the disease can be prevented by vaccination of chickens with a related herpesvirus of turkeys. The significance lies in the prevention of a neoplastic disease by immunization against the causative agent.

Human herpesviruses have been associated with human tumors. The evidence for a causal relationship is very good for EBV and less well established for HSV-2 and HSV-1. In the case of EBV, viral antigens especially the nuclear antigen EBNA is found in the cells of African Burkitt's lymphoma. The cells also contain EBV DNA. Cell-free EBV is capable of transforming B-lymphocytes into continuously replicating lymphoid cell lines. All the cells in these lines carry EBNA and EBV DNA. Some cells can be induced to express other EBV antigens such as EA and VCA. Cell-free EBV can cause lymphomas in marmosets and autologous lymphocytes transformed by EBV cause disseminated lymphomatous disease in squirrel monkeys. EBV is also linked to nasopharyngeal carcinoma occurring in Southeast Asia and southern China. In the case of this tumor, EBNA is found in the epithelial cells of the tumor.

HSV-2 has been linked epidemiologically with cervical carcinoma and HSV-1 with squamous cell carcinoma of the head and neck. Both of these viruses can affect transformation of cells in vitro when they are partially inactivated so as to inhibit lytic growth. Recent reports have demonstrated viral DNA and antigens in human tumors.

RNA TUMOR VIRUSES

The RNA tumor viruses belong to the subfamily Oncornaviridae of the Retroviridae. There are three suggested genera in the subfamily differentiated on the basis of antigenicity and morphology of the virion. They are the B type, C type, and D type viruses. B type viruses mature by the envelopment at the plasma membrane of a precursor particle (A type particle) found within the cytoplasm of the infected cell. Type C viruses bud from the membrane but no percursor nucleoid is apparent in the cell and maturation of this structure occurs during budding. The formation of the type D virion is similar to type B, however, the nature D particle has a central nucleoid whereas the type B nucleoid is eccentric within the virion.

All retroviruses have enveloped virions 100 nm in diameter with an RNA genome of two identical subunits. They also contain an RNA directed DNA polymerase called reverse transcriptase.

Classification of RNA Tumor Viruses. Several ways of classifying the RNA tumor viruses are used. Each is based on specific aspects of the biology of the viruses and find application in different types of study.

The viruses can be classified according to their usual mode of transmission. Exogenous strains are those transmitted horizontally among individuals of a susceptible population. Mature virions are transferred to the new individual and infect the cells of the new host. On the other hand, endogenous strains are those that do not produce virions but are transferred to progeny by the germ cells. These strains usually exist only as a provirus segment of DNA integrated into cellular DNA. Under special circumstances endogenous viruses can be induced to produce viral gene products and sometimes virions.

Another way to classify the RNA tumor viruses is according to their species of origin. This method of classification correlates well with antigenic classification (see below). Exogenous and endogenous strains of a given species are not always similar in antigenicity or nucleic acid homology, however. This is interpreted as indicating an interspecies crossing of the virus during the evolutionary history of the species carrying the virus.

Classification by antigenic similarity has been used. The most specific determinants are type specificities. They define the different viruses within a group. Group-specific determinants are found on all (or most) viruses infecting a given species. Interspecies antigens are found on viruses infecting several different species. Most of the proteins of the RNA tumor viruses have all three types of determinants, but the proportion differs greatly. For example, the major envelope glycoproteins contain mostly type-specific determinants while the major capsid protein bears mostly group-specific determinants.

Host range is another basis of classification. Among the avian viruses, host range is determined by the presence of receptors for the viral glycoproteins on cell surfaces. Among the murine viruses, receptors are also important but other factors are also operative. One system of host range classification among the murine viruses is the NB classification. Inbred strains of mice are classified as N or B on the basis of alleles at a single gene locus, Fv-1. N-tropic viruses infect N mice, B-tropic viruses infect B mice. Some viruses are NB-tropic, infecting both types. The basis of this tropism is not the receptor on the cell but some event during replicative cycles.

Oncogenicity is another way to classify the RNA tumor viruses. Sarcoma viruses cause solid tissue tumors in vivo and transform fibroblasts in vitro. Acute leukemia viruses cause rapid lymphoproliferative diseases and transform fibroblast and lymphoid cells in vitro. In this group are avian myeloblastosisvirus, murine erythroid leukemia (Friend and Raucher viruses), and the Abelson virus that causes B-cell lymphoma. Lymphatic leukemia viruses cause leukemias and lymphomas in vivo and do not transform cells in vitro. Similarly, mammary tumor viruses cause adenocarcinomas in vivo and do not transform in vitro.

Replicative Cycle of Nondefective RNA Tumor Viruses. Replication of RNA tumor viruses differs in several significant aspects from replication of conventional RNA and DNA viruses (Fig. 5-22). The virion interacts with specific receptors on the cell surface and the RNA genome is introduced into the cytoplasma of the cell. The reverse transcriptase makes a DNA copy of the genome that is transferred to the nucleus of the cell. The viral DNA is integrated into the cellular DNA. From this integrated site, the genome is transcribed by cellular RNA polymerase producing genome length viral RNA for packaging into virions and polyadenylated mRNA molecules. Three species of mRNA are produced from the genome which has four genes (Fig. 5-23). The sequence of genes from the 5′ end is *gag, pol, env,* and *src.* The largest mRNA molecule contains the entire sequence and is polyadenylated at the 3′ end. Translation of this molecule occurs through the *gag* sequence and occasionally through *gag* and *pol.* The product of these translations is a polyprotein precursor that is proteolytically cleaved in four internal virion proteins and from the product of the *gag pol* translation, reverse transcriptase. The middle size mRNA species contains the *env* and *src* sequences and is produced by excision of the *gag* and *pol* species. Translation of this molecule produces a protein that is later cleaved and glycosylated to produce two glycoproteins found in the viral envelope. Though

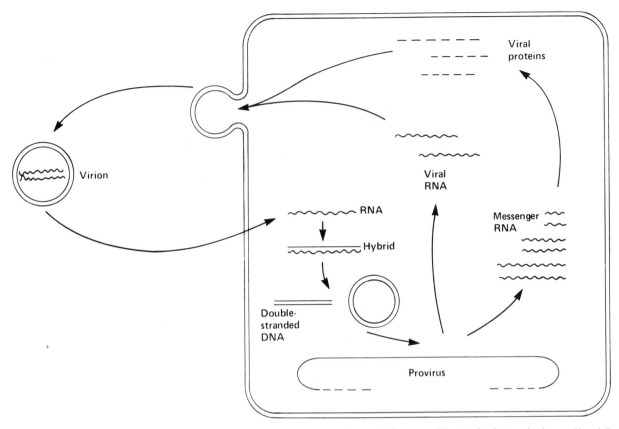

Fig. 5-22. Replicative cycle of a nondefective RNA tumor virus. (Milgrom F, Flanagan TD: Medical Microbiology. Churchill Livingstone, New York, 1982.)

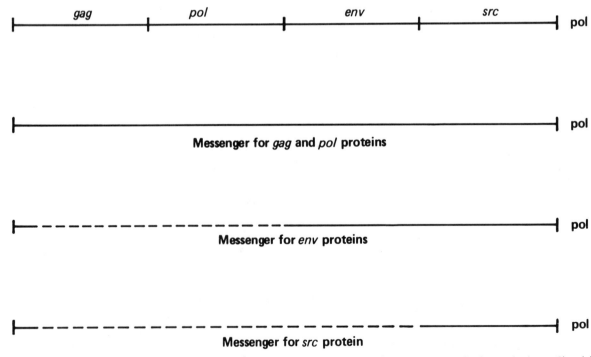

Fig. 5-23. Transcription of the nondefective RNA tumor virus genome. (Milgrom F, Flanagan TD: Medical Microbiology. Churchill Livingstone, New York, 1982.)

the mRNA contains the *src* sequence, this portion is not translated. The smallest mRNA contains only the *src* gene and is produced by excision of the preceding sequences. Translation produces the 60 K *src* phosphoprotein. This protein plays a role in transformation. Progeny virions are assembled at the plasma membrane of the cell with the *env* glycoproteins present in the membrane and the nucleocapsid composed of the *gag* and *pol* proteins in the adjacent cytoplasm. The virion matures by budding and the released particle continues to undergo maturation.

Genetics of RNA Tumor Viruses. RNA tumor viruses contain three or four genes. In the case of the sarcoma viruses, there are *gag, pol, env,* and *src* genes; whereas in lymphocytic leukemia viruses there are only *gag, pol,* and *env.* All murine and some avian sarcoma viruses are defective in that they lack one or more of the *gag, pol,* or *env* sequences thus cannot direct the production of virions. A frequent defect in these viruses is the absence of the *env* sequence a situation in which complementation of the defective sarcoma virus with a nondefective leukemia virus. This results in the production of pseudotypes with the host range and specificity of the leukemia virus but the transforming capacity of the sarcoma virus.

RNA tumor viruses undergo high rates of recombination. This apparently occurs by crossing over between genes of the integrated proviruses. Recombination can occur between exogenous viruses and endogenous viruses and can also be a means of incorporating cellular genes into the viral genome. Some RNA tumor viruses carry cellular genes analogous to the *src* sequence of sarcoma viruses.

Transformation by RNA Tumor Viruses. The transformation of cells by sarcoma viruses is apparently due to the *src* gene product. Evidence for this comes from several sources. Transformation-defective mutants of sarcoma viruses do not produce the smallest mRNA species which is found abundantly in transformed cells. Temperature sensitive mutations in the *src* or analogous sequences cause transformation at permissive temperatures but the cells revert to the nontransformation phenotype at restrictive temperatures. The *src* gene product of Rous sarcoma virus is a 60 K phosphoprotein with an associated protein kinase activity. Such activity is closely associated with the control of cellular enzyme activity. Normal cells have proteins similar to the *src* product but transformed cells have much higher levels. Other sarcoma viruses and acute leukemia viruses carry cellular genes that code for phosphoproteins or other proteins with protein kinase activity.

Lymphatic leukemia viruses do not carry an analogous gene to the *src* sequence of sarcoma viruses. They are noncytopathic and do not affect transformation in vitro. In vivo they cause disease after very long incubation periods. During the incubation period the virus is constantly present. Disease expression is dependent on the presence of an intact thymus. Thymectomized animals do not develop disease. Certain preleukemic changes occur such as disappearance of lymphocytes from the thymus mark the onset of disease. It is postulated that the transformation that occurs is a result of recombination of the leukemia virus with some resident gene sequence in the thymus. The resident sequence could belong to an endogenous virus since antigenic changes in thymocytes are detected in the preleukemic stage.

MEDICAL PARISITOLOGY

Protozoa

All members of the phylum *Protozoa* are single-cell organisms consisting of a nucleus and a cytoplasm (Table 5-21). Many specialized organelles are seen among the various species. For example, organelles of locomotion include cilia, flagella, undulating membranes, and pseudopodia. The limiting membrane may contain cytostomes (alimentary openings) and cytopyges (excretory openings). In the cytoplasm there may be various vacuoles and inclusions.

The life history of protozoa often consists of several stages occurring in two distinct phases, sexual and asexual (Fig. 5-24). Not all protozoa have all stages; some organisms may have but two or three. The trophozoite is the vegetative stage, reproducing asexually in a process called schizogony. A trophozoite may differentiate into a highly resistant cyst form which can in turn return to the trophozoite form. The reproducing form of the trophozoites is the merozoite. On occasion, merozoites may differentiate into gametocytes and thus enter the sexual stage of the life cycle, gametogony. Union of macrogametocytes (female) and microgametocytes (male) gives a zygote that differentiates into an oocyst. The oocyst gives rise to many sporants in the stage of sporogony. These forms eventually differentiate into trophozoites.

Trypanasoma and Leishmania

The genera *Trypanasoma* and *Leishmania* of the family Trypanasomatidae contain species pathogenic for humans. All pathogens have two hosts, a mammalian host and an insect host which acts as a vector. Four morphologic forms of the trophozoite are seen, the amastigote, the promastigote, the epimastiogote, and the

Table 5-21. Taxonomy of the Major Pathogenic Protozoa

Subphylum	Class	Order	Family	Genus	Species	Disease
Sarcomastigophra	Mastigophora (Zoomastigophora)[a]	Protomastigida	Trypanosomatidue	*Trypanosoma*	*gambiense*	Trypanosomiasis (*sleeping sickness*)
					rhodesiense	Sleeping sickness
					cruzi	Chagas' disease
				Leishmania	*tropica*	Cutaneous leishmaniasis (Oriental sore)
					brasiliensis	Mucocutaneous leishmaniasis (espundia)
					(pifanoi)	Cutaneous leishmaniasis
					(peruanta)	Uta
					(mexicana)	Chiclero disease (buba, forest yaws)
					(guyanensis)	?
					donovani	Kala-azar
		Polymastigida	Hexamitidae	*Giardia*	*lamblia*	Giardiasis
		Trichomonadida	Trichomonadidae	*Trichomonas*	*vaginalis*	Trichomoniasis (vaginitis)
					hominis	Diarrhea (?)
	Sarcodina	Rhizopoda	Dimastigamoebidae	*Acanthoamoeba*		Amebiasis (meningoencephalitis)
				Naegleria	*fowleri*	Primary amebic meningoencephalitis
			Entamoebidae	*Entamoeba*	*histolytica*	Amebiasis
				Dientamoeba	*fragilis*	Diarrhea (?)
Apicomplexa	Sporozoa	Eucoccidia (Eimerina)		*Isospora*	*hominis*	Isosporosis
				Sarcocystis	*lindemann*[b]	Sarcocystosis
				Toxoplasma	*gondii*	Tosoplasmosis
				Pneumocystis	*carinii*	Interstitial atypical pneumonia
		Haemosporina		*Plasmodium*	*vivax*	Malaria (tertian)
					ovale	Malaria (tertian)
					malariae	Malaria (quartan)
					falciparum	Malaria (malignant)
	Piroplasmea	Piroplasmida	Babesiidae	*Babesia*	*bovis*	Babesiosis
					divergens	Babesiosis
Ciliophora	Ciliatea	Spirotrichida	Bursaridae	*Balantidium*	*coli*	Balantidiasis (colitis)

[a] Subunits are given in parentheses.
[b] *Sarcocystis lindemanni* is sometimes considered a developmental stage of *Isospora hominis*.
(Milgrom F, Flanagan TD: Medical Microbiology. Churchill Livingstone, New York, 1982.)

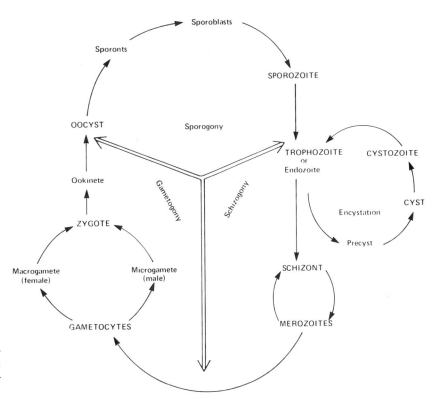

Fig. 5-24. Composite life cycle of protozoan parasites. (Milgrom F, Flanagan TD: Medical Microbiology. Churchill Livingstone, New York, 1982.)

mature form, the trypomastigote. No sexual stage has been described for the trypanosomes or the leishmania.

Trypanosoma gambiense and *T rhodesiense* cause sleeping sickness. *T gambiense* is found in western and central Africa. The vector is the tsetse fly, *Glossima palpalis*. *T rhodesiense* is found in sparsely populated regions of central and eastern Africa. It is spread by the tsetse fly, *G morsitans*. The reservoir for the parasites is wildlife. Disease caused by *T gambisense* is a chronic generalized infection called African sleeping sickness. It is characterized by a protracted, irregular series of periodic attacks of fever, lymphadenopathy, and neurologic signs. The usual course leads to encephalitis and death. *T rhodesiense* causes a more acute disease leading to death within a few weeks as contrasted to the course of several years in disease caused by *T gambiense.*

T cruzi causes Chagas' disease. The reservoir for this parasite is a variety of mammalian species. The organisms occurs over a wide range of semi arid areas of South and Central America and occasionally in the Southwest United States. The vector is one of a number of species of triatomid bugs. Chagas' disease manifests in five distinct clinical forms, acute, latent, cardiac, digestive, and congenital. Acute disease, usually seen in children, manifests as fever, lymphadenopathy, and hepatosplenomegaly. Symptoms subside in two to three months in 90 percent of cases which then become latent. The remaining 10 percent of cases are usually fatal. The

acute and latent forms may evolve into cardiac or digestive forms of the disease. The congenital form results from invasion of the placenta causing damage to the fetus often leading to premature delivery or stillbirth.

Leishmania tropica causes a skin disease known as Oriental sore. The disease occurs in North Africa, Mediterranean Europe, Turkey, and into Central Asia and India. The reservoir for the organism consists of wild rodents, dogs, and humans. The female sandfly *(Phlebotomus)* serves as the vector. The initial lesion manifests as a discrete reddish indurated papule that eventually ulcerates and heals within one year. A more chronic form occurs, especially in the Middle East, wherein central healing of the lesion follows a centrifical spread of the active lesion. This form, called leishmalia lupoid, may persist for years.

L brasiliensis causes four distinct forms of leishmaniasis distinguished on the basis of geographic distribution, antigenic characteristics of the causative strain, and clinical features. The forms are Chiclero ulcer, caused by the *L mexicana* variant, Espundia, caused by *L brasiliensis,* Uta, caused by *L peruana,* and diffuse cutaneous leishmaniasis, the cause of which is not known. The diseases are all characterized by small initial lesions that heal spontaneously within 2 years. There are metastatic lesions in Espundia that manifest at the mucocutaneous junctions. Chiclera ulcer, Espundia, and diffuse cutaneous leishmaniasis are characterized by granuloma formation, tissue destruction, and scarring. The vectors for the agents are various species of *Phebotomus*.

L donavani causes kala-azar, a generalized reticuloendotheliosis that has a 90 percent case fatality rate in untreated cases. Four epidemiologic forms are recognized, Indian, Mediterranian, African, and American. The reservoir for the Indian form is human and the vector is the sandfly. The Mediterranean and American forms have canine species as the reservoir and the disease is also spread by sandflies. In the African form, rodents serve as the reservoir and the vectors are species of sandfly.

Giardia Lamblia

G lamblia is a cosmopolitan parasite found predominantly in children. The trophozoite is a heart-shaped cell with two nuclei separated by an axostyle. Four pair of flagella emerge from different sites along the axostyle. The life cycle is apparently an alternation of the trophozoite and cyst forms. The cyst is infective by ingestion and releases two trophozoites on reaching the intestine. Giardiasis is the clinical expression of a high parasite load. It manifests as diarrheal disease accompanied by upper gastric pain and steatorrhea. *G lamblia* infection is also associated with the so-called gay bowel syndrome wherein sexual transmission of trophozoites may occur.

Trichomonas Vaginalis

The trophozite form is the only form of *T vaginalis* that has been described. It is an oval form with a single nucleus, an axostyle, four flagella originating from a pole of the axostyle, and an undulating membrane. The organism lives in the acid environment of the vagina, prostrate, and urethra. It is transferred during coitus, however, nonsexual modes of transfer both direct and indirect are apparently possible. The principal clinical manifestation of infection is vaginitis although bartholinitis, cystitis, urethritis, and prostatitis have been reported. About 20 percent of infected persons are symptomless.

Entamoeba Histolytica and Other Sarcodinae

E histolytica is the cause of amebic dysentery. The trophozoite is an amebic cell containing a single nucleus and a variety of ingested particles including erythrocytes and bacteria. The cyst is a rounded cell devoid of cytoplasmic inclusions but containing four nuclei. The cyst is the infectious form, it can remain infectious for 12 days in the environment. The parasite has cosmopolitan distribution, commonly infecting pigs, dogs, and monkeys

as well as humans. The cyst is ingested and matures in the intestine releasing a metacystic trophozoite that divides into four trophozoites. The trophozoites colonize the cecum and subsequently invade the mucosa. The principal manifestation of infection is amebic dysentery (amebic colitis). The disease is characterized by episodes of diarrhea, cramps, nausea, and malaise. Complications often arising from amebic infection are peritonitis, hepatitis, pericarditis, and lesions in the lung, brain, and skin. Diagnosis is accomplished by demonstration of the trophozoites in fluid stool, biopsies, and sputum or cysts in formed stools. The organisms must be differentiated from nonpathogenic amebae. Amebic dysentery must be differentiated from bacillary dysentery because of the seriousness of extraintestinal complications. The treatment of the two diseases is of course different.

Other members of the class Sarcodina are occasionally encountered as pathogens. Two ill-defined genera of the Dimastigamoebidae, *Hartmannella* and *Acanthamoeba,* cause fulminating infections characterized by microabscess formation. The aquatic organism *Naeglaria fowleri* has been documented as the cause of a fatal meningoencephalitis. The organism apparently gains entry through the nasal mucosa.

Parasites of the Class Sporozoa

A number of important parasites are found in the Sporozoa.

Toxoplasma gondii is a cosmopolitan parasite whose definitive hosts are members of the family Felidae. For humans, the domestic cat is a source of infection as is undercooked meat. Ingestion of the oocyst in food contaminated with cat feces or of cysts from various sources can initiate infection of humans. Transplacental infection of fetuses is also an important route of acquisition. Occasionally infection can be acquired from blood transfusion or tissue transplantation. The principal manifestation of toxoplasmosis is lymphadenitis with or without fever. This may be accompanied by headache, myagia, pharyngitis, hepatosplenomegaly, and atypical lymphocytosis. The lymphadenopathic form is usually self-limiting although persistence or recurrence is not uncommon. About 1 percent of toxoplasmosis cases have ocular involvement. Chorioretinitis is the principal manifestation. Thirty-five percent of cases of chorioretinitis are caused by *T gondii*. One-third of all women acquiring acute toxoplasmosis during pregnancy will deliver an infected infant. The frequency of infection early in gestation (1st trimester) is low but the consequences are severe, often leading to spontaneous abortion. The frequency of fetal infection late in pregnancy is high but the severity of the infection in the fetus is mild. Immunosuppressive therapy and disease states predispose to toxoplasmosis. The infection may be exogenous but many cases are reactivation of latent infection. Brain involvement is prominent (about 50 percent) in cases in immunocompromised patients.

Pneumocystis carinii, an organism that is not classified with certainty, is the cause of interstitial pneumonia in newborns, malnourished infants, and patients who are immunosuppressed. The mode of spread of the organism in nature is unknown but it has been suggested that it occurs by airborne droplets containing cysts or trophozoites.

Plasmodium

The genus *Plasmodium* has four species, *P vivax, P ovale, P malariae,* and *P falciparium.* All of these organisms cause human malaria. *P vivax* and *P ovale* cause tertain malaria. *P malaria* causes quatran malaria and *P falciparium* causes malignant or subtertian malaria.

The parasites have a complex life cycle in which the asexual stage (schizogony) takes place in the human host and the sexual stage (gametogony) begins in the human and is completed in the female anophelian mosquito. The *P vivax* cycle, is typical for the species *P ovale* and *P malariae,* except that *P malariae* takes 4 days in the erythrocytic stage (Fig. 5-25).

Macrogametocytes and microgametocytes present in the blood of a human host are ingested at a blood meal by female anophelian mosquitos. They transform into macrogametes and microgametes, respectively, and merge to form a zygote. The zygote transforms into a motile ookinete that migrates through the gut wall and forms an oocyst. Sporozoites emerge from the oocyst and migrate to the salivary glands; there to be injected into a human host at a blood meal. In the human host, the sporozoites invade the endothelial cells of the liver to initiate the extraerythrocytic schizogony phase of the cycle. The sporozoite transforms into a schizont, a form that eventually segments into many (10^4) small spherical merozoites. These are released on rupture of the cell either to invade erythrocytes or to invade other hepatic endothelial cells, reinitiating the sequence. In the erythrocyte, the invading merozoites transform into trophozoite or schizonts which divide into 8 to 24 merozoites. Trophozoites may differentiate into macrogametocytes or microgametocytes. Merozoites released from erythrocytes go on to invade other erythrocytes.

The life cycles for *P ovale* and *P malariae* are similar to the cycle for *P vivax.* The most obvious difference is in the length of the erythrocytic schizogony of *P malariae* which is 68 to 72 hours while the other organisms have cycles about 48 hours. All three species differ from *P falciparum* in that they have a continuing extraerythrocytic schizogony.

The clinical manifestations of malaria are sudden onset of fever, chills, headache, tachycardia, and tachypnea. These coincide with the rupture of erythrocytes in erythrocytic shizogony. The attacks last several hours and end with a fever crisis. As attacks occur coincident with the rupture of erythrocytes, the disease caused by *P vivax* and *P ovale* is called tertian (every 3 days) while *P malariae* causes quartran malaria. *P falciparum* causes a more irregular disease pattern, sometimes called subtertian. This disease is also more severe with high fatality in untreated cases.

Diagnosis of malaria is based on the clinical picture and demonstration of the parasites in blood smears. Chloroquine sulfate and hydroxychloroquine are the primary drugs for both treatment and prophylaxis.

Metazoa

Metazoan parasites of humans belong principally to the phyla Platyhelminthes and Nemathelminthes. In addition there are some members of the Antropoda. Among the Platyhelminthes are the classes Trematoda (flukes) and Cestoidea (tapeworms).

Trematoda

Humans are parasitized by several kinds of flukes, among them are blood flukes, lung flukes, and liver flukes. Occasionally humans may be infested by intestinal flukes that are primarily parasites of other species such as pigs. All flukes have snails as the intermediate host in which the asexual phase takes place.

Blood flukes belong to the genus *Schistosoma* and three species are parasites of humans, *S mansoni, S japanicum,* and *S hematobium.* These flukes have male and female forms. The male worm is a flattened cylinder rolled up to form a groove, called the gynocophoric canal, in which the longer and more slender female worm lays. This union is permanant and the female produces large numbers of ova for periods of years.

S mansoni is found in Africa and South and Central America including the Caribbean basin. In Africa the intermediate hosts are several snails of the genus *Biomphalaria* while in the Americas, a single species *B galbrata* serves. The life cycle of *S mansoni* begins with the deposition of ova by female worms in tissues of the infected human host. The ova mechanically and enzymatically move through the tissue and enter the intestine where they exit with feces. If the ova reach fresh water, they hatch producing ciliated miracidia. Miracidia actively seek snails and penetrate the soft tissues of the host. They shed their ciliated coat, they elongate, and they differentiate into mother sporocysts. Mother sporocysts give rise to daughter sporocysts which produce

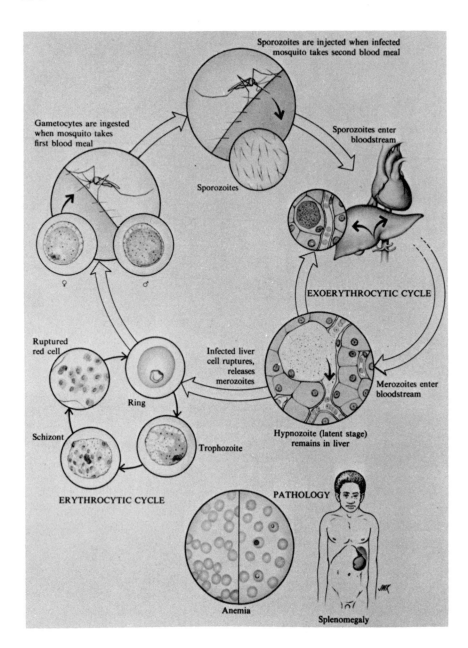

Fig. 5-25. Life cycle of *Plasmodium vivax*. (Katz, Despommier, Gwadz: Parasitic Disease. Springer-Verlag, New York, 1982.)

fork-tailed cercariae. Cercariae are periodically released from the snail into the water. They actively swim seeking a human host. Cecariae directly penetrate the human skin or mucosa. The cercariae lose their tails and undergo changes in surface properties. The resultant schistosomule enters the circulation and eventually the liver where they grow and mature into adult worms. Adult worms couple and migrate to the mesenteric veins of the small and large intestines and sometimes the veins of the urinary bladder. In these sites the worms produce the ova that penetrate the vessel walls and move through the tissues. Host response is directed to the ova and the principal pathology of the infection is associated with this response. Humoral immunity is also directed to the cer-

cariae and schistosomule stages. The adult worms avoid the response by acquiring surface characteristics of human cells. Control of *S mansoni* is attempted by control of the snail population and education of the human population regarding the need to keep water free of feces and urine.

Similar life cycles are seen in *S japonicum* and *S hematobium* except different snail species act as intermediate hosts. *S japonicum* can use several vertebrates as definitive hosts while *S hematobium*, like *S mansoni*, infect humans primarily.

Clinical manifestations of schistosomiasis include dermatitis resulting from the penetration of cercariae, onset of fever and chills when eggs are deposited in the mesenteric vessels, and severe gastrointestinal distur-bance accompanied by abdominal cramps. Disease due to *S japonicum* often is characterized by cirrhosis and has a high fatality rate. *S hematobium* generally causes the least severe disease. Diagnosis of schistosomiasis is carried out by demonstration of the ova in feces or urine. *S mansoni* ova are characterized by a prominent lateral spine while *S japonicum* ova are small and do not have well developed spines. The ova of *S hematobium* have a terminal spine.

The lung fluke, *Paragonimus westermani,* exists as an encysted hemaphroditic adult in lung tissue. Occasion-ally a cyst will burst, liberating ova that are expelled in sputum. Swallowed sputum brings the ova to the ali-mentary tract and they exist in the feces. Miracidia pene-trate snails wherein they produce several generations of rediae. The last generation of rediae form cercariae. The cercaviae penetrate various crustaceans where they en-cyst. If these animals are eaten raw, the young flukes are released, penetrate the intestinal mucosa, and some eventually reach the lung.

The lung disease caused by *P westermani* occurs in places where crayfish and crabs are commonly eaten raw. The symptoms are similar to tuberculosis. Diag-nosis may be made by demonstration of ova in sputum or feces.

The liver fluke most frequently causing human infec-tion in the United States is *Fasciola hepatica.* The orga-nism is a parasite of several species including domestic cattle, sheep, goat, and horses. Humans acquire the in-fection by ingestion of encysted cercariae on aquatic veg-etation such as watercress. The metacercariae penetrate the intestinal wall and migrate to the liver where they locate in biliary ducts. Adult worms produce ova which enter the bile and are shed in the feces. The intermediate hosts are various snails. Control is directed to the inter-mediate host.

CESTOIDEA

In the definitive host, tapeworms are characterized by a scolex (an attachment organ) and a stroblia (a chain or ribbon of segments). The segments of the stroblia are termed proglottids and contain both male and female reproductive organs. The youngest proglottids are found adjacent to the scolex and the oldest at the distal end of the stroblia. Sexual maturity occurs about midworm and the older proglottids are often filled with ova (gravid proglottids). Ova may be released in the intestinal envi-ronment of the worm or proglottids containing the ova may be shed. Intermediate hosts of cestodes carry the larval form of the parasites. Most often the larvae are bladder-like in form with a scolex on the inner surface. This form is called a cysticerum. Some larvae have sev-eral inward oriented scoleces within a bladder; these are called cenurii. The most elaborate form is the hyatid cyst. This form consists of a large bladder with a germinal layer that gives rise to many daughter cysts (brood cap-sules) each of which has numerous scolices.

The organism *Taenia solium* or pork tapeworm uses pigs as both definitive and intermediate hosts. Humans are more frequently definitive hosts but occasionally act as intermediate hosts. In the pig, the larvae occur as cysticerci in the muscle and other tissues. Human infec-tion is initiated by ingestion of viable cysticerci in under-cooked meat. The bladder-form larva everts and the sco-lex attaches to the intestinal wall by means of suckers (4) and hooks (25–30). The stroblia develops as many as 800 proglottids. Symptoms of infection vary widely but are generally mild. More serious infection occurs when humans act as intermediate hosts, a condition called cysticercosis. Cysticerci in muscles may cause mechani-cal problems, however more serious consequences can result from invasion of the eye, brain, or spinal cord.

The beef tapeworm, *T saginata,* is the most common human tapeworm. It is usually acquired by ingestion of undercooked beef. The cycle is similar to that of *T so-lium,* however humans do not serve as intermediate hosts. The adult worm has a scolex with four suckers. The stroblia can attain lengths of 4 to 5 m and have up to 1,000 proglottids. Infection can often be unnoticed and symptoms are usually mild.

Echinococcus granulosus is a minute tapeworm of dogs and other canines. Humans function as interme-diate hosts with the development of hyatid cysts. Close association with dogs can provide the opportunity for human infection. Developing hyatid cysts can become quite large and may be mistaken for tumors. Surgical removal of the cyst may be preceded by chemical treat-ment to inactivate the germinal layer of the cyst and thus prevent metastatic spread of the parasite.

The fish tapeworm *Dibothriocephalus latum* (for-merly *Diphyllobothrum latum*) uses humans and other species as a definitive host and various species of fish as an intermediate host. The worm is acquired by inges-tion. Adult worms can reach 10 m in length and have 3,000 to 4,000 proglittids. Symptoms are weakness, ab-dominal pain, and weight loss. Severe anemia can result as the worms absorb vitamin B_{12} at high rates.

Nemathelminthes

Human nematode parasites can be broadly divided into groups that infect the alimentary canal and those that invade other tissues. Unlike the platyhelminths, ne-matodes have a complete digestive tract and a true body cavity. They have simple life cycles and usually do not require intermediate hosts.

The whipworm *Trichuris trichura* is a parasite of many mammalian species including humans. Adult worms are about 4.5 cm in length with a slender anterior end containing the head and esophagus and a thicker posterior end containing the reproductive organs. Infection is acquired by ingestion of oval eggs that hatch and the embryos burrow into the intestinal mucosa. After maturation, the adult worms migrate to the cecum where they remain for several years continuously producing eggs. Infection is more common in children. Severity of symptoms is related to the worm load. A few worms will produce no noticeable symptoms whereas a large worm load will produce weakness, bloody stools and diarrhea. Diagnosis is carried out by demonstration of the typical football-shaped ova.

Human trichinosis results from the ingestion of uncooked meat containing encysted larvae of *Trichinella spiralis.* The larvae give rise to adult worms which mate in the intestine. The female burrows into the intestinal wall. Embryos leave the female uterus, enter the lymph and blood, and are disseminated throughout the body. They enter the tissues, favoring striated muscle, and encyst. Symptoms result from migration of the larvae and the consequent response. The severity of disease is dependent upon the number of cysts that develop. Control of trichinosis is attempted by educating people to cook fully pork and other meats (bear) and by prohibiting the feeding of pigs with uncooked garbage and scraps.

Diagnosis is often difficult as symptoms are irregular and variable in severity. Periorbital edema is a fairly constant finding. Demonstration of cysts in biopsy is difficult but possible. Serologic tests can provide some guidance.

Two species, *Necator americanus* and *Ancylostoma duodenale* are the principal causes of human hookworm infection. The worms are similar in morphology and life cycle. *N americanus* predominates in the Western hemisphere but is not restricted to that locale. Also *A duodenale* predominates in the Eastern hemisphere but is not restricted there. Hookworms flourish in most tropical and subtropical regions of the world.

Adult hookworms reside in the small intestine of the human host. They fasten tightly in place by their mouth parts, sucking blood and tissue juices. *N americanus* is about 1 cm in length with sharp cutting plates in the mouth, while *A duodenale* is about 1.2 cm with six sharp teeth in the mouth. Females of both species can produce up to 10,000 eggs per day. Larvae emerge from the eggs in the soil under proper conditions of temperature and humidity. The first larval stage, rhabditiform larvae, are free living, feeding on soil bacteria. A second stage ensues, strongiliform and finally, the infective stage, filariform. The latter can penetrate intact skin and subsequently migrate through the subcutaneous tissues to the blood. They pass through the right heart and are trapped in the capillaries of the lung. They penetrate the alveolar air sacs and are swept up by the trachea. They are then either expectorated or swallowed. The swallowed larvae burrow into the intestinal mucosa where they molt and develop the buccal teeth that characterize the adult. After an additional molt, they become sexually mature and egg production begins. Adult worms live several years.

Symptoms of hookworm infection are associated with the various stages of pathogenesis. Skin irritation occurs as a result of the penetration of the filariform larvae. Pulmonary symptoms along with fever, headache, and eosinophilia characterize the migration through the lungs. The intestinal phase causes nausea, abdominal pain, and diarrhea. Diagnosis is dependent upon finding eggs in feces and sometimes the rhabditiform larvae. Management of anemia is the principal clinical problem. Drugs for elimination of the worms are available.

Strongyloides stercolalis causes human infection similar to hookworm infection. The life cycle of the parasite is incompletely known. The female worm (males have not been described) burrows into the intestinal mucosa and eggs are produced. Eggs and rhabditiform larvae are shed in the stool. In addition filariform larvae also develop that are capable of reinitiating infection in the host (autoinfection). Shed forms in the feces can develop into free living adult forms. These produce more larvae, some of which as filariform larvae, are infectious by direct penetration of skin. A route of migration through the right heart and lungs occurs as is seen with hookworm infection.

Similar symptoms occur as in hookworm infection. Diagnosis depends on the demonstration of rhabditiform larvae in the stool. Treatment is prolonged and autoinfection is a principal problem in management.

Ascaris lumbricoides, the human roundworm, is a large nemetode. Females are 25 to 30 cm long and 2.5 cm in diameter. Males are somewhat shorter and more slender. Adult worms live in the small intestine where they may attach to the mucosa occasionally to suck nutrients. They also live unattached and utilize partially digested nutrients in the intestinal contents. Ascaids produce up to 2×10^5 eggs per day. These are passed with the feces and under favorable conditions of temperature and moisture become infectious after 1 week. Infection of the human host is most often affected by ingestion of the infectious embryo. The larvae that hatch penetrate the mucosa, enter the blood, and pass through the right heart to the lungs. They travel to the intestine by swallowing of sputum. They mature into adult forms and they reside in the intestine.

Symptoms due to larval migration are principally pulmonary, fever, cough, and pneumonitis. A few adult worms cause no intestinal symptoms, however a large worm load can cause nausea, vomiting, and abdominal discomfort. Heavy worm loads are serious, causing malnutrition or intestinal obstruction. Complications can result from migration of adult worms into ducts and body cavities. Diagnosis depends on demonstration of ova. Effective drug treatment is available, however it must be properly monitored as migration of worms increases during treatment.

Enterobius vermicularis, the pin worm, is the most common human nemetode parasite. It is cosmopolitan in distribution, primarily found in temperature zones, and occurs more frequently in Caucasians. Adult worms live in the cecum. Females migrate to the rectum and at night migrate out the anus and deposit eggs in the perianal area. Eggs are disseminated in the environment and remain viable for several days. Infection is usually acquired by ingestion of eggs from fingers or food contaminated with the eggs. Autoinfection is common, particularly among children. Adult worms live 1 to 2 months.

Symptoms appear in about one-third of cases. Intense itching of the perinanal area is the most prominent symptom. Restlessness, nervousness, and inability to concentrate are often seen. Worms may invade other body sites such as the vagina of young girls and occasionally other sites including the peritoneum. Diagnosis is carried out by the observation of eggs or worms in the perianal regions. Effective treatment is available but management must include family contacts as the organisms can readily reestablish infection.

MEDICAL MYCOLOGY

There are over 10^5 species of fungi of which only about 50 are pathogenic for humans. The classification of the fungi is based principally on morphology (Table 5-22). The genera in which human pathogens are found are indicated in Table 5-22.

Clinically, fungi can be classified by the type of disease they cause in the human host. The groups are (1) those causing infection of the superficial layers of the skin, (2) those causing infection of the skin, hair and nails, (3) those causing infections of the subcutaneous tissues and (4) those causing systemic infections (Table 5-23). This grouping, illustrated in Table 5-23, pertains to those agents causing disease in normal individuals and does not address the long list of fungi that can cause opportunistic infections.

Identification of Fungi

COLONIAL MORPHOLOGY

Fungi form two types of colony on solid laboratory media, a yeast colony or a mold colony. Yeast colonies are similar in some respects to bacterial colonies. They are frequently larger and usually opaque. Pigmentation is frequent. Microscopic examination of material from yeast colonies shows spherical or ovoid cells considerably larger than the bacterial coccus. Mold colonies are made up of the filamentous mass of hyphae called the mycelium. That part of the mycelium that penetrates the solid medium is called the vegetative mycelium while the portion above the medium is called the aerial mycelium. The aerial mycelium gives rise to the various structures on which the spores are borne. Mold colonies have a range of appearance, cottony, wooly, fluffy, or powdery. They also have a variety of pigments.

Types of Spores

Identification of mold fungi is based on the morphology of their asexual spores. Individual species of fungi may have one or more of the spore types and an individual spore type may have an appearance unique for that species.

Table 5-22. Classification of Fungi and Bacteria of Related Interest That Are the Principal Etiologic Agents of Human Disease

Fungi
  Zygomycetes—nonseptate; sexual and asexual spores
    Mold fungi: *Rhizopus, Mucor, Absidia*
  Ascomycetes—septate; sexual and asexual spores
    Yeast and molds
    Includes some pathogenic fungi with sexual stages
  Basidiomycetes—septate hyphae; have clamp connection for sexual reproduction
    Includes mushrooms and toadstools, and possibly some pathogenic fungi with sexual stages
  Deuteromycetes (fungi imperfecti)—septate; asexual spores only
    Yeast fungi: *Candida, Cryptococcus*
    Dimorphic fungi: *Histoplasma, Coccidioides, Blastomyces, Paracoccidioides, Sporothrix*
    Mold fungi:
      Dermatophytes (Microsporum, Trichophyton, Epidermophyton)
      Aspergillus
      Producing mycetoma *(Petriellidium, Madurella)*
      Chromoblastomycotic agents *(Fonsecaea, Phialophora, Cladosporium)*

Bacteria
  Funguslike bacteria
    Actinomyces
    Nocardia

(Milgrom F, Flanagan TD: Medical Microbiology. Churchill Livingstone, New York, 1982.)

Table 5-23. Clinical Types of Fungus Infections

Type	Disease	Causative Organism
Superficial infections	Pityriasis versicolor Piedra	*Malassezia furfur* *Trichosporon beigelii* (white) *Piedraia hortai* (black)
Cutaneous infections	Ringworm of skin, hair, and nails	Dermatophytes (*Microsporum* spp., *Trichophyton* spp., *Epidermophyton floccosum*)
	Candidiasis of skin, mucous membranes, and nails	*Candida albicans* and related species
Subcutaneous infections	Sporotrichosis Chromomycosis Mycotic mycetoma	*Sporothrix schenckii* *Fonsecaea pedrosoi* and related organisms *Petriellidium boydii, Madurella* spp. (Funguslike bacteria: *Nocardia*)
Systemic infections	Opportunistic fungus infections Candidiasis, systemic Cryptococcosis Aspergillosis Mucormycosis Pathogenic fungus infections Histoplasmosis Coccidioidomycosis Blastomycosis Paracoccidioidomycosis	 *Candida albicans* *Cryptococcus neoformans* *Aspergillus fumigatus*, etc. *Rhizopus* spp., *Mucor* spp., *Absidia* spp. *Histoplasma capsulatum* *Coccidioides immitis* *Blastomyces dermatitidis* *Paracoccidioides brasiliensis*

This table is intended not as a complete list of fungi pathogenic for humans but as a list of the more important microorganisms divided according to their major sites of infection.
(Milgrom F, Flanagan TD: Medical Microbiology. Churchill Livingstone, New York, 1982.)

Cutaneous Infections

DERMATOPHYTOSES

Dermatophytic infections involve the skin, hair, and nails. Infection is limited to the cornified layers of the skin but pathologic changes can occur in living tissues as a result of host response or toxic effect of metabolic products. The disease caused by the dermatophytes is called tinea or ringworm because of the typical appearance of the centifugally spreading lesion. All infections begin in the cornified layer of the epidermis. In those infections that involve the hair or nails, invasion of these structures follow. On the skin, host reaction may be limited to patchy scaling or may proceed to a toxic eczemaform eruption. Apparent resolution usually occurs but a carrier state may be established in which exacerbation of the infection occurs upon provocation (stress, trauma).

Three genera of dermatophytes cause human (and other) infections. They are *Microsporum, Trichophyton,* and *Epidermophyton*. Species of these genera infect the hair and skin. *Trichophyton* also infect the nails. *M audouinii* is the most common cause of tinea capitis in school children; however, in certain locals *T tonsurans*

causes more disease. The principal agents of tinea pedis (athlete's foot) are *T mentagrophytes* and *T rubrum*.

CANDIDIASIS

Primary and secondary infections caused by the genus *Candida* occur in three basic clinical forms, acute cutaneous and mucocutaneous, chronic mucocutaneous, and acute systemic candidiasis. In addition to infections, *Candida* may cause allergic reactions. The most common pathogen is *C albicans* (Fig. 5-26). Acute cutaneous or mucocutaneous candidiasis is a localized and self-limiting infection usually occurring on the oral or vulvar mucosa or the nails. These infections are associated with local changes such as water immersion or sweating, physiological changes such as pregnancy, changes in the microbial flora as affected by antibiotics, or changes caused by steroid therapy. Chronic mucocutaneous infections also occur on the oral or vulvar mucosa or the nails, however the lesions are spreading and chronic in nature. Systemic spread is not seen. Patients have underlying defects in cell mediated immunity. Acute systemic candidiasis is characterized by dissemination of lesions in viseral organs, meninges, the endocardium, kidney,

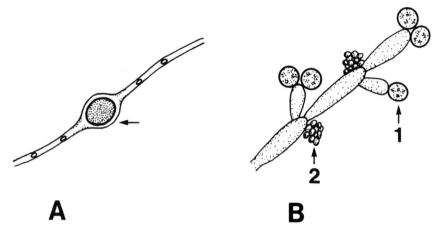

Fig. 5-26. (A) Chlamydospore formation within hyphal strand (×400). (B) Terminal chlamydospores of *Candida albicans*. (1) Terminal chlamydospore. (2) Clusters of yeast cells (×300). (Milgrom F, Flanagan TD: Medical Microbiology. Churchill Livingstone, New York, 1982.)

brain, and other sites. This form of infection is associated with introduction of yeasts by catheters, or intravenous drug use. Debilitated patients or those with lymphoproliferative disease are particularly vulnerable.

Subcutaneous Infections

Introduction of certain soil fungi into subcutaneous tissues can result in infection. These infections are usually associated with trauma. They are most often localized or, if spreading, do so along lymphatics. Hematogeneous spread or systemic disease is rare.

SPOROTRICHOSIS

The chronic nodular infection caused by *Sporothrix schenkii* is called sporotrichosis. The organism is a common soil inhibitant and gains entry by trauma. The initial cutaneous or subcutaneous lesion spreads along lymphatics causing secondary lesions. These often ulcerate and drain. Spread may continue to muscle, bone or other sites. Resolution of the lesions is prolonged.

CHROMOMYCOSIS

Infection with a group of dematiaceous or pigmented fungis is referred to as chromomycosis. Several clinical forms are recognized including chromoblastomycosis (a condition resembling sporotrichosis), keratomycosis (ulcers on the cornea), and mycetoma. The principal characteristics of these infections is chronicity and hyperplasia leading to verrucoid, warty nodules.

MYCETOMA

Mycetoma is characterized by tumifaction, draining sinuses, and granules in the draining exudate. It often involves the destruction of connective tissue, muscle, and bone. Etiologically about 50 percent of cases are caused by bacteria such as *Nocardia, Streptomyces,* and *Actinomandura.* The most important causes of eumycotic mycetoma are *Petriellidium* and *Manduella.* The lesions develop after traumatic introduction of the organisms. The foot and the hand are the most frequently affected sites. The lesion develops as a soft subcutaneous swelling that ruptures to the surface forming sinus tracts and burrowing into deeper tissues. Drainage is characterized by granules of the causative agent. These are useful in determining etiology. Resolution of the lesions is followed by development of masses of fibrotic tissue resembling a tumor. This often leads to disfigurement.

Systemic Fungal Infections

Systemic fungal infections are caused by two groups of agents, those that are opportunistic and those that are frankly pathogenic. The opportunists are agents of low virulence that produce disease almost exclusively in patients whose defense mechanisms are impaired. The pathogens cause disease in normal persons providing the infecting dose is sufficient. Pathogens cause exaggerated disease in debilitated patients. Among the opportunists are the yeasts *Candida albinicans* and *Cryptococcus neoformans* and the molds of *Aspergillus* spp. and *Mucor* spp. Two other characteristics of the opportunists are that they are always present in the environment and they

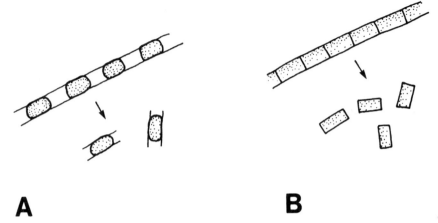

Fig. 5-27. (A) Barrel shaped arthrospores of *Cocidioides immitis* (×100). (B) Rectangular arthrospores of *Geotrichum candidum* (×500). (Milgrom F, Flanagan TD: Medical Microbiology. Churchill Livingstone, New York, 1982.)

have no particular geographic distribution (Figs. 5-27 and 5-28).

The pathogenic fungi (except *Coccidioides immitis*) show a temperature dependant dimorphism when grown in the laboratory. At 37°C the organisms grow as yeasts; whereas, at 22°C, they grow as molds. This reflects morphologic forms found in tissues. (*C immitis* occurs as a spherule in tissue, but no corresponding yeast is seen in laboratory cultures at 37°C.) All of the pathogens are soil organisms and disease results from the entry of the spores of the organisms by the respiratory route. The distribution of the pathogenic fungi is geographically restricted and factors such as moisture, wind, alkalinity, and the soil microbial flora all play a role in the epidemiology of their diseases.

CRYPTOCOCCOSIS

C neoformans is a fungus found in association with bird droppings. The alkaline substrate apparently provides the proper environment for the organism. In the United States and Europe pigeon droppings are a frequent source of human infection. The fungus is an opportunistic pathogen causing disease in compromised patients. While the portal of entry is the respiratory tract, symptoms of respiratory infection are usually subclinical or transitory in normal persons. In compromised persons the primary respiratory infection becomes rapidly systemic. The organism has a prediliction for the central nervous system and meningitis is the principal expression of infection. Other forms of disseminated disease, cutaneous, mucocutaneous, osseus, and viseral, are infrequently seen in the United States. Diagnosis can be aided by the demonstration of the yeast cells in CSF. They have a large prominent capsule readily observed in

India ink preparations. The organism grows as a yeast on Sabouraud's dextrose agar (SDA) regardless of temperature. Additionally, *C neoformans* is urease positive and develops a brown pigmentation when grown on niger

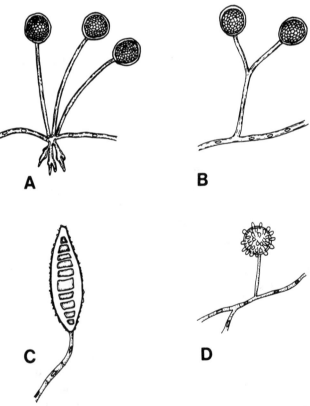

Fig. 5-28. (A) Conidiospores (conidia) of *Aspergillus niger* (×100). (B) Conidia of *Sporothrix schenckii* (×500). (C) Macroaleuriospores of *Microsporum canis* (×250). (D) Macroaleuriospores of *Histoplasma capsulatum* (×550). (Milgrom F, Flanagan TD: Medical Microbiology. Churchill Livingstone, New York, 1982.)

MICROBIOLOGY AND IMMUNOLOGY

283

seed agar. Serologic detection of capsular antigen in CSF is also a useful aid to diagnosis.

ASPERGILLOSIS

Members of the genus *Aspergillus* are ubiquitous fungi that are opportunistic pathogens. Three forms of pathogenesis are recognized; allergic, colonizing, and invasive. The allergic form results from hypersensitivity responses to the antigens of the fungus. The disease may become chronic and progressive. The colonizing forms are those in which the organism develops and grows in cavitations present as a result of some other disease process such as tuberculosis or sarcoidosis. The *Aspergillus* often grows into a macroscopically visible "fungus ball." Invasive disease can develop from other forms and is almost universally fatal. Clinically, pneumonia is the most prominent component, however, the organism can be found in many organs.

ZYGMYCOSIS (MUCORMYCOSIS)

Infection with various ubiquitous members of the class *Zygomycetes* usually *Mucor* spp., *Rhizopus* spp., and *Absidia* spp., is referred to as zygmycosis. Infections occur in patients with various debilitating diseases such as diabetes mellitus, leukemia, lymphoma, malnutrition, and those treated with various cytotoxic drugs. The rhinofaciocranial form of the disease is most often seen in diabetic patients, frequently running a fatal course in 10 days. Direct demonstration of large, aseptate hyphae in clinical material is diagnostic.

HISTOPLASMOSIS

Histoplasma capsulatum is a dimorphic pathogenic fungus and the cause of histoplasmosis. It is a soil organism often found in association with bird and bat droppings. It is distributed in several areas throughout the world. In the United States the Ohio-Mississippi valley regions are the most highly endemic for the organism. It is estimated that 200,000 new infections occur yearly in the United States but about 95 percent are subclinical.

The organism enters by the respiratory route and pulmonary infection ensues. Flu-like symptoms of variable severity are the most common manifestation. X-ray pictures reveal multiple lesions similar to tuberculosis, a disease from which histoplasmosis must be differentiated. Dissemination to other tissues can occur but it is usually benign. Diagnosis can be made by demonstration of yeast cells within RES cells in sputum or tissue specimens. However, this is not a sensitive method. Cultural demonstration of the organism by growth on SDA at 37°C and 22°C is reliable. Serology can also be useful

both for diagnosis and prognosis. Immunodiffusion of standard reference serum against histoplasmin results in two precipitin lines, H and M. The presence of the H line in a serum usually indicates recent infection. The reaction is often present up to a year after recovery. The M line is indicative of past infection but is also present during the active disease. It can also result from skin-testing with histoplasmin, a test which reveals delayed hypersensitivity to the fungus.

COCCIDIOIDOMYCOSIS

Coccidioides immitis is a soil organism found in dry, semiarid soils of Southwest United States and other areas in Central and South America. The organism causes a mild to severe respiratory disease called San Joaquin fever. It also causes a systemic disease known as desert rheumatism. Allergic manifestations also contribute to the disease picture caused by *C immitis*.

Primary coccidioidomycosis varys from clinically inapparent infection to moderately severe pulmonary disease. Recovery ensues and strong resistance to reinfection develops. Secondary coccidioidomycosis is a disseminated disease occuring as a chronic progressive process or as an acute rapidly fatal process.

Allergic manifestations are seen in 5 to 10 percent of primary infections, often occurring as raised nodules on the lower extremities, especially around the knees. These "desert bumps" are pathognomonic for the infection.

Diagnosis can be accomplished by demonstration of spherules in sputum or tissue. The organism grows only in a mold phase on laboratory media.

BLASTOMYCOSIS

Blastomyces dermatitidis is the cause of a chronic granulomatous, supparative pulmonary disease. The agent is a soil saprophyte that grows dimorphically at 37°C and 22°C on laboratory media. It commonly occurs in North America but is found in Africa and the Middle East as well.

The infection is acquired by the airborne route and primarily manifests as a pulmonary infection. Inapparent infection does not seem to occur as with other systemic mycoses. The lesions resemble those of tuberculosis and histoplasmosis. As the lesions heal, macrophages engulf and transport the organism to other sites. A cutaneous form of disease results from this dissemination. Cutaneous blastomycosis is the most common form of extrapulmonary disease, manifesting as subcutaneous or cutaneous nodules then often ulcerate and evolve to verrucous granulomas.

Direct examination of sputum or lesion material reveals yeasts with broad-based buds. Demonstration of these forms usually suffices for diagnosis. The organism grows on SDA and the dimorphism can be demonstrated.

REFERENCES

Braude A (ed): Medical Microbiology and Infectious Disease. Vol 2. WB Saunders, Philadelphia, 1981
> A comprehensive text emphasizing the clinical aspects of microbiology and immunology.

Davis B, Delbecco R, Eisen H, et al: Microbiology. 4th Ed. Harper and Row, New York, 1984
> A comprehensive text with excellent treatment of more basic microbiology and immunology.

Joklik W, Willert R, Amos S (eds): Zinsser Microbiology. 18th Ed. Appleton Century Crofts, East Norwalk, 1984
> A comprehensive text covering most medically significant bacteria, fungi and viruses. Up-to-date treatment of immunology.

Milgrom F, Flanagan TD (eds): Medical Microbiology. Churchill Livingstone, New York, 1982
> A concise presentation covering all areas of medical microbiology.

MULTIPLE CHOICE QUESTIONS

1. The poliovirus genome
   A. Is composed of four segments of single stranded RNA
   B. Requires transcription to mRNA
   C. Is double stranded DNA
   D. Requires transcription to DNA to be expressed
   E. Is directly translated on host ribosomes

2. Early adenovirus mRNA is
   A. Transcribed by a virion transcriptase
   B. Transcribed from one entire DNA strand
   C. Translated into products active in DNA synthesis
   D. Translated into virion proteins
   E. Translated into a 75 K protein found on the 3′ end of the DNA strands

3. Replication of influenza A virus gene segments is a function of
   A. The HA protein
   B. The N protein
   C. The M protein
   D. The P1, P2, and P3 proteins
   E. The NS, P1, P2, and P3 proteins

4. In herpes virus replication, β synthesis is characterized by the following *except*
   A. Initiates gamma transcription
   B. Products are active in DNA synthesis
   C. Modulates α synthesis

   D. Products that terminate γ translation
   E. Modulation by products of γ synthesis

5. Changes in the antigenicity of influenza A viruses that result in 1 to 3 year epidemic cycles are due to
   A. Reassortment of the N gene
   B. Mutation in the NS gene
   C. Reassortment of the M gene
   D. Mutation in the H gene
   E. Reassortment of the P1 gene

6. Which of the following concerning the Paramyxoviridae is incorrect
   A. Protection against respiratory syncytial virus is engendered with a live vaccine virus
   B. Measles virus does not have neuraminidase activity
   C. Mumps is a systemic disease
   D. Parainfluenza virus type 1 is immunologically distinct from influenza A
   E. The rash of measles appears when antibodies are present

7. Which of the following concerning syphilis is incorrect?
   A. The causative agent cannot be grown on laboratory media
   B. Spirochetes are present in the primary and secondary lesions
   C. Anticardiolipin antibodies are present in the secondary stage
   D. Syphilis is caused by *Treponema pallidum*
   E. Effective treatment causes loss of antitreponemal antibody

8. Which of the following is spread to humans by lice
   A. *Leptospira interrogans*
   B. *Borrelia recurrentis*
   C. *Borrelia hermsii*
   D. *Treponema pertenue*
   E. *Treponema pallidum*

9. Which of the following concerning mycoplasma is incorrect
   A. Form colonies on lifeless media
   B. Are insusceptible to penicillin
   C. Cause primary atypical pneumonia
   D. Pass through filters with 5 μm pores
   E. Can revert to "bacterial form"

10. The etiologic agent of Rocky Mountain spotted fever is
    A. *Rickettsia rickettsii*
    B. *Rickettsia prowazeki*

C. *Rickettsia akari*
D. *Rickettsia typhi*
E. *Coxiella burnetti*

11. Direct human-to-human spread can occur with
    A. *Rickettsia rickettsii*
    B. *Rickettsia prowazeki*
    C. *Rickettsia akari*
    D. *Rickettsia typhi*
    E. *Coxiella burnetti*

12. Which of the following would not be used in the formal classification of a virus?
    A. Presence of an envelope
    B. Symmetry of the capsid
    C. Numbers of capsomers
    D. Segmentation of the genome
    E. Tissue tropism

13. Concerning T-4 bacteriophage, contractile properties are associated with
    A. Head protein
    B. Tail pins
    C. Tail fibers
    D. Tail sheath
    E. Collar protein

14. Vaccination against whooping cough is carried out using
    A. Capsular polysaccharide from *Haemophilus influenza* type B
    B. Killed phase 1 cells of *Bordetella pertussis*
    C. Live phase 4 cells of *Bordetella bronchoseptica*
    D. Killed phase 4 cells of *Bordetella parapertussis*
    E. A cell wall preparation of *Bordetella bronchoseptica*

15. The leading cause of bacterial meningitis in children under 4 years is
    A. *Haemophilus influenzae*
    B. *Streptococcus pneumoniae*
    C. *Neisseria meningitidis*
    D. *Streptococcus pyogenes*
    E. *Streptococcus agalactiae*

16. Primary atypical pneumonia is associated with the following except
    A. *Chlamydia trachomatis*
    B. *Legionella pneumophilia*
    C. *Mycoplasma pneumonia*
    D. *Chlamydia psittaci*
    E. *Streptococcus pneumoniae*

17. Replication of *Mycobacterium tuberculosis* within macrophages is controlled by
    A. Lymphokine activation of the macrophages
    B. Natural killer cell-mediated cytolysis
    C. Antibody-mediated cellular cytoxicity
    D. Complement mediated bacteriolysis
    E. IgE-induced mediator release

18. The generation time for growth of *Mycobacterium tuberculosis* in culture is
    A. 20 to 30 minutes
    B. 4 to 6 hours
    C. 12 to 18 hours
    D. 48 to 72 hours
    E. 10 to 14 days

19. *Nocardia* may be differentiated from *Actinomyces* on the basis of
    A. Gram stain
    B. Cellular morphology
    C. Branching of filaments
    D. Growth in air
    E. Lack of motility of nocardiae

20. Anaerobic organisms frequently involved in brain abcesses belong to the genus
    A. *Staphylococcus*
    B. *Bacteroides*
    C. *Clostridium*
    D. *Bacillus*
    E. *Fusobacterium*

21. A principal factor in the pathogenicity of *Neisseria gonorrhoeae* is
    A. Hemolysin
    B. Leukocidin
    C. Antiphagocytic factor
    D. Flagella
    E. Fimbriae

22. Vaccine against *Neisseria meningitidis* is composed of
    A. Live bacterial cells
    B. Formalin-killed bacterial cells
    C. Disrupted bacterial cells
    D. Cell wall material
    E. Capsular polysaccharide

23. Immune status to diphtheria is clinically determined by injection of
    A. Toxin
    B. Toxoid
    C. Heat-inactivated toxin

D. *Corynebacterium diphtheriae* (heat-killed)

E. Antiserum to toxin

24. Food poisoning resulting from ingestion of pre-formed toxin is caused by the following *except*
    A. *Bacillus cereus*
    B. *Clostridium botulinum*
    C. *Staphylococcus aureus*
    D. *Clostridium perfringens*
    E. *Salmonella enteridis*

25. Which of the following is nonmotile
    A. *Escherichia coli*
    B. *Salmonella typhi*
    C. *Shigella sonnei*
    D. *Vibrio cholerae*
    E. *Proteus mirabelis*

26. Enterotoxigenic strains of *Escherichia coli* (ETEC) cause
    A. Dysentery
    B. Travellers diarrhea
    C. Diarrhea of newborns
    D. Cholera
    E. Septicemia

27. The etiologic diagnosis of typhoid fever can be accomplished by
    A. Serology in the first week
    B. Stool culture in the first week
    C. Blood culture in the first week
    D. Urine culture in the first week
    E. Detection of capsular antigen in serum throughout the course of the infection.

28. The effector cell of delayed hypersensitivity in humans is
    A. A natural killer cell
    B. A null cell
    C. A T-lymphocyte bearing the T4 marker
    D. A T-lymphocyte bearing the T5 and T8 markers
    E. A B-lymphocyte

29. Children of a blood group A father and a blood group B mother may have genotype(s)
    A. AB only
    B. OO only
    C. AB and OO only
    D. AO, BO, AB, and OO only
    E. AA, AO, BB, BO, AB, and OO

30. Which of the following genotype pairs of parents would most likely produce a pregnancy leading to hemolytic disease of the newborn

	Father	Mother
A.	cde/cde	cde/cde
B.	cde/cde	cDe/CDe
C.	cDe/CDe	CDe/cde
D.	CDe/cde	cDE/cDE
E.	CDe/CDe	cde/Cde

31. Abcess formation of *Staphlococcus aureus* is attributed in part to the action of
    A. Hyaluronidase
    B. Exfoliatin
    C. Enterotoxin
    D. Coagulase
    E. DNAase

32. Which of the following is regarded as the most significant cause of meningitis during the newborn period
    A. *Streptococcus pyogenes*
    B. *Streptococcus agalactiae*
    C. *Streptococcus pneumoniae*
    D. *Haemphilus influenzae*
    E. *Neisseria meningiditis*

33. Among the immunopathologic sequelae to Group A β hemolytic streptococcal infection is
    A. Rheumatic fever
    B. Scarlet fever
    C. Toxic shock syndrome
    D. Scalded skin syndrome
    E. Kawasaki disease

34. Specificity of an Ig molecule for an antigenic determinant
    A. Is a property of the carboxy terminus of the heavy chain
    B. Results from "instruction" of the Ig by antigen
    C. Is dependant upon the conformation of C domains
    D. Is a property associated with the Fc fragment
    E. Is due in part to VDJ sequences in immunoglobulin heavy chain genes

35. The least sensitive method for the detection of antibody is
    A. Agglutination
    B. Precipitation
    C. Radioimmunoassay
    D. Enzyme immunoassay
    E. Complement fixation

36. C5 convertase activity resides in
    A. Properdin
    B. C14a2b
    C. C14a2b3b

D. C5b67
E. C3bBb

37. The genes of the MHC
    A. Code for immunoglobulins
    B. Have a small number of alleles at each locus
    C. Code for intracellular enzymes
    D. Code for products involved in cell-cell recognition
    E. Code for nonantigenic surface molecules

38. The change in isotype of Ig of a B-cell during ontogeny is mediated by
    A. J sequences of immunoglobulin genes
    B. D sequences of immunoglobulin genes
    C. V sequences of L chain genes
    D. S sequences of immunoglobulin genes
    E. C sequences of H chain genes

39. Which of the following is *not* a lymphokine
    A. IgA
    B. Interferon
    C. Macrophage migration inhibition factor
    D. Macrophage activating factor
    E. Leukocyte activating factor

40. Associative recognition refers to the requirement for MHC compatibility
    A. Between antibody and cell surface antigens
    B. In blood transfusion
    C. Between donor and recipient cells
    D. Between target cell and effector T-lymphocyte
    E. Between target cell and natural killer cell

41. Anaerobic respiration uses all of the following as an electron receptor *except*
    A. Carbonate
    B. Nitrate
    C. Oxygen
    D. Sulfate
    E. NAD

42. Daughter DNA molecules segregate to new bacterial cells as a result of
    A. Cytoplasmic streaming
    B. Repulsive forces between the molecules
    C. The action of actin-like strands
    D. Membrane biosynthesis between attachment sites
    E. Centriole activity

43. Regulation of bacterial genes by induction depends upon
    A. Inhibition of repressor synthesis

B. Activation of the repressor gene
C. Attachment of the inducer to the operator site
D. Inhibition of repressor attachment by the inducer
E. Synthesis of inducer

44. Illegitimate recombination is
    A. Site specific
    B. Mediated by Tn sequences
    C. Mediated by *rec A, rec B*, and *rec C*
    D. Mediated by IS
    E. Dependant on sequence homology of the exogenote and endogenote

45. Endogenotes are protected from endogenous nuclease activity by
    A. Methylation of critical bases
    B. Lack of appropriate base sequences
    C. Temperature optima of the enzymes
    D. Membrane attachment of the chromosome
    E. Circularity of the chromosome

46. Acquisition of an exogenote by transformation requires
    A. Competence of the recipient cells
    B. An F plasmid
    C. A temperate prophage
    D. A conjugation bridge
    E. The Hfr state

47. Transfer of bacterial genes by a bacteriophage is
    A. Conjugation
    B. Plasmid directed
    C. Transformation
    D. Sexduction
    E. Transduction

48. Resistance to antimicrobic drugs occurs by the following mechanisms *except*
    A. Loss of a drug binding site
    B. Change in permeability
    C. Development of an alternative metabolic pathway
    D. Production of an enzyme that destroys the drug
    E. Antimicrobic-directed mutation

49. Bacterial endospores will remain viable when
    A. Pasteurized
    B. Antoclaved
    C. Ultraviolet irradiated
    D. Treated with ethylene oxide
    E. Treated with microwaves

50. The source of lymphocytes is hematopoietic tissue of the
    A. Liver
    B. Spleen
    C. Thymus
    D. Bone marrow
    E. Lymph nodes

51. The differentiation of B cells into plasmacytes is
    A. Thymus dependent
    B. Antigen stimulated
    C. Accompanied by a change in isotype of immunoglobulin
    D. Accompanied by acquisition of surface class II molecules
    E. Suppressed by T4-bearing lymphocytes

52. Which of the following would most likely be a T-independant antigen
    A. Bovine serum albumin
    B. Glucosamine
    C. Pneumococcal capsular polysaccharide
    D. Tetanus toxoid
    E. Lipoteichoic acid

53. Immunoglobulin M
    A. Is the major secretory Ig
    B. Is the principal Ig in the primary response
    C. Is found on the surface of all mature B memory cells
    D. Has a molecular weight of 150,000
    E. Is composed of two identical four chain units

54. Ig isotypes are detected by
    A. The molecular weight of the molecule
    B. The electrophoretic migration
    C. Solubility in water
    D. Antigenicity of the light chain
    E. Antigenicity of the heavy chain

55. A constituent common to both gram-positive and gram-negative cell wall is
    A. Lipoteichoic acid
    B. Peptidoglycan
    C. KDO
    D. Teichoic acid
    E. LPS

56. Bacterial LPS differ among species by the structure of their
    A. Lipid A
    B. Ketodeoxyoctonate
    C. Heptose residues
    D. O-specific side chains
    E. Hydrophobic regions

57. The following structures are found on the surfaces of bacterial cells *except*
    A. Mesosomes
    B. Flagella
    C. Fimbriae
    D. Capsules
    E. Sex pili

58. The phase of the bacterial growth curve in which the rate of cell division equals the rate of cell death is the
    A. Lag phase
    B. Logarithmic phase
    C. Stationary phase
    D. Decline phase
    E. Death phase

59. Initiation of a bacterial culture with cells from a culture growing logarithmically results in an immediate lag in growth if
    A. The new culture medium has the same nitrogen source
    B. The new culture medium has a different carbon source
    C. Metabolites are transferred with the inoculated cells
    D. The temperature of growth is the same for both cultures
    E. The new culture is kept in the dark

60. Fermentations that produce a single end product are
    A. Aerobic
    B. Photosynthetic
    C. Homolactic
    D. Oxidative
    E. Reductive

61. Coxsackie B viruses are frequently associated with
    A. Reye's syndrome
    B. The common cold
    C. Hand, foot, and mouth disease
    D. Paralytic poliomyelitis
    E. Pericarditis

62. Viruses of the Reoviridae are distinguished from other viruses by
    A. A segmented genome
    B. A double-stranded RNA genome
    C. Lack of an envelope
    D. Icosahedral shape
    E. Possession of a virion transcriptase

63. The serologic finding most suggestive of potential for infectiousness of hepatitis B is
    A. anti-HBs
    B. HB$_s$Ag
    C. HB$_s$Ag and anti-Hb$_c$
    D. HB$_s$Ag-anti-HB$_s$ complexes
    E. HBsAg, anti-HB$_c$, and HB$_e$

64. Which of the following predisposes to HSV infection from exogenous sources
    A. Burns
    B. Sunlight
    C. Menses
    D. Emotional stress
    E. Fever

65. Mental retardation is significantly associated with
    A. Cytomegalic inclusion disease
    B. CMV mononucleosis
    C. EBV mononucleosis
    D. Postnatal CMV infection of newborns
    E. Chronic EBV infection

66. Infection with *Necator americanis* is acquired by
    A. Ingestion of rhabidiform larvae
    B. Invasion by filariaform larvae
    C. Ingestion of ova
    D. Invasion by adult worms
    E. Ingestion of adult worms

67. Acute systemic candidiasis
    A. is an allergic manifestation to *Candida albicans* antigens
    B. is acquired from soil
    C. occurs in immune compromised patients
    D. affects the mucosae principally
    E. is associated with steroid therapy

68. Dimorphic growth is a characteristic of
    A. *Candida albicans*
    B. *Aspergillus niger*
    C. *Crytococcus neoformans*
    D. *Coccidiodes immitis*
    E. *Histoplasma capsulatum*

69. *Sporothrix schenkii* is typically associated with
    A. Mucocutaneous infections
    B. Infections of the skin and hair
    C. Subcutaneous infections
    D. Chronic infections of the lung
    E. Infections of the skin, hair, and nails

70. The cause of Chaga's disease is
    A. *Leishmania donovani*
    B. *Trypanosoma cruzi*
    C. *Leishmania braziliensis*
    D. *Trypanosoma gambiense*
    E. *Trypanosoma rhodesiense*

71. Chorioretinitis is an important complication of infection with
    A. *Trichamonas vaginalis*
    B. *Pneumocystis carinii*
    C. *Entamoeba histolytica*
    D. *Toxoplasma gondii*
    E. *Giardia lambia*

72. The initiation of gametogony of Plasmodia takes place in
    A. The liver of the human host
    B. The salivary glands of the mosquito
    C. The gut of the mosquito
    D. The human blood stream
    E. The human spleen

73. Human shistosomal infection results from
    A. Ingestion of ova
    B. Invasion by miricidae
    C. Ingestion of adult flukes
    D. Invasion by cercariae
    E. Ingestion of shistosomules

74. Paul-Bunnell antibodies are a characteristic of
    A. HSV encephalitis
    B. Zoster
    C. CMV mononucleosis
    D. EBV mononucleosis
    E. Burkitt's lymphoma

75. Prophylaxis against rabies in humans is
    A. Carried out with a live virus vaccine
    B. Carried out after possible exposure
    C. Employs a nerve tissue source of virus antigen
    D. Not practiced
    E. Ineffective

76. Retroviruses are characterized by the following *except*
    A. Dimeric RNA genome
    B. Reverse transcriptase
    C. Neuraminidase
    D. A DNA intermediate in the replicative cycle
    E. An envelope

77. Transformation of fibroblasts in vitro
    A. Can be affected by lymphatic leukemia viruses
    B. Results from the activities of the *gag* gene products

C. Results from the activities of the *pol* gene product
D. Results from the activities of the *env* gene products
E. Results from the activities of the *src* gene product

Answers to Multiple Choice Questions

1 E	2 C	3 E	4 D	5 D
6 A	7 E	8 B	9 E	10 A
11 E	12 E	13 D	14 B	15 A
16 E	17 A	18 C	19 D	20 B
21 E	22 E	23 A	24 E	25 C
26 B	27 C	28 C	29 D	30 E
31 D	32 B	33 A	34 E	35 B
36 C	37 D	38 D	39 A	40 D
41 C	42 D	43 D	44 D	45 A
46 A	47 E	48 E	49 A	50 D
51 B	52 C	53 B	54 E	55 B
56 D	57 A	58 C	59 B	60 C
61 E	62 B	63 E	64 A	65 A
66 B	67 C	68 E	69 C	70 B
71 D	72 D	73 D	74 D	75 B
76 C	77 E			

Pathology

Stephen A. Geller and Alberto Marchevsky

Pathology is the specialty of medicine that, in the broadest sense, is concerned with the study of disease. Disease can be regarded as any deviation from the normal state. Pathology combines the methods of the basic sciences with the pragmatic approach of the practice of medicine in order to effectively contribute to the understanding of mechanisms of disease while participating in the evaluation and therapy of the patient with disease. Pathologists, to a great degree, still concern themselves with the whole body and its illnesses and in this way tend to function as generalists. The breadth of the pathologist's approach combined with highly technical methodology, however, does contribute to pathology having a critical role in both the education of the physician and the care of the patient.

The scope of pathology is too broad for any single individual to claim mastery of all aspects. The traditional responsibilities of the pathologist are anatomic pathology and clinical pathology. Anatomic pathology includes autopsy pathology, surgical pathology, neuropathology, pediatric pathology, cytopathology, forensic pathology, electron microscopy, and immunopathology as well established subspecialty areas. In recent years, there has been a tendency for pathologists to identify themselves with separate organ systems, so that there are many other subspecialties, such as dermatopathology, hematopathology, gynecologic pathology, etc. Clinical pathology includes the disciplines of clinical chemistry, urinalysis, hematology, blood banking (immunohematology), coagulation, toxicology, blood gas evaluation, radioimmunoassay, enzymology, endocrinology, nuclear medicine, medical bacteriology, parasitology, mycology, virology, rickettsiology, hospital epidemiology, serology, pregnancy testing, sterility testing, cytogenetics, and laboratory computerization. Another major area of interest is experimental pathology, which includes almost as many disciplines as there are experimental methods. Emphasis is often placed on experimental pathogenesis and subcellular biochemistry and morphology.

This chapter will first review the major disease processes in broad terms of injuries and host reactions. The sections devoted to the individual organ systems will then summarize the most important conditions, emphasizing pathophysiologic features, but including, where appropriate, key clinical manifestations and laboratory tests. This chapter cannot replace one of the standard texts and will be most effective if the student preparing for a medical licensing examination has had the opportunity to complete a course in pathology.

INJURY

Cell Injury

Cells can be injured by numerous agents including ischemia, chemicals, and infections. These various injurious agents act on intracellular systems that are particularly vulnerable to damage such as aerobic respiration, cell membranes, enzymes, structural proteins, and the genetic apparatus of the cell. The results of cell injury depend on the type of noxious agent, and the duration and severity of exposure. The type, state, and adaptability of a particular cell also play important roles in the pattern of injury that ensues after exposure to noxious agents. For example, ischemic injury depends on the degree of occlusion of blood vessels nourishing a particular area, the duration of ischemia, and the organ affected (i.e., neurons die 5 minutes after ischemia while renal tubular necrosis occurs after 30 minutes).

CAUSES OF CELL INJURY

Injuries induced by hypoxia, physical agents (cold, heat, radiation), chemicals, infectious organisms (bacteria, virus, fungi, parasites), nutritional imbalance, genetic defects, and immune mechanisms are the causes of cell injuries.

PATHOGENESIS OF CELL INJURY

The precise biologic and biochemical cellular mechanisms involved in reversible and irreversible cell injury are frequently difficult to unravel. The cell has so many biochemical systems that are potentially vulnerable to injury that it is often difficult to distinguish the primary targets of the injurious agent from secondary ripple effects. The precise chemical mechanisms of hypoxic, chemical, and physical injuries have been studied in experimental models.

Hypoxia. The cellular mechanisms of aerobic respiration such as oxidative phosphorylation are attacked by hypoxia. As the intracellular oxygen tension decreases, the mitochondrial production of adenosine triphosphate (ATP) progressively diminishes. The ATP loss is associated with intracellular accumulations of adenosine monophosphate (AMP) which stimulate anaerobic glycolysis to maintain alternate energy sources for cellular metabolism. Glycogen is rapidly depleted and the intracellular milieu becomes acidotic due to the accumulation of lactic acid and inorganic phosphates. The ATP-dependent sodium pump fails and potassium diffuses extracellularly while sodium and water accumulate intracellularly. As a result, the cell swells ("low amplitude swelling"). This phenomenon of acute cellular swelling is rapidly followed by the detachment of ribosomes from the rough endoplasmic reticulum, dissociation of polysomes, increased membrane permeability, decreased mitochondrial enzymatic functions, loss of microvilli on the cell surface, and the formation of intra- and extracellular myelin figures. The latter are phospholipid complexes that follow membrane damage. All of these changes are potentially reversible and the cell is capable of restoring its morphology and metabolic capabilities if oxygen supply is restored. When hypoxia persists, however, the cell undergoes irreversible damage. Mitochondria become severely vacuolized with loss of cristae ("high amplitude swelling"), lysosomes swell and leak their enzymes into the cytoplasm, and the cellular membranes fragment. The cell dies and is degraded into large masses of phospholipids that are phagocytosed by macrophages.

Chemical Injury. Numerous chemical agents can cause tissue damage. They injure cellular membranes by lipid peroxidation or by direct covalent binding of one of the metabolites of the chemical to macromolecular components of the membrane such as proteins or lipids. Carbon tetrachloride (CCl 4) poisoning is a well studied example of chemical injury by the second mechanism. This halogenated hydrocarbon is not itself toxic but is converted in the liver into a highly toxic free radical, carbon trichloride (CCl 3). This free radical has unpaired electrons and is electrically uncharged, a physical property that accounts for its great potential to form chemical bonds with various intracellular macromolecules. CCl 3 causes autooxidation of fatty acids in membrane phospholipids, oxidative decomposition of lipids, and formation of organic peroxides. The latter also act as free radicals. These activities, within the hepatocyte, cause destruction of mitochondria, endoplasmic reticulum, and cell membranes.

Tissue responses to injury include manifestations of reversible injury, termed degenerations, and consequences of irreversible damage in various forms of cell necrosis.

Cell Degeneration. Two light microscopic patterns of cell degeneration can be recognized: hydropic degeneration (cellular swelling) and fatty change (steatosis). Hydropic degeneration is the common early pattern of ischemia and is an increase in cell size due to the accumulation of water in the cytoplasm. Fatty change is due to a derangement of lipid metabolism, as either increased intracellular synthesis, decreased degradation, or impairment in the mechanisms of lipid transport from the cell into the blood. It is a common morphologic pattern of chronic ischemic or chemical injury.

Cell necrosis or cell death follows various physical, chemical, or biologic injuries and manifests as increased cytoplasmic eosinophilia, nuclear pyknosis (shrinking), and karyorrhexis (disintegration). Cell necrosis usually elicits an acute inflammatory response with accumulation of polymorphonuclear leukocytes and other inflammatory cells. Coagulation necrosis is usually the result of ischemia and is characterized by transformation of the cell into a shrunken, hypereosinophilic mass with nuclear loss. This occurs most frequently in the heart, kidney, adrenal glands, and liver. Liquefaction necrosis usually results from the action of hydrolytic enzymes, often from polymorphonuclear leucocytes. The affected tissues progressively soften and liquefy. This pattern of damage may follow ischemia and infections by pyogenic bacteria. Fat necrosis is a distinctive type of cell death, most often following acute pancreatitis where lipases contact adipose tissue. These enzymes catalyze the degradation of triglycerides to produce free fatty acids that complex with calcium to form soaps. Areas of fat necrosis appear grossly as foci of soft, white-yellow friable tissue. Caseous necrosis is a specific type of cell death characteristic of mycobacterial or fungal infections. It appears grossly as soft, white, chalky areas. Histologically, caseous necrosis is a part of a granuloma with central areas of acellular, eosinophilic, granular, necrotic tissue. Gangrenous necrosis is a clinical term that generally refers to coagulative necrosis, usually of a lower extremity in response to ischemia. It is classified as dry gangrene when coagulative necrosis is not complicated and as wet gangrene when the tissues demonstrate the combined changes of coagulative and liquefactive necrosis, usually when infection supervenes.

Abnormal intracellular accumulations occur as a response to injury. There can be excessive accumulation of lipids, proteins, or carbohydrates, and of pigments such as hemosiderin, lipofucsin, melanin, hematin, bilirubin, and of abnormal molecules such as the carbohydrate-lipid complexes present in storage diseases.

Tissue calcification may occur in dead or normal tissue, with the accumulation of calcium salts and other minerals. Calcification occurring in the presence of normal levels of serum calcium is known as dystrophic calcification, and affects injured or dead tissues. Mineralization of tissues can also be the result of markedly elevated levels of serum calcium, a phenomenom known as metastatic calcification. The latter condition appears as a consequence of abnormalities in the calcium metabolism and can affect any normal tissue, often affecting areas of high acid-base activity, such as pulmonary alveoli, gastric mucosa, and renal tubules.

ACUTE INFLAMMATION

The acute inflammatory response is one of the most basic of host reactions to injury, and is the process by which cellular and serum elements attempt to remove or destroy injurious agents. Inflammation is defined by the specific etiologic agent, by the intensity and severity of the initiating insult, and by the types of cells or serologic factors able to respond.

Acute inflammation is characterized by the accumulation of polymorphonuclear (PMN) leukocytes at the site of injury. This depends on the elaboration of chemotactic factors, the release of chemical mediators of inflammation from circulating cells, plasma, and tissue elements, and the subsequent effects on vascular permeability and the migration of inflammatory cells to the site of injury. Acute inflammation can follow mechanical injury, chemical injury, injury by physical agents (i.e., radiation), ischemic injury (i.e., compromise of blood supply), and injury from the effects of living organisms (i.e., bacterial infection).

The chemotactic factors are not completely understood. PMN chemotaxis can be stimulated by products of microorganisms such as bacteria, plasma factors (i.e., complement system, kinin system, clotting system), tissue factors (i.e., prostaglandins, collagen fragments), and by cell products (i.e., neutrophil-derived factor, lymphocyte-derived factor). Chemotaxis can be inhibited by certain drugs, such as steroids, colchicine, and quabain. Chemotaxis may be initiated by activation of specific receptors on the PMN surface, leading to microtubule and microfilament stimulation. Phagocytosis may be controlled by the same receptor elements.

Chemotaxis is characterized by the migration of PMN's to blood vessels at the site of injury, initially accompanied by increased blood velocity. Blood velocity slows and there is vasodilation at the injury site, leading to local vascular stasis, accumulation of PMNs at one area (pavementing), and increase of hydrostatic forces. Vascular permeability increases, due to alterations of endothelial cell junctions, increased transcellular transport, or both. Vascular permeability may be due to plasma factors, such as kinins (e.g., bradykinin, C kinin, leukokinin), complement factors, (e.g., anaphylatoxins, C3a, C5a), and clotting factors (e.g., fibrinopeptides, fibrin degradation products) and to tissue factors, such as vasoactive amines (e.g., histamine, 5-hydroxytryptamine), SRS (slow-reacting substance of anaphylaxis), prostaglandins (e.g., PGE1, PGE2), and others.

The kinins are among the most potent vasodilator substances known. They also increase capillary permeability. Their action may require activation of prostaglandins. Indeed, antiinflammatory drugs such as indomethacin and aspirin block bradykinin activity by inhibiting prostaglandin production. The kinin, clotting, complement, and fibrinolytic systems all interact in the inflammatory response. Hageman factor, for example, activates the kinin system, which then stimulates complement activity, which then activates the clotting cascade, which can then further augment Hageman factor activity. A rare hereditary disorder is characterized by deficiency of the Cl esterase inhibitor. Formation and activity of Kallikrein (Kinin system) and plasmin (fibrinolytic system) are repressed, and there is unrestricted formation of bradykin, C kinin, C3a, and C5a, with clinical manifestations of episodes of edema (increased vascular permeability) affecting the skin, larynx, and intestinal tract, often initiated by emotional stress. This condition may be fatal.

Histamine also causes vessel dilation, and increased capillary permeability. Histamine is found in tissue mast cells or circulating basophils, and is released whenever tissue damage has occurred, either by mechanical, chemical, or immunologic means. Prostaglandins are a complex group of substances with a variety of functions.

PGE1 has been shown to be as potent as bradykinin in producing increased capillary permeability in experimental animals. Prostaglandins can cause vasodilation (PGE) and vasoconstriction (PGF). Other factors active in the inflammatory process include a variety of lysosomal products which act to increase vascular permeability, augment chemotaxis, degrade basement membranes, collagen, and fibrin, stimulate complement activity, and release kinins. Lymphocyte products may have similar activities.

The release of fluid and inflammatory cells into an area of injury, as an exudate, functions to dilute the injurious agent, to form a fibrin scaffold as means of connecting injured tissues, stopping bleeding, and aiding phagocytosis, and to release natural antibacterial substances, such as opsonins and immunoglobulins.

Phagocytosis follows chemotaxis and migration of inflammatory cells. Phagocytosis is characterized by (1) contact, recognition, and attachment to foreign material, (2) ingestion of foreign material by cell with formation of phagosomes and degranulation, and (3) breakdown of foreign material or microbiocidal effects. The PMN phagosome contains many potentially antimicrobial agents including an acid medium, cationic proteins, superoxide anion, and hydrogen peroxide. A variety of conditions may affect chemotaxis and phagocytosis. They may clinically manifest as frequent, repeated, severe, and prolonged infections, or as impaired responses to antibiotics. There may be an absolute deficiency in the numbers of PMNs, as in leukemias, the rare condition cyclic neutropenia, or in drug-induced agranulocytoses. Chemotaxis may be affected, as in the Chediak-Higashi syndrome. This autosomal recessive disorder is characterized by giant azurophilic (peroxidase-containing) granules. Both chemotaxis and lysosomal degranulation are impaired, and patients suffer from increasing susceptibility to infection. Deficiencies of the various chemotactic factors, such as complement, may produce similar effects. The PMNs of patients with diabetes mellitus show poor chemotactic responsiveness. Phagocytosis may be limited because of defective attachment, associated with immunoglobulin or complement deficiencies as well as impaired degranulation. Microbiocidal mechanisms may also be faulty. An example of this is chronic granulomatous disease (CGD) of childhood. This inherited disorder almost always affects males only and manifests as multiple skin and systemic infections. The disease is due to deficiency of the hydrogen peroxide-myeloperoxidase-halide system of PMNs. A diagnostic test is to evaluate the ability of PMNs to phagocytose nitro-blue tetrazolium granules.

Fever is a hallmark of the acute inflammatory response. Pyrogens may be released from neutrophils or other inflammatory cells and act on the hypothalamic regulatory center. The number of circulating PMNs is increased (leucocytosis).

Acute inflammation may be followed by tissue destruction (i.e., necrosis, abscess formation, ulceration), by spread to adjacent or distant organs (i.e., cellulitis, lymphadenitis, blood stream invasion), by organization of the exudate and subsequent fibrosis, by chronic inflammation, and, in some cases, by complete resolution.

Other inflammatory cells (e.g., monocytes, eosinophils, basophils, lymphocytes) may also take part in the acute inflammatory reaction.

CHRONIC INFLAMMATION

Chronic inflammation can be defined as a temporal event, in which case the inflammatory cell component may be defined as variable, or, as is usually done, in terms of the cellular reaction. Chronic inflammation is characterized by the accumulation of macrophages, lymphocytes, or plasma cells at the site of injury, and is usually associated with residual acute inflammation and/or persistence of the injurious agent.

Chronic inflammation may follow the same type of injuries that cause acute inflammation, but generally indicates inability of the host defenses to effectively deal with the etiologic factor. Healing responses often coexist with the inflammatory reaction. As example, a chronic pneumonia may show accumulations of macrophages, lymphocytes, and granulation tissue response. The hyperemic response may persist.

Chronic inflammation may be followed by complete resolution, by resolution with fibrosis (scarring), by continued chronicity (e.g., sinus formation), or by reactivation of the acute inflammatory response.

GRANULOMATOUS INFLAMMATION

Granulomatous inflammation is a special form of chronic inflammation, thought, in most instances, to be related to a cell-mediated immune response, and characterized by nodular collections of specially activated macrophages (epithelioid cells), as well as multinucleated giant cells, and, with varying frequency, lymphocytes, fibroblasts, and necrosis.

Tuberculosis is the prototype of this type of reaction. The initial tissue response to the tuberculosis organism is a PMN infiltration. This occurs within 12 hours of infection. It is ineffective and is followed by macrophage accumulation. In 3 to 4 days, these macrophages transform to large, oval-to-polyhedral, eosinophilic epithelioid cells. Within 10 to 12 days, coincident with the onset of the tissue hypersensitivity response, there is caseation type of necrosis. After 2 to 3 weeks, the typical granuloma forms with macrophages, epithelioid cells, fused epithelioid cells (giant cells), lymphocytes, and fibroblasts, surrounding the necrotic zone.

The macrophage (mononuclear phagocyte) system is diverse. Promonocytic cells reside in the marrow. The circulating blood form is the monocyte. The tissue forms include histiocytes (connective tissues), Kupffer cells (liver), alveolar macrophages (lung), microglia (brain), osteoclasts (bone), Langerhans' cells (epidermis), pleural and peritoneal macrophages, and lymphoid macrophages. These cells have the potential for both pinocytosis and phagocytosis, and are able to respond chemotactically to a variety of stimuli (C5, activated T-lymphocytes, kinins, neutrophil lysosomal cationic protein, etc.), although the response is slower than that of the neutrophil. Maturation of the monocyte to the macrophage is accompanied by enhanced microbiocidal potential, greater phagocytic and degradative capacity, and increased synthetic potential. The epithelioid cell has a large volume of granular, eosinophilic cytoplasm, eccentric nucleus, intertwining filamentous cell processes, little or no phagocytic capacity, but increased lysosomal hydrolases and greater synthetic excretory and microbiocidal capacity. Mature epithelioid cells cannot divide. Epithelioid cells can transform into small lymphocyte-like cells which can then retransform to macrophages, or can fuse to form multinucleate giant cells, of the foreign body or Langhans type. The type of cellular reaction formed depends on the nature and intensity of the injurious agent, on the presence and degree of immune response, on the responsiveness of the bone marrow for macrophage mobilization, and on the longevity of the macrophages.

Macrophage activity includes release of lysosomal enzymes, secretion of complement, interferon production, secretion of pyrogens, prostaglandins, tissue thromboplastin, and increased microbiocidal and antitumor activity.

The delayed hypersensitivity response can augment and accelerate the development of the mature granuloma. However, not all epithelioid granulomas are the result of a hypersensitivity response. They can be initiated by antigen-antibody reactions, by inert substances (zirconium, beryllium), by chemicals without prior sensitization, and can develop in thymectomized animals. They also occur, in humans, in diseases such as sarcoidosis where a cell-mediated immune response cannot be demonstrated.

The granulomatous response is a response to an injurious agent which cannot be handled by the usual inflammatory reaction.

IMMUNOPATHOLOGY

The disciplines of medical immunology and immunopathology have considerable overlap, and relevant material is covered in other sections of this book. Here we will review certain disease entities but will not discuss mechanisms in detail.

Immunodeficiency diseases can be categorized as inherited and acquired disease states, and can affect the immune system at multiple levels as illustrated by the following:

Inherited disorders
    Severe combined immune deficiency
        Autosomal recessive
        Lack of both T- and B-cells
        Lack of common lymphoid stem cells
        Defect in adenosine deaminase
    Lack of T-cell immunity
        Thymic dysplasia
        DiGeorge's syndrome
    Lack of B-cell immunity
        Bruton's disease
Acquired disorders are
    Lack of T-cell immunity
        AIDS
        Hodgkin's disease
        Episodic lymphopenia
    Lack of B-cell immunity
        Acquired agammaglobulinemia
        Selective dysgammaglobulinemia
Immune deficiencies associated with other diseases
    Cushing's disease
    Ataxia telangiectasia
    Wiskott-Aldrich's syndrome
Therapeutically induced (iatrogenic) immune deficiencies
    Corticosteroid treatment
    Cancer chemotherapy
    Immunosuppression for transplantation

Immediate hypersensitivity diseases usually manifest within minutes after exposure to an allergen, are associated with mast cell and basophil activity, and are mediated by the release of histamine, slow-reacting substance (SRS-A), kinin, serotin, prostaglandins, eosinophil chemotactic factor (ECFA), and platelet activating factor (PAF). The major atopic diseases are allergic rhinitis, bronchial asthma, urticaria, and atopic dermatitis (infantile eczema). The most dramatic, and potentially fatal, form of reaction is systemic anaphylaxis in which "target" organs may be the lungs, larynx, intestinal tract, skin, and cardiovascular system. Patients may have laryngeal edema, bronchospasm, shock, cardiac arrythmias, urticaria, and brain edema.

Immune complex diseases are the result of the deposition of circulating immune complexes (CiC) in tissues following a complicated series of events based on the quantity or quality of CiC, the release of complement-dependent and complement-independent vasoactive amines, reticuloendothelial (RES) system activity, hemodynamic forces, and the structural and physiologic characteristics of the tissues. Human diseases that are most likely of immune complex origin are systemic lupus erythematosus (SLE), acute glomerulonephritis, chronic glomerulonephritis, vasculitis, rheumatoid arthritis, and hypersensitivity pneumonitis. SLE is a multisystem disease which mostly affects young adult women and seems to be increasing in frequency of occurrence. Immune complexes may have polynucleotides and DNA as antigens, and the disease is remarkably similar to the spontaneously occurring NZB/NZW disease of mice. The disease may be induced by certain drugs. Characteristics of the disease are polyserositis (pericarditis, pleuritis, peritonitis), nonbacterial verrucous (Libman-Sacks) endocarditis, glomerulonephritis, arteritis, skin rash classically showing a malar ("butterfly") distribution, cerebritis, and arthritis. Antinuclear antibodies are clinically demonstrable and evidence of phagocytosis of nuclear protein is seen as the LE cells of the peripheral blood, and the hematoxylin bodies seen in tissues.

Diseases of cell-mediated immunity (delayed hypersensitivity reactions) are due to the action of sensitized lymphocytes on target cells, with the associated elaboration of a number of lymphocyte products. Participating in the reaction may be variable numbers of lymphocytes, monocytes, macrophages, histiocytes, and transformed monocyte-macrophages (epithelioid cells, multinucleated giant cells). The cell-mediated immune (CMI) response is the basis of diagnostic skin tests to confirm infection with tuberculosis, leprosy, brucellosis, histoplasmosis, coccidioidomycosis, dermatomycosis, leishmaniasis, and echinococcosis. Human diseases related to CMI include contact hypersensitivity and the various conditions characterized by the formation of granulomas, such as tuberculosis, sarcoidosis, schistosomiasis, and various fungal disorders. CMI may also contribute to autoimmune diseases, homograft rejection, tumor immunity, and drug allergies.

Autoimmune disease results from the reaction of antibodies or immunologically competent cells produced by the host which react with the host's own tissue. A true autoimmune response is exceedingly rare as a cause of human disease, although such conditions as SLE, Goodpasture's syndrome, and myasthenia gravis are often used as illustrations. Chronic thyroiditis, with thyro-globulin as the principal antigen, may be the best example. Other conditions in which autoimmune reactions have been implicated are pernicious anemia, Addison's disease, phagoanaphylaxis, sympathetic ophthalmia, pemphigus vulgaris, pemphigoid, rheumatic heart disease, hemolytic anemia, chronic glomerulonephritis, idiopathic thrombocytopenia (ITP), male infertility, thyrotoxicosis, postrabies-vaccination encephalomyelitis, multiple sclerosis, ulcerative colitis, Sjögren's syndrome, chronic active hepatitis, primary biliary cirrhosis, sprue, dermatitis herpetiformis, and diabetes mellitus.

VASCULAR INJURIES AND REACTIONS

Thrombosis is a common pathologic condition characterized by the presence of coagulated blood within the lumen of blood vessels or the heart. Thrombi consist of a fibrin network binding together platelets, leukocytes, and erythrocytes.

The fluidity of circulating blood depends on the integrity of several physiologic mechanisms: (1) laminar blood flow, (2) integrity of the endothelium, (3) presence in plasma of inhibitors of coagulation such as antithrombins, heparin and fibrin split products, and (4) fibrinolytic systems. Thrombosis results from disturbance of one or more of these mechanisms. For example, loss of laminar blood flow secondary to external compression of a blood vessel results in thrombosis. Abnormalities of the endothelium in atherosclerosis are frequently accompanied by thrombus formation.

Thrombi can (1) become larger and occlude the entire lumen of a blood vessel, (2) resolve as a result of fibrinolytic enzymes, (3) become organized and recanalized, or (4) become dislodged and/or fragmented and embolize to distant blood vessels.

Embolism is the pathologic condition in which there is partial or complete vascular occlusion by a solid or gaseous mass that has been carried to a blood vessel by the circulation from another site. The transported material, or embolus, can be a detached thrombus (thromboembolus), adipose tissue, tumor cells, air, bacteria (septic embolus), parasites, foreign bodies, amniotic fluid, or bone marrow material. The pathologic effects of embolism depend on the size, number, and nature of the emboli and the site of embolization. For example, massive embolization to the pulmonary artery results in sudden death, whereas septic embolization of blood vessels of an extremity leads to gangrene.

Infarction is the term given to death of tissues, usually due to an impairment of blood supply. The most common cause of infarction is the sudden occlusion of an artery or vein by a thrombus or embolus. Similar vascular occlusion may also ensue as a result of large atherosclerotic plaques, external compression of the vessel wall by tumor or fibrosis, and/or twisting of the blood vessel (e.g., torsion of a testis). The extent of necrosis is dependent on several physiologic parameters including degree of vascular obstruction, general status of the cardiovascular system, efficiency of collateral circulation and vulnerability of a particular tissue to ischemia.

Most infarcts are pyramidal with the base at the periphery of the organ and the apex at the obstructed blood vessel. They appear as pale, anemic areas ("anemic infarct") when the necrosis is secondary to arterial obstruction and as red, hemorrhagic areas when the infarct follows venous obstruction. Arterial infarcts in soft organs like the lung can also be hemorrhagic, due to hemorrhage from collateral vessels. Histologically, infarcts show changes of ischemic coagulative necrosis such as loss of normal tissue architecture, hypereosinophilia of parenchymal cells, nuclear pyknosis, and infiltration by polymorphonuclear leukocytes and macrophages as well as hemorrhage in infarcts due to venous occlusion. Eventually the necrotic area becomes infiltrated by granulation tissue and is transformed into a scar.

Vascular Responses to Injury

The homeostasis of the organism depends on a normal blood supply and an adequate fluid environment. In many conditions, these supporting systems are altered in response to injurious agents such as chemicals, radiation therapy, or infections. Vascular abnormalities can also be the primary event leading to a variety of pathologic processes, such as myocardial infarction and pulmonary thromboembolism.

Hyperemia or congestion are pathologic terms that indicate the presence of an increased volume of blood within blood vessels in a part of the body. Active hyperemia is the increased flow of blood into an organ due to dilatation of functioning microvessels, usually venules or arterioles. This vasodilatation is followed by dilatation of previously inactive capillaries that open up to the circulation. Active hyperemia occurs in acute inflammation, as a heat response, certain immunologic reactions, blushing, exercise, and other conditions. Passive hyperemia refers to a decreased outflow of blood from an organ due to an interference with the venous drainage. The venous return may be impaired by a mass compressing veins extrinsically (e.g., the pregnant uterus) or intrinsically (e.g., venous thrombosis). It can also be secondary to cardiac failure.

Edema is the excessive accumulation of fluids in intercellular tissue spaces or body cavities. It can be classified according to distribution as local, generalized (anasarca), ascites (in peritoneal cavity), hydrothorax (in pleural cavity, pulmonary, etc. There may be varied etiology, such as cardiac, angioneurotic, inflammatory, hypoalbuminemic, nephrotic, etc. In composition, it may be an exudate (i.e., inflammatory with high protein content), or a transudate (i.e., noninflammatory, with low protein content).

Edema results from imbalances between physiologic factors that control the movement of water between the vascular and extravascular spaces. It can result from increased microvascular permeability with escape of colloids from the plasma into interstitial fluids through interendothelial gaps, with the accumulation of fluids in tissues. Vascular permeability increases in inflammation, anaphylactic reaction, hypoxia, and chemical poisoning, and is modulated by chemical mediators of inflammation such as histamine, bradykinin, prostaglandins, complement factors, such as C5, C3, and anaphylaxotoxins, and by various substances such as drugs, toxins, and venoms. Edema can also result from increased intravascular hydrostatic pressure, which occurs frequently in heart failure, mechanical obstruction of veins (extrinsic or intrinsic), and excessive administration of intravenous fluids. Edema can also be due to: (1) decreased plasma oncotic pressure due to a decrease in plasma protein (malnutrition, nephrotic syndrome, cirrhosis, malabsorption syndromes), (2) increased osmotic pressure in tissues due to increased sodium concentration (sodium retention in nephrotic syndrome, acute glomerulonephritis, congestive heart failure), and (3) lymphatic obstruction due to trauma, surgery, neoplastic infiltration, inflammation, and radiation therapy.

Edematous organs, when enlarged, are pale and heavier than normal. Their surface is usually glistening and they ooze fluid on pressure. The pressing finger also induces a depression in edematous tissues ("pitting edema"). Histologically, edematous tissues have a granular acidophilic precipitate in interstitial spaces.

Shock is a pathophysiologic syndrome characterized by an acute and persistent hypoperfusion of tissues, usually resulting from a disparity between the blood volume and the capacity of the vascular system. Primary (neurogenic) shock results from sudden vasodilatation following pain, emotional reactions, or injury to the central or peripheral nervous systems. Secondary shock can occur with a normal volemia (normovolemic shock) or with loss of blood volume (hypovolemic shock). Normovolemic shock is due to an impairment in the capacity of the heart to displace a normal stroke volume (cardiogenic shock) or to vasodilatation due to the action of bacterial endotoxins (endotoxic shock). Hypovolemic shock is the loss of blood which can follow acute hemorrhage, or fluid losses in burns, dehydration, or ascites.

The pathogenesis of shock is complex and incompletely understood. The main pathogenetic factor is a disproportion between the capacity of the vascular bed and the blood volume, resulting in hypoperfusion of tissues with resulting hypoxia and cell injury (Fig. 6-1).

Shock is manifested by signs of hypoperfusion such as weakness, cold pale skin, rapid weak pulse, low blood pressure, shallow respiration, blood acidosis, oliguria, and changes in the hematocrit (decreased in shock secondary to hemorrhage, increased in shock due to dehydration). The point at which irreversible shock is reached is hard to define. In its clinical evolution, shock may become refractory to therapy and the patient dies. This irreversibility of shock may be due to (1) failure to control the primary etiologic agent (e.g., severe gram-negative bacterial infection), (2) marked tissue acidosis resulting in decreased sensitivity to vasoactive amines, (3) failure to detoxify endotoxins, and (4) the development of multiple thrombi in small vessels. The latter phenomenon has been recognized as an important factor in the development of irreversible shock and is thought to be due to a local hypercoagulable state in small blood vessels following stasis and neutralization of heparin by acidic catabolites.

Shock leads to the morphologic changes of ischemia in multiple organs, including acute tubular necrosis in the kidney, centrolobular necrosis in the liver, myocardial necrosis, lipid depletion in the adrenal cortex, and ulcerations and mucosal hemorrhages in the gastrointestinal tract.

HEALING AND REPAIR

Healing refers to those processes in which there are varying combinations of regeneration and repair, to maintain or restore body tissues to structural and/or functional integrity.

Regeneration is the process of tissue restoration by multiplication of cells. In man, only certain tissues have the capacity to regenerate. These are generally the short-lived, labile cells such as epidermis, gastrointestinal epithelium, genitourinary epithelium, and hematopoietic cells. These cells generally undergo continuous multiplication, and usually have mitoses obvious even in their normal state. Other tissues may show regeneration after injury, but are normally long-lived and show few mi-

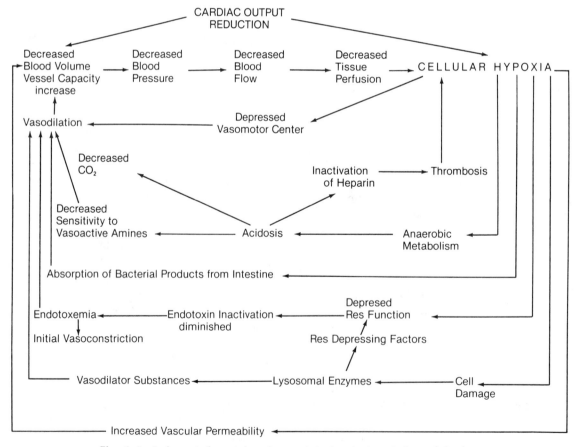

Fig. 6-1. Pathogenic factors that play a role in the physiopathology of shock.

toses. These are liver, kidney, endocrine and exocrine glands, bone, and cartilage. Some tissues are composed of permanent cells which do not multiply, even after injury. Examples are the nervous system, sensory organs, and, to a great extent, skeletal and cardiac muscle.

Regeneration is enhanced by factors released from damaged or necrotic cells, by functional needs (e.g., decreased serum proteins after hepatectomy), relative youth, certain chemical agents, and, perhaps, hormone-like agents released at wound sites (trephones). Regeneration is inhibited by poor nutrition, impaired blood supply, anemia, old age, hormone deficiencies (e.g., hypothyroidism), and bacterial infections. Chalones may also be active.

Repair refers to those tissue responses which particularly act to return or improve structural integrity, and includes those cellular responses which act to remove damaged or dead tissues, and subsequently, to replace or join the injured tissues. Tissue removal is mainly accomplished by macrophages. Structural restoration generally follows the development of granulation tissue.

Granulation tissue is the basic element of healing by repair. It is affected by the site of injury, the injurious agent(s), time, and host responses. The early stage of the granulation tissue response is inflammatory, and may include PMNs, macrophages, and lymphoid and plasma cells. Granulation tissue itself consists of two major elements, endothelial cells and fibroblasts. Endothelial cells proliferate to form delicate, highly permeable capillaries which mature to form arterioles and venules. Fibroblasts grow in from the wound margins and derive from fibrocytes (resting cells). The fibroblasts, in turn, form two major elements, matrix (ground substance), consisting of acid mucopolysaccharides, and collagen. Collagen fibrils increase in size and number as the matrix decreases. As the (700 Å periodicity) collagen contracts through aggregation and cross-linking, the wound gains in tensile strength.

Restoration is the process of healing with return of normal structure and little or no granulation tissue retention. This occurs when the injury is relatively limited in size, when the injurious agent is effectively and rapidly removed, and where the inflammatory component is relatively modest and completely resorbed. A superficial gastric ulcer will heal in this way. In contrast, organization occurs when the proliferative granulation tissue response becomes dominant. The granulation tissue elements increase as the inflammatory response decreases, and a scar (fibrosis) evolves. Skin wounds heal in this way.

The healing of a skin wound may be by primary union (primary intention) or by secondary union (secondary intention). Primary union occurs when the wound edges are regular, clean, and easily brought together. Inflammatory cell infiltration is modest, blood supply is adequate, and there is relatively little need for granulation tissue as a bridge between wound edges. Epithelialization is usually complete and complete restoration may occur. This occurs following an uncomplicated surgical incision. Secondary union follows an irregular, poorly apposed wound, in which the wound edges are only brought together by the formation of a large cellular and fibrinous exudate with relatively abundant granulation tissue response and heavy inflammatory cell infiltration. Epithelialization may be incomplete and a scar may be prominent. This type of repair follows, for example, a traumatic laceration.

Nutritional, hormonal, and vascular factors, age, and the presence of infections affect wound repair. Poor nutrition inhibits repair. In particular, vitamin C is needed for adequate collagen synthesis. Bacterial infections, particularly, limit repair.

PIGMENTS AND DEGENERATIONS

This section will emphasize processes that usually occur in association with a variety of disease entities but are distinct and relatively common.

A variety of pigments may affect tissue. Endogenous pigments may be hemoglobin- or nonhemoglobin-derived. Hemoglobin-derived pigments include bilirubin, hematoidin, hemosiderin, and hematin.

Bilirubin is a product of hemoglobin breakdown. Bilirubin is normally conjugated, by liver cells, with glucuronic acid. It accumulates with hemolysis (unconjugated), hepatocyte destruction, as in hepatitis (conjugated and unconjugated), and obstruction of biliary tree (conjugated).

Hematoidin is chemically indistinguishable from bilirubin, and forms in tissues with diminished oxygen supply (infarcts). Hematoidin is not demonstrable with usual tissue stains for iron pigment.

Hemosiderin is a golden-brown pigment containing loosely-bound iron formed by excessive hemoglobin-breakdown in the tissues or bloodstream, or it follows excessive intake of iron which stains with the Prussian blue method. Hemosiderin may be localized, as in an area of hemorrhage, or after chronic pulmonary congestion ("heart-failure" cells), or may be generalized (hemosiderosis), as a reflection of systemic iron overload (after multiple transfusions, long-standing hemolytic anemia). Hemosiderin deposits in the reticuloendothelial system (RES) (Kupffer cells of liver, littoral cells of spleen) first, then, when the RES becomes overloaded, in parenchymal cells. Primary (idiopathic) hemochromatosis is a rare disorder of iron metabolism, usually affecting middle-aged men, due to excess absorption of iron from normal diet, and is characterized by systemic deposition of iron in parenchymal and RES cells. It manifests as hepatic cirrhosis, diabetes mellitus (pigment in islets of Langerhans), and increased skin pigmentation (activation of melanocytes); clinically it is recognized as the syndrome of "bronze diabetes." It may be familial.

Hematin (malarial pigment) is a brownish, granular pigment formed by acid or alkali acting on hemoglobin. The iron is firmly bound and does not stain with Prussian blue. Malarial pigment is formed by the parasite.

Nonhemoglobin derived pigments include melanin, lipochromes, and other substances.

Melanin is formed by oxidative metabolism from tyrosine, and is found in the skin, choroid layer of eye, and leptomeninges. Increased pigmentation occurs after sun exposure, in Addison's disease (adrenal insufficiency) due to secondary increase of melanocyte-stimulating hormone from the pituitary, as localized lesions such as lentigo (freckle), and benign (nevus) and malignant (melanoma) tumors. Decreased pigmentation may be localized (vitiligo; idiopathic or secondary to lesions such as burn or infection) or generalized (albinism; congenital deficiency of tyrosinase).

Ochronosis is a genetic defect of phenylalanine and tyrosine metabolism, in which a melaninlike pigment localizes in cartilage.

Melanosis (pseudomelanosis) coli consists of brown or black discoloration of colonic mucosa, due to accumulation of pigment in lamina propria macrophages. The complex pigment is thought to be related to ingestion of cascara alkaloids in laxatives.

Lipochromes (lipofuscins) are yellow, lipid-containing pigments accumulating in old age, or after chronic, debilitating diseases ("wear-and-tear" pigment). Lipochromes are normally found in the seminal vesicles, adrenal cortex, ganglion cells, corpus luteum, and may be associated with loss of tissue mass in the heart and liver ("brown atrophy").

Exogenous pigments include anthracotic (environmental) pigment, silver, lead, and other substances. Anthracosis (environmental pigment) is a black pigment accumulating in the lungs and pulmonary lymphatic system. It is a carbon-based residue, but usually not true anthracotic (coal-derived) material, and it is more prevalent in city dwellers and cigarette smokers. Argyria is due to absorption of organic or inorganic silver compounds with deposition in mucus membranes and skin. There are no functional alterations, even in severe cases where pigment may be in the kidney and liver. "Lead line" refers to the deep blue pigment at the junction of the

teeth and gums in lead poisoning (plumbism). Tattoos leave various pigments in dermal macrophages.

Degenerations are forms of cellular reaction to injury which do not necessarily interfere with cell integrity or function.

Amyloidosis is a relatively uncommon condition in which a characteristic, amorphous, proteinaceous substance accumulates between cells, usually unaccompanied by an inflammatory response. It is not a single disease, but is a group of disorders. When deposits are massive, they can be perceived macroscopically as waxy, firm infiltrations. Amyloid interferes with tissue or organ function. Amyloid stains with Lugol's iodine at the macroscopic level, is eosinophilic and hyalinelike in standard hematoxylineosin histologic sections, and has histologic affinity for the Congo red reagent. Congo red positive tissues characteristically demonstrate "apple-green" birefringence with polarizing filters. Amyloid may have variable protein composition. Some forms derive from light chain immunoglobulin material. All forms show same ultrastructural appearance, with fine, branching 10 nm fibrils. Amyloid A (secondary amyloid) is seen after long-standing chronic inflammatory conditions such as rheumatoid arthritis, tuberculosis, osteomyelitis, syphilis, chronic bronchiectasis, Crohn's disease, and leprosy, and generally involves parenchymal organs such as the liver, spleen, kidneys, and adrenals (type II pattern). Amyloid B (primary amyloid) is seen in patients with myeloma and other plasma cell dyscrasias, and in the elderly in the absence of a specific disease (senile amyloidosis), and generally involves mesenchymal tissues such as the heart, skeletal muscle (especially tongue), and gastrointestinal tract, skin, and nerves (type I pattern). Amyloid is also associated with hereditary disorders, such as familial Mediterranean fever and Portugese familial amyloidosis, and may also be seen as a local deposit in the islets of Langerhans, in patients with diabetes mellitus, and as a component of certain tumors, particularly medullary carcinoma of the thyroid.

Gout is the clinical condition associated with hyperuricemia. Deposition of uric acid crystals in joints causes chronic arthritis, in renal tubules leads to kidney stones (nephrolithiasis), and in soft tissues causes deforming, sometimes painful nodules (tophi). Gout may be primary, with etiology not known but with a familial tendency, involving mostly males, or secondary, associated with abnormal uric acid metabolism from an acquired disorder, especially conditions in which there is high cell turnover, such as leukemia. Gout may also be due to impaired renal excretion of uric acid, from primary genetic defect, in certain metabolic conditions such as diabetic ketoacidosis, and as a manifestation of renal toxicity, as with thiazide diuretics, and lead poisoning.

DISTURBANCES OF GROWTH

Growth disturbances may occur during development, during embryogenesis, or during the pre- and postnatal periods. Growth disturbances may follow certain injuries, or alterations in work demands on the host, and may also reflect abnormalities of growth factors. Neoplasia can also be considered a form of growth disturbance, but will be separately discussed in another section.

A variety of growth factors have been identified. Some of these affect a single cell or organ, whereas others may affect the entire body. Some important growth factors are insulin, somatotropin (growth factor), thyroxine, glucocorticosteroids, platelet-derived growth factor (PDGF), nerve growth factor (NGF), epidermal growth factor (EGF), erythropoietin, lymphopoietins, and various colony stimulating factors. Growth inhibitors (chalones) have been identified in experimental settings, but have not been proven in humans.

Hypertrophy and hyperplasia may each follow a stimulus to growth. Hypertrophy is growth due to an increase in the size of cells, and hyperplasia is growth due to an increase in the number of cells. In most instances, both processes take place to some extent, and the classification reflects the dominant process. Cardiac and skeletal muscle responses to "injury" (increased work demands) are entirely hypertrophy-type reactions, however, since these muscles, in the mature individual, have lost the capacity to divide. An example of hormone-induced growth is benign prostatic hyperplasia (often mistakenly called hypertrophy), in which there are increased numbers of prostatic epithelial and stromal cells.

Aplasia is the failure of a tissue or organ to develop at all. Hypoplasia is the failure of a tissue or organ to develop to full size. Renal agenesis is an example of organ aplasia and is, by necessity, unilateral.

Atrophy is a decrease in tissue or organ size after attainment of normal size. Atrophy usually involves a decrease in the size of cells, but may, occasionally, be associated with decrease in the number of cells. Atrophy may be due to a decreased work-load (immobilized or paralyzed limb), decrease in the blood supply (brain in old age), decrease in endocrine stimulation (adrenal glands in patients treated with exogenous corticosteroids), inadequate nutrition, and aging (brown atrophy of heart, liver).

Metaplasia is the reversible replacement of one adult cell type with another. An example is the replacement of pseudostratified, ciliated epithelium by stratified squamous epithelium in the respiratory tract of long-term smokers.

Dysplasia is a highly atypical form of hyperplasia, characterized by increased cell production and defective maturation. The changes of dysplasia are potentially reversible, but are often the precursor to malignancy. Dysplasia manifests as increased mitotic activity, pleomorphism (variation in cell size and shape), and increase of nucleus-to-cytoplasm ratio, with increased nuclear size and nuclear hyperchromatism. In addition, the architecture of the tissue is disturbed with loss of the usual maturation pattern.

Neoplasia is a persistent, abnormal, relatively or completely autonomous proliferation of cells which reflects a cellular defect that is transmissible from parent cells to their progeny. Neoplasia may be characterized as benign or malignant. These will be discussed in a subsequent section.

Anaplasia is the term to describe the growth process in which cells become completely undifferentiated; this term is restricted to the description of malignant cells.

ENVIRONMENTAL INJURIES

We are only beginning to understand the diverse way in which environmental factors can affect us. In some instances, the effect will be directly toxic and clearly proven. At other times, the evidence for injury will be circumstantial. In other settings, the environmental factor will not, itself, cause injury but will add to an already existing disease. The manifestations of injury may be quite remote from the time of exposure as in the case of the chronic interstitial lung disease or the malignant mesothelioma that follows asbestos exposure. Substances may be passed across the placenta, to cause mutations or birth defects. In this regard, it is worth noting that thalidomide had undergone extensive animal testing before being released for clinical usage. Some of the environmentally related conditions, such as the lung diseases that follow cigarette smoking, will be discussed in the setting of the various systems.

Ionizing Radiation

All radiation is potentially injurious, depending on the intensity, its intrinsic energy, and the susceptibility of cells and tissues. The shorter the wave length, the greater the potential for injury. Exposure comes from the sun and cosmic space, from radioactive substances in the earth, and, more significantly, from man-made devices such as x-ray machines, atomic weapons, and nuclear reactors.

The effects of radiation on cells are exceedingly variable. In general, mammalian cells are very sensitive, particularly the nuclei. Radiation induces significant damage, in the form of breaks, in the DNA chain. The mechanism of radiation injury is thought to be by the production of unstable radicals which combine with water or oxygen to produce peroxides which are highly toxic to the cell. Another theory suggests that ionizing radiation directly alters molecules, affecting both structure and function. The effects usually do not become manifest at the time of injury; there is a period of latency. The greatest effect of radiation is in dividing cells. Consequently, rapidly growing tissues or tissues with a high rate of replacement are most sensitive (embryonal cells, hematopoietic cells, intestinal and bladder epithelium, germ cells of the ovary and testis, and certain malignancies). Vascular injury is important. Endothelial cells, especially of small arterioles and arteries, are sensitive, and radiation may lead to intimal scarring with subsequent compromise of the lumen, and ultimately, decrease of blood supply to tissues.

The clinical manifestations of radiation injury include radiodermatitis, radiation pneumonitis, radiation gastroenteritis, radiation osteitis, and radiation chrondritis as relatively acute phenomena in the therapeutic setting. Total body radiation can be lethal, at doses of 500–600 rads, or can cause severe illness with doses as little as 75–100 rads. The acute radiation syndrome begins with nausea, vomiting, anorexia, and apathy, which abate. They are followed by more specific dose dependent manifestations such as hematopoietic system depression, hemorrhage (thrombocytopenia), infections (granulocytopenia), and severe anemia, after 2 to 3 weeks. With a dose of 2,000 rads, the latent period is short, 1 to 2 hours, manifestations are mainly cerebral (confusion, convulsions, and coma), and death occurs in 12 to 36 hours.

Late effects of radiation injury include aplastic anemia, leukemia, tumors of various organs, eye cataracts, and, in children, developmental defects.

Radiotherapy is based on the principle that cancer cells are more susceptible to radiation injury than normal cells.

HEAVY METALS

All metals are potentially toxic if taken in high enough doses. This section will briefly summarize the most important heavy metals and their effects.

Arsenic may come from smelting or ores, insecticides, and paints, formerly was used therapeutically, and in warfare, and enters by inhalation (arsine gas) and ingestion. There may be fulminant poisoning, with vasomotor paralysis, peripheral vasodilation, and shock. Acute poisoning is characterized by CNS depression (death within 24 hours), vascular and intestinal necrosis with hemorrhages, severe diarrhea, vomiting, and CNS hemorrhages, and edema. Chronic poisoning is complicated by chronic dermatitis, weight loss, and perhaps, lung cancer. Arsenic leads to inhibition of respiratory enzymes.

Mercury poisoning may occur from tool manufacturing, electric batteries, pesticides, insecticides, accidental food contamination (Murimata), skin ointments, and diuretics. Routes of entry include inhalation, skin absorption, and suicidal ingestion. Manifestations may be acute or chronic. Acute toxicity may include CNS after inhalation, and the kidney and gastrointestinal tract after ingestion. Chronic mercurialism includes dermatitis, gingivitis, gastroenteritis, renal failure, and neurologic and mental disorders (tremors, aphasia, or memory loss). Mercury acts by protein precipitation and cytochrome oxidase inactivation.

Lead poisoning derives from paints, automobile exhaust, water pipes, "moonshine," cookware, and gunshots. Entry is by inhalation, or ingestion (especially children). Lead accumulates in the body, especially the bones. In acute toxicity, there is anemia (inhibition of heme synthesis), edema and degeneration of brain neurons and basal ganglia (ataxia, convulsions, confusion), demyelinization of peripheral nerves (wrist- and foot-drop), and renal tubular damage. Chronic toxicity may lead to anemia, abdominal colic and constipation (autonomic ganglia degeneration), "lead line" (gums, bones), renal aminoaciduria (Fanconi syndrome; enzyme inhibition with decreased ability to resorb glucose, phosphorus, and amino acids), premature arteriosclerosis, and hypertension.

Platinum is usually given, therapeutically, intravenously, and may lead to renal tubular necrosis and marrow depression.

Cadmium toxicity may occur in zinc refining, aerospace industry, battery manufacturing, cigarette smoke, automobile tires, oil and coal combustion, and from antique utensils, following inhalation or ingestion. In acute poisoning, there is pulmonary edema, intra-alveolar hemorrhage, and death. Chronic toxicity leads to emphysema, renal tubular defects, "Itai-Itai" disease (osteomalacia, osteoporosis, bone deformities, renal tubular defects; from contaminated rice), hypochromic anemia, and, possibly, hypertension and/or cancer.

Drug-Related Disorders

As many as 5 percent of hospital admissions may be for drug-related injuries, and as many as 15 percent of hospitalized patients will have an adverse drug reaction. Selected conditions will be discussed in the organ system portions of this chapter. Drug-related injuries may be due to direct toxicity (phenacitin-induced renal injury, streptomycin-induced acoustic nerve dysfunction), an acute idiosyncratic reaction (acute hemolytic anemia in glucose-6-phosphate dehydrogenase deficient individuals given primaquine, sulfonamides, analgesics, etc.), immunologic reaction (penicillin reaction, halothane hepatitis), hormonal stimulation (estrogen-induced endometrial hyperplasia and carcinoma), inhibition of normal host defences (opportunistic infections in immunosuppressed individuals, pseudomembranous enteritis in clindamycin-treated individuals), and, in some instances, the mechanisms of injury may not be well understood.

AGING

Aging is a progressive and irreversible biologic process which begins at maturity and is associated with or is responsible for an ever increasing susceptibility to disease and death. Senescence is defined as a constellation of deteriorative changes in the structure and function of an organism with progressive decline in the efficiency of homeostasis and in successful reactions to injury.

All members of a species accumulate progressive physiologic and morphologic changes after reaching sexual maturity that lead to an increase in their likelihood of dying. In addition to the well known external morphologic changes that appear with aging, there are histologic and biochemical changes in tissues that are characteristic of senescence. In the extracellular matrix there is an increase in cross-linking of collagen. In the cytoplasm of parenchymal cells, there is accumulation of lipochrome (lipofuscin) pigment, derived from the lipid peroxidation of membrane fragments.

The process of aging is still incompletely understood. There are several theories of pathogenesis as is illustrated by the following:

1. Genetic: The process of aging is encoded in DNA
2. Error: Aging results from a progressive breakdown in the accuracy of replication, transcription, and translation of DNA
3. Mutation: Aging results from damage or alteration to DNA
4. Free radicals: The progressive accumulation of damage due to free radical reactions in cells is a major contributor to the aging process
5. Progressive loss of self recognition: By the immune system as a result of mutations or defects in protein specificity

Syndromes of premature aging include (1) progeria (senile nanism, Hutchinson-Gilford syndrome) characterized by severe growth retardation, normal intelligence and premature senescence with fulminant atherosclerosis and death in the teens, and (2) Werner's syndrome (progeria adultorum or progeria of late onset) characterized by onset between the ages of 15 and 30 years old, short stature, early cataracts, early gonadal involution, generalized atherosclerosis, increased incidence of diabetes mellitus, and neoplasia.

Common diseases of old people include heart disease, the major cause of death in elderly patients, hypertension, malignancy, cerebral vascular disease, chronic skeletal disorders (osteoarthritis, osteoporosis), prostatic gland hyperplasia in men, chronic obstructive pulmonary disease, diabetes, and others.

NEOPLASIA

Neoplasia can be defined as a process of uncoordinated and autonomous new growth. In contrast to the normal, the neoplastic cell does not function for the well-being of the host, does not participate in host repair or defense, and does not respond to host requirements, and is, instead, parasitic and often deleterious.

The names of tumors serve as a form of shorthand to communicate, besides morphology, behavior and host response (prognosis), therapeutic considerations, etiologic or pathogenetic factors, location, mode of presentation, and histogenesis. However, much about neoplasia is not well understood and some names are illogical. A few eponyms prevail because of tradition (e.g., Paget's disease of the nipple), because a more scientifically exact name is not yet available (e.g., Hodgkin's disease), or because modern terminology is complex and not easily accepted (e.g., Warthin's tumor v papillary cystadenoma lymphomatosum of the salivary gland).

The classification of tumors usually is based on the cell or origin (epithelial, mesenchymal, neural), the histologic appearance, and the clinical behavior. The names of most benign tumors end with *oma* (with important exceptions such as the malignant tumors hypernephroma, lymphoma, hepatoma, mesothelioma, and even nonneoplastic swellings or masses, such as hematoma). The names of most malignant epithelial tumors end with *carcinoma* and the names of most malignant nonepithelial tumors end with *sarcoma*. The tumor name is often modified in terms of the type and degree of differentiation (e.g., well differentiated mucus-producing adenocarcinoma), or even in terms of the macroscopic appearance (e.g., papillary, cystic, medullary, etc.).

Teratomas are complex, illogical tumors containing tissues from more than one germ layer. They may be benign or malignant, although the most common teratoma (ovarian cystic teratoma or dermoid cyst) is almost always benign. A hamartoma is a nodular mass of cells or tissues normal to the organ in which it occurs (e.g., pulmonary hamartoma consists of cartilage and respiratory epithelium) and is most likely developmental, rather than neoplastic.

Choristoma is the term for normal cells or tissues in abnormal places (e.g., pancreatic tissue in the stomach wall).

Tumor growth is modified by nutrition of the host, by vascular supply, by host reactions (?immunologic) to the tumor, and, for certain tumors, by hormonal influences. The terms *benign* and *malignant* indicate certain characteristics, but the distinctions may be arbitrary.

Mitotic figures provide an index of tumor growth. Malignant tumors often have abnormal mitotic figures, or abnormal hyperchromatic nuclei, with an increase of the nuclear-cytoplasmic ratio. There may be marked variation in cell size and shape (pleomorphism). Differentiation implies an ability of a tumor to produce an organized growth form and, in general, varies inversely with the rate of growth of the tumor.

Most cancer patients die from metastatic disease and not from the primary tumor. Metastasis requires that a tumor be able to extend from the primary site into adjoining tissues, into body cavities, or into vessels. Tumor cells must then detach and must have the ability to reattach at the secondary site, where they can invade. In general, epithelial cancers (carcinoma) metastasize via lymphatics, and mesenchymal cancers (sarcomas) metastasize via blood vessels. Tumor cells can freely pass between blood and lymph channels, but the cell membrane characteristics of the tumor cell determine where the detached cells will survive and invade.

Histologic grading of tumors (Broder's index) is illustrated by the following:

Grade 1: More than 75 percent differentiated cells (well-differentiated)

Grade 2: 50–75 percent differentiated cells (moderately well differentiated)

Grade 3: 25–50 percent differentiated cells (poorly differentiated)

Grade 4: Less than 25 percent differentiated cells (undifferentiated)

Staging refers to the procedure to determine the extent of disease by a variety of diagnostic techniques. The World Health Organization (WHO) standard staging nomenclature useful for most tumors is the following:

T signifies the extent of the primary growth
- T0   no primary tumor present
- TIS   carcinoma in situ
- T1   tumor local, <2 cm diameter
- T2   tumor 2–5 cm
- T3   tumor >5 cm diameter
- T4   tumor not local, involves adjacent structures

N signifies the condition of the regional lymph nodes
- N0   no apparent spread
- N1   movable, homolateral node involvement
- N2   movable, contralateral or bilateral node involvement
- N3   fixed (spread into surrounding tissues), contralateral or bilateral

M signifies distant metastases
- M0   no evidence of distant spread
- M1   evidence of distant spread

The causes of tumors are varied and, to a large extent, still unknown. A number of associations are, however, well recognized. The associations are illustrated by the following:

1. Hereditary disorders. A number of tumor syndromes are potentially inherited (familial polyposis coli, retinoblastoma, neurofibromatosis, medullary carcinoma of the thyroid). Some cancers consistently demonstrate abnormal, nonrandom chromosomal abnormalities (chronic myelogenous leukemia, retinoblastoma), whereas others irregularly show a variety of (random) chromosomal abnormalities. A number of human disorders (xeroderma pigmentosum, ataxia telangiectasia, Fanconi's anemia, Cockayne's syndrome, Bloom's syndrome) show enhanced sensitivity to the induction of genetic damage and an increased incidence of malignancy.

2. Ionizing radiation. Increased incidence of malignancy in uranium miners, atom bomb survivors, individuals subjected to medical irradiation for diagnostic (mammography, thorium dioxide) and therapeutic ("thymic enlargement," acne, ankylosing spondylitis) indications. Skin cancers are more common in individuals exposed to intense sunlight (melanoma particularly common in Australia).

3. Oncogenic viruses. There is strong evidence that certain viruses cause cancer in animals, both naturally and experimentally. With the exception of the recently identified T-cell lymphoma virus thought to be responsible for a lymphoma occurring mostly in Japan, there is no unequivocal evidence of the viral etiology of human tumors, although there is strong circumstantial evidence for some (Epstein-Barr virus and Burkitt's lymphoma, epidermiologic evidence of the transmissibility of Hodgkin's disease).

4. Chemicals. Carcinogenic chemicals can act directly by reacting irreversibly with electron-rich regions of cell components (nitrogen mustard, epoxides, halo-alkanes)

or indirectly requiring metabolic activation into chemically reactive, carcinogenic derivatives (polycyclic aromatic hydrocarbons, aromatic amines, azo dyes, nitrosamines, mycotoxins).

Complications of neoplasia may be local (replacement and destruction of normal tissue with loss of specific function, local circulatory disturbances due to pressure on or infiltration of blood vessels, bleeding, thrombosis of vessels, obstruction of tubular structures, pressure on nerves) or general (cachexia, anemia, fever, increased susceptibility to infection, hypogammaglobulinemia, paraproteinemia, intravascular coagulopathy, inappropriate hormone elaboration, other paraneoplastic syndromes).

Diagnostic approaches, in addition to careful history and examination, radiographic studies, and morphologic evaluations, may include certain biochemical determinations which can be useful in establishing the diagnosis or in following the course of the disease. The substances are not themselves abnormal and can be found, to varying degrees, in normal people. Some of these are the following:

Carcinoembryonic antigen (CEA): GI tract, pancreas, lung, breast
Alpha-fetoprotein (AFP): Hepatocellular carcinoma, embryonal carcinoma of testis
Alkaline phosphatase: Osteogenic sarcoma, metastatic tumor to bone
Acid phosphatase: Prostatic carcinoma
Serotonin (5-OH-tryptamine): Carcinoid
Chorionic gonadotropin (HCG): trophoblastic tumors
B-12 binding protein: Myelogenous leukemia
Lysozyme: Monocytic leukemia
Calcitonin: Medullary carcinoma of the thyroid
Catecholamines: Neuroblastoma
Various hormones: Endocrine and extraendocrine tumors

Prognosis of the patient with cancer depends on the basic biology of the tumor, tumor site, size, differentiation (grading), degree of spread (staging), and response to therapy by the tumor.

TUMOR IMMUNOLOGY

Tumor antigens may be individually specific (tumor specific transplantation antigens (TSTA)) or may demonstrate cross reactivity to antibodies formed against other tumors (group specific). Chemical carcinogens have been shown to induce TSTA, whereas viral induced tumor antigens are group specific.

Tumor specific antigens have not been convincingly demonstrated in human tumors. Group specific antigens have been demonstrated, as a part of a humoral antibody reaction, in humans with Burkitt's lymphoma, nasopharyngeal carcinoma, melanoma, and osteogenic sarcoma, and, with detection by sensitized lymphocytes (cell-mediated immune response) in neuroblastoma, melanoma, and a large group of epithelial tumors. Oncofetal antigens, such as CEA, AFP, HCG, calcitonin, and others are examples of group specific antigens.

Immunity plays a part in host response to tumors, but the mechanisms and their significance are not clearly understood. Experimentally, cytolytic T-lymphocytes, natural killer cells, null or K cells, macrophages, and B-lymphocytes have all been shown to participate in host responses to tumors. There is considerable evidence of host response in humans, also. Indirect evidence includes the increased incidence of tumors in either congenital or acquired immune deficiency states (Bruton type agammaglobulinemia, ataxia telangiectasis, Wiskott-Aldrich syndrome, immunosuppressive therapy, AIDS). Both humoral and cell-mediated immune reactions have been demonstrated, and serum factors may either block or unblock lymphocytotoxicity. T-cells, natural killer cells, and "armed macrophages" (macrophages with cytophilic antibody fixed to their surface by an Fc receptor) may be cytotoxic to tumor cells. Recently, antibody-dependent lymphocytotoxicity has been shown; its significance is not clear. Finally immunotherapy of tumors, utilizing several approaches (immunization with tumor specific antigens, passive transfer of sensitized cells, injection of transfer factor, passive transfer of cytotoxic antibody, nonspecific stimulation of cell mediated immunity, and topical application of macrophage arming factor), has been successful, but only when the number of tumor cells have been reduced by surgery or other therapy.

INFECTIOUS DISEASES

This section cannot discuss, in detail, the majority of infectious diseases. Infectious diseases, as a group, remain the major cause of morbidity and mortality throughout the world and the student should have a firm foundation for the evaluation of the patient who may have an infectious condition.

Pyogenic Infections

Pyogenic (pus-forming) infections evoke suppurative exudates, consisting primarily of PMNs, dead cells, necrotic debris, and various tissue breakdown products including lecithin, fats, soaps, nucleic acids, and enzymes released from injured and dead cells. The most common pus-producing organisms are certain gram-positive and gram-negative cocci, although many other organisms including fungi can also evoke a pyogenic response.

Staphylococcal infections can affect any organ or tissue and characteristically cause abscess formation. Furuncles ("boils") are focal, superficial abscesses of skin and subcutaneous tissue, whereas carbuncles are more extensive, deep-seated infections. Both commonly begin in hair follicles (folliculitis). Other forms of infection include pneumonia, which is particularly serious because of the destructive nature of the process, pharyngitis, tonsillitis, sinusitis, enteritis, endocarditis, and osteomyelitis. Food poisoning occurs due to a toxin produced by the organism in contaminated food. The abscess itself contributes to resistance to antibiotic therapy, as the crowding of organisms, within a semipermeable pyogenic membrane, causes decreased bacterial metabolic activity and, subsequently, decreased sensitivity to chemotherapy. Effective therapy usually requires that the abscess be opened and left to drain freely ("I and D"; incision and drainage). A variety of exotoxins are produced by *Staphylococcus aureus* (hemolysins, hyaluronidase, coagulase, staphylokinase, leucocidin); not all have been shown to be important in human disease.

Streptococcal infections are most often due to β-hemolytic *Streptococcus pyogenes* and may express as local infection (e.g., tonsillitis), spreading infection (e.g., cellulitis or lymphangitis), hematogenous dissemination, exanthematous disease (i.e., Scarlet fever) due to elaboration of an erythrogenic toxin, and poststreptococcal hypersensitivity disease (rheumatic fever, poststreptococcal glomerulonephritis). Impetigo contagiosa is a highly contagious, autoinnoculable skin infection, usually in children. Erysipelas is a rapidly spreading, erythematous skin infection, often accompanined by lymphangitis, bacteremia, and metastatic infection.

α-Hemolytic *Streptococcus viridans,* usually found in the mouth and generally not virulent; may cause endocarditis, especially in individuals with chronic rheumatic valvulitis.

Pneumococcal infections are caused by *Diplococcus pneumoniae.* The principal disease is lobar (pneumococcal) pneumonia, which characteristically is not destructive and not usually followed by fibrosis. Pleuritis is common. Other pneumococcal infections include endocarditis, pericarditis, peritonitis, arthritis, meningitis, otitis, and sinusitis.

Meningococcal infections (Neisseria meningitidis) may express as nasopharyngitis, meningococcal meningitis, and meningococcemia. Meningococcemia may be an acute fulminating disease with high fever and widespread petechiae and ecchymoses due to acute vasculitis of small vessels with subsequent thrombosis and suppurative necrosis. Massive adrenal hemorrhage may lead to acute adrenal insufficiency and profound circulatory collapse (Waterhouse-Friderichsen's syndrome); this may be a form of disseminated intravascular coagulopathy (DIC).

Gonococcal infections, due to Neisseria gonorrheae, are usually venereal. Exceptions are *ophthalmia neonatorum* in newborns delivered from an infected birth canal, and epidemic vulvovaginitis, usually occurring in infants. In the male, gonorrhea causes acute urethritis characterized by painful micturition and the flow of pus from the penile urethra. This clears spontaneously or may progress to posterior urethritis and epididymitis as well as prostatitis. There may be hematogenous dissemination with arthritis or endocarditis. The major complications are urethral stricture and sterility. Females may have urethritis, vulvovaginitis, and cervicitis, with the fallopian tubes as the site of major involvement. This may lead to pyosalpinx and then hydrosalpinx or tubal obliteration and sterility. The endometrium, during reproductive years, is resistant. Many cases of "pelvic inflammatory disease" (PID) are due to gonococcal infection.

Other Bacterial Infections

Some of the most important bacterial infections will be briefly discussed.

Escherichia coli is usually a noninvasive enteric commensal which may cause serious disease when it is in other than its usual site, or in predisposed adults and infants. *E coli* may cause suppuration or may cause disease by the elaboration of toxins. The most common form of disease is urinary tract infection, including cystitis and pyelonephritis, and, in contrast to other enteric bacilli, may infect when there is no cause for urinary stasis. *E coli,* along with Enterobacteriaceae and *Proteus,* may cause infection within the abdominal cavity, as in such common conditions as acute appendicitis, cholecystitis, cholangitis, and diverticulitis, and may be complicated by gram-negative bacteremia which is characterized by uncontrollable febrile reactions, DIC, shock, and, in as many as 50 percent of cases, death. Severe illness may also be caused by the elaboration of enterotoxins, as in epidemic diarrhea of the newborn or traveller's diarrhea.

Typhoid fever is the most serious of the Salmonelleae, and is contracted by the ingestion of contaminated water or food. Typically, a bacteremia occurs and fever develops about 2 weeks after exposure, perhaps due to an endotoxin. Organisms collect, and proliferate, in Peyer's patches of the terminal ileum. Histologically, phagocytic and reticuloendothelial cells proliferate and contain bacteria, cellular debris, and, characteristically, engulfed red cells (erythrophagocytosis). Other reticuloendothelial organs, such as the spleen, liver, and lymph nodes, also show nodules of phagocytic cells with erythrophagocytosis ("typhoid nodules"). Recurrent chills accompany the bacteremia and there is colicky abdominal pain, severe diarrhea, and skin rash ("rose spots"). Patients have bradycardia and leukopenia. Complications include intestinal hemorrhage, intestinal perforation, splenic rupture, and pneumonia.

Bacillary dysentery, due to *Shigella* infection, affects the colon mostly. A fibropurulent exudate forms an extensive pseudomembrane. Abrupt diarrhea, high fevers, nausea, vomiting, headache, and crampy abdominal pain ensue. Death, particularly in infants, may follow.

Diphtheria is an acute, highly communicable disease, characterized by severe local membranous inflammation, usually in the upper respiratory tract with systemic dissemination of an exotoxin. The membrane, necrotic epithelium, and coagulated fibrinosuppurative exudate, contain the organism. Corynebacterium diphtheriae tenaciously adheres to the tracheobronchial mucosa. The exotoxin interferes with the fatty acid transport activity of carnitine, causing toxic myocarditis, fatty change of other organs, and polyneuritis.

OPPORTUNISTIC INFECTIONS

Infections may occur when treatment or a disease itself contributes to impairment of the host humoral and/or cellular immune system, and are often severe and potentially fatal. In addition to common pathogens, the infective agent may be an organism that is usually of low virulence or even saprophytic. Susceptible patients include those with natural or acquired immune deficiency, with neoplastic disorders, particularly those affecting the hematopoietic system, and those patients that are severely debilitated. Fungal and protozoal organisms are particularly prevalent.

Candidiasis (moniliasis) is most often a sequel to antibiotic therapy, although it may also occur in untreated individuals, particularly diabetics, and in pregnancy. In these latter conditions, the nature of the immunologic defect is unknown. Cutaneous candidiasis occurs particularly in the moist folds beneath the breasts of women and as a vulvovaginitis. Healthy newborns may develop oral candidiasis (thrush). In contrast to these relatively mild infections, acute generalized candidiasis occurs in (1) patients with malignant disorders, especially leukemia, who have been given immunosuppressives and corticosteroids, (2) patients undergoing intestinal surgery who receive antibiotics to suppress intestinal flora, (3)

patients with long-term intravenous catheters, (4) those with cardiac abnormalities or prosthetic devices, (5) intravenous narcotic addicts (who may develop right-sided endocarditis), and (6) individuals with the acquired immune deficiency syndrome (AIDS). In this latter group, a chronic, less aggressive form of candidiasis may develop.

Aspergillosis organisms may affect otherwise healthy farmers or pigeon feeders. In addition, preexisting lung cavities favor the development of intracavitary aspergillus "fungus balls." Aspergillus fumigatus, the most common species, is ubiquitous. Immunosuppressed patients are particularly prone to a highly virulent, often fatal, form of the disease. Abscesses develop and vigorously invade blood vessels with subsequent thrombosis and infarction. The disease may be localized or disseminated, and any organ may be affected.

Mucormycosis (phycomycosis) is due to the phycomycetes group of fungi, and occurs most often with diabetes mellitus, hematologic malignant disease, immunosuppression, after thermal burns, and, occasionally, after surgery.

The ubiquitous fungi grow rapidly and, consequently, the course may be remarkably rapid, with extensive necrosis and destruction, largely due to fungus growth within blood vessels, with resultant thrombosis and infarction. *Mucor* organisms are somewhat larger than aspergillus, which also grows intravascularly, and, in addition, are nonseptate and have "right angle" (90 degree) branching. A rhinocerebral type of involvement is especially common in diabetics. Organisms enter through the nose with subsequent destruction of antrum and/or orbit. Pulmonary mucormycosis mostly affects leukemics. The infection affects any organ and may be disseminated.

Pneumocystosis is a pulmonary infection by the protozoa *Pneumocystis carinii,* and occurs primarily in (1) premature and debilitated malnourished individuals when transplacentally-passed maternal immunoglobulins have decreased, (2) adults with disease-impaired immunity (e.g., Hodgkin's disease), (3) after immunosuppressive therapy (e.g., chemotherapy for neoplasia or immunosuppressive therapy in a transplant patient), and (4) patients with AIDS, in whom the pneumocystosis is often fatal. The ubiquitous organism is inhaled. Insidious in onset, the disease has rapid development of severe dyspnea and cyanosis, with a characteristic "ground-glass" opacification of lung fields seen on x-rays. Only lungs are affected. There is interstitial inflammation by plasma cells and other mononuclears, and alveoli become filled with foamy eosinophilic, relatively acellular exudate in which the characteristic cysts can be demonstrated with the aid of special stains.

CARDIOVASCULAR SYSTEM

The cardiovascular system includes the heart and great vessels, all of which can be affected by degenerative, inflammatory, traumatic, and, to a lesser extent, neoplastic conditions. Congenital malformations are of particular importance in this system.

Arteriosclerotic Disorders

Arteriosclerosis is the group of degenerative diseases of the large arteries, including atherosclerosis, which is characterized by the deposition of lipids, complex carbohydrates, and blood and its products, in vessel walls, with subsequent complicating fibrosis, calcification, and other sequelae. Arteries tend to degenerate because of constant tension, relative lack of intramural capillaries which limits repair, and an inability to "rest."

Atherosclerosis

The early lesions are (1) fatty dot and streak, present in most infants after age one, but not in typical adult distribution, (2) gelatinous elevations, mostly of intimal edema (insudate), and (3) small mural thrombi. These probably contribute to the atheromatous plaque, the basic lesion of atherosclerosis, which is a smooth, yellow or white, slightly raised intimal lesion. Initially discrete, the atheromatous plaque eventually merges with other plaques. Microscopically, there is accumulation of lipids with smooth muscle and connective tissue proliferation. The complicated lesions are fibrous plaques, ulcers, calcifications, and intimal hemorrhages.

Atherosclerosis may be severe with few sequelae. In many cases, however, there may be (1) stenosis with resultant ischemia, (2) complete occlusion due to severe intramural hemorrhage, thrombosis, or embolism, with resultant death, of the tissue (infarction) or the individual, or without effect, if collateral circulation is adequate, (3) aneurysm formation, (4) rupture and hemorrhage, and (5) embolism.

Particular sites have the following special features:

Aorta: Ascending and descending thoracic aorta relatively spared, with most prominent lesions in arch and below renal arteries, where confluent lesions are most likely.

Coronary arteries: Site of most devastating effects of atherosclerosis and often basis of death. Left anterior descending coronary most severely affected, especially 1–3 cm from ostium.

Cerebral arteries: Thrombosis, aneurysm, hemorrhage all contribute to cerebrovascular accident ("stroke," "apoplexy"). Second only to coronaries in importance.

Femoral, popliteal, tibial arteries: Commonly affected and third major syndrome. Occlusions and stenosis impair blood supply to lower extremities, with resultant pain following activity and relief with rest. In male, accompanied by impotence (Leriche's syndrome).

Carotid arteries: Advanced lesions particularly at point of bifurcation.

Vertebral arteries: Importance increasingly recognized as one cause of cerebral ischemia.

Suggested mechanisms for atherosclerosis are (1) mechanical injury, because of high hydrostatic tension, variations of vessel direction and caliber, and varying fluid dynamics, (2) injurious agent in circulating blood causing initial damage and impeding repair, (3) disordered subendothelial metabolism causing accumulation of lipids or other substances, and (4) neoplasticlike proliferation of smooth muscle cells, caused by a "carcinogen" in the circulating blood. Two or more of these factors may be active.

Cystic Medial Necrosis

Cystic medial necrosis is cystic, mucoid degeneration of media, with loss of elastic and muscle fibers, and accumulation of mucopolysaccharidelike material. It may be familial, and is often associated with Marfan's syndrome. Its major complication is dissecting aneurysm, usually of the thoracic aorta.

DISSECTING ANEURYSM

With the decline of syphilis, dissecting aneurysm is the most frequent thoracic aortic aneurysm. Most cases are in sixth to seventh decade, men affected 3 : 1, and hypertension is commonly found. Symptoms often follow physical exertion, with a sudden stabbing or tearing pain in the chest. Dissections may vary in length, even involving the entire length of aorta. Death results from rupture and exsanguination, or impairment of blood flow to a vital area. May occur *de novo* without cystic medial necrosis, and may follow trauma.

Syphilitic aortitis occurs more than 10 years after primary infection. It mostly affects the aortic valve ring (dilatation with aortic regurgitation) and the ascending aorta (mostly media destruction with aneurysm formation).

Syphilitic myocarditis is rare.

Myocardial Infarction

Coronary artery disease may cause myocardial ischemia. This may result from (1) atherosclerotic narrowing with partial or complete obstruction, (2) thrombosis, (3) hemorrhage into a preexisting plaque, (4) rupture of plaque into the lumenal space, and, rarely, there may be (5) embolism, either from a thrombus in the heart or from an aortic valve vegetation or (6) narrowing of coronary artery ostia from nonatherosclerotic causes, such as aortitis or arteritis. Thrombosis may also be the result of myocardial ischemia. Thrombi may recanalize.

Coronary artery atherosclerosis is usually diffuse, but the most significant site of occlusion is the proximal 1–2 cm. Two or more coronary arteries are usually affected. Infarction does not always follow when intercoronary anastomotic circulation is adequate, and infarcts may occur without occlusion, as after a hypotensive episode.

Myocardial infarction occurs when the oxygenation of the heart is not sufficient for viability. Pain is usually immediate, but may not occur in all patients. Electrocardiographic changes are seen within a minute of injury. Ultrastructural alterations (loss of glycogen, edema, endoplasmic reticulum vacuolization, mitochondrial swelling and dissolution, myofilament separation, and loss of striations) begin within 5 minutes. Light microscopic changes may not be obvious for as long as 12 hours, although evidence of loss of contractability of fibers ("wavy-lines") may be seen after 10 minutes.

Microscopic findings are the following:

10 minutes:	"Wavy-line" phenomenon
6 hours:	Eosinophilia (cellular dehydration) progression to coagulative necrosis
2 days:	Beginning leukocytic infiltration
4 days:	Marked leukocytic infiltration
5 days:	Phagocytosis of necrotic muscle
6 days:	Granulation tissue
12 days:	Early collagen
4 weeks:	Mature collagen

Microscopic evidence may not be seen until 6 hours after ischemia. Pallor and dryness are followed by slight swelling. Firmness increases as necrosis and leukocytic infiltration proceed with associated peripheral hyperemia. Redness means granulation tissue forms. Myocardium may be depressed when phagocytosis is marked. Later, a firm, gray, contracted scar is seen. The infarction may be subendocardial or transmural, and the site varies with the vessel involved. The vessels include the following:

Left anterior descending: Anterior left ventricle or anteroseptum; bundle of His; right bundle branch.

Circumflex: Posterior or lateral left ventricle; atrioventricular (AV) node; rarely, sinoatrial (SA) node.

Right coronary: Posterior left ventricle or posteroseptum; posterior right ventricle; SA node, AV node; bundle of His.

Diffuse, (i.e., hypotensive): Extensive subendocardial ischemia.

General manifestations include, in addition to pain, fever, and leukocytosis, elevation of serum enzymes as follows:

1–2 days	CPK
2–6 days	GOT, GPT
2–14 days	LDH

Complications include death, cardiogenic shock, arrhythmias, cardiac failure, intracardiac thrombosis and thromboembolism, pericarditis, cardiac rupture, and ventricular aneurysm.

Pericardial Diseases

Pericarditis may be purulent (pneumonia, sepsis), fibrinous (rheumatic fever, systemic lupus erythematosus, viral, uremic), and fibrotic (tuberculosis, idiopathic).

Hemopericardium may be due to a ruptured aortic aneurysm, trauma, or ventricular rupture. Death follows cardiac tamponade.

Hydropericardium is accumulation of transudate in excess of usual 30–50 cc, due to cardiac failure, hypoproteinemia, uremia, and myxedema. If accumulation is gradual, there may be minimal compromise in function. Rapid accumulation may lead to tamponade.

Tumors may present as acute pericarditis or chronic stricture. Primary tumors are exceedingly rare. Secondary tumors (lung, breast, esophagus, lymphomas) are more common.

Myocardial diseases

Myocarditis may be due to infection, immunologic injury, metabolic disorders, toxicity, and trauma. Clinical manifestations may be similar. Heart failure is most common, due to poor contractility, impaired outflow, impaired filling, disturbances of conduction, or, often, combinations of these. Occasionally, sudden death is the presenting phenomenon. Macro- and microscopic features vary. In general, however, the hearts are pale, dilated, and flabby.

INFECTIOUS MYOCARDITIS

Viral. Coxsackie myocarditis is the prototype, may have associated peri- and endocarditis. Rarely fatal. Arrhythmias, cyanosis, and heart failure. Occurs in epidemics. Histopathology includes focal necrosis, with interstitial accumulations of lymphocytes, plasma cells, histiocytes.

Bacterial. Usually complication of infection at another site. May be staphylococcal, pneumococcal, tuberculosis, syphilis; all uncommon today. Diphtheritic myocarditis is due to exotoxin, and not direct infection.

Protozoal. Chagas' disease is one of the most worldwide important causes of heart failure. In late stage, organisms are not detectable in the heart. Ventricular aneurysms characteristically develop.

Fungal. Usually occur in an immunosuppressed patient. Candidiasis, aspergillosis, mucormycosis; usually associated with extracardiac infection.

Degenerative and metabolic conditions include the following:

1. Brown atrophy: Common postmortem finding, associated with cachexia, rarely clinically significant.
2. Fatty degeneration: Common postmortem finding, associated with toxic states, sepsis, long-standing anemia.
3. Amyloidosis: Most often idiopathic (primary); increased incidence with age ("senile amyloidosis"). Extracellular deposition of amyloid around individual muscle fibers in endocardium and vessel walls causes intractable restrictive heart failure. Heart is usually enlarged with a "waxy" appearance and texture.
4. Glycogenoses: Especially α-glucosidase deficiency (Pompe's disease) leads to massive glycogen infiltration with cardiomegaly and heart failure. Death occurs in infancy.

Chemical and physical agents such as carbon monoxide, irradiation, and drugs (arsenic, adriamycin, isoproterenol, digitalis) may cause myocardial injury.

Acute idiopathic myocarditis (Fiedler's myocarditis; giant cell myocarditis) is a rare condition, possibly due to multiple causes. Usually affects myocardium only with interstitial infiltration of lymphocytes, plasma cells, and variable numbers of eosinophils and multinucleated giant cells.

Idiopathic cardiomyopathy, typically has cardiomegaly due to hypertrophy and dilatation; may also have endocardial thickening, mural thrombi, and myocardial scars. Histologic changes are nonspecific. A possible variant is idiopathic hypertrophic subaortic stenosis (IHSS), a rare condition in which there is asymmetrical, often subaortic, hypertrophy with a characteristic whorling pattern of myocardial fibers in the affected area.

Sarcoidosis affects the heart in 10–20 percent of generalized cases. Often, cor pulmonale is the result of severe pulmonary involvement. Rarely, the myocardium itself may have sarcoid granulomas, with resultant arrhythmias, scarring, and, occasionally, aneurysm formation.

Alcoholic cardiomyopathy may be clinical (abrupt onset of right-sided heart failure) or subclinical (radiologic or electrocardiographic cardiomegaly). Cardiomegaly, dilatation, and mural thrombi are common. Alcoholic cardiomyopathy may be thiamine-therapy-independent or dependent (alcoholic beriberi).

Ischemic cardiomyopathy results from slow, progressive coronary artery stenosis with diffuse myocardial fibrosis. Congestive heart failure occurs unrelated to myocardial infarction.

Hypertensive cardiomyopathy is characterized by concentric hypertrophy of left ventricular muscle.

Endocardial Disease

Infective endocarditis is fatal, if untreated. Manifestations may be similar, whether the infecting organism is a bacteria, fungus, rickettsia, or protozoa, and depend on the site and complications of the infection. Predisposing conditions include rheumatic heart disease, congenital heart disease, arteriosclerosis, surgery, and the presence of artificial substances (pacemakers, catheters, synthetic vessels, prostheses). Normal hearts may also be affected. Portals of entry include dental infections and manipulations, urinary tract instrumentation, skin infections, respiratory infections, postpartum infections, infected burns, cardiac surgery, and intravenous (iatrogenic and narcotics abusers). Clinical manifestations include fever, anemia, new or changing heart murmur, leukocytosis, splenomegaly, heart failure, embolism and infarction, immune phenomenon such as glomerulonephritis, and allergic vasculitis (Osler's nodes of the tips of fingers and toes, Janeway lesions of the palms of the hands and soles of the feet, Roth's spots of the retina, and splinter hemorrhages under the nails). Macroscopically, there may be vegetations of varying sizes, on the lines of closure of the valves, or at any site in the cardiovascular system. Most often the left heart is affected. In intravenous drug abusers, the right heart, especially the tricuspid valve, may be affected. The value surface of lesser pressure (semilunar ventricular, and atrioventricular atrial) is first involved. Vegetations may interfere with function because of their location, they may be destructive, causing perforations, and they may embolize. If incompletely treated, they cause scarring and deformity. Histologically, they are usually characterized by an acute inflammatory response. Pathogenesis varies with the infecting agent, but it may be that all forms are preceeded by intimal or valvular injury with deposition of fibrin as a nidus for infection.

Nonbacterial thrombotic endocarditis (NBTE). Formally called "marantic endocardiosis" because of its association with wasting conditions and cachexia, is thought to be a form of disseminated intravascular coagulation syndrome (DIC). Delicate, friable excrescences, consisting of fibrin and platelets without inflammatory cells, necrotic debris, or infective agents, form. NBTE is rarely diagnosed during life. NBTE may embolize with resultant ischemia of distant organs.

Nonbacterial verrucous endocarditis (Libman-Sacks disease) is, in modern times, exceedingly rare. It is seen only in systemic lupus erythematosus, it affects undersurface of mitral and tricuspid valves, and it consists of fibrin with evidence of organization. Emboli are not seen.

Carcinoid heart disease is most likely due to the effects of serotonin (5-hydroxy-tryptamine) on the endocardium. It is associated with metastasis to the liver because monoamine oxidase in the liver and lung interferes with serotonin activity; consequently, the right heart valves are affected. The valves become fibrotic and insufficiency results.

Endocardial fibroelastosis may be congenital, secondary to other cardiac disease (cardiomyopathy), or, possibly, infective (Davies' disease of Uganda). Fibrous tissue thickens the endocardium.

Rheumatic Heart Disease

Rheumatic fever is an immunologically mediated inflammatory disease which occurs as a delayed sequel to pharyngitis caused by group A β-hemolytic Streptococci. The acute form of the disease is a diffuse, nonspecific inflammatory process principally involving the heart and affecting all layers (pericarditis, myocarditis, and endocarditis) with a range of clinical manifestations that may reflect this. In addition, the joints, central nervous system, skin, and subcutaneous tissues may display evidence of involvement (migratory polyarthritis, Sydenham's chorea, erythema marginatum, subcutaneous nodules). Fever is almost always present, and patients may die, usually from heart failure and/or arrhythmias. The chronic form of the disease consists primarily of scarred, deformed heart valves with associated noninflammatory cardiomyopathy.

Prevailing evidence supports the concept that a preceeding infection with a β-hemolytic streptococcus causes the development of an antibody which initially reacts with the bacteria, but also "attacks" the sarcolemmal membranes of heart muscle which are antigenically similar to the M-protein of the Streptococcus cell wall. Disease usually affects children and develops 2 to 4 weeks after the initial infection, when bacteria are no longer recoverable.

Acute rheumatic fever is a systemic disease resembling acute serum sickness reaction, and may include acute arteritis, synovitis, meningoencephalitis, and glomerulitis. Cardiac involvement is characterized by the presence of a unique, pathognomonic granulomatous reaction, the Aschoff nodule. The granuloma follows fibrinoid necrosis of collagen and degeneration of cardiac and vascular smooth muscle, with accumulation of characteristic multinucleated giant cells, lymphocytes, plasma cells, and Anitschkow cells. Aschoff nodules occur mostly in the endocardium and in myocardial neurovascular areas, but may be found at any site of involvement. The endocarditis is characterized by fibrinoid necrosis, and fibrin verrucae may be present. Fibrinous epicarditis may lead to chronic adhesive pericarditis. Chronic rheumatic fever becomes manifest 10 to 20 years after the acute episode, and typically consists of deformed, fibrotic valves which show collagenization, increased vascularity, and, in late stages, calcification and ossification. Typically, there is fusion of commissures, and thickening, shortening, and fusion of chordae tendinae. The mitral valve is most often involved (48 percent), and combined mitral and aortic involvement is second most common (42 percent). Valve deformities lead to stenosis and/or insufficiency, with the clinical sequelae of murmurs, hypertrophy, and dilatation, depending on disease site and severity.

Complications include congestive heart failure, bacterial endocarditis, often associated with an organism of low virulence, such as the α-hemolytic *Streptococcus viridans* (subacute bacterial endocarditis), and mural thrombosis, especially in the left atrium in cases of severe mitral stenosis with atrial fibrillation.

There is no specific diagnostic test for acute rheumatic fever. Diagnosis is based on the signs and symptoms and history of preceeding streptococcal infection with supporting evidence provided by the demonstration of antibodies to the Streptococcus. The antistreptolysin-*O* assay is positive in approximately 90 percent of patients with acute rheumatic fever. The diagnosis of chronic rheumatic fever is established by the presence of left-sided valvular disease in association with a history of past acute rheumatic fever.

Congenital Heart Disease

Congenital cardiovascular anomalies are the most common cause of heart disease in infancy and are at least equal in importance to rheumatic heart disease in childhood. Cardiac anomalies constitute about 25 percent of all congenital malformations, and there are approximately 32,000 babies born each year with congenital heart disease.

Prognosis varies according to the type and severity of the anomaly, but in general, there are serious cardiac malfunctions which may impair normal growth and development. In infancy, the major complications are heart failure, systemic hypoxemia, frequent respiratory infections, growth retardation, and pulmonary hypertension. In childhood, there may be pulmonary hypertension, infective endocarditis, brain abscess, and "paradoxical" emboli.

Most of the anomalies reflect abnormalities of partitioning of the vascular tube during embryonic development. This chapter cannot discuss, in detail, the cardiac anomalies and students are referred to textbooks of pathology. It is important, however, to emphasize that the cardiac anomalies contribute to (1) disturbances of cardiac function, in terms of overwork due to abnormal shunts, regurgitations and obstruction, insufficient output due to overwork, hypooxygenation, and inadequate contractile capacity, and arterial oxygen unsaturation (cyanosis) because of abnormal shunts; (2) pulmonary arterial hypertension, because of increased pulmonary artery flow from left to right shunts, and increased pulmonary resistance from obstructions; and (3) impaired development of the individual as a whole.

Major anomalies include the following:

Ventricular septal defect: Most common anomaly. May be complicated by congestive heart failure, especially in infancy, pulmonary infections, pulmonary vascular obstruction, and infective endocarditis.

Atrial septal defect: May be combined with mitral stenosis (Lutembacher's syndrome), may be combined with ventricular septal defect and incomplete mitral and/or tricuspid valves (endocardial cushion defect).

Patent ductus arteriosus: May be persistent, narrow ductus ("classical") or wide and short. The latter is associated with onset, during infancy, of cardiac failures, pulmonary hypertension, and many respiratory infections. The classical form may not require early surgery, but may be complicated by infective endocarditis.

Tetralogy of Fallot: Combined right ventricular outflow obstruction, ventricular septal defect, biventricular origin of the aorta, and, secondarily, right ventricular hypertrophy. Associated right-to-left shunt.

Complete transposition of the great vessels: Cardiac architecture normal, but vessels arise from opposite ventricle. Due to inverted development of truncus swellings.

Coarctation of the aorta: May be preductal (fetal type) or postductal (adult type). Preductal often associated with patent ductus and hypoplastic heart and has poor prognosis. Postductal may be associated with patent ductus and/or ventricular septal defect, with left to right shunt. With closed ductus, there is no systemic pulmonary shunt and there is upper extremity hypertension and left ventricular hypertrophy. Coarctation may be complicated by dissecting aneurysm proximal to coarctation, infective endocarditis, cerebral (hypertensive) hemorrhage, and heart failure.

Tumors of the Heart

Primary tumors are extremely rare. Most frequent are myxomas, which usually affect the left atrium, and which may manifest as syncopal attacks, cardiac insufficiency, and sudden death. Rhabdomyomas and rhabdomyosarcomas are exceedingly rare.

Secondary tumors occur much more frequently, as a consequence of hematogenous dissemination, lymphatic spread, and direct extension from an intrathoracic tumor. They may be clinically silent or manifest as a pericarditis.

Disorders of Veins

Varicose veins affect 10–20 percent of the adult population. Contributing factors include familial, obesity, age, pregnancy, pelvic masses or tumors, intravascular thromboses, and, perhaps most importantly the upright position. Complications include dependent edema, trophic skin changes, thrombosis, inflammation (phlebitis), and, most importantly, embolism.

Hemorrhoids are, along with appendicitis and carcinoma of the colon, most likely due to the Western low-fiber diet. Excess straining during defecation causes varicosity of the hemorrhoidal veins, which may be painful ("external" hemorrhoids), may bleed ("internal" hemorrhoids), and may thrombose (both).

HEMATOPOIETIC SYSTEM

The hematopoietic system can be considered to include the circulating blood, blood marrow, spleen, lymph nodes, thymus, and liver; many of the disorders of the blood involve these organs directly or indirectly. A clear understanding of the normal structure and function of these organs is necessary to fully comprehend the related diseases and should be reviewed.

Red Blood Cell Disorders

The anemias are a heterogeneous group of disorders as follows:

Decreased production
    Iron deficiency
        Dietary
        Blood loss
        Chronic inflammation
    Marrow insufficiency
        Toxic injury
        Marrow replacement
        Intrinsic marrow disease
    Erythropoietin deficiency
        Renal disease
        Hyperoxygenemia
        Reduced oxygen need
Abnormal maturation
    Microcytic
        Iron deficiency
        Sideroblastic
    Normocytic
        Myelofibrosis
    Megaloblastic
        B_{12} deficiency
        Folate deficiency
        Intrinsic marrow disease
Hemolytic
    Reticuloendothelial phagocytosis (extrinsic)
        Autoimmune
        Hypersplenism
    Red cell membrane disorders (intrinsic)
        Inherited
            Hereditary spherocytosis
            Hereditary elliptocytosis
    Acquired
        Paroxysmal nocturnal hemoglobinuria
    Metabolic defects
        Glucose-6-phosphate dehydrogenase
(G6PD) deficiency
    Hemoglobinopathies
        Sickle cell disease and trait
        Thallasemias
        Unstable hemoglobin (Heinz body)
anemia
    Red cell fragmentation
        Disseminated intravascular coagulopathy
(DIC)
        Vasculitis
        Endocarditis
        Vascular prostheses

    Intravascular hemolysis
        Water
        Hyperthermia
        Exotoxins (C. welchii)
        Favism
        Autoimmune

Iron deficiency anemia may follow reduced dietary intake, either from malnutrition or impaired absorption, or may be due to excess blood loss as in intestinal or excess uterine bleeding. Fatigue, dyspnea on exertion, palpitations, headaches, and dizziness may occur, and there may be marked pallor. These signs and symptoms occur in all chronic anemias, and their severity and mode of onset depend on the etiology and extent and rate of decline of hemoglobin levels. There may be associated epithelial changes affecting nails (koilonychia), tongue (glossitis), mouth (angular stomatitis), hair (dry, brittle), esophagus (postcricoid web with dysphagia), and stomach (atrophic gastritis). Patients with the association of chronic iron-deficiency anemia, dysphagia due to an esophageal web, and glossitis (Plummer-Vinson syndrome) are at increased risk for the development of upper esophageal or pharyngeal carcinoma.

Megaloblastic anemias are almost always due to a deficiency of vitamin B_{12} and/or folate and may reflect the following:

Diminished dietary intake
Diminished absorption
    Absence of intrinsic factor
        Pernicious anemia
        Postgastrectomy
    Antiepileptic drugs
Acquired intestinal structural disorders
    Gastrocolic fistula
    Blind loop with bacterial overgrowth
Fish tapeworm
Folic acid antagonists (methotrexate)
Increased demand
    Megaloblastic anemia of pregnancy
    Chronic hemolytic anemia

Pernicious anemia patients characteristically have atrophy of the mucosa of the body and fundus of the stomach, resulting in diminished secretion of intrinsic factor and, consequently, impaired vitamin B_{12} absorption. The majority have antibodies to intrinsic factor or gastric parietal cells, or both. Many also show antithyroid antibodies. The classical patient is elderly, pale, and prematurely gray. The onset is insidious and there may be slight jaundice. In addition to profound anemia, there may be demyelination of the brain and cord with associated neurologic abnormalities, mental disturbance, peripheral neuritis, and about half of the patients have a severe glossitis. Patients also have weight loss, gastrointestinal symptoms such as indigestion and diarrhea, and there is an increased incidence of gastric adenocarcinoma. White cells are also affected and there may be neutropenia characteristically with hypersegmentation of the polymorphonuclear leucocytes. The marrow shows marked erythroid hyperplasia, which can be misinterpreted as acute leukemia.

Hemolytic anemias are the result of increased red cell destruction and shortening of the normal 100 to 120 day life span of the red blood cell. The wide range of diseases that can cause hemolytic anemia have little in common except the end result. Diagnosis can be made by recognizing characteristic abnormal red cell forms (spherocytes, sickle cells), demonstrating free hemoglobin in the plasma or urine, demonstrating reduced amounts of plasma haptoglobin, or, in some cases, detecting plasma methemalbumin.

Hereditary spherocytosis occurs as an autosomal dominant disorder mostly in Northern Europeans. Anemia is usually slight; jaundice is common and there may be gallstones. There is moderate splenomegaly. The red cells show increased lysis in hypotonic saline.

Hereditary elliptocytosis is an uncommon, autosomal dominant defect which causes a severe anemia which can be lessened by splenectomy.

Paroxysmal nocturnal hemoglobinuria (PNH) is a rare, acquired chronic hemolytic anemia in which the red cell membrane is abnormal, showing excess sensitivity to complement and tendency to lysis. There may be associated aplastic anemia. Red cells lyse when incubated in fresh (complement-rich) ABO compatible serum acidified to pH 6.5 – 7 (Ham' test). PNH may be fatal, or may be complicated by the development of leukemia.

G6PD deficiency is an X-linked disorder with a recessive pattern of inheritance. There is a Mediterranean variant and a less severe African (A type) variant. Anemia usually does not become manifest unless there is a provoking episode, due to drugs (antimalarials, sulfonamides, phenacetin, vitamin K analogs), chemicals (naphthalene mothballs), or ingestion of fava beans. There may be neonatal jaundice which, in susceptible infants, can be accentuated by the administration of a vitamin K analog. Rarely, there may be chronic hemolysis in the absence of a provoking substance.

Sickle cell anemia may manifest as an acute hemolytic episode, as an aplastic crisis, as painful infarcts, or, particularly in infants, as a sequestration crisis in which there is sudden pooling of red cells in the spleen with consequent acute, profound systemic anemia. The diagnosis can be made by recognizing the sickle cells in blood smears, by inducing the sickling phenomenon by suspending red cells in a reducing solution, or by demonstrating, by hemoglobin electrophoresis, the abnormal hemoglobin. A less severe form of disease occurs as sickle cell-hemoglobin C disease. Approximately 20 percent of Africans and 8 percent of North American blacks have the sickle cell trait and may never demonstrate hemolysis unless subjected to reduced oxygen concentration because of accident during anesthesia, high-altitude flying in unpressurized aircraft, or increased oxygen demand as in a septic state.

The thallasemias are a heterogenous group of disorders which are characterized by a lack or insufficient synthesis of either the α or β-globin chain of hemoglobin A. The pathologic consequences, however, are due to the relative excess of the other chain. As example, β-thallasemia is a deficiency of β-globin chain, but the manifestations are due to excess of α-globin. Unstable hemoglobins aggregate within mature erythrocytes and erythroid precursors, often appearing as inclusions, damaging the cells and rendering them more susceptible to phagocytosis and destruction. Thallasemia is an autosomal dominant condition. In homozygous β-thallasemia there is marked microcytic hypochromic anemia, with dramatic expansion of the red marrow with resultant thinning of the cortical bone and reactive new bone formation of the outer surface. Similar changes in the long bones make them more vulnerable to fracture. Splenomegaly and hepatomegaly reflect reticuloendothelial hyperplasia with marked erythrophagocytosis and extramedullary hematopoiesis. This form of thallasemia is often fatal. Thallasemia minor is the heterozygous state of both α- and β-thallasemia and is characterized by variable degrees of anemia, marrow hyperplasia, and siderosis.

White Blood Cell Disorders

The leukemias are a heterogenous group of malignant disorders of white blood cells. The leukemias have been increasing in incidence and are the basis of as many as 15,000 deaths per year. Although any of the white cells can autonomously proliferate as a leukemia, most of the cases are either lymphocytic or granulocytic. The relative frequency of leukemias in the United States is as follows:

Chronic lymphocytic	25 percent
Chronic granulocytic	22 percent
Acute lymphocytic	20 percent
Acute granulocytic	20 percent
Acute myelomonocytic	10 percent
Chronic myelomonocytic	3 percent

Etiology is unknown, but multiple factors, environmental and genetic, may contribute.

The clinical features of acute leukemias reflect the replacement of normal bone marrow by the leukemia cells, with the resultant characteristic triad of anemia, infections, and thrombocytopenic bleeding. Onset is abrupt and, without treatment, death may occur within weeks. Acute lymphocytic (lymphoblastic) leukemia is mostly a disease of children, whereas acute granulocytic (myelocytic, myeloid, myeloblastic) leukemia mostly affects adults.

The chronic leukemias are less fulminant, but may still lead to death. The manifestations develop insidiously and organ enlargement (hepatomegaly, splenomegaly) may be prominent. Chronic lymphocytic leukemia is relatively benign, occurring mostly in the sixth and seventh decades, particularly affecting men, in whom anemia may be the most significant problem. Progression is usually slow, but it may become more aggressive. Chronic granulocytic leukemia, in contrast, affects men and women equally, and occurs in the fifth and sixth decades. A characteristic chromosomal abnormality (Philadelphia chromosome) is found in most patients. Hepatosplenomegaly may be marked, and the problems of anemia, infections, and bleeding, more severe. Although prolonged survivals may occur, most patients with this disorder are dead within 4 years.

Monocytic leukemia is relatively uncommon, and usually acute or subacute. Hairy cell leukemia is an unusual disorder of lymphoreticular cells characterized by insidious onset, marked splenomegaly with pancytopenia, and characteristic cells which have numerous cytoplasmic extensions, best seen in the peripheral blood. The cells also infiltrate the marrow and parenchymal organs.

The myeloproliferative disorders are characterized by proliferation of cells of granulocytic, megakaryocytic, or erythrocytic series, or, in many cases, more than one cell line. Stromal elements may produce marked marrow fibrosis. The marrow characteristically shows a panmyelosis. Polycythemia vera is the condition in which the excess production of red blood cells is dominant, patients are plethoric, circulation time is decreased because of increased blood viscosity, and thromboses occur. Erythroleukemia (Di Guglielmo disease) is not characterized by the presence of a panmyelosis and is most likely a variant of acute myelogenous leukemia. In myeloid metaplasia all cell lines are proliferative and there may be extramedullary hematopoiesis, particularly in myelofibrosis. Idiopathic thrombocythemia is especially rare. The conditions may all terminate as a myelogenous leukemia, further emphasizing their similarity.

Nonneoplastic Lymphoreticular Disorders

Many nonneoplastic conditions affect lymph nodes, spleen, and, usually to a lesser degree, the liver. These organs may react locally or systemically to a variety of inciting stimuli, and the pattern of reaction is often characteristic.

Lymph nodes may be affected by acute or chronic lymphadenitis. Acute lymphadenitis usually occurs locally as a secondary response to an infection. Special variants include cat-scratch disease in which there is a macrophage-granulomatous response with formation of a characteristic stellate zone of necrosis. Many conditions cause chronic lymph node enlargement; these may sometimes be confused with malignant processes. Infectious mononucleosis is a sporadic viral infection affecting children and young adults. There may be lymphadenopathy and splenomegaly, along with sore throat, headache, skin rash, and, less commonly, hepatitis. Antibodies to Epstein-Barr virus are demonstrable. Chronic lymphadenitis may be due to toxoplasmosis, various granulomatous infections such as tuberculosis and sarcoidosis, and nonspecific causes. Forms of lymphadenopathy often simulate lymphoma. Postvaccinial lymphadenitis may be the sequel to vaccination against smallpox, tetanus, diphtheria, and other agents. Dilantin lymphadenopathy may be accompanied by other manifestations of hypersensitivity, such as skin rash, fever, and arthritis, and, because of a mixed cellular infiltrate, may be misdiagnosed as Hodgkin's disease.

The spleen similarly responds to a variety of infectious, immunologic, and hematologic stimuli. Hypersplenism causes anemia, leukopenia, and thrombocytopenia. It is associated with splenomegaly from a variety of causes, such as portal hypertension of cirrhosis. The basis for the hematologic effects is unknown, but may be due to reticuloendothelial hyperplasia causing increased phagocytosis of blood elements. Most instances of splenomegaly, however, are not associated with hypersplenism. Other causes of splenomegaly are passive congestion, storage diseases, and amyloidosis. Some of the largest spleens that occur are in patients with malaria and leishmaniasis (kala-azar).

Neoplastic Lymphoreticular Disorders

Hodgkin's disease is a fatal disease of unknown cause, characterized by the proliferation of atypical histiocytic cells, including characteristic giant (Sternberg-Reed) cells, in association with variable numbers of histologically and functionally normal lymphocytes, neutrophils, plasma cells, eosinophils, and fibroblasts. The disease occurs at any age, but mostly affects those in the early adult years and, to a lesser degree, those in the fifth and sixth decades. There is usually progressive, painless enlargement of a lymph node, most often cervical, with progression to other node areas as well as to other organs. Because, in most patients, the progression is predictable, spreading from one lymphoid area to the anatomically closed lymphoid area (usually from the neck), a staging approach has proven particularly useful for determining therapy. The clinical stages are the following:

I: Involvement of a single lymph node region (I) or single extralymphatic organ or site (IE).

II: Involvement of two or more lymph node regions on the same side of the diaphragm (II) or localized involvement of an extralymphatic organ or site and or one or more lymph node regions on the same side of the diaphragm (IIE).

III: Involvement of lymph node regions on both sides of the diaphragm (III) which may also be accompanied by localized involvement of an extralymphatic organ or site (IIIE) or by the involvement of the spleen (IIIS) or both (IIISE).

IV: Diffuse or disseminated involvement of one or more extralymphatic organs or tissues with or without associated lymph node enlargement.

Patients with Hodgkin's disease may also have a variety of constitutional manifestations, such as fever, anemia, weight loss, night sweats, and itching, and the staging may be modified to indicate their absence (A) or presence (B). A patient who is stage IIB, will not have as good a prognosis as one who is stage IIA.

The lymph nodes are enlarged, with loss of normal architecture, tend to be discrete, rubbery, homogenous tan, and show variable necrosis and/or fibrosis. The spleen may be focally involved, or massively infiltrated; removal of the spleen is an important part of the evaluation because of the difficulty in documenting splenic involvement by clinical means.

Histologic diagnosis of Hodgkin's disease requires the recognition of the Reed-Sternberg cell in an appropriate background. This large (15–45 μm) cell has abundant, slightly basophilic cytoplasm with a multilobed nucleus in which there are particularly prominent, amphophilic nucleoli. For prognostic purposes, a histologic classification has been devised, with the most favorable form listed first as is illustrated by the following:

Lymphocyte predominance: Consists mostly of small lymphocytes and benign-appearing histiocytic cells with only rare Reed-Sternberg cells.

Nodular sclerosis: Interconnecting bands of fibrous tissue divide the lymph node into cellular nodules, in which there are lymphocytes, reactive histiocytes, relatively inconspicuous Reed-Sternberg cells, and distinctive atypical histiocytic cells sitting in spaces formed by shrinkage artifact (lacunar cells). This variant, in contrast to the other forms, mostly affects women and may arise in the mediastinum rather than the neck. Progression is less predictable than the other forms of the disease, and the tumor is especially radiosensitive.

Mixed cellularity: Usually shows a wide variety of cells, including eosinophils, plasma cells, lymphocytes, histiocytes, and many Reed-Sternberg cells. Necrosis may be seen.

Lymphocytic depletion: Lymphocytes are particularly reduced in number, and there are mostly highly atypical histiocytic cells, with variable numbers of Reed-Sternberg cells as well as necrosis and fibrosis.

Defective cellular immunity is characteristic of Hodgkin's disease, manifesting as cutaneous anergy, impaired homograft rejection, and increased sensitivity to opportunistic infections. The etiology remains unknown, but recent evidence has suggested that the disease is transmissable.

The nonHodgkin's lymphomas are a heterogeneous group of malignant lymphoid disorders, whose pathogenesis is not well understood. Few areas of medicine are as confused as this, mostly because there have been a plethora of classifications, in recent years, which have attempted to combine scientific accuracy, reproducibility, and clinical applicability. To a considerable degree, none has succeeded. The most widely used classification is that of Rappaport which, because of its ease of understanding, will be used here. The important concept to remember is that these disorders are all of tumors of lymphocytes which may derive from either B- or T-cells, and which may manifest with close resemblance to normal cells (well differentiated) or may manifest as completely undifferentiated cells ("histiocytic"). The designation "histiocytic" is inaccurate, since lymphomas arising from histiocytes are exceedingly rare, and the "histiocytic," or "large cell" tumors might best be regarded as very poorly differentiated lymphocytic lymphomas. A particularly important morphologic feature is the presence of a pattern of growth, within the lymphoma, which mimics the normal lymphoid follicle, but which consists of malignant cells rather than the variety of cells found normally. This "nodular" pattern is associated with a better prognosis than the "diffuse" pattern. It is also important to note that the spread of the non-Hodgkin's lymphomas is not as predictable as that of Hodgkin's disease, and a staging classification has not been universally utilized. The Rappaport classification is the following:

Nodular
　　Poorly differentiated lymphocytic
　　Mixed lymphocytic-"histiocytic"
　　"Histiocytic"
Diffuse
　　Well differentiated lymphocytic
　　Poorly differentiated lymphocytic
　　Mixed lymphocytic-"histiocytic"
　　"Histiocytic"

Other variations have been recognized, but they are rare.

The diffuse lymphomas are all characterized by complete effacement of the usual architecture and replacement by a generally homogenous population of cells. In the well differentiated lymphocytic lymphoma, the cells resemble normal, "mature" lymphocytes. In the poorly differentiated lymphocytic lymphoma, the cells are larger than normal lymphocytes, and show nuclear pleomorphism, with angulations and indentations. In the "histiocytic" (very poorly differentiated lymphocytic) lymphomas, there is considerable pleomorphism, often with prominent nucleoli, mitoses, and necrosis.

The nonHodgkin's lymphomas occur at all ages, most often in males. These progressive, fatal disorders may initially present with lymphoid or extralymphoid involvement, and complications may reflect involvement of a variety of organs.

The majority of adult lymphomas, including all of the nodular variants, demonstrate cytologic markers of B-lymphocytes. In childhood, most of the lymphomas show either T-cell markers or fail to show markers ("null").

A number of malignant lymphoreticular disorders are less common.

Extranodal lymphomas may develop in the intestinal tract, lungs, bone marrow, skin, or virtually any organ. Primary intracerebral lymphomas are very rare, but occur with greater frequency in immunosuppressed patients.

Angioimmunoblastic lymphadenopathy occurs in elderly patients and is accompanied by hemolytic anemia, fever, and polyclonal gammopathy. There is proliferation of immunoblasts with effacement of the normal architecture of the lymph nodes. Some patients have a relatively benign course, some have a severe hemolytic anemia, some develop severe infections, and some progress to an immunoblastic ("histiocytic" with prominent central nucleoli) lymphoma.

Mycosis fungoides is a chronic, slowly progressive, eczematoid skin disorder in which there is infiltration of the skin by lympho-"histiocytic" T-cells, with particular involvement of the epidermis (Pautrier abscess). Eventually, disseminated lymphoma may develop.

Sézary's disease is a chronic progressive dermatosis due to infiltration of the skin by atypical, mostly "histiocytic" T-cells in which the cells also circulate in the blood.

Burkitt's (African childhood) lymphoma is a unique neoplasm, of B-lymphocytes, that typically affects children living in the equatorial portions of Africa at less than 4,000 feet above sea level. Epstein-Barr virus has been strongly incriminated as a causative agent. The lymphoma typically affects facial structures, such as the orbit and the jaws, and consists of sheets of lymphoblasts in which there are scattered, benign macrophages, imparting a "starry-sky" appearance. Another unique feature is the exquisite sensitivity to certain chemotherapeutic agents. A histologically similar tumor occurs in our population, but does not affect facial structures and generally has a poor prognosis.

Plasma Cell Neoplasms

Since plasma cells derive from B-lymphocytes and are responsible for the synthesis and secretion of antibodies, it is not surprising that neoplasms of these cells commonly produce large amounts of immunoglobin.

Multiple myeloma (myeloma, myelomatosis) affects the elderly, especially men, and is characterized by the proliferation of a clone of plasma cells at multiple sites in the bone marrow. More than 85 percent of patients will demonstrate an abnormal immunoglobulin. The tumor areas appear as gel-like red nodules scattered throughout the bone, with marked osteolysis which may cause fractures of long bones and collapse of vertebrae. These areas are seen as "punched-out" lesions on radiographs. Virtually any bone can be affected. The tumors consist of sheets of plasma cells, in varying stages of differentiation. Bone resorption and osteoporosis lead to hypercalcemia, hypercalciuria, and hyperphosphaturia. The increased levels of immunoglobulins cause rouleaux formation, increased erythrocyte sedimentation rate, and increased blood viscosity. Anemia follows marrow replacement; there may also be thrombocytopenic bleeding. Renal dysfunction may be due to the hypercalcemia-induced nephrocalcinosis. In addition, the presence of light-chain immunoglobulin material may cause tubular obstruction, with epithelial cell proliferation and casts ("myeloma kidney"). There may also be immunologic deficiency and amyloidosis. Death usually occurs in 2 to 5 years, generally from anemia, renal failure, amyloidosis, or infection. IgG myeloma is most frequent (50 percent). Next most common is myeloma producing light-chain (Bence Jones) material; this is particularly associated with myeloma kidney.

Waldenström's macroglobulinemia mostly affects men over the age of 50. The disease most often presents as a chronic disorder with a monoclonal IgM gammopathy, and without recognizable tumor. There may be, however, extensive proliferation of cells which have light and electron microscopic features of both lymphocytes and plasma cells. Patients are weak, easily fatigued, have weight loss, increased susceptibility to infections, spontaneous hemorrhages, and varying degrees of hepatosplenomegaly and lymphadenopathy.

Franklin's (heavy-chain) disease is a rare, neoplastic condition with infiltration of tissue by lymphoid cells associated with the presence of a protein identified as the Fc fragment of the immunoglobulin heavy chain.

A summary of cell surface markers in lymphoreticular neoplasms is the following:

    B-lymphocytic
        Chronic lymphocytic leukemia
        Most adult nonHodgkin's lymphomas
        All nodular lymphomas
        Burkitt's lymphoma
    T-lymphocytic
        Lymphoblastic lymphoma of childhood
        Mycosis fungoides
        Sezary's disease
        Adult T-cell lymphoma of Japan
    Variable B, T, or null
        Mixed lymphoma, diffuse
        "Histiocytic" lymphoma
    Monocytic
        True histiocytic lymphoma
        Malignant histiocytosis

RENAL PATHOLOGY

The kidneys can be the site of origin of numerous neoplastic, inflammatory, and degenerative diseases. It is customary to describe these pathologic entities according to the anatomic portion of the organ primarily involved (i.e., glomerular, tubular, vascular disease). Not infrequently, however, several renal components may be affected by one renal disease.

Glomerular Diseases

Proteinuria is a common sign of glomerular disease, defined by the presence of excessive amounts of protein in the urine (over 150 mg/24 hrs). Normally, plasma proteins that are smaller in molecular weight than 70,000 daltons are filtered through the glomerulus and almost completely reabsorbed by the tubules, while larger molecules are retained in the circulation. Any disease that damages the glomerular filter may result in abnormal filtration of these large proteins into the urine. Some functional conditions, such as fever, physical or emotional stress, and exposure to heat or cold may lead to proteinuria. When proteinuria exceeds 4 g over 24 hours it is considered massive and results in depletion of serum proteins such as albumin.

Nephrotic syndrome, a common manifestation of renal disease, is characterized by massive proteinuria, hypoproteinemia, and hypoalbuminemia with peripheral edema due to decreased osmotic blood pressure. This syndrome can be the result of many diseases that damage the glomerulus, including the following:

    Lipoid nephrosis ("nil" disease, minimal change disease)
        Focal sclerosis
        Membranous nephropathy
        Diabetes mellitus
        Amyloidosis
        Mesangiocapillary glomerulonephritis
        Lupus nephritis

Lipoid nephrosis ("nil" disease, minimal change disease) is a common cause of nephrotic syndrome that affects mostly male children, but may affect adults. Its etiology is uncertain, but it occasionally follows exposure to drugs (tridione), allergens (bee venom), and tumors (Hodgkin's disease). Patients present with the nephrotic syndrome and frequent infections. Their urine has large amounts of small molecular weight proteins, such as albumin, and low molecular weight globulins ("selective proteinuria"). The kidneys are enlarged and pale yellow due to the accumulation of proteins and lipids in tubular cells and the presence of protein casts in the lumina of renal tubules.

On light microscopy and on immunopathologic studies, the glomeruli appear normal. Ultrastructurally, however, the glomeruli have characteristic findings of fusion or effacement of epithelial foot processes. The epithelial cells form a continuous cytoplasmic layer closely apposed to the basement membrane. It is not known whether proteinuria results from this podocyte fusion or from other mechanisms.

Patients usually have a benign course without disease progression. In 10–20 percent of instances, however, the disease progresses to focal sclerosis and later on to diffuse glomerular sclerosis with renal failure. This occurs most frequently in adults.

Focal and segmental glomerulosclerosis (focal sclerosis) affects older children and adults. Patients present with massive nonselective proteinuria, other manifestations of the nephrotic syndrome, and microscopic hematuria. The kidneys appear grossly as in lipoid nephrosis. On light microscopy, selected glomeruli (focal distribution) show small solid areas of sclerosis which may affect one or two lobules of each affected glomerulus (segmental distribution). Ultrastructurally, mesangium is expanded and capillaries are collapsed. In addition, all glomeruli show diffuse loss of foot processes. Immunofluorescence studies of renal biopsies from patients with focal sclerosis show deposits of IgM and C_3 in segmental and focal distribution, which are thought to represent nonspecific trapping of large molecules, rather than a true immunologic phenomenom. Prognosis is generally poor with gradual progression to renal failure and only limited response to steroid treatment.

Membranous nephropathy affects adolescents and middle aged adults. Patients present with nonselective massive proteinuria and other manifestations of the nephrotic syndrome. Etiology is unknown, but occasionally the disease follows exposure to drugs or heavy metals (gold, mercury), systemic lupus erythematosus, malaria, secondary syphilis, diabetes mellitus, malignant tumors, or hepatitis-B antigenemia.

The kidneys grossly resemble lipoid nephrosis. Histologically, the glomerular capillary walls show characteristic thickening with "spikes" of basement membrane, revealed by apical stains (silver impregnation). Ultrastructurally, the glomeruli show characteristic changes, including deposits of protein between the capillary basement membrane and the fused foot processes of epithelial cells as well as progressive thickening of the epithelial basement membrane. The latter begins as projections (spikes) of basement membrane material between the protein deposits that later surround and incorporate the deposits into the basement membrane. Immunofluorescence reveals granular deposits of immunoglobulins (IgG and IgM) and complement along glomerular capillary walls. The nature of these protein deposits in membranous nephropathy is unknown, but it is suspected that they constitute antigen-antibody complexes, probably formed in situ, and possibly consisting of a variety of proteins that are capable of crossing the basement membrane, but not the epithelial cell layer.

Proteinuria may diminish and there may be recovery from the nephrotic syndrome as the basement membrane becomes progressively thickened causing decreased glomerular permeability. However, the markedly thickened basement membrane impairs the passage of small molecules, becomes also impaired, and, as the capillary lumina become narrowed by the thickened capillary walls, renal failure ensues. In general, the disease does not respond well to available therapy. Some patients recover in the early stages of membranous ne-

phropathy, but most individuals with more advanced disease have nephrotic syndrome for many years or die of renal failure.

Amyloidosis may cause nephrotic syndrome. The kidneys appear enlarged, pale, firm, and have a typical "waxy" appearance. Histologically, deposits of amyloid material are in the glomerular mesangium and capillary walls as acidophilic amorphous deposits. The prognosis of renal amyloidosis is variable. In a small portion of cases, the disease progresses to renal failure.

Diabetes mellitus frequently affects the kidney. The clinical manifestations of renal disease due to diabetes include hematuria, hypertension, pyelonephritis, nephrotic syndrome, and renal failure. The gross appearance is variable. Kidneys may be enlarged, normal, or reduced in size, and are usually pale and firm. Surfaces are smooth in early stages and become granular as the disease progresses. The histologic changes are variable. Mesangium may be diffusely widened (diffuse glomerulosclerosis). There may be hyaline nodules in the peripheral lobules of the capillary tuft (nodular glomerulosclerosis or Kimmelstiel-Wilson syndrome), acellular hyaline material may deposit in the urinary space of glomeruli or on the glomerular Bowman's capsule (hyaline or exudative lesions), and there may also be capillary aneurysms, compression of glomerular capillaries, hyaline arteriolosclerosis, thickening of tubular basement membrane, arteriosclerosis of renal arteries, and necrosis of renal papillae and/or pyelonephritis. A characteristic finding is diffuse thickening of capillary basement membranes. Diabetic nephropathy is generally progressive. Renal failure is the leading cause of death in long-standing diabetes, particularly patients with early onset diabetes. Nephrotic syndrome is relatively uncommon in diabetes mellitus but may be a manifestation of the Kimmelstiel-Wilson syndrome.

Glomerulonephritis

Diseases that are characterized by glomerular inflammation constitute the largest group of renal pathologic entities. They present in a variety of ways, but often have the so-called nephritic syndrome (i.e., hematuria with red blood cell casts in urine, preoteinuria, azotemia, and hypertension.

Glomerulonephritis can be classified on the basis of pathologic findings into diffuse and focal forms, as is illustrated by the following:

Diffuse glomerulonephritis
    Proliferative glomerulonephritis (post streptococcal)
    Crescentic (extracapillary, rapidly progressing) glomerulonephritis

Mesangiocapillary (membranoproliferative) glomerulonephritis

Sclerosing (chronic) glomerulonephritis

Focal glomerulonephritis

Intrinsic renal (benign recurrent hematuria, IgA disease)

Associated with systemic disease (anaphylactoid purpura, bacterial endocarditis, systemic lupus erythematosus, Wegener's granulomatosis)

Diffuse proliferative glomerulonephritis (DPG) is the most common form of the disease and includes 95 percent of cases of acute glomerulonephritis. DPG affects mostly children, although any age group can be involved. Patients present clinically with acute signs of the nephrotic syndrome. The pathogenesis of DPG has been thoroughly studied and it is thought to be an example of immune-complex disease. Most cases follow infections by group A hemolytic Streptococci (most frequently of the serologic types 12, 4, and 1). Some cases follow infection by Staphylococci, pneumococci, and viruses. Antibodies such as antistreptolysin-*O* and anti-streptokinase appear in the plasma. Circulating soluble immune-complexes are deposited in glomeruli, where inflammation ensues. The inflammatory response is modulated by chemotactic factors of activated complement.

The kidneys appear enlarged and pale with occasional petechiae. Histologically, most glomeruli are involved by the disease (diffuse involvement) and show variable infiltration by polymorphonuclear leukocytes within capillaries. This exudative phase is followed by proliferation of mesangial cells and increases in the mesangial matrix that can be detected as eosinophilic, periodic acid-Schiff (PAS)-positive material (proliferative phase).

The center of glomerular lobules become enlarged, capillaries are compressed and pushed to the periphery and glomerular filtration decreases. Immunofluorescence studies show granular deposits of immunoglobulins and complement along glomerular capillary walls. Ultrastructurally, the glomeruli show a finding very characteristic of DPG (i.e., dense deposits or "humps" between the epithelial cells and the basement membrane). DPG has a good prognosis, 90 percent of children and 50–60 percent of adults with the disease recover. The other patients with DPG remain with slight disturbances in urine output or progress to renal failure.

Crescentic extracapillary glomerulonephritis (CG) is a less frequent form of acute glomerulonephritis (5 percent of cases) that affects patients older than those with DPG. It is characterized by a rapid progression to anuria and renal failure. The etiology is unknown but is probably viral. Approximately half the patients develop serum antibodies against basement membrane and may present with associated hemoptysis and pulmonary hemorrhages (Goodpasture's syndrome). Cross reaction between glomerular and alveolar basement membranes contributes to the combined renal and pulmonary damage. The kidneys in CG have glomeruli with large, cellular crescents in the Bowman's spaces composed of proliferating epithelial cells. These crescents compress the glomerular lobules and capillaries and are thought to be the result of fibrinous exudates into Bowman's spaces that stimulate epithelial proliferation. Glomeruli become fibrotic with a few weeks or months following the fibrinous exudation. Immunofluorescent studies are diagnostic, showing linear deposition of immunoglobulins, complement, and fibrinogen. Similar deposits may be found in pulmonary alveolar walls. Ultrastructurally, glomeruli breaks into glomerular basement membranes but there are no deposits.

Mesangiocapillary glomerulonephritis (MCG) is an unusual form of glomerulonephritis that presents with insidious onset of proteinuria, hematuria, hypertension, and the nephrotic syndrome. More than half the patients have low serum complement levels. The kidneys are large, smooth, or finely granular, and pale yellow. Histologically, the glomeruli are enlarged, and hypercellular, with increases in mesangial matrix. The lobules become thickened ("membranoproliferative"). The capillaries have a characteristic thickening of their walls with splitting of the basement membrane. They appear ultrastructurally as areas of mesangial ingrowth between the endothelium and basement membrane. In addition, there are subendothelial, mesangial, or intramembranous deposits. Immunofluorescent studies show granular deposits of complement in the periphery of glomerular lobules.

Chronic sclerosing glomerulonephritis (CSG) is the end result of a number of types of progressive glomerulonephritis. However, in only few instances is there a well documented history of a previous attack of acute glomerulonephritis. Most cases are probably the result of repeated episodes of subclinical glomerulonephritis. Patients with CSG present with nephrotic syndrome or renal failure with azotemia. Grossly the kidneys appear small, pale, and with granular surfaces. Histologically, most glomeruli are abnormal and exhibit distortion of glomerular lobules by fibrous adhesions, cellular proliferation, and fibrosis. The tubules are focally atrophic and blood vessels show all stages of arteriosclerosis.

Focal glomerulonephritis includes forms of glomerulonephritis characterized by the inflammatory involvement of only a certain number of glomeruli (focal) or portions of glomeruli (segmental). Focal glomerulonephritis can appear as a primary kidney disease, often following nonstreptococcal respiratory infections. Focal glomerulonephritis can also be the result of systemic diseases such as bacterial endocarditis, Schönlein-Henoch disease and Wegener's granulomatosis. Patients present with intermittent hematuria. Histologically, biopsies show focal mesangial and epithelial proliferation with thrombosis and/or necrosis. These changes are followed by sclerosis.

A special form of focal glomerulonephritis is Berger's disease (IgA disease). Glomeruli show focal proliferation. Immunofluorescent studies in Berger's disease, however, show diffuse deposits of IgA and IgG in the mesangium, seen as dense deposits on electron microscopy.

Lupus nephritis occurs in as many as 90 percent of kidneys, seen at autopsy in patients with systemic lupus erythematosus (SLE). The manifestations are due to the formation of immune complexes, including antigens such as native DNA. These immune complexes localize in multiple organs, including the kidneys and blood vessels. The renal manifestations vary from hematuria and mild proteinuria to renal insufficiency, with 20 percent of SLE patients presenting with the nephrotic syndrome.

The pathologic manifestations of SLE are also varied and include five types of glomerular lesions (i.e., minimal, mesangial, focal glomerulonephritis (GN), diffuse GN, and membranous GN) and even mixed types. Characteristic but infrequent findings include the fibrinoid thickening of capillary walls ("wire loops"), hematoxylin staining bodies (purple homogeneous clumps of nuclear material that are the tissue counterparts of LE cells in blood), and fibrinoid necrosis of arteries. Immunofluorescent studies show granular, often lumpy, deposits of immunoglobulins and complement along glomerular capillary walls and mesangium and the presence of immune complexes in wire loops.

Ultrastructurally, the characteristic features are (1) electron dense deposits between endothelial cells and the basement membrane corresponding to the wire loops seen on light microscopy, (2) mesangial and subepithelial deposits, and (3) tubuloreticular structures resembling myxoviruses in endothelial cells. The prognosis depends on the degree of renal involvement by the disease. Mild forms never pose a serious clinical problem, whereas, severe cases progress to renal failure.

Vascular Diseases of the Kidney

Essential hypertension is a very common condition, thought to be inherited, and characterized by diastolic pressures above 90 mm Hg in the absence of a specific hypertensogenic factor. Patients may have either benign or malignant nephrosclerosis.

Benign nephrosclerosis appears in older patients, many of whom have generalized arteriolosclerosis and diabetes mellitus. Blood pressure is moderately increased. Death generally results from congestive heart failure or a cerebrovascular accident, and seldom from significant renal disease. At autopsy, the kidneys are finely granular with linear v-shaped scars. Histologically, there is prominent arteriolonephrosclerosis, arterionephrosclerosis, thickening of glomerular Bowman's capsule, and focal tubular atrophy.

Malignant nephrosclerosis appears in younger individuals, especially males 30 to 50 years old. They present with diastolic pressures over 130 mm Hg, papilledema, hematuria, proteinuria, and renal failure. The kidneys are small and may be indistinguishable from chronic glomerulonephritis or chronic pyelonephritis. Histologically, there is a characteristic hyperplastic arteriosclerosis, consisting of onion-skin concentric thickening of the intima. There is also arteriolar fibrinoid necrosis with little inflammatory reaction and focal fibrinoid necrosis of glomeruli. Hyperplasia of juxtaglomerular apparatus may also be seen. Patients usually die from uremia and cardiovascular problems.

Secondary hypertension can be caused by renal diseases (pyelonephritis, SLE, polyarteritis nodosa, etc.), endocrine tumors (pheochromocytoma, cortical adenoma of adrenal glands, etc.), neurogenic disorders, coarctation of the aorta, etc. It can also be secondary to stenosis of the renal artery, generally due to arteriosclerosis in older patients, to intimal fibroplasia, or medial hyperplasia and fibroplasia, with aneurysms, in young women.

Renal infarcts, wedge-shaped necrotic zones, are common in the kidney and result from emboli, renal vein thrombosis, polyarteritis nodosa, sickle cell anemia, or malignant hypertension.

Renal cortical necrosis is thought to be mediated by vasomotor disturbances or by a Shwartzman reaction. Massive bilateral cortical necrosis with sparing of the renal medulla can be a complication of abruptio placentae, septicemia, peritonitis, burns, trauma, thrombocytopenic purpura, hemolytic uremic syndrome, and diethylene glycol poisoning.

Thrombotic microangiopathy is a manifestation of DIC. Intravascular coagulation and/or endothelial damage with thrombosis in the microcirculation of glomerular capillaries and other blood vessels is accompanied by microangiopathic hemolytic anemia with fragmentation of red cells and thrombocytopenia. This may be a complication of hemolytic uremic syndrome, thrombotic thrombocytopenic purpura, malignant hypertension, SLE, periarteritis nodosa, and scleroderma.

Renal vein thrombosis is an unusual cause of hemorrhagic infarcts of the kidney and the nephrotic syndrome. Renal vein thrombosis can be primary or secondary to inferior vena cava obstruction, or glomerulonephritis (membranous nephropathy, amyloidosis, etc.).

Vasculitis frequently affects renal blood vessels (Table 6-1).

Tubular Diseases of the Kidney

The renal tubules can undergo necrosis, degeneration (cloudy swelling, fatty degeneration, hyaline droplet degeneration, etc.) or atrophy in response to different injuries. Most commonly tubular disease is secondary to glomerular and vascular diseases which cause acute or chronic ischemia. It may also be secondary to toxic substances, which are concentrated in the tubules (e.g., heavy metals), accumulation of toxins, failure of extra-renal regulatory mechanisms (e.g., inappropriate antidiuretic hormone secretion), or congenital defects (renal glycosuria, cystinuria, Hartnup disease, vitamin D resistant rickets, nephrogenic diabetes insipidus, renal tubular acidosis, etc.).

Acute Renal Failure

Renal tubules may undergo acute tubular necrosis (ATN) manifested clinically by a marked decrease in urine production and uremia. The etiology of acute tubular necrosis can be prerenal (shock with marked decrease in renal blood supply), renal, and postrenal (obstruction in the lower urinary tract). Renal causes of acute renal failure include vascular obstruction (embolism), glomerular damage (acute glomerulonephritis), toxic injury to tubules (heavy metals, sulfurs), severe infections (malaria), etc. Histologically, there are necrotic tubules with hypereosinophilic cytoplasm and pyknotic nuclei, hemoglobin casts, focal rupture of basement membranes, and signs of epithelial regeneration, such as mitotic figures and the presence of double-nucleated tubular cells.

The mechanisms of oliguria are unclear. There may be mechanical tubular blocking by casts, nonselective reabsorption of glomerular filtrate through damaged cells or through breaks in the basement membrane, glomerular ischemia due to constriction of efferent arterioles, or decreased total renal blood flow.

Cystic Diseases of the Kidney

Cystic lesions may occur as congenital or developmental anomalies or as sporadic, acquired disorders. Renal cysts can be single or multiple and may appear in any age period. Renal cystic disease is classified by Potter's scheme, based on microdissection studies into four major types: (1) infantile polycystic disease, (2) adult type polycystic disease, (3) renal dysplasia, and (4) obstructive renal displasia.

Infantile polycystic disease differs in clinicopathologic manifestations depending on the age of the individual. In infants, the disease is inherited as an autosomal recessive disorder and is characterized by multiple, bilateral cysts in the kidney, liver (bile duct cysts), pancreas, and/or lung. The cysts are thought to represent tubular ectasia in the cortex and medulla, and are lined by cuboidal epithelium. The disease is usually fatal; anuria occurs during the neonatal period or early infancy. Infantile polycystic disease has a slightly better prognosis when it presents in childhood. Renal failure may occur but it is not present in all patients and children usually survive the manifestations of renal insufficiency or of hepatic fibrosis and portal hypertension until adolescence or, rarely, adult life.

Adult polycystic disease has no known etiology and is transmitted as an autosomal dominant disorder with high penetrance. Patients present with bilateral enlargement of the kidneys, due to multiple cysts in the cortex and medulla. One-third of patients have cysts in the liver and some individuals have associated cerebral artery aneurysms. Patients develop hypertension, cerebral hemorrhages, heart failure, or uremia. Average age at death is 50-years-old.

Renal dysplasia is a rare condition where abnormalities of parenchymal development result in the formation of unilateral or bilateral cysts accompanied by persistence of primitive structures derived from the uretic bud. Dysplastic kidneys vary in size and shape and usually have no normal landmarks. The pelvis and calyces are often absent, the ureter is hypoplastic and may have no lumen, and the blood supply is abnormal. Clinical manifestations depend on the degree of involvement (e.g., bilateral renal dysplasia is fatal).

Urinary tract infection (pyelonephritis). Urinary tract infections (UTI) are among the most common infections seen in clinical practice. Approximately 20 percent of women are affected by UTI at least once during their lifetime. Most instances of UTI are limited to the urinary bladder and urethra and, in the absence of renal anomalies, rarely result in severe renal impairment. In patients with renal anomalies, however, UTI is a significant cause of end stage kidney. Pyelonephritis affects the renal pelvis and parenchyma, and is due to an infectious agent. It should be distinguished from interstitial nephritis, an inflammatory process involving the renal interstitium and tubules. Interstitial nephritis is secondary to noninfectious conditions such as chemicals (e.g., methicillin, sulfonamides), radiation, and autoimmune disorders (e.g., systemic lupus erythematosus). Chronic interstitial nephritis can also appear as a hereditary condition or in certain geographic areas (e.g., Balkan nephropathy).

Bacteria can reach the kidney through hematogenous, or lymphatic routes. However, most intances of pyelonephritis are the result of ascending infections that extend

Table 6-1. Clinical, Histological, and Immunofluorescent Findings in Five Types of Systemic Necrotizing Angiitis

	Periarteritis Nodosa	Hypersensitivity Angiitis	Granulomatous Angiitis	Wegener Granulomatosis	Malignant Nephrosclerosis
Clinical Features					
Allergic history	Occasional	Frequent	Frequent	Rare	Rare
Preceding bacterial infections	Occasional	Occasional	Occasional	Always	Occasional
Initial events	Various (arthralgia, GI symptoms, renal failure)	Various (arthralgia, purpura, albuminuria)	Asthma, respiratory infections	Ulceration and necrosis in respiratory system	Hypertension, retinopathy, renal and cardiac failure
Hypertension	Frequent	Occasional	Occasional	Frequent	Always
Eosinophilia	Rare	Occasional	Frequent	Absent	Rare
Response to steroid	Occasional	Frequent	Frequent	Rare	?
Common cause of death	Uremia, congestive heart failure	Various	Cardiac failure, cerebral hemorrhage, uremia	Uremia	Uremia
Histological Features					
Type of vessels involved	Muscular arteries	Venules, arterioles, small arteries	Veins, arterioles, capillaries	Small artery and veins	Arterioles and arteries
Site of lesions	Mesentery, gastrointestinal tract, liver, gallbladder, kidney, pancreas, muscles, testis	All organs, skin, joints, muscles, kidney, heart, peripheral nerves	Lungs, cardiovascular system, skin	Upper and lower respiratory tract and kidney	Kidney, gastrointestinal tract, gallbladder, pancreas, adrenal
Stage of lesions	Acute and healing	Acute or healing	Acute or healing	Acute	Acute
Inflammatory reaction	Neutrophils	Neutrophils, eosinophils	Neutrophils, eosinophils, histiocytes	Neutrophils	None
Renal glomerular involvement	Frequent	Frequent	Frequent	Always	Always
Immunohistochemical Localization in Vessels of					
Immunoglobulins	Frequent	Frequent	Frequent	Negative	Frequent
Complement	Frequent	Frequent	Frequent	Negative	Frequent
Fibrinogen	Frequent	Occasional	Occasional	Frequent	Occasional

The antigen involved is not known in most cases. In some patients with periarteritis nodosa, Australia (HBsAG) in the serum, and mild hepatitis, Australia antigen, immunoglobulins, and complement have been demonstrated in the vessel wall.

In some form of vasculitis, bacterial antigens have localized in affected vessels.

from the lower urinary tract. Several factors favor the development of ascending UTI such as (1) urethral colonization by enteric bacteria, (2) instrumentation (catheter insertion, cystoscopy), (3) urethral trauma ("honeymoon" cystitis), (4) bladder wall abnormalities (fistula, invasive cancer, radiation necrosis of bladder, etc.), (5) urinary stasis (bladder atony, diverticula, extrinsic compression of bladder or ureters by tumors or fibrosis, neurogenic bladder, etc.), and (6) vesicoureteral reflux. Women are more prone to UTI than males because they have shorter urethrae and lack bacteriostatic prostatic secretions. Vesicoureteral reflux is a major factor. The normal ureter has a long segment within the bladder wall and the bladder muscle provides a competent functional valve during micturation, preventing reflux. However, in patients with ectopic ureters, ureterocele, abnormal implantation of the ureters, bladder tumors, or cystitis, this functional valve becomes inefficient, resulting in urinary reflux and migration of bacteria to the normally sterile upper urinary tract.

Conditions commonly associated with UTI are (1) diabetes mellitus, because of impaired antibacterial defense mechanisms, vascular damage to the kidney, glucosuria, autonomic neuropathy with bladder dysfunction, and frequent urethral catheterization, (2) pregnancy, because of dilation of the pelvis and ureter with reduced ureteral peristalsis, and mechanical compression of the bladder by the uterus, and (3) immune-deficiency states.

Acute pyelonephritis usually occurs in the presence of urinary obstruction (i.e., due to calculi). The kidneys are enlarged, congested, and have scattered, localized or confluent subcapsular cortical abscesses. The cortex and medulla also exhibit yellow streaks corresponding histologically to pus-filled tubules. The pelvic mucosa is markedly congested, has hemorrhagic foci, and is covered by inflammatory exudates. Histologically, tubules contain acute inflammatory infiltrates which may extend to the interstitium with microabscess formation. Glomeruli, arterioles and arteries are resistant to infection. Severe acute pyelonephritis can progress to perirenal abscess, usually in cases due to *Staphylococcus aureus* infection, generalized sepsis, and pyonephrosis, a condition where the pelvis is transformed into a dilated pus-filled cavity. Acute papillary necrosis may also develop.

Papillary necrosis is a serious renal condition characterized by necrosis of the distal portions of the renal papilla, associated with diabetes mellitus, phenacetin abuse, urinary tract obstruction, and sickle cell anemia. The necrotic papilla appear yellow or gray-red and may be sloughed off and passed into the urine. Necrotic areas may become calcified.

Chronic pyelonephritis can follow acute pyelonephri-

tis. More often, however, it presents as renal failure, proteinuria, or hypertension. The kidneys are small, with irregularly scarred surfaces, containing coarse, broad, u-shaped cortical scars. The corticomedullary junctions are blurred and the papilla are blunted, retracted, and distorted. The pelvic mucosa is dull and granular. Histologically, there is periglomerular fibrosis which may progress to global sclerosis. The most important findings are in the pelvis (chronic inflammation), blood vessels (medial and intimal thickening), interstitium (focal scars with chronic inflammation in subcapsular areas), and tubules (atrophy resembling thyroid tissue, the so-called thyroidization). Rarely chronic pyelonephritis is secondary to tuberculosis or fungal disorders such as candidiasis, histoplasmosis, mucormycosis, and others.

Tumors of the Kidney

The kidney can be the site of benign and malignant tumors of epithelial or mesenchymal origin. Epithelial tumors can arise from renal tubules or from the pelvic (transitional) epithelium.

Renal cell carcinoma (hypernephroma) is the most common carcinoma in adults, especially in males over 40 years. Patients present with varied clinical manifestations such as hematuria, costovertebral pain, weight loss, and erythrocytosis. Often, however, the initial manifestation of the disease is related to a metastasis to the lung, bone, brain, or liver. Hypernephroma has been called the "great simulator." Macroscopically, hypernephromas are large, well circumscribed, yellow-brown tumors that tend to infiltrate the renal capsule and invade the renal vein. They can be very hemorrhagic. Microscopically, they consist of nests, trabeculae, and papillary structures with clear or oncocytic (eosinophilic, granular) cuboidal cells. Those cells exhibit only moderate degrees of pleomorphism in most instances, but occasionally undergo dedifferentiation and appear as spindle cell pseudosarcomas. Hypernephromas disseminate hematogenously. Lymphatic spread is less frequent.

Renal cell adenoma is usually detected incidentally at autopsy or in kidneys removed for other reasons. They are round, yellow, renal cortical nodules, usually smaller than 2–3 cm. Histologically, they are identical to well differentiated hypernephromas and can be distinguished only on the basis of their small size.

Wilms' tumor (nephroblastoma), the most common renal tumor in infants and the most common malignant tumor in infants and young children, presents as hematuria, large abdominal mass, and pain. Wilms' tumor is composed of renal epithelium which abnormally recapitulates different stages of development of the nephrons and collecting systems. Histologically, these abortive epithelial structures appear as abnormal glomeruli, tubules, and solid cords of immature renal epithelium. Nephroblastomas also show malignant proliferation of the renal stroma. Sarcomatous elements, such as striated muscle fibers (rhabdomyosarcoma), cartilage (chondrosarcoma), spindle cells, and small round cells appear admixed with epithelial elements. The proportion of epithelial to stromal elements is extremely variable. Wilms' tumors are very aggressive and disseminate rapidly through the bloodstream to the lungs, brain, bone, liver, and other organs. A rare variant of nephroblastoma, congenital mesoblastic nephroma, in newborns and infants, usually behaves in a benign fashion.

Stromal tumors of the kidney include angiomas, lipomas, myomas, or fibromas. These elements can appear in one neoplasm or as angiomyolipoma, which occurs more frequently in patients with tuberous sclerosis. Malignant stromal tumors, such as angiosarcoma, rhabdomyosarcoma, and liposarcoma have also been described.

Surface tumors of the urinary passages arise from the transitional cell epithelium lining the renal pelvis, ureters, urinary bladder, and urethra. They are often multicentric. The transitional cell epithelium undergoes hyperplasia and squamous metaplasia in response to carcinogens such as occupational exposure to β-naphtylamine, tobacco smoke, and other mechanical irritation (i.e., chronic inflammation and schistosomiasis). Transitional cell neoplasms present with painless hematuria and are more frequent in males older than 40 years. They appear as benign papillomas, as malignant papillary transitional cell carcinomas, or as flat ulcerating lesions composed of pleomorphic cells arranged in trabeculae. Flat, ulcerating carcinomas are more aggressive.

Transitional cell carcinomas behave biologically according to their histologic degree of differentiation and their clinical stage, as determined by the extent of tumor, depth of infiltration of the wall, and presence of metastasis. Well differentiated papillary carcinomas, limited to the surface epithelium, have a good prognosis and, although they can recur locally, they rarely metastasize. Poorly differentiated tumors extend through the muscular layer of the bladder or ureter, tend to disseminate through lymphatic spread, and metastasize to the liver and lungs.

MALE GENITOURINARY TRACT

Diseases of the Testis

A number of congenital anomalies of the testis occur, including variations in number, position, and morphology. Rarely, both testes are absent (anorchidism). The patients are phenotypically female, the penis is poorly developed, the serum 16-ketosteroids are low, and gonadotropins are elevated. More frequently, one testis is absent (monorchidism) and the penis, prostate, and other genital organs are normal, hypoplastic, or absent. There may be more than two testes (polyorchidism). The extra gonad may be in the scrotum, in the inguinal canal, mesentery, or retroperitoneum, and give rise to a testicular tumor.

Variations in the position are more frequent. Undescended testes are present in 4 percent of full term infants and 33 percent of prematures. The right testis is more likely to remain ectopic (cryptorchidism) and can be arrested in the abdomen (15 percent), inguinal canal (60 percent), and superficial inguinal area (25 percent). The mechanism is unknown, but may be due to inherent abnormalities of the gonad, hormonal insufficiency, or mechanical interference with descent.

Testicular maldevelopment or hypogonadism can be the result of chromosomal abnormalities or appear as dysgenesis of unknown etiology. Klinefelter's syndrome is an example of testicular hypogonadism associated with the presence of a supernumerary X chromosome (XXY pattern). Young men with this syndrome present with infertility, azoospermia, eunochoidism, small firm testes, gynecomastia, subnormal intelligence, and elevated serum levels of gonadotropins. Buccal smears show cells with Barr bodies indicating two X chromosomes. Ullrich-Turner's syndrome is an example of dysgenesis of unknown etiology. Male patients present with short stature, webbed neck, low set ears, shieldlike chest, cryptorchidism with decreased spermatogenesis, ocular and cardiovascular anomalies, mental retardation, gynecomastia, and variable lymphedema. Only 20 percent of these patients have sex chromosome abnormalities.

Hermaphroditism is the presence of ovarian and testicular tissue in the same individual. This unusual condition can have male or female phenotypic manifestations. Pseudohermaphroditism is a more common condition. The external genital organs of a patient resemble those of the opposite sex. This syndrome results from hormonal abnormalities that stimulate an abnormal development of external genitalia. Chromosomal studies, however, reveal the true sex of the patient. An example is testicular feminization syndrome characterized by male chromosomes, poorly formed testes located in the abdominal cavity or inguinal canal, and external female characteristics (enlarged clitoris, gynecomastia). This syndrome is thought to be related to Leydig's cell abnormalities.

Acquired gonadal insufficiency, with or without impotence, can be the result of irradiation, toxic injury (chemotherapy for the treatment of malignant diseases), estrogen therapy, chronic liver disease (cirrhosis) pituitary insufficiency, Addison's disease, myxedema, vascular insufficiency, neurogenic, myotonia dystrophica, chronic inflammation (mumps), diabetes mellitus, etc. Acquired gonadal insufficiency can also be idiopathic.

INFLAMMATORY CONDITIONS OF THE TESTIS

Orchitis may be the result of nonspecific spread of bacterial infections from the lower genitourinary system or from septicemia. It can also be secondary to viral infections such as mumps. Orchitis appears in 20–30 percent of adult males with mumps, but is unusual in children with the disease. Testes are tender and swollen with marked edema, mononuclear infiltrates, and epithelial damage. Rarely, mumps orchitis result in infertility. Orchitis can also be secondary to syphilis and tuberculosis.

Tumors of the testis. The testis can be the site of origin of numerous benign and malignant epithelial and mesenchymal tumors. These neoplasms are relatively infrequent (0.5 percent of all malignant tumors in males) but are important because they are usually malignant and affect young males. The different histologic types of testicular tumors are the following:

> Germ cell tumors
> > Seminoma
> > Embryonal cell carcinoma
> > Endodermal sinus tumor (yolk sac tumor)
> > Teratoma
> > Choriocarcinoma
> Nongerminal tumors
> > Interstitial Leydig's cell tumors
> > Sertoli's cell tumors
> Connective tissue tumors
> > Fibromas, leiomyomas, rhabdomyomas, sarcomas
> Lymphoid tumors
> Metastatic
> > Prostate, lung, malignant melanoma

Germ cell tumors comprise 90–95 percent of testicular tumors and are invariably malignant. They include seminomas, embryonal cell carcinomas, teratomas, choriocarcinoma, and combined tumors showing more than one histologic pattern. Seminomas are the most frequent histologic variant of germ cell tumors of the testis (40–50 percent of cases). They appear as solid, firm, gray-white, irregularly lobulated nodules in 30 to 50-year-old males. Histologically, they are composed of large, round cells with a central spherical nucleus organized into cords, alveolar groups, or sheets. Seminomas

disseminate through lymphatic route, and can metastasize to the lungs. However, 80 percent of patients with seminoma survive 5 years following surgical ablation and radiotherapy. Other histologic variants of germ cell tumors of the testis are (1) embryonal cell carcinoma (20 percent of germ cell tumors, affects patients younger than 30-years-old), (2) endodermal sinus tumor (yolk sac tumor), a variant of embryonal cell carcinoma that predominates in infants, (3) teratoma, composed of tissues derived embryologically from more than one germ layer, and (4) choriocarcinoma. These tumors are highly malignant, disseminate hematogenously, and metastasize to the lungs and other organs. Germ cell tumors are frequently accompanied by the presence of biochemical tumor markers in serum. For example, embryonal cell carcinoma is accompanied by elevated serum levels of α-fetoprotein, and choriocarcinoma by elevated levels of gonadotropins. Serum cell tumors can be treated successfully with modern chemotherapeutic drugs and serial measurement of the serum levels of these serum markers is useful to follow the progress of the disease.

Diseases of the Epididymis and Spermatic Cord

Epididymal and spermatic cord conditions are (1) cysts (appendix epididymis, hydatid of Morgagni) that are rarely important clinically, (2) spermatocele (cyst containing spermatozoa, often the result of chronic inflammation and fibrosis), (3) acute infections (epididymitis, frequently secondary to gonorrhea, tuberculosis, or syphilis, and filarial infections), (4) torsion, (5) varicocele (varicosity of veins of pampiniform plexus), and (6) tumors, adenomatoid (benign small fibrous tumor of mesothelial origin), adenoma, adenocarcinoma, lipomas, myxoma, etc.

Diseases of the Penis

Penile disorders include syphilitic lesions (primary chancre), phimosis (inadequate preputial orifice that fails to permit retraction of prepuce over glans), hypospadias (imperfect closure of urethral groove with abnormal urethral opening along the undersurface of the penis), Peyronie's disease (a fibrositis involving Buck's fascia and resulting in scarring with painful curvature of the penis on erection), and tumors (usually squamous cell carcinoma).

Diseases of the Prostate

The prostate can be affected by inflammatory conditions (prostatitis), hyperplasia, and carcinoma. Acute and chronic prostatitis may follow instrumentation or

PATHOLOGY

local surgery or be secondary to granulomatous infections such as tuberculosis.

Nodular (fibroadenomatoid) hyperplasia of the prostate is a common process that affects older males. The gland becomes enlarged and nodular and compresses the urinary bladder causing urinary obstruction. Nodular hyperplasia is most likely due to endocrine stimulation. Histologically, there is hyperplasia of smooth muscle and prostatic glands that often have a papillary lining.

Prostatic carcinoma is a very common malignancy in the elderly male. Most cases, however, are found incidentally at autopsy or at surgery for removal of fibromuscular adenomatous prostatic tissue. Carcinomas are more common in the posterior lobe of the prostate where they appear as hard, irregular nodules. They are often yellow and may extend locally into the seminal vesicles, urethra, and bladder. They also can metastasize widely and give osteoblastic bone metastasis. Patients are treated with surgery and hormonal therapy (orchiectomy, estrogens).

PITUITARY GLAND

Inflammatory conditions can affect the pituitary. The anterior lobe may be acutely inflamed as a result of septicemia or by direct spread from neighboring structures such as the meninges or sinuses. It can also be the site of chronic inflammation in patients with sarcoidosis, tuberculosis, syphilis (congenital and gummatous), mycotic infections, and autoimmune disorders (e.g., lymphocytic autoimmune hypophysitis in patients with Hashimoto's thyroiditis, autoimmune adrenalitis, etc.).

Vascular Disturbances

The pituitary can undergo vascular disturbances. Hemorrhage and infarction may be due to trauma, cerebrovascular accidents, or tumors. Rarely, the gland suffers massive postpartum necrosis with acute hypofunction after severe hemorrhage at parturition (Sheehan's syndrome). If the patient survives, the gland undergoes scarring with chronic pituitary insufficiency (Simmonds' disease).

Infiltrations and metabolic disorders, including amyloidosis, Hunter-Hurler syndrome (mucopolysaccharidosis), and Hand-Schüller Christian disease may affect the pituitary.

Empty sella syndrome is a rare cause of pituitary insufficiency related to the effects of increased intracranial pressure transmitted via the diaphragma sellae. It may also follow therapeutic ablation of the gland.

Benign and malignant tumors can arise from the pituitary and appear clinically with symptoms related to: 1 the presence of hormonal insufficiency or hyperfunction, 2 pressure on adjacent structures (optic atrophy), and 3 increased intracranial pressure (headache, vomiting, papilledema). Tumors of the pituitary include the following:

Tumors arising in developmental rests or anomalies
    Parapituitary epithelial residues
    Rathke's pouch cysts
    Craniopharyngioma
Glandular neoplasms
    Chromophobe adenoma
    Acidophil adenoma
    Basophil adenoma
    Pluriglandular adenomatosis
Secondary neoplasms
    Metastatic tumors from lung, breast, etc.

Craniopharyngioma, a benign tumor arising from displaced remnants of embryonic hypophyseal duct, occurs in childhood and adolescence, and usually presents as a solid or cystic tumor in the suprasellar region and causes ocular disturbances due to optic chiasm compression. It consists of islands of squamous cells resembling primitive tooth structures and is usually calcified.

Chromophobe adenoma is the most frequent pituitary tumor (65 percent of tumors). It occurs in adults 30 to 50 yers of age and varies from small tumors found incidentally at autopsy to large nodules that compress the normal gland and cause hypogonadism.

Acidophil adenomas are less frequent (30 percent of pituitary tumors) and are usually confined to the sella turcica. Patients present with acromegaly or gigantism due to hypersecretion of growth hormone and galactorrhea due to prolactin secretion.

Basophil adenomas are associated with Cushing's syndrome due to hypersecretion of ACTH. They may appear after adrenalectomy (Nelson's syndrome – increased ACTH and prolactin production, and hyperpigmentation of the skin).

FEMALE GENITAL TRACT

Congenital anomalies of the vulva are related to chromosomal sex aberrations and hormonal abnormalities. The most frequent abnormality is clitoral hypertrophy usually secondary to congenital adrenal hyperlasia.

The vulva can present with different inflammatory conditions usually infectious in nature including venereal bacterial diseases such as gonococcal infection of the vulva, vagina and Bartholin's gland, syphilis, granuloma inguinale, lymphogranuloma venereum, and chancroid. Viral infections of the vulva are becoming more frequent. Indeed herpes simplex type 2 infection is the most common cause of external genital infection affecting 30–40 percent of the female population. Patients have vulvar vesicles, ulcerations, edema, and lymphadenopathy. Histologic study demonstrates typical intranuclear inclusions in epithelial cells and multinucleated cells. Serum titers for specific antibodies are elevated. Other viral disorders, such as condyloma accuminatum and molluscum cotagiosum as well as fungi (*Candida species*) and parasites (trichomonas) can also infect the vulva.

A variety of skin diseases such as Behcet's syndrome, Fox-Fordyce disease (hidradenitis suppurativa), and benign pemphigus may affect the vulva.

Leukoplakia is a descriptive term for a variety of conditions affecting the vulva and other mucosal surfaces. Characterized by white plaques, leukoplakia may be due to vitiligo, scarring with hyperkeratosis, lichen sclerosus et atrophicus (kraurosis vulvae), and epithelial dysplasia. The latter is usually premalignant.

Neoplasms of the vulva can be benign, such as Bartholin's gland cysts, fibromas, angiomas, granular cell tumors, and hidradenomas, or malignant, such as Bowen's disease, extramammary Paget's disease, squamous cell carcinoma, adenocarcinoma of Bartholin's gland or minor vestibular glands, and malignant melanoma. The vulva can also be infiltrated by sarcomas and metastatic lesions including uterine and cervical malignancies, choriocarcinoma, and ovarian tumors.

Squamous cell carcinoma is the most common malignant tumor of the vulvar representing approximately 4 percent of all female genital malignancies, and occurs in postmenopausal women. Squamous cell carcinoma presents as nodular or ulcerated lesions with elevated margins, most often in the anterior $\frac{2}{3}$ of the vulva. Histologically, these tumors are usually well differentiated and produce keratin, but may be poorly differentiated or exhibit glandular formation (adenosquamous carcinoma). Adjacent vulvar skin frequently shows other lesions such as dysplasia and/or carcinoma in situ. Spread is lymphatic with metastasis to inguinal and femoral lymph nodes.

The Vagina

Inflammatory conditions include gonoccocal vaginitis, a form of vaginitis that occurs in children and postmenopausal women in which the vaginal epithelium is thin and immature. Adult vaginal mucosa is resistant to this infection because the mature epithelium is thick stratified squamous and because the acid pH of vaginal secretions impairs the growth of the microorganisms. Hemophilus vaginitis is the most common etiologic agent of nonspecific sexually transmitted vaginitis. Vaginal smears show characteristic "clue cells" containing numerous intracytoplasmic gram-negative bacilli. Trichomonas vaginalis is another common etiologic agent of vaginitis and affects about $\frac{2}{3}$ of pregnant women. It is sexually transmitted and presents clinically with a typical green-yellow foamy discharge. Candidiasis is frequent in diabetics and postmenopausal women, and is characterized by pruritus and white discharge. Herpes simplex virus can also infect the vagina.

Neoplasms can be benign (congenital cysts of Gardner's duct, fibroepithelial polyps, fibroleiomyoma, and granular cell tumor) or malignant (squamous cell carcinoma, embryonal rhabdomyosarcoma, clear cell carcinoma and metastatic lesions from the cervix, uterine corpus, colony, urinry bladder, and other primary sites).

Squamous cell carcinoma is the most common primary vaginal malignancy (95 percent of cases) and presents with ulcerating, infiltrating lesions, most often in the upper third. Embryonal cell rhabdomyosarcoma is a disease of children and adolescents and presents as nodular or papillary masses, usually in the anterior wall. It has a very poor prognosis.

DES-related changes occur in daughters of women given diethylstilbesterol (DES) for threatened abortion, 15 to 30 years after the administration and transplacental passage. Pathologic abnormalities include vaginal adenosis (presence of abnormal glandular epithelium in the squamous epithelium of the vagina) and clear cell carcinoma of the vagina and/or cervix. It is not yet clear whether women exposed in utero to DES also have higher incidences of other genital malignancies such as squamous cell carcinoma of the uterine cervix or endometrial carcinoma.

Uterine Cervix

Congenital anomalies include hypoplasia, duplication and stenosis of the cervical os, and are often associated with other genital tract anomalies.

Cervicitis is the most frequent disorder affecting the uterine cervix. It can be acute or chronic, is almost invariably associated with vaginitis, and presents as leucorrhea (white discharge). Cervicitis can be due to specific pathogens such as bacteria (gonorrhea, syphilis, chancroid, tuberculosis), fungi (candidiasis), viruses (herpes), and others (chlamydial, helminthic, mycoplasmal). Frequently, however, the etiology remains unknown. This is more frequent in pregnancy, after gynecological instrumentation, and in patients with hormonal imbalances (hypoestrinism, steroid therapy, anticontraceptive pill usage).

Cervical polyps are protrusions of the endocervical mucosa that usually follow chronic cervicitis. They are not true neoplasms and may produce irregular vaginal bleeding.

The most important neoplasm is invasive squamous cell carcinoma, a highly malignant disease that has declined in frequency in the United States in the past 3 decades, due to its early detection and treatment. Its histogenesis is of great interest.

The junctional area between the endocervical columnar epithelium and the exocervical squamous epithelium is a site of competitive growth during the reproductive years. Eversion of the columnar epithelium into the exocervix is a common phenomenon followed by squamous metaplasia, necessary to protect the tissues from the acid pH of the vaginal secretions. Squamous metaplasia of endocervical epithelium can also follow chronic cervicitis of various etiologies. The metaplastic squamous epithelium can undergo abnormal growth changes and become dysplastic. Dysplastic epithelium is characterized cytologically by cells growing in a disorganized pattern. The severity of dysplasia may be mild to severe. Severe dysplasia can progress to a frank carcinoma in situ (CIS) of the cervix, and ultimately to invasive carcinoma. The histogenetic progression of dysplasia to CIS has become controversial, as pathologists have not always been able to distinguish accurately between severe dysplasia and CIS. This has led to the concept that the epithelium undergoes progressive changes of abnormal growth (cervical intraepithelial neoplasia or CIN). According to the concept of CIN, the abnormal growth patterns vary from that showing a few dyskeratotic epithelial cells in the epithelial layers close to the basement membrane (CIN I) to completely disorganized epithelium suggesting an in situ neoplasm (CIN III). The CIN concept considers that the natural history of the precursor stages of cervical carcinoma includes a spectrum of intraepithelial lesions that begin as a well differentiated intraepithelial neoplasia and end with invasive carcinoma.

The etiologic factors involved in these changes are under intense investigation. Associations include cervicitis, herpes simplex type 2 infections, a history of early sexual intercourse with multiple partners and multiple pregnancies, and low socioeconomic status. Jewish and Moslem women and nuns are rarely affected. The viral genome is present in the nucleus of cervical epithelial cells and may induce DNA mutations leading to malignant growth of the infected cells.

Carcinoma in situ (CIN III) progresses to invasive carcinoma in many instances. Malignant cells break through the epithelial basement membrane and infiltrate the underlying stroma. It has been demonstrated that lesions with early invasion (less than 1 – 2 mm in thickness, microinvasive) have a better prognosis than those with further tissue extension.

Infiltrating squamous carcinoma consists of ulcerating, infiltrative or fungating masses composed histologically of keratinizing or nonkeratinizing squamous cells. This tumor infiltrates locally to involve structures including the bladder rectum, and pelvic wall, and frequently metastasizes to the parametrial paracervical, hypogastric, obturator, and external iliac lymph nodes. Hematogenous spread may also occur and distant metastasis are present in 40 percent of patients at autopsy. The prognosis is closely related to the stage with 100 percent survival after simple hysterectomy. Lesions confined to the cervix (stage I) have an 80 – 90 percent 5 year survival after radical hysterectomy. Lesions infiltrating the parametrium and/or upper vagina (stage II), pelvic wall or lower third of the vagina (stage III), or extending into the pelvic wall or other pelvic organs (stage IV) have progressively worse prognosis. Death is most often due to urinary infections and renal failure from urinary tract obstruction because of extension to the bladder and ureters.

Papillary or glandular adenocarcinomas of the cervix are less frequent (5 percent). They may, however, grow undetected and have a worse prognosis than squamous cell carcinoma.

Benign neoplasms include condyloma acuminatum (venereal wart) and papilloma, a lesion of mature squamous epithelium. Mesenchymal tumors, such as leiomyomas, also occur.

Uterine Corpus

The uterine corpus may be affected by endometrial and/or myometrial disorders.

Functional abnormalities of the endometrium are common. Menorrhagia (abnormal endometrial bleeding) is one of the most frequent gynecologic signs of disease and is usually due to abnormalities in the ovulatory cycle. Following anovulatory cycles the endometrium grows in the proliferative phase unopposed by progesterone and exhibits pathologic changes including cystic hyperplasia, polyp formation, and adenomatous hyperplasia. These changes reverse after ovulation or when the patient is treated with progesterone.

Inflammatory conditions of the endometrium are unusual because of the periodic shedding of the endometrium. Acute endometritis, usually due to Streptococcal or staphylococcal infections, follows delivery or abortion. Chronic endometritis is usually due to mycoplasma, chlamydia, or other infections (i.e., tuberculosis, brucellosis, etc.).

Benign endometrial tumors are uncommon; most are malignant and epithelial (adenocarcinoma).

Endometrial adenocarcinoma has increased in incidence during the last decades. It affects most frequently postmenopausal women that are nulliparous, obese, and/or diabetic. The development of endometrial adenocarcinoma appears to be endocrine-related. Women with estrogen producing ovarian tumors, adrenocortical hyplerplasia, longstanding anovulatory cycles causing hyperplastic endometrium, and those who received prolonged estrogen therapy are at highest risk. Over the course of several years the endometrium undergoes proliferative and hyperplastic changes when exposed to unopposed estrogenic stimulation. The endometria become hyperplastic and cystic (cystic hyperplasia, "swiss-cheese" pattern) and later on develop adenomatous hyperplasia with epithelial proliferation and nuclear crowding with pluristratification. Endometrial glands and atypical adenomatous hyperplasia, with cellular atypia then develops. This premalignant condition is frequently followed by adenocarcinoma.

Endometrial adenocarcinoma presents as a polypoid, superficially spreading or ulcerating mass that frequently infiltrates the uterine wall. The histologic patterns range from well differentiated endometrial glands with papillary structures to anaplastic sheets of undifferentiated tumor cells. The tumor infiltrates the cervix and then the pelvis and metastasizes to regional lymph nodes. Staging is important for the management of patients: stage 0: Carcinoma in situ, stage 1: Carcinoma confined to the uterine corpus, stage 2: Carcinoma involving the cervix, stage 3: Carcinoma growing beyond the uterus but within the pelvis, and stage 4: Carcinoma that extends beyond the pelvis or into the bladder and/or rectal wall.

Infrequently, the endometrium is involved by sarcomas or by malignant tumors composed of epithelial and mesenchymal elements; mixed mesodermal or mixed mullerian tumors. The latter neoplasm contains, in addition to malignant glands, a variety of sarcomatous elements including rhabdomyosarcoma, osteosarcoma, chondrosarcoma, and fibrosarcoma. Mixed mullerian tumors are usually polypoid, affect women in the fifth to sixth decades, and have a very poor prognosis.

Leiomyoma (fibroleiomyoma, fibroid) of the myometrium is the most common tumor in females and affects about 40 percent of women over 35-years-old. It is more common in black women and its growth is estrogen dependent. For example, leiomyomas increase in frequency and size during pregnancy while they involute after the menopause. Leiomyomas present as well circumscribed, nonencapsulated firm nodules with a whorled appearance on section. They can be in the uterine wall (intramural) or protrude into the endometrial cavity (submucosal) or the peritoneum (subserosal). They may undergo degenerative changes including hyalinization, necrosis, calcification, and cystic change. They seldom become malignant.

Adenomyosis (endometriosis interna) is characterized by the presence of endometrial tissue (glands and stroma) in the thickened myometrium. Adenomyosis may be associated with endometriosis at other sites (ovaries, pelvis, etc.). The glands in adenomyosis, however, usually do not undergo cyclic menstruation changes, as they are not hormone responsive.

Endolymphatic stromal myosis is an unusual disease characterized by the presence of islands of endometrial stroma growing into lymphatic vessels and the myometrium. Endolymphatic stromal myosis has a low grade malignant potential.

Leiomyosarcoma is the malignant counterpart of leiomyoma. Most leiomyosarcomas, however arise *de novo* and not from a preexistent myoma. These sarcomas are highly malignant neoplasms that metastasize through the blood stream into the lungs and other organs.

Fallopian Tubes

Inflammatory conditions may follow a variety of etiologic factors. Acute salpingitis is secondary to infections by Neiserria gonorrhoea. Streptococci, mycoplasma, chlamydia, cocksackie B group virus, and fungi. Chronic salpingitis may be due to any of these agents, but most often follow gonorrheal and mycoplasmal infections. It can result from tuberculosis, dissemination through the hematogenous route from the lungs, actinomycosis, schistosomiasis, Crohn's disease, and sarcoidosis. Chronic salpingitis often results in sterility or ectopic pregnancy. Sequelae include mucosal fold adhesions, distorsion of the lumen, adhesions to other pelvic organs (pelvic inflammatory disease), pyosalpinx (distension by purulent material), and hydrosalpinx (distension by clear fluid after resorption of pus).

Primary neoplasms of the fallopian tubes are infrequent and include adenomatoid tumors and benign tumors of mesothelial origin and tubal adenocarcinoma. The fallopian tubes are more frequently involved by metastatic tumors, usually from the ovary or endometrium.

Ovaries

Diseases of ovarian development include (1) gonadal agencies (dysgenesis) or Turner's syndrome, a disorder with karyotypic (45 chromosomes XO or mosaicism with 45/46, 45/47, XO/XY or XO/XX), phenotypic (streak gonads with absent germ cells, infantile uterus and external genitalia) and somatic abnormalities (short stature, webbed neck, cardiac malformations); (2) testicular feminization syndrome, a disorder in which the karyotype is 46 XY (male) but in which the patient has phenotypic characteristics of a female due to a yet undefined androgen insensitivity; patients have immature testes and lack ovaries and female internal genitalia, they have, however, a small vagina and hypoplastic vulva; and (3) true hermaphroditism, characterized by the presence of both ovarian and testicular tissue in a patient that usually has ambiguous external genitalia. The karyotype is 46 XX in 50 percent of instances and exhibits mosaicism in the others. The testis and ovaries can be separate or combined into one structure (ovotestis).

Neoplastic ovarian cysts are quite common. Follicular cyst is an abnormal enlargement of a graafian follicle due to the accumulation of fluid in its cavity. Cysts, may be multiple (polycystic ovaries) in patients with anovulatory cycles and amenorrhea (Stein-Leventhal syndrome). Lutein cysts can be single or multiple and result from the resorption of blood from the center of a corpus luteum. Multiple lutein cysts are usually secondary to excess gonadotropin secretion of placental or tumoral origin (hydatidiform mole, choriocarcinoma).

Endometriosis of the ovary frequently appears as single or multiple dark-blue cysts filled with dark brown tenacious material (chocolate cyst), frequently associated with endometriosis in the fallopian tubes, pelvis, and other organs. The ectopic endometrial glands and stroma undergo cyclic changes with menstruation.

The ovary tumors may be benign, of borderline malignancy, and malignant, and may be of epithelial or mesenchymal origin (Table 6-2). They are generally classified according to their presumed histologic and biologic behavior. The concept of "borderline" malignancy

refers to ovarian neoplasms that are capable of local recurrence and extension into the peritoneal cavity, without distant metastasis. Borderline tumors have prognosis intermediate between benign and frankly malignant neoplasms.

Serous cystadenoma is a frequent (23 percent of cases) benign ovarian neoplasm that occurs in young women, is bilateral in 20 percent and consists of uni- or multilocular cysts lined by columnar epithelium, sometimes with papillary projections and psammoma bodies (laminated calcified structures). Occasionally the epithelial component is combined with fibrous proliferation (cystadenofibroma).

Mucinous cystadenoma accounts for 20 percent of benign ovarian tumors and occurs in women in the fourth to fifth decade, is bilateral in 5 percent, and is composed of multilocular cysts lined by mucinous epithelium of intestinal or endocervical type. Rupture of these cystic tumors may produce peritoneal dissemination and ongoing proliferation (pseudomyxoma peritonei).

Brenner tumor is a benign neoplasm of young women that presents as a solid, white, unilateral nodule, usually asymptomatic. These tumors are composed of nests of epithelial cells resembling transitional epithelium. They may rarely undergo malignant transformation.

Sex cord tumors are infrequent (5 percent of ovarian tumors) and are derived from the specialized stroma of the genital ridge. These tumors can be hormonally active and present with manifestations of hypertrinism or hy-

Table 6-2. Neoplasms of the Ovary

Origin	Benign	Borderline	Malignant
Germinal epithelium	Serous cystadenoma	Serous papillary cystadenoma, borderline	Papillary cystadenocarcinoma
	Papillary cystadenofibroma		
	Mucinous cystadenoma	Mucinous cystadenoma, borderline	Mucinous cystadenocarcinoma
	Endometrioma		Endometrioid carcinoma
			Clear cell carcinoma
	Brenner tumor	Proliferating Brenner tumor	Malignant Brenner tumor
			Anaplastic carcinoma
Sex cord stroma	Fibromathecoma		Granulosa cell tumor (low malignancy)
			Granulosa-theca cell tumor
			Sertoli-Leydig cell tumor
	Hilus cell tumor		
Germ cells	Benign cystic teratoma (dermoid cyst)		Dysgerminoma
			Teratocarcinoma
			Embryonal cell carcinoma
			Choriocarcinoma
Metastatic			Krukenberg tumor
			Malignant lymphoma
			Burkitt's lymphoma
			Others

perandrogenism. Neoplasms in this category include granulosa cell tumor, an estrogen producing ovarian neoplasm of low malignant potential; fibromathecoma, a benign tumor occasionally associated with pleural effusion (Meig's syndrome); and arrhenoblastoma (Sertoli-Leidig cell tumor), a tumor that may be associated with virilization and hilus cell tumor.

Papillary serous cystadenocarcinoma is the most frequent (40 percent of cases) malignant ovarian neoplasm. Bilateral in 50 percent, these tumors are composed of solid and cystic areas with solid sheets of anaplastic columnar cells. They metastasize widely through the peritoneal cavity and may have lymphatic and hematogenous spread. Prognosis is related to the degree of histologic differentiation and to the clinical stage.

The staging system of ovarian tumors recommended by the International Federation of Gynecology-Obstetrics (IFGO) is the following:

    Stage I: Growth limited to ovaries
        One ovary, no ascites
        Both ovaries, no ascites
        One or both ovaries with malignant ascites
    Stage II: Growth involving one or both ovaries and the pelvis
        Uterus, fallopian tube, other genital organs
        Other pelvic organs
    Stage III: One or both ovaries with widespread intraperitoneal metastases
    Stage IV: One or both ovaries with distant metastases

Mucinous cystadencarcinoma represents 3–10 percent of ovarian malignancies, is frequently bilateral, and is composed of mucin producing cells.

Endometrioid carcinoma accounts for 20 percent of ovarian malignancies and is composed of solid and cystic areas containing cells identical to those of endometrial adenocarcinoma, sometimes mixed with benign squamous epithelium (adenocanthoma) or malignant squamous cell carcinoma (adenosquamous carcinoma).

Germ cell tumors are derived from primitive germ cells. They include dysgerminoma, the female counterpart of seminoma; benign teratomas (dermoid cysts) very common neoplasms consisting of adult tissues derived from all three germ layers; malignant teratomas; embryonal carcinoma, yolk sac (endodermal sinus) tumor; and choriocarcinoma.

Metastatic tumors to the ovary are often found. The most common are carcinomas from the colon, breast, stomach, and pelvic organs (endometrium, cervix). A peculiar form of bilateral metastatic disease to the ovary is the Krukenberg tumor in which both ovaries are involved by mucinous adenocarcinoma, usually of gastric

origin. Malignant lymphomas can also involve the ovaries.

Diseases of Pregnancy

The placenta is a fetal organ which develops in intimate relationship with the maternal tissues and blood. It can become implanted in abnormal intrauterine or extrauterine sites. Abnormal intrauterine implantation sites include the lower uterine segment (placenta praevia), uterine horn (cornual placenta), and the cervix. Extrauterine sites of placental implantation (ectopic pregnancy) include the fallopian tubes, ovaries, and, very rarely, other abdominal organs. Placenta accreta is the condition of abnormal adherence of the placenta to the uterine wall with associated deficient decidual formation.

Trophoblastic tumors may be locally invasive or systemically aggressive. The trophoblast develops from the outer layer of the blastocyst and is composed of two layers (i.e., the cytotrophoblast and the syncytiotrophoblast). These cells can undergo neoplastic changes to form hydatidiform mole, chorioadenoma destruens (invasive mole), and choriocarcinoma. The first two lesions are locally aggresive and tend to recur if incompletely excised. Hydatidiform mole consists of multiple cysts lined by edematous, vascular chorionic villis with atypical trophoblastic cells, and is usually limited to the endometrium. Chorioadenoma destruens is an agressive form of hydatidiform mole in which the myometrium may be infiltrated extensively. Choriocarcinoma is a highly malignant tumor with the capacity to metastasize hematogenously to the lungs and other organs. These trophoblastic tumors secrete abnormal levels of chorionic gonadotropin (HCG) allowing for their detection and also for monitoring the effects of therapy.

Breast

Anomalies are rare and generally do not contribute to significant morbidity. There may be amastia with complete absence of breast tissue on one or both sides as well as polymastia, in which accesory breast tissue may be found anywhere along the milk line, especially near the axilla or just below the breast; may be mistaken for tumor, and subject to all breast disorders.

Inflammatory disorders may affect the breast and may mimic carcinoma. Acute mastitis, a suppurative infection, occurs mostly during lactation. Tuberculosis is uncommon, and is virtually always secondary to a pulmonary focus or involvement of an axillary lymph node. Mammary duct ectasia (plasma cell mastitis, comedomastitis) is of uncertain pathogenesis, but most likely noninfectious. Microscopically, there is ductal dilatation with chronic inflammation. Fat necrosis is usually traumatic in origin, especially in large breasts, and usually simulates carcinoma with induration, fixation, skin retraction, and, in chronic stages, calcification which is seen on mammography. Foreign body inflammatory reaction may be due to injection of paraffin, silicone, or other cosmetic material.

Fibrocystic disease is the most common breast disorder, occurring mostly during reproductive years. Cysts may be lined by flattened cuboidal epithelium, eosinophilic columnar cells (apocrine metaplasia), or there may be epithelial proliferation (papillomatosis, and adenosis). Dense collagenous fibrous tissue proliferation may compress and obliterate epithelial elements. Sclerosing may be difficult to distinguish from carcinoma, both clinically and microscopically. Fibrocystic disease may be associated with increased incidence of breast cancer.

Tumors of the breast are common. Fibroadenoma is a benign tumor characterized by proliferation of both epithelial and stromal elements. Most often during reproductive years. This painless, firm, ovoid, encapsulated, mobile tumor is slow-growing, with more rapid growth during pregnancy and with contraceptive pills. The tumor may be present during puberty and tends to regress in menopause. Cystosarcoma phyllodes is a variant of fibroadenoma in which there is marked stromal proliferation, with the tumor typically being quite large. Approximately 10–20 percent are malignant (only mesenchymal element). Intraductal papilloma occurs in major mammary ducts and contributes to bloody nipple discharge, and subareolar mass.

Approximately 7 percent of American women develop breast cancer, with 90,000 new cases, and 33,000 deaths, yearly. Risk factors include (1) female (99 percent of breast cancers), (2) age over 40, (3) family history, (4) nulliparous or late first pregnancy, (5) previous breast cancer, (6) fibrocystic disease, (7) immunosuppression, (8) prior breast irradiation, (9) Western hemisphere, (10) temperate zone, (11) Caucasian, (12) higher socioeconomic group, (13) early menarche, (14) anovulatory cycles, and (15) history of endometrial carcinoma. Approximately 50 percent of cases occur in the upper, outer quadrant of breast. More than 90 percent arise in mammary ducts.

Intraductal carcinoma accounts for 3–5 percent of breast cancer. It may be papillary or solid with central necrosis (comedocarcinoma) often with nipple discharge. A mass may not be palpable and the tumor may be multifocal.

Infiltrating duct carcinoma is the most common (75 percent breast cancer). Dense fibrosis (cirrhous carcinoma) contains nests, cords, and ductlike structures composed of malignant epithelial cells. Paget's disease is

a variant of duct carcinoma in which the cells migrate via the lactiferous duct epithelium to involve in the skin, producing an eczemalike clinical picture. Medullary carcinoma is uncommon (5–10 percent). The tumors tend to be bulky with little or no fibrosis, sheets of tumor cells, and frequent lymphocytic infiltration. Prognosis is generally better than duct carcinoma. Tubular (well differentiated) carcinoma consists of regular, small tubular structures lined by single rows of uniform cells in a fibrous stroma. Distant spread is infrequent. This variant is uncommon. Lobular carcinoma arises from acinar elements, and consists of small, uniform cells which typically infiltrate dense stroma in a single file pattern. Precursor lesions are thought to be lobular neoplasia (lobular carcinoma in situ) which is frequently multifocal and bilateral, and consists of clusters of enlarged lobules filled with uniform, bland-appearing cells, with obliteration of acinar lumina. As many as 35 percent of patients with lobular neoplasia develop carcinoma within 20 years of diagnosis.

Favorable prognostic factors for breast cancer include small size, few or no regional lymph nodes affected, sinus histiocytosis of nodes, and high concentration of estrogen receptor protein in tumor tissue. Spread is to regional nodes (axillary for lateral tumors, internal mammary for medial), bones, lungs, liver, ovaries, and adrenals; 60 percent of cases involve lymph nodes at times of diagnosis.

Male breast disorders are less common. Gynecomastia may be unilateral or bilateral, with ductal and stromal proliferation, occurring at puberty, during senescence, and in association with hormonally active testicular tumors, cirrhosis, therapy with estrogens and other drugs (digitalis, isoniazid), and in Klinefelter's syndrome. Carcinoma is infrequent, occurring with cirrhosis, estrogen therapy, and Klinefelter's syndrome.

RESPIRATORY SYSTEM

Nasal Cavity, Paranasal Sinuses, and Oral Cavity

Nasal polyps are not true neoplasms but soft, pink inflammatory protrusions of the nasal mucosa. Histologically they exhibit an edematous stroma with many eosinophils and lymphoplasmacytic cells. They are most often associated with allergy but may follow local infection, trauma, chemical irritation, and cystic fibrosis.

Nasal papilloma (Scheneiderian papilloma) is a benign tumor of the nasal mucosa composed of a fibrovascular core of connective tissue usually covered by transitional (Scheneiderian) respiratory or squamous epithelium. They tend to recur locally in as many as 50 percent of cases and 15 percent become malignant, usually after several recurrences.

Juvenile nasopharyngeal angiofibroma is an unusual benign tumor of the nasopharynx that occurs almost exclusively in adolescent and young adult males. They are polypoidal, posterior nasal cavity tumors that tend to bleed profusely after biopsy. The tumors regress after puberty. The pathogenesis of the tumor is unknown but is probably hormonal. Histologically, angiofibromas are composed of large blood vessels admixed with a fibrous stroma.

The oral mucosa can be the site of origin of numerous malignant tumors including squamous cell carcinoma (the most frequent primary malignancy), adenocarcinoma, tumors from minor salivary gland origin (mixed tumor, adenoid cystic carcinoma, mucoepidermoid carcinoma), melanoma, plasmacytoma, malignant lymphoma, lymphoepithelioma, and rhabdomyosarcoma.

Laryngeal polyps and nodules are a form of noninflammatory reactions of the laryngeal mucosa to injury. They are not true neoplasmas but degenerative conditions. Laryngeal nodules predominate in singers ("singers' nodules") and in women. They cause hoarseness and seldom become malignant.

Squamous papilloma is a true neoplasm of the squamous mucosa lining the true vocal cords. It can be multiple in children and is probably due to a viral infection. Squamous papillomas tend to recur locally and may cause respiratory difficulties when they are multiple. The childhood form tends to disappear at puberty. Malignant change has been reported in papillomas treated with radiotherapy.

Squamous cell carcinoma is the most common laryngeal malignancy and the most frequent neoplasm of the upper respiratory tract (7.5/100,000). Squamous cell carcinoma affects males (7:1), usually older than 40 years of age, especially alcoholics, and those smoking more than 20 cigarettes/day for more than 10 years. Chronic inflammation is followed by metaplasia and dysplasia of the epithelium. The latter changes are premalignant. Patients present with hoarseness, pain, dysphagia, dyspnea, and hemoptysis. The tumors are more frequent in the true vocal cords where they appear as exophytic, ulcerated masses. They invade local structures and metastasize through lymphtic channels to regional lymph nodes and the lungs.

The Lungs

Vascular diseases of the lung may reflect abnormalities of the lungs' dual blood supply (i.e., the bronchial circulation that contributes to the nutritional needs of airways, and the pulmonary circulation, involved with gas exchange). The pulmonary circulation can be affected by various inflammatory, degenerative, and neoplastic pathologic processes including pulmonary edema, hypertension, and thromboembolism.

Pulmonary edema is the abnormal accumulation of fluid and solutes in the extravascular tissues and spaces of the lung. Under physiologic conditions the movement of fluid and solutes across the endothelial barrier is controlled by factors expressed in Starling's law. They include (1) the capillary infiltration coefficient, that depends upon capillary permeability and surface area; (2) factors that tend to move fluid and solutes from the blood vessel into the tissues (hydrostatic pressure in capillaries and oncotic pressure in tissues); and (3) factors that tend to expel fluid from tissues (hydrostatic pressure in tissues and oncotic pressure in blood vessels). Pulmonary edema occurs because of alterations in these mechanisms. For example, altered alveolar epithelial or pulmonary capillary endothelial permeability results in pulmonary edema. Altered permeability can be secondary to viral infections, toxic inhalants (ozone, NO_2 SO_2, paraquat), oxygen toxicity, circulating toxins (endotoxins, alloxan, α-naphthylthiourea), vasoactive substances (histamine, serotonin, kinins), drug reactions (busulfan, methotrexate, hydralazine), radiation therapy, aspiration of acid fluids, and smoke inhalation. Pulmonary edema can also follow (1) increases in pulmonary hydrostatic pressure in heart failure, pulmonary veno-occlusive disease, and overinfusion of fluids, (2) decreases in capillary oncotic pressure (hypoalbuminemia), and (3) increased negative interstitial pressure (rapid removal of pneumothorax or large pleural effusion). Edema can also be the result of unknown mechanisms in patients suffering from neurologic conditions such as hypothalamic lesions.

The lungs characteristically are heavy, pale, airless, and on section exude frothy pink proteinaceous fluid. There frequently is an accompanying pleural effusion, further reducing pulmonary reserve.

Patients show multiple physiologic abnormalities, including marked decreases in vital capacity, total lung capacity, functional residual capacity, and diffusing capacity for carbon monoxide, decreases in pulmonary static compliance, and arterial hypoxemia with increased alveolar-arterial oxygen gradients. Pulmonary edema resolves when the pathogenic factor has been removed. Ocassionally however, it persists as the adult respiratory distress syndrome. Pulmonary edema also predisposes to infections in the form of bronchopneumonia.

Pulmonary hypertension present when the resting systolic-diastolic pressure in the pulmonary artery exceeds 30/15 mm of Hg or when the mean pressure exceeds 25 mm of Hg, except during the first 2 weeks of extrauterine life, when high pulmonary artery pressures are normal.

Pulmonary arterial pressure is regulated by the volume of blood flow per unit of time and the resistance to flow. Pulmonary hypertension can thus appear in situations of increased resistance in precapillary vessels, impaired pulmonary venous outflow, or sudden increase in blood volume (overhydration). From an etiologic viewpoint pulmonary hypertension can be classified as idiopathic and secondary. Idiopathic pulmonary hypertension is a rare disorder that afflicts mostly young women and results in progressive dyspnea, chest pain, syncope and right side heart failure. Secondary pulmonary hypertension is more common and results from pulmonary and cardiac abnormalities, including congenital heart disease with longstanding left to right shunting of blood (patent ductus arteriosus, atrial septal defect, ventricular septal defect), pulmonary venous hypertension (mitral valve stenosis and/or regurgitation, left ventricular failure), pulmonary embolism, interstitial fibrosis, musculoskeletal abnormalities (thoracoplasty, poliomyelitis, kyphoscoliosis), and alveolar hypoventilation (obesity with pickwickian syndrome).

Morphologicaly the pulmonary vessels show intimal proliferation and fibrosis, medial elastosis and fibrosis, thrombosis, recanalization, and aneurysm formation. Histologic changes are graded on a 1 to 6 scale.

Pulmonary embolism (PE) is the impaction in the pulmonary vascular bed of a previously detached thrombus or foreign matter, as a complication of thrombosis of leg or pelvic veins, or from tumors. PE is found in approximately 15 percent of all autopsies and is second only to pneumonia as the most common acute pulmonary lesion. Pulmonary embolism results in a reduction in cardiac output due to increased pulmonary blood flow, congestion behind the area of obstruction, impairment of pulmonary function (decreased pulmonary capillary perfusion and ventilation), and frequently, but not invariably, pulmonary hemorrhagic necrosis (infarct).

There is no clear agreement as to the degree of pulmonary vessel obstruction necessary to kill a patient. Experimental animals can tolerate 60–70 percent obstruction, while patients probably can survive sudden occlusion of 50 percent. Embolism completely occluding the main pulmonary artery or its primary branches, however, is lethal within a few minutes or hours. Massive pulmonary embolism is accompanied by acute right sided heart failure with dilatation of the pulmonary artery and the right ventricle.

Pulmonary infarcts present as wedge-shaped areas of consolidation located subpleurally. They are hemorrhagic and undergo organization into a fibrous scar. Thrombosis does not usually cause infarction unless the bronchial (aortic) circulation is also compromised, as in left heart failure.

Chronic obstructive lung disease (COPD) is a common functional disorder of airways characterized by obstruction to expiratory airflow. This condition is diagnosed clinically under the names of emphysema, chronic bronchitis, and chronic obstructive lung disease to asthmatic bronchitis. COPD is divided into disorders affecting primarily the large conducting airways (chronic bronchitis) and those involving bronchioles and lung parenchyma (emphysema).

Chronic bronchitis is a form of COPD diagnosed clinically in the presence of chronic cough with excessive sputum production and wheezing persisting for more than 3 months, a year, 2 or more consecutive years, and cannot be attributed to other causes such as tuberculosis or bronchiectasis. A common disorder affecting primarily men in their fifth or sixth decade; it is usually associated with a history of cigarette smoking for 20 to 30 years. It is controversial whether air pollution also plays a role. Patients suffer from frequent respiratory infections, usually in the winter. They also develop dyspnea secondary to bronchial obstruction. Functional studies of these patients show findings typical of large airway obstruction (i.e., reduced vital capacity and expiratory flow rates, hyperinflation of the lungs due to an increase in residual volume, normal compliance, normal total lung capacity, and normal diffusion capacity of carbon dioxide). Blood gases determinations reveal hypoxia ("blue puffers") and hypocapnia due to hyperventilation. The lungs have characteristic changes including marked hyperplasia of bronchial glands, metaplasia of the ciliated epithelium, and chronic peribronchial inflammation. The lumina of major airways is frequently filled with thick, inspissated mucous that impairs the normal flow of air.

Emphysema is a form of COPD characterized by the presence of airspace enlargement with destruction of lung parenchyma. It is common in men with a history of heavy smoking. Patients present primarily with dyspnea that at first is noticed only after exertion, but usually progresses until the individual can only perform, with difficulties, simply physical tasks. Although these individuals are usually not cyanotic, they appear weak and cachectic. Physical examination demonstrates marked lung hyperinflation and markedly decreased breath sounds. Chest roentgenograms show depressed diaphragmatic domes, attenuated lung and vascular markings in the periheral lung fields, and increased radiolucency in the space located between the sternum and the base of the aorta and heart. Functional studies reveal findings of airway obstruction similar to those described in chronic bronchitis. However, increased total lung capacity and decreased diffusion capacity of CO and lung compliance are also found. Blood gas determinations reveal hypoxia usually less severe than that seen in patients with chronic bronchitis ("pink puffers") and hypocapnia due to hyperventilation.

The pathologic changes include an abnormal enlargement of airspaces distal to the terminal bronchioles, caused by tissue destruction but without significant fibrosis. Based on the anatomic distribution, emphysema can be classified as centriacinar or centrilobular, panacinar or palobular, focal, irregular or paracicatricial, and unilateral or lobular. Pulmonary blood vessels show significant changes, marked decrease in the number of small vessels present in the parenchyma as a result of destruction of alveolar septa, and subsequent pulmonary hypertension that leads to right ventricular hypertrophy (cor pulmonale). Longstanding, severe emphysema frequently leads to right sided heart failure.

Bullous emphysema develops in subpleural areas as large air filled spaces lined by ragged lung tissue (bullae). Bullae can be single or multiple, and may occasionally rupture into the pleural cavity with the development of pneumothorax.

α-1 Antitrypsin deficiency may be associated with emphysema in young individuals who are not heavy smokers. This form of bilateral, severe, panlobular emphysema is associated with the absence of α-1 antitrypsin in serum. This enzymatic inhibitor is normal in serum. Its presence is determined genetically. Severe deficiency states are transmitted as an autosomal dominant trait. As many as 5 percent of the general population may have a modest deficiency of the protein and are at a greater risk of developing emphysema.

Bronchial obstruction can be secondary to intrinsic factors (foreign body aspiration, endobronchial neoplasms such as bronchial carcinoids, mucous plugs, etc.) or extrinsic airway compression (i.e., enlarged lymph nodes, tumor pleural effusion, etc.). It can also be the result of bronchial collapse because of loss of mural support and thickening of the bronchial mucosa due to marked edema and inflammation. The consequences of airway obstruction are either atelectasis or hyperinflation. Atelectasis, or pulmonary collapse, is the result of complete obstruction of a relatively large bronchus (i.e., segmental bronchus). In this situation the obstruction is too great for the lung parenchyma to be ventilated from collateral spaces through pores of Kohn and canals of Lambert. Hyperinflation of the lung parenchyma usually follows partial obstruction of a bronchus. The obstructed area acts like a valve that impairs the outflow of air from the lung.

Immunologic diseases of the lung may be due to systemic or local immunologic disorders, and may be mediated through different mechanisms (Table 6-3).

Respiratory atopy develops when predisposed individuals establish contact with specific allergens from the environment. They are associated with the development of reaginic antibodies (IgE immunoglobulins) and include allergic rhinitis, bronchial asthma, and angioneurotic edema with laryngeal involvement.

Bronchial asthma is a state of altered reactivity of the lower respiratory tract in which there is smooth muscle spasm, mucous hypersecretion, and increased capillary permeability with mucosal edema. Clinically, there are frequent attacks of acute dyspnea with diffuse expiratory wheezing of paroxysmal nature. These reactions are usually reversible. The sputa of these patients show eosinophils in mucous plugs, numerous desquamated epithelial cells, Curschmann's spirals, Charcot-Leyden crystals, rounded clumps of bronchial epithelial cells (Creola bodies), and masses of fibrin.

Asthma can be classified as extrinsic asthma, in which there is a clear allergic etiology and intrinsic asthma in which there is no clear allergic etiology. In extrinsic asthma, skin tests for different antigens are positive. The sputum shows Creola bodies and abundant eosinophils. This form of asthma usually starts in childhood and has a benign clinical course. Skin tests are negative in intrinsic asthma. The clinical course is chronic and symptoms are refractory to therapy. Pathogenesis probably relates to infections and noxious inhalants as well as psychosomatic factors.

Extrinsic allergic alveolitis (acute granulomatous in-

Table 6-3. Classification of Pulmonary Hypersensitivity Disease[a]

Type I	Cell-fixed IgE antibody interacting with free antigen to cause release of vasoactive mediators	Bronchial asthma, respiratory atopy, anaphylaxis
Type II	Circulating antibody plus complement, interacting with cell-fixed antigen to cause cytotoxicity	Possibly Goodpasture's disease
Type III	Circulating antibody interacting with free antigen	Extrinsic allergic alveolitis
Type IV	Cellular hypersensitivity	Granuloma formation rejection phenomena
Type V	"Stimulatory" hypersensitivity	Long-acting thyroid stimulator (LATS)

[a] Based on the Gell and Coombs classification of immune reactions.

terstitial pneumonitis) is a group of diseases related to the inhalation of particulate organic antigens and characterized by the presence of circulating precipitating antibodies that mediate immunologic reactions of the Gell and Coombs type III. The most common forms of the syndrome and the proposed organic antigens involved in their etiology are summarized (Table 6-4).

Farmer's lung is an acute illness occurring in agricultural workers a few hours after exposure to the dust of moldy hay. Patients present with chills, fever, malaise cough, cyanosis, and dyspnea. Symptoms subside in a few days although there may be persistent cough and dyspnea. Pulmonary function tests show hypoxia and findings of an obstructive defect with increased residual lung volume and decreased expiratory flow rates. Farmer's lung represents a hypersensitivity reaction to antigens produced by thermophilic actinomycetes that grow in hay. Histologically the lungs show numerous interstitial noncaseating epithelioid cell granulomata. In many instances the disease progresses to a chronic form with interstitial fibrosis and honeycombing.

Pulmonary drug reactions follow exposure to nitrofurantoin, methotrexate, sulfas, and other drugs. Bleomycin, as example, can induce severe pulmonary interstitial fibrosis.

Pulmonary infiltration with eosinophilia may be due to several syndromes which are often transient and migratory. They represent hypersensitivity reactions to helminths (tropical pulmonary eosinophilia), intestinal parasites, drugs and inhalants (Löffler's syndrome), and aspergillus (bronchopulmonary aspergillosis).

Systemic collagen diseases involve the lungs with variable frequency. They include rheumatoid arthritis (pleuritis, pulmonary nodules, interstitial fibrosis), systemic lupus erythematosus (pleural effusion, rarely interstitial fibrosis), scleroderma and dermatomyosis

Table 6-4. Extrinisic Allergic Alveolitis Acute Granulomatous Interstitial Pneumonitis

Syndrome	Antigen Involved in the Pathogenesis
Farmer's lung	Thermophilic, anaerobic actinomycetes; micropolyspora faeni; and thermoactinomycetes vulgaris
Maple bark stripper's disease	Fungal spores of *Cryptostroma corticale*
Pigeon's breeder disease	Pigeon's feces
Bagassosis	Bagasse (dried fiber residue from sugar cane)
Byssinosis (brown lung disease)	Fine particles of cotton

(progressive interstitial pulmonary fibrosis), and Goodpasture's syndrome (pulmonary hemorrhages and renal failure due to deposition of antibasement antibodies in the lung and kidneys). Polyarteritis nodosa seldom involves the pulmonary vasculature.

Angiitis and granulomatosis occurs in the lung in several diseases that may represent hypersensitivity reactions to yet undetermined antigens. They include (1) Wegener's granulomatosis involving the lungs, upper airways and kidneys, (2) localized Wegener's granulomatosis involving the lungs only, and (3) lymphomatoid granulomatosis. The latter is premalignant angiocentric lymphoreticular proliferation and granulomatous disease involving the lung, brain, skin, and kidneys. Patients frequently develop malignant lymphomas.

PATHOLOGY OF THE PNEUMONIAS

Pneumonias are defined as inflammatory exudative consolidations of lung parenchyma. They can be classified according to their etiologic agent (bacteria, virus, fungus, protozoa) and anatomic distribution (lobar, lobular bronchopneumonia, interstitial).

Bacterial Pneumonia

Bacterial pneumonia is a major cause of death (present in up to 50 percent of cases at autopsy). Common etiologic agents are the following:

Gram-positive cocci: Streptococcus pneumonia (Diplococcus pneumonia), *Staphylococcus aureus, Streptococcus pyogenes* (Group A, β-hemolytic)

Gram-negative bacilli: Klebsiella pneumoniae (Friedländer's bacillus), *Pseudomonas aeruginosa* (namely P pseudomallei), Proteus: *Pasteurella tularensis, P pestis, E coli* (usually neonatal)
Hemophilus influenzae

Mixed flora: responsible for aspiration and some neonatal pneumonias

There are several defense mechanisms in the normal respiratory system that protect against bacterial infections. They include the filtering function of the nasopharynx, epiglottal reflex, cough reflex, mucus and ciliary action alveolar macrophages, and IgG-IgA antibodies. Pneumonia may result from impairment of these defense mechanisms, low host resistance, or unusually virulent infections (e.g., *P pestis*). For example, loss of the cough reflex in patients with coma or anesthesia predisposes to the development of aspiration pneumonia.

Lobar Pneumonia

Lobar pneumonia is characterized by consolidation of one or more lung lobes. The inflammatory process starts subpleurally and spreads through airways and the pores of Kohn to involve the whole lobe. This variant occurs most commonly in debilitated old people and it is uncommon in infancy. Males are affected more commonly. Most cases are due to pneumococcal infectious types 1, 3, 7, and 2. About 50 percent of cases are preceded by upper respiratory infections (URI). Patients present with sudden onset of fever, cough, purulent or bloody sputum, and pleuritic chest pain. On physical examination, there is tachycardia, rales, dullness to percussion, decreased breath sounds, and occasionally a pleural rub. Chest x-ray reveal localized lobar opacity with air bronchograms, and laboratory findings include leukocytosis.

PATHOLOGIC FEATURES

Laennec described the four stages of lobar pneumonia as the following:

1. Congestion (1 to 2 days) gross pathology: Red, "wet" lobe, exuding edema, fluid
Microscopic: Alveolar capillary engorgement, and fluid in alveoli
2. Red hepatization (2 to 4 days) gross pathology: Lobe is red, firm (liver-like), airless. There is an acute fibrinous pleuritis.
Microscopic: The alveolar spaces are filled with fibrin, red blood cells gives the red color on gross exam and neutrophils containing engulfed bacteria
3. Gray hepatization (4 to 8 days) gross pathology: Lobe is firm, yellow-gray, and dry with pleuritis on its surface
Microscopic: Fibrin, deteriorating red blood cells and neutrophils
4. Resolution (8 to 10 days): If the outcome is favorable the lung parenchyma and the pleura are restored to their normal stage. The exudate is digested by enzymes and is transferred into a granular debris that is either resorbed, ingested by macrophages, or coughed up

The complications include lack of normal fibrinolysis followed by organization of the exudate into fibrinous tissue, progression to necrosis and abscess formation (especially *Staphylococcus* and *Klebsiella*), local dissemination (pericarditis, empyema, followed by organization of pleural exudate and fibrothorax), and systemic dissemination (sepsis with endocarditis, meningitis, arthritis,

metastatic brain, and kidney abscesses). The mortality of pneumonia is about 5 percent.

Bronchopneumonia

Bronchopneumonia is characterized by patchy consolidation of the lung. The affected lobules are interspersed with normal ones. Bronchopneumonia usually represents an extension of a preexisting bronchitis or bronchiolitis, occurs most commonly in infancy and old age, and is very common at autopsy as a terminal episode in patients with cancer and chronic debilitating diseases (e.g., congestive heart failure). Etiologic organisms include gram-positive cocci (*Staphylococcus*, streptococcus, pneumococcus) and gram-negative bacilli (*Pseudomonas aeruginosa, H influenza, E coli, Proteus, Legionella pneumophilia*), etc.

Patients with bronchopneumonia frequently have a history of confinement to bed, an underlying serous disorder, or alcoholism. They present with fever of 39.5°C, cough, expectoration, expiratory rales, and multiple focal opacities on chest roentgenograms. The process is frequently bilateral and involves the lower lobes because of the tendency for secretions to gravitate into the basal portions of the lung.

The pathology of bronchopneumonia is very characteristic; bronchi are red and filled with exudate; there are multiple gray red to yellow, poorly demarcated round areas of consolidation interspersed with congested nonconsolidated foci in the lung parenchyma. These areas show acute alveolitis on microscopic examination.

Lung abscess is a localized area of suppuration with necrosis of pulmonary parenchyma and central cavitation. It may develop at any age but is more frequent in young male adults. Predisposing conditions include oropharyngeal surgical procedures, sinusitis, dental sepsis, bronchiectasis, and alcoholism.

The most common etiologic agents are gram-positive cocci (e.g., staphylococcus, streptococcus), gram-negative bacilli (e.g., klebsiella and mixed infections), and anaerobes (e.g., bacteroids).

Lung abscess can follow (1) inhalation (aspiration) of gastric or foreign infective material, especially in comatose, alcoholic, convulsing, or anesthetized individuals or with esophageal or pyloric obstruction or from oral or tonsilar infection; (2) as a complication of pulmonary infection (pneumonia, bronchiectasis, etc.); (3) bronchial obstruction by tumor or mucus plug; (4) septic embolism in systemic trombophlebitis (usually of legs or pelvis), right sided endocarditis, intravenous injections, infected cannulas or osteomyelitis; (5) cystic disease of lung or bronchiectasis; and (6) trauma or extension of infection from an adjacent structure (i.e., rupture of liver abscess through diaphragm.).

In 25 percent of cases no predisposing factor can be identified. Lung abscesses are usually close to the pleura and may be multiple. The cavity usually contains pus. The wall of the cavity is usually ragged, gray, and firm. The surrounding parenchyma is usually consolidated. The overlying pleura shows a fibrinous exudate. Lung abscesses may result in bronchopleural fistula, hemorrhage, or empyema or gangrene of the lung, and they may disseminate (brain abscess, meningitis). Rarely, they are associated with secondary amyloidosis.

The commonest functional disorder in pneumonias is an imbalance of ventilation-perfusion (V/Q), which is the consequence of sustained perfusion of poorly ventilated areas of the lung. Obstructed airways, shallow breathing, and local hyperventilation secondary to pleural pain can aggravate the V/Q imbalance.

Primary atypical pneumonia is an acute febrile respiratory disease characterized by interstitial pneumonitis (inflammatory infiltrates in the alveolar septa and pulmonary interstitium) with little intra-alveolar exudate. In about 50 percent of cases, no etiologic agent is isolated. The most frequent etiologic agent is Mycoplasma pneumoniae (Eaton agent). Other causes include influenza A-B, parainfluenza, respiratory syncytial virus (common in infants), rhinovirus, measles, and coxsackie. In immunosuppressed patients, herpes simplex, Zoster-varicella, and cytomegalovirus are often found.

Patients present with vague symptoms including fever, headache, muscle aches, pains in the legs, no cough or only dry, unproductive cough, and no clear physical signs. Chest roentgenograms show peribronchial opacities and diffuse reticular or multinodular opacities.

In fatal cases, the lungs are bulky, heavy, and plumcolored. These changes mainly involve the lower lobes. Microscopically, the respiratory tract epithelium (bronchi and bronchioles) shows destructive and regenerative changes consisting of necrosis and sloughing of ciliated and mucous cells causing ulceration of bronchial mucosa.

There is also regeneration of the respiratory epithelium, variable squamous metaplasia mononuclear inflammatory infiltration of bronchi and bronchioles, and hyalin membranes in terminal bronchioles and alveoli. The most characteristic pathologic change in the presence of interstitial inflammation by mononuclear inflammatory cells (lymphocytes, macrophages, and occasional plasma cells). Occasionally intracytoplasmic and/or intranuclear inclusions are seen at some stage in viral pneumonias, such as measles, CMV, adenovirus, and coxsackie. Atypical primary pneumonias usually resolve completely, but they may organize and result in interstitial fibrosis.

Interstitial

Interstitial lung disease includes many pulmonary diseases that involve the interstitium of the lungs. The etiologic agents are diverse and in many instances remain unknown. Patients with interstitial lung disease often present with characteristic clinical, pathologic, and radiologic features. They have various degrees of dyspnea and tachypnea, small lungs with coarse respiratory rales on physical examination, and characteristic roentgenographic findings including bilateral diffuse involvement of lung fields by fine nodular, reticular and/or linear patterns. Chest radiographs can also show patchy, "alveolar type" infiltrates. Functionally patients with interstitial lung disease exhibit loss of lung volumes (decreased total lung capacity, decreased vital capacity), decreased flow rates, and impaired diffusion of CO_2 due to loss of vascularity in fibrous areas. Interstitial lung disease can be classified according to the duration of disease, etiology, and clinicopathologic manifestations.

Acute exudative interstitial disease is usually secondary to viral infections, uremia, chronic pulmonary venous hypertension, mitral stenosis, pulmonary venous thrombosis, oxygen toxicity, and shock ("shock lungs"). Patients present with the adult respiratory distress syndrome (ARDS) and develop progressive dyspnea, hypoxia, and diffuse bilateral infiltrates on chest roentgenograms. The lungs are edematous, heavy, and exhibit necrosis of alveolar lining cells with exudation of proteinaceous edema fluid into alveolar spaces. These exudates resemble hyaline membranes present in newborn premature infants. In later stages, the alveoli show pneumocyte proliferation. There may be progression to chronic interstitial disease with fibrosis or reversal if the etiologic agent is removed at an early stage.

Subacute interstitial fibrosis usually follows infections or granulomatous diseases including sarcoidosis, tuberculosis, pneumocystis carinii pneumonia, farmer's lung and related extrinsic allergic alveolitis as well as eosinophilic granuloma of lung and related histiocytoses.

Chronic diffuse interstitial disease is a severe and usually irreversible condition. It can follow many multiple etiologic events. In 50 percent of cases, the etiology remains unknown. Originally described as the Hamman-Rich syndrome, the disorder is characterized by the rapid progression of interstitial disease, usually in young females, leading to fibrosis and death within a few months of onset. Genetic or familiar factors may be important in some patients. However, not all patients follow the rapid subacute course described as the Hamman-Rich syndrome. Some patients may have a chronic, protracted clinical course leading to respiratory failure after years of onset. Currently patients with idiopathic forms of diffuse interstitial disease are classified on the basis of morphologic findings as (1) usual interstitial pneumonitis (UIP), including cases described as classical Hamman-Rich syndrome; (2) desquamative interstitial pneumonitis (DIP), a form with extensive exudation of macrophages into alveolar spaces; and (3) lymphoid interstitial pneumonitis (LIP). DIP appears to have a less aggressive clinical course and responds better to corticosteroid therapy. LIP is an inflammatory condition frequently associated with autoimmune disorders such as Sjögren's syndrome, LIP may also be a precursor of malignant lymphoma of the lung.

The other 50 percent cases of chronic interstitial disease are secondary to various specific etiologic agents, such as (1) industrial particulate and fume exposures (pneumoconiosis), including asbestosis, berylliosis, mercury vapors, metallic aluminum, and cadmium; (2) allergic alveolitis and hypersensitivity diseases, such as farmer's lung, pigeon fanciers lung, mushroom workers lung, pituitary snuff takers lung, and maple bark strippers lung; and (3) collagen type disorders including rheumatoid arthritis, systemic sclerosis, lupus erythematosus, and Caplan's syndrome (rheumatoid arthritis and pneumoconiosis).

End stage disease may follow any of the clinicopathologic forms of interstitial lung disease. The pulmonary architecture is severely distorted by extensive fibrosis, and the lungs are small, firm and shrunken or large, with multiple cystic spaces lined by fibrous tissue ("honeycomb" lung). Histologically, end stage lungs show extensive fibrosis, squamous metaplasia of the epithelium of bronchi and bronchioles, smooth muscle hyperplasia, and marked thickening of blood vessel walls. Patients with these forms of terminal interstitial lung disease often develop pulmonary hypertension and cor pulmonale. They are also at a higher risk for the development of lung cancer.

Pneumoconiosis

The respiratory system has continuous and active contact with the environment; occupational exposures particularly provide varied opportunities for intense and/or prolonged exposure to injurious substances resulting in various lung diseases. Occupational lung diseases include the following:

> Dust macules
> Pulmonary fibrosis
>   Silicosis
>   Diatomaceous earth pneumoconiosis
>   Silicatosis
>   Coal worker's pneumoconiosis
>   Asbestosis

> Pulmonary infiltration of immunologic origin
>   Extrinsic allergic alveolitis
>   Beryllium diseases
>   Occupational asthma
>   Byssinosis
>   Industrial bronchitis
> Toxic injury
>   Effects of irritant gases
>   Chemical injury
> Cancer

The pneumoconioses are a group of diseases in which the prolonged exposure to irritating substances is accompanied by the development of chronic interstitial inflammation and fibrosis. These diseases usually result from chronic exposure to industrial dusts, particules, and fumes. The most common injurious element in dust is silica. Several physical factors influence the deposition of dust in the lungs of which the most important is particle size. For example, particles larger than 5 μm have a low probability of reaching the alveoli as they are trapped in the nose or are cleared by the mucociliary apparatus of the bronchial tree.

The chemical nature of the inhaled particle is also important and substances such as carbon or bismuth are inert and produce no disease while others such as asbestos induce extensive fibrosis.

Silicosis

Silicosis results from exposure to silica in many occupations including coal mining. Usually, exposure causes focal zones of fibrosis containing silica crystals in lung and hilar lymph nodes. These 3–13 mm, spherical nodes have no clinical significance and are distributed throughout both lungs with no sites of predilection. Occasionally, simple silicosis progresses to a clinically significant disease, complicated silicosis, usually in patients with secondary tuberculosis. In addition to silicotic nodules, interstitial fibrosis develops and results in hypoxemia, carbon dioxide retention, and cor pulmonale. Diffuse interstitial fibrosis can also follow exposure to silica flour, a different crystalline form of the chemical. This form of disease has a rapid, severe clinical course resulting in fatal impairment of respiratory function due to severe fibrosis. Another form of silicosis is conglomerate silicosis, developing after tuberculosis and characterized by multiple coalescent silica nodules resulting in a fibrotic mass in the lung. This can undergo cavitation, caseous necrosis calcification, and other tuberculous changes may simulate a neoplasm.

COAL WORKER'S PNEUMOCONIOSIS

Coal worker's pneumoconiosis occurs in coal miners who show deposition of coal dust around bronchioles (macules) with minimal or no fibrosis. Airspace enlargement (focal emphysema) usually surrounds these macules. Patients with simple coal worker's pneumoconiosis are asymptomatic and have no functional abnormalities. In patients with tuberculous superinfections, this pneumoconiosis can lead to progressive massive fibrosis in which there is a large fibrous and pigmented mass, usually in the upper lobes. It can simulate a neoplasm and induces restrictive and obstructive physiologic changes.

ASBESTOSIS

Asbestosis occurs in ship yard workers, pipe fitters, insulation workers, and others and has been shown to be related to higher incidence of various neoplasms such as lung cancer, malignant mesothelioma, gastrointestinal adenocarcinomas, and pulmonary fibrosis. The disease is characterized by diffuse nonnodular interstitial fibrosis involving particularly the lateral and basal portions of both lungs. It is almost invariably accompanied by dense fibrous pleural thickening often in the form of plaques which may calcify. Asbestos bodies (elongated $20-50 \mu$m bodies composed of asbestos fibers, iron, and proteins) are found within fibrotic areas in the lungs. Asbestosis lead to a small shrunken lung or honeycomb lung.

BERYLLIOSIS

Berylliosis can be a serious and acute respiratory affliction within 72 hours of a heavy exposure. Patients present with cough, dyspnea, hemoptysis, and weakness. The disease progresses during 1 to 4 months and may regress completely or progress to interstitial fibrosis (chronic berylliosis). Microscopically the lungs show varying degrees of interstitial inflammation, fibrosis, and noncaseating epithelioid cell granulomas.

CARCINOMA OF THE LUNG

Carcinoma of the lung is the most common malignancy in men (approximately 100,000 new cases in 1982) and the sixth most common in women. It is a very aggressive form of cancer with a 5 year survival rate of 9 percent. Lung cancer occurs most often between ages 40 and 70.

Epidemiologic and experimental studies have demonstrated a close relationship between cigarette smoking and the development of lung cancer. Atmospheric pollution may also be related but evidence in this regard is less convincing. Occupational exposure to a diverse group of substances including asbestos, uranium, nickel, chromates, coal, mustard, gas, arsenic, beryllium, iron, and gold has also been shown to be important.

A few cases of lung cancer are diagnosed on routine x-ray but most patients are symptomatic and are discovered at a late stage of the disease. They may have symptoms due to the primary tumor (cough, expectoration, hemoptysis, wheezing, dyspnea, fever, and weight loss) from tumor extension to adjacent tissues (chest pain, shoulder pain, hoarseness due to involvement of recurrent laryngeal nerve, superior vena cava syndrome with edema of head, neck, and extremities, erosion of ribs with pain (Pancoast's syndrome), dysphagia due to compression or invasion of the esophagus and pleural effusion with pleurisy, and dyspnea and pericarditis with cardiac arrhythmias), and from distant metastases (e.g., headache due to brain metastases). In addition, there may be systemic syndromes without metastases (paraneoplastic syndromes). They include endocrinopathies (gynecomastia, Cushing's syndrome, inappropriate secretion of ADH, hypercalcemia with secretion of ADH, hypercalcemia with secretion of PTH and carcinoid syndrome); neuromuscular disorders (myasthenia, peripheral neuropathy and cerebellar degeneration); connective tissue disorders (clubbing of fingers and toes, pulmonary hypertrophic osteoarthropathy, dermatomyositis, and acanthosis nigricans); and vascular disorders (thrombophlebitis purpura with decrease in platelets and thrombocytosis).

The different histologic types of lung carcinoma are the following:

1. Benign
   Papillomas
     Squamous
     Transitional
   Adenomas
     Pleomorphic
     Monomorphic
     Others
2. Dysplasia – carcinoma in situ
3. Malignant
   Squamous cell carcinoma (epidermoid ca)
     Spindle cell carcinoma
   Small cell carcinoma
     Oat cell carcinoma
     Intermediate cell type
     Combined oat cell carcinomas

Adenocarcinoma
    Acinar adenocarcinoma
    Papillary adenocarcinoma
    Bronchioloalveolar carcinoma
    Solid carcinoma with mucus formation
Large cell carcinoma
    Giant cell carcinoma
    Clear cell carcinoma

Squamous Cell Carcinoma. Centrally arising from the mucosa of a major bronchus, close to the hilus, squamous cell carcinoma frequently exhibits areas of necrosis, focal hemorrhages, and cavitation. Microscopically, the tumor is composed of nests of cuboidal or polygonal cells with different degrees of pleomorphism. Intercellular bridges and abnormal keratin formation in the form of keratin pearls and dyskeratosis are the main diagnostic criteria. Adjacent bronchial mucosa usually shows areas of in situ carcinoma. Squamous cell carcinoma extends locally into the pleura, nerves, pericardium, and chest wall, and spreads through lymphatics, bronchial, tracheal, and mediastinal nodes. Hematogenous spread is less frequent but not uncommon and explains distant metastases, particularly to brain, bone, adrenals, kidneys, and liver.

Adenocarcinoma. Usually presenting as a peripheral, subpleural, firm, gray mass with abundant anthracotic pigment, adenocarcinoma has a thick and retracted (pleural puckering) overlying pleura. Microscopically, the tumor forms glandular spaces lined by pleomorphic cells that usually secrete mucin with varying degrees of desmoplastic stromal reaction. Adenocarcinomas grow slower than squamous carcinoma but the ultimate prognosis is slightly worse.

Bronchioloalveolar cell carcinoma is a distinct form of adenocarcinoma that originates in bronchiolar cells (Clara cells) or alveolar cells (type II pneumocytes). The tumor can be single or multiple and is composed of round, soft, gray nodules with only focal anthracotic pigment and abundant mucus on its surface. Microscopically, they exhibit very well differentiated tall, columnar cells lining preserved alveolar walls. Bronchioloalveolar cell carcinoma has a better prognosis than adenocarcinoma, especially if the tumor is peripheral and smaller than 2 cm in diameter.

Tumors that are believed to originate from Kulchitsky (neuroendocrine cells) (APUD cells) include carcinoid tumors and "oat-cell" carcinomas.

Bronchial Carcinoid Tumors. Comprising 5 percent of pulmonary neoplasms, bronchial carcinoid tumors arise mostly from main stem bronchi, but also from smaller bronchi or bronchioles. Grossly, they present as endobronchial pedunculated polyps. They are highly vascular and can bleed easily. Microscopically,

they are composed of ribbons and festoons of small, monotonous polygonal cells. Silver stains reveal argyrophyllic granules. Ultrastructurally, they exhibit characteristic neurosecretory type cytoplasmic granules.

Oat Cell Carcinomas. Highly malignant tumors that in most instances have already metastasized to the regional lymph nodes by the time the diagnosis is made are oat cell carcinomas. It is not unusual to establish the diagnosis from a metastasis. Frequently associated are endocrine paraneoplastic syndrome (Cushing's syndrome, inappropriate ADH secretion, carcinoid syndrome, etc.). Oat cell carcinoma presents as large, bulky, white-gray, soft masses, usually with central necrosis. Mediastinal lymph nodes almost invariably are enlarged. Microscopically, they are composed of sheets and nests of round to oval or spindle small cells with dark hyperchromatic nuclei and scanty cytoplasm. They may differentiate to form rosettes, trabeculae, or tubules. Oat cell carcinomas metastasize early and are usually not resectable at the time of diagnosis. The prognosis of these tumors has improved with modern chemotherapy.

Metastatic Tumors. Accounting for 20–40 percent of all lung cancers are metastic tumors. They are very common and they occur by lymphatic or hematogenous spread and may stimulate a primary tumor on clinicoradiologic examination and even on pathologic examination when they present as a solitary nodule. However, most metastatic tumors are multiple. Breast carcinoma and gastrointestinal tract carcinoma (colon, pancreas, stomach, etc.) are the most common, but virtually any tumor can involve the lungs.

PLEURA

Pleural diseases are usually secondary to underlying pulmonary parenchymal disease, a pathologic process originating in an adjacent structure, such as the chest wall, a systemic disease, or trauma.

Pleuritis can be fibrinous, serous, serofibrinous, suppurative (empyema), and hemorrhagic. In fibrinous pleuritis the surfaces are covered by fibrin. In serous pleuritis the pleural cavity contains fluid (effusion) that can be a transudate (clear, watery, with a specific gravity of less than 1.012 and a protein content of less than 3 g/dl; with mesothelial cells and a few lymphocytes) or an exudate (yellow, sometimes slightly viscous, with a specific gravity greater than 1.016 and a protein content of more than 3 g/dl; variable numbers of white blood cells). In serofibrinous pleuritis there is a combination of both features. The same pathologic processes can cause a serous, fibrinous and/or serofibrinous pleuritis. Contributing factors may be bacterial (M. tuberculosis), fungi (histoplasmosis, coccidioidomycosis, blastomycosis, actinomycosis), viroles (Coxsackie), mycoplasma, and chlamydial as well as connective tissue disorders (systemic lupus erythematosus, rheumatoid arthritis, diffuse systemic sclerosis), rheumatic fever, pulmonary infarct, uremia, acute pancreatitis, splenic injury, pleural asbestosis, and sarcoidosis. In empyema (suppurative pleuritis) the pleural cavity contains pus. It is usually secondary to pneumonia or lung abscess and can be secondary to subdiaphragmatic or liver abscesses or dissemination from a distant source of infection. Empyema rarely resolves unless drained surgically. The exudate usually organizes with the formation of dense fibrous adhesions that obliterate the pleural space (fibrothorax). The fibrous tissue can become calcified. Hemorrhagic effusions must be differentiated from hemothorax. They are usually secondary to metastatic tumors to the pleura, tuberculosis, pulmonary infarction, acute pancreatitis, rickettsial diseases, and hemorrhagic diatheses.

Noninflammatory processes can result in pleural fluid collections. Hydrothorax is characterized by the presence of a transudate in the pleural cavity. It may be uni- or bilateral and is usually secondary to heart failure, cirrhosis, or renal failure. Chylothorax is the accumulation of fluid with high lipid content and "milky" character. It results from leaks in the thoracic duct system, most often due to duct obstruction by neoplasm such as lymphoma. It may also follow trauma. Hemothorax (blood in pleural space) should be distinguished from hemorrhagic effusions. It results from trauma, dissecting aneurysm, hemorrhagic diseases, and spontaneous pneumothorax. Pneumothorax is the presence of air or gas in pleural cavity. It can be spontaneous, traumatic, or therapeutic. Spontaneous pneumothorax can be due to a variety of diseases that lead to alveolar rupture, especially emphysema, asthma, and tuberculosis. It can also be secondary to congenital cysts of the lung, or sarcoidosis. Idiopathic pneumothorax occurs in young adults without demonstrable pulmonary pathology.

Pleural fibrosis, either patchy or diffuse, occurs in a wide variety of conditions. Pleural fibrosis can be secondary to inflammation and pneumoconioses (pyogenic infections, tuberculosis, etc.).

Pleural cysts are usually located on parietal pleura. They can be mesothelial parasitic *(Echinococcus, Paragonimus westermani)* or neoplastic (cystic lymphangioma).

The most important pleural tumor is malignant mesothelioma, an unusual malignant tumor that has considerably increased in prevalence in recent years, attributable to the greatly augmented use of asbestos since the early part of the 20th century. Malignant mesothelioma presents with extensive pleural involvement and tumor encasement of the lung. The pleura is diffusely thickened, and the tumor invades contiguous structures (lung, parenchyma, chest wall, mediastinum, pericardium and diaphragm, and peritoneum). In approximately half of the cases, metastases are present at autopsy (regional and distant lymph nodes, contralateral pleura, lungs, liver, adrenals, kidneys, thyroid, bone, and brain). Microscopically, malignant mesotheliomas can be (1) epithelial (most frequent), forming tubular, papillary or combined pattern, (2) sarcomatoid or mesenchymal, and (3) mixed or biphasic (epithelial and sarcomatous). The cells of malignant mesothelioma secrete acid mucopolysaccharide (hyaluronic acid) which may be demonstrated within their cytoplasm or in tubular lumina by staining sections with alcian blue or colloidal iron, or in effusion fluid by chemical methods. The negation of these reactions by hyaluronidase pretreatment confirms the identity of the substance. These histochemical stains are useful to distinguish mesotheliomas from carcinomas.

Submesothelial fibroma ("localized mesothelioma") is an unusual benign tumor with no known relationship to asbestos exposure. It may reach a giant size and presents characteristically as a pedunculated mass on the visceral pleura.

Carcinomas of the lung and breast are the most common metastatic malignancies to the pleura. Other carcinomas (stomach, colon, kidney, etc.), lymphomas, and sarcomas can also involve the pleura.

THE MEDIASTINUM

The mediastinum is the site of origin of numerous neoplasms. They can be classified according to their location as illustrated by the following:

Superior
   Thymoma
   Thymic cyst
   Malignant lymphoma including Hodgkin's disease
   Thyroid and parathyroid lesions
Posterior
   Neurogenic tumors
      Neuroblastoma
      Neurofibroma
      Paraganglioma
   Gastroenteric cyst
   (Aneurysm of aorta)
Middle
   Pericardial cyst
   Bronchogenic cyst
   Malignant lymphoma

Anterior

Same as superior mediastinum plus germ cell tumors (seminomas, teratomas, etc.)

Thymomas are the most common tumors of the anterior mediastinum. They present as slowly enlarging masses that are usually discovered radiographically. In 25 percent of cases the patient, usually 40 to 60 years old, present with pressure symptoms (chest pain, cough, dyspnea). Thymomas can also be associated with a variety of syndromes including myasthenia gravis (30 percent of thymomas patients; 9 percent of myasthenia gravis patients have an associated thymoma), hypogammaglobulinemia, erythroid hypoplasia (red cell aplasia), collagen diseases, myositis, and myocarditis. They also have an increased incidence of carcinomas. Thymomas are large (5–10 cm), lobulated, gray-yellow, well encapsulated tumors, that can become cystic. Microscopically, they are composed of epithelial cells admixed with lymphocytes. Most thymomas are well encapsulated and rarely (2 percent) recur after surgery. They may, however, infiltrate the surrounding tissues. These invasive tumors are more aggressive, tend to recur locally, implant in the pericardial and pleural surfaces, and can rarely metastasize (malignant thymomas). Histologically, this variety is indistinguishable from benign thymomas except for the presence of local infiltration.

Malignant lymphomas are the most common middle mediastinal tumors. They may compress the superior vena cava and give superior mediastinal syndrome. The most common lymphomas in the mediastinum are nodular sclerosing Hodgkin's disease and lymphoblastic lymphoma.

Metastatiac neoplasms include oat cell carcinoma of the lung, breast, esophageal and other carcinomas. They may simulate a primary mediastinal neoplasm.

Nonneoplastic cysts are rare and include (1) the thymic cyst, lined by squamous or columnar epithelium; (2) pericardial cysts, lined by mesothelium, usually at the right cardiophrenic angle; (3) bronchogenic cysts, lined by respiratory epithelium, usually posterior to the carina; and (4) others, including gastric, enteric, and lymphatic (cystic hygroma) cysts.

Mediastinitis may be acute or chronic. Acute mediastinitis is a severe condition usually resulting from traumatic perforation of the esophagus. Chronic mediastinitis can be due to tuberculosis and fungal (histoplasmosis) infections. It presents as an area of fibrosis and chronic inflammation, with or without granulomata in the anterior mediastinum. Chronic mediastinitis can compress the superior vena cava and simulate a malignant process.

GASTROINTESTINAL TRACT

Oral Cavity

Inflammations of the mouth may be due to a variety of infectious agents (Vincent's bacillus, herpes virus, moniliasis, tuberculosis, syphilis, actinomycosis) or may be idiopathic (aphthous stomatitis). Vitamin C deficiency (scurvy) may lead to gingivitis, and vitamin B complex (niacin, riboflavin) deficiency may lead to glossitis, gingivostomatitis, and angular cheilosis. Pyorrhea is a progressive inflammatory gingivitis involving peridontal tissues, and destruction of the tooth-supporting bone.

Atrophic glossitis may be associated with iron-deficiency anemia. Gum hyperplasia may be seen in leukemia and with diphenylhydantoin-treated epileptics. Pigmentations of the gum may be indicative of heavy metal (arsenic, bismuth, lead, mercury, silver) toxicity. Melanotic spots may be seen in Addison's disease and Peutz-Jeghers syndrome.

Tumors of the mouth, including the tongue, buccal mucosa, and pharynx, are not uncommon. They are almost always squamous cell carcinoma, occur mostly in men, and are associated with age, smoking, iron-deficiency anemia (Plummer-Vinson syndrome), and, in India, betel nut chewing. They may be preceded by leukoplakia. In general, squamous cell carcinoma has extensive local infiltration, and metastasizes to cervical lymph nodes and, eventually, distant sites. Five-year survival rates are the following: anterior tongue, 20 percent; posterior tongue, 12 percent; floor of mouth, 17 percent, cheek and palate, 14 percent; and pharynx and tonsil, 10 percent. A rare pharyngeal tumor, lymphoepithelioma (Schmincke tumor), consists of undifferentiated tumor cells with an intense lymphocytic background, occurs most often in the third and fourth decades, and may metastasize widely despite a small, often clinically inconspicuous hypopharyngeal primary. Tumors of the mouth may also arise at sites of minor salivary glands.

Salivary Glands

Salivary glands may be nonspecifically inflamed (acute or chronic sialoadenitis). They are also the site of infection with mumps virus, tuberculosis, or actinomycosis. Infants with disseminated cytomegalovirus infection may have salivary gland involvement. Chronic sialoadenitis may be associated with salivary duct stone formation (sialolithiasis).

Benign lymphoepithelial lesion (Sjögren's syndrome, Mikulicz's disease) is thought to be an autoimmune disorder. Salivary gland enlargement is due to lymphocytic infiltration of the salivary glands with glandular atrophy and replacement of intralobular ducts by epimyothelial islands. Middle-aged females are most often affected. Rarely, there may be subsequent tumor development.

A variety of tumors may affect the salivary glands. Most common is the pleomorphic adenoma ("mixed" tumor) which usually affects the parotid. The tumor is firm, encapsulated, and often has a glistening, semitranslucent (chondroid) cut surface. Histologically, epithelial and mesenchymal elements, with abundant ground substance, are seen. Adenolymphoma (papillary cystadenoma lymphomatosum, Warthin's tumor) almost always occurs in the parotid, and has cysts of varying size lined by papillary adenomatous tissue with lymphocytic infiltration, including germinal centers, in the stroma. The tumor is completely benign. Mucoepidermoid carcinoma consists of mucus-secreting and squamous epithelial elements and may be of low- or high-grade malignancy. Acinic cell tumor is rare, affects mostly males, and consists of epithelial cells resembling the salivary serous cells. These tumors all have malignant potential, and many recur locally. Adenoid cystic carcinoma (cylindroma) is an infiltrative malignant tumor with a characteristic cribriform pattern, and a hyaline stroma. The tumor is relatively more common in the submandibular gland and may affect minor salivary glands. Tumor growth is usually slow and metastases occur late.

Esophagus

Developmental anomalies in the esophagus are uncommon and, because they cause regurgitation immediately after feeding, are usually discovered in the newborn, Agenesis is very rare. More common are atresia and fistula formation, with the fistula almost always developing between the esophagus and the tracheobronchial tree (tracheo-esophageal fistula). Abnormal narrowing with at least partial lumen maintenance (stenosis) may be congenital, but occurs most often as an acquired phenomenon secondary to chronic esophagitis. Trauma (chemical or radiation), scleroderma, or tumor.

Achalasia is a disorder of esophageal motility characterized by progressive dysphagia in the absence of an obstructing lesion, and is due to loss of normal peristalsis in the lower esophagus and failure of the cardioesophageal sphincter to relax. Myenteric ganglia are absent in the body of the esophagus. The etiology is not known, but, in endemic areas, Chagas' disease may cause a similar condition. In Chagas' disease, however, other organs may show similar changes (megaesophagus, megaduodenum, megacolon, megaloureter). Patients with idiopathic achalasia are at higher risk for the development of esophageal carcinoma.

Esophageal webs are anular narrowings, often as circumferential mucosal folds, almost always affecting individuals over the age of 40. In the upper esophagus, they usually occur in women with severe iron-deficiency anemia, and may be associated with atrophic glossitis, and oral mucus membrane leukoplakia. The combination of anemia, atrophic glossitis, and dysphagia is known as the Plummer-Vinson syndrome, and is associated with a high risk of carcinoma.

Esophageal diverticula occur above the upper esophageal sphincter (Zenker's or pulsion variety), near the midpoint of the esophagus (epibronchial or traction variety), and immediately above the lower esophageal sphincter (epiphrenic). They are symptomless when small, but when larger may contribute to regurgitation, dysphagia, or the sensation of a mass.

Hiatus hernia is a saclike dilatation of the stomach which protrudes above the diaphragm, is usually congenital, and may be found in as many as 5 percent of "normal" individuals.

Esophagitis occurs most often because of reflux of gastric contents, with or without hiatus hernia. Esophagitis may also be due to prolonged gastric incubation, chemical injuries, radiation injury, and viral and fungal infections (especially in immunologically debilitated patients). Long-standing reflux esophagitis may lead to reepitheliazation of the esophagus by a columnar, rather than stratified squamous, epithelium (Barrett's esophagus); patients with this condition have a higher risk of developing esophageal adenocarcinoma.

Rupture (Boerhaave's syndrome) may occur after prolonged vomiting, overdistension, or abdominal trauma. Laceration (Mallory-Weiss syndrome) occurs as a linear tear in the long axis of the esophagus, usually in alcoholics after prolonged vomiting. Both conditions may lead to mediastinitis.

Esophageal varices are due to longstanding portal venous obstruction, usually from cirrhosis. They are asymptomatic until they rupture, at which time massive hemorrhage often precipitated by minor trauma or esophagitis, may occur.

Benign tumors are rare. The major tumor of the esophagus is squamous cell carcinoma, occurring mostly in men in the sixth decade, and associated with chronic alcoholism, smoking, achalasia and strictures. Approximately 50 percent occur in the middle third, 30 percent in the lower third, and 20 percent in the upper third. They may be polypoid, ulcerating, or diffusely infiltrating, and tend to spread by direct continuity, although they do metastasize. Insidious and progressive dysphagia is the usual mode of presentation, but involvement of adjacent structures may also cause pain, dyspnea, hoarseness (laryngeal nerve involvement), hemorrhage, and pneumonia (fistula to tracheobronchial tree). Adenocarcinoma is uncommon, usually associated with gastric gland origin in lower third or Barrett's esophagus. A dysphagia-inducing tumor at the cardioesophageal junction is most likely to be adenocarcinoma of the gastric cardia. Other malignant tumors which may affect the esophagus include melanoma, lymphoma, and leiomiosarcoma.

Stomach and Duodenum

Developmental anomalies of the stomach are exceedingly rare. The stomach is affected when there are diaphragmatic defects permitting herniation of the stomach, and other abdominal contents, into the thorax. Congenital hypertrophic pyloric stenosis occurs in as many as 1 in 300 live births, almost always affects males, and generally manifests after the second or third week of life. The genetic basis has not been well established.

Gastric dilatation occurs with intestinal obstruction, either organic or functional. Gastric rupture is rare, usually associated with blunt trauma, and often leads to death.

Gastritis is a nonspecific term used for a variety of acute and chronic conditions, some of which may not be, in the strict sense, inflammations. Acute gastritis may be associated with chronic aspirin ingestion, excess alcohol consumption, heavy smoking, severe stress, certain drugs, systemic infections, shock, food poisoning, uremia, irradiation, and other factors, most of which seem to have in common the ability to alter the gastric mucosal barrier. Changes may vary from slight edema to severe hemorrhagic erosive gastritis. There may be ulcers. Chronic gastritis includes a variety of changes from superficial gastritis to atrophic gastritis, with the end stage of gastric atrophy, characterized by increasing severity of inflammatory cell infiltration and gastric gland atrophy. Associated with these changes are progressively more marked epithelial atypia and dysplasia, leading to an increased incidence of gastric adenocarcinoma. This pattern is especially true in patients with pernicious anemia (PA), whose gastritis may be a reflection of an autoimmune disorder, with antibodies to both parietal cells and intrinsic factor demonstrable. In PA the usual mucosa becomes atrophic and may be replaced by a small intestinal type of epithelium. There may also be megaloid changes of individual cells as well as the intense lymphocytic and plasmacytic infiltration.

Chronic hypertrophic gastritis (giant rugal hypertrophy of the stomach, Menetrier's disease) occurs in patients with excess gastrin production, as in the Zollinger-Ellison (Z-E) syndrome. The mucosal hypertrophy is preceded by hyperchlorydia. This condition may be confused radiologically with gastric lymphoma or diffuse infiltrative carcinoma.

Eosinophilic gastritis is thought to be a hypersensitivity reaction in which there may be eosinophil-rich granulomatous inflammation, sometimes with vasculitis. Granulomatous gastritis may occur in association with systemic disorders in which granulomas occur (sarcoidosis, Crohn's disease, tuberculosis), but may also be found as a nonspecific inflammatory response, sometimes in patients with peptic ulcers.

Peptic ulcer disease may affect the stomach or the duodenum, and can be regarded as a more advanced stage of acute erosive gastritis, with the same antecedent conditions as described above. Gastric acidity, but not necessarily hyperacidity, is always present, and the mucosal barrier is most likely disturbed. Acute ulcers are often multiple, especially in the stomach. In contrast, chronic peptic ulcers are generally solitary and occur at any site exposed to prolonged effects of acid-peptide juices. Most occur in the duodenum or stomach, but they may be in the esophagus, at the margins of a gastroenterostomy, in a Meckel's diverticulum with heterotopic gastric mucosa, and in the jejunum in the Z-E syndrome. Impaired mucosal resistance, due to altered mucosal blood flow, gastric stasis, mucosal defects, bile regurgitation, or gastritis seem to be most important in the pathogenesis of gastric ulcers. In contrast, duodenal ulcers are mostly due to relative or absolute hypersecretion of acid and pepsinogen, due to increased numbers of cells, increased responsiveness of mucosal epithelium, and decrease of acid-inhibitory factors. Gastric ulcers occur mostly in the antrum, but may be found in any part of the stomach. Duodenal ulcers are almost always in the first part, close to the pylorus. Peptic ulcers are typically sharply punched-out round areas, but almost always less than 3 cm in diameter, with relatively straight walls, and varying degrees of cellular necrosis, inflammatory response, and healing. Complications include bleeding, perforation, obstruction, and, in the case of gastric but *not* pyloric ulcers, malignant transformation.

Benign tumors of the stomach include polyps, leiomyomas, and lipomas. Polyps may be hyperplastic, adenomatous, or hamartomatous. Adenomatous polyps resemble those of the colon and, similarly, have malignant potential. Leiomyomas and lipomas usually present as small submucosal tumor masses which become clinically manifest when the overlying mucosa ulcerates and bleeds. Heterotopic pancreas may be found in the stomach and may mimic a tumor, both radiologically and endoscopically.

Adenocarcinoma is the most important tumor of the stomach. Far less common, are lymphomas, leiomyosarcomas, and carcinoids (argentaffinomas). Gastric adenocarcinoma is one of the most common and one of the most lethal of human malignancies, with dramatic inter- and intra-country variations in incidence. There is a 2:1 male predominance, and a 10 percent increase in individuals with blood group A. The major pathogenetic factors, however, are thought to be environmental, with implicated factors including diet, low socioeconomic class, urban living, trace metals in the soil, and occupation. No specific factor has been identified, although nitrates, used in the preservation of foods, have been strongly incriminated. Precancerous lesions that are well recognized include adenomatous gastric polyps and chronic atrophic gastritis (pernicious anemia). Carcinomas can occur anywhere in the stomach, but about half are in the pyloric region. They may be macroscopically classified as nodular, ulcerative, diffuse (linitis plastica), polypoid, or superficial, although it is not clear that these designations have prognostic import in and of themselves. More important is the pattern of infiltration. The diffusely infiltrating tumors are less amenable to resection than those with solid, cohesive, expanding masses of cells. Histologically, gastric carcinoma may be of the intestinal goblet or gastric mucus type cell with all stages of cellular differentiation. Spread of gastric carcinoma is to local lymph nodes (as many as 70 percent of patients at time of resection), remote lymph nodes (Virchow's), Blumer's (rectal) shelf, ovaries (Krukenberg tumor), and liver. Favorable signs at time of resection are that they are superficially absent of nodal involvement, and have clear resection margins, features usually not present in most patients. Early gastric cacinoma, confined to mucosa or mucosa and submucosa, has best prognosis. Clinical features include weight loss, pain, vomiting, anorexia, and early satiety. Gastric acid studies may be useful. In the presence of an ulcerating lesion, achlorhydria is almost diagnostic of adenocarcinoma, but the presence of acid does not preclude against it. Almost all patients will have occult blood in the stool. In many patients, elevated levels of carcinoembryonic antigen (CEA) may be detectable. Endoscopy, radiography, cytology, and, of course, biopsy can help to establish the diagnosis.

Small Intestine

Developmental anomalies include atresia, stenosis, and reduplications as well as diverticula, a special variant of which is Meckel's diverticulum. Atresias and stenosis may occur singly or at multiple sites and lead to intestinal obstruction with persistent vomiting and secondary fluid, electrolyte, and nutritional deficiencies. Multiple jejunal and ileal diverticula may occur along the line of entry of mesenteric nerves and vessels. They

may be the site of inflammation with bleeding and perforation. Stasis of bacterial contents may lead to bacterial overgrowth and excess utilization of vitamin B12, producing a PA-like syndrome. Meckel's diverticulum is the omphalomesenteric duct remnant. This usually occurs about 25 cm proximal to the ileocecal valve. It may contain heterotopic gastric mucosa, with subsequent peptic ulceration and bleeding. Heterotopic pancreatic mucosa may cause a Z-E syndrome. Inflammation may cause an appendicitislike episode.

Intestinal obstruction may be caused by extrinsic lesions, such as hernias, intestinal adhesions, intussusception, and volvulus, and by intrinsic conditions, such as atresia and stenosis, tumors, vascular insufficiency, and neurogenic disorders. Hernias are weaknesses or defects of the peritoneal cavity wall which bulge out, with persistent intraperitonenal pressure, to form saclike structures within which loops of bowel can be trapped (incarcerated). If the volume in the sac or in the bowel lumen increases, the vascular supply may be compromised (strangulated) causing infarction. Hernias can be inguinal, femoral, diaphragmatic, intraperitoneal, or at the site of a previous abdominal wound (incisional).

Mesenteric thrombosis and intestinal infarction may be due to arterial occlusion or insufficiency from embolic occlusion, local, usually atherosclerotic, thrombosis, or prolonged hypotension in a patient with compromised arteries, and to venous thrombosis, from postoperative trauma, peritonitis, portal hypertension, venous compression by tumor, polycythemia vera, and contraceptive pills. The sequel is hemorrhagic infarction in both cases with severe abdominal pain, obstruction, bloody diarrhea, shock, and, if untreated, death.

Infectious enteritides are covered in the microbiology section. Major intestinal infections are cholera and salmonellosis, including typhoid fever, shigellosis, actinomycosis, and tuberculosis. Cholera is a diarrheal disease of high mortality with few anatomic changes and no bowel ulcerations. Watery diarrhea contains flecks of mucus ("rice-water" stool) and fatalities result from dehydration, acidosis, hypokalemia, and shock. Typhoid fever is the most important of the salmonellosis. Organisms proliferate in Peyer's patches, causing characteristic enlargement and secondary ulceration of overlying mucosa. The ulcers follow the long axis of the bowel. Histologically, there is marked reticuloendothelial proliferation, with characteristic erythrophagocytosis. Similar changes may be seen in the spleen, lymph nodes, and liver, and death may occur from intestinal hemorrhage or perforation, splenic rupture, or pneumonia. Bradycardia and leukopenia may accompany the higher fever, abdominal pain and distension, severe diarrhea, and typical skin rash ("rose spots"). Shigellosis causes colonic disease primarily with dysentery associated with fever, headache, nausea, and vomiting. Abdominal actinomycosis is usually due to colonic or appendiceal disease. Penetration of the mucosa causes abscesses and internal and external fistula formation. Intestinal tuberculosis may develop from the ingestion of infected milk or from the spread of pulmonary tuberculosis by the swallowing of infective sputum. The ileum is the usual site and disease begins in the lympoid tissue, with later mucosal ulceration, which tends to be circumferential. Two conditions which may resemble intestinal tuberculosis are Yersinia infection and Crohn's disease, both of which typically affect the ileum. Yersinia generally causes an acute mesenteric lymphadenitis, particularly in children and young adults, with the formation of necrotic granulomas. Because of the clinical resemblance to appendicitis, diagnosis is usually made after appendectomy.

Crohn's disease (regional enteritis, granulomatous enteritis) may affect the small and large bowel commonly, and the stomach rarely. The etiology is unknown, but there are genetic and familial predispositions; Jews are affected three times more often than non-Jews. The macroscopic features directly reflect the microscopic. Single or multiple separate and well demarcated lesions occur. The bowel wall shows inflammation of all layers and the intestine appears thickened, with narrowing of the lumen. The serosal fat is hypertrophied and the mesentery is thickened. The serosal inflammation causes adhesions. The earliest lesion is thought to be the "aphthous" ulcer, which then dissects through the bowel layers as fissures which may lead to intra- and extramural abscesses, sinus tracts, and fistula. When the large bowel is involved, the rectum is usually spared, but the anus is affected. Sarcoidlike granulomas are seen in less than half of the cases, and may also be found in lymph nodes. The inflammation and fistula may involve adjacent structures, such as the abdominal wall, urinary bladder, and vagina, by contiguity. Manifestations include nausea and vomiting because of strictures, protein-losing enteropathy and malabsorption due to mucosal involvement, weight loss, fluid and electrolyte loss, and, in children, failure to thrive. Systemic complications or associations include migratory polyartheritis, ankylosing spondylitis, uveitis, amyloidosis, and carcinoma.

Malabsorption syndrome is characterized by abnormal fecal fat excretion (steatorrhea) and variable malabsorption of fats, fat-soluble vitamins, proteins, minerals, carbohydrates, and water. It is due to disturbance of digestion of nutrients into molecules small enough to be transported across the intestinal mucosal, reduction in the ability of the bowel mucosa to transport, or reduction in the absorptive capacity, in general. Combinations of these may also occur. Clinically, the malabsorption syndromes resemble each other, although the etiologic factors may differ greatly. Sprue (celiac disease, gluten-sensitive enteropathy, nontropical sprue) appears to be due to hypersensitivity to gluten, and is characterized by loss of small intestinal villi and consequent reduction of absortive surface area. The blunted villi may completely disappear, and there may be a marked lymphocytic and plasmacytic infiltration. The epithelial cells themselves become quite atypical. Gluten restriction leads to prompt restoration of mucosal integrity. Sprue patients may have an increased incidence of intestinal lymphoma. Tropical sprue may be morphologically indistinguishable from sprue, but is most likely due to an infectious agent; many patients respond to antibiotic therapy, although a specific etiology has not been confirmed. Whipple's disease is a rare systemic disorder in which the small intestine is infiltrated by characteristic foamy, glycoprotein-rich (periodic-acid-Schiff reaction-positive) histiocytes, within which rod-shaped bacilli can be recognized. The epithelial cells are not affected. The macrophages distend the villi and macroscopically the bowel resembles a shaggy rug. In addition to diarrhea, abdominal cramps, distension, steatorrhea, and fever, patients may have involvement of the lymph nodes, spleen, heart, liver, kidney, lung, and central nervous system. Antibiotic therapy may be effective. Other causes include intestinal lymphoma, eosinophilic (allergic) enteritis, abetalipropoteinemia, disaccharidase deficiency Crohn's disease, scleroderma, radiation enteritis, congenital lymphangiectasia, extensive metastatic carcinoma, and various infections, including tuberculosis, histoplasmosis, strongyloidiasis, giardiasis, and cryptosporidiosis. The latter two infections have been increasingly recognized in patients with AIDS.

Tumors of the small intestine are uncommon. Benign tumors include leiomyomas, lipomas, and heterotopic pancreatic rests as well as hamartomatous polyps. Carcinomas are distinctly unusual. Lymphomas also occur. Carcinoid tumors (argentaffinomas, apudomas) may arise anywhere in the intestinal tract, biliary tract, pancreas, or bronchial tree. Generally more indolent than carcinomas, they do have a malignant potential. They often occur as small yellow or tan, submucosal elevations found, in decreasing order of frequency, in the appendix (35–45 percent), small intestine (20–25 percent), rectum, bronchi, and large bowel. They may produce a variety of polypeptide hormones including serotonin, histamine bradykinin, prostaglandins, ACTH, insulin, glycagon, ADH, gastrin, VIP, somatostatin, and others. Histologically, the tumors tend to consist of monotonous round to oval, finely stippled cells arranged in nests, cords, sheets, and acini. Patients with heptatic metastases may have the symptom complex known as the carcinoid syndrome, in which there is vasomotor disturbance, intestinal hypermotility, bronchoconstrictive attacks, and right-sided cardiac fibrosis.

Appendix

Developmental anomalies of the appendix are rare. Diverticula do, however, occur. Appendiceal diverticulitis is often the basis of acute periappendicitis without lumenal involvement, but with the typical clinical manifestations of acute appendicitis.

Acute appendicitis is the most important appendiceal disease and an extremely common condition that occurs at any age, but is most frequent in the most industrialized countries of the world. This condition, along with colonic diverticulosis and colonic adenocarcinoma, is thought to be related to a fiber-poor diet. Appendicitis is probably preceded by obstruction of the ostium with subsequent increase of intralumenal pressure, relative compromise of bloody supply, and ischemia of the mucosa permitting invasion and proliferation of bacteria. The morphologic changes are those of an acute pyogenic response with accumulation of polymorphonuclear leukocytes. Complications include peritonitis, periappendiceal abscess, pylephlebitis with portal venous thrombosis, liver abscess, and generalized sepsis. Chronic appendicitis is a controversial concept, clinically and morphologically difficult to prove.

Mucocele refers to the accumulation of mucus within the lumen with spherical or fusiform enlargement of the organ, usually due to lumenal obstruction without bacterial growth. The appendix may rupture and mucus-elaborating cells may be dispersed throughout the peritoneal cavity, causing pseudomyxoma peritonei.

Adenocarcinoma may cause a mucocelelike condition and, when ruptured, can also appear as pseudomyxoma peritonei. Carcinoids have been discussed. Other tumors are exceedingly rare.

Large Intestine

Congenital anomalies of the colon are infrequent. There may be malrotations and reduplications. More common and clinically significant are Hirschsprung's disease and imperforate anus. Hirschsprung's disease is due to failure of development of Meissner's and Auerbach's plexuses. The anorectal junction regions are always involved and the defect may, in a retrograde and contiguous fashion, involve variable lengths of bowel. The absence of ganglion cells prevents normal peristalsis, causing a functional obstruction with dilatation proximal to the site of defect. The results may be complete obstruction, or degrees of constipation. Megacolon usually results. Diagnosis depends on confirmation of the absence of plexuses in the rectum. Acquired mega-

colon may be due to obstruction from other reasons, such as inflammatory disease or tumor, or from acquired loss of ganglia as in Chagas' disease. Imperforate anus occurs in 1 in 5,000 births and may vary from a thin membrane at the entodermal-ectodermal anal junction to varying lengths of rectal canal atresia or agenesis.

Diverticular disease is particularly common in industrialized countries. Diverticulosis occurs as herniations of colonic mucosa at points of weakness in the muscle wall, usually at the point of penetration by segmental blood vessels, and is thought to be induced by excess intralumenal pressure, most likely related to relatively low fiber content in the diet. Most diverticula occur in the sigmoid, but they may be throughout the colon. The small, saclike protrusions are filled with stool. Diverticulitis may follow the obstruction of a diverticulum, with subsequent increase of pressure, relative mucosal ischemia, and permeability to bacteria. Diverticulitis may cause an appendicitis-like condition, often left-sided, may lead to perforation and peritonitis, or, after repeated episodes with muscular hypertrophy and fibrosis, may lead to obstruction.

Hemorrhoids are also more common in Western societies, and are usually due to chronic constipation associated with diet, but may follow venous obstruction from other causes, such as tumor compression, pregnancy, or from portal hypertension. Hemorrhoids are varicela dilatations of anal and perianal venous channels. They may become thrombosed. Those that develop in the inferior hemorrhoidal plexus, below the anorectal line (external hemorrhoids) are usually painful; those in the superior hemorrhoidal plexus, above the anorectal line (internal hemorrhoids) are not painful; both may bleed. Ischemic colitis may occur at any part of the large bowel and may be pathogenically and morphologically similar to small bowel ischemia. The area of the splenic flexure is particularly susceptible because of its position at the terminus of two major arteries.

Infectious colitides are discussed in the microbiology section. Cholera, the salmonellosis, and shigellosis usually affect the colon as well as the small intestine. Amebiasis is an infection primarily of the colon, which may secondarily spread to the liver, lungs, and brain. The cecum and ascending colon are most often affected, with the sigmoid and rectum frequently involved. In fulminant cases, the entire colon may be infected. The amebae invade the crypts of the colonic glands and cause tissue destructions by spreading laterally in the lamina propria typically causing, in cross-section, an Erlenmeyer flasklike ulcer. Inflammatory cell response is usually slight, unless there is secondary bacterial invasion. Perforation, and peritonitis, may occur. Amebic abscesses may perforate the diaphragm to involve the thorax either from peritonitis or directly after liver abscesses form from venous spread. Antibiotic-associated (pseudomembranous) colitis has been associated with a variety of antibiotics, and is thought to be due to the suppression of normal bacterial flora and the elaboration of a toxin of *Clostridium difficile*. Characteristically, there are multiple plaquelike foci which microscopically have a distinct appearance of superficial necrosis in which the necrotic debris and acute inflammatory cells seem to be explosively streaming from the surface. Specific antibiotic (vancomycin) therapy is usually curative. A pseudomembrane may also form in staphylococcal colitis. Anorectal lymphogranuloma venereum has become more important in recent years as recognized infection of male homosexuals. Diagnosis is confirmed serologically. It is important to note that the classical feature of "bubos" (large, draining sinuses from infected inguinal lymph nodes) are virtually never seen in these individuals in whom the deep rectal nodes are affected. This population group may also present with anorectal syphilis or gonorrhea, and they also have a higher than expected incidence of amebiasis. The group of proctitides is often referred to as the "gay bowel syndrome" and does not necessarily indicate the presence of immunodeficiency (AIDS). Colorectal infections that are associated with AIDS include cytomegalovirus and cryptosporidiosis.

Idiopathic ulcerative colitis is a chronic disorder of unknown etiology characterized by extensive colonic mucosal ulceration and inflammation, typically beginning in the rectum and spreading contiguously, in a retrograde manner, to involve the entire colon. Unlike Crohn's disease, the anus and small intestine are not involved and there are no spared segments. The inflammation is almost always limited to the lamina propria, except in fulminant cases when it may spread beyond the muscularis mucosae. Histologically, ulceration and acute inflammation are the hallmarks, including characteristic, but *not* phathognomonic "crypt abscesses." In contrast to Crohn's disease, there are no granulomas, fissures, sinus tracts, fistulas, serositis, or involvement of adjacent structures, and healing does not lead to fibrosis and thickening of the bowel. As the ulceration develops, small areas of mucosa may remain viable. These may form polypoid extensions ("inflammatory polyps"). As in most forms of colitis, there is usually diarrhea, bleeding, and lower abdominal pain. In ulcerative colitis, the diarrhea is often mucoid. Bleeding may be so severe as to require transfusion. In some patients, an episode may be fulminant and life-threatening, particularly when inflammation extends beyond the muscularis mucosa, and the bowel segment (transverse colon) becomes dilated ("toxic megacolon"). These patients may pool enormous amounts of blood and other fluids in the dilated segment, causing fluid and electrolyte disturbances,

shock, and, if untreated, death. In long-standing disease, the bowel becomes atrophic and considerably shortened. With long-term disease there is considerable risk of malignancy, especially in patients who have had relatively active disease for more than 10 years and in whom the entire large intestine is affected. Ulcerative colitis usually affects teenagers and young adults. When it begins in older adults, it often affects the left colon only ("ulcerative proctitis"). These patients are at less risk for the development of cancer. In recent years, a precancerous mucosal change has been recognized. This epithelial dysplasia allows for surveillance, by biopsy, of susceptible patients.

Tumors of the colon, benign and malignant, are among the most common forms of neoplasia in man. Colorectal adenocarcinoma is a disease primarily of industrial societies. Considerable evidence suggests that colorectal carcinoma virtually always arises from preceding benign neoplastic polyps and that diet is a major factor in its development. It also seems clear that diet does not cause the development of polyps. Polyps of the colon may be hyperplastic, neoplastic, hamartomatous, or inflammatory. Hyperplastic polyps are typically minute mucosal mounds consisting of exaggerations of normal colonic mucosa. Their major significance seems to be as precursors of neoplastic polyps, although this is not universally agreed upon. Adenomatous (neoplastic) polyps may vary in their growth pattern. They may be on a stalk (pedunculated) or broad-based (sessile). They may consist of branching acini ("tubular adenoma") or slender fingerlike projections covered by a single layer of columnar epithelial cells ("villous adenoma"), or combinations of the two patterns ("tubulovillous adenoma"). The terms "tubular adenoma," "tubulovillous adenoma," and "villous adenoma" do not represent differences in pathogenesis, but only imply different growth patterns. The villous pattern is more likely to be present in larger polyp, and has a greater likelihood of malignant change. As many as 50 percent of adenomatous polyps greater than 2 cm diameter show malignant change. This change is only biologically significant, however, if the carcinoma has spread beyond the muscularis mucosa since the lymphatics are not present in the lamina propria. Familial (multiple) polyposis is an autosomal dominant condition characterized by innumerable colonic polyps developing in late childhood of adolescence, with carcinoma occurring in virtually 100 percent of cases within 20 to 30 years after the appearance of the polyps. It has been suggested that all neoplastic polyps are genetically determined to some degree and that carcinoma cannot develp, despite the diet, if the precursor of the polyp is not present. Polyps have been recognized in population groups in whom there is almost no colonic carcinoma. Furthermore, a few studies in the United

States have shown that the risk of carcinoma is dramatically reduced in susceptible individuals if the polyps are all excised.

There are more than 125,000 new cases of colonic adenocarcinoma each year in the United States, and approximately 60,000 deaths. Any part of the colon may be affected, but the left colon has the most tumors. On the left side the tumors are often circumferential ("napkin-ring") and may obstruct relatively early. Right sided lesions, where the fecal stream is more liquid, tend to be large, exophytic tumors which rarely obstruct. The overwhelming majority are well differentiated glandular cancers. The depth of invasion (Duke's classification) of the tumor has proven to be of greater prognostic significance than the site or the histologic differentiation (Table 6-5). Other malignant tumors include carcinoid, lymphoma, leiomyosarcoma, and, in the anorectum, squamous cell carcinoma, cloacogenic (basaloid) carcinoma, and melanoma.

Pancreas

The most important developmental anomaly of the pancreas, heterotopic pancreatic tissue, is rarely symptomatic, but may be seen as a submucosal nodule in the stomach, duodenum, or a Meckel's diverticulum. The gland may be absent (agenesis) or hypoplastic. The head of the pancreas may completely surround and occasionally obstruct the duodenum (annular pancreas). The separate ducts of the embryonic pancreas (Wirsung and Santorini) may persist and, if unrecognized, can be traumatized during duodenal or common duct surgery.

The pancreas may be the site of excess iron-pigment deposition in hemochromatosis. Considerable fatty infiltration may occur as a nonspecific response to injury, without dysfunction to the pancreas. In juvenile diabetes mellitus, beta cell necrosis may be seen; usually, there are no recognizable changes. Some adult diabetics may have amyloid change of the islets.

Atrophy may be ischemic, most often follows pancreatic duct obstruction, or is congenital or acquired. In

uremia, ducts and acini dilate and are filled with inspissated material.

Acute hemorrhagic pancreatitis may follow bile reflux, obstruction, excess alcohol ingestion, duodenal reflux, shock, and hypercalcemia. There is edema, hemorrhagic necrosis, and fat necrosis, to varying degrees. Acute hemorrhagic pancreatitis may be complicated by DIC syndrome, and has a high mortality rate, if untreated. If patients survive, complications include abscess, pseudocyst formation, and duodenal obstruction. Chronic pancreatitis does *not* invariably follow acute pancreatitis. It is most common in men, especially with alcoholism, biliary tract disease, hypercalcemia, and hyperlipidemia. Familial cases are known. Edema and mild interstitial inflammation may progress to severe inflammation and, ultimately, atrophy with fibrosis and calculous filled ducts.

Cysts of the pancreas may be congenital or acquired. Small cysts may develop with duct obstruction. The clinically important pseudocyst almost always follows hemorrhagic pancreatitis and presents as an abdominal mass, with a fibrotic wall contiguous with the pancreas.

Benign tumors are generally small and become manifest when they are hormonally active (insulinoma, glucagonoma, gastrinoma, somatostatinoma, vipoma, etc). The hormonally active tumors may be indistinguishable from carcinoid tumors and may also behave in a malignant fashion. In the Z-E syndrome, more than 50 percent of the tumors are islet cell carcinoma. Specific secretory granules are identified ultrastructurally or immunohistochemically. Nonfunctional tumors are rare and usually present as a mass.

Adenocarcinoma is the most important tumor of the pancreas, arising, in most cases, from duct cells. Carcinoma of the head obstructs common bile duct to cause obstructive jaundice and dilated (Courvoisier's) gallbladder. Carcinoma of the tail remains "silent" and is more widespread at the time of diagnosis. There is high mortality, whatever the site, with metastases common at diagnosis. Adenocarcinoma is also associated with DIC syndrome. Histologically, usually seen are tall columnar and mucus-secreting malignant cells, with marked fibroblastic reaction.

Liver

The liver is subject to a large number of morphologic and functional injuries. Patients with liver diseases, however, tend to display similar signs and symptoms. Jaundice and hepatic failure are the most common expressions of major liver injury.

Jaundice (icterus) is the yellow-green cutaneous and scleral discoloration due to billirubin accumulating in blood, tissues, and interstitial fluids. Jaundice may fol-

Table 6-5. Depth of Invasion of the Tumor (Duke's Classification)

	Duke's Stage	5 Year Survival
A	Mucosa	100%
B1	Into muscularis propria — nodes	65%
B2	Through entire wall — nodes	55%
C1	Limited to wall + nodes	43%
C2	Through the entire wall + nodes	22%
D	Distant metastases	10%

low an increased rate of production of bilirubin, a decreased uptake of bilirubin in liver cells, defective conjugation of bilirubin, and impaired canaliculi and biliary tract (Table 6-6).

Cholestasis is the accumulation of bile substances, particularly bile acids, in plasma. Usually, there is conjugated hyperbilirubemia. Intrahepatic cholestasis occurs most often as a result of liver cell injury, due to infection, toxin, or other factors. Extrahepatic cholestasis is due to mechanical obstruction of extrahepatic or large intrahepatic ducts. The characteristic microscopic features of cholestasis are bile plugs in canaliculi, particularly centrolobular, and bile pigment in hepatocytes ("feathery degeneration") and, eventually, Kupffer cells. Intrahepatic cholestasis may be due to cytoskeletal disturbance, faulty bile salt formation, canalicular membrane alterations, decreased bile salt flow across membranes, or subsequent bile salt bilirubin retention. In addition to the changes described, extrahepatic cholestasis leads to dilatation of intrahepatic bile ducts, portal tract edema, bile ductule proliferation, and fibroblast proliferation. Eventually, extrahepatic cholestasis leads to fibrosis in portal tracts, periductal and intraductal infiltration by polymorphonuclear leukocytes ("cholangitis"), and, as diagnostic features, extravasation of bile from ducts, with resultant, usually periportal, hepatocellular necrosis ("bile infarct"). Since bile duct and ductule epithelium is rich in alkaline phosphatase, this enzyme is generally elevated in extrahepatic cholestasis in addition to the hyperbilirubinemia. The critically important differentiation between intra- and extrahepatic cholestasis is usually made on clinical and biochemical, rather than morphologic, grounds.

Hepatic failure may follow extensive ("massive"), usually acute, necrosis of the liver or may be the result of chronic liver disease, particularly, cirrhosis. Rarely, hepatic failure may be seen in conditions in which hepatocellular necrosis is minimal, and the significant cellular changes are seen at the ultrastructural level (Reye's syndrome, tetracycline toxicity, fatty liver of pregnancy). Major, usually life-threatening, sequelae are hepatic encephalopathy and hepatorenal syndrome, in which se-vere central nervous system or renal disturbances occur, often in the absence of recognizable morphologic alteration of those organs. Pathogenesis is not well understood for either condition. The encephalopathy is thought to be due to elaboration of a thus far unidentifed "neurotoxin," whereas the renal failure most likely reflects vasospastic shunting of blood from outer cortical to juxtamedullary nephrons.

Developmental anomalies of the liver are exceedingly rare and generally of no clinical import. In contrast, circulatory changes are extremely common, and, because liver cells are extremely sensitive to anoxia, may be clinically important. The primary cause may be extrahepatic and the hepatic vessels themselves may be affected. In chronic passive congestion the liver is enlarged and the central veins and sinusoids are engorged with blood. The central zone is especially sensitive to anoxic changes and, if congestion is slightly prolonged, central hemorrhagic necrosis may occur. A similar lesion is seen in shock. Chronic heart failure may lead to fibrosis around the central veins ("cardiac sclerosis"). This has become distinctly uncommon as therapy for heart failure has become effective. Cirrhosis, on the basis of chronic passive congestion, probably does not occur. Indeed, the hepatic changes of congestion rarely cause liver failure. Infarcts of the liver are rare, since the liver is supplied by the hepatic artery and portal vein. Among the causes of hepatic infarcts are arteriosclerotic disorders, periarteritis nodosa, and shock. Portal vein obstruction usually does not cause infarcts, but will cause acute congestive splenomegaly. Causes include trauma, inflammation such as peritonitis, and tumor. Hepatocellular carcinoma has a particular propensity for invading portal veins. The liver is usually not enlarged and there may not be ascites or jaundice. In contrast, hepatic vein obstruction may lead to an enlarged, tender liver, intractable ascites, acute portal hypertension, and acute liver failure (Budd-Chiari syndrome). This has been associated with hypercoagulable states such as DIC and polycythemia vera, oral contraceptive use, radiation effect, tumor involvement and, in most cases, no definable cause is identified. Initially, centrolobular congestion is severe

Table 6-6. Mechanisms of Jaundice

Mechanism	Example	Hyperbilirubinemia
Increased production	Hemolytic anemias	Unconjugated
Decreased uptake	Gilbert's syndrome	Unconjugated
Defective conjugation	Crigler-Najjar syndrome	Unconjugated, conjugated
Impaired excretion	Dubin-Johnson syndrome	Conjugated
	Rotor's syndrome	Conjugated
	Cholestasis	Conjugated, unconjugated

and accompanied by hepatocellular necrosis. Later, fibrosis and regeneratory changes may be seen.

Metabolic and degenerative changes have been discussed elsewhere. Changes often seen affecting the liver are lipofuscin deposition with aging ("brown atrophy"), hemosiderosis, amyloidosis, fatty changes, and glycogen accumulation.

Inflammatory conditions of the liver are particularly important. Hepatitis might be defined, in the broadest sense, as a hepatocytic injury with resulting inflammatory response. In reality, hepatitis is a complex group of disorders which vary greatly in etiology and clinical import, but which are similar in terms of pathophysiology and clinical manifestations. Hepatitis may be due to viruses, other microorganisms, toxins, including alcohol, drugs and various chemicals, and may also reflect immunologic injury. Characteristically, there is (1) abnormal hepatic function with decreased bile secretion, (2) release of liver cell substances, many of which are diagnostically useful, into the blood, (3) decreased ability to secrete various normal products, and (4) impaired ability to metabolize. Patients usually display malaise and easy fatigability, and they may have anorexia or jaundice.

Acute viral hepatitis is most often due to viruses A, B, non-A non-B (NANB), and Delta agent. There are no major histopathologic differences between these. The liver is swollen, and slightly pale. Histologically, there is ballooning degeneration, due to hydropic swelling. This may lead to cell death, with complete loss of cell water and the formation of acidophilic (Councilmanlike) bodies. Typically, there is marked variation of size, shape, and staining characteristics of hepatocytes, and focal necrosis, with a few neutrophils in lobules, portal tracts, and infiltrating central veins. Kupffer cells are hypertrophied and hyperplastic. There is usually mild cholestasis, although this may be absent, and signs of regeneration (mitoses, 2-cell thick plates, multinucleation). In acute cholestatis viral hepatitis, cholestasis and neutrophil infiltration are marked. In submassive necrosis there is severe centrolobular necrosis and parenchymal collapse, linking central veins with portal tracts ("bridging necrosis"). This often leads to hepatic failure or cirrhosis. Massive necrosis is marked by a small, shrunken, flabby, congested liver, in which there is extensive loss of almost all hepatocytes, collapse of reticulin framework of the liver, marked sinusoidal congestion, and many pigment-ladden macrophages. Death usually ensues in days.

Hepatitis B is particularly varied in its clinical expressions as is illustrated by the following:

Acute hepatitis
 Anticteric
 Icteric
 Fulminant
Chronic hepatitis
 Persistent
 Aggressive
 Cirrhosis
Extrahepatic diseases
 Glomerulonephritis
 Papular acrodermatitis
 Other rashes
 Arthritis
 Vasculitis
Carrier state
 Transplacental
 Postnatal from mother
 Posttransfusion
 Family contact
 Institutional exposure
 Immunosuppression (disease, medication)
 Drug abuse

Serologic markers of hepatitis B are illustrated (Table 6-7).

Chronic hepatitis has been defined as hepatocellular damage accompanied by chronic inflammatory reaction and/or fibrosis, continuing without improvement for 6 months or longer. The etiology is not always identified.

Table 6-7. Serological Markers of Hepatitis B

	Prodrome Phase	Acute Hepatitis	Convalescent Phase	Carrier State	Chronic Hepatitis
HBsAg	++	++	+−	+	+
HBsAb	−(+)	−	+−	+ or −	+ or −
HBcAg	−(+)	−	−	+ or −	+ or −
HBcAb	−	++	++	+	+
HBeAg	++	+−	−	+ or −	+ or −
HBeAb	−−	++	+++	+ or −	+ or −
Polymerase	++	+−	−	+ or −	+ or −

Some cases follow hepatitis A or NANB, and possibly Delta agent. It may follow drug, including alcohol, injury. In some cases, there is an immune component; many cases remain cryptogenic. Two major histopathologic forms of chronic hepatitis are recognized (Table 6-8).

Chronic persistent hepatitis (CPH) is a mild disease, with good prognosis, and no progression to cirrhosis. Patients are asymptomatic or have vague symptoms. Laboratory tests are usually normal, except for slight elevations of aminotransferase activity. Diagnosis is made by liver biopsy. HBV may be present or absent. Chronic active hepatitis (CAH) is generally more severe, depending on the etiology. HBV-positive CAH progresses slowly, and usually has a low mortality. HBV negative ("autoimmune") CAH generally progresses rapidly to cirrhosis, with portal hypertension and liver failure, and high mortality. Many patients show hyperbilirubinemia, increased aminotransferase, hypergammaglobulinemia, and antinuclear and antismooth muscle antibodies. However, hepatocellular carcinoma is rare in HBV-negative CAH, but common in HBV-positive CAH.

Drug-induced and toxic hepatitides are heterogenous groups of disorders, both in terms of precipitating factors and clinical and morphologic manifestations. In our society, the most important liver disorder is alcoholic liver disease. Ethanol, or its metabolite acetaldehyde, is hepatotoxic. In addition, liver injury may be amplified by the primary malnutrition that is often an integral part of the alcoholism syndrome as well as by the secondary malnutrition that is caused by ethanol-induced intestinal damage and the inefficient nutrient utilization that follows the injury. Initially, the liver may be enlarged because of fatty change and accumulation of export protein in hepatocytes. Further injury may lead to alcoholic hepatitis with hydropic swelling of hepatocytes, cytoplasmic accumulation of alcoholic hyalin ("mallory body," intermediate type filaments, prekeratin), and often with necrosis and neutrophilic reaction. Fibrosis of the central

vein ("central hyaline sclerosis") develops. This change is diagnostically useful and probably prognostically significant in terms of later cirrhosis. Cholestasis is sometimes seen. Alcoholic hepatitis often presents as an acute illness, with hepatomegaly, hepatic tenderness and pain, jaundice, ascites, anorexia, and liver failure. In the chronic stages of alcoholic liver disease, the fibrosis extends from centrolobular zones to involve portal tracts and cirrhosis follows. Some patients show features of chronic hepatitis.

Drug effects on the liver may be classified as predictable or as unpredictable (idiosyncratic). The histopathologic changes that occur are extremely variable as is illustrated by the following:

Viral hepatitislike
    Halothane
    Isoniazid
    α-Methyldopa
    Imipramine
Chronic hepatitislike
    Isoniazid
    α-Methyldopa
    Oxyphenisatin
    Nitrofurantoin
    Sulfonamides (?)
Cholestatic hepatitis
    Phenothiazines
Cholestasis
    Oral contraceptives
    Anabolic steroids
Steatosis
    Tetracyclin
    Corticosteroids
    Antituberculosis agents
    Methotrexate
Hepatocellular damage
    Acetaminophen
    Mithramycin C

Table 6-8. Histopathologic Forms of Chronic Hepatitis

	Chronic Persistent Hepatitis	Chronic Active Hepatitis
Chronic inflammatory cell (lymphocytes and plasma cell) infiltrate	Portal	Portal and adjacent lobule
Hepatocellular necrosis	Little focal	Piecemeal necrosis, sometimes bridging or multibolular necrosis
Fibrosis	Little	Progressive, at first portal
Lobular architecture	Preserved	Distorted

Granulomata
  Quinidine
  BCG
  Alluporinol
  Diphenylhydantoin
  Sulfonamides
  Phenylbutazone

Primary biliary cirrhosis (PBC) is a unique inflammatory liver disease, affecting mostly middle-aged women, presenting initially as pruritis and later as painless jaundice, hypercholesterolemia, with associated xanthomata, and with hyperbilirubinemia and hyperalkaline phosphatemia. Serum IgM is high, antimitochondrial antibodies are demonstrable, and there may be the other immunologic abnormalities, such as rheumatoid arthritis, Sjögren's syndrome, arteritis, thyroiditis, progressive systemic sclerosis, SLE, glomerulonephritis, and lymphoma. Inflammation is primarily portal, with many plasma cells infiltrating, associated with bile duct destruction and, sometimes, granulomata (stage I). With progression there is bile ductular proliferation (stage II), portal fibrosis (stage III), and, finally, cirrhosis with cholestasis (stage IV). Characteristically, the liver has markedly increased copper content.

Cirrhosis can be the end-result of many liver injuries, and should be thought of in physiologic as well as morphologic, terms. The key morphologic features of cirrhosis are (1) connective tissue septa linking portal tracts and central veins and (2) regenerating nodules. The septa include vascular channels which serve to bypass the usually sinusoidal pathway, resulting in (1) limitation of the interaction of blood with metabolically-active hepatocytes, (2) increasing portal vein pressure (i.e., portal hypertension), (3) reduction of effective hepatic blood flow, particularly after gastrointestinal hemorrhage, augmented by increasing sinusoidal fibrosis, and (4) shunting of bacteria and bacterial toxins from intestinal tract into systemic circulation because of bypass of Kupffer cells. Portal hypertension may be (1) postsinusoidal, from compression of hepatic vein branches by regenerating nodules, and obliteration by fibrosis, (2) parasinusoidal, if hepatic artery to portal vein anastomoses develop, and (3) presinusoidal, from portal tract fibrosis, portal vein thrombosis, or disease of intrahepatic portal vein branch (e.g., schistosomiasis). Portal hypertension causes (1) the development of collaterals between portal vein and vena cava systems (esophageal varices, hemorrhoids, dilated abdominal veins), (2) hypersplenism, and (3) ascites (when postsinusoidal). The pattern of cirrhosis may be micronodular (Laennec, portal, nutritional), macronodular with parenchymal collapse (postnecrotic) or without collapse (posthepatitic). The pattern of cirrhosis does not always reflect the etiol-

ogy. Cirrhosis may follow the hepatitides, toxic injuries, drugs, alcohol, hemochromatosis, Wilson's disease, α-1-antitrypsin deficiency, chronic right heart failure, parasitic infections, and may be cryptogenic.

Tumors of the liver are particularly common. The overwhelming majority of these are metastatic. Adenoma of the liver is well defined, highly vascular, single tumor mass, occurring almost exclusively in women who have taken oral contraceptives for relatively long periods of time, which regresses when the contraceptive is no longer used. Hepatocellular carcinoma (hepatoma) is less common in the United States than in parts of Asia and Africa. In most cases there is a preceding cirrhosis. Hepatitis B infection and aflatoxin ingestion have been incriminated as significant contributing factors. Other causative influences include thorium dioxide (thorotrast), a radioactive substance used in the past, liver fluke infestation (cholangiocarcinoma), and, possibly, oral contraceptives and androgenic-anabolic steroids. Typically, there are multiple nodules in a cirrhotic liver. They may be yellow-white, or green, with varying amounts of bile production. Histologically, the more differentiated tumors resemble liver cells, and may mimic the pattern of liver cords. α-Feto-protein levels may be greatly elevated. Cholangiocarcinoma arises from intrahepatic bile ducts and resembles biliary tree and pancreatic carcinoma, usually evoking a marked fibroblastic response. Hepatoblastoma usually occurs in infancy and childhood, and consists of undifferentiated epithelial and mesenchymal elements. Prognosis is better than that of hepatocellular carcinoma. Angiosarcoma is extremely rare, but has recently been recognized in workers involved with the polymerization of monomeric vinyl chloride to polyvinyl chloride.

GALLBLADDER

Congenital anomalies include agenesis, hypoplasia, and reduplication as well as similar anomalies of the bile ducts.

Cholelithiasis may occur without preceding inflammation, and is thought to be mostly due to abnormalities of bile composition. Gallstones may contain cholesterol, calcium bilirubinate, and/or calcium carbonate. Almost all gallstones are mixed in composition, but pure bilirubin stones may form in patients with hemolytic anemia. Gallstones have been incriminated in the pathogenesis of cholecystitis, obstructive jaundice, cholangitis, cholecystointestinal fistula, gallstone ileus, and carcinoma of the gallbladder.

Cholecystitis may be acute or chronic. Acute cholecystitis may show all the usual inflammatory cellular reactions, and may progress to gangrene and perforation. Chronic cholecystitis may not always be preceded by acute cholecystitis. There may be chronic inflammation, fibrosis, accentuation of the glands (Rokitansky-Aschoff sinuses), and variable numbers of gallstones. Cholesterolosis is a frequent, but not inevitable, accompaniment of cholecystitis and consists of collections of lipidrich histiocytes distending mucosal folds and imparting a bright-yellow speckled mucosal pattern. Hidrops (mucocele) may occur in a normal or previously inflamed gallbladder and is due to total cystic duct obstruction with resorption of bile and retention of a clear mucinous fluid within a distended gallbladder.

Tumors are relatively uncommon. Papillomas, adenomas, myomas, and carcinoids occur, but the clinically most significant and most frequent tumor is adenocarcinoma. These tumors may be infiltrating or fungating and are frequently found incidentally during cholecystectomy for other reasons. They may spray extensively to the liver and biliary tree, if clinically undetected, in which case there is a high mortality. Chronic inflammation and gallstones are thought to be contributing factors. Bile duct and ampulla of Vater adenocarcinomas are rare and usually present early, before there is extensive dissemination, because of obstruction of bile flow. A distinct variant occurs at the junction of the hepatic ducts (Klatskin tumor) and similarly may present early and have a good prognosis if surgically resected.

ADRENAL GLAND

Congenital hyperplasia of the adrenal cortex is transmitted as an autosomal recessive abnormality and is usually accompanied by oversecretion of androgens with undue virilization of males or pseudohermaphroditism in females (Adrenogenital syndrome). Three major types of congenital hyperplasia include (1) partial 21-hydroxylase deficiency (macrogenitosomia preacox in the male and pseudohermaphroditism in the female), (2) complete 21-hydroxylase deficiency (virilization with Addison's like syndrome and death in early infancy), and (3) 11-hydroxylase deficiency (virilization with associated hypertension).

Waterhouse-Friderichsen syndrome is characterized by the presence of acute bilateral and generally fatal adrenal hemorrhages associated with meningococcemia or other bacterial and viral infections. It is characterized clinically by the sudden onset of purpura, circulatory collapse, and intravascular coagulation syndrome.

Addison's disease is characterized by chronic adrenocortical insufficiency from a variety of pathologic processes that destroy the adrenal cortex. They include tuberculosis, amyloidosis, hemochromatosis, neoplasms, venous thrombosis, emboli, periarteritis nodosa, and fungal and viral infections (blastomycosis, coccidiodomycosis, histoplasmosis, herpes, cytomegalovirus). In most instances, however, the etiology of Addison's disease remains unclear (idiopathic adrenal cortical atrophy) and is thought to be due to circulating antiadrenal mitochondrial and microsomal antibodies. Autoimmune thyroiditis may also accompany the adrenal disease (Schmidt's syndrome). Patients present with weakness, weight loss, anorexia, pigmentation of skin and mucous membranes, hypotension, hypoglycemia, hyponatremia, hyperkalemia, and tendency to dehydration. They frequently develop acute adrenal insufficiency ("crisis") following infections, trauma, or surgery.

Adrenal cortical hyperactivity results in syndromes characterized by hypersecretion of corticosteroids (Cushing's syndrome), aldosterone (Conn's syndrome), or androgens (adrenogenital syndrome).

Cushing's syndrome is the result of hypersecretion of corticosteroids by the adrenal cortex in response to excessive pituitary ACTH output or ectopic ACTH production by bronchogenic carcinoma, pancreatic islet cell tumors, thymomas, and other neoplasms. It can also be the result of primary diseases of the adrenal gland (Cushing's disease) including diffuse or nodular hyperplasia (70 percent of cases), adenomas or carcinomas. Cushing's syndrome is also frequently secondary to exogenous, therapeutic administration of corticosteroids.

Patients have a characteristic habitus including moon facies, buffalo hump, truncal obesity, striae of skin, acne, hirsutism, amenorrhea and muscle weakness. They also have diabetes, polycythemia, osteoporosis, and systemic hypertension.

Hyperaldosteronism is usually associated with a cortical adenoma (Conn's syndrome) and less often with bilateral hyperplasia. Patients with this syndrome present with hypertension, muscle weakness, hypernatremia, hypokalemia, alkalosis hyperaldosternemia, and decreased serum renin levels.

Tumors of the adrenal cortex include adenomas, carcinomas, and metastatic lesions of the lung, breast, and other primary sites. Adrenal cortical adenomas are a common finding at autopsy. They are usually small (less than 5 cm) and present as rounded yellow-brown nodules. Clinically they may be functional and present with Cushing's syndrome, adult virilization, or Conn's syndrome. Frequently, however, they are nonfunctional.

Adrenal cortical carcinomas are uncommon. They present as large tumors with areas of hemorrhage, necrosis, and calcification and tend to metastasize widely. In 90 percent of cases, the lesion is functional (Cushing's syndrome, virilization, feminization, and/or aldosteronism).

Pheochromocytoma is an encapsulated, hemorrhagic tumor arising from the adrenal medulla (80 – 90 percent of cases) or extraadrenal paraganglion tissues located in the retroperitoneum, mediastinum, organ of Zuckerkandl, urinary bladder, middle ear, etc. They may be multiple and can be associated with neurofibromatosis, Von-Hipple-Lindau disease, Sturge-Weber syndrome, and Sipple's syndrome. Pheochromocytoma can metastasize widely but behaves in a benign manner in most cases (90 percent). They store and secrete norepinephrine and epinephrine, producing episodic or persistent systemic hypertension which may lead to death.

Neuroblastoma is a malignant adrenal tumor composed of primitive small dark round neural cells arranged in rosettes. It is almost always a tumor of children younger than 4 years and frequently metastasizes to the liver, lungs, and bones. Neuroblastoma is usually functional and is accompanied by elevation in blood levels of various catecholamines and their metabolites.

THYROID GLAND

Adenomatous hyperplasia or nodular enlargement of the thyroid (nodular goiter) frequently represents a form of work hypertrophy of the gland to compensate for an absolute correlative insufficiency of iodine. The latter can be secondary to dietary deficiency, is usually endemic, and can result from marked increased in body demands for iodine in pregnancy and female adolescence or from the genetic enzymatic defects of drugs. Chronic cyclic hyperplasia and regression of the thyroid tissues result in an enlarged, multinodular gland. Occasionally one of the nodules grows suddenly as a result of hemorrhage, necrosis, or cystic degeneration and simulates a thyroid tumor.

Diffuse thyroid hyperplasia (Graves' disease) is usually a disease of women. Diffuse enlargement of the gland (diffuse goiter) is accompanied by clinical manifestations of hyperthyroidism (tachicardia, increased body temperature, hyperactivity, exophthalmus, and pretibial myxedena). Graves' disease is thought to be an autoimmune disorder and is frequently associated with other autoimmune diseases including pernicious anemia, Hashimoto's thyroiditis, systemic lupus erythematosus, and rheumatoid arthritis. The thyroid is enlarged diffusely with hyperplastic follicular cells forming papillary projections in thyroid follicles. The amount of colloid is decreased. Interstitial lymphoid infiltrates characteristic of lymphocytic thyroiditis are also present and may be the histologic manifestation of autoimmune activity.

Graves' disease may be secondary to increase secretion of extrapituitary hormones that stimulate thyroid hormone production and secretion, such as the long acting thyroid stimulator (LATS). It may also result from autonomous hyperactivity of the gland.

Hashimoto's thyroiditis is a form of chronic diffuse thyroiditis that is more frequent in women. It is probably an autoimmune disease related to autosensitization to thyroglobulin. The serum of patients with this form of thyroiditis contains circulating antibodies to thyroglobulin and to cytoplasmic and nuclear components of the thyroid epithelium. Pathologically the gland is diffusely infiltrated by mononuclear cells, plasma cells, and lymphocytes with prominent germinal centers. The follicular epithelium is degenerate with formation of metaplastic cells with abundant eosinophilic cytoplasm (Askanasi cells).

Granulomatous thyroiditis (de Quervain's thyroiditis) is a form of subacute thyroiditis with granulomas that mostly affects women. It is usually a self-limited disease and most likely of viral origin.

Riedel's struma is a form of chronic thyroiditis that affects both sexes equally and is characterized by a small fibrotic thyroid gland that is firmly adherent to adjacent structures. Patients present with hypothyroidism and may have associated fibromatosis at other sites (mediastinum, peritoneum, etc) Riedel's struma probably represents an end stage of previous acute or subacute thyroiditis.

The thyroid gland may be the site of nodular lesions that appear clinically as neoplasms. They include cystic degenerated colloid nodules, localized thyroiditis, benign adenoma, malignant tumors (primary or metastatic), and nodules due to amyloidosis.

Follicular adenoma is a benign usually solitary thyroid nodule surrounded by a distinct capsule. Clinically self-limited, it may reach a large size. Histologically follicular adenoma consists of thyroid follicles of varying sizes (micro, macro, and fetal). The cells may be eosinophilic granular cells showing prominent mitochondria on ultrastructural studies (Hürthle cell adenoma).

Thyroid carcinoma may appear in any age group.

Papillary carcinoma is the most common type of thyroid cancer and is occasionally associated with a history of exposure to ionizing radiation. As example, incidence was greater in Japanese people that survived the atomic bomb attacks. Grossly these carcinomas present as small to large, white, firm, nonencapsulated nodules that infiltrated the adjacent parenchyma. Histologically they are composed of papillary structures with focal laminated calcific nodules (psammoma bodies). These tumors have a low malignant potential and tend to metastasize to regional lymph nodes. They rarely metastasize to distant sites and seldom result in fatal carcinomatosis.

Follicular carcinomas present as well circumscribed masses composed of follicular cells with vascular and capsular invasion. They have a low grade malignant potential and usually metastasize through the blood stream to distant sites such as bone and lung.

Medullary carcinoma of the thyroid is a special variant of cancer composed of endocrine cells derived from parafollicular (C type) cells. The tumors are usually small, may be multiple and may be familiar. Histologically, there are trabeculae and solid nests of endocrine cells with prominent amyloid stroma. A variety of hormones, including calcitonin, histamine, serotonin, and prostaglandins, may be produced. Medullary carcinomas usually metastasize to regional lymph nodes, the lungs, bones, and liver. Approximately 50 percent of patients survive 5 years.

Undifferentiated (anaplastic) carcinoma occurs in older patients (seventh decade) and is the most malignant form of thyroid cancer. Most patients die within 6 months with widespread bloodborne metastasis. Histologically these tumors can be quite variable, with giant, small, squamous, and/or spindle cells.

PARATHYROID GLANDS

Parathyroid glands enlarge in response to different stimuli and any or all of the usual cellular elements (chief, oxyphil, water-clear cells) may participate.

Primary (autonomous) hyperplasia appears in 15 percent of patients with primary hyperparathyroidism. Patients present with enlargement of hypercalcemia due to elevated serum levels of parathormone, bony lesions due to reabsorption of bony trabecular (osteitis fibrosa), cystica, osteomalacia, nephrocalcinosis, renal calculi, pyelonephritis secondary to nephrocalcinosis, metastatic calcifications in various organs (lungs, stomach, pituitary, etc.), peptic ulcer, pancreatitis, and for psychotic episodes. Water-clear cells are most often involved.

Secondary (physiologic) hyperplasia occurs in response to prolonged hypocalcemia secondary to long standing renal diseases, malabsortive states, or vitamin D deficiency. The four glands are enlarged. Removal of the cause of hypocalcemia in most instances leads to a return to a normal parathyroid state.

Tertiary hyperparathryroidism results from prolonged secondary hyperplasia of the parathyroids. The glandular hyperplasia becomes autonomous and does not improve after removal of the initial hyperplastic stimulus.

Most instances of primary hyperparathyroidism are secondary to benign adenomas of the parathyroids (80 percent of cases). These tumors are usually solitary but may be associated with endocrine neoplasms in other organs (multiple endocrine neoplasm syndrome or MEN). Rarely hyperparathyroidism is secondary to a parathyroid carcinoma (3–4 percent of cases). These

tumors are adhered to other neck structures, are slow growing, and tend to recur locally. They can metastasize to regional lymph nodes.

Hyperplasia or neoplasia of multiple endocrine glands can present with a wide range of clinical and pathologic manifestations. These unusual syndromes are often familial and are accompanied by elevations in the serum levels of various polypeptide hormones. Patients present with tumors at various separate anatomical sites. These neoplasms are thought to be derived from neuroendocrine cells with biochemical characteristics of amine precursor uptake and decarboxylase (APUD) cells. These APUD cells have an ectodermal or endodermal embryologic origin and are normally present in many parts of the body including pancreatic islet cells, pituitary cells, thyroid parafollicular cells, endocrine cells in the gastrointestinal tract (more than 11 different types of cells producing various polypeptide hormones), Feyrter cells in the lung, and Merkel's cells in the skin. The two most common pluriendocrine syndromes are the Wermer's syndrome (MEN I) and Sipple's syndrome (MEN 2), as is illustrated by the following:

Wermer's syndrome (MEN I)
    Pituitary adenoma
    Islet cell tumor of pancreas
    Parathyroid hyperplasia or adenoma
    Renal cortical adenoma
    Thyroid hyperplasia or adenoma
    Carcinoid
Sipple's syndrome (MEN II)
    Medullary carcinoma of thyroid
    Pheochromocytoma
    Parathyroid adenoma or hyperplasia
    Mucosal neuromas

DIABETES MELLITUS

Diabetes mellitus is a disorder of carbohydrate metabolism present in 5 percent of the population. A detailed description of its clinical and physiopathologic manifestations is beyond the scope of this chapter.

Diabetes mellitus can be classified from a pathogenetic view into (1) hormonal diabetes which results from the secretion of hormones with insulinlike activity by tumors or hyperplastic processes, including pituitary and adrenal cortical lesions, pheochromocytoma, tumors of pancreatic islets, and carcinomas of the lung and pancreas; (2) diabetes due to parenchymal pancreatic pathology resulting from pathologic processes that destroy the pancreatic parenchyma, including acute and chronic pancreatitis, cystic fibrosis, pancreatic lithiasis, malignant tumors, and hemochromatosis; (3) surgical diabetes resulting from pancreatectomy with removal of substantial portions of the gland; and (4) idiopathic diabetes, the most common form, with two distinct clinicopathologic forms. Maturity onset diabetes occurs in adult patients and often can be controlled with oral hypoglycemic drugs. Patients are not prone to develop ketosis. Juvenile diabetes occurs in young patients who may have severe hyperglycemia and ketosis. These patients are dependent on insulin treatment.

The pathology of idiopathic diabetes mellitus is disappointing. Frequently there is no clear correlation between the severity of clinical manifestations and the morphologic findings at autopsy. The pancreas of patients with diabetes of the adult onset form may show hyalinization of islets of Langerhans due to amyloid deposition and fibrosis. The pancreas of patients with juvenile onset diabetes shows lymphocytic infiltrates in islets of Langerhans, perhaps related to a viral infection or an autoimmune reaction. Beta cells have hydropic degeneration and insulin granules. The total islet volume, proportions of beta to alpha cells, and levels of extractable insulin are also lower in the pancreas of diabetics.

Diabetes mellitus is a systemic disease with abnormalities of carbohydrate, lipid, and protein metabolism that are reflected in pathologic abnormalities in multiple organs. For example, there is excessive glycoprotein deposition in the basement membrane of many organs, changes in large blood vessels (macroangiopathy and capillaries, microangopathy), and accumulations of fat in multiple cells such as the liver and kidney. As a result of these abnormalities, diabetics have a higher incidence of myocardial infarction, gangrene of extremities, aortic aneurysm, cerebral infarction and hemorrhage and retinopathy with loss of vision. Diabetics have also a higher incidence of infections, especially when the levels of blood glucose and electrolytes are controlled poorly. Hyperglycemia is associated with in vitro abnormalities decreased leukocyte phagocytosis, chemotaxis, adherence to fiberglass, and intracellular killing capacity. Opportunistic infections such as mucormycosis develop in diabetics and are accompanied by a very high mortality.

SKELETAL SYSTEM

Developmental disorders of bone can be congenital and/or familial. Some of these conditions are the result of gene mutations (osteogenesis imperfecta, achondroplasia, multiple exostoses). Others are related to metabolic abnormalities that result in the accumulation of abnormal metabolites in bone marrow histiocytes.

As example, mucopolysaccharidoses are due to the absence of an enzyme for the breakdown of certain polysaccharides resulting in their accumulation in reticuloendothelial cells. For example, Morquio's syndrome results from a deficiency of the enzyme acetylhexosaminidase accompanied by dwarfism and other skeletal abnormalities. Gaucher's disease is a deficiency of beta-galactosidase leading to the accumulation of glucocerebrosides in reticuloendothelial cells with skeletal, hematopoietic, and hepatic abnormalities.

Rickets and osteomalacia are two bone disorders characterized by the presence of soft, demineralized bones. Rickets occurs in children and osteomalacia occurs in adult patients. They are both associated with dietary deficiency of vitamin D, intestinal malabsorption, renal tubular abnormalities, and renal failure. The basic mechanism involved in the development of rickets and osteomalacia is insufficient serum calcium necessary to stimulate bone resorption to maintain homeostasis. Osteomalacia can also be the result of endocrine abnormalities including hyperpituitarism, hypopituitarism, hyperparathyroidism, hypoparathyroidism, and hyperthyroidism.

Osteoporosis is a bone disorder of unknown etiology characterized by reduced amounts of bone secondary to abnormal matrix deposition. It may be related to disuse, aging, use of corticosteroids, genetic factors, and decreased estrogen serum levels in postmenopausal women.

Paget's disease of the bone is a degenerative disorder of the skeleton of unknown etiology that affects mostly men older than 55 years of age. It affects the lumbosacral spine, pelvis, skull, femur, tibia, clavicle, and other bones. Initially the lesions are osteoclastic (bone resorption) but later becomes osteoblastic (new bone formation) resulting in enlargement and deformity of the affected bones. Rarely Paget's disease is monostotic. Histologically, at an advanced stage, there is abnormal mineralized bone. This disease is associated with an increased risk of bone tumor development (osteogenic sarcoma, chrondroblastoma, etc.).

The skeleton can be the site of numerous benign and malignant neoplasms as is illustrated by the following:

Tumors of cartilaginous origin
    Osteochondroma
    Multiple osteocartilaginous exostoses
    Enchondroma
    Enchondromatosis
    Chondrosarcoma
Tumors of osteoblastic origin
    Osteoid osteoma
    Osteosarcoma
Tumors of marrow origin
    Ewing's sarcoma
    Plasma cell myeloma
Tumors of uncertain origin
    Giant cell tumor

Fibrous cortical defect and nonossifying fibroma
    Solitary bone cyst
    Aneurysmal bone cyst
    Fibrous dysplasia
    Eosinophilic granuloma of bone

Osteochondroma, the most common benign tumor of bone, involves long bones of extremities. It is characterized by the presence of cartilage capped bony projections arising from the cortex of a long tubular bone. Rarely osteochondromas can be multiple and familial (multiple osteocartilaginous exostoses). A small percentage of patients develop chondrosarcoma, usually affecting adults in the fourth to sixth decades. The tumor is more frequent in the bones of the pelvis, femur, humerus, and tibia, it recurs locally, but may metastasize to the lungs and other organs.

Enchondroma is a malignant tumor arising *de novo* or from a preexisting cartilaginous neoplasm, usually affecting adults in the fourth to sixth decades. The tumor is more frequent in the bones of the pelvis, femur, humerus, and tibia, but may metastasize to the lungs and other organs.

Osteogenic sarcoma (osteosarcoma) is the most common malignant tumor of bone origin. It affects mostly men between 10 and 25 years of age and it is most frequent at the metaphysis of long bones (femur, tibia, humerus). Lesions present with irregular bone destruction and bone formation, destruction of the cortex, and soft tissue extension with periosteal bone formation. Histologically the tumors show evidence of atypical bone production as well as cartilagenous fibroblastic and vascular formation by malignant tumor cells. Osteogenic sarcomas are aggressive tumors that metastasize widely through the blood stream to the lungs, bones, and other organs. Prognosis has improved in recent years with combined surgery and chemotherapy.

Rheumatoid arthritis is an autoimmune chronic systemic disease characterized by deformity and pain of joints of the hands, feet, and other sites. The joint involvement tends to be symmetrical and bilateral and can include large joints such as the knee. The disease affects mostly young women in the third and fourth decades of life and often results in severe deformities. The involved joints usually show chronic hypertrophic villous synovitis and severe chronic inflammation with plasma cell infiltrates. The characteristic pathologic lesion of rheumatoid arthritis is the rheumatoid nodule, present only in 20 percent of cases. This rheumatoid nodule is a necrotizing granuloma with central fibrinoid necrosis. Rheumatoid arthritis is accompanied by characteristic laboratory findings including elevation of the rheumatoid factor in serum and synovial fluid. Extra-articular

sites (lungs, sclera, subcutaneous tissues) may be affected.

Other arthritides include (1) clinicopathologic variants of rheumatoid arthritis such as juvenile rheumatoid arthritis, ankylosing spondylitis (Marie-Strümpell disease), a disease involving the sacroiliac, hip, and intervertebral joints, psoriatic arthritis, and Reiter's syndrome (arthritis, uveitis, urethritis), (2) bacterial arthritis including gonococcal, staphylococcal, and streptococcal arthritis, (3) tuberculous arthritis, and (4) luetic arthritis.

Osteoarthritis (degenerative joint disease) is a common, noninflammatory progressive disorder of the joints, affecting mostly older adults. It is more frequent in women. Osteoarthritis involves joints that are subjected to extensive stress during life including those of the knee, hip, hands, and vertebral column. These joints exhibit deformity and painful limitation of motion due to softening, fibrillation, and erosion of articular cartilage, osteosclerosis with bony exostosis, and joint destruction and deformity.

Gout is a metabolic disease characterized by hyperuricemia, recurrent attacks of acute arthritis, and deposits of urate crystals (tophi) in tissues. The disease is inherited as an error of purine metabolism, leading to hyperuricemia secondary to overproduction or decreased renal excretion of uric acid. Gout affects males (sex-linked disorder) in the fourth and fifth decades, and may lead to destructive articular deposits.

The term soft tissues applies to the supporting connective tissue structures of many organs, particularly, those in the limbs and body wall. These tissues present a variety of inflammatory, proliferative, and neoplastic lesions.

Fibromatoses are a group of benign proliferative fibroblastic lesions of unknown etiology characterized by the presence of tumorlike proliferations of fibrous tisue that may stimulate a malignant neoplasm. Different clinicopathologic forms of fibromatoses include Dupuytren's contracture, nodular fasciitis, juvenile fibromatoses, juvenile aponeurotic fibroma, and desmoid tumor.

There are many different pathologic types of benign and malignant soft tissue tumors. A discussion of their varied clinical and pathologic characteristics is well beyond the purpose of this chapter. The most common soft tissue tumors are the following:

Tumors and tumorlike conditions of fibrous tissue
    Juvenile aponeurotic fibroma
    Nodular and proliferative fasciitis
    Focal and proliferative myositis
    Elastofibroma
    Fibromatosis
    Fibrosarcoma

Tumors of probable histiocytic origin
  Histiocytoma
  Fibrous histiocytoma
Tumors of peripheral nerves
  Neuroma
  Neurilemoma
  Neurofibroma
  Malignant schwannoma
Tumors of adipose tissue
  Lipoma
  Lipoblastomatosis
  Liposarcoma
  Hibernoma
Tumors of blood and lymph vessels
  Hemangioma
  Glomus tumor
  Hemangiopericytoma
  Angiosarcoma
  Lymphangioma
  Lymphangiosarcoma
Tumors of smooth muscle
  Leiomyoma
  Leiomyosarcoma
Tumors of striated muscle
  Rhabdomyoma
  Rhabdomyosarcoma
Tumors of synovial tissue
  Synovial sarcoma
Tumors of pluripotential mesenchyme
  Mesenchymoma
Tumors of probable extragonadal germ cell origin
  Teratoma
Tumors of neurogenic origin
  Pigmented neuroectodermal tumor of infancy
  Other neurogenic tumors
Tumors of uncertain origin
  Fibrous hamartoma of infancy
  Myxoma
  Granular cell tumor
  Alveolar soft part sarcoma
  Clear cell sarcoma of tendons and aponeuroses
  Epithelioid sarcoma
  Malignant giant cell tumor of soft parts
  Extraskeletal Ewing's sarcoma

Myositis ossificans is an unusual condition characterized by localized areas of soft tissue, chronic inflammation, and bone formation, usually at one site. In the generalized form of the disease, areas of ossification occur in multiple tendons, ligaments, and joint capsules. Patients have respiratory complications from immobilization and involvement of thoracic muscles and joints by the calcifying process.

SKIN

Erythema multiforme is an uncommon inflammatory dermatosis, usually related to hypersensitivity to drugs (sulfas, penicillin, oral contraceptives, etc.) or infections (herpes virus, mycoplasma histoplasmosis, coccidioidomycosis, leprosy, etc.). It can also appear in patients with carcinomas, lymphomas, and collagen vascular diseases. Erythema multiforme is characterized by the presence of multiple macules, papules, vesicles, bullae and the so-called target lesions (red macule with pale center) in the skin of the extremities. The disease is self-limiting and lasts 2 to 6 weeks. One of its forms, the Stevens-Johnson syndrome, is accompanied by extensive mucosal lesions, fever, prostration, and respiratory symptoms. The mucosal lesions frequently become infected with subsequent development of sepsis.

Panniculitis refers to a group of diseases characterized by inflammation of the subcutaneous fat. The inflammatory process may affect primarily the connective tissue septae separating fat lobules (erythema nodosum), the septa, lobules, and blood vessels (erythema induratum), or the fat lobules only (Weber-Christian disease). Erythema nodosum is the most common form of panniculitis and may be associated with drugs (sulfonamides) or infections (beta hemolytic streptococci, tuberculosis, histoplasmosis, coccidioidomycosis, leprosy, etc.). In many cases the etiology remains unknown. Patients with erythema nodosum exhibit painful erythematosus plaques and nodules on extremities.

Lichen planus is a common disorder of the skin and mucous membranes characterized by the presence of itchy, violaceous, flat papules with white dots and lines (Wickman's striae). Histologically these papulae show vacuolarization of the epithelial basement membrane, hyperplasia of the stratum granulosum, and a bandlike mononuclear inflammatory infiltrate in the upper dermis. Etiology of lichen planus is unknown but occasionally the lesions are associated with drug ingestion (atabrine, chloroquine) or exposure to color film developers. The mucosal lesions may evolve into a squamous cell carcinoma of the oral mucosa in 1–4 percent of cases.

Psoriasis includes a group of dermatoses characterized by the presence of scaly erythematous plaques and epidermal epithelial proliferations. The etiology and pathogenesis is unclear but there appears to be an inherited predisposition. The lesions frequently follow exposure to precipitating factors such as trauma, infection, and endocrine changes. For example, psoriasis frequently appears in women after parturition. Patients may have associated arthritis that resembles rheumatoid arthritis, myopathy, enteropathy, and spondylitic heart disease.

Pemphigus is a group of dermatoses characterized by

vesicles and bullae in the skin. On histologic examination, these lesions exhibit acantholysis (rupture of intercellular junctions between keratinocytes). Immunopathologic studies show the presence of autoantibodies (IgG) directed against epidermal lesions in the acantholytic areas.

The disease has several clinical forms of which pemphigus vulgaris is the most common. It affects the skin and mucosa of patients in their fifth to seventh decade.

Dermatitis herpetiformis is an unusual dermatosis characterized by itchy papulovesicular lesions and the presence of IgA at the dermoepidermal junction of the skin. Dermatitis herpetiformis affects mostly adults 25 to 50 years old but it may appear in children and it follows a protracted clinical course with remissions and exacerbations. It is frequently associated with glutensensitive enteropathy and both diseases appear to be more frequent in individuals with the HLA antigens B8 and DW3.

Porphyrias are an unusual group of inborn or acquired disturbances of the metabolism of porphyrins, pigments normally present in hemoglobin, myoglobin, and cytochromes. The major types of porphyria are erythrohepatic protoporphyria, acute intermittent porphyria, porphyria cutanea tarda, and mixed porphyria.

Most of these forms present with urticarial lesions and vesicles that heal with scarring of the skin. These lesions frequently appear after exposure to light (photosensitivity). Porphyria cutanea tarda occasionally follows ingestion of drugs such as hexachlorobenzene.

Benign tumors of the skin are quite common and are of greatest clinical significance only when they mimic malignant tumors. Only a few of the more common tumors will be discussed.

Squamous cell papilloma is a papillary overgrowth of squamous mucosa, which may be pigmented or nonpigmented. It occurs more often in older people.

Seborrheic keratosis occurs as sharply circumscribed, yellow or brown, roughened surface lesions, which may be single or multiple, most often on the trunk, face, and arms of elderly individuals. It may resemble basal cell carcinoma or, when pigmented, melanoma. Microscopically, there is hyperkeratosis, basal cell proliferation, keratin-filled ("horn") cyst, and variable melanin pigmentation.

Senile keratosis appears on the face and hands of elderly people as small, hard, scaly lesions on an erythematous base. There is hyperkeratosis and dyskeratosis, with atypical prickle cells, including some mitoses. This lesion may progress to squamous cell carcinoma.

Nevi are pigmented tumors arising in neuroectodermal-derived nevus cells. The nevus is present in almost all individuals and is a flat or raised, brown or black, scaly, hairy, sometimes inflamed, sometimes hyperkera-

totic growth, usually confined to the dermis as an intradermal nevus. In some cases, there is accompanying proliferation of the nevus cells in the basal epidermis, in which case the name compound nevus is applied. Where there is only proliferation of the melanocytes at the epidermal-dermal junction, the lesion is called a junctional nevus.

Juvenile (Spitz) nevus is a distinctive tumor, usually occurring in children, but which may occur at any age, in which there is proliferation of nevus cells usually in association with spindle cells and even giant cells. In contrast to other nevi, the lesion may not be well circumscribed and can be misinterpreted as a malignant melanoma.

Benign tumors, apparently arising from the various dermal appendages, such as the sebaceous and sweat glands and the hair follicles, occur but are relatively uncommon. In addition, there may be cutaneous tumors arising in all of the supporting structures of the skin, such as lipomas, fibromas, angiomas, and leiomyomas.

Malignant tumors of the skin are also quite common.

Bowen's disease is usually a single, slightly thickened, brown or keratotic lesion which histologically shows hyperkeratosis, parakeratosis, and, particularly, marked atypia of the prickle cell layer with loss of polarity, single-cell keratinization, mitotic activity, and bizarre forms. This lesion does not penetrate the basement membrane, is in situ, and is definitely malignant.

Squamous cell carcinoma is probably the single most common malignancy, but is only a rare cause of death. Most cases occur in older men, particularly on the exposed parts of the face, neck, and hands. They are more common in fair skinned individuals in sunny climates, as are the other major skin tumors, basal cell carcinoma, and melanoma. In addition, squamous cell carcinoma is more frequent in individuals exposed to carcinogenic hydrocarbons over a prolonged period of time, in people who have had irradiation, in arsenic workers, and after long standing chronic ulcerations or burns. The lesions usually appear as somewhat indolent, poorly healing ulcers with raised, rolled, nodular, and everted edges, and induration of the base. They may be well differentiated, with clearly developed prickle cell and basal layers, but including atypia and dyskeratosis, or they may be completely dedifferentiated and appear as anaplastic or even spindle cell malignancies. They usually infiltrate locally, but may rarely metastasize.

Basal cell carcinoma occurs mostly in the elderly, particularly in the upper face often above a line connecting the angle of the mouth and the ear. Sunlight, irradiation, and prolonged arsenic contact are all predisposing factors. Early, the tumors are pearly nodules. They slowly grow and eventually ulcerate. Histologically, there are solid sheets of dark cells (resembling basal cells) with mitoses, varying degrees of melanin pigmentation, cystic change, and, at the periphery, a characteristic palisade arrangement of cells. They spread by direct infiltration and may be destructive of subjacent bone or cartilage, but rarely metastasize.

Malignant melanoma is an uncommon, highly malignant tumor which occurs at any age but only rarely before the age of 30. Any part of the body may be involved. Melanoma may be confined to the epidermis, or may infiltrate deeply. Metastases are frequent and may occur via blood or lymphatic spread, or both. There are four major types of melanoma: (1) Lentigo malignant melanoma begins as a preinvasive lesion, known as lentigo maligna, which is usually an irregular, tan, macular lesion on the face of people over age 50, and may be related to chronic sun exposure. It may remain preinvasive for 15 to 20 years. (2) Superficial spreading melanoma occurs in somewhat younger individuals as flat or slightly raised, irregular, multicolored lesions, often showing zones of tumor regression, at any site of the body, but occurring most often on the upper back or legs. They tend to grow radially for a period of time before developing dermal invasion and nodular masses. (3) Nodular malignant melanoma are dark brown or black dome-shaped neoplasms without a radial growth phase or lateral spread. This pattern is associated with the worst prognosis. (4) Acral-lentiginous melanoma is an initially flat lesion of the hands and feet which spreads laterally before invasion occurs. Prognosis can be evaluated by determining the depth of invasion of the tumor. Two methods are used. The Clark levels are based on invasion depth in terms of normal structures, as is illustrated by the following:

Clark level
I   Confined to epidermis (in situ)
II   Extends into papillary dermis
III Extends to junction of papillary and reticular dermis
IV Extends into reticular dermis
V   Extends into subcutis

The Breslow method requires measurement of the depth of invasion from the granular layer of the epidermis to the base of the neoplasm.

Kaposi's sarcoma is a rare disease usually presenting as multiple hemorrhagic nodules and plaques, most often in elderly Jewish and Italian men, typically affecting the lower extremities. The course is indolent and dissemination may not occur for 5 to 10 years. Microscopically, the dermis is infiltrated by proliferating vascular channels, which usually lack endothelial-lining cells, and which are separated by atypical spindle cells. In recent years, a more aggressive variant of this disorder has been recognized in individuals with (AIDS).

REFERENCES

Cawson RA, McCracken AW, Marcus TB: Pathologic Mechanisms and Human Disease. CV Mosby Co., St. Louis, 1982
   This highly readable, soft cover textbook has a summary of discussions of major conditions and is very useful as a review text.
Damjanov I: General Patholgy. Medical Examination Publishing Co., New Hyde Park, 1976
   This concise textbook, in soft cover edition, covers the basic areas of general pathology and provides a well illustrated, well written review of major topics of tissue injury and response. Each chapter is followed by a long list of questions, but there are no included answers. In spite of this, it is a useful guide to understanding general pathology.
King DW, Fenoglio CM, Lefkowitch JH: General Pathology. Lea & Febiger, Philadelphia, 1983
   This is a major textbook of general pathology which is well written and extremely well illustrated. It is an up-to-date reference source with a comprehensive list of references.
Robbins SL, Cotran RS, Kumar V: Pathologic Basis of Disease. 3rd Ed. WB Saunders, Philadelphia, 1984
   This is the single best, most easily read textbook of pathology. It is characterized by high quality illustrations and excellent clinical correlations.
Symmers WStC: Systemic Pathology. 2nd Ed. Vols. 1–6. Churchill Livingstone, London, 1976–1980
   This superb set of pathology textbooks, devoted only to discussion of the various systems, does not include principles of pathology but is a fine reference source for specific organ injuries.

MULTIPLE CHOICE QUESTIONS

Each question below contains four suggested answers of which one or more is correct. Choose the answer:

  A. 1 and 3 are correct
  B. 2 and 4 are correct
  C. 1, 2, and 3 are correct
  D. Only 4 is correct
  E. All are correct

1. The principal subcellular effects of anoxia are
  1. glycogen depletion
  2. ribosomal detachment
  3. lactic acidosis
  4. release of lysomal enzymes

2. The sequence of progression of histopathologic changes in a myocardial infarction is
  1. "Wavy-line" phenomenon, granulation tissue, polymorphonuclear leukocytic infiltration
  2. "Wavy-line" phenomenon, polymorphonuclear leukocytic infiltration, collagen formation
  3. Collagen formation, increased eosinophilia, granulation tissue
  4. Granulation tissue, collagen formation, increased eosinophilia

5. Increased eosinophilia, granulation tissue, polymorphonuclear leukocytic infiltration

3. Membranous nephropathy is characterized by
   1. Foot process fusion
   2. Nephrotic syndrome
   3. Granular deposits of immunoglobulins and complement
   4. Hypertension

4. Periarteritis nodosa is characterized by
   1. Venous inflammation common
   2. Complement deposition
   3. Frequent allergic history
   4. Lesions in variable stages

5. Emphysema is characterized by
   1. Tissue eosinophilia
   2. Fibrosis
   3. Bronchiolar dilatation
   4. Airspace enlargement

6. Ulcerative colitis is characterized by
   1. Multiple, discontinuous ("skip") lesions
   2. Fibrosis and stricture
   3. "Aphthous" ulcers
   4. Inflammation of lamina propria

7. Hashimoto's thyroditis is associated with
   1. Circulating antithyroid antibodies
   2. Lymphocytic and plasmacytic infiltration
   3. Metaplastic follicular epithelial cells ("Askanasi cells")
   4. Granulomas

8. An acute injury may manifest as
   1. Coagulation necrosis
   2. Fat necrosis
   3. Liquefactive necrosis
   4. Caseous necrosis

9. Thrombosis may follow
   1. Disturbances of blood flow
   2. Endothelial injury
   3. Alterations of plasma components
   4. Loss of heparin inhibitors

Choose the one best answer for each of the following questions.

10. The most common breast disorder is
    A. Fibroadenoma
    B. Intraductal carcinoma
    C. Infiltrating duct carcinoma
    D. Medullary carcinoma
    E. None of the above

11. Principle features of chronic active hepatitis are
    A. Portal and lobular inflammation, fibrosis, granulomata
    B. "Piecemeal" necrosis, fibrosis, granulomata
    C. Granulomata, bile-duct destruction, fibrosis
    D. Portal and lobular inflammation, "piecemeal" necrosis, fibrosis
    E. "Piecemeal" necrosis, Councilmanlike bodies, increased copper content

12. In a Clark's level III malignant melanoma, the tumor
    A. Is confined to epidermis
    B. Extends into papillary dermis
    C. Extends to junction of papillary and reticular dermis
    D. Extends into reticular dermis
    E. Extends into subcutis

13. Of the following normal tissues, which will be most sensitive to radiation injury?
    A. Skeletal muscle
    B. Liver
    C. Adrenal glands
    D. Small intestinal mucosa
    E. Skin

14. The most important histologic feature in determining prognosis in a lymph node involved by malignant lymphoma is
    A. Capsule infiltration
    B. Total node effacement
    C. Fibrosis
    D. "Nodular" pattern
    E. All of the above are equally important

15. The most common tumor of the uterus is
    A. Adenomyosis
    B. Mixed mesodermal tumor
    C. Squamous cell carcinoma
    D. Adenocarcinoma
    E. Leiomyoma

Answers to Multiple Choice Questions

1 E	2 D	3 C	4 B	5 D
6 D	7 C	8 C	9 E	10 E
11 D	12 C	13 D	14 D	15 E

7

Pharmacology

Dennis W. Schneck

GENERAL CONCEPTS

The term receptor refers to a cellular macromolecule with which a drug interacts. An agonist causes biological effects as a result of this interaction. Compounds that are devoid of activity but that inhibit the action of a specific agonist (e.g., by competition for binding sites) are antagonists. The dose response curve defines the relationship between dose administered and intensity of effect. Potency refers to the location of a drug's dose-effect curve on the dose axis. Efficacy refers to the maximal effect produced by a drug. No drug produces a single effect but rather a spectrum of effects. The relationship between the doses of a drug required to produce undesired and desired effects is termed its therapeutic index. The dose of a drug required to produce a specified intensity of effect in 50 percent of individuals is known as the median effective dose (ED_{50}). If death is the end point the ED_{50} becomes the median lethal dose (LD_{50}).

Pharmacokinetics relates to the absorption, distribution, biotransformation, and excretion of drugs and the time course of drug effects. Exponential elimination kinetics (first-order process) means that a constant fraction of drug is eliminated per unit time. The half-life ($t\frac{1}{2}$) refers to the time required for 50 percent completion of an elimination process. Zero-order kinetics means that a constant amount of drug is eliminated per unit time and indicates saturation of a process. The distribution volume of a drug (Vd) can be defined as the relationship between the amount of drug in the body relative to the concentration of drug in the plasma. The clearance (Cl) of a drug is defined as the volume of blood cleared of drug by metabolism and excretion per unit time. The $t\frac{1}{2}$ is related to Vd and Cl by the following formula:

$$t\tfrac{1}{2} = \frac{0.693 \, Vd}{Cl}$$

When a drug is given repeatedly or continuously, the total body store (or plasma concentration) increases exponentially to a plateau with a half-time of increase equal to $t\frac{1}{2}$. Thus 50 percent of the plateau is achieved in one $t\frac{1}{2}$ and 93.7 percent of the plateau in four half-lives. Similar arguments apply when a drug is discontinued. The average plasma concentration when the plateau is reached following oral administration is given by:

$$Cp = \frac{1.44 \, t\tfrac{1}{2} \, f \, D}{Vd\pi}$$

where D = dose, f = systemic availability of the drug, and π = dose interval. If a prompt effect is required, a loading dose may have to be given.

Additional definitions of value in the study of pharmacology include the following. Tolerance has developed when increasingly larger doses are required to produce the effects seen with the original dose. Physical dependence refers to an altered physiological state produced by the repeated administration of a drug that necessitates the continued use of the drug to prevent the appearance of a withdrawal syndrome. Drug abuse refers to the use of any drug in a manner socially unacceptable. Addiction means a behavioral pattern of drug use characterized by overwhelming involvement with the use of a drug, the securing of its supply, and a high tendency to relapse after withdrawal.

CARDIOVASCULAR DRUGS

Inotropic Drugs

Digitalis glycosides increase myocardial contractility. They are also useful for ventricular rate control in patients with atrial fibrillation or flutter. Digoxin and digitoxin are the most commonly used glycosides.

The cardiac glycosides enhance cardiac contractility

by inhibition of Na^+-K^+ stimulated membrane adenosinetriphosphatase (ATPase). As a result intracellular Na^+ increases producing a Ca^{++} influx in exchange for intracellular Na^+. The increased intracellular Ca^{++} activates the contractile proteins. The increase in cardiac output, decreases in heart size, venous pressure, blood volume, and diuresis are based on this action. Cardiac glycosides increase cardiac vagal activity by a variety of mechanisms including stimulation of central vagal nuclei. This effect causes a decrease in the rate of impulse conduction in the atrioventricular (AV) node, decreases in the rate of impulse generation in the sinoatrial (SA) node and automaticity of atrial conducting fibers, the action potential duration and effective refractory period are shortened in atrial fibers, and the effective refractory period is prolonged in the AV node. Direct effects of cardiac glycosides in AV nodal tissue include depression of conduction velocity and prolongation of effective refractory period. The cardiac glycosides can cause an increase in the automaticity of atrial and ventricular conducting fibers and can initiate the development of delayed after potentials in these fibers.

The most important toxic manifestations of digitalis are cardiac arrhythmias. These include premature ventricular beats, ventricular tachycardia, ventricular fibrillation, AV junctional tachycardia, atrial tachycardia with block as well as second and third degree heart block, sinus bradycardia, and SA block. Other adverse effects include anorexia, nausea and vomiting, headache, neuralgia, confusion, fatigue, delirium, and visual disturbances. Factors that enhance toxicity include hypokalemia, hypomagnesemia, hypercalcemia, hypoxia, hypercarbia, and alkalosis. Risk of toxicity increases substantially when serum levels exceed 2 ng/ml. Infants may tolerate higher serum levels than adults.

Oral digoxin is almost completely absorbed (60 to 80 percent, as tablet, 85 percent as elixir). Digoxin has a large distribution volume. The drug is removed from the body primarily by glomerular filtration and renal tubular secretion. The half-life averages 1.5 days with normal renal function and increases with impairment of kidney function. The elimination rate and distribution volume of digoxin is reduced in older patients.

Digitoxin is completely absorbed. It is bound >90 percent to plasma albumin. The distribution volume is similar to digoxin. Hepatic metabolism is primarily responsible for elimination and the half-life is 5 to 7 days. Therapeutic levels lie between 15 and 25 ng/ml.

Dopamine increases myocardial contractility and heart rate by stimulating β_1 receptors. Higher doses will activate α_1 receptors. Stimulation of dopamine receptors in the renal and mesenteric circulations produces vasodilation. Dopamine is rapidly eliminated following discontinuation of the intravenous infusion. The principal adverse effect is the development of cardiac arrhythmias.

Dobutamine stimulates cardiac β_1 receptors to augment cardiac contractility. Dobutamine exerts a more prominent inotropic than chronotropic action as compared to isoproterenol. Dobutamine produces less peripheral arterial effects and tachycardia than other sympathomimetic amines at dose levels that produce similar increases in contractility. Dobutamine does not activate dopamine receptors. It is rapidly eliminated following discontinuation of the infusion. The major side effect is the production of cardiac arrhythmias.

Organic Nitrates

Nitroglycerin and other organic nitrates such as isosorbide dinitrate, pentaerythrital tetranitrate, and erythrityl tetranitrate are of value in the treatment of angina pectoris, congestive heart failure, and may be effective in the treatment of acute myocardial infarction. Nitroglycerin interacts with nitrate receptors in vascular smooth muscle to cause relaxation. Peripheral veins are more sensitive than arterioles. Venous capacitance increases causing reduced myocardial preload. Relaxation of arteries and arterioles results in a decrease in mean blood pressure and a reduction in myocardial afterload. Ventricular wall tension decreases resulting in a reduction in myocardial oxygen demand. A reflex increase in heart rate and myocardial contractility may occur. Nitroglycerin may increase coronary blood flow to ischemic subendocardium.

The biotransformation of organic nitrates is the result of reductive hydrolysis by the hepatic enzyme glutathione-nitrate reductase. Large oral doses of oral nitroglycerin and other nitrate esters produce pharmacologic effects by saturating hepatic nitrate reductase. Nitroglycerin ointment has sustained antianginal efficacy. Several other transdermal delivery systems are available for nitroglycerin. These systems consist of a nitroglycerin reservoir sandwiched between an impenetrable backing and a porous membrane that controls the rate of nitroglycerin absorption or a special nitroglycerin-containing matrix which controls the rate of flow of drug to the skin. Nitroglycerin is well-absorbed through skin.

Adverse reactions include headache, dizziness, and syncope secondary to postural hypotension. Nitroglycerin is readily degraded by light, heat, air, and moisture.

Calcium Entry Blockers

These drugs are useful in treating vasospastic and effort-induced angina. Intravenous verapamil is the drug of choice in treating paroxysmal supraventricular tachycardia unresponsive to vagal maneuvers. Verapamil is useful in decreasing ventricular rate in patients with atrial fibrillation or atrial flutter.

Proteins that traverse the lipid bilayer of the cell membrane and selectively permit ions to move from one side of this barrier to the other are referred to as channels. Depolarization of the membrane region containing the Ca^{++}-channel causes the "gate" to open permitting Ca^{++} to enter the cells. The "gate" closes when the interior of the cell has again become electronegative. $Beta_1$ agonists in cardiac muscle and α receptor agonists in vascular smooth muscle can also increase Ca^{++} influx via the slow inward current. The influx of Ca^{++} during depolarization or receptor stimulation leads to activation of the contractile apparatus. This current is primarily responsible for conduction through the atrioventricular mode.

There are significant differences between the pharmacologic properties of verapamil, diltiazem, and nifedipine. Nifedipine appears to reduce the number of available Ca^{++} channels without affecting the time course of activation or recovery from inactivation. In contrast, verapamil influences the rates of activation and recovery after inactivation of the slow current. Diltiazem is more similar to verapamil than to nifedipine. They are all potent peripheral and coronary vasodilators. Nifedipine has minimal direct depressant effects on sinus frequency or AV conduction. At the doses used clinically, the peripheral vascular effects of nifedipine dominate and a reflex trachycardia and an enhancement of cardiac contractility can occur.

All of the Ca^{++} blockers are rapidly and completely absorbed after oral administration. Their plasma protein binding is 80 to 90 percent. Nifedipine and verapamil are eliminated by hepatic metabolism and diltiazem is removed 60 pecent by metabolism and 40 percent by renal excretion. The half-lives vary from 4 to 7 hours. The major adverse effects of nifedipine include hypotension, headaches, flushing, leg edema, and constipation. Similar side effects can occur with verapamil and diltiazem. AV conduction disturbances can also occur with the latter two drugs.

Beta-Adrenergic Blocking Drugs

Beta-Adrenoceptor blocking drugs are effective in the treatment of angina pectoris, hypertension, paroxysmal supraventricular trachycardia, atrial flutter, and atrial fibrillation. Administration of these drugs to patients who survive a myocardial infarction will reduce subsequent mortality rate and possibly re-infarction rate. Other therapeutic indications include migraine prophylaxis, benign action tremors, anxiety, possibly schizophrenia, narcotic and alcohol withdrawal, and for ophthalmic administration in the treatment of open-angle glaucoma (timolol maleate). Propranolol reduces the risk of bleeding from esophageal varices in patients with cirrhosis.

Two distinct types of adrenergic receptors exist. These are classified as α- and β-receptors. Beta-Receptors are further divided into β_1-receptors in the heart and β_2-receptors in the bronchi and blood vessels. Beta-blocking drugs are competitive inhibitors of the effects of catecholamines at β-receptor sites (Table 7-1). Blockade of cardiac β_1-receptors reduces heart rate and myocardial contractility. Myocardial oxygen consumption is decreased as a result of reductions in heart rate, ventricular systolic pressure, and contractility. Beta-blockers can prolong systolic ejection and cause dilation of the ventricle. These effects tend to increase oxygen requirements. However, the oxygen-sparing effects predominate. Beta-Adrenergic blocking drugs slow conduction in the atria and in the AV node. Automaticity is suppressed. Peripheral resistance initially rises when β-adrenergic blocking therapy is started in the treatment of hypertension. In some patients resistance falls with prolonged β-blockade. Beta-blockers with intrinsic sympathomimetic activity (ISA) such as pindolol reduce blood pressure to the same degree as those without ISA. However, heart rate and cardiac output decrease less in hypertensive patients and peripheral resistance is reduced to a greater extent than with non-ISA drugs. Some investigators claim that ISA protects against heart failure, bradycardia, and asthma.

Renin levels usually fall promptly after β-blocker therapy. Activation of β_1 receptors in adipose tissue results in increased cyclic AMP levels and subsequent release of fatty acids. Stimulation of pancreatic β_2 receptors results in insulin release and activation of liver and muscle β_2 receptors causes glycogenolysis with release of glucose and lactate. In low doses, selective blockers inhibit cardiac β_1 receptors but exert little influence on bronchial,

Table 7-1. Pharmacologic Properties of β-Adrenoreceptor Blocking Drugs

Drug	β-Blockade Potency (Propranolol = 1)	Cardioselectivity	Membrane-stabilizing Activity	Partial Agonist Activity
Propranolol	1	0	++	0
Metoprolol	1	+	±	0
Nadolol	2–4	0	0	0
Timolol	6	0	0	±
Atenolol	1	+	+	0
Pindolol	6	0	+	+++

vascular, and metabolic β_2 receptors. Cardioselectivity is diminished at larger doses.

Membrane-stabilizing activity ("quinidine-like" effect) is unrelated to competitive inhibition of catecholamine action. The antiarrhythmic effects of these drugs have been shown to be due to β-blockade.

A summary of the pharmacokinetic properties of the various β-blockers is shown (Table 7-2).

The major adverse reactions to β-blockers include bradycardia, hypotension, heart failure, slowing of AV conduction, and asthma. Other adverse reactions include fatigue and vivid dreams. Propranolol and other β-blockers increase lidocaine plasma levels in subjects receiving intravenous infusions of lidocaine. Abrupt discontinuation of β-blockers may rarely induce "an acute withdrawal" syndrome characterized by tachycardia, hypertension, and angina.

Beta-Adrenergic Agonists

Isoproterenol produces marked β_1 and β_2 receptor stimulation. This results in increased heart rate, myocardial contractility, and reductions in peripheral vascular resistance. The latter further augments tachycardia by reflex sympathetic stimulation. Isoproterenol causes bronchodilation by stimulation of β_2 receptors. Several selective β_2 agonists are available for relief of bronchospasm. These include metaproterenol, isoetharine, terbutaline, and albuterol. Administered by aerosol inhalation at doses that produce equivalent bronchodilatation as compared to isoproterenol, these drugs produce substantially less cardiac β_1 stimulation. Higher doses stimulate β_1 receptors. Terbutaline, metaproterenol, and albuterol can be administered by the oral route. Terbutaline is also administered subcutaneously. Terbutaline has been administered intravenously to delay premature labor. However, cardiac effects are common at the doses used. Adverse effects include cardiac stimulation, tremor, nervousness, insomnia, dizziness, nausea, and paradoxical increase in bronchospasm.

Alpha-Adrenergic Antagonists and Agonists

Phenoxybenzamine irreversibly blocks α_1 and α_2 receptors in smooth muscle and exocrine glands. As a consequence, blood pressure is significantly reduced in standing subjects, hypovolemic subjects, and in subjects with excessive sympathetic activation. Reflex tachycardia is noted. Phentolamine also blocks α receptors but also has sympathomimetic, parasympathomimetic, histamine-like, and antiserotonin effects. Other α blockers include tolazoline and prazosin.

Agonists such as phenylephrine and methoxamine are relatively selective for the α_1 receptor. Drugs such as ephedrine, metaraminol, mephenteramine, tyramine, and amphetamine release norepinephrine from adrenergic nerve terminals. These drugs may also have variable direct α/β receptor activity properties. Thus, doses of ephedrine that increase blood pressure cause tachycardia whereas doses of phenylephrine that increase blood pressure cause bradycardia due to reflex vagal activation. Other actions of these drugs include mydriasis, piloerection, and sweating. Insulin secretion is reduced. Prolonged therapy with these agents may lead to reduced blood volume and myocardial necrosis.

Sympatholytics

Seveal drugs effective in the treatment of hypertension act primarily by reducing the outflow of sympathetic nervous system activity from the central nervous system. These drugs include clonidine, α-methyldopa, and quanabenz.

Clonidine stimulates central presynaptic (α_2) receptors leading to a reduction in sympathetic vasoconstrictor tone to the heart, kidneys, and peripheral vasculature. Bradycardia and a reduction in total peripheral resistance is noted. The cardiac response to exercise is preserved. No significant change in renal blood flow or glomerular filtration is noted. Clonidine reduces plasma renin activity.

Table 7-2. Pharmacokinetic Properties of β-Blockers

Drug	Absorption (% of dose)	Bioavailability (% of dose)	Plasma Proteins (% Binding)	Liver (% Elimination)	Kidney (% Elimination)	Elimination Half-life (hour)
Propranolol	>90	30	90–95	>95	< 5	2–6
Metoprolol	>95	50	12	>95	< 5	3–4
Nadolol	30	30	30	<25[a]	>75	20–24
Timolol	>90	55	—	80	20	2–3
Atenolol	50	50	10	<10	>90	6–7
Pindolol	>90	100	40	60	40	3–4

[a] Biliary excretion. Nadolol and Atenolol require modification of dose schedule when renal function is significantly impaired.

Clonidine is readily absorbed after oral administration. Plasma $t\frac{1}{2}$ is 12 to 16 hours. Forty to 60 percent of a dose is excreted unchanged in the urine. High doses of clonidine may produce mild hypertension due to peripheral α-adrenergic stimulation. An occasional patient may develop nervousness, headache, tachycardia, nausea, and marked increases in blood pressure following abrupt withdrawal of clonidine. This withdrawal syndrome can be readily treated by administration of clonidine or phentolamine. Other side effects include dry mouth and sedation.

Within brain neurons methyldopa is converted to α-methylnorepinephrine. This metabolite stimulates central α_2 receptors leading to inhibition of the vasomotor center in the medulla.

Absorption of methyldopa is only 50 percent after oral administration. Alpha-methyldopa is metabolized in the liver and the metabolites are excreted in the urine. Methyldopa has a short plasma $t\frac{1}{2}$ (2 hours) but the active metabolite formed in brain neurons is retained resulting in an antihypertensive effect that persists after the parent drug has been eliminated.

The major side effects include sedation, decreased intellectual drive, forgetfulness, sexual dysfunction, depression, hepatotoxicity, and drug fever. Twenty percent of patients on methyldopa therapy develop a positive direct Coombs test, but only 5 percent have a raised reticulocyte count and less than 2 percent develop hemolysis.

Guanabenz stimulates central α_2 receptors leading to reduced sympathetic outflow. About 75 percent of an oral dose is absorbed. The $t\frac{1}{2}$ is 6 hours with liver metabolism being the major mechanism of elimination. Side effects are similar to clonidine.

Reserpine blocks the transport of norepinephrine into storage granules so that less transmitter is released upon stimulation. The decrease in sympathetic tone leads to a decrease in peripheral vascular resistance. Reduction of myocardial catecholamine stores leads to a reduced cardiac output and bradycardia. Adverse effects include nasal stuffiness, increased gastric secretion, and depression.

Guanethidine is taken into adrenergic nerves by a specific pump mechanism. Inside the adrenergic neuron guanethidine releases stored norepinephrine and blocks release of norepinephrine during nerve stimulation. These actions result in decreased peripheral resistance and a reduction in cardiac output. These effects are much more pronounced in the upright position. The response to oral guanethidine gradually increases and persists for many days following discontinuation of the drug. Adverse effects include postural hypotension, fluid retention, diarrhea, and failure of ejaculation. Tricyclic antidepressants antagonize guanethidine's action by inhibiting guanethidine transport into the adrenergic neuron.

Bethanidine acts similarly to guanethidine. The main difference is a shorter duration of action (8 to 12 hours).

Vasodilators

Vasodilators are used to treat hypertension, usually in combination with a diuretic and adrenergic blocker, and as "unloaders" for the treatment of severe heart failure.

Hydralazine produces direct relaxation of vascular smooth muscle; the effect on arterioles is greater than on veins. Peripheral vascular resistance decreases and blood pressure drops. As a consequence, reflex increases in heart rate and stroke volume occur.

Hydralazine is well absorbed from the intestine. Peak plasma levels occur within 30 minutes of drug administration and the $t\frac{1}{2}$ for elimination is 0.5 to 1 hour. Slow acetylators have higher hydralazine levels following oral administration than rapid acetylators. Despite the rapid clearance of hydralazine, the blood pressure lowering effect persists for several hours. Hydralazine pyruvic acid hydrazone is a major metabolite of hydralazine following intravenous administration and forms from nonenzymatic coupling with pyruvic acid in the vascular compartment. This metabolite is inactive.

Headache and palpitation are the most common adverse effects. Angina may be increased unless β-adrenergic blockers are also administered. Drug-induced lupus may occur in 10 percent of patients receiving high doses. Slow acetylators are more prone to this reaction.

Minoxidil is a very effective direct dilator of arterioles. This action triggers reflex sympathetic activation that is more pronounced relative to hydralazine.

Minoxidil is well-absorbed after oral administration. Peak plasma levels occur within 1 hour and the plasma $t\frac{1}{2}$ is 4 hours. Minoxidil is cleared from plasma primarily by hepatic metabolism.

Salt and water retention can be profound especially in patients with pre-existing cardiac dilatation and renal disease. Large doses of furosemide may be required to control the edema. Pericardial effusion has been noted. Hypertrichosis is a troublesome side-effect.

Prazosin lowers blood pressure by reducing both peripheral vascular resistance and venous tone. Thus a reduction in both afterload and preload is noted. Little increase of reflex release of norepinephrine is observed. Heart rate and plasma renin activity do not change as much as that seen with other vasodilators. Prazosin acts primarily as a blocker of peripheral α_1 receptors which mediate vasoconstriction. Presynaptic α_2 receptors function in an inhibitory feedback loop by which norepinephrine regulates its own output. Prazosin blocks the α_1

receptor while leaving the α_2 feedback receptor unblocked.

Prazosin is well-absorbed from the gut with peak plasma levels occurring in 2 to 3 hours. Prazoxin is cleared by hepatic metabolism and a significant first pass effect is noted. The drug is highly bound to plasma proteins (>90 percent) and the $t\frac{1}{2}$ of elimination is 3 to 5 hours.

After the first dose of prazosin some patients feel weak and diaphoretic. Syncope can occur. The nature of this reaction is presumed to be postural hypotension.

Captopril is a specific inhibitor of the enzyme that converts angiotensin I to II and which also inactivates bradykinin. Following captopril administration plasma renin activity increases due to removal of feedback inhibition by angiotensin II. Plasma levels of angiotensin II, aldosterone, and converting enzyme activity decrease. Plasma potassium levels may initially rise slightly but often return to normal with continued therapy. Captopril lowers blood pressure by dilating the peripheral vasculature. Cardiac output, heart rate, and body fluid volumes change little if any. Renal blood flow increases and glomerular filtration may remain unchanged or increase. Captopril causes reduced preload and afterload in patients with heart failure.

About 70 percent of a single dose is rapidly absorbed from the gut and lowers blood pressure within 15 minutes with the maximal effect seen at 60 to 90 minutes. Food may diminish its absorption. Twenty-five to 30 percent of the circulating drug is bound to plasma proteins. Forty to 50 percent is excreted in the urine as unchanged drug and the rest as metabolites. The $t\frac{1}{2}$ is less than 2 hours. Excretion rates are reduced in patients with impairment of renal function.

The most common adverse effect is a pruritic skin rash. Other adverse effects reported include transient loss of taste, aphthous ulcers in the mouth, proteinuria and nephrotic syndrome, and leukopenia.

Nitroprusside is the most effective parenteral agent for rapidly lowering blood pressure in severely hypertensive patients. It is also effective in severe refractory congestive heart failure. Other uses include dissecting aortic aneurysm and to produce controlled hypotension during certain surgical procedures in normotensive patients. Nitroprusside relaxes both arteriolar and venous smooth muscle. Cardiac preload and afterload are reduced. Cardiac output usually changes little unless the patient is in heart failure in which case the cardiac output may increase. Heart rate may increase in normal or hypertensive patients but may decrease in patients with cardiac failure.

Nitroprusside has a rapid onset and offset of action. Cyanide formed from nitroprusside is rapidly converted to thiocyanate by red blood cells and other tissues. High prolonged infusion rates can produce thiocyanate toxicity characterized by weakness, aphasia, psychoneurosis, slurred speech, and muscle twitching. These effects usually do not occur below a serum thiocyanate level of 10 mg percent. The most common adverse effect is excessive hypotension. Cyanide toxicity and methemoglobinemia is rare.

Diazoxide is effective in lowering blood pressure in severely hypertensive patients when administered parenterally. Its major action is on resistance vessels rather than on capacitance vessels. Accompanying the reduction in peripheral vascular resistance is a reflex increase in heart rate and cardiac output.

Diazoxide is 90 percent bound to plasma albumin. The $t\frac{1}{2}$ of elimination is 24 hours with about one-third of its clearance due to renal excretion and the remainder due to hepatic metabolism.

Diazoxide can cause salt and water retention, nausea, and vomiting. Prolonged oral treatment of hypoglycemia can produce hyperglycemia, hypertrichosis, and extrapyramidal effects.

Antiarrhythmic Drugs

Lidocaine is indicated for intravenous therapy of ventricular arrhythmias. The efficacy of lidocaine is related to decreases in automaticity in Purkinje fibers and reduced conduction velocity in diseased tissues. The elimination $t\frac{1}{2}$ of lidocaine is 90 to 110 minutes and its clearance is dependent on hepatic metabolism. Following bolus injection, lidocaine is rapidly distributed to well-perfused organs (heart, brain, lung, liver, kidney). Liver disease impairs lidocaine clearance but does not change distribution volume (Vd). Heart failure decreases both Vd and clearance. Beta-blocking drugs may impair lidocaine clearance. Therapeutic plasma levels are 1.5 to 5 μg/ml. Toxicity includes paresthesias, somnolence, giddiness, nervousness, confusion, and seizures. Myocardial depression and conduction block can occur in patients with severe heart disease.

Quinidine is useful in the treatment of atrial and ventricular arrhythmias. Quinidine decreases automaticity, membrane responsiveness, and conduction velocity in Purkinje fibers. The action potential duration and effective refractory period is prolonged and the ratio of effective refractory period to action potential duration is increased. Quinidine blocks the effect of vagal stimulation on cardiac tissue. These effects can increase heart rate and AV nodal conduction. Therapeutic plasma concentrations (1.5 to 5 μg/ml) produce a small increase in the P-R, QRS, and Q-T intervals. The QRS interval progressively widens as the cardiac concentration of quinidine rises. Quinidine also blocks α-adrenergic receptors.

Quinidine sulfate is well absorbed with peak levels occurring 2 to 4 hours. The elimination $t\frac{1}{2}$ ranges from 3 to 19 hours with a mean of 7 hours. The drug is 75 percent bound to protein in plasma and hepatic metabolism accounts for 60 percent of elimination and the remainder occurs by renal excretion of unchanged drug. Quinidine clearance and Vd is reduced in the elderly. Phenytoin and phenobarbital can induce hepatic metabolism.

Common adverse reactions include nausea and diarrhea. Cardiac toxicity includes heart block, ventricular arrhythmias, and hypotension. Other adverse effects include syncope, thrombocytopenia, granulomatous hepatitis, and cinchonism.

The effects of procainamide on the electrical properties of the heart are similar to those produced by quinidine. The anticholinergic action of procainamide is less than that of quinidine and procainamide does not produce α-adrenergic blockade. High doses can produce ganglionic blockade.

Absorption is rapid after oral administration. The $t\frac{1}{2}$ of elimination is 3.5 hours. About 20 percent is bound to plasma protein. The hepatic enzyme N-acetyltransferase contributes to the elimination of procainamide. The activity of this enzyme is genetically determined and has a polymorphic expression. Up to 40 percent of a dose of procainamide is converted to N-acetylprocainamide in rapid acetylators whereas slow acetylators may convert only 15 percent to the metabolite. This metabolite has antiarrhythmic activity and is eliminated via the kidney with a $t\frac{1}{2}$ of 7 hours. Forty to 60 percent of procainamide is excreted unchanged in the urine. The usual therapeutic plasma concentration of procainamide is 4 to 10 μg/ml.

Adverse effects include nausea, diarrhea, hypotension, and heart block. Long-term procainamide therapy can induce lupus erythematosus. After a year almost all patients develop antinuclear antibodies and about 20 percent will develop symptoms. Both rapid and slow acetylators are at risk although it takes longer for rapid acetylators to develop the equivalent titer of antinuclear antibodies.

Disopyramide is effective in the treatment of ventricular and atrial arrhythmias. Disopyramide has electrophysiological properties similar to those of quinidine and procainamide.

About 90 percent of an oral dose is absorbed. About 55 percent of a dose is excreted unchanged in the urine and the remainder metabolized in the liver. The $t\frac{1}{2}$ varies from 4 to 10 hours and is prolonged up to 18 hours in the presence of renal insufficiency. Plasma protein binding of disopyramide decreases with increasing plasma drug concentrations.

The anticholinergic action of disopyramide can produce dry mouth, constipation, blurred vision, urinary hesitancy, and retention. Myocardial depression and conduction defects have been noted.

Bretylium is indicated when other antiarrhythmic drugs prove to be ineffective. The drug increases the threshold for ventricular fibrillation and prolongs refractoriness in Purkinje and ventricular muscle fibers. It is taken up and concentrated in adrenergic nerve terminals. Initially norepinephrine is released and subsequently norepinephrine release following nerve stimulation is impaired.

The most troublesome adverse effect is orthostatic hypotension. Some arrhythmias may worsen following initial doses.

Diuretics

Many analogues of the benzothiadiazide class of diuretics are available. Their basic pharmacological actions are similar. Thiazide diuretics are useful in the treatment of hypertension, induction of diuresis in congestive heart failure and cirrhosis, prevention of calcium nephrolithiasis, and reduction of renal excretion of water in diabetes insipidus. Thiazides directly inhibit sodium reabsorption in the cortical diluting segment of the ascending limb of the loop of Henle. A significant kaliuresis is noted. Magnesium ion excretion is also increased whereas the excretion of calcium and uric acid is reduced. Blood glucose, cholesterol, and triglyceride may be raised by thiazides. Plasma volume decreases and cardiac output falls following acute administration. With chronic use, plasma volume returns to near normal values but peripheral vascular resistance decreases. Plasma renin, aldosterone, and norepinephrine levels rise during diuretic therapy.

Thiazides are rapidly absorbed from the gut and diuresis is usually noted within an hour of administration. Thiazides are highly protein bound and are secreted in the proximal tubule and most compounds are eliminated within 3 to 6 hours. Chlorthalidone resembles the thiazides in pharmacological effects but the drug has a long half-life.

High-ceiling diuretics (furosemide, ethycrynic acid, bumetanide) affect a diuresis far greater than the thiazides. Their site of action is the ascending segment of the loop of Henle where they inhibit chloride reabsorption and secondarily sodium reabsorption. Other effects include increased potassium, magnesium, and calcium excretion. Uric acid excretion is reduced and glucose tolerance may be diminished. Plasma renin activity is raised. In the treatment of hypertension, these drugs are less effective than thiazides.

The loop diuretics are generally well-absorbed, highly protein bound, and rapidly acting. The drugs are actively secreted into the urine and have short half-lives. Diuretic synergism may be noted when metolazone and benzothiadiazide diuretics are added to furosemide. Side effects include hypovolemia, hypokalemia, and ototoxicity.

Potassium sparing diuretics (spironolactone, triamterene, amiloride) are used principally in combination with other agents. As natriuretics they are only 10 percent as effective as furosemide. Spironolactone competitively inhibits aldosterone mediated potassium-hydrogen exchange in the distal convoluted tubule. Triamterene and amiloride act on the distal tubule to inhibit potassium excretion independent of aldosterone action. The major side effect of these drugs is the danger of hyperkalemia especially when renal decompensation is present. Spironolactone can cause gynecomastia.

DRUGS AFFECTING THE ACTIONS OF ACETYLCHOLINE

Parasympathomimetics

Acetylcholine (Ach) is the neurotransmitter at autonomic ganglia, parasympathetic nerve terminals, and the neuromuscular junction. The receptors at autonomic ganglia and at the neuromuscular junction are labeled nicotinic and those at other parasympathetic nerve terminals muscarinic. Although similar, the receptors are not identical in structure and furthermore, nicotinic receptors at autonomic ganglia are slightly different from nicotinic receptors on skeletal muscle cells. These drugs activate muscarinic receptors causing arterial vasodilatation, bradycardia, and enhanced bowel motility. Higher doses produce bronchoconstriction, heart block, salivation, lacrimation, urination, and defecation. The choline ester bethanechol has more pronounced effects on the urinary bladder and gastrointestinal tract than on the cardiovascular system. Other agents of this class are methacholine and carbechol. Carbechol and bethanechol are resistant to hydrolysis by pseudocholinesterase and by acetylcholinesterase. Methacholine is hydrolyzed slightly by acetylcholinesterase. The natural alkaloids pilocarpine and muscarine have similar actions as the choline esters. Muscarine acts almost exclusively at mucarinic receptors and pilocarpine has a dominant muscarinic action.

Anticholinesterases

Inhibitors of Ach cholinesterase block the activity of the enzyme that catalyzes hydrolysis of Ach resulting in accumulation of the neurotransmitter at synaptic sites. Pharmacological effects include diaphoresis, salivation, lacrimation, respiratory secretion, bronchospasm, bradycardia, hypertension (adrenomedullary discharge, ganglionic stimulation), miosis, contraction of nonvascular smooth muscle, and stimulation of voluntary muscle. Edrophonium is effective following intravenous administration but its action is short-lived. It is useful for diagnosis of myasthenia gravis and for terminating paroxysmal atrial tachycardia. Pyridostigmine, neostigmine, and ambenonium are useful in the long-term management of myasthenia as they can be given orally. Physostigmine has been used to reverse the central anticholinergic syndrome associated with overdosage of phenothiazines and tricyclic antidepressants.

Neuromuscular Blocking Drugs

The major action of these drugs is to interrupt transmission of the nerve impulse at the skeletal neuromuscular junction. The competitive agents include D-tubocurarine, alcuronium, β-erythroidine, gallamine, and pancuronium. The depolarizing agents include decamethonium and succinylcholine. Benzoquinonium has dual actions. The competitive agents combine with the cholinergic receptor sites on the postsynaptic membrane and block the actions of Ach. The depolarizing agents depolarize the membrane in the same manner as Ach but, since they persist at the receptor site, their action is long-lasting. A brief period of muscular fasciculation is followed by block of neuromuscular transmission. The effect of these drugs when given in sufficient dose is to produce flaccid muscle paralysis. D-tubocurarine produces some ganglionic blockade. Gallamine selectively blocks the cardiac vagus nerve. Pancuronium and alcuronium have lower degrees of ganglionic blockade. D-tubocurarine releases histamine and heparin from mast cells. Succinylcholine also has this effect but to a lesser degree. Benzoquinonium has some anticholinesterase activity. The brief duration of action of succinylcholine is due to rapid hydrolysis by pseudocholinesterase in plasma. Some individuals have prolonged apnea after succinylcholine. This is due to an inherited defect in the pseudocholinesterase which results in slow hydrolysis of succinylcholine. Malignant hypothermia has rarely been noted with a combination of halothane and succinylcholine. The main use of neuromuscular blocking agents is to obtain skeletal muscle relaxation during surgery.

Ganglionic Blocking Drugs

Ganglionic blocking drugs are competitive antagonists of Ach at the nicotinic receptor of the postsynaptic neuron. This action leads to disruption of neurotransmission in both sympathetic and parasympathetic ganglia. The net effect observed depends on the relative role of each system on the organ system affected. Thus, arteriolar and venodilatation and decreases in myocardial contractility and bradycardia are the effects observed on the circulation. Other effects include cycloplegia, mydriasis, constipation, urinary retention, xerostomia, and anhydrosis. Drugs of this class include *hexamethonium, pentolinium, mecamylamine,* and *trimethaphan.* Only trimethaphan still has application in the treatment of hypertensive emergencies, especially dissecting aortic aneurysm. The drug's effect is highly posture-dependent. It has some direct relaxant action on vascular tissue, and can cause the release of histamine and catecholamines. High doses can cause neuromuscular blockade and tolerance has developed to its antihypertensive actions.

Parasympatholytics

These drugs are competitive inhibitors of Ach at muscarinic receptors on a variety of cells including smooth and cardiac muscle cells, exocrine gland cells, and certain neurons. Scopolamine has a more potent action on the iris, ciliary body, secretory glands, and CNS. Atropine is more potent on heart, intestine, and bronchial muscle. Scopolamine is effective in preventing motion sickness. This action probably reflects an effect on the maculae of the utricle and saccule. CNS effects include drowsiness, euphoria, and higher doses produce central excitation with restlessness, disorientation, hallucinations, and delerium. Eye changes include mydriasis and cycloplegia. If vagal tone is high, significant increases in heart rate and AV conduction will be seen. Low doses of atropine can cause slight bradycardia and higher doses can produce AV dissociation and atrial arrhythmias. The motor activity of the gut and urinary tract is diminished. Lower doses of atropine reduce the secretions of the bronchial track and the sweat and lacrimal glands. Larger doses produce the full spectrum of pharmacological effects. Toxicity includes the above effects with marked CNS excitation and psychosis, fever, and flush. Acute angle glaucoma can be precipitated in susceptible patients.

CHEMOTHERAPEUTIC AGENTS

Antibiotics

Penicillin G inhibits a cell wall transpeptidase. This action leads to increased activity of membrane bound autolysins that destroy the structural integrity of the cell. Cell lysis is dependent on bacterial cell replication and an intact β-lactam ring in the penicillin molecule. The penicillins are bactericidal agents.

Most gram-positive and gram-negative cocci, gram-positive bacilli, anaerobic bacteria, actinomycetes, and spirochetes are susceptible to penicillin. Staphylococci are often resistant, particularly those strains isolated in hospitals. Gonococci are sensitive to penicillin G although strains have been isolated that are resistant due to production of a β-lactamase. *Bacteroides fragilis* may be resistant to penicillin. Gram-negative bacilli are usually resistant because their cell walls are impermeable to penicillin and they produce a variety of β-lactamases.

Penicillin G is hydrolyzed in acid and is ineffective when given orally. Sixty percent is protein-bound and 90 percent of a dose is secreted unchanged into the urine by the organic acid transport system. The half-life is 30 minutes with normal renal function and is 6 to 10 hours in anuric individuals. Penicillin enters most tissues including bone and abscesses. Penetration into the cerebrospinal fluid and aqueous humor is improved with inflammation. Combining penicillin G with procaine or with an ammonia base (benzathine penicillin G) delays absorption from intramuscular injection sites. Allergic reactions are common to penicillin. Patients who have a positive skin test to the minor determinant mixture of penicillin are most likely to develop anaphylaxis. Other adverse reactions include thrombocytopenia, pancytopenia, interstitial nephritis, pseudomembranous colitis, glossitis, and CNS toxicity.

Penicillin V is more stable in an acidic medium than penicillin G and is therefore better absorbed from the gut. The antimicrobial spectrum is similar to penicillin G.

Methicillin, nafcillin, cloxacillin, dicloxacillin, and oxacillin are effective against staphylococci that produce penicillinase. They are less active than penicillin toward penicillin sensitive organisms. About 1 percent of staphylococci are methicillin-resistant.

Methicillin and nafcillin are acid labile whereas cloxacillin, dicloxacillin, and oxacillin are acid stable. All are greater than 90 percent protein-bound except methicillin which is 35 percent bound. Half-lives range from 0.5 to 2 hours. The renal acid transport system secretes these drugs into the urine. About 50 percent of oxacillin and nafcillin are metabolized in the liver and excreted in the bile.

Besides immunologic adverse reactions, interstitial nephritis and neutropenia have been noted. Hemorrhagic cystitis has been associated with methacillin.

The aminopenicillins ampicillin and amoxicillin penetrate cell walls better than penicillin G. This property accounts for their action against 80 percent of strains of *Hemophilus influenzae,* enterococci, *Escherichia coli, Shigella* and *Salmonella* organisms, and *Proteus mirabilis.* Their susceptibility to β-lactamases makes them inactive against staphylococci, *B fragilis,* and most other

374 BURNSIDE'S EXAMINATION REVIEW

gram-negative aerobic bacilli. Aminopenicillin resistance in *H influenzae* ranges from 5 to 15 percent.

The aminopenicillins are acid-stable and well-absorbed from the gut. Both drugs are about 20 percent protein-bound in plasma. The half-life for each is 1 hour which increases to 10 to 20 hours in anuric patients. About 80 percent of each drug is secreted in the urine and 20 percent metabolized in the liver.

Skin rashes are common especially in patients receiving allopurinol or who have viral illnesses such as infectious mononucleosis. Other adverse reactions include nausea, diarrhea, pseudomembranous colitis, moniliasis, agranulocytosis, and interstitial nephritis.

Carbenicillin and ticarcillin penetrate bacterial cell walls that are impermeable to other penicillins. They are effective against many gram-positive and gram-negative bacteria including *Pseudomonas aeruginosa* and indole-positive proteus. Both drugs are synergistic with aminoglycosides against *P aeruginosa*. Acquired resistance can develop rapidly due to plasmid-mediated production of β-lactamases.

Both are acid-labile and have kinetic profiles similar to the other penicillins. The lower sodium load with ticarcillin may be of benefit in patients with heart failure or chronic renal failure.

Hypokalemia, platelet dysfunction, granulocytopenia, and neurotoxicity have been reported. They inactivate gentamicin when mixed together in intravenous solutions.

Piperacillin and Mezlocillin have a broad spectrum of activity against many gram-negative organisms including strains of *Pseudomonas, Klebsiella, Enterobacter, Serratia,* and *Proteus.* They are effective against several gram-positive organisms and anaerobic bacterii including *Bacteroides fragilis.* Synergism may be seen with aminoglycosides in the treatment of *Streptococcus faecalis* and *Pseudomonas aeruginosa* infections. Side-effects include those typical of penicillin plus bleeding abnormalities characterized by prolongation of prothrombin time and disturbance of platelet aggregation.

Cephalosporins inhibit bacterial cell wall synthesis in a manner similar to penicillin. In general these drugs are resistant to penicillinase but may be susceptible to other β-lactamases called cephalosporinases. Cephalothin and cefamandole are most resistant to these enzymes. Cefoxitin differs from cefamandole in its susceptibility to β-lactamases. These differences may contribute to differences in bacterial susceptibility among different cephalosporins.

Cephalosporins inhibit the growth of most gram-positive cocci, including *Staphlococcus aureus, Streptococcus pneumoniae,* and β-hemolytic streptococci. These agents also inhibit the growth of gram-negative bacilli including *Escherichia coli, Klebsiella pneumoniae, Proteus mirabilis,* and *Neisseria gonorrhoeae.* Differences in bacterial susceptibility exist among the different drugs. Cefoxitin is more active than cefamandole against *Proteus vulgaris* and *Serratia marcescens.* Cefamandole is more active against *Enterobacter.* Cefoxitin and cefamandole are active against *Hemophilus influenzae* and *Providencia.* These drugs are ineffective against enterococci, *Acinetobacter,* and *Pseudomonas aeruginosa.* However, cefotaxime has demonstrated activity in vitro against isolates of *P aeruginosa.* Cefoxitin is the most active against anaerobic organisms including *Bacteroides fragilis.* None of the available cephalosporins can be recommended for the treatment of meningitis with possibly the exception of cefotaxime and moxalactam. Moxalactam has a broad spectrum of activity against gram-negative bacteria including *Serratia marcesens* and *Pseudomonas aeruginosa.* It is also active against *Bacteroides fragilis* but the enterococcus and *Listeria monocytogenes* are resistant. It is weakly bound to plasma proteins and is eliminated via the kidney with a half-life of 2 hours. Adverse effects include those noted with other cephalosporins plus a disulfiram-like reaction in subjects who drink alcohol while being treated and an increased prothrombin time and thrombocytopenia.

Cephalothin, cephaloridine, cefoxitin, cephapirin, cefazolin, and cefamandole are available as parenteral preparations only. Cephalexin, cephradine, cefadroxil, and cefaclor are available in oral dosage forms.

The half-life of most cephalosporins varies from 30 to 90 minutes. These agents are excreted by glomerular filtration and the acid transport system in the kidney. About 40 percent of cephalothin is deacetylated in the liver. Because cephalosporins are eliminated via the kidney, dosage should be reduced in patients with severe renal impairment.

Most of the adverse effects to this group of antibiotics are characterized by urticaria and other skin eruptions. The majority of patients with a history of penicillin allergy can be given cephalosporins without risk of serious reactions. Nephrotoxicity has been reported in patients taking cephaloridine. Concomitant use of cephalothin increases the risk of aminoglycoside nephrotoxicity.

Aminoglycosides are bactericidal agents. They are transported across the bacterial cell membrane and bind to the 30 S ribosomal subunit leading to inhibition of bacterial protein synthesis.

Gentamicin is effective against most gram-negative bacteria including *Pseudomonas aeruginosa* although many strains of *Proteus, Providencia, Alcaligenes, Serratia marcescens,* and *Pseudomonas* are resistant. A synergistic effect of penicillin and gentamicin is noted against most enterococci. *Tobramycin* is about 3 times more active on a weight basis than gentamicin against

Pseudomonas aeruginosa. The spectrum of antibacterial activity of amikacin is the broadest of the group and its resistance to aminoglycoside — inactivating enzymes is greatest. Netilmicin may be active against many bacterial strains resistant to other aminoglycosides. Neomycin is used to "sterilize" the gut in patients with hepatic encephalopathy. Streptomycin is used to treat tuberculosis, brucellosis, yersinia infections, and tularemia. The action of aminoglycosides against most gram-positive bacteria is limited. Most strains of *Staphlococcus aureus* and *Staphlococcus epidermidis* are sensitive in vitro to aminoglycosides. Anaerobic bacteria are resistant.

Aminoglycosides are poorly absorbed from the intestine but are well-absorbed following intramuscular injection. Aminoglycosides are not protein-bound. They are excreted unchanged in the urine with a half-life in normal adults of 2 to 4 hours. Dosage adjustment is necessary in patients with abnormal renal function. Levels in renal tissue may be 10- to 20-fold higher than those in serum, and this observation may be related to nephrotoxicity. Peak levels of gentamicin, tobramycin, and netilmicin should lie between 5 and 12 μg/ml. The corresponding values for amikacin are 20 and 40 μg/ml.

Both vestibular and auditory damage can follow administration of any of the aminoglycosides. Furosemide and ethycrynic acid potentiate this effect. Gentamicin is the most nephrotoxic of the aminoglycosides. Prolonged therapy, excessively high plasma trough concentrations, and patient age correlate with the severity of renal damage. Neuromuscular blockade can occur in susceptible patients.

Vancomycin is a bactericidal agent that inhibits biosynthesis of essential cell wall mucopeptides. Vancomycin is effective against gram-positive organisms including methicillin resistant *Staphlococcus aureus* and *Staphlococcus epidermidis.* Vancomycin is effective in treating pseudomembranous colitis caused by *Clostridium difficile.*

Vancomycin is not absorbed from the gut. It is excreted unchanged in the urine with a half-life of 6 hours in patients with normal renal function which increases to 9 days in anuric patients. The most serious adverse effects are ototoxicity and nephrotoxicity.

Erythromycin acts by binding to the 50 S ribosomal subunit to inhibit protein synthesis. Erythromycin can be either bactericidal or bacteriostatic depending on the concentration of the drug and the susceptibility of the organism. Resistance is usually due to poor penetration of the bacterial cell wall.

Most gram-positive bacteria are sensitive including penicillinase producing *Staphlococcus aureus, Staphlococcus epidermidis, Clostridium, Corynebacterium, Listeria monocytogenes,* and Enterococci. *Mycoplasma pneumoniae, Rickettsia,* chlamydiae, *Treponema palli-*

dum, and atypical mycobacteria may be sensitive. Erythromycin is the most active drug for treating pneumonia caused by *Legionella pneumophilia.* Erythromycin is also effective for treating brucellosis, actinomycosis, amebiasis, and gonorrhea.

Erythromycin base is acid-labile and must be administered as an enteric coated tablet. Various esters (stearate, succinate, propionate, estolate) have been prepared that are stable to gastric acid. However, they must be converted to the free base following absorption to be effective. The stearate ester is hydrolyzed in the gut prior to absorption as the base. The base is about 75 percent protein-bound and the half-life is 1.5 hours. Greater than 90 percent is N-demethylated in the liver and excreted in the bile. The drug does not penetrate the CSF well even in the presence of inflammation. It enters prostatic fluid well.

Adverse reactions include epigastric distress, nausea, and diarrhea. The estolate ester may cause cholestatic hepatitis.

Chloramphenicol acts by binding to the 50 S ribosomal subunit in bacteria resulting in inhibition of protein synthesis. Protein synthesis in mammalian mitochondria is also inhibited. In general chloramphenicol is bacteriostatic.

Chloramphenicol has a broad spectrum of activity including many gram-positive and gram-negative organisms. *Bacteroides fragilis* and most other anaerobes are susceptible. This drug is useful for treatment of *Hemophilus influenzae* infections caused by ampicillin-resistant strains and in individuals hypersensitive to penicillin. It is effective in the treatment of Typhoid fever. A variety of nonbacterial organisms are also sensitive including *chlamydiae, Mycoplasma, Actinomyces,* and *Rickettsia.* Resistance to chloramphenicol is transmitted via R-factors resulting in the production of an acetyl-transferase that inactivates chloramphenicol.

Chloramphenicol is readily absorbed from the gut with peak plasma levels occurring 1 to 2 hours after the dose. The half-life varies from 1 to 4 hours. Hepatic glucuronidation is responsible for 80 to 90 percent of chloramphenicol clearance. About 70 percent is protein-bound.

Two types of bone marrow toxicity occur; a reversible depressant effect on erythropoiesis and an irreversible aplastic anemia. The former is dose-related and is more common when chloramphenicol serum levels exceed 25 μg/ml. The aplastic anemia may develop weeks to months after therapy with an incidence of about 1 : 30,000 and a mortality rate of 80 percent. A syndrome of pallid cyanosis, irregular respiration, hypothermia, and vasomotor collapse has been noted particularly in infants less than 3 months of age. It is seen with plasma levels in excess of 50 μg/ml. These infants do not conjugate the drug effectively. Because of its inhibitory effect on hepatic microsomal enzymes, chloramphenicol reduces the clearance of tolbutamide, phenytoin, phenobarbital, and dicoumerol. Phenobarbital may lower chloramphenicol levels and a disulfiram effect has been noted in patients consuming alcohol.

Tetracyclines are bacteriostatic agents that bind reversibly to the 30 S ribosomal subunit of bacterial cells resulting in an inhibition of protein synthesis. Passive diffusion and active transport move tetracyclines into bacterial cells. Resistance to tetracyclines is plasmid-mediated and involves the formation of proteins that interfere with the transport of the drug into the cell.

Although there are specific differences between the tetracyclines, they are in the main similar. This class of antibiotics includes tetracycline, Chlortetracycline, Oxytetracycline, Demeclocycline, Methacycline, Doxycycline, and Minocycline.

Most strains of *Streptococcus pneumoniae, Streptococcus pyogenes, Listeria monocytogenes, Clostridium, Neissevia meningitidis, Neissevia gonorrhoeae, Hemophilus influenza, Mycoplasma pneumoniae, T mycoplasma,* and chlamydiae are inhibited. *Brucella, Pasturella, Borrelia recurrentis, Vibrio cholerae, Rickettsia, Actinomyces, Nocardia,* and atypical mycobacteria are usually susceptible. High urinary levels inhibit about 70 percent of *Escherichia coli, Klebsiella pneumoniae,* and enterobacterorganisms. Enterococci, *Serratia, Shigella,* and *Pseudomonas aeruginosa* are resistant.

Doxycycline and Minocycline are one- to twofold more active than tetracycline against susceptible organisms. Minocycline has greater activity against *Staphlococcus aureus, Bacteroides fragilis,* and *Nocardia.*

Most of the tetracyclines are adequately but incompletely absorbed from the gut. Doxycycline and minocycline are 95 to 100 percent absorbed. Absorption is impaired by milk products, aluminum hydroxide, sodium bicarbonate, calcium and magnesium salts, and iron preparations. The plasma protein binding of these drugs varies from 20 to 40 percent (oxytetracycline) to 80 to 95 percent (doxycycline). The plasma half-life of these drugs varies from 10 hours (tetracycline) to 20 hours (minocycline). The majority of tetracycline (40 to 60 percent) is excreted unchanged in the urine. About 50 percent of doxycycline is excreted in the urine and the remainder is unchanged in the feces. Only 10 percent of minocycline is excreted in the urine, 30 percent in the feces, and the rest metabolized.

Tetracyclines are useful for the treatment of syphilis and gonorrhea in patients sensitive to penicillin. They are useful in exacerbations of bronchitis, prostatitis, malabsorption due to bacterial overgrowth, and acne. They may be useful for the treatment of Rickettsia, Chlamydia infection, and nonspecific urethritis. Mino-

cycline may be used prophylactically to eliminate the meningococcal carrier state because it is excreted in saliva and tears. Doxycycline is used to prevent traveller's diarrhea.

Adverse effects include nausea, vomiting, glossitis, proctitis, diarrhea, pseudomembranous colitis, phototoxicity, and esophageal ulceration. Large doses can cause severe hepatic damage characterized by fatty infiltration. Pregnant and postpartum women are particularly susceptible to this reaction. Tetracyclines worsen azotemia in patients with abnormal renal function. Administration of tetracycline to pregnant women can discolor the teeth of offspring. Administration of tetracycline to children can cause discoloration and hypoplasia of the teeth enamel.

TRIMETHOPRIM – SULFAMETHOXAZOLE

Sulfamethoxazole inhibits the incorporation of p-aminobenzoic acid into dihydrofolate and trimethoprim inhibits the formation of tetrahydrofolate from dihydrofolate. Bacterial dihydrofolate reductase is much more susceptible to inhibition by trimethoprim than the mammalian enzyme. In addition bacteria rely on production of dihydrofolate whereas man absorbs it from food. These drugs are synergistic in vitro and effectively kill bacteria.

Most strains of *Escherichia coli, Proteus mirabilis, Salmonella, Shigella, Hemophilus influenzae, Streptococcus pneumoniae, Staphlococcus aureus* (methicillin-sensitive), and *Chlamydiae* are susceptible to the combination. Proteus (indole-positive), *Seratia, Klebsiella, Enterobacter, Yersinia, Bacteroides fragilis, Neisseria, Streptococcus fecalis, S Pyogenes, S aureus* (methicillin-resistant), *Nocardia,* and *Pneumocystis carinii* are variably susceptible. *Pseudomonas aeruginosa, Treponema pallidum,* and *M tuberculosis* mycoplasma are resistant.

This antibiotic combination has been useful for the treatment of chronic urinary tract infections, chronic bronchitis, gonorrhea, meningitis, shigellosis, typhoid fever, and *Pneumocystis carinii* pneumonia.

Trimethoprim and sulfamethoxazole are well-absorbed from the gut. Trimethoprim's half-life is 12 hours and is excreted unchanged in the urine. Sulfamethoxazole's half-life is 9 hours and is acetylated and glucuronidated in the liver. The metabolites are then excreted in the urine. When creatinine clearance is less than 20 ml/min dosage modification needs to be made.

Adverse reactions include skin rash, nausea, diarrhea, stomatitis, and glossitis. Patients with folate or vitamin B_{12} deficiency may develop megaloblastic anemia, neutropenia, or thrombocytopenia. Rarely nephrotoxicity and hemolysis in glucose-6-phosphate dehydrogenase-deficient patients occurs. Coumadin's action may be enhanced. Phenytoin clearance may be decreased and the effects of oral hypoglycemic agents increased.

Clindamycin inhibits bacterial protein synthesis by binding to the 50 S ribosomal subunit. It is bacteriostatic or bactericidal depending on concentration and organism tested.

Clindamycin is usually active against anaerobic bacteria including *Bacteroides fragilis, Fusobacterium,* and *peptostreptococcus* and is also useful for the treatment of gram-positive infection in patients sensitive to penicillin.

Clindamycin is well-absorbed from the intestine. About 80 percent is bound to plasma protein. The half-life is 3 hours and hepatic metabolism is the principal mechanism of elimination. Clindamycin does not enter the cerebrospinal fluid well.

Adverse reactions include skin rash and diarrhea. Pseudomembranous colitis occurs in 2 percent of patients.

Isoniazid (INH) inhibits synthesis of mycolic acids which are essential cell wall components of mycobacteria. Sensitive bacteria concentrate the drug and it is effective against bacilli growing within cells. Resistant strains emerge in vivo when INH is used as a single agent.

INH is well-absorbed orally. It is not protein-bound in plasma. INH is metabolized in the liver to acetylisoniazid, isonicotenic acid, and acetylhydrazine. Slow acetylators have a half-life of 3 hours and rapid acetylators $1\frac{1}{2}$ hours.

Hepatitis occurs in about 1 percent of patients. It appears to be due to toxic effects of acetylhydrazine. Rapid acetylators, alcoholics, and elderly patients are more susceptible. Peripheral neuritis and optic neuritis are more common in slow acetylators and is prevented by pyridoxine. Memory disturbance, psychosis, seizures, and coma can develop at high serum levels and is also reversible by pyridoxine. Other adverse effects include drug-induced lupus erythematosis. INH inhibits phenytoin and warfarin metabolism.

Rifampin kills bacteria by inhibiting the activity of DNA-dependent RNA polymerase. Rifampin readily penetrates phagocytic cells and kills intracellular bacteria. When used as a single agent, resistant organisms emerge rapidly. Rifampin is also effective against gram-positive and gram-negative cocci and bacilli.

Rifampin is well-absorbed orally. It is 80 percent protein-bound and penetrates most tissues well including the cerebrospinal fluid. The half-life is 2 to 4 hours. Rifampin and deacetylated metabolites are excreted in the bile.

Rash occurs in 5 to 8 percent of patients. Rarely severe allergic reactions characterized by fever, rash, eosinophilia, and Stevens-Johnson syndrome occur. Hepatitis can develop. Immunoglobulin light-chain proteinuria has been noted. Red coloration of saliva, tears, urine, and feces may develop. Rifampin induces hepatic microsomal metabolism and may enhance the clearance of corticosteroids, oral contraceptives, oral anticoagulants, oral hypoglycemics, and digitoxin.

Ethambutol inhibits actively dividing mycobacteria and may interfere with cell wall synthesis.

About 75 percent of an oral dose is absorbed. About 25 percent is protein-bound and the half-life is 4 hours. The drug is excreted unchanged in the urine (55 percent) and the rest metabolized in the liver.

The most important adverse effect is optic neuritis resulting in a decrease of visual acuity and loss of the ability to perceive the color green.

Metronidazole is effective against *Trichomonas vaginalis, Ento histolyticum, Giardia lamblia, Clostridium perfringens, Bacteroides fragilis,* and most other anaerobes.

Metronidazole is well-absorbed orally and has a wide tissue distribution including the CSF. Less than 5 percent is protein-bound and the plasma half-life is about 9 hours. Hepatic metabolism is responsible for elimination.

The major adverse effects include nausea, vomiting, and metallic taste. Other effects include reddish discoloration of urine, reversible leukopenia, disulfiram-like activity, sensory neuropathy, and seizures.

Antifungal Agents

Amphotericin binds to ergosterol in the fungal cell membrane resulting in increased permeability and loss of essential cell contents. *Aspergillus, Blastomyces, Candida, Coccidioides, Paracoccidioidomycosis, Cryptococcus, Histoplasma, Sporotrichum,* and *Mucor* species are usually sensitive. Amphotericin is synergistic with flucytosine, rifampin, and minocycline. Amphotericin is the preferred treatment for serious systemic fungal infections.

Amphotericin is given by the intravenous route and concentrates in the liver, spleen, lung, and kidney, but penetrates the cerebrospinal fluid and eye poorly. Following distribution, the plasma half-life is about 24 hours followed by a terminal half-life of 15 days. The drug is probably eliminated in the bile.

Adverse effects are common and include fever, chills, headache, nausea, vomiting, thrombophlebitis, hypertension, hypokalemia, hypomagnesemia, and nephrotoxicity.

Flucytosine is taken up by fungi and converted to 5-fluorouracil. 5-Flurouracil is incorporated into fungal RNA and causes abnormal protein synthesis. Fungal DNA synthesis is also inhibited following conversion to 5-fluorouridine.

Flucytosine inhibits most *Candida albicans, Cryptococcus neoformans,* and *Torulopsis glabrata.* Most *Aspergillus, Histoplasma,* and *Coccidioides* are resistant. In general, it should not be used as a single agent due to the development of resistant fungi.

Flucytosine is orally effective. It penetrates most tissues and its half-life is 4 to 6 hours. It is eliminated unchanged in the urine and dosage needs modification in the presence of renal failure.

Adverse effects include diarrhea, elevation of serum glutamic-oxaloacetic transaminase (SGOT) and alkaline phosphatase, neutropenia, and thrombocytopenia.

Ketoconazole damages fungal membranes by interfering with ergosterol synthesis. It may also increase intracellular hydrogen peroxide which damages the fungal cell.

Ketoconazole has been effective in treating dermatophytoses, pityriasis versicolor, onychomycosis, oral and vaginal candidiasis, and chronic mucocutaneous candidiasis. Ketoconazole may also be effective in treating systemic fungal infections.

Ketoconazole is well-absorbed orally but requires gastric acid. Absorption is reduced in achlorhydria patients and in patients receiving cimetidine or antacids. It is widely distributed in various tissues including sebum although penetration of CSF is low. It is highly bound to plasma albumin. Ketoconazole is eliminated by hepatic metabolism. The half-life varies from 6 to 9 hours.

Adverse reactions include nausea, anorexia, skin rash, and hepatotoxicity (5 percent). Males may develop gynecomastia, decreased libido, oligospermia, and loss of hair due to inhibition of testosterone synthesis. Ketoconazole also produces a dose-dependent reduction in serum cortisol. As yet no clinical consequences have been reported.

Antiviral Agents

Adenine arabinoside (ara-A) is a purine nucleoside most effective against DNA viruses including herpesvirus, poxvirus, and indovirus. It is rapidly taken up by cells and phosphorylated to ara-ATP, which inhibits viral replication.

Ara-A must be given by intravenous infusion and is rapidly converted to ara-hypoxanthine, an active metabolite. The metabolite readily penetrates the CSF. Ara-A has been used to treat a variety of serious herpesvirus infections including herpes encephalitis, herpes labialis, herpes zoster, and CMV encephalitis. The best success has been in herpes encephalitis.

Nausea and vomiting occur in 30 percent of patients. Other adverse effects include neutropenia, thrombocytopenia, and CNS toxicity at high doses.

Acyclovir is a purine nucleoside analogue with inhibitory activity against herpes simplex, varicella-zoster, Epstein-Barr, and cytomegalovirus. Acyclovir is converted to the triphosphate derivative in virus infected cells and the latter can interfere with viral DNA replication.

The half-life is about 3 hours in patients with normal renal function and this increases to 20 hours in anuric patients. The drug is administered by the intravenous route to treat initial and recurrent mucosal and cutaneous herpes simplex infections in immunocompromised patients and for severe initial clinical episodes of herpes genitalis in patients who are not immunocompromised. No evidence of clinical benefit has been demonstrated in cases of recurrent herpes infections.

The most common adverse effects include rash, transient elevation of serum creatinine, and phlebitis at injection sites. Serious CNS toxicity has occurred in a few patients.

Amantidine inhibits replication of most strains of influenza A virus and has prophylactic value when administered to humans who have had contact with an active case of influenza A. Amantidine also releases dopamine from neurons which accounts for its use in the treatment of parkinsonism. It is excreted unchanged in the urine. Toxicity includes nervousness, confusion, hallucinations, seizures, and coma.

Anti-Neoplastic Drugs

ALKYLATING AGENTS

Alkylating drugs exert their effects through the formation of reactive alkyl groups that covalently bind to nucleic acids and proteins essential for cell growth and function. Bifunctional agents form inter- and intrastrand bridges within and between DNA and RNA strands. These bridges prevent DNA replication and RNA translation.

Nitrogen mustard (mechlorethamine) is used for the treatment of Hodgkin's disease and other lymphomas. Mechlorethamine avidly combines with water and cell constituents. Severe local tissue damage results if extravasation occurs.

Toxic manifestations include nausea, vomiting, leukopenia, thrombocytopenia, menstrual irregularities, impaired spermatogenesis, and rarely hemorrhage due to hyperheparinemia.

Cyclophosphamide has a broad clinical spectrum of activity including various lymphomas, leukemias, and multiple myeloma.

The drug is well absorbed orally and is converted to several toxic metabolites in the liver which mediate the drugs actions. The half-life of cyclophosphamide is 6 to 7 hours. Phenobarbital enhances the rate of metabolism and its leukopenic effects. Allopurinol and chloramphenicol may enhance the effects and bone marrow toxicity. Cyclophosphamide is a potent immunosuppressant.

Adverse effects include nausea, vomiting, diarrhea, alopecia, leukopenia, thrombocytopenia, and gonadal suppression. Hemorrhagic cystitis may result from the presence of reactive metabolites in the urine.

Chlorambucil is effective in the treatment of chronic lymphocytic leukemia, Waldenstrom's macroglobulinemia, and Hodgkin's and non-Hodgkin's lymphomas.

Chlorambucil is absorbed following oral administration. The plasma half-life is 90 minutes. Adverse effects include bone marrow suppression and hyperuricemia. Nausea, vomiting, and alopecia are not common.

L-phenylalanine mustard (L-PAM, melphalan) is effective in multiple myeloma, ovarian cancer, and breast cancer. Plasma melphalan levels are highly variable following oral dosing. The half-life is 100 minutes. The major toxic effects are leukopenia, thrombocytopenia, oligospermia, and amenorrhea. Acute lymphatic leukemia may develop following therapy of multiple myeloma. Secondary malignancies have also developed following therapy with the other alkylating agents. Acute myelocytic leukemia has been the most common tumor.

Busulphan is used to treat chronic myelogenous leukemia. It is well-absorbed following oral administration and disappears rapidly from blood following intravenous administration. Leukopenia, thrombocytopenia, and anemia can be severe. Rarely lung damage characterized by irreversible interstitial pneumonitis and fibrosis develops.

NITROSOUREAS

The most widely used agents include carmustine (BCNU), lomustine (CCNU), and semustine (methyl CCNU). They are all highly lipid-soluble which facilitates entry into the brain. They alkylate nucleic acids and protein and also carbamylate proteins. These actions cause inhibition of DNA, RNA, and protein synthesis.

The half-lives of nitrosoureas are very short due to non-enzymatic and hepatic enzymatic decomposition. BCNU is administered intravenously and CCNU and methyl CCNU are given orally. Because these drugs (or metabolites) penetrate the blood-brain barriers, they have been useful in treating malignant gliomas. CCNU and BCNU are active in Hodgkin's and non-Hodgkins lymphomas. Me CCNU has shown activity in colo-rectal cancer. The most important adverse reaction to these drugs is delayed myelosuppression characterized by leukopenia and thrombocytopenia which can be severe.

Streptozacin contains a nitrosourea group. It has been effective in the treatment of metastatic islet cell tumors of the pancreas. Streptozocin causes little myelosuppression but can cause nephrotoxicity, nausea, and vomiting.

ANTIMETABOLITES

Methotrexate (MTX) inhibits dihydrofolate reductase which is required for the reduction of dihydrofolate to tetrahydrofolate. Single carbon fragments are then added to tetrahydrofolate and these can be transferred in specific reactions. The dominant cytotoxic effect of MTX is blockade of thymidylate synthesis which involves transmethylation of uridylate. Since thymidylate is an essential component of DNA, DNA synthesis is inhibited. MTX is active against acute lymphocytic leukemia, squamous cell carcinoma of the head and neck, adenocarcinoma of the breast, and choriocarcinoma. It is administered intrathecally for the treatment of meningeal neoplasms. It is also used for the treatment of severe psoriasis. The role of high-dose MTX followed by tetrahydrofolate in the treatment of malignancies is uncertain.

MTX is well absorbed orally. It is 50 percent bound to plasma protein. Its half-life is 2 to 3 hours and is excreted via the acid transport system of the kidney. MTX enters cells by active transport.

Toxicity includes myelosuppression, nausea, vomiting, stomatitis, diarrhea, and intestinal ulceration. Hepatic toxicity can occur. Interstitial pneumonitis and renal damage have been noted. Probenecid and salicylates reduce MTX renal excretion. Salicylates, sulfonamides, phenytoin, phenylbutazone, tetracycline, and chloramphenicol displace MTX from plasma albumin.

5-Fluorouracil (5-FU) is converted intracellularly to 5-fluorodeoxyuridylate, which is the active moiety. The latter compound inhibits thymidylate synthetase and thus thymidylate formation and DNA synthesis.

5-FU is rapidly cleared from the body following intravenous administration. Both hepatic metabolism and urinary excretion of unchanged drug take place. Oral absorption is unpredictable and incomplete. Infusion into the hepatic artery has been performed in patients with liver metastases. 5-FU is useful in the palliative management of carcinoma of the colon, rectum, pancreas, stomach, and breast. Toxic effects include myelosuppression, nausea, vomiting, diarrhea, and stomatitis. Alopecia is uncommon. Cerebellar ataxia rarely occurs.

Cytosine arabinoside (Ara-C) inhibits DNA polymerase and is incorporated into both DNA and RNA. These actions lead to an impairment of DNA synthesis. Ara-C is activated to the triphosphate by deoxycytidine kinase. It is deactivated by a deaminase enzyme. Ara-C is rapidly metabolized following intravenous administration. It is not effective orally. Ara-C is indicated for the treatment of acute myelocytic leukemia, acute lymphocytic leukemia, and for intrathecal use in meningeal leukemia. Toxicity includes myelosuppression, nausea, vomiting, diarrhea, stomatitis, and fever.

6-Mercaptopurine (6-MP), azathiopine, and 6-thioguanine (6-TG) are purine antimetabolites and are similar in their pharmacologic actions. These drugs inhibit DNA and RNA synthesis by inhibiting enzymes in the de novo pathways of purine synthesis as well as by incorporation into the DNA and RNA molecules leading to strand breaks and nonsense messages. These agents require activation to the corresponding nucleotide by the enzyme hypoxanthine-guanine phosphoribosyl transferase (HGRTase).

These drugs are readily absorbed after oral ingestion. They are degraded in the liver. Azathioprine is converted to 6-MP in vivo. 6-MP and azathioprine (but not 6-TG) are converted by xanthine oxidase to 6-thiouric acid (inactive). Allopurinol inhibits their degradation and potentiates their toxic effects. 6-MP is used during the maintenance phase of childhood acute lymphocytic leukemia. 6-TG is used in the treatment of acute granulocytic leukemia in combination with Ara-C. Azathioprine is used as an immunosuppressive agent for organ transplantation and in a variety of immune disorders. Adverse effects to these agents include myelosuppression, nausea, vomiting, stomatitis, and intestinal ulceration. Hepatotoxicity can occur.

NATURAL PRODUCTS

Vincristine and vinblastine cause metaphase arrest in actively dividing cells. They bind avidly to tubulin, a key protein of cellular microtubules. This binding results in disruption of the microtubular array (mitotic spindle) necessary for chromosome separation. This action leads to cell death. In addition, disturbances of microtubular structures necessary for maintaining cell shape and motility may contribute to their activity.

Both drugs are administered by the intravenous route and are cleared from the circulation primarily by hepatic metabolism. Disturbances in liver function alter their metabolism and dosage modification needs to be made. Vincristine is active in acute lymphocytic leukemia, Hodgkin's and non-Hodgkin's lymphoma, breast and testicular cancer, soft tissue sarcomas, Wilm's tumor, and neuroblastoma. Vinblastine is active in the treatment of Hodgkin's disease, non-Hodgkin's lymphoma, testicular cancer, trophoblastic tumors, and breast carcinoma. A lack of cross-resistance between the vinca alkaloids has been noted.

Toxicity includes myelosuppression especially leukopenia with vinblastine. Alopecia is frequent. Nausea, vomiting, and stomatitis occur. Neurotoxicity is the

major adverse effect of vincristine and also occurs with vinblastine. Foot or wrist drop, cranial nerve palsies, severe muscle weakness and autonomic neuropathy can develop. Inappropriate release of anti-diuretic hormone has been described. Extravasation produces considerable irritation.

ANTIBIOTICS

The antibiotics doxorubicin (Adriamycin) and daunorubicin exert their effects by intercalating into the DNA helix leading to inhibition of DNA and RNA synthesis.

Both Doxorubicin and daunorubicin are metabolized in the liver. The half-life of doxorubicin is 17 hours and daunorubicin is 18 hours. Dose reduction is necessary if liver function is depressed. Daunorubicin is used to treat acute non-lymphocytic leukemias particularly in combination with Ara-C. Doxorubicin is useful for the treatment of several solid tumors including breast cancer, lung cancer, carcinoid tumors, and gastric, testicular, endometrial, and ovarian carcinomas.

Toxic effects include myelosuppression, stomatitis, nausea, vomiting, alopecia, and soft tissue necrosis if extravasation occurs. Cardiotoxicity is a unique reaction to these drugs and is characterized by cardiomegaly and congestive heart failure.

Mithramycin is a highly toxic antibiotic that binds to DNA and inhibits DNA directed RNA synthesis. Mithramycin lowers serum calcium by interfering with osteoclast function. The drug is used as a secondary choice in the treatment of advanced germ cell tumors. It has been used for the treatment of Paget's disease of bone. Toxicity includes myelosuppression, hepatotoxicity, renal tubular dysfunction, nausea, vomiting, and consumptive coagulopathy.

Dactinomycin (Actinomycin D) is a chromopeptide that binds to double-helix DNA to form a stable complex which leads to an inhibition of RNA polymerase directed DNA transcription. This drug has been used in the treatment of Wilm's tumor, rhabdomyosarcoma, methotrexate-resistant choriocarcinoma, and testicular and uterine cancer. Toxicity includes severe soft tissue necrosis if extravasation occurs, nausea, vomiting, stomatitis, diarrhea, myelosuppression, alopecia, and rash.

MISCELLANEOUS AGENTS

Bleomycin is a mixture of glycopeptides that fragment single-stranded DNA. Inhibition of DNA, RNA, and protein synthesis has been observed.

Bleomycin is administered parenterally and high concentrations are localized in the skin and lung, the major cities of toxicity. The half-life is about 9 hours and the kidney is primarily responsible for its elimination. Bleomycin has activity against lymphomas, testicular cancer, and squamous cell carcinoma of the head and neck.

Adverse effects include cutaneous toxicity characterized by erythema, edema, desquamation, and ulcers. A diffuse interstitial pneumonitis is the most dangerous toxic effect. A few patients with lymphoma may experience severe hyperpyrexia and hypotension.

Procarbazine (PCB) depolymerizes DNA. PCB also methylates guanine and adenine residues. These effects lead to an inhibition of DNA, RNA, and protein synthesis.

The drug is well-absorbed following oral administration and crosses the blood-brain barrier readily. PCB is eliminated following hepatic metabolism. PCB is used primarily in combination with other drugs for the treatment of Hodgkin's disease.

Toxicity includes myelosuppression, nausea, vomiting, and CNS effects (depression, somnolence, lethargy, agitation). A disulfiram-like reaction may be seen with ethanol. Foods rich in tyramine may cause severe hypertension since PCB has MAO inhibitory properties.

The chloride ions are removed from cisplatin intracellularly resulting in the formation of a reactive species which causes inter- and intrastrand cross-linking of DNA. The binding of platinium complexes to DNA results in disruption and unwinding of the double helix.

After intravenous administration, the drug has an initial half-life in plasma of 25 to 50 minutes. The subsequent terminal half-life is 60 to 75 hours. Greater than 90 percent is bound to plasma proteins. Poor penetration of the CNS is noted. The primary route of excretion is via the kidney. Cisplatin (Cis-diamine dichloroplatinum, CDPP) is active in tumors of the testis, ovary, squamous carcinoma of the head and neck, tumors of the bladder and cervix, and Hodgkin's disease.

CDPP can cause acute tubular necrosis. Nausea and vomiting are often severe. Ototoxicity and peripheral neuropathy may occur. Anaphylaxis has occurred.

Asparaginase contains the enzyme L-asparagine amido-hydrolase. Some malignant cells cannot synthesize asparaginine and require exogenous asparagine for survival. Rapid depletion of asparagine in these cells by asparaginine leads to cell death. This enzyme has been used in patients with acute lymphoblastic leukemia.

Anticoagulants

Heparin is effective in the treatment of venous thrombosis, pulmonary and systemic embolization. It is used to anticoagulate patients during cardiopulmonary bypass, arterial surgery, hemodialysis, and for the treatment of disseminated intravascular coagulation. Heparin is a heterogeneous group of anionic mucopolysac-charides that are strongly acidic in nature. The anticoagulant effect of heparin is immediate. Heparin accelerates the interaction of antithrombin III with thrombin to form an irreversible inactive complex. The subsequent inhibition of thrombin activity prevents conversion of fibrinogen to fibrin. This results in the prolongation of whole blood clotting time and activated partial thromboplastin time. Heparin releases tissue bound lipoprotein lipase and stabilizes it. This action accounts for the stimulation by heparin of triglyceride hydrolysis from chylomicrons.

Heparin is inactivated by the liver enzyme heparinase. The half-life is about 1 hour at usual doses. Heparin can be given by the intravenous or subcutaneous routes.

The main adverse effect of heparin is hemorrhage. Hypersensitivity reactions, thrombocytopenia, alopecia, and osteoporosis have been observed.

Protamine sulfate is strongly basic and complexes with heparin to inactivate it. Rapid intravenous injection may cause dyspnea, flushing, bradycardia, and hypotension.

Warfarin is the prototype and the most widely used oral anticoagulant. The anticoagulant effects of the other oral agents differ only quantitatively. Warfarin inhibits the hepatic synthesis of vitamin K-dependent clotting factors (II, VII, IX, and X). Vitamin K is required for the conversion of the precursors of these proteins to their active forms. During this reaction, vitamin K is inactivated but is reactivated by an enzyme requiring NADH. Warfarin inhibits this reaction. The S(−) warfarin isomer is more potent than the R(+) isomer. Both the prothrombin time and partial thromboplastin time is prolonged.

Warfarin is well-absorbed orally. The drug is highly bound to plasma albumin (> 97 percent). The half-life is about 40 hours. Warfarin is eliminated by hepatic metabolism. The S(−) isomer is cleared more rapidly than the R(+) isomer. Warfarin readily crosses the placenta. Hereditary resistance to warfarin action has been noted. This is an autosomal trait.

Hemorrhage is the principal adverse effect. Drugs that increase the response to warfarin include aspirin and NSAID, which inhibit platelet aggregation. Phenylbutazone displaces warfarin from albumin and inhibits the S(−) isomer's metabolism. Several other drugs inhibit warfarin metabolism. These include chloramphenicol, allopurinol, disulfiram, metronidazole, clofibrate, nortriptyline, cimetidine, and trimethoprim-sulfamethoxazole. Drugs that increase the activity of warfarin metabolizing enzymes include barbiturates, phenytoin, rifampin, spironolactone, and oral contraceptives. The potential for drug interaction needs to be reviewed carefully for each drug administered concomitantly with warfarin.

Anti-Inflammatory Drugs

The prostaglandins and leukotrienes are derived from arachidonic acid. Arachidonic acid is released from cell membranes by the action of phospholipases which are activated by a variety of stimuli such as norepinephrine, thrombi, bradykinin, and trauma. The liberated arachidonic acid is rapidly converted in the presence of oxygen to endoperoxides by the enzyme cyclo-oxygenase. A variety of different prostaglandins can be made by a series of different enzymes from the endoperoxide intermediates. Thus, endothelial cells form prostacyclin (PGI_2), which is a potent vasodilator and inhibitor of platelet aggregation. The platelet makes thromboxane A_2, which is a potent vasoconstrictor and promoter of platelet aggregation. PGE_2 is a vasodilator and $PGF_{2\alpha}$ a vasoconstrictor. PGI_2 stimulates platelet adenylcyclase increasing cyclic AMP levels. Inhibitors of phosphodiesterase that degrade cyclic AMP potentiate the antiplatelet effect of PGI_2. This action might explain the mechanism by which the phosphodiesterase inhibitors sulfinpyrazone and dipyridamole inhibit platelet aggregation.

Nonsteroidal anti-inflammatory (NSAID) compounds, such as aspirin and indomethacin are potent inhibitors of cyclo-oxygenase. This action probably accounts for the anti-inflammatory, antipyretic, and analgesic properties of these drugs. Aspirin binds irreversibly to cyclo-oxygenase rendering it inactive. New synthesis of enzyme is required to restore the enzyme's activity. The other NSAID are reversible inhibitors of this enzyme.

Leukotrienes are also formed from arachidonic acid. The enzyme 5-lipoxygenase converts arachidonate to 5-hydroperoxy-6,8,11,14-eicosatetraenoic acid (5-HPETE) from which LTC_4, LTD_4, and LTE_4 are made. The latter three substances are potent constrictors of bronchial smooth muscle particularly in small airways. They constitute the slow reactive substance of asthma. These substances also increase vascular permeability with loss of fluid. These compounds may play important roles in the pathogenesis of a variety of disorders including asthma and inflammatory diseases.

Aspirin is rapidly hydrolyzed to salicylic acid following absorption. Aspirin can irreversibly inhibit cyclo-oxygenase and salicylic acid is a reversible inhibitor. Aspirin relieves pain of low intensity such as headache, myalgia, and arthralgia which arise from integumental structures. Salicylates are effective antipyretics.

Salicylate is eliminated by renal excretion of unchanged drug and by a variety of hepatic enzymatic reactions. Saturation of the liver enzymes at higher doses results in "dose-dependent" elimination. Thus, a low-dose salicylate has a half-life of 4 hours and at higher doses this is increased to 15 to 30 hours. Urinary excre-

tion of unchanged salicylate is increased by alkalinizing the urine. Therapeutic plasma levels of salicylate in connective tissue disorders are 200 to 300 μg/ml.

Other effects of salicylate include inhibition of renal urate excretion at low doses and enhanced urate excretion at high doses. Bleeding time is prolonged. Common adverse effects include abdominal pain, nausea, and vomiting. Gastric hemorrhage is a possibility. Other toxic effects include tinnitus, respiratory alkalosis, metabolic acidosis, and hepatotoxicity. Angioneurotic edema, urticaria, bronchospasm, and hypotension can occur in sensitive individuals. (Other NSAID can also produce this syndrome.)

Acetaminophen is an effective analgesic-antipyretic but has only weak anti-antiflammatory activity. It is only a weak inhibitor of prostaglandin biosynthesis. The drug is rapidly absorbed and has a half-life of 1 to 4 hours. Hepatic metabolism is responsible for elimination. High doses can produce serious hepatotoxicity due to formation of reactive metabolites leading to liver necrosis. A plasma half-life greater than 4 hours and a serum value greater than 300 μg/ml at 4 hours after ingestion are associated with extensive hepatic damage. N-acetylcysteine may be effective in reducing the hepatic necrosis.

A great number of NSAIDs are available for use in the United States. Some of these include *ibuprofen, naproxen, sulindac, piroxicam, fenoprofen, tolmetin, meclofenamate, indomethacin, phenylbutazone,* and *diflunisal.* These NSAIDs are structurally different but possess similar pharmacologic properties to aspirin and all inhibit prostaglandin synthesis. Gastrointestinal intolerance is the most common adverse effect despite claims they are better tolerated than aspirin. They do cause less microbleeding from the gut than aspirin. These drugs approach aspirin in effectiveness but none is superior. Considerable interest and debate has recently developed concerning the potential of these drugs to produce serious hepatic and renal toxicity. Indomethacin is not suitable for chronic administration due to a high incidence of gastrointestinal complaints including bleeding and CNS effects characterized by frontal headache, dizziness, and confusion. Phenylbutazone is also poorly tolerated and can cause agranulocytosis and significant edema due to sodium retention.

Gold salts such as gold sodium thiomalate can suppress experimental arthritis. Although the anti-inflammatory action of these salts is not well understood, they have been found to inhibit lysosomal enzymes of leukocytes, decrease rheumatoid factor, impair mitogen-induced proliferation of lymphocytes, and to suppress cellular immunity. Gold is given by intramuscular injection and the pharmacokinetics are complex. The half-life is about 1 week after an initial dose and can be weeks or months after prolonged therapy. The excretion is 40 to 60 percent renal and 10 to 40 percent by biliary excretion. Skin and mucous membrane lesions are common. Serious blood dyscrasia and nephrotoxicity can develop. Gold salts are used in the treatment of severe rheumatoid arthritis.

Penicillamine has been effective in some patients with severe rheumatoid arthritis. This action does not appear related to the metal chelating properties of this drug. Adverse reactions include skin rash, leukopenia, thrombocytopenia, anorexia, vomiting, and nephrotoxicity.

Chloroquine and hydroxychloroquine possess anti-inflammatory properties that make them useful for the treatment of rheumatoid arthritis and discoid lupus erythematosis. Long-term therapy can produce retinopathy characterized by loss of central visual acuity which may be irreversible.

Colchicine is effective in the treatment of gout. It reduces inflammation either by inhibiting leukocyte microtubule formation from tubulin or by preventing the leukocyte production of crystal-induced chemotactic factor. The drug is useful for the acute attack of gout and for prophylaxis. The principal toxic effects are hyperperistalsis, cramping, nausea, vomiting, and diarrhea.

Allopurinol is useful for the therapy of the primary hyperuricemia of gout and that secondary to hematological disorders or antineoplastic therapy. Both allpurinol and its metabolite oxypurinol are inhibitors of xanthine oxidase which forms uric acid from hypoxanthine and xanthine.

Allopurinol is well-absorbed. It is rapidly metabolized to oxypurinol which has a long half-life. A maculopapular rash occurs in 3 percent of patients. Occasionally serious hepatic reactions occur. Allopurinol inhibits the metabolism of 6-mercaptopurine and azathioprine and other drugs, such as dicoumerol.

Probenecid inhibits the reabsorption of uric acid in the proximal tubule of the nephron. Probenecid is rapidly absorbed, is 90 to 95 percent bound to plasma proteins, has a half-life of 4 to 12 hours, and is largely eliminated via hepatic metabolism and to a lesser extent via renal excretion. Probenecid inhibits the tubular secretion of many drugs including penicillins and cephalosporins. Toxicity includes gastrointestinal symptoms and skin rash.

Narcotic Agonists and Antagonists

The opioids are used as analgesics and for the induction and maintenance of anesthesia. They interact with a variety of closely related opiate receptors to mediate their effects. They share the properties of certain endogenous peptides that are important neurotransmitters which act on opiate receptors. These peptides include the pentapeptides met-enkephalin and leu-enkephalin. The

31 amino acid peptide β-endophin is a potent opiate agonist. Both spinal and supraspinal sites of action are involved in the production of opiate analgesia. The main pharmacological effects of narcotic drugs include analgesia, respiratory depression, nausea, vomiting, cough suppression, vasodilation, constipation, miosis, and biliary smooth muscle contraction. The most commonly used potent narcotics are morphine, hydromorphine, and methadone. Intermediate potency drugs include meperidine (demerol), oxycodone, and pentazocine. Codeine has weak analgesic activity compared to the other opiate agonists.

With most opioids, including morphine, the effect of a given dose is less after oral than after parenteral administration, due to significant first-pass metabolism in the liver. The half-life of morphine is 2 to 3 hours and the major metabolic pathway is glucuronidation in the liver. Meperidine has a half-life of about 3 hours and is metabolized chiefly in the liver. Methadone because of a long half-life (15 hours) and reasonable oral bioavailability can achieve pain control on a twice daily regimen following oral administration. Codeine is also well-absorbed orally.

The development of tolerance and physical dependent with repeated use is a characteristic feature of all opioid drugs.

Propoxyphene is an analgesic drug that acts by binding to opiate receptors in the brain. Propoxyphene is effective for the relief of mild to moderate pain but is no more effective than usual doses of aspirin, acetaminophen, or codeine. Evidence is conflicting as to whether there is an additive effect with aspirin or acetaminophen. Propoxyphene is well-absorbed, has a half-life of 12 hours, is eliminated by hepatic metabolism, and extensive first-pass metabolism is noted. Habituation and rarely addiction can occur. Overdosage causes seizures, coma, respiratory depression. Pulmonary edema, cardiac arrhythmias, and hypotension have been reported.

Naloxone is an opioid competitive antagonist that acts at the opioid receptor which mediates supraspinal analgesia, respiratory depression, euphoria, and physical dependence. It has no agonist activity. Nalorphine also prevents or abolishes opiate-induced CNS effects. It does have weak agonistic properties. These drugs are used to treat opioid-induced respiratory depression and in the diagnosis of physical dependence on opioids.

Anticonvulsant Drugs

Phenytoin reduces the development of maximal seizure activity and inhibits the spread of the seizure process from an active focus. Phenytoin is useful in most forms of epilepsy except absence seizures. It has also been used to treat trigeminal and related neuralgias and ventricular arrhythmias.

Absorption of phenytoin after oral ingestion can be slow, variable, and incomplete. Peak plasma levels occur 2 to 12 hours after administration. Phenytoin should not be given by intramuscular injection since it precipitates in muscle. Phenytoin can be given intravenously but only in saline or lactated Ringers solution since the drug precipitates in dextrose solutions. Phenytoin is highly bound to plasma proteins. In uremia the free fraction is increased 2 to 3 fold. Phenytoin is eliminated via biotransformation to hydroxylated inactive metabolites. This process is saturable at therapeutic plasma levels (10 to 20 μg/ml). As a consequence there is a disproportionate increase in plasma levels relative to dose increases.

Adverse effects include nystagmus, ataxia, diplopia, confusion, and drowsiness. Other side-effects include gingival hyperplasia, hirsutism, nausea, osteomalacia, rash, leukopenia, megaloblastic anemia, and lymphadenopathy.

Phenobarbital limits the spread of seizure activity and elevates seizure threshold.

Oral absorption of phenobarbital is complete but slow. Plasma protein binding is 40 to 60 percent. Elimination is primarily by hepatic metabolism (75 percent) and by pH-dependent renal excretion (25 percent). The half-life is 90 hours. Plasma concentrations of 15 to 40 μg/ml are usually therapeutic.

Major adverse effects include sedation, nystagmus, and ataxia. Other side-effects include rash, megaloblastic anemia, osteomalacia, and precipitation of acute porphyria. Hemorrhage in neonates of phenobarbital-treated mothers has occurred. Phenobarbital induces the metabolism of many drugs including warfarin, phenytoin, hydrocortisone, prednisone, and phenobarbital itself.

Carbamazepine limits seizure propagation. It is useful in treating temporal lobe and grand mal epilepsy. It has some success in the treatment of trigeminal neuralgia and lightening tabetic pains.

Carbamazepine is well-absorbed after oral administration. Peak levels occur in 2 to 6 hours and plasma protein binding is 80 percent. Carbamazepine is eliminated via hepatic metabolism. The 10,11-epoxide metabolite is active as an anticonvulsant. The half-life of carbamazepine is 13 to 20 hours and the drug induces its own metabolism. Therapeutic serum levels range from 5 to 12 μg/ml.

Toxicity include diplopia, drowsiness, ataxia, nausea, vomiting, and skin rash. The most serious toxicity includes leukopenia, thrombocytopenia, and anemia. Acute oliguria with hypertension, thrombophlebitis, left ventricular failure, and cardiovascular collapse has been described as has cholestatic jaundice.

Primidone is effective for treatment of all types of epilepsy except absence seizures. It resembles phenobarbital in its actions. Primidone is well-absorbed orally. The half-life is 8 hours and elimination is 60 percent via hepatic metabolism. Two active metabolites, phenobarbital and phenylethylmalonamide, are formed. Therapeutic levels are 5 to 15 μg/ml for parent compound and 15 to 40 μg/ml for phenobarbital.

Adverse effects include sedation, vertigo, ataxia, nystagmus, and nausea. Serious reactions include leukopenia, thrombocytopenia, lupus erythematosis, lymphadenopathy, hemorrhagic disease in the neonate, megaloblastic anemia, and osteomalacia.

Valproic acid may act by increasing γ-aminobutyric acid (GABA) in the brain by inhibiting neuronal re-uptake and by inhibition of GABA breakdown. Valproic acid is particularly effective in absence seizures. The drug has also been shown to be effective in a variety of other types of epilepsy including myotonic and grand mal seizures.

Valproic acid is rapidly absorbed following oral administration. Peak blood levels occur within 1 to 4 hours and plasma protein binding ranges from 80 to 95 percent. Hepatic metabolism accounts for elimination and the half-life is 15 hours. Therapeutic levels range from 10 to 100 μg/ml. The most common adverse effects are anorexia, nausea, and vomiting. Several deaths from hepatic failure have been associated with valproate therapy. Valproic acid inhibits phenobarbital metabolism. A decrease in total serum phenytoin levels may occur and phenobarbital and phenytoin induce valproic acid metabolism.

Ethosuximide is probably the drug of choice for absence seizures. Peak blood levels occur 1 to 7 hours after dosing. It is not bound to plasma proteins and is primarily eliminated by hepatic metabolism. The half-life is 30 hours in children and about 60 hours in adults. Therapeutic levels vary from 40 to 100 μg/ml. The most common side-effects are gastrointestinal (nausea, vomiting, and anorexia) and CNS effects (drowsiness, dizziness, headache). Bone marrow depression is a serious but uncommon adverse reaction.

Anti-Parkinsonian Drugs

Dopamine is formed from levodopa by L-amino acid decarboxylase. Pyridoxine is a cofactor for this reaction. Parkinsonism appears to results from a deficiency of striatal dopamine. Studies indicate that the dopamine forming and storage capacity of nerve terminals of the nigrostriatal fibers is not completely lost in parkinsonism. Thus, the striatal concentrations of dopamine are enhanced when levodopa is administered. Bradykinesia and rigidity responds better than does tremor. About 95 percent of oval levodopa is decarboxylated in the periphery to dopamine and large doses are required to significantly increase the brain concentrations of dopamine.

Levodopa is absorbed from the small bowel by a transport system for aromatic amino acids. Enzymes in the gastric mucosa can degrade the drug. The plasma half-life is 1 to 3 hours. The principal metabolites are derived from dopamine and include 3,4-dihydroxyphenylacetic acid (DOPAC) and 3-methoxy-4-hydroxy-phenylacetic acid (HVA).

Common early adverse effects include nausea and vomiting, orthostatic hypotension (mechanism poorly understood), and cardiac arrhythmias. Serious long-term effects include involuntary movements such as tics, grimacing, bobbing, and various oscillatory movements. Behavioral disturbances such as confusion, delerium, paranoia, mania, hallucinations, sexual arousal, and depression can occur especially in older patients.

Carbidopa is an inhibitor of L-amino acid decarboxylase. The advantages of combining levodopa with carbidopa are the following: the dose of levodopa can be reduced by 75 percent and a larger portion of levodopa enters the brain; nausea and vomiting is reduced; pyridoxine antagonism is avoided; and cardiovascular effects are greatly reduced.

Bromocriptine is a dopamine agonist and its neuroendocrine effects include inhibition of prolactin secretion. It transiently increases blood levels of growth hormone in normal subjects but reduces it in patients with acromegaly. Bromocriptine is useful for treatment of amenorrhea/galactorrhea associated with hyperprolactinemia not associated with pituitary tumors. It can prevent physiological lactation and has been found useful in the management of Parkinson's disease. Side-effects include drowsiness, dizziness, faintness, and hypotension.

The deficiency of dopamine in the striatum of patients with parkinsonism enhances the excitatory effects of the cholinergic system within the striatum. Anticholinergics blunt this component of the nigrostriatal pathway. Trihexyphenidol is the prototype of this group of drugs. Other drugs include benztropine, procyclidine, and biperiden. These drugs are more effective in relieving tremor than rigidity and bradykinesia. The peripheral anticholinergic effects are less than those seen with atropine although they can occur especially in aged patients. CNS side-effects include confusion, drowsiness, delerium, and hallucinations.

Benzodiazepines

Benzodiazepines reduce anxiety, produce sedation and sleep, have anticonvulsant effects, and cause muscle relaxation. These drugs bind with high affinity to a receptor in the CNS which is concentrated at synaptoso-

mal membranes. Binding to this receptor potentiates the inhibitory actions of the neurotransmitter γ-aminobutyric acid (GABA). It has been suggested that the benzodiazepine and GABA receptors are coupled and that together they modulate Cl^- conduction across neuronal membranes. Benzodiazepine binding to the above receptor is best correlated to the anxiolytic and anticonvulsant effects. It is possible that different benzodiazepine receptors mediate the sedative and muscle relaxant effects.

Benzodiazepines are well-absorbed from the gastrointestinal tract with peak levels occurring in 30 to 90 minutes. Only lorazepam is effectively absorbed following intramuscular injection. The benzodiazepines can be divided into two categories. The first includes those having a long duration of action due to slow elimination of parent compound and/or active metabolites. These benzodiazepines include diazepam, chlordiazepoxide, chlorazepate, prazepam, and flurazepam. The half-lives of parent compounds vary from 15 to 70 hours. A key active metabolite formed from several benzodiazepines is N-desmethyl diazepam which has a half-life of 50 to 100 hours. This metabolite is formed from diazepam, chlorazepate, prazepam, and to some extent chlordiazepoxide. Chlorazepate and prazepam are "pro" drugs in that chlorazepate is rapidly converted to desmethyldiazepam in the stomach and prazepam in the liver. Multiple dose therapy with these drugs takes several days to reach steady state levels of parent drug and metabolite(s). Intermediate and short-acting benzodiazepines include *lorazepam* (half-life 10 to 20 hours), oxazepam (half-life 5 to 10 hours), *halazepam* (half-life 14 hours), alprazalam (half-life 12 to 15 hours), temazepam (half-life 9 to 12 hours), and triazolam (half-life 2 to 3 hours). These drugs do not accumulate to a great extent and are appropriate to allay acute, short-lived anxieties and for use as hypnotics. Some studies suggest that several weeks of night use of rapidly eliminated benzodiazepine hypnotics may lead to increased wakefulness during the last third of the night and increased signs of day-time anxiety. Drug discontinuance may result in "rebound" insomnia.

Benzodiazepines are effective treatment for anxiety, insomnia, muscle spasm, alcohol withdrawal, and seizures. They are also used to produce sedation and anterograde amnesia for cardioversion, endoscopy, and induction of anesthesia. Because of profound sedation at anticonvulsant doses, benzodiazepines are only useful in the acute treatment of seizures. Clonazepam has been used to treat absence, akinetic, and myoclonic seizures.

Tolerance to the long-term administration of benzodiazepines rarely occurs in clinical practice. The incidence of benzodiazepine dependence is probably present in a small minority of patients receiving these drugs. The withdrawal syndrome following discontinuation of drug includes insomnia, agitation, anxiety, tachycardia, diaphoresis, anorexia, and nausea. Hallucinations, psychosis, and seizures may occur but are rare. Greater dependence potential may be associated with short-acting benzodiazepines. Other factors implicated include prolonged usage at high doses.

The most common adverse reactions to benzodiazepines are somnolence, increased appetite, fatigue, and weakness. Ataxia and nystagmus can occur. Elderly patients are more sensitive to these drugs and eliminate the desmethyldiazepam metabolite less rapidly than younger patients. Cimetidine may inhibit the metabolism of diazepam and chlordiazepoxide.

Antidepressants

The tricyclic antidepressants are effective in the treatment of endogenous depression and probably effective in the treatment of reactive or neurotic depression. They may have some value for treatment of phobias and chronic pain syndromes such as neuralgias and migraine. Imipramine has been used to treat enuresis in children over 6 years of age.

The tricyclic agents include the tertiary amines imipramine, amitriptyline, doxepin, and the secondary amines desipramine, nortriptyline, and protriptyline. Amoxapine is a more recently available tricyclic. Maprotiline is a tetracylic antidepressant and trazodone is unrelated chemically to tri- and tetracyclic antidepressants.

Tricyclic antidepressants have antihistamine and anticholinergic actions, and the ability to block presynaptic neuronal uptake of norepinephrine and serotonin. The tertiary tricyclic amines are more potent inhibitors of serotonin uptake whereas the secondary amines are more potent inhibitors of norepinephrine uptake. Trazodone inhibits serotonin uptake and maprotiline exclusively inhibits norepinephrine re-uptake. Amoxapine inhibits both the re-uptake of serotonin and norepinephrine and may also block dopamine receptors. The effect of antidepressants on neuronal amine uptake is thought to be the pharmacologic basis of their efficacy.

The tricyclic antidepressants are well-absorbed orally, are highly protein-bound, and have a wide tissue disbribution. Tricyclics are metabolized in the liver by ring hydroxylation and subsequent glucuronidation and by demethylation. Monodemethylation of a tertiary amine forms a pharmacologically active secondary amine (e.g., amitriptyline to nortriptyline). Imipramine has a half-life of 10 to 20 hours and protriptyline 80 hours. The other agents have intermediate values. Amoxapine has a half-life of about 8 hours. Maprotiline is slowly but completely absorbed with a half-life of about 48 hours. Tra-

zodone is well-absorbed, metabolized in the liver, and has a half-life of 6 to 9 hours.

Adverse effects are common and include sedation, weakness, muscle tremors, fatigue, anticholinergic effects, and orthostatic hypotension. EKG changes include T wave flattening and inversion, and prolonged QRS, Q-T, and P-R intervals. Overdosage results in neuromuscular irritability, delerium, hyperpyrexia, hypotension or hypertension, and bowel and bladder paralysis. Cardiotoxicity with arrhythmias, conduction abnormalities, and depressed contractility can be serious. Amoxapine and maprotiline may have less anticholinergic effects. Trazodone has no anticholinergic effects. Trazodone and doxepine may have less cardiotoxicity.

Tricyclic antidepressants inhibit the antihypertensive effect of guanethidine, methyldopa, and clonidine. Since monoamine oxidase inhibitors prevent degradation of amines tricyclics should not be given for 2 to 3 weeks after a monoamine oxidase inhibitor. Alcohol and benzodiazepines enhance the motor impairment and sedative properties of tricyclics.

Monoamide oxidase inhibitors (MAO) block oxidative deamination of monoamines. These drugs are used when tricyclic antidepressants are ineffective. Certain neurotic illnesses with depressive features and some phobias may respond. These drugs include tranylcypramine, phenelezine, and isocarboxazid. The potential for toxicity is great with these agents. The most serious reactions are orthostatic hypotension, agitation, hallucinations, seizures, and hepatotoxicity. Because of their interference with various enzymes the MAO inhibitors alter the actions of numerous other drugs. They prolong and intensify the action of central depressant agents such as sedatives, anticholinergic agents, and tricyclic antidepressants. Hyperpyrexia can be induced with meperidine. Hypertensive crisis can be precipitated if patients consume food rich in tyramine. The tyramine releases large amounts of endogenous catecholamines since the breakdown of tyramine is inhibited by the MAO inhibitor.

Lithium carbonate is effective in the treatment of acute mania and in the prophylaxis of cyclic manias. Lithium's onset of action is slow in mania and concomitant initial therapy with a major tranquilizer may be required.

Lithium absorption from the gastrointestinal tract is complete and not impaired by food. Lithium is excreted by renal elimination and its half-life is about 24 hours. Lithium plasma levels should be drawn in the morning 12 hours after the evening dose. Therapeutic levels range from 0.9 to 1.4 mEq/l. Toxicity appears at plasma levels greater than 1.5 mEq/l. Adverse reactions include tremor, polyuria, mild thirst, and nausea. More serious toxicity includes ataxia, confusion, hypothyroidism, cardiotoxicity, and kidney damage, including diabetes insipidus. Sodium restriction, dehydration, renal failure, and diuretic therapy may elevate lithium plasma levels.

Antipsychotic Agents

These drugs have been shown to be effective in the treatment of schizophrenia, organic psychoses, and the manic phase of manic-depressive illness. In addition, they have sedative and anxiolytic actions. It has been suggested that their antipsychotic effects are mediated via antagonism of dopamine receptors in the limbic, mesocortical, and hypothalamic systems. The extrapyramidal effects are thought to be due to antagonism of dopamine in the basal ganglia. Several of these drugs have anti-nausea and anti-vomiting activity mediated by anti-dopamine actions at the chemoreceptor trigger zone. Other actions include anticholinergic and adrenergic blocking effects.

These drugs are well-absorbed following oral administration although erratic patterns of absorption have been noted. They are lipophilic, have large distribution volumes, are highly bound to plasma proteins, and are eliminated by hepatic metabolism including oxidation and glucuronidation. In some cases metabolites are active. The usually stated half-lives vary from 10 to 20 hours although a long terminal phase of elimination exists (half-life > 60 days). The biological effects last about 24 hours.

Adverse effects include orthostatic hypotension, with extrapyramidal symptoms including dyskinesia, parkinsonism, and akathisia. The most important side-effect is tardive dyskinesia. This syndrome consists of involuntary buccal, facial, and mandibular movements, such as sucking or smacking of the lips. This abnormality develops after prolonged therapy and may not become apparent until therapy is discontinued. Other effects include electrocardiographic changes characterized by prolongation of Q-T and P-R intervals, T wave blunting, and S-T segment depression. Anticholinergic effects include dry mouth, blurred vision, constipation, and urinary retention. Endocrine abnormalities include weight gain, gynecomastia, lactation, oligomenorrhea, and glucose intolerance. These abnormalities are thought to be due to either increased release of prolactin or decreased release of insulin or gonadotropic hormones. Bluish skin pigmentation and lens deposits have been noted. Skin rash including photosensitivity reactions are common. Rarely cholestatic jaundice and agranulocytosis develop. These drugs can potentiate the actions of sedatives and analgesics including alcohol.

The antipsychotic drugs share many pharmacological effects and therapeutic applications. However, differences in side-effect profiles are noted. Thus low-potency drugs such as chlorpromazine, triflupromazine, and thioridazine have greater sedative and hypotensive effects. High-potency drugs such as haloperidol, fluphenazine, and trifluoperazine have less sedative, hypotensive, and anticholinergic effects. However, the extrapyramidal effects may be pronounced. Loxapine and molindone may have less hypotensive, sedative, and extrapyramidal effects than many of the other drugs.

Endocrine Pharmacology

ANTITHYROID DRUGS

Thionamides comprise the group of commonly used antithyroid drugs. These drugs include propylthiouracil, methimazole, and carbimazole. These drugs inhibit the incorporation of iodine into tyroxyl residues of thyroglobulin and they inhibit the coupling of these iodotyroxyl residues to form iodothyronines. These are both peroxidase-dependent reactions.

These drugs are well-absorbed orally. Propylthiouracil has a half-life of 2 hours and methimazole 6 hours. Carbimazole is converted completely to methimazole.

Adverse reactions include skin rash, hypothyroidism, cholestatic jaundice, lupus-like syndromes, and rarely agranulocytosis.

GLUCOCORTICOIDS

Glucocorticoids enter target cells by diffusion, and combine with cytosolic receptors. The complex is transferred to a specific acceptor site on chromatin in the nucleus leading to an increase in RNA and protein synthesis. The physiological actions of the glucocorticoids are predominantly anti-insulin. They increase hepatic glycogen content and promote heart gluconeogenesis. These actions result from the mobilization of glycogenic amino acids from tissues such as bone, skin, muscle, and connective tissue due to protein breakdown as well as inhibition of protein synthesis and amino acid uptake. Glucocorticoid-induced hyperaminoacidemia stimulates glucagon secretion. Pharmacological doses of glucocorticoids produce hyperglycemia and glucosuria. Glucocorticoids enhance activation of cellular lipase by lipid-mobilizing hormones (e.g., catecholamines). Large doses lead to an alteration in fat distribution with deposition of fat in the back of the neck, supraclavicular area, face, and a loss of fat from the extremities. Glucocorticoids inhibit nucleic acid synthesis in most tissues but increase liver RNA synthesis. Glucocorticoids increase the number of polymorphonuclear leukocytes in the blood while the number of lymphocytes decrease, particularly those derived from the thymus. Cortisol suppresses the secretion of antidiuretic hormone, enhances glomerular filtration rate, and reduces water uptake by cells. Glucocorticoids suppress all facets of inflammation. Pharmacological doses retard growth in children.

Toxicity from glucocorticoids include increased susceptibility to infection, possibly peptic ulceration, myopathy, behavioral changes, cataracts, osteoporosis, osteomalacia, glucose intolerance, and hypertension. Acute adrenal insufficiency results from rapid withdrawal of corticosteroids after prolonged therapy.

The glucocorticoids are divided into three groups according to the duration of biologic activity. Short-acting preparations have a biologic half-life less than 12 hours and include cortisol and cortisone. Intermediate preparations have a half-life between 12 and 36 hours and include prednisone, prednisolone, methyl prednisolone, and triamcinolone. Long-acting preparations have a half-life greater than 48 hours and include betamethasone and dexamethasone.

MINERALOCORTICOIDS

Minealocorticoids act on the distal tubules of the nephron to enhance the reabsorption of sodium ions and to promote excretion of potassium and hydrogen ions. They also affect ion transport in other tissues (salivary, sweat, exocrine, pancreas, intestine) in a fashion similar to that noted in the nephron. Aldosterone is the most potent mineralocorticoid and is the hormone of physiological significance.

ORAL HYPOGLYCEMIC AGENTS

The commercially available sulfonylureas are tolbutamide, acetohexamide, tolazamide, and chlorpropamide. They lower blood sugar primarily by stimulating the pancreas to secrete insulin. Peripheral tissues develop an increased sensitivity to insulin possibly due to an increase in the number of insulin receptors.

The sulfonylureas are readily absorbed from the gut. Tolbutamide is carboxylated in the liver. Its half-life is about 6 hours. Acetohexamide is converted in the liver to hydroxyacetamide, an active metabolite. The half-life of the parent compound is 1.5 hours and the metabolite 6 hours. Tolazamide is slowly absorbed with onset of activity at 4 to 6 hours. It is metabolized to a number of active metabolites in the liver. Chlorpropamide is excreted unchanged in the urine with a half-life of 36 hours.

Adverse effects include myelosuppression, rash, photosensitivity, cholestatic jaundice, disulfiram-like reaction, and severe hypoglycemia. Chlorpropamide may impair free water clearance. Fears that sulfonylureas might increase deaths from heart attacks, prompted by reports of the University Group Diabetes Program, have largely dissipated because of questions about the design of that study. Noninsulin-dependent diabetes that cannot be controlled by dietary management often responds to sulfonylureas. However, patients with signficant hyperglycemia improve but do not approach normality. As a result a higher percentage of these patients are being treated with insulin since more rigorous control may delay the development of diabetic complications.

Miscellaneous Agents

Theophylline is effective for the treatment of bronchospastic disorders and respiratory apnea in neonates. Theophylline relaxes bronchial and various other smooth muscle cells. The effect on the circulation is complex and includes the net result of direct chronotropic and ionotropic actions, stimulation of central vagal nuclei, peripheral vasodilation, and release of catecholamines. Tachycardia, increased cardiac output, and cardiac arrhythmias can be observed. The cerebral circulation is constricted. Theophylline stimulates the CNS, including the respiratory center. It induces a diuresis secondary to inhibition of sodium reabsorption in the kidney. It is known that the drug inhibits phosphodiesterase which leads to intracellular accumulation of CAMP and it is a potent antagonist of adenosine receptors. It also affects translations of intracellular calcium. To what extent these actions contribute to the different effects observed is not known.

Theophylline is well-absorbed orally. It is 15 percent protein bound. The half-life of elimination varies from 3 to 10 hours. Hepatic metabolism is responsible for elimination. Patients with hepatic disease and heart failure require a reduction in dose. Smoking enhances theophylline metabolism and macrolide antibiotics such as erythromycin inhibit its metabolism. Therapeutic plasma levels range from 5 to 20 μg/ml. Adverse effects include nausea, vomiting, diarrhea, and headache. Serious toxicity includes focal and generalized seizures and cardiac arrhythmias. The latter may be enhanced by simultaneous administration of sympathomimetic drugs.

Cromolyn sodium is of value for the treatment of chronic asthma. Cromolyn blocks the release of chemical mediators (histamine, serotonin, leukotrienes) by acting on the mast cell membrane to prevent the effects of antigen-antibody (IgE) reactions that would release these mediators. It may do this by preventing calcium influx into the cells which is required for mediator release. It also blocks the release of mediators in response to nonimmunological stimuli such as exercise. It is of no value for the acute asthmatic attack but is effective when used in a prophylactic fashion. Cromolyn is administered as a powder by inhalation. Throat irritation, hoarseness, acute cough, and chest tightness are minor adverse effects.

Cimetidine is a competitive inhibitor of histamine (H_2) receptors. This action reduces gastric acid secretion induced by histamine, acetylcholine, and gastrin. Clinical application of this drug centers on its capacity to inhibit gastric acid secretion in hypersecretory states.

Food delays absorption and reduces peak levels but does not reduce the amount absorbed. About 20 percent is protein-bound and 70 percent is eliminated via the kidney and the remainder by hepatic metabolism. The half-life is 2 hours, which is prolonged to 5 hours with severe renal disease.

Adverse effects include nausea, diarrhea, and skin rash. Cimetidine can cause mental confusion and coma. Patients with renal disease and the elderly are more susceptible to this reaction. Myelosuppression has been reported. High doses produce a weak antiandrogen effect with gynecomastia and reduced sperm counts in men. Cimetidine inhibits the metabolism of a wide variety of drugs such as warfarin, diazepam, and theophylline, leading to clinically significant drug interactions.

Histamine occurs in mast cells and basophils. It stimulates gastric secretion of acid and pepsin, relaxes vascular smooth muscle, contracts nonvascular smooth muscle, and increases capillary permeability. These effects result in flushing, headache, hypotension, wheals, sympathoadrenal activation, bronchiolar constriction, increased intestinal motility, and increased salivation. Increased capillary permeability, contraction of nonvascular smooth muscle, and vasodilation are mediated by H_1 receptors. They are blocked by diphenhydramine, tripelenamine, promethazine, chlorpheniramine, and hydroxyzine. Gastric acid secretion is mediated via H_2 receptors that are blocked by cimetidine, which is discussed elsewhere. Most antihistamines (H_1 blockers) possess some anticholinergic potency. The principal use of anti H_1-histamines is in the management of allergic rhinitis and conjunctivitis. The major side effects of H_1-antihistamines are sedation and dry mouth. Most antihistamines are metabolized in the liver.

REFERENCES

Gilman AG, Goodman LS, Gilman A, eds: The Pharmacological Basis of Therapeutics. 6th Ed. MacMillan Publishing Co., Inc., 1980
    Useful for in-depth discussion of selected drugs.
Goth A: Medical Pharmacology. 10th Ed. The CV Mosby Company, St. Louis, Toronto, London, 1981
    Standard text book for medical pharmacology.
Katcher BS, Young LY, Koda-Kimble MA, eds: Applied Therapeutics. 3rd Ed. Applied Therapeutics, Inc., San Francisco, Spokane, 1983
    Good discussion of drug action in relationship to the clinical setting of the drugs used.
Notari RE: Biopharmaceuticals and Clinical Pharmacokinetics. 3rd Ed. Marcel Dekker, Inc., New York, Basel, 1980
    Excellent and readable introduction to clinical pharmacokinetics.
Robertson D, Smith GR: Manual of Clinical Pharmacology, Williams and Wilkins, Baltimore, 1981
    Brief résumé of basic and applied pharmacology of most drugs in use today. Excellent for a rapid review of a drug's pharmacology.

MULTIPLE CHOICE QUESTIONS

1. The plasma concentration of phenytoin is 10 μg/ml on a dose of 300 mg daily. The dose is increased to 400 mg daily and the plasma concentration was 20 μg/ml. This observation is explained by:
   A. First-order kinetics
   B. Zero-order kinetics
   C. Change in distribution volume with dose
   D. Change in plasma protein binding
   E. Change in the biovailability of phenytoin with increased dose.

2. Factors which alter the bioavailability of drugs include:
   A. Extent of absorption from the intestine
   B. Intestinal metabolism of drugs
   C. Extensive hepatic metabolism
   D. Physical characteristics of the drug formulation
   E. All of the above

3. Which of the following drugs have been effective in the treatment of severe heart failure:
   A. Hydralazine
   B. Captopril
   C. Nitroprusside
   D. Nitroglycerin
   E. All of the above

4. Bone marrow toxicity has been caused by which of the following drugs:
   A. Chloramphenicol
   B. Carbamezepine
   C. Carmustine (BCNU)
   D. Propylthiouracil
   E. All of the above

5. Nephrotoxicity has been associated with:
   A. Gentamicin
   B. Cephaloridine
   C. Vancomycin
   D. Rifampin
   E. All of the above

6. Which of the following sequences correlates with the anti-inflammatory potency of steroid drugs.
   A. Cortisol > deoxycorticosterone > prednisone > betamethasone
   B. Dexamethaxone > prednisolone > 9-α fluorocortisol > cortisol
   C. Prednisone > cortisol > aldosterone > triamcinolone
   D. Betamethaxone > 9-α fluorocortisol > prednisone > cortisol

Match the following to the drugs below:

7. Conversion of paroxysmal atrial tachycardia (PAT) to sinus rhythm
8. Intrinsic sympathomimetic activity
9. Reduction of cardiac preload
10. Reflex increase in heart rate
11. Bronchospasm
    A. Verapamil
    B. Nitroglycerin
    C. Propranolol
    D. Pindolol
    E. Nifedipine

Match the following to the drugs below:

12. Muscarinic receptor
13. Nicotinic receptor—neuromuscular junction
14. β_1-receptor
15. Nicotinic receptor—ganglia
16. Dopamine receptor
    A. Trimethaphan
    B. Atropine
    C. Nadolol
    D. Pancuronium
    E. Haloperidol

Match the following to the drugs below:

17. β_1 receptor agonist
18. Inhibitor of dopa decarbonylase
19. α_1 receptor antagonist
20. Inhibitor of norepinephrine re-uptake
21. Tardive dyskinesia
    A. Maprotiline
    B. Prazosin
    C. Dobutamine
    D. Carbidopa
    E. Fluphenazine

Match the following to the drugs below:

22. Cell wall transpeptidase
23. Dihydrofolate reductase
24. DNA-dependent RNA polymerase
25. 50 S ribosomal subunit
26. 30 S ribosomal subunit
    A. Penicillin
    B. Amikacin
    C. Clindamycin
    D. Trimethoprim-sulfamethaxazole
    E. Rifampin

Match the characteristic adverse effects to the drugs below:

27. Dyspnea, cough, basilar rales
28. Orthopnea, edema
29. Footdrop
30. Hematuria
31. Severe nausea, vomiting, proteinuria
    A. Daunorubicin
    B. Vincristine
    C. Cyclophosphamide
    D. Bleomycin
    E. Cisplatin

Match the following to the agents below:

32. Suppression of intestinal absorption of Ca^{++}
33. Formation by renal mitochondria
34. "C" cells of the thyroid
35. Hepatic microsomes
36. Distal tubular Ca^{++} reabsorption.
    A. PTH
    B. Calcitriol
    C. Glucocorticoids
    D. Calciferol
    E. Calcitonin

Match the following to the drugs below:

37. Inhibition of Na^+ conductance
38. Depression of AV nodal conduction
39. Decrease in automaticity
    A. Lidocaine
    B. Verapamil
    C. Both
    D. Neither

Match the following to the drugs below:

40. Increased urinary Ca^{++} excretion
41. Increased urinary K^+ excretion

42. Increased urinary Na^+ excretion
   A. Furosemide
   B. Hydrochlorothiazide
   C. Both
   D. Neither

Match the following to the drugs below:

43. Effective against tinia capitis
44. Effective against systemic candidiasis
45. Effective against P carinii
   A. Amphotericin
   B. Griseofulvin
   C. Both
   D. Neither

Match the following to the drugs below:

46. Tolerance
47. Dependence
48. Respiratory depression
   A. Morphine
   B. Prazosin
   C. Both
   D. Neither

Match the following to the drugs below:

49. Effective for the treatment of schizophrenia
50. Effective for the treatment of mania
51. Effective as an hypnotic agent
   A. Lithium
   B. Lorazepam
   C. Both
   D. Neither

Each question below contains four suggested answers of which one or more is correct. Choose the answer:

   A   if 1, 2, and 3 are correct
   B   if 1 and 3 are correct
   C   if 2 and 4 are correct
   D   if 4 is correct
   E   if 1, 2, 3, and 4 are correct

52. Hepatotoxicity results from the formation of reactive metabolites with which drugs:
   1 Acetaminophen
   2. Oral contraceptives
   3. Isoniazid
   4. Tetracycline

53. Which of the following drugs are dopamine antagonists:
   1. Metoclopramide
   2. L-dopa
   3. Chlorpromazine
   4. Imipramine

54. Which of the following drugs interact with warfarin:
   1. Ibuprofen
   2. Cimetidine
   3. Phenobarbital
   4. Diazepam

55. Which of the following drugs may alter serum digoxin levels:
   1. Quinidine
   2. Verapamil
   3. Erythromycin
   4. Furosemide

56. Drugs that involve the action of the neurotransmitter GABA include:
   1. Diazepam
   2. Phenytoin
   3. Valproic acid
   4. Haloperidol

57. Inhibition of cyclo-oxygenase by NSAID would be expected to:
   1. Reduce prostacyclin formation
   2. Reduce thromboxane A_2 formation
   3. Reduce PGE_2 formation
   4. Reduce LTC_4 formation

58. Which of the following drugs inhibits the peripheral conversion of T_4 to T_3:
   1. Propylthiouracil
   2. Methinazole
   3. Propranolol
   4. Cimetidine

59. Lack of response to methotrexate might result from:
   1. Impaired transport of methotrexate into cells.
   2. Production of altered forms of dihydrofolate reductase that have decreased affinity for MTX.
   3. Increased concentrations of intracellular dihydrofolate reductase.
   4. Concurrent administration of folic acid.

Answers to Multiple Choice Questions

1 B	2 E	3 E	4 E	5 E
6 D	7 A	8 D	9 B	10 E
11 C	12 B	13 D	14 C	15 A
16 E	17 C	18 D	19 B	20 A
21 E	22 A	23 D	24 E	25 C
26 B	27 D	28 A	29 B	30 C
31 E	32 C	33 B	34 E	35 D
36 A	37 A	38 B	39 A	40 A
41 C	42 C	43 B	44 A	45 D
46 C	47 A	48 A	49 D	50 A
51 B	52 B	53 B	54 A	55 A
56 B	57 A	58 B	59 A	

8

Physiology

Lois W. Forney

PART 1 _____

Integration of Function

THE CELL

Human physiology is the study of the dynamic inter-relationships between the tissues and organ systems that make man a viable being. Life goes on at the level of the organ system, but an understanding of the basic cellular components of specialized tissues is of fundamental importance. The failure of a major system such as the respiratory, cardiovascular, or central nervous system can mean death. In a complex organism the demise of a tissue may not be life threatening, but the quality of life is compromised. The cell is the basic unit of life, the cornerstone of health.

Cells connect to form tissues by surface modifications in which cell membranes can fuse in tight junctions by intercellular bridges of fine filaments called desmosomes or by merely overlapping junctions. Each individual cell is bound by the plasma membrane, a complex lipid and protein structure, which serves as a barrier to the cell's environment, the interstitial fluid. The plasma membrane encloses the cell contents, the salts, minerals, organic molecules, and organelles, which are suspended in a gelatinous soup, the cytoplasm. The organelle substructures are also membrane bound and include the mitochondria, sites of cell respiration and energy production; the endoplasmic reticulum, site of protein synthesis; the nucleus, site of mitosis and genetic control; and the golgi apparatus, a packaging system for export of

cell products. Each membrane serves as a permeability barrier which maintains the electrochemical integrity of the organelles, just as the plasma membrane serves this function for the cell.

Membrane Architecture

The cell membrane is a mosaic of proteins and lipids, with the lipid architecture presenting an ideal barrier against an aqueous environment. The typical membrane is tripartite, a sandwich in which hydrophobic regions are on the interior and hydrophilic regions are exposed to the cytoplasm and to the extracellular medium. The major lipid component is phospholipid, with two fatty acyl chains and the phosphorylated polar head group attached to a glycerol backbone. Cholesterol molecules are found intercalated as packing between and parallel to chains of fatty acids, which arrange themselves in bilayer leaflets.

Biological membranes are symmetric. In red blood cells, for example, phosphatidylcholine and sphingomyelin are found primarily within the outside (extracellular) leaflet of the lipid bilayer, while phosphatidylethanolamine and phosphatidylserine are found primarily within the inner (cytoplasmic) leaflet. These particular phospholipids are typical membrane components.

The membrane is a fluid mosaic. Proteins and lipids can move laterally across the membrane via conformational changes. However, the cell's cytoskeleton, a scaffolding of protein attached to the cytoplasmic surface, restricts the movement of integral membrane proteins so that a flip-flop from extracellular to cytoplasmic surface is not possible. Lipid membrane components may flip-flop, but at an extremely slow rate. Additionally, proteins form microfilaments, microtubules, and intermediate filaments which insert upon the plasma membrane.

Evidence for a fluid mosaic model is obtained by freeze fracture experiments in which cleavage of frozen membranes results in fractures between lipid leaflets. The inner hydrophobic surface is studded with particles thought to be the hydrophobic regions of integral proteins.

Permeability Properties

The cell membrane is a semipermeable barrier which maintains cell homeostasis, a steady state condition where there is no net molecular movement of any consequence except for substrate entry and product exit. Water is in osmotic equilibrium, easily diffusing back and forth across the membrane. However, solutes are not free to move and the barrier maintains approximately equal but drastically different electrolyte concentrations on opposing sides of the membrane. The cell is rich in potassium, phosphates, and proteins, which are negatively charged at physiological pH. The extracellular fluid contains large amounts of sodium chloride and very little protein. Extracellular and intracellular osmolalities are balanced at about 310 mosm. Membrane channels permit the diffusion of small molecules and ions in response to concentration and electrochemical charge gradients; proteins are restrained. There is a negative potential across the plasma membrane (intracellular negative/extracellular positive) caused primarily by the tendency for K^+ to diffuse out of the cell down its concentration gradient. Na^+ diffuses into the cell but is actively pumped out by an adenosine triphosphate (ATP) driven ion pump coupled to the return of leaked K^+ to the interior of the cell (Fig. 8-1).

The Donnan Equilibrium

If two compartments, I and II, are filled with water and are separated by a membrane permeable to K^+ and Cl^-, K^+ and Cl^- will diffuse through the membrane until the concentrations are equal. However, if an impermeant charged solute (A^-) is placed into compartment I, K^+ will diffuse from II to I while Cl^- will diffuse from I to II to maintain electrical neutrality. Thereby a concentration gradient will be formed by which the concentration of K^+ on side I is greater than on side II and the concentration of Cl^- on side I is less than on side II. K^+ and Cl^- will distribute so that equilibrium exists as the following:

$$[K^+]_1[Cl^-]_1 = [K^+]_2[Cl^-]_2$$

The Donnan equilibrium operates in cells where the im-

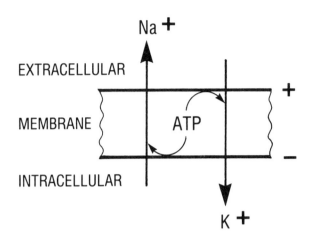

Fig. 8-1. Membrane ATP ion pump.

permeant intracellular anion is a protein and the positively charged counter ion is K^+.

The Resting Membrane Potential

The membranes of most cells are electrically charged with clouds of positive and negative ions spread over their surfaces. There is a net excess of positive charges on the outer side of the membrane and negative charges on the inner cytoplasmic side. This separation of charge gives rise to the membrane potential, mV. The most important factors in the development of a membrane potential and its magnitude are the permeabilities of the membrane to Na^+ and K^+ and the concentration gradients of these ions across the membrane. The separation of charges is maintained by ATP ion pumping and the Donnan equilibrium.

Membrane channels permit diffusion of certain small ions, notably K^+, Na^+, and Cl^-. These channels can open and close rapidly resulting in large changes in membrane potential. Hydrated Na^+ has a larger ionic radius; in resting membranes the Na^+ channel is largely closed. As a result Na^+ does not diffuse as rapidly as K^+. K^+ mobility is 100 times faster than Na^+ and the K^+ channel is open. This imbalance in charge movement causes an excess of negative charges inside the cell, an opposing force to the concentration gradient which serves as a deterent to further passage of K^+. The membrane becomes charged with a resting or steady state potential of -90 to -60 mV and acts as a capacitator with the movement of K^+ generating a potential difference across the membrane (inside negative to outside). The potential at which the force of the concentration gradient is balanced by the force of the membrane potential is called the equilibrium potential of an ion (E_K or E_{Na}). The resting potential is the value of the membrane potential that corresponds to zero net charge flux and is neither E_K nor

E_{Na}. In this steady state, ionic charges (Na^+) moving into the cell equal ionic charges (K^+) moving out of the cell.

Control of Cell Volume: Osmosis

Because of the semipermeable nature of the cell membrane, osmotic forces regulate cell volume. The cell behaves as a tiny osmometer, with water equilibrating rapidly. In a hypotonic extracellular environment, the nondiffusible cell contents attract water (water moves to dilute the higher solute concentration). Osmotic pressure is the hydrostatic pressure which must be applied to prevent the movement of solvent and is dependent on the number of dissolved particles. The osmotic effect of a molar Na^+Cl^- solution (two ions) is twice that of a non-electrolyte such as glucose which does not dissociate. The term osmolality is used to describe the osmotic effects of solute concentrations, with the term osmole (osm) replacing mole.

The response of red blood cells to osmotic pressure generated by internal impermeant molecules can be observed with the light microscope. If red cells are placed in distilled water, a hypotonic medium, water rapidly enters the cells causing them to swell and burst. In hypertonic 5 percent saline, water is pulled from the cells causing them to shrink. In 0.9 percent physiologic saline, an isotonic medium, cell volume is undisturbed.

Movement Across the Cell Membrane

Molecules get in and out of cells by simple diffusion, facilitated diffusion, and active transport.

Diffusion across the membrane barrier is governed by Fick's first law of diffusion which states that the rate of flux is directly proportional to the cross-sectional area, the permeability constant, and the concentration gradient, and that the rate of flux is inversely proportional to the membrane thickness. The membrane is highly permeable to lipid soluble molecules such as O_2, CO_2, alcohol, and fatty acids which dissolve in the membrane and diffuse freely through it. Lipophobic small molecules, such as water, diffuse through 8 Å wide membrane pores. The ability of a molecule to pass through these pores is inversely proportional to its hydrated diameter.

Facilitated diffusion requires transport proteins which are integral membrane proteins. Transport molecules share many characteristics with enzymes, due to the presence of specific binding sites, including stereospecificity, saturability, competitive inhibition, and hormonal control. Facilitated diffusion requires no metabolic energy from the cell and is able to equilibrate substrate concentrations across the membrane.

Active transport is similar to facilitated diffusion, but requires the expenditure of energy (ATP) and is capable of moving a substrate against its concentration gradient. In both facilitated diffusion and active transport a conformational change in a carrier protein is thought to be involved in translocation of the substrate.

REGULATORY MECHANISMS

The regulatory systems of the body maintain the homeostasis or steady state of blood pressure, cardiac output, and neural and other functional activities. The steady state is maintained by the input of metabolic energy and differs from the equilibrium condition in which materials are distributed so that the electrical and chemical forces are balanced and no energy is expended. In the steady state, energy is expended to maintain gradients of ions across the membrane in which energy that can be used for generation of electrical potentials is stored.

Chemical Messengers

In a complex organism, systems must respond to outside stimuli quickly, and internal regulation must be precise. Homeostatic control occurs at the cellular level with the response synchronized and amplified to tissues and organs. Chemicals are used as messengers in the body by the central nervous system and the endocrine system. Many of these messengers are impermeable to the cell and response involves binding to membrane proteins known as receptors.

The nervous system employs anatomical connections, known as synapses, between axons and the effector cells. Messages are relayed via the spinal cord to the brain which functions as a computer bank to analyze and integrate external and internal stimuli for the appropriate response. Regulation of internal organs and of the blood pressure occurs by means of a system of autonomic ganglia which is partially independent of central control. Neurotransmitters are chemical messengers elaborated by the nervous system. Some neurotransmitters are hormonal in nature.

HORMONES

The endocrine system releases chemical messengers called hormones directly into the systemic circulation where they affect target tissues, frequently at distant sites. Insulin, a prime regulator of carbohydrate metabolism, is a polypeptide hormone produced in the islet cells of the pancreas in response to rising blood sugar levels. Insulin lowers blood sugar to maintain steady state levels by accelerating glucose transport into muscle and adipose tissue cells.

Functional overlaps of chemical messengers occur.

For example, norepinephrine and oxytocin act as both neurotransmitters and hormones. Structurally similar hormones may have different actions. Oxytocin causes uterine contractions and milk ejection, while vapopressin causes arteriolar constriction and water absorption in the kidney. In some instances, the same messenger may have varied functions. Somatostatin differs in action depending on the site of release. When released from the hypothalamus into the anterior pituitary, it suppresses growth hormone secretion. The production of the hormone in pancreatic D cells suppresses the release of insulin and glucagon.

The Role of the Target Cell in Regulation

Intercellular regulators include membrane impermeable neurotransmitters and peptide hormones which bind to receptors on the surface of the cell to modify intracellular adenosine $3':5' =$ cyclic phosphate (cAMP) or Ca^{++} levels, which are important to a large number of physiologic processes within the cell. While over long periods of time both the hormone and the receptor can be internalized in the cell, the most important factor in regulation is the binding of the hormone to the receptor. Steroid hormones pass readily through the cell membrane, bind to receptors in the cell cytosol, and are transferred to the nucleus to affect gene expression.

Peptide hormones exert their effects by changing the levels of cAMP or Ca^{++} in the cell. The hormone binds to a membrane receptor that penetrates through to a nucleotide binding protein which exists in stimulatory and inhibitory forms which are dependent on the binding of guanosine triphosphate (GTP). If GTP is bound to the activating nucleotide along with the receptor-hormone complex, adenylate cyclase is activated and cAMP is produced. However, if the inhibitory nucleotide is involved, adenylate cyclase is inactivated and no cAMP is produced.

Catecholamines act in the same manner. For example, epinephrine elevates the blood sugar in times of stress by influencing phosphorylase, the regulatory enzyme in the breakdown of liver glycogen stores, via cAMP.

Cyclic AMP appears to be an almost universal second messenger which effects metabolic control by stimulating (or inhibiting) regulatory enzymes in a cascade response to the primary chemical message.

Intracellular regulators include steroids, cAMP, and Ca^{++} which function directly within the cell. Steroids are lipid soluble cholesterol derivatives which are carried in the blood by specific proteins. They dissolve in the cell membrane and move into the cell to function. Steroids regulate by modifying the forms and amount of enzymes produced by the cell. The steroid penetrates the membrane, binds to a receptor inside the cell, and moves to the nucleus, where it changes DNA transcription and results in different types and/or amounts of mRNA coding for enzyme protein.

Catecholamines also act to regulate physiologic processes such as glycogen metabolism in the liver and the breakdown of triglycerides in adipose tissue. Two nucleotide binding receptor proteins in the cell membrane bind catecholamines to modulate adenylate cyclase activity in the production of cAMP. β receptors are stimulatory; α receptors are inhibitory. cAMP production influences the phosphorylation of certain enzymes to catalyze a physiologic response. This action involves a cascade effect in which cAMP binds to a regulatory subunit of a protein kinase causing the release of the catalytic subunits.

Some cells, such as fat cells, have both stimulatory and inhibitory receptors so that the relative amounts of hormone bound to each receptor will regulate how much cAMP is produced by the cell. The release of catecholamines by the adrenal medulla can be regulated by a feedback system sensitive to inhibitory receptors.

The Role of Ca^{++} as a Regulator

Most of the intracellular calcium is sequestered in the endoplasmic reticulum or in the mitochondria, with the free Ca^{++} level as only about 0.1 μm in the cell. Certain stimuli influence the liberation of bound intracellular Ca^{++} or accelerate movement of Ca^{++} into the cell to raise free Ca^{++} levels. Free Ca^{++} can bind to calmodulin, a Ca^{++} dependent regulatory protein present in the cytoplasm. Protein kinases, stimulated by Ca^{++} in the presence of calmodulin, phosphorylate specific enzymes to alter activity. For example, the Ca^{++}-calmodulin complex activates phosphorylase kinase and regulates adenylate cyclase and phosphodiesterase which are involved with cAMP formation and degradation. Ca^{++} plays a role in regulating blood pressure in a cascade effect involving adrenergic receptors which activate a kinase that controls the contraction of smooth muscle cells of arterioles. In muscle contraction, for example, Ca^{++} binds to troponin, a Ca^{++} binding protein that is closely related to calmodulin.

THE COMMUNICATIONS NETWORK: NEURAL TRANSMISSION

The Action Potential

Signaling by the nevous system must be extremely rapid for survival, and chemical messengers alone are too slow for this task. The functional unit of the nervous system is the neuron, the individual nerve cell. Signals are received by the synapses, terminal contacts located on the cell body and the nearby dendrites. Signals are analyzed and integrated in this area with an efferent response transmitted electrically via the cablelike axon. The axon is a long process insulated by the myelin sheath that is interrupted at nodes of Ranvier. A large part of the neuronal surface is covered by satellite cells called glia or Schwann's cells.

The nerve axon has a typically different ion composition inside than in the extracellular fluid. The resting potential can be measured by the use of KCl filled microelectrodes attached to a voltmeter. When one electrode is inserted into a nerve cell, the voltmeter will immediately show a potential difference between inside and outside of $\sim -60mV$ (Fig. 8-2). The resting potential will remain constant until disrupted. If a positive current is added to the cell through a second electrode, the positive charge will cause depolarization of the cell membrane, moving the membrane potential toward zero. The positive charge is added as short bursts of current given at time intervals, called square waves. Small depolarizations (~ 20 mV) cause small membrane potential fluctuations, with the membrane potential dropping back to the resting potential. Cells can also be hyperpolarized by adding more negative charge. In the hyperpolarized state, the membrane potential becomes more negative.

Depolarization of 20 to 30 mV causes an action potential. In an action potential, the membrane potential rises past zero to approximately 50 mV, reversing polarity (Fig. 8-3). The action potential fires the neuron, propagating the nerve impulse as a wave of electrical depolarization. At the end of the current pulse (2 ms), the membrane potential rapidly falls to the initial steady state level.

The threshold potential is the minimum depolariza-

tion necessary to generate an action potential. At this point partial depolarization of the membrane becomes amplified automatically by increased Na^+ conductance (Hodgkin, 1958). Na^+ enters the fiber, increasing the positive charge and reinforcing depolarization. Increased permeability to Na^+ becomes explosive. At the peak of the action potential, the membrane becomes very permeable to sodium, so that the equilibrium potential for Na^+ is almost reached. The Na^+ conductance reinforces the impulse, enabling transmission down the fiber without loss of voltage. This is vital in a biological system in which the conducting axoplasm has a high electrical resistance and poor insulation. The movement of K^+ and Cl^- restore the displaced potential to its initial level.

THE ALL OR NONE LAW

Passage of the impulse leaves the neuron in a refractory state in which the nerve cannot conduct another impulse for 1 ms or more. In addition, it takes several milliseconds to recover to full strength transmission. Thus, the conductance of the nerve impulse is an all or none event in which an electrical signal of fixed amplitude is transmitted in response to threshold stimulation.

SYNAPTIC TRANSMISSION

The propagation of the nerve impulse occurs as a wave of successive depolarization and repolarization of the membrane as the impulse travels to the terminal end of the neuron, a distance frequently measured in meters. Here the neuron will synapse with another neuron or muscle fiber. Synaptic transmission can be electrical or chemical.

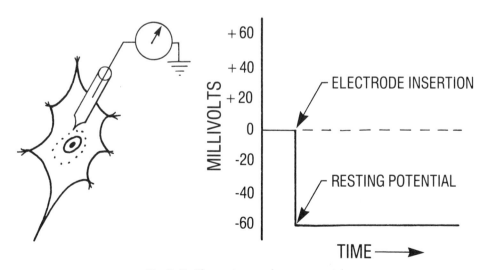

Fig 8-2. The resting membrane potential.

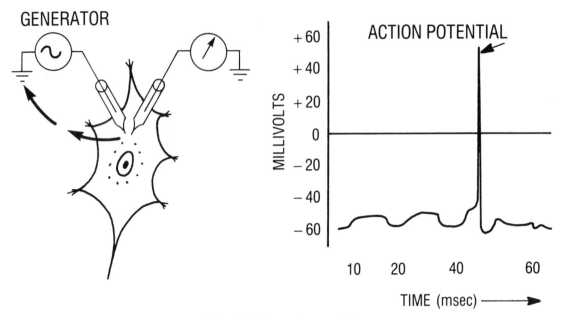

Fig. 8-3. The action potential.

THE ELECTRICAL SYNAPSE

Electrical synapses are best known in the heart, where interconnected muscle fibers contract as a synchronized unit with no significant delay in contractile activity. Both pre- and postsynaptic membranes are lipid bilayers separated by an extracellular space which is only about 10 percent that of synapses using neurotransmitters. A pore called the connexon (composed of the protein connexin) allows substances of up to molecular weight 1000 to penetrate the lipid bilayers. The electrical synapse is called the bridge synapse or gap junction.

The Neuromuscular Action Potential

INNERVATION OF SKELETAL MUSCLE: THE CHEMICAL SYNAPSE

At the neuromuscular junction, cable transmission is replaced by quantal secretion of a chemical transmitter, acetylcholine. Efferent impulses travel down the axon to the motor end of the nerve fiber. This terminus is bound by a presynaptic membrane in close apposition to the postsynaptic membrane of the end-plate of the muscle fiber to be innervated. The membranes are separated by a synaptic cleft, a space across which the action potential must be transmitted. The arrival of the action potential depolarizes the presynaptic membrane and effects the release of the neurotransmitter acetylcholine, specific for skeletal muscle. Acetylcholine is synthesized by the mitochondria of the nerve terminal and stored in vesi-

cles at the presynaptic membrane. Acetylcholine diffuses into the presynaptic cleft and combines with receptor sites on the postsynaptic membrane at the end-plate of the muscle cell. This causes a transient increase in Na^+/K^+ permeability which depolarizes the membrane. The resulting potential is called the end-plate potential (EPP). This potential change initiates a postsynaptic action potential in the muscle which propagates in both directions, leading to contraction coupled with the development of tension in the muscle fiber.

Acetylcholine is subsequently broken down by acetylcholine esterase, with most of the choline taken up across the presynaptic membrane and recycled by the mitochondria for acetylcholine synthesis.

The Reversal Potential

The resting end-plate potential is normally about -90 mV. Depolarization by a chemical transmitter or other stimulus causes a transient increase in both the Na^+ and K^+ permeability. The membrane potential shifts to a level somewhere between the equilibrium potentials of the permeant ions, Na^+ and K^+. Depolarization of the cell membrane progressively diminishes the amplitude of the end-plate potential. Somewhere between -15 and -30 mV, the synaptic potential completely disappears, a point called the reversal potential. This is the point at which further depolarization will reverse the direction of current flow and is roughly halfway between the equilibrium potentials of Na^+ and K^+. At the reversal potential, Na^+ and K^+ currents flow in opposite directions.

Miniature End-plate Potentials

Motor nerve terminals at rest are in a state of intermittent secretory activity. The spontaneous release of transmitter from a few presynaptic vesicles occurs chronically resulting in small changes in postjunctional membrane potentials. These miniature end-plate potentials are of insufficient magnitude to activate the muscle.

Summation and Facilitation

Summation and facilitation are phonomena in which the magnitude of the response to stimuli is enhanced. Summation occurs when two independent stimuli occur simultaneously so that the magnitude of the response is doubled. Facilitation occurs when the response to two related stimuli is greater than the sum of the independent responses. If one nerve impulse follows shortly after another, the second postsynaptic potential change is greater than the sum of the two. Facilitation results in the growth of individual changes in end-plate potentials toward a peak.

The Role of Ca^{++} in Chemical Synapses

Calcium ions must be present in the synaptic cleft for a neural action potential to effect the release of acetylcholine. If a motor axon is stimulated and Ca^{++} is deposited in the synaptic cleft simultaneously, a postsynaptic potential of a given magnitude is produced. However, if the motor axon is stimulated without the deposition of Ca^{++}, or if deposition of Ca^{++} follows stimulation, a diminished postsynaptic potential is observed. Therefore, Ca^{++} must be deposited at the same time the action potential reaches the terminal end of the neuron.

The mechanism for facilitation appears to involve the uptake of Ca^{++} into the presynaptic fiber in response to a neural action potential. Ca^{++} is thought to combine with specific sites on the inner surface of the membrane, increasing acetycholine release. Synaptic facilitation occurs when the Ca^{++}-membrane complex persists from one neural action potential to the next.

Muscle Contraction

FUNCTIONAL ANATOMY

Muscle cells contain myofibrils that are made up of contractile proteins that are activated by the action potential. Skeletal muscle comprises most of the somatic muscle mass and is characterized by cross striations. Cardiac muscle also has cross striations, but cells exhibit a

synctial, integrated response to stimulation controlled by pacemaker cells. Smooth muscle lacks cross striations.

The individual muscle fiber cell is the functional unit of muscle. The muscle fiber has a plasma membrane called the sarcolemma. The contractile elements of the muscle fiber are the myofibrils, which are surrounded by a cytoplasm called the sarcoplasm. Flattened double membrane vesicles, the sarcoplasmic reticulum, surround the myofibrils. The sarcoplasmic reticulum maintains a high internal Ca^{++} concentration, release of which triggers contraction. Continuous with the plasma membrane are transverse tubules which pass through the muscle fiber, lace themselves between myofibrils, and contact the sarcoplasmic reticulum.

Skeletal muscle viewed in the polarizing microscope demonstrates a striated pattern of dark A bands (anisotropic) and light I bands (isotropic). The light bands contain only actin filaments while the dark bands contain myosin filaments plus any overlapping actin filaments. The region in which actins do not overlap the myosin filaments forms a lighter region within the A band termed the H band. The Z disk passes from myofibril to myofibril, attaching myofibrils to each other. The portion of a myofibril that lies between two Z lines is called a sarcomere (Fig. 8-4). At rest, the length of the sarcomere is 2.0 μm.

Actin overlap with the myosin cross-bridges is proportional to tension in the muscle. Where there is no overlap, there is no tension developed. When the sarcomere is shorter, the actin filament overlaps the myosin filament to a greater extent until the sarcomere length reaches 2.2 μm, the point of maximum cross-bridge overlap. The sarcomere maintains full tension until shortened to 2 μm. Below 2 μm, the actin filaments begin to overlap and tension decreases. At 1.65 μm, the Z lines are pulled up against the myosin filaments and further shortening of the sarcomere causes the ends of the myosin filaments to crumple, with tension dropping precipitously.

MOLECULAR CHARACTERISTICS OF THE CONTRACTILE FILAMENTS

The myosin filament is composed of about 200 myosin molecules. Myosin (MW 460,000) contains two heavy chains which wind around each other into a helical structure. The thick filaments consist of longitudinally bundled myosin molecules. The body of the filament is composed of the rod portion (light meromyosin) from multiple myosin molecules. The heavy meromyosin portions protrude from all sides of the myosin filament and constitute the cross-bridges. The heads of the

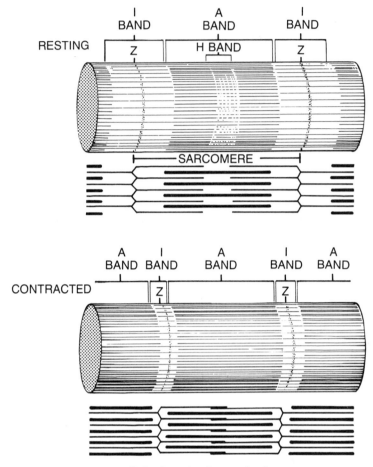

Fig. 8-4. Skeletal muscle: Contractile elements.

cross-bridges lie in apposition to the actin filaments, whereas the helix portions act as hinged arms, allowing the heads to move toward or away from the body of the myosin filament.

The actin filament is composed of actin and the accessory proteins tropomyosin and troponin. G (globular) actin is polymerized to F (fibrous) actin in the presence of ATP. Two strands of F-actin are coiled together into a helix which is the backbone of the thin filament. The accessory proteins regulate the ability of myosin to bind actin filaments. Tropomyosin molecules are arranged in the shallow grooves of the coiled F-actin filaments and block the myosin binding site on actin in the absence of Ca^{++}. Troponin is a regulatory protein with three subunits. Tn-C binds Ca^{++}, Tn-I (inhibitory) binds actin, and Tn-T binds tropomyosin. When Ca^{++} binds to Tn-C, a conformational change occurs in Tn-I and Tn-C which drives tropomyosin deeper into the groove of the actin helix, exposing the active binding site for the myosin head groups.

When the myosin head group binds to the actin filament, the head group tilts with the expenditure of ATP.

This tilting causes a power stroke which slides the actin filament, causing contraction.

EXCITATION-CONTRACTION COUPLING

The initial event in contraction of a muscle is the arrival of an action potential in the terminals of a motor neuron, releasing acetylcholine which binds to a receptor on the sarcolemma, generating a second action potential which travels down the sarcolemma of the muscle cell. The depolarization is spread rapidly into the muscle fiber along the T-tubules. Ca^{++} is released from the sarcoplasmic reticulum and diffuses into the myofilaments. Ca^{++} binds to Tn-C, uncovering the myosin binding sites on actin. Cross-bridges form between actin and myosin, and sliding of thin or thick filaments produces shortening.

Relaxation begins as Ca^{++} is pumped back into the sarcoplasmic reticulum against a concentration gradient by a Ca^{++}-dependent ATPase. Ca^{++} is released from troponin-C and the interaction of actin and myosin is once again blocked by the troponin-tropomyosin complex.

THE MUSCLE TWITCH

A single action potential causes a brief contraction followed by relaxation, a response called a muscle twitch. Depolarization and repolarization are complete in about 5 ms. The duration of the twitch varies with the type of muscle. Skeletal muscle fibers are characterized as red or slow (type I) and white or fast (type II).

Muscle Mechanics

THE ENERGY SOURCE: ATP

Skeletal muscle utilizes ATP to energize myosin-actin cross-bridge formation during contraction, for active pumping of Ca^{++} into the sarcoplasmic reticulum, and for maintenance of intra- and extracellular K^+ and Na^+ concentration. Muscle contains sufficient ATP to maintain full contraction for less than a second. ATP is rapidly regenerated by rephosphorylation of adenosine diphosphate (ADP) by energy rich creatine phosphate:

$$phosphocreatine + ADP \longrightarrow creatine + ATP$$

However, the combined energy stores of ATP and creatine phosphate in muscle are capable of causing maximal contraction for only a few seconds. Ultimately, ATP is regenerated by glycolysis and respiration. In red or slow muscles, the chief source of ATP is oxidative phosphorylation; in white or fast muscles, glycolysis is the chief ATP source.

TYPES OF MUSCLE CONTRACTION

The two types of muscle contraction are described as isotonic and isometric. Isometric contraction causes tension development within the muscle, while the muscle length remains constant. In isotonic contraction there is constant tension during contraction and shortening of the fibers. In an isometric twitch, the action potential peaks in 1.5 ms, then decays rapidly. At about 7 ms, muscle tension rapidly drops (latency relaxation), reaching a minimum at 11.5 ms. It then reverses sign and within 3.5 ms returns to its initial value. From this point tension increases to the full isometric twitch tension. The time course of isometric contraction differs greatly among different muscles.

TETANUS

If a muscle fiber is stimulated repeatedly at a fast frequency, a smooth sustained contraction called a tetanus results. In tetanus individual twitches cannot be detected. Tetanus tension is much greater than the maximal tension of a single twitch and is maintained at a constant level as long as stimulation is continued or until the muscle becomes fatigued.

CONTRACTILE AND ELASTIC COMPONENTS

The muscle can be represented as a contractile component in parallel with an elastic component (sarcolemma, connective tissue) and in series with a second elastic component (tendon, connective tissue). As the contractile component shortens in response to an impulse, it stretches the series elastic component while tension is developed and transmitted to the external load. Contraction is isometric at this point. When the tension developed in the series elastic component equals the weight of the load, the muscle begins to shorten and lifts the load. The contraction becomes isotonic. Thus, an active and passive component to the total tension develops in contraction. At maximum tension during an isometric contraction, the series elastic components stretch by an amount equivalent to 2 percent of the muscle length. The contractile component shortens by an equivalent amount and therefore, the external length remains constant.

LENGTH-TENSION RELATIONSHIP

Both the tension that a muscle develops when stimulated to contract isometrically (total tension) and the passive tension exerted by the unstimulated muscle vary with the length of the muscle fiber. The amount of tension actually generated by the contractile process is the active tension. The length of a muscle at which the active tension is maximal is often near the resting length. When the muscle fiber contracts isometrically, the tension developed is proportional to the number of cross-linkages between the actin and myosin molecules (maximum at resting length).

In isotonic contraction as the load is increased the muscle needs more time to develop adequate tension to lift the weight. The muscle also shortens less with greater loads.

FORCE-VELOCITY RELATIONSHIPS

In a series of isotonic contractions starting at resting length, the velocity drops as the force required to lift the load increases. If the load is made sufficiently heavy, there is no external shortening and the contraction is isometric. The velocity is maximal at zero load. The tendency for the actin filaments to slip backward against the production of force by cross-bridge activity should increase as the load is raised.

SMOOTH MUSCLE

Smooth muscle fibers are small spindle-shaped cells which are far smaller than skeletal muscle fibers. Smooth muscle may be multiunit or visceral. Multiunit smooth muscle is composed of discrete muscle fibers which operate independently and are often innervated by a single nerve ending (as occurs for skeletal muscle). Multiunit smooth muscle fibers are controlled almost entirely by nerve signals. They rarely exhibit spontaneous contractions.

Visceral smooth muscle fibers are usually arranged in sheets or bundles with the cell membranes contacting each other at multiple points to form gap junctions. The fibers form a functional syncytium with integrated contraction. The action potential generated in one area of the muscle electrically excites the adjacent fibers without secretion of any neurotransmitter.

CONTRACTION IN SMOOTH MUSCLE

Smooth muscle contains actin and myosin filaments, but without cross striation. Myosin filaments (about 1 per 12 actin filaments) contain cross-bridges and are in close proximity to the actin filaments. Contraction occurs by a sliding filament mechanism. Isometric contraction of smooth muscle is far slower than skeletal muscle, apparently because of the slowness of the biochemical reactions which cause contraction. Only about 1/500th as much energy is required to sustain the same tension of contraction in smooth muscle as in skeletal muscle, presumably due to decreased myosin ATPase activity and the formation of "latch" bridges.

MEMBRANE POTENTIALS AND ACTION POTENTIALS

The membrane potential in smooth muscle varies, but averages about 30 mV less negative than skeletal muscle. Action potentials in visceral smooth muscle occur either as spike potentials similar to those in skeletal muscle or as action potentials with plateaus. In the plateau, the onset is similar to the spike potential, but repolarization is delayed for several hundred milliseconds. Ca^{++} permeability probably increases on depolarization causing delayed repolarization. The plateau lasts for the prolonged periods of contraction that occur in some types of smooth muscle (ureter, uterus in some conditions, some vascular smooth muscle).

SLOW WAVE POTENTIAL IN VISCERAL SMOOTH MUSCLE

Some smooth muscles are self-excitatory, exhibiting a slow wave rhythm of the membrane potential caused by waxing and waning of the pumping of Na^+ outward.

When the slow wave potential rises above threshold potential, an action potential develops, spreading over the visceral smooth muscle and causing contraction. This promotes a series of rhythmical contractions of the smooth muscle mass, with the slow waves frequently called pacemaker waves. Once an action potential begins, it spreads rapidly through the muscle fibers via the gap junctions.

EXCITATION-CONTRACTION COUPLING

Ca^{++} activates the contractile process in smooth muscle. Since smooth muscle contains limited sarcoplasmic reticulum, most of the Ca^{++} enters from the extracellular fluid after an action potential. Smooth muscle fiber does not contain T-tubules as in skeletal muscle, but the small size of the cells allows Ca^{++} to rapidly diffuse. In many types of smooth muscle the onset of depolarization is caused by the influx of Ca^{++} rather than Na^+.

To cause relaxation, Ca^{++} is pumped either into the sarcoplasmic reticulum by a Ca^{++} pump which is much slower than its skeletal muscle counterpart or back into the extracellular fluid. Therefore, the duration of contraction of smooth muscle is on the order of seconds rather than tens of milliseconds.

Since the concentration of troponin is low or nonexistent in smooth muscle, the role of Ca^{++} in contraction differs from skeletal muscle. In smooth muscle Ca^{++} appears to function in activation of the myosin ATPase activity.

SMOOTH MUSCLE TONE

Smooth muscle can maintain a state of long-term, steady contraction called tonus contraction or smooth muscle tone. Tone allows prolonged or indefinite continuance of smooth muscle function. Tonic contractions can be caused by summation of individual contractile pulses (similar to tetanic contractions in skeletal muscle) or by prolonged direct smooth muscle excitation without action potentials. The latter is usually caused by local tissue factors or circulating hormones.

SENSORY PERCEPTION

Sensory Receptors

Sensation is a fragile link with reality which enables us to perceive the environment around and within ourselves. Information reaches the CNS via afferent sensory neurons which have specialized areas capable of generating a neural action potential. The sense organ is a specialized receptor, such as the light sensitive rods and cones of the eye, with associated nonneural cells. Sensory receptors transduce various forms of energy into localized changes in membrane potential that result in formation of action potentials. Sensations, received initially by a specialized receptor, cause a local change in the membrane potential in the terminal portion of the receptor which is conducted to the first node of Ranvier where a train of action potentials are formed in the sensory nerve. Sensory modalities, which are initially processed by separate afferent information channels, converge in the spinal cord, project to the thalamus, and finally reach the somatic sensory cortex of the cerebrum. The modalities of sensation include touch-pressure, temperature, pain, and position. Receptors also monitor blood pressure, blood sugar levels, and other bodily functions.

There are several classifications of somatic receptors. Exteroceptive receptors are sensitive to stimuli from the external environment and consist of the sensations of touch-pressure, position of limbs, environmental temperature, and pain. Proprioceptive receptors are involved in the sensation of the position of body segments and the body in space. Interoceptive receptors are sensitive to internal signals, such as blood pressure and blood sugar levels. Pain receptors sensitive to damaging or noxious stimuli are often called nociceptors, while chemoreceptors are stimulated by changes in the environmental chemistry.

CORRELATION OF PERCEPTION OF SENSATION WITH NEURONAL FUNCTION

The absolute sensory threshold is defined as the lowest stimulus intensity a subject can detect. In practice, it is that stimulus intensity at which there is a 50 percent probability of detection. As the stimulus intensity increases, the probability of detection increases sigmoidally. Difficulties in the measurements of absolute sensory threshold include subject reporting and recording of action potentials in the sensory nerve.

SENSORY TRANSDUCTION

The function of somatic receptors is to convert (transduce) natural stimuli into electrical impulses. Vibrational phenomena, for example, are detected by pacinian corpuscles which are located in connective tissue below the surface of the skin. Pacinian corpuscles consist of a nerve fiber surrounded by layers of connective tissue lamina. The terminal portion of the nerve is unmyelinated. Myelin begins within the corpuscle and the first node of Ranvier is inside the corpuscle.

Sensory transduction involves production of a generator potential. In the case of the pacinian corpuscle, the generator potential is produced in the terminal unmyelinated portion of the nerve fiber due to pressure on the corpuscle. The depolarization caused by the generator potential is passively conducted to the first node of Ranvier where the action potential is initiated, provided the threshold potential is achieved. The generation potential is a local, nonpropagating, depolarizing potential which is restricted to the receptor membrane. The generator potential is due to an increase in conductance of Na^+ and K^+ and is nonpropagating because there are no Na^+ gates open in the adjacent portion of the membrane prior to the first node of Ranvier. Therefore, the potential does not spread at the same level along the membrane, but decays as the first node is approached.

Once the magnitude of the generator potential brings the first node of Ranvier to threshold and action potentials are formed, the frequency of the action potentials decrease as the strength of the generator potential decreases. Thus, the force applied to the receptor is transduced into the frequency of impulses conducted to the dorsal root of the spinal cord. The larger the generator potential, the more frequent are the action potentials. The frequency is a code in which the strength of the stimulus is converted into the number of impulses.

ADAPTATION

Adaptation is a property whereby the generator potential decreases in amplitude in response to a maintained stimulus. The degree and speed of adaptation is determined by the type of receptor (e.g., the pacinian corpuscle adapts rapidly).

CONDUCTION VELOCITY

Each individual nerve has only one type of sensory receptor on its branches, and there are various sizes of nerve fibers which go into the spinal cord. Nerve size is directly related to conduction velocity, with the largest diameter fibers conducting the most rapidly. A sensory nerve from muscle has four types of nerve fibers. Type I fibers (largest) conduct very rapidly and are related to sensation of the length and tension of the muscle. Smaller fibers, types II and III, are involved with pain and thermal sensation. The smallest fibers, type IV (in cutaneous nerves, C fibers), conduct impulses related to pain.

Pain is mediated by nociceptors. The sensation of pain as fast or slow relates to fiber size and is significant because a delayed response can cause tissue damage if conduction velocity is slow in reaching the brain. Pain fibers have free nerve endings rather than specialized structures and respond best to a pinch or needle tip as compared to a blunt stimulus.

THERMAL SENSATION

Thermal sensation is mediated by discrete cold and warm receptors. The frequency of action potentials generated is proportional to the rate and extent of temperature lowering. Cold receptors respond to cold temperature ($\sim 30\,^{\circ}$C or less) and somewhat to hot temperature ($\sim 45\,^{\circ}$C or more). The response of cold receptors to hot stimuli is called paradoxical cold, and is only perceived when a single cold receptor is stimulated. Paradoxical cold is an example of the labelled line code, in which a receptor will transmit one type of signal to the dorsal root regardless of the type of stimulus. Thus, a cold receptor interprets a heat stimulus as cold.

Sensations respond to the following codes in identifying the type and intensity of the stimulus: (1) frequency code (frequency of impulses), (2) population code (number of receptors stimulated), and (3) labelled line code (the particular receptor stimulated).

POSITION SENSE

Position receptors sense the length and tension of muscle. Each muscle spindle consists of several muscle fibers enclosed in a connective tissue capsule. The ends of the spindle capsule are attached to the tendons at either end of the muscle or to the sides of the contractile fibers which are attached to the tendons. The contractile units of muscle are called extrafusal fibers. The intrafusal fibers are in parallel to the extrafusal fibers and act as a length guage. Intrafusal fibers do not extend from tendon to tendon.

Intrafusal fibers are of two types. The nuclear bag fibers have central nuclei with some myofilaments at the ends. They are innervated by dynamic motor neurons which influence afferent response to phasic stretch. The nuclear chain fibers have nuclei scattered along the fiber. Efferent innervation is by static motor neurons, which influence afferent response to static stretch. Afferent fibers are differentiated by the size of the nerve fibers and the intrafusal fibers they innervate. Primary (group IA) afferents are the larger fibers which innervate both types of intrafusal fibers. Secondary (group II) afferents are smaller fibers which innervate only the nuclear chain fibers.

The Golgi tendon organs sense muscle tension and are located in the tendon at the end of the extrafusal fiber.

FUNCTION OF MUSCLE RECEPTORS

The afferent response of muscle spindle (intrafusal fibers) and the Golgi tendon organ is induced by the stretching of the muscle which produces action potentials in both. However, the spindle afferents characteristically cease firing on contraction of the extrafusal fibers because the muscle shortens while the spindle does not. The result is the disappearance of action potentials from the intrafusal fibers and an increase in action potentials from the Golgi tendon organ which responds to the increased tension of extrafusal fiber contraction.

STATIC AND DYNAMIC MOTOR NEURONS

In normal contraction of a muscle, while the muscle is changing in length (the dynamic phase) and after the muscle has reached its new length (static phase), a certain response is recorded from the primary afferent neuron. If the motor fibers are stimulated, a change in the frequency of action potentials produced by the primary afferent neuron results. Stimulation of the static motor neuron modulates the sensitivity of perception of the static position of the muscle, while stimulation of the dynamic motor neuron allows the rapid sensing of changes in muscle length. Sustained tension elicits steady firing of the primary afferent and when the muscle contracts, the primary afferent stops firing. However, if a static motor neuron is stimulated during contraction, the intrafusal fiber contracts, preventing the muscle from going slack. In this situation the primary afferent continues to respond rather than cease firing. Thus, the threshold for sensing tension is changed by the contraction of the intrafusal fiber.

Spinal Reflexes

THE REFLEX ARC

The reflex arc is the integral unit of neural activity and involves a sensory receptor, an afferent neuron, one or more CNS synapses, an efferent (motor) neuron, and an effector. The cell bodies of afferent neurons lie in the dorsal root (sensory) ganglia of the spinal cord or in the homologous ganglia of the cranial nerves. Communication takes place within the spinal cord or the brain, with efferent fibers leaving via the ventral root (motor) ganglia and the motor cranial nerves. Cell bodies supplying efferent neurons originate in the ventral root.

The simplest reflex arc involves a single synapse between afferent and motor neurons. The stretch reflex of skeletal muscle is the only monosynaptic reflex in the body. This reflex originates in muscle stretch, with the contraction response sensed by the muscle spindle and conducted to the spinal cord by fast afferents which synapse directly with motor neurons innervating the same muscle.

Most reflex arcs are polysynaptic, with afferent fibers terminating on one or more interneurons. Interneurons form the majority of neurons in the CNS and serve as integrators, since they are able to process information from several sources simultaneously. Interneurons also act as amplifiers of strength, amplifiers in time, and signal inverters.

Amplification of strength occurs when the sensory neuron synapses with a motor neuron cell body (MCB) and also has a branch which synapses with an interneuron. This permits multiplication of the amount of excitatory transmitter released to the MCB, increasing the probability that an action potential will be initiated. In addition, interneurons may distribute an incoming volley to widely separate groups of motor neurons.

Interneurons act as amplifiers in time when a sensory neuron synapses with an interneuron which synapses with and excites the original sensory neuron, causing the interneuron to fire again (after some time delay).

Interneurons act as signal inverters when a sensory neuron releasing excitatory transmitter excites an interneuron to release its inhibitory transmitter.

TIME COURSE OF FACILITATION

Facilitation and summation occur within the CNS when two afferent nerve branches enter a dorsal root from a single muscle. Facilitation produces a greater response from two simultaneous stimuli than the algebraic sum of the two independent stimuli. This occurs when the one stimulus causes a subthreshold amount of excitatory transmitter to be released. When the second stimulus is fired more transmitter is released, facilitating an action potential. If the second stimulus is fired at increasingly longer time delays after the firing of the first (millisecond range), the response reflects the time delay because the transmitter from the first stimulus has partially been hydrolyzed, taken back up into the nerve terminal, or diffused away.

TIME COURSE OF INHIBITION

All responses from sensory neurons are excitatory and the interneuron is therefore required for the release of inhibitory transmitter. The time course of inhibition can be modulated if sensory neurons from two separate antagonistic muscles converge to stimulate the same interneuron. If one of the stimuli causes inhibitory transmitter to be deposited at the motor neuron, the response to the excitatory stimulus will be weaker. The minimum response occurs after only a slight delay because the stimuli must go through an interneuron requiring some time for the synapse. Only when inhibitory and excitatory transmitters reach the motor neuron at the same time does the minimum response (maximum inhibition) occur. As the synapse delay is increased, the response increases until it returns to the original maximum value where only the effect of the excitatory transmitter is felt at the motor neuron.

THE EXCITATORY POSTSYNAPTIC POTENTIAL

Stimulation of a dorsal root afferent by a single stimulus causes a depolarization of the postsynaptic cell membrane immediately under the active synaptic knob. This depolarizing response, called the excitatory postsynaptic potential (EPSP), reaches its peak about 2.5 – 3 ms after stimulation and then declines exponentially. During this period (about 6 ms), the excitability of the neuron to other stimuli is increased. The EPSP is similar to the end-plate potential in that it is not conducted all the way down the fiber, but extends only to the axonal hellock, dependent on cell membrane properties.

SPATIAL AND TEMPORAL SUMMATION

The depolarization produced by each of the active synaptic knobs is capable of summation. Since there is no refractory period in the EPSP, temporal as well as spatial summation can occur. In spatial summation as the strength of afferent stimuli increase more of the sensory fibers which synapse with the MCB release excitatory transmitter, and the EPSP increases until enough sensory fibers are involved to reach threshold and initiate an action potential. Temporal summation occurs when different afferent stimuli cause new EPSPs before the previous EPSPs have decayed. The EPSP is, therefore, not an all or none response but is proportional to the number and frequency of the afferent stimuli.

A transient increase in both Na^+ and K^+ conductance follows depolarization of the synaptic knob to produce the EPSP. A reversal potential, similar to that of muscle end-plate potential, can also be elicited. The reversal potential is nearly halfway between E_K and E_{Na}.

THE INHIBITORY POSTSYNAPTIC POTENTIAL

The release of inhibitory transmitter at the presynaptic membrane by an interneuron can cause hyperpolarization of the postsynaptic membrane. During this hyperpolarization, known as the inhibitory postsynaptic potential (IPSP), the response of the motor neuron to stimuli is decreased. Both spatial and temporal summation of IPSP occurs. If an EPSP and IPSP simultaneously stimulate a motor neuron, the response is somewhere between the independent responses. Interneurons and motor neurons integrate information within the CNS by this mechanism.

Facilitation is the structural possibility that one neuron can synapse with more than one postsynaptic membrane. Occlusion is the response to simultaneous stimulation of two neurons which is less than the summed response if the neurons are stimulated separately.

Excitation in the motor neuron pool is related to the number and strength of the presynaptic stimuli. If there are no stimuli (zero strength), there are no motor neurons with EPSPs or action potentials. If the strength is increased slightly, some motor neurons may have sub-threshold EPSPs, though none discharge action potentials. A further increase in stimulus strength will cause some motor neurons to discharge action potentials and more subthreshold EPSPs will occur in other neurons. Even at maximum strength not all motor neurons will be in the discharge zone, and some subthreshold EPSPs will remain.

Central excitatory and inhibitory states describe prolonged states in which excitatory or inhibitory stimuli radiate to many somatic (or autonomic) areas of the spinal cord in reverberating circuits with amplification in time. Central excitatory mechanisms may also involve the prolonged effects of synaptic mediators. Some mediators, such as acetylcholine, produce fast EPSPs, while others produce slow EPSPs with excitatory effects that last for extended periods of time (minutes).

Sensitization is a response to damaging stimuli which is more rapid because increased Ca^{++} uptake results in increased release of transmitters. Habituation is the opposite effect in which a slower response is mediated to repeated nondamaging stimuli.

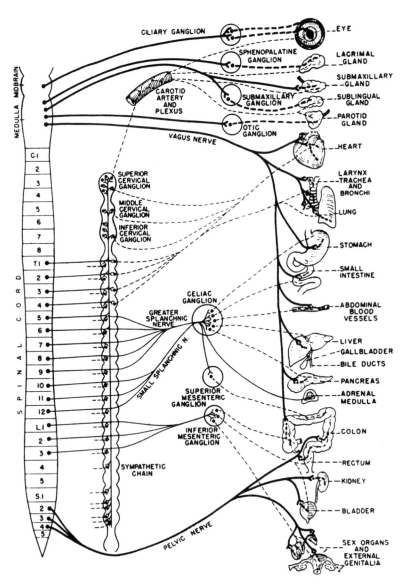

Fig. 8-5. Efferent autonomic pathways. Heavy lines are the parasympathetic division; light lines, the sympathetic division; continuous lines represent preganglionic fibers; and broken lines, postaganglionic fibers. (Reprinted with permission from Youmans WB (ed): Fundamentals of Human Physiology for Students in the Medical Sciences. 2nd Ed. Copyright © 1962 by Year Book Medical Publishers, Inc., Chicago.)

The Autonomic Nervous System

The autonomic nervous system regulates the normally involuntary visceral processes of the body and is under the control of centers within the CNS. Autonomic reflexes are similar to those of the somatic nervous system, with simple refexes, such as bladder contraction, integrated in the spinal cord. More complex reflexes are regulated by the medulla oblongata, the hypothalamus, and higher centers of the brain (Fig. 8-5).

Afferent autonomic pathways relay impulses from the viscera to the CNS where they are integrated and a response is transmitted via efferent pathways to visceral effectors. The peripheral efferents are oganized into preganglionic and postganglionic neurons. The preganglionic cell bodies are found in the gray matter of the spinal cord or the homologous efferent nuclei of the cranial nerves. Preganglionic fibers are generally myelinated B type fibers, slower than somatic efferent fibers. Their axons form branches which synapse on the cell bodies of postganglionic neurons outside the CNS. The axons of postganglionic neurons innervate visceral effectors and are generally unmyelinated slower conducting C fibers with a longer refractory period.

SYMPATHETIC DIVISION

The autonomic nervous system is divided by anatomy, function, and pharmacology, into two main divisions, the sympathetic and parasympathetic systems. The cells of origin of the sympathetic system are found in lateral horns of the spinal cord from the first thoracic to the third lumbar rgions. This region constitutes the only outlet for sympathetic impulses. The axons of sympathetic preganglionic neurons are each connected to a paravertebral ganglion by the white ramus communicantes. At this point, a preganglionic fiber may pursue one of three pathways. The fiber may synapse with cells in the ganglion it first enters, it may pass up or down the sympathetic trunk for some distance to terminate at a segment different than its origin, or it may pass through the ganglion to prevertebral ganglia, such as the celiac, where it synapses with a ganglion cell. The preganglionic fibers from a particular segment will connect with several ganglia, usually from 1 to 5 and in some cases as many as 32, accounting for the diffuse nature of the sympathetic discharge. The axons of some of the postganglionic neurons transmit the impulses to innervate the viscera directly.

PARASYMPATHETIC DIVISION

The cells of origin of the paraympathetic fibers are found in the midbrain, the medulla oblongated, and the sacral region of the spinal cord. Parasympathetic fibers are preganglionic and postganglionic in nature, with ganglion cells lying within or in close proximity to the target organ.

CHEMICAL TRANSMISSION IN THE AUTONOMIC SYSTEM

The involvement of acetylcholine in transmission at the somatic neuromuscular junction has already been noted. Acetylcholine also mediates impulses at all autonomic ganglia, all parasympathetic postganglionic terminations, and sympathetic postganglionic terminations at the sweat glands. All nerves in which transmission is mediated by acetylcholine are termed cholinergic.

Norepinephrine is the chemical transmitter which mediates impulses at most sympathetic postganglionic nerve endings. Such nerves are termed adrenergic because they release norepinephrine. Epinephrine is the major substance secreted by the adrenal medulla. The catecholamines norepinephrine, epinephrine, and dopamine are secreted by neurons in the brain (Table 8-1).

Other neurotransmitters of importance are certain amino acids and peptides. The gut-brain peptides were identified originally as hormones (glucagon and cholecystokinin). Other families of peptides, the enkaphalins and β-endorphins, bind to opiate receptors in the brain and are the natural painkillers of the brain.

SYNTHESIS OF NEUROTRANSMITTERS

All of the enzymes essential for the synthesis of peptide neurotransmitters are found in the nerve cell body. Neurotransmitters are packaged in vesicles in the golgi and are transported down the axon (at a rate of about 40 cm per day) to the nerve terminal. After release of the neuro-

Table 8-1. Neurotransmitters

Transmitter	Source
Acetylcholine	Motor neurons of the spinal cord, autonomic nervous system, basal ganglia of brain
Biogenic amines	
Dopamine	Substantia nigra, midbrain, hypothalamus, sympathetic ganglia
Norepinephrine	Locus cerulus, sympathetic nervous system
Serotonin	Brain stem
Histamine	Hypothalamus
Amino Acids	
GABA (γ-aminobutyric acid)	Basal ganglia, cerebellum, spinal cord
Glutamate	Cerebellum, spinal cord
Glycine	Spinal cord (inhibitory transmitter)

transmitter, vesicle membranes are transported back to the cell body for recycling. Small neurotransmitters such as acetylcholine and norepinephrine are synthesized in the nerve terminal.

PART 2

The Cardiovascular System

THE SYSTEM

The cardiovascular system is designed to produce blood flow to all tissues of the body. The system consists of the heart that is made up of four pumps, arteries, capillary networks, and veins. Blood flow is maintained by ventricular pressure developed by the pumping action of the heart. The left ventricle develops a peak pressure of 120 mm Hg during contraction (systole), with intraventricular pressure dropping to near 0 during relaxation (diastole). As blood is forced into the aorta, the aortic pressure also rises to peak at 120 mm Hg. The pressure in the aorta usually does not drop below 80 mm Hg because of vessel elasticity and prevention of backflow of blood into the ventricle by the one-way aortic valve. The pressure in the aorta is then about 120/80. The mean aortic pressure of 93 mm Hg is the driving pressure for the systemic circulation. Vessels branch progressively and once blood gets to the arteriole level, resistance to flow is highest and the pressure drops very rapidly. Arteriolar resistance can be regulated by the autonomic nervous system, circulating hormones, and/or metabolic products.

The capillary beds supplying the tissues form a microcirculation which is the essence of the system. When blood passes from the arterioles through the capillaries to venules, the pressure of the heart beat is largely lost and venous blood pressure is low (approximately 15 mm Hg).

Blood Volume Distribution in the Systemic Circulation

The arterial system contains about 20 percent of the total blood volume, a fairly constant amount. Increased pumping does not increase arterial volume but does increase arterial pressure. This is because the relatively thick-walled arteries do not stretch sufficiently to accommodate an increase in blood volume. The venous system contains about 75 percent of total blood volume. The capacity of the venous sytem can vary dramatically by venous constriction or dilation. The venous system is a thin-walled, low pressure, high volume system. The capillary networks contain about 5 percent of the total blood volume.

Functional Anatomy of the Heart

The heart has four muscular chambers which are separated from each other by septa and valves. Atrial muscle is thin and translucent, while the ventricles are thick-walled (i.e., composed of three muscular layers). The heart also has a fibrous skeleton composed of four fibrous rings which serve as a base for the attachment of atria, ventricles, and leaflets of tricuspid, mitral, aortic, and pulmonary valves. The fibrous skeleton also forms a nonconducting electrical barrier between the atria and the ventricles. This is important in the coordination of atrial and ventricular contraction. Cardiac muscle has no motor innervation and is supplied by fibers from the autonomic nervous system. The heart is nourished by coronary arteries terminating in a rich capillary bed.

Characteristics of Cardiac Muscle

Both cardiac muscle and smooth muscle have gap junctions located in the intercalated disk portion of cardiac muscle and on the longitudinal surface of smooth muscle cells. Gap junctions permit ionic conductance of impulses from one cell to another, integrating a network of cells into electrical comnunincation, a phenomenon called a syncytium.

Both cardiac and smooth muscle cells have action potentials of long duration, much longer than is found in nerve and skeletal muscle. Both cardiac and smooth muscle also have a less extensive sarcoplasmic reticulum and are dependent on extracellular Ca^{++} for contraction (unlike skeletal muscle). Therefore, contraction of cardiac (and smooth) muscle requires both extracellular and sacroplasmic reticulum Ca^{++}.

NATURE OF THE SYNCYTIUM

If one cardiac muscle fiber is stimulated, the impulse will spread through gap junctions to all the fibers in the muscle mass which act as one large contracting cell, a functional syncytium. Two functional cardiac syncytia exist. Both atria act as one syncytium and will contract almost simultaneously with the stimulation of either one. Both ventricles act as the other syncytium.

An electrical impulse will spread between atria and

ventricles through a special conductive pathway, such as the bundle of His. The two syncytia are otherwise electrically separated from each other by the nonconducting fibrous connective tissue barrier.

MYOCARDIAL EXCITATION AND RELAXATION

Cardiac muscle has a very well developed T-tubule system. Excitation occurs in much the same way as in skeletal muscle, except that in cardiac muscle, as the action potential spreads over the sarcolemma, Ca^{++} is released into the cell both across the sarcolemma (extracellular source) and from the sarcoplasmic reticulum. Ca^{++} binds to troponin C which moves tropomyosin out of the groove on actin and allows cross-bridge formation between actin and myosin. Contraction results. Removal of Ca^{++} causes relaxation. Ca^{++} is removed by longitudinal vesicles of the sarcoplasmic reticulum and by movement back into the extracellular space by transport processes.

FORCE OF CONTRACTION

The force of contraction from any stimulation is proportional to the amount of Ca^{++} released into the intracellular environment and to the amount of troponin C that is complexed with Ca^{++}. Thus, a main way to increase the force of contraction is to increase intracellular Ca^{++}.

ELECTRICAL PROPERTIES OF THE HEART

Cardiac action potentials involve ionic changes in which depolarization occurs due to a rapid massive influx of Na^+. The cardiac muscle action potential has a long duration. While the upswing of depolarization is the same as with skeletal muscle, a plateau region occurs which can be accounted for by a constant influx of Ca^{++} and a maintained, but lower, influx of Na^+. These two factors keep the membrane depolarized during the plateau stage of the action potential.

The slow influx of Na^+ and Ca^{++} occur via a slow Na^+ and Ca^{++} channel present in cardiac muscle. Therefore, two types of channels exist for the influx of positive ions in cardiac muscle, the rapid Na^+ channel for the initial depolarization and the slow Na^+ and Ca^{++} channel for the plateau stage. Repolarization of the membrane potential is due to an increased K^+ efflux while Na^+ and Ca^{++} influx is decreased.

The influx of extracellular Ca^{++} is partly the source of Ca^{++} needed for contraction. Clinically, cardiac function is modulated by controlling the rate of Ca^{++} influx with drugs, such as digitalis, and Ca^{++} blocking agents.

Increased intracellular Ca^{++} yields a greater force of contraction. However, unlike skeletal muscle, greater contractile force cannot be obtained by recruiting more motor units because cardiac muscle acts as a functional syncytium. Also, unlike skeletal muscle, contractile force cannot be increased by a summation of the contractile response because the duration of the action potential is too prolonged.

LACK OF SUMMATION IN CARDIAC MUSCLE

In cardiac muscle the duration of the action potential is about the same as the contractile response. Therefore, with multiple stimuli summation does not occur. In addition, cardiac muscle has a relatively long refractory period. Since another action potential is precluded in the refractory period, summation of contractile response is not possible. This is of physiologic importance since the heart chambers need to relax in order to refill. If summation were possible, the heart might never relax, a situation destructive to its function as a pump.

The Conduction System of the Heart

Specialized cardiac fibers, which generate or conduct electrical activity, coordinate the pumping activity of the heart. The sinoatrial node is a small patch of such cells and is the normal pacemaker of the heart. The structures that make up the conduction system are the sinoatrial (SA) node, the internodal atrial pathways, the atrioventricular (AV) node, the bundle of His with its branches, and the Purkinje system (Fig. 8-6).

Normally the SA node spontaneously generates its own action potential which sets the rate of the heart beat. The SA nodal fibers have a low resting membrane potential which exhibits very rapid spontaneous decay. The autonomic nervous system influences only the rate of this spontaneous decay and does not elicit the action potential as in skeletal muscle. (There are no neuromuscular junctions.) The AV node can also generate action potentials. However, since the SA node generates action potentials at a more rapid rate than the AV node, it is the heart's pacemaker.

The AV node and the bundle of His form the only electrical connection between the two functional syncytia (atrial and ventricular). Impulses generated in the SA node pass through the internodal atrial pathways to the AV node, then to the bundle of His and its branches via the Purkinje system to the ventricles. The heart then normally contracts rhythmically to promote atrial systole, followed by ventricular systole, and then by diastole in which all four chambers are relaxed.

If the dominant pacemaker, the SA node, becomes

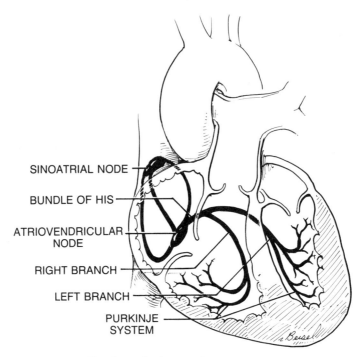

SINOATRIAL NODE

BUNDLE OF HIS

ATRIOVENDRICULAR
NODE

RIGHT BRANCH

LEFT BRANCH

PURKINJE
SYSTEM

Fig. 8-6. Cardiac conductance system.

inactive, a subordinate pacemaker could assume the pacemaker role, as its membrane potential would eventually decay to threshold. Any cell in the heart is potentially capable of becoming the pacemaker. In pathologic conditions, premature contractions called ectopic beats can be caused by a single cell somewhere in the ventricles or atria that becomes irritated and has a spontaneous decay in membrane potential (ectopic focus), generating an impulse which spreads throughout the heart. However, conduction through the AV node is normally unidirectional from atrium to ventricle.

VELOCITY OF CONDUCTION

The velocity of conduction through atrial muscle is relatively fast. Longitudinal velocity increases with cell diameter. Conduction is most rapid in the Purkinje fibers which are the largest, and slowest at the AV node where fibers are the smallest. The conductance delay at the AV node serves an important function. Once the action potential gets by the AV node it is conducted very rapidly by the Purkinje fibers. Both atria contract almost simultaneously, with a delay from the AV node to the Purkinje system of about 0.16 s. This delay is approximately the same as the duration of the action potential in the atria. This means that the atria can contract completely before the action potential is spread to cause contraction of the ventricles. The delay in conductance at the AV node, therefore, is essential if the heart is to act as

a pump, emptying the atria before contracting the ventricles.

CONTROL OF THE HEART RATE

Both SA and AV nodes have an abundant supply of parasympathetic and sympathetic nerve fibers which can have antagonistic effects. As has been noted, the SA node is the normal pacemaker. The intrinsic heart rate is set by the SA node and depends on the spontaneous decay in the resting membrane potential and the balance between sympathetic and parsympathetic nervous influences. Parasympathetic regulation is via the vagus nerve and depends on release of acetylcholine which increases the permeability of the SA nodal membrane to K^+. This slows conductance because the hyperpolarization caused by increased K^+ conductance offsets the rise in the action potential. Therefore, it takes longer for the membrane to depolarize to threshold and fire an action potential. This pacemaker activity slows down the rest of the heart. Experimentally, stimulation of the vagus nerve can completely stop membrane depolarization.

Effects of the sympathetic nervous system are mediated by norepinephrine which effects both SA and AV nodal regions. At the SA node, norepinephrine increases the heart rate by increasing Na^+ conductance, allowing the cell to reach threshold earlier. At the AV node, conduction velocity is increased by the same mechanism. Norephinephrine causes an increase in conduction through the slow Na^+ channels. Ca^{++} also enters via these channels and the force of contraction increases with an increase in intracellular Ca^{++}.

In comparison parasympathetic regulation, via vagal release of acetylcholine, slows the heart rate and has no effect on ventricular contraction.

Sympathetic regulation, via norepinephrine, speeds up the heart rate and increases the force of ventricular contraction.

Electrical Activity in the Heart

THE ELECTROCARDIOGRAM

The electrocardiogram (EKG) measures the three dimensional current flow produced by the heart in a volume conductor, the electrolyte fluids of the body. The transmembrane potential is about -80 mV, with the action potential reflecting changes in the Na^+ conductance in which the membrane potential becomes positive in respect to the extracellular fluid. Repolarizaton restores the membrane potential as Na^+ influx is reversed and K^+ efflux is restored.

The voltage change measured depends on the placement of the electrodes. The greatest charge recorded will be found when the electrodes are arranged on either side of a line separating the activated and resting tissue (the maximum separation of charges); the further away from this dipole, the smaller the charge measured. The EKG records on a millivolt and time scale the algebraic sum of the thousands of tiny electrical vectors over the entire heart produced by fluctuations in cardiac potential.

In a unipolar EKG recording, an active (exploring) electrode is connected to an indifferent electrode at zero potential. Bipolar recording involves two active electrodes. In volume conductance, the sum of the potentials at the points of an equilateral triangle with the current source in the center is zero. Placement of electrodes on both arms and the left leg approximates a triangle with the heart as its center and is referred to as Einthoven's triangle.

The P wave records the movement of depolarization as it starts at the SA node and spreads radially through all of the atrial muscle fibers. When half of the atrial mass is depolarized, the peak of the P wave is achieved. As the wave spreads across the entire atrium, the potential returns to zero. Atrial depolarizaion is completed in about 0.1 s. The atrial action potential is over before the QRS complex occurs (Fig. 8-7).

The QRS complex represents ventricular depolarization. The Q wave records depolarization as it starts from the left bundle branch moving via the interventricular septum from left to right through the muscle mass at the top of the septum.

The wave of depolarization spreads via the Purkinje fibers through the endocardial surface of both right and left ventricles. The endocardial surface becomes negative relative to the epicardial surface (especially the left ventricle). The direction of the vector is from the AV node to the apex of the left ventricle. This is recorded as a large positive deflection called the R wave.

The S wave is a negative deflection which records the depolarization of the lateral wall of the ventricle. The plateau interval following is the period when all of the

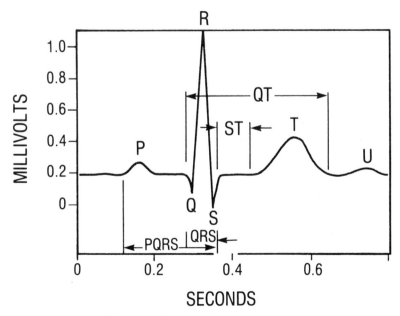

Fig. 8-7. Electrocardiogram conventions.

ventricle muscle cells are depolarized and no current is flowing.

The entire QT segement of the EKG records generation of the action potential and contraction in the ventricular muscle cells. The appearance of the T wave records ventricular repolarization.

ABNORMAL ELECTROCARDIOGRAMS

Premature atrial contractions involve stimulation of the AV node before the wave of depolarization gets through the entire atrium and are recorded as a shortened interval between the P wave and the QRS complex.

Atrial paroxysmal tachycardia (intermittent fast heart beat with atrial source) is indicated by a very close P wave and QRS complex. In AV nodal paroxymal tachycardia, the P wave occurs during the QRS complex. In ventricular paroxymal tachycardia, the QRS wave is inverted. There is no P wave.

In atrial fibrillation, the muscle cells of the atria are not contracting together. There is no organized P wave and no regular rhythm for the QRS complex. However, the heart will continue to pump.

In ventricular fibrillation, the heart stops working and there are no organized QRS or P waves.

Heart block usually occurs in the AV nodal area. In first degreee block, there is a delay between the P wave and QRS complex. Second degree heart block involves delay extended to the point where only a portion of the P waves gets through to produce the QRS complex (with two P waves for each QRS). In third degree heart block, the atria and ventricles beat independently

THE CARDIAC CYCLE

The heart functions to transfer blood from the low pressure venous system (mean pressure 1 mm Hg) to the high pressure arterial system (mean pressure 100 mm Hg). Cardiovascular flow depends on a pressure gradient to overcome resistance. The heart develops a left ventricular peak pressure of about 120 mm Hg as opposed to a right heart peak pressure of about 25 mm Hg. The arterial pressure generated is dissipated to energize flow from one system to the other.

Cycle Phases

The cardiac cycle is the orderly sequence of pressure changes and flow in the four heart pumps and in the blood vessels. The five phase cycle begins in late diastole, followed by atrial systole, ventricular contraction (isovolumetric), ventricular ejection, and ventricular relaxation (isovolumetric).

In late diastole, the atria and ventricles are relaxed.

The mitral and tricuspid valves between the two chambers are open and the aortic and pulmonary valves are closed. Venous blood is flowing into the heart throughout diastole through the atria to the ventricles via a pressure gradient. In later diastole, pressures in the right atrium and right ventricle equalize ($\sim$0 mm Hg) but there is higher pressure in the pulmonary artery ($\sim$11 mm Hg at the end of diastole). In the left heart, blood is returning from the pulmonary veins to the left atrium and into the left ventricle. The pressure in the aorta at this time is about 80 mm Hg. At this stage in late diastole, when the ventricle is relaxed, the pulmonary and aortic valves support pressure in the pulmonary artery and aorta, respectively. This is the afterload, the load that cardiac muscle senses only when it begins to contract.

In atrial systole, the P wave of the EKG represents initiation of atrial depolarization, which is shortly followed by atrial contraction. The atrial pressure increases 3–4 mm Hg and results in an additional flow of blood into the ventricle, raising the ventricular pressure.

Isovolumetric ventricular contraction then occurs. The QRS complex occurs after atrial contraction and represents ventricular deporlarization. Ventricular contraction initiates shortly thereafter (near the end of the R wave of the EKG). Because aortic and pulmonary pressures are so much higher than pressure in the ventricles at the beginning of contraction, initial ventricular contraction is isovolumetric and does not result in ejection of blood from the ventricles (the sarcomeres contract and stretch the series elastic elements in the muscle, but the muscle itself does not shorten). The force of developing ventricular contraction is exerted on the blood, and ventricular pressure increases to meet the afterload, until the aortic and pulmonary pressures are exceeded. At this point ($\sim$80 mm Hg in the aorta), the aortic and pulmonary valves open.

In the ventricular ejection phase, there is rapid ejection of blood into the arterial system as ventricular contraction continues to develop pressure. Aortic pressure increases as the wall of the aorta bulges from incoming blood and peaks at about 120 mm Hg. When the ventricles have ejected about 50 percent of their volume, the pressure drops in the ventricles, aorta, and pulmonary arteries, and the aortic and pulmonary valves close.

In the right heart (the low pressure side), as the pulmonary valve opens, the ventricle ejects fluid until peak pressure is reached at about 25 mm Hg.

There is rapid flow in both aorta and pulmonary arteries early in systole. The rate is much faster in the aorta because of higher pressure in the left ventricle. This period of ejection is the plateau stage in the action potential of the ventricle and is important in pump function. The duration of the action potential maintains contraction so that the ventricle has time to eject fluid into the aorta.

Isovolumetric ventricular relaxation is indicated by the T wave on the EKG which signals the repolarization of the ventricles. Pressure drops rapidly as the ventricles relax. When left and right ventricular pressures get below aortic and pulmonary pressure, respectively, the aortic and pulmonary valves close. Valve closure occurs because of the tendency of blood to back flow into the ventricles. As the valves stop the momentum of backflow, a slight rise in aortic pressure results (the dicrotic notch in aortic pressure tracings). There is no volume change in the ventricles until the pressure drops below the respective atrial pressures (isovolumetric relaxation). All valves are closed.

In early diastole, ventricular pressures fall below atrial pressures, creating a small pressure gradient. The atrioventricular valves open and the ventricles begin to refill rapidly. The ventricles are about two-thirds full when the atria contract.

With a normal heart rate of about 75 beats per minute, the complete cardiac cycle occurs in about 0.8 s. Ventricular systole takes about 0.3 s; ventricular diastole, about 0.5 s. Diastole shortens as the heart rate increases. The total ventricular volume is normally about 130 ml. During contraction the ejection volume (i.e., the stroke volume per beat) is about 70 ml. The ventricles never empty completely, and the normal reserve volume at the end of systole is about 60 ml.

Heart Sounds

Two heart sounds which occur at the beginning and end of ventricular systole, respectively, can be heard with the stethoscope. The first heart sound (S1, lubb) is caused by the closure of mitral and tricuspid valves as the ventricles begin to contract. Opening of the aortic and pulmonary valves also occurs at this time. This sound is caused by the vibrations resulting from the closing of the valves and the rapid rush of blood. The second heart sound (S2, dupp) occurs at the end of ventricular systole and is caused by closure of aortic and pulmonary valves. Opening of the atrioventricular valves also occurs at this time. Sound 3 is caused by turbulence as blood rushes from the atria into the ventricles when ventricular pressure is very low. This sound is normally not audible but can be electronically recorded. Sound 4 is caused by turbulent vibrations as the atria contract and blood is ejected from the atria into the ventricles. This sound is sometimes heard immediately before the first sound.

Factors Regulating Cardiac Output

Cardiac output is the output of the heart per unit of time. The stroke volume (i.e., the amount of blood pumped out of the ventricles per beat) is about 70 ml. The cardiac output averages about 5.0 L/min (70 ml ×

69 beats/min). Factors controlling the cardiac output include the heart rate, stroke volume, intrinsic preload and afterload factors, and contractility.

The cardiac rate and stroke volume are controlled by antagonistic sympathetic and parasympathetic influences. The inhibitory action of acetylcholine is termed a negative chronotropic action. The action of norepinephrine to increase contractility is termed a positive inotropic effect. Stroke volume varies also with the length of the muscle fibers, an effect independent of sympathetic innervation.

INTRINSIC CONTROL OF CARDIAC OUTPUT

Preloading and afterloading are internal mechanisms which control the force of cardiac contraction. Preload is the extent to which the myocardium is stretched before contraction. The afterload is the resistance the blood meets when it is expelled.

The Starling law of the heart describes the length-tension relationship in cardiac muscle. According to this law the following occurs:

1. Within limits the heart will intrinsically adjust to and pump out all blood returned to it by the venous system.
2. With increased venous return, the heart will adjust and pump the extra blood back into the arterial side of the circulation.
3. If the arteriole pressure drops, the heart will adjust the force of contraction to maintain stroke volume against the higher afterload (higher resistance to pumping).

The force of cardiac muscle contraction is proportional to the initial length and tension of the fiber. Since direct measurements of length and tension are impractical, related volume/pressure relationships are useful in this area. Pressure is related to tension by the Laplace law: $T = Pr/2h$ (P = ventricular pressure; r = radius of ventricle cavity; h = thickness of ventricle muscle). Volume is directly proportional to length as defined in the relationship: $V \sim 1$ (1 = initial fiber length; v = ventricular volume).

Initial fiber length is determined by the end diastolic ventricular (preload) volume (EDVV). Ventricular function, as represented by cardiac output, stroke volume, etc., increases with longer initial fiber length. EDVV determinants include preload and afterload considerations. Ventricular filling pressure is set by both the pressure of blood entering the ventricle and the atrial contraction pressure. These determine the end diastolic ventricular pressure (EDVP) which determines EDVV and thus initial fiber length.

Small pressure changes cause great volume changes. If ventricular volume increases, subsequent contraction will be more forceful and caridac output greater.

Other factors which influence EDVV include the duration of diastole, ventricular compliance (distensibility), and afterload. The ventricular volume can be decreased by short diastoles (shorter filling times), which reduce preload. The ventricular compliance, the ease with which the ventricle can be stretched, can compromise cardiac output since stiff ventricle muscles require greater filling pressures to increase volume. An increase in the arterial end diastolic (afterload) pressure effects cardiac output for only the first few heartbeats as stroke volume decreases and EDVV goes up. Thereafter the heart contracts more forcefully to maintain the cardiac output. Other important factors influencing afterload adaptation are total blood volume, venous tone, intrathoracic pressure, and contraction of skeletal muscle on the vasculature.

EXTRINSIC CONTROL OF CARDIAC OUTPUT

A change in contractility for any ventricular volume will produce corresponding changes in other cardiac parameters such as stroke volume, peak pressure, etc., without a change in preload. Therefore, extrinsic control is independent of preload and consequently of the Starling law. The sympathetic nervous system, via norepinephrine, is the major control of contractility. The frequency of action potentials in the sympathetic nerves to the heart is regulated by aortic pressure that is perceived by aortic arch and carotid sinus pressoreceptors. Norepinephrine release stimulates the pacemaker, increases heart rate, and increases contractility. As the rate increases, the diastolic period is shortened, with less time for Ca^{++} to be sequestered by the sacroplasmic reticulum. Thus, free Ca^{++} build-up leads to overall increase in Ca^{++} bound to troponin C. Contractility can be depressed artificially by β-blockers and Ca^{++} blockers which inhibit slow Na^+/Ca^{++} channels. Parasympathetic nervous control also produces cholinergic depression of the contractility of the atria, but has no effect on the ventricles.

Measurements of contractility must be made under constant preload, afterload, and heart rate. These measurements are used to construct ventricular function curves.

Studies of muscle mechanics are also used to measure contractility. An increase in preload will cause cardiac muscle to develop a much greater maximum tension. The velocity of contraction at any given preload is inversely proportional to the afterload. If these measurements are extrapolated to zero load, the maximum velocity of contraction is obtained and can serve as an index of contractility.

The pressure-volume loop is another method of measuring contractility (Fig. 8-8). This diagram illustrates changes in ventricular volume and pressure over the entire cardiac cycle. The loop begins in the lower left corner. At this point, atrial contraction forces the mitral valve open, leading to an increase in ventricular volume, with very little pressure change. As the mitral valve closes systole begins. As ventricular pressure builds all valves are closed so there is no change in ventricular volume (isovolumic contraction). When the pressure in the ventricle exceeds the pressure in the aorta, the aortic valve opens the blood is ejected. Thus, ventricular volume drops while the pressure increases slightly due to the resistance against the fluid ejection. The aortic valve closes. Ventricular volume remains constant while ventricular pressure falls (isovolumic relaxation).

If the aorta is clamped, the subsequent contraction of the ventricle will be isovolumic. A greater volume results in a greater pressure when the ventricle contracts. Pressure-volume relationships can be plotted to obtain an isovolumic pressure line (IVL). All movements along this line can be explained according to the Starling law. Increased volume stretches the muscle fibers and leads to a greater force of contraction proportionate to greater pressure.

Addition of norepinephrine to a system increases contractility and generates a new IVL. For a given initial volume, an increase in the end diastolic volume after constant load generates a new loop. However, when the loop reaches the point of aortic valve closure, this point will coincide with the original IVL.

If the afterload is changed, the ventricular pressure required to eject blood will also change. For example, increasing the aortic pressure (afterload), increases ventricular pressure. However, the end of the eject phase still falls on the same IVL.

Heart Failure

Cardiac pathology (ischemia, thrombosis, etc.) leads to a decline in contractility. For any given left ventricular diastolic volume, the cardiac output of the ischemic heart is lower than that of the normal heart. The heart attempts to compensate for the reduced cardiac output by increasing the stroke volume (i.e., increasing left ventricular volume) and thereby working harder.

According to Laplace's law, when the ventricular volume increases, the ventricle stretches and its radius is increased. In order to maintain pressure and cardiac output in an ischemic heart (and not burst), the wall tension must also increase, requiring a higher O_2 consumption. By attempting to increase cardiac output, the damaged heart creates a self-defeating need for greater O_2 consumption. Therapy involves alteration of the contractility of the damaged heart to produce a more

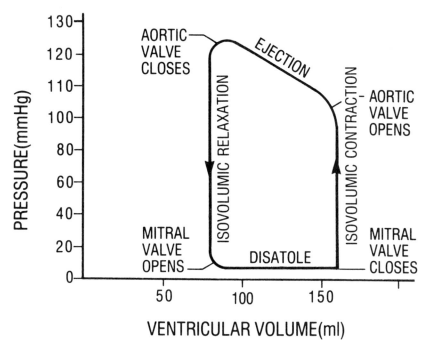

Fig. 8-8. Pressure-volume loop.

normal ventricular function curve where pressure and O_2 consumption are lower.

EFFECTS OF BODY POSITION, EXERCISE

Body position effects ventricular volume. Reclining causes greater venous return, resulting in greater filling of ventricles and high ventricular volume. Standing causes less venous return with diminished ventricular volume due to pooling of blood in the extemities.

Exercise stimulates the sympathetic nervous system with release of norepinephrine mediating an increase in contractility. Cardiac output rises, primarily as a result of increases in heart rate and contractility.

Energy Metabolism of Heart Muscle

The energy requirements of cardiac muscle are enormous. There is a 6–7 percent ATP turnover per contraction. Myocardial energy metabolism is totally dependent on oxidative production of ATP and the heart extracts about 70 percent of arterial oxygen for this task. The major substrates used are fatty acids, glucose, and lactate. Free fatty acids are the primary energy source, are preferred over glucose, and account for about 70 percent of the oxidative substrate. The remainder is chiefly glucose (15–20 percent) and lactate (15–20 percent). An adequate supply of free fatty acids actually suppresses glucose utilization by blockage of glucose transport and inhibition of key enzymes in glucose metabolism. An-

aerobic sources of ATP (glycolysis) account for only 1–3 percent of ATP requirements. Pyruvate, ketone bodies, and amino acids are substrates of minor importance.

Because lipids cannot be anaerobically metabolized, oxygen deficit produces a rapid decrease in cardiac function. Free fatty acids are transported in the blood as lipoprotein. The cardiac muscle cell transports fatty acids across the cell membrane and activates them to acyl CoA derivatives for transport across the mitochondrial membrane by the acylcarnitine mechanism. In the mitochondria, fatty acids are degraded by β-oxidation to regenerate ATP via oxidative phosphorylation in the respiratory chain. Fatty acids are oxidized completely to CO_2 and H_2O.

MYOCARDIAL OXYGEN CONSUMPTION

The rate of ATP hydrolysis by muscle contraction is determined by the force generated by sarcomere shortening and the rate at which actin-myosin cross-bridges form. For the intact heart, the major determinants of oxygen consumption are wall tension and heart rate. Contractility and fiber shortening have less influence on oxygen consumption.

CARDIAC EFFICIENCY

The heart performs useful work in imparting potential and kinetic energy to the blood during the ejection phase of systole. The energy which must be expended to maintain the vitality of cardiac muscle cells as well as the heat liberated from friction, etc. is wasted energy. The quantity of wasted energy exceeds the useful work about four-fold. The efficiency of myocardial contraction (useful work/total energy release) varies considerably, but averages about 23 percent.

OXYGEN EXTRACTION: CONTROL OF CARDIAC BLOOD FLOW

Cardiac muscle extracts the largest percent (~ 70) of arterial oxygen of any tissue. Oxygen consumption cannot be increased by increased extraction. Fortunately, the normal heart has a large reserve capacity to increase its coronary flow and oxygen delivery to cardiac tissue. The major control of coronary flow is mediated by local metabolic autoregulation. Most coronary flow occurs during diastole when the external pressure on the vascular bed due to myocardial contraction is absent. Adenosine appears to be very important in this control. Arterial oxygen content plays a role as well as the autonomic nervous system which influences demand for oxygen by affecting myocardial contraction. In addition, autonomic control produces some adrenergic vasoconstriction or cholinergic vasodilation.

THE SYSTEMIC CIRCULATION

From the left ventricle the heart pumps blood through the arteries, which branch to the arterioles which feed the capillary beds. Blood drains from the capillaries into venules, which merge into larger veins for return to the right atrium. The right ventricle pumps blood into the pulmonary circulation for oxygenation and removal of CO_2. Freshly oxygenated blood is returned to the left atrium, flowing into the left ventricle to repeat the cycle. The lymphatics return excess tissue fluids and drain via the thoracic duct and right lymphatic duct into the venous system.

Mechanics of Blood Flow

Blood flows through all parts of the system with ease except for the arterioles where the major resistance to blood flow occurs. Flow is normally laminar in nature as planes of fluid flow over one another with the greatest velocity in the center of the vessel. Viscosity increases resistance to flow and depends chiefly on the hematocrit (i.e., the percentage of red cells per volume of blood). Velocity and temperature also influence viscosity (inversely). In the blood vessels, red cells tend to accumulate in the center of the blood stream so that blood at the vessel sides has a lower hematocrit. As vessels branch, a

process of "plasma skimming" occurs in which a disproportionate amount of side blood enters the branching vessels, resulting in a lower hematocrit.

The factors which influence laminar blood flow in a vessel are expressed mathematically by Poiseuille's law

$$F = \Delta P \times \tfrac{1}{8} \times 1/n \times \pi r^4/L$$

where F = flow, n = viscosity, P = pressure drop, and L = length.

Poiseuille's law illustrates the opposing forces which influence flow. Flow is directly related to the pressure (pressure causes flow) and the radius. If the radius is doubled, flow is increased by a factor of 16. However, pressure in a vessel is related to the difference between the height of the column of fluid at various points. As flow proceeds along the vessel, the pressure drops. While flow is the same everywhere in a vessel, a longer vessel has a greater pressure change as a driving force. If a vessel is constricted, the pressure no longer drops at a uniform rate. In a compliant system, increased pressure causes increased vessel radius. Sympathetic innervation also affects blood flow. The vascular bed can be constricted by sympathetic stimulation or dilated by removal of the stimulus, altering the flow pressure curve.

The rate of flow can become high enough to produce turbulence at the critical velocity at which eddy currents develop. This happens normally only during the phase of most rapid ejection into the aorta.

The factors of pressure and flow interact to produce a stable vessel diameter. The total energy of blood flowing in a vessel equals the sum of the kinetic energy of flow and the pressure and is a constant (Bernoulli's principle). According to this principle, the greater the velocity of flow in a vessel, the less the lateral pressure on distending walls. When a vessel is narrowed in diseased states, the velocity of flow increases and the distending pressure is reduced on the sides of the vessel so that the vessel diameter can narrow further to the point of collapse.

Venous Flow

In going from arteries to veins, there is a large increase in the cross-sectional area at the capillaries. The velocity decreases dramatically because of the large number of individual branches in parallel.

The venous system is a low pressure system with a fast rate of flow and tendency to collapse easily. The pressure drops from 12–18 mm Hg in the venules to only about 5.5 mm Hg in the large veins. While venous blood flow is aided by the pumping action of the heart, the negative intrathoracic pressure during inspiration as well as the contractions of skeletal muscle to compress the veins have a pumplike action to effect venous return. The hydrostatic pressure of blood can become a problem in the veins. Quiet standing, for example, will cause pooling of blood in the legs.

Peripheral Vascular Control

Systemic arterial pressure and blood flow are determined by the relationship between caridac output and peripheral resistance as is illustrated by the following equation:

$$\text{Cardiac output (flow)} = \frac{P\left(\begin{array}{c}\text{mean}\\\text{arterial}\end{array}\right) - P\left(\begin{array}{c}\text{right}\\\text{atrial}\end{array}\right)}{\text{TPR (total peripheral resistance)}}$$

The total peripheral resistance (TPR) is the important factor in overall control of blood flow. The hydrostatic pressure head is normally 120/80 mm Hg and does not drop below 60/40 mm Hg. The mean arterial pressure (100/60 mm Hg) is maintained within narrow limits both at rest and during activity. Cardiac output is continuously adjusted to compensate for changes in peripheral resistance which adjust the flow of blood to tissue requirements. Changes in resistance to flow occur throughout the vascular system but are greatest in the arterioles. Changes in TPR are due mainly to small arteriole dilation or constriction.

Cardiac output is determined by the product of heart rate and stroke volume. Since the left ventricle does not always fill or empty completely, stroke volume can be regarded as the difference between diastolic and systolic ventricular volumes. Stroke volume is influenced by the ventricular filling pressure which depends on the total volume of the blood and the distensibility (compliance) of ventricular walls.

Blood flow per unit time is determined by the pressure gradient from the arteries to the veins and the resistance of the vascular bed as controlled by constriction in the smaller branches.

REGULATION OF BLOOD VOLUME

The mean arterial volume is dependent on the total blood volume in the cardiovascular system, the venous capacity, the total peripheral resistance, and the effectiveness of the heart as a pump. Sympathetic stimulation of the venous circulation, which serves as a reservoir for blood, causes venoconstriction, redistributing blood to the arterial side. An increase in total peripheral resistance essentially "holds" blood on the arterial side.

REGULATION OF BLOOD FLOW

The peripheral circulation is controlled by a number of mechanisms (local, neural, and humoral) which effect smooth muscle contraction or relaxation primarily at the level of the arterioles.

Local Factors. Vasodilation occurs primarily at the local level. The oxygen demand theory postulates a negative feedback mechanism in which precapillary sphincters respond to increased tissue oxygen tension by constriction. The vasodilator theory suggests that end products of metabolism (CO_2, lactic acid, adenosine, K^+, etc.) play a feedback role to cause precapillary sphincter dilation. There is evidence to support both these theories.

Autoregulation is a special aspect of local control in which flow rate is correlated with mean arterial pressure. Over the autoregulatory range, pressure changes result in little or no change in flow rate. However, at the autoregulatory breakthrough point (above the autoregulatory range) flow depends directly on pressure. Below the autoregulatory range, flow is again pressure dependent. Autoregulation helps to maintain a constant flow over a fairly wide range of pressures.

Autonomic Regulation. The autonomic nervous system exerts overall coordination by rapid, simultaneous control of large portions of the circulatory system. Both sympathetic and parasympathetic fibers terminate on vascular smooth muscle in large and small arteries (secondary control) and in arterioles and precapillary sphincters (primary control). The venules and veins (reservoir system) are also subject to autonomic influences.

Vasoconstriction (tone) is accomplished by increased sympathetic stimulation of the α-adrenergic smooth muscle receptors via norepinephrine. In the normal state, resting sympathetic tone exists when some of the receptors are stimulated, producing a partial vasoconstriction. If α-adrenergic receptors are blocked, 1-epinephrine produces vasodilation, presumably by acting on β-adrenergic receptors. Many tissues have both α- and β-adrenergic receptors so that a response of vasodilation or vasoconstriction depends on the ratio of the receptors and receptor sensitivity. The parasympathetic system also produces vasodilation via acetylcholine.

Humoral Agents. Other humoral vasoactive agents include angiotensin II, the most powerful vasoconstrictor known, vasopressin, which also produces vasoconstriction to decrease blood flow, and histamine, which is released during tissue injury or an antigen-antibody reaction to produce vasodilation and increased blood flow. Angiotensin production from plasma precursors is initiated by the release of renin by the kidney in response to decreased blood pressure.

REGULATION OF BLOOD PRESSURE

When resistance changes, the mean arterial pressure is held fairly constant by two broad classes of pressure regulatory mechanisms. A rapid control mechanism consists of nervous and hormonal mechanisms, some of which are identical to those involved with regulation of blood flow (angiotensin, etc.). Slow regulation is related to kidney function and blood volume, involving pressure-volume relationships.

Neural Mechanisms. Baroreceptors are found in most large arteries and are highly concentrated at the bifurcation of the common cartoid artery and the aortic arch. These receptors are directly sensitive to stretch rather than pressure. An increase in blood volume causes a pressure increase which stretches the arterial wall. The baroreceptors sense the increased stretch and send impulses to the medulla via Hering's nerve and the glossopharyngeal nerve. The medullary response can result in (1) excitement of the cardioinhibitory center which increases vagal stimulation to decrease heart rate and blood presure and (2) inhibition of the vasomotor center which leads to vasodilation, decreasing contractility as well as heart rate and ultimately blood pressure.

The baroreceptors are extremely sensitive and discharge is rapid in response to changes in blood pressure. During systole, baroreceptor firing increases, while diastole decreases discharge. The system is not only sensitive to the absolute blood pressure value, but also to the status of the blood pressure. If the blood pressure is 150 mm Hg and increasing, receptor discharge is greater than that for a constant blood pressure of 150 mm Hg. If the blood pressure is 150 mm Hg and falling, receptor discharge is less than that for a constant pressure.

The system adapts over a period of time. An initial increase in blood pressure effects increased baroreceptor discharge. However, after a period of time, the receptor discharge rate tends to return to the original level. In hypertension, the blood pressure increases chronically and the baroreceptors will respond in time by escaping to their normal discharge rate. Essentially, new set points for the baroreceptors are established. This system also adapts to hypotension and therefore is not effective in long range regulation of blood pressure.

The frequency of baroreceptor impulses is greatest over the normal mean arterial pressure range so that greatest sensitivity to changes in blood pressure occurs over this range. This allows for tight regulation of blood pressure since a very slight change in blood pressure will elicit a response.

CNS Ischemic Response. The medullary vasomotor center is stimulated by increased arterial CO_2 tension to produce a powerful vasoconstriction effecting increased venous return and cardiac output. The mechanism of this response appears to be sensitive to increased H^+ of the cerebrospinal fluid caused by hydration of CO_2 to H_2CO_3 and subsequent dissociation of the acid.

Chemoreceptors. Located near the baroreceptors in the carotid bifurcation, chemoreceptors are sensitive to decreases in O_2 tension and increases in CO_2 tension and H^+ concentration. This is not a functionally powerful reflex since the oxygen tension seldom gets low enough to increase the rate of afferent firing.

Low Pressure Receptors. Located on the venous side of the circulation, low pressure receptors respond in a manner similar to the baroreceptors of the arterial side. These receptors respond to changes in pressure in both atria and the pulmonary arteries.

Specific Hormonal Mechanisms. The epinephrine-norepinephrine mechanism discussed in the regulation of blood flow acts via vasoconstricton and ultimately leads to an increase in blood pressure.

The renin-angiotensin II mechanism is initiated by the release of renin in response to decreased blood pressure. Correction is by vasoconstriction, leading to elevation of pressure. Although not as fast acting as neural mechanisms, this is a rapid system which has a long term effect on blood volume, which influences blood pressure.

Vasopressin also acts rapidly to produce vasoconstriction, leading to increased blood pressure. This is a fairly rapid mechanism with the same long-term effect as the renin-angiotensin II mechanism.

In summary, the rapid acting systems for blood pressure regulation exhibit a time course over a period of seconds or minutes. They are not efficient over the long-term since they tend to adapt over a period of time, but are important short-term regulators.

The long acting systems exhibit a time course over a period of hours to days to produce lasting long-term changes in blood pressure. Long-term regulation is accompanied by renal retention of water and electrolytes, with decreased urinary output. The accompanying increase in blood volume increases venous return and cardiac output, so that ultimately blood pressure increases.

The Microcirculation

The cardiovascular system serves as a conduit for transport of oxygen, nutrients, and regulatory metabolites to the tissues and removal of waste products and export metabolites. The microcirculation is the essence of the system, the site of exchange. While only 5 percent of the total blood volume is in the capillaries, they permeate every tissue and are rarely more than 0.1 mm from any cell. Capillary length averages about 500 μm, with a diameter of about 6 μm, sufficient for a single red blood cell to squeeze through. Transit time in the capillary bed is about 1 s with 500 μm/s velocity. The capillaries have the greatest cross-sectional area of any part of the vascular system, about 2,000 cm^2, with a surface area of about 700,000 cm^2.

The microcirculation consists of the arterioles, capillaries, and venules. Tissue demands vary greatly and blood flow is controlled via precapillary constriction or dilation. Resting muscle, for example, may have 90 percent of the capillaries closed and only 10 percent open. In vigorous exercise, muscle capillaries may be completely dilated, and splanchnic capillaries may constrict to provide more blood to skeletal muscle.

Blood flow in the arterioles may travel through three pathways as follows:

1. Blood may supply a capillary bed. Arterioles may branch into metarterioles which terminate in precapillary sphincters. The walls of these structures contain smooth muscle and are innervated with sympathetic fibers. The precapillary sphincters are control points to the true capillary beds, the actual site of exchange, which drain into venules.
2. Blood flow may bypass the capillary bed via a thoroughfare channel. The arteriole will join a metarteriole, but at the sphincter blood will be routed via a preferential channel directly to the venule.
3. Blood may be shunted via AV anastomoses directly to the venules. AV anastamoses are short channels that act as direct conduits from arterioles to venules and are regulated by sphincters.

The capillary bed is an ideal exchange area, possessing the requisites for maximum rates (i.e., high surface area, an ultrathin barrier, and regulated flow). The capillaries present about 400 m^2 of surface area, which increases with vasodilation to modulate the total ability to exchange metabolites. The barrier thins in progressing from arterioles to true capillaries. The arterioles, metarterioles, and sphincters function as resistance vessels, strengthened for vasomotor control, with relatively thick walls containing muscle fibers, elastin, and collagen. Regulation is neural, hormonal, and chemical. True capillaries, the exchange vessels, have a high surface area/volume ratio, with absence of muscle, elastin, or collagen and ultrathin endothelial walls for rapid exchange. The collecting vessels, the venules, have a high volume/surface area and are larger vessels, with thin walls containing a little muscle and connective tissue. The venules and veins are distensible and serve as reservoirs for blood.

CAPILLARY TYPES

The endothelial type capillary consists of single epithelial layer wall architecture with continuous tight junctions which act as permeability barriers. Exchange occurs through tight junctions, which are attached to tissue by a basement membrane. This type is found in skeletal muscle, heart, skin, CNS, and adipose tissue. The fenestrated capillary possesses pores about 0.1 μm in diameter through which exchange occurs and which are closed by a thin diaphragm. The discontinuous type capillary exhibits larger holes between cells and is found in bone marrow, liver, and spleen.

EXCHANGE MECHANISMS: DIFFUSION

Materials are exchanged by diffusion in response to concentration gradients. The rate of diffusion is directly related to the product of the permeability factor and the difference between blood and tissue concentrations.

$$D = CPF \times (C_B - C_T)$$

The capillary permeability factor (CPF) is dependent on the thickness of the capillary wall and the solubility and the molecular weight of the solute (permeability decreases with increasing molecule weight). For small molecules (glucose, water, etc.), exchange (not net movement) is limited by perfusion not diffusion since diffusion occurs very rapidly. For molecules in a range of about 10,000 MW, diffusion becomes the rate limiting step. For molecules above 50,000 MW, such as albumin, exchange is restricted by diffusion. The capillary membrane acts as a dialyzing membrane, permitting small molecules and ions (crystalloid substances) to diffuse freely, but restraining macromolecules and cells. While the cell membrane is selectively permeable to small ions (K^+, Na^+, etc.), the capillary wall is not.

PINOCYTOSIS

The endothelial cell can form a pinocytic vesicle around material in the blood. This pinosome may migrate through the cell wall to either the blood or tissue side. Pinosomes are utilized to transfer large materials, such as immunoglobulins.

FILTRATION

Net filtration (F) is determined by the balance between the effective capillary pressure ($P_c - P_t$) and the effective osmotic pressure ($\pi_c - \pi_t$), and the capacity filtration coefficient (CFC), which depends on the specific properties of the capillary bed. Starling's law summarizes this relationship.

$$F = CFC[(P_c - P_t) - (\pi_c - \pi_t)]$$

The capillary hydrostatic pressure (P_c) is normally 17–25 mm Hg, a force which pushes fluid out of the capillary. The tissue hydrostatic pressure (P_t) is about -6 mm Hg and tends to pull fluid from the capillary. The capillary colloidal osmotic (oncotic) pressure is about 28 mm Hg and is a force which pulls fluid into the capillary. The tissue oncotic pressure (~ 5 mm Hg) is an opposing force pulling fluid into the tissue.

Capillary pressure may be measured directly by cannulating the capillary. Tissue oncotic pressure can be measured by means of a porous sphere implant. The oncotic pressure is caused by nondiffusible macromolecules (proteins). The oncotic pressure may be calculated from the amount of protein in the capillary fluid or interstial fluid (ISF) (7.3 g/100 ml plasma; 1.8 g/100 ml ISF).

The Donnan effect causes osmotic pressure to be greater than expected because proteins are anions which attract cations. Since the osmotic effect is dependent on the number of particles in solution, a high molecular weight substance, such as β-globulin has fewer molecules/100 g than a lower molecular weight substance, such as albumin. Thus, globulins exert less osmotic pressure than albumin when both are present in equal concentrations (g/100 ml). The normal plasma osmotic pressure is the sum of the pressure exerted by all proteins present.

If the effective capillary pressure equals the effective osmotic pressure there is no net exchange of material across the capillary. The effective capillary pressure changes as the capillary is traversed due to changes in pressure. At the arteriole end there is filtration because the effective hydrostatic pressure (P_c) is greater than the effective osmotic pressure. At the venous end there is reabsorption because the effective hydrostatic pressure is less than the effective osmotic pressure. Other variables remain the same.

Pressures differ in various capillary beds. In the lung, for example, capillary pressure is ~ 7 mm Hg, lower than in the systemic circulation. Such capillaries allow protein to pass through their walls, increasing the tissue osmotic pressure. In the kidney, capillary pressure is ~ 60 mm Hg, providing a powerful driving force for glomerular filtration.

The volume of tissue fluid is controlled by the balance between reabsorption and filtration. Normally, these parameters are equal but various factors can cause change.

Increased protein in the ISF increases osmotic pressure and can interfere with fluid return. Increased hydrostatic pressure favors net filtration and reduces reabsorption. Both can result in the edema characteristic of excess interstitial fluid.

PART 3

Respiratory Physiology

The task of delivering oxygen to the mitochondria and removing carbon dioxide produced by metabolism is one of unbelievable magnitude. Gas exchange across the blood gas barrier is the primary function of the lungs in the process of external respiration. The conducting airway (trachea, bronchi, and bronchioles) is anatomic "dead space" in which gas exchange does not occur. The conducting zone branches until bronchioles terminate in the alveolar ducts and alveoli, the bubblelike air sacs which form the respiratory zone. Here gases are exchanged across alveolar and capillary membranes. The pulmonary capillaries form a dense network around the alveolar walls, a moving film of blood in ultrathin vessels the diameter of a single red blood cell. About three hundred million alveoli are packed into an area which extends only about 5 mm distal to the terminal bronchioles. The alveoli present a surface area of 70 m², with 70 ml of blood traversing the pulmonary capillaries at any given moment. Diffusion of gases takes place very rapidly because of the thin endothelial barrier (0.5 mm) and large area. Ventilation and perfusion must be matched for sufficient gas exchange to occur. There is a 1:1 ratio between alveolar ventilation and pulmonary blood flow under normal conditions (cardiac output, 5.0 L/min; alveolar ventilation, 5.25 L/min.)

INTRAPLEURAL PRESSURE

The lungs lie free in the thoracic cavity in a pleural space bounded by the visceral pleural membrane (in contact with the lungs) which is normally in contact with the parietal pleural membrane (in contact with the chest wall). The pressure in the potential intrapleural space is negative (below atmospheric). Both the chest cavity wall and the lung itself are structures with elastic properties. At rest, the elastic recoil of the lungs tends to pull the chest wall inward against the opposing force of the chest wall tending to pull the lungs outward. The retracting force of the lungs on the chest wall is the basis of the negative pressure in the intrapleural space. Introduction of air into the intrapleural space (pneumothorax) increases pressure causing immediate collapse of the lungs (atelectasis).

The Gas Laws

THE IDEAL GAS LAW

The behavior of lung gases is governed by the physical principles embodied in the gas laws. Boyle's law states that gases are compressed in response to an increase in pressure (P) and expand when pressure is decreased (Volume $\propto 1/P$, temperature constant). Charles' law states a direct relationship of volume and absolute temperature, when pressure remains constant ($V \propto T$, °K) The ideal gas law combines both Boyle's and Charles' laws ($V \propto nRT/P$) where n is the number of moles, R the gas constant, and T the absolute temperature.

DALTON'S LAW OF PARTIAL PRESSURES

Inspired air is a mixture of gases (20.98 percent O_2, 78.06 percent N_2, 0.04 percent CO_2 with trace amounts of rare gases. The character of lung air changes as O_2 is exchanged for CO_2 in the alveoli. Lung gas may also contain traces of the intestinal gas methane and alcohol or acetone if these are present in the blood. Each gas behaves independently exerting the same pressure that it would if present alone. The total pressure of a mixture of gases is equal to the sum of the partial pressures, p, of the component gases. A statement of Dalton's law of partial pressures is $pA + pB + pC = ptotal$.

The partial pressure of a gas in solution, also described as the gas tension, is the partial pressure exerted by the dissolved gas in equilibrium in solution.

HENRY'S LAW

Gases have characteristic solubilities in water at a given temperature. Henry's law states that the concentration of a gas in solution at equilibrium is directly proportional to the partial pressure of the gas phase (i.e. [Gas]aq $\propto$ pGas). Thus the solubility of gases in the body fluids increases with pressure as described by Henry's law.

GRAHAM'S LAW OF DIFFUSION

Graham's law states that in the gas phase, at a given temperature and pressure, the rate of diffusion of a gas is inversely proportional to the square root of its molecular weight: $D \propto 1/\sqrt{MW}$. The use of low molecular weight helium to replace nitrogen in helium/oxygen breathing mixtures is an application of Graham's law.

In the liquid phase, the rate of diffusion of a gas is also related to solubility, so that the gas diffusion constant (permeability coefficient) is derived as $D \propto Sol/\sqrt{MW}$.

FICK'S LAW

Fick's law describes the rate of diffusion of a gas through a tissue slice as proportional to the area (A) and thickness (T) of the tissue, the diffusion constant of the gas, and the partial pressures of the gas on opposing sides of the tissue:

$$V_{gas} \propto \frac{A}{T} D(P_1 - P_2)$$

The Mechanics of Breathing

The flow of air in and out of the lungs is a mechanical process accomplished by the contraction and relaxation of the diaphragm and intercostal muscles. Contraction expands the thorax, making alveolar pressure less than atmospheric pressure. Lung inflation occurs as air flows into the lungs in response to this gradient. In exhalation, the opposite events occur. The diaphragm and intercostals relax, increasing alveolar pressure so that atmospheric pressure is exceeded. Increased pressure of lung gas exceeds atmospheric pressure; long deflation occurs as lung gas is expelled. Thus, the activity of the respiratory muscles causes compression and distention of the lungs as gas pressure in the alveoli rises and falls.

At the start of normal inspiration, the intrapleural pressure is about −3 mm Hg, which decreases to about −6 mm Hg as the lungs further expand, pulling open the alveoli and ducts. Expiration is passive and is the result of the elastic recoil of the lungs and the thoracic cage when the muscles relax. During expiration the pressure becomes slightly positive, about 3 mm Hg, to compress the alveoli. The integration of the activity of the muscles of respiration is controlled by the respiratory center of the brain located in the lower medulla and influenced by apneustic (inspiratory) and pneumotaxic (deflationary) centers in the pons. The Hering-Breuer reflex is a regulator of lung inflation and deflation. Impulses, stimulated by lung stretch, are carried by vagal afferents to terminate inspiration (apneusis). As the lungs deflate, vagal afferent impulses are absent, leaving inspiratory neurons free to fire again. This relfex is of particular importance in infants and when tidal volumes become large as in exercise.

Lung Volumes

STATIC VOLUMES

The tidal volume (500 ml) is the air inhaled and exhaled during each normal breath. The volume of gas remaining in the lung after a normal expiration is called the functional residual capacity (3.0 L). The vital capacity (4.5 L) is the maximal amount of air which can be expelled from the lungs after a maximal inspiration followed by a maximal expiration and represents a pulmonary reserve. After maximal expiration, a residual volume (1.5 L) will remain in the lungs. This residual volume is the smallest volume to which the lung can be compressed voluntarily. Both tidal volume and vital capacity can be measured by means of a spirometer, while functional residual capacity and residual volume are measured indirectly by dilution techniques or a body plethysmograph. Other lung volumes of importance include the inspiratory capacity (3.0 L), which is the total lung capacity minus the functional residual capacity, the anatomic dead space, and alveolar volumes. The alveolar volume may be calculated from the tidal volume (500 ml) minus the dead space volume (150 ml) and is normally about 350 ml. The total lung capacity is about 6 L (vital capacity 4.5 L + residual volume 1.5 L). Each inhalation brings a volume of gas into the lungs that is less than 10 percent of the total lung capacity.

DYNAMIC (MINUTE) VOLUMES

Total ventilation is measured by the minute respiratory volume (i.e., the amount of tidal air moved out of the lungs each minute). A normal tidal volume of 500 ml $\times$ 15 breaths/min equals a minute volume of 3 L, the total minute ventilation. This includes the volume of the dead space unavailable for aeration as well as the gas volume of the alveolar space. The alveolar ventilation at 15 breaths/min $\times$ 350 ml is normally about 5.25 L/min. Increased rate and depth of respiration during stress can increase total ventilation 20 to 30 times the normal rate.

Compliance

Excised lung placed in a bell jar responds to a reduction in pressure by inflation. However, in deflation the volume at a given pressure is greater than that for infla-

tion, a phenomenon called hysteresis. Compliance of the lung is the relationship between volume and pressure changes and is a measure of the distensibility of the lung. Compliance is equal to the volume change in liters per unit pressure change in centimeters of water. Normal compliance is about 200 ml/cm water. Compliance decreases with inflation pressure (i.e., as the lung inflates a progressively greater force is required for a unit volume change). The closer to vertical the P/V curve, the more distensible the system; the more horizontal the curve, the stiffer the lung tissue. Fibrotic lung is less compliant, for example, than lung with deteriorating tissue as seen in emphysema. The specific compliance is the normal compliance adapted to the patient's size and age. Specific compliance should be approximately equivalent whether infant, child, or adult.

Elastic Properties of Lung

Other factors which influence the distensibility and stability of the lung are the elastic properties of lung tissue, mutual alveolar support, and surface tension. Stretching of lung tissue to provide the capacity for filling is limited by the elastic protein components of lung tissue, collagen, and elastin. In addition, the degree of stiffness of alveoli is influenced by neighboring alveoli which can impede inflation. Finally, alveloar surface tension developed across the air interface of the liquid film lining the alveoli acts as a collapsing tendency. The bubblelike alveoli would collapse from this force except that surface tension forces are very low due to the secretion of surfactant, a complex lipoprotein rich in lecithin, by type II cells of the alveoli. Low alveolar surface tension makes the lung easier to fill and promotes alveolar stability. The respiratory distress syndrome charcterized by hyaline membrane disease is caused by lack of surfactant. Infants with this disease have difficulty inflating their lungs, and the lung tissue exhibits collapsed alveoli and distended airways.

Dynamics of Air Flow

Air flow in smooth vessels is described by Poiseuille's law as laminar. However, the airways are not smooth but are irregular ducts with rough walls where flow becomes transitional or turbulent. Turbulence increases with resistance to flow. The nature of flow is directly related to vessel radius, velocity, and density, and inversely related to viscosity (Reynold's number: RE = 2 rvd/viscosity). At low tidal volumes and velocities flow is more nearly laminar with turbulence increasing as the volume increases. At high volumes, a greater unit pressure change is required for a smaller unit volume change. Respiration requires more work at higher tidal volumes where flow is turbulent.

Resistance to breathing is inversely related to airway radius ($R \propto 1/r^4$). As the radius (r^4) is halved, resistance increases 16 fold. As the bronchial tree branches into a multitude of progressively more narrow bronchioles, resistance increases. The resistance is greatest at the level of the segmental bronchi, rather than at the level of the narrower bronchioles, because the smaller airways are so much more numerous. These small airways are a "silent zone" in which disease may be undetected. Their numbers are an advantage in that limited small airway destruction may result in little impairment of function.

Bronchial smooth muscle tone affects resistance since increased constriction decreases the radius of the airway. Sympathetic stimulation causes dilation, while parasympathetic stimulation causes constriction of bronchial tubes. Epinephrine relieves asthmatic bronchiole constriction for this reason.

At low lung volumes, airway resistance becomes a very important factor in air flow since there is a high dependence of resistance on volume. Persons with high airway resistance tend to breathe at high lung volumes, where resistance is relatively lower, a functional advantage.

Nonuniform Ventilation

There are uneven resistances to air flow and uneven compliances in different parts of the lungs which result in regional differences in ventilation. Uneven resistance to airflow may be caused by obstruction of the airways as in asthmatic bronchial constriction, airway collapse as in emphysema, or compression of the airway by tumors, edema, etc. Uneven compliance can result from emphysema in which elastic recoil is lost, fibrosis, lack of surfactant, congestion or edema, tumors or cysts which compress lung tissue, etc.

Nonuniform ventilation resulting from a mismatch of ventilation and perfusion is responsible for most of the gas exchange problems in pulmonary disease. Ideally, the PO_2 of arterial blood should be the same as alveolar gas. However, diffusion from alveolus to blood is never absolutely complete. Breathing low PO_2 oxygen mixtures insufficient to match perfusion tension, such as that which occurs at high altitudes, can be one cause of uneven matching.

Vascular shunts in which blood bypasses ventilated alveoli is a common cause of mismatched ventilation and perfusion. A shunt will cause systemic arterial hypoxemia because poorly oxygenated venous shunted blood mixes in the pulmonary veins with fully oxygenated blood. In an absolute shunt, venous blood bypasses well ventilated alveoli and cannot be oxygenated no matter how high the alveolar PO_2. Blood shunted through areas where alveoli are collapsed or filled with exudate also will not be oxygenated. Areas of pathologic alveoli where gas exchange cannot occur are referred to as physiologic dead space.

Gas Transport

HEMOGLOBIN

Oxygen is only slightly soluble in the plasma water. Freshly oxygenated blood leaving the lungs contains only 0.3 vol percent dissolved oxygen. This slight solubility is insufficient to supply the needs of the tissues. Delivery of oxygen is dependent on the oxygen carrying protein of the blood, hemoglobin. The hemoglobin molecule consists of four iron containing heme subunits attached to the polypeptide chains of the protein globin. Each hemoglobin molecule can carry four oxygen molecules, which bind to the ferrous irons. Oxyhemoglobin can be represented as $Hb_4O_8^{-4}$ or simply HbO_2^-. The dissociation curve of this complex exhibits sigmoidal kinetics indicating that the oxygenation of one of the four heme groups enhances the oxygenation of the other three. This superb oxygen carrier is also abundant. Each 100 ml of blood normally contains 15 g of hemoglobin, with an oxygen carrying capacity of 20.1 vol percent. Hemoglobin is normally 97 percent saturated.

BUFFER FUNCTION

Hemoglobin also has an important function as a buffer for carbonic acid. HbO_2^- is a stronger acid than reduced hemoglobin, which functions as a weak acid (or stronger base) to bind protons as HHb. The activity of the buffer pair HbO_2^-/HHb may be represented as follows:

$$HbO_2^- + H^+ \rightleftharpoons HHb + O_2$$

In unloading oxygen at the tissues, hemoglobin binds available protons to protect the pH of the extracellular fluid. Gas exchange at the lungs also involves this equilibrium.

Although CO_2 is 20 times more soluble in the plasma than oxygen, dissolved CO_2 represents only 5 percent of the total carried by the blood. Most of the CO_2 (90 percent) is hydrated to carbonic acid, a reaction catalyzed in the red cell by carbonic anhydrase, and is present in the blood as bicarbonate formed from the forced dissociation of this weak acid. Another 5 percent is carried bound as carbaminohemoglobin.

Oxyhemoglobin and bicarbonate transport enormous quantities of oxygen and CO_2 but are not directly involved in gas exchange. Only the tensions of gases in simple solution generate the pressure gradients necessary for movement of gas. Oxyhemoglobin and bicarbonate serve as carriers which unload oxygen at the tissues and CO_2 at the lungs to maintain the gas tensions.

Gas Exchange

ALVEOLAR/BLOOD GAS TENSIONS

The composition of alveolar air is constantly changing as inspired air delivers oxygen to replace that which diffuses into the blood and to dilute and carry away carbon dioxide diffusing from the blood. Nitrogen is an inert gas which is neither consumed nor produced by metabolism. A sample of lung air taken at the end of a normal expiration would be more like alveolar air. In the steady state the composition of alveolar gas remains quite constant. Lung gases are saturated with water vapor, a factor which must be taken into consideration when calculating partial pressure (called tension when referring to dissolved gases). At body temperature the aqueous tension (pH_2O) is 47 mm Hg. Alveolar gas is about 5.6 percent CO_2. The aqueous tension must be subtracted from the atmospheric pressure in calculating the PCO_2.

$$PCO_2 = 5.6/100(760 - 47) = 40 \text{ mm Hg}$$

Compare the tensions of blood and alveolar gases (for inspired air the PO_2 is 157 mm Hg; the PCO_2, 0.3 mm Hg).

Gas Tension	Alveolar	Blood Gases	
mmHg	Gas	Venous	Arterial
PO_2	100	40	100
PCO_2	40	46	40

EVENTS AT THE LUNGS

Venous blood is oxygen poor and has taken on considerable CO_2. The oxygen tension is a low 40 mm Hg compared to an alveolar O_2 tension of 100 mm Hg. The difference, 60 mm Hg is the driving force for rapid diffusion, equalizing pressures across the blood/gas barrier. The elements of this barrier are the alveolar membrane with surfactant film, a very thin interstitial space, the capillary endothelium, and plasma red cell hemoglobin. In a fraction of a second venous blood becomes arterial blood as hemoglobin becomes saturated with the fresh oxygen load as is represented by the following:

$$HHb + O_2 \longrightarrow HbO_2^- + H^+$$

The CO_2 tension of venous blood is only 46 mm Hg compared to an alveolar CO_2 tension of 40 mm Hg. However, the rate of diffusion of a gas through a liquid is also dependent on solubility (Henry's law) and CO_2 is 20 times more soluble than oxygen. A rapid rate of diffusion attributed to solubility acts in concert with the 6 mm Hg driving force of the pressure gradient. CO_2 equilibrates rapidly. An amount of CO_2 removed is almost equivalent to the oxygen absorbed.

CO_2 carried as bicarbonate takes on the proton released from the dissociation of oxyhemoglobin to form carbonic acid. Assisted by the enzyme carbonic anhydrase, carbonic acid breaks down to CO_2 and water.

$$HHb + O_2 \longrightarrow HbO_2^- + H^+HCO3^- \longrightarrow$$
$$H_2CO_3 \longrightarrow CO_2 + H_2O$$

The CO_2 is then eliminated by simple diffusion.

EVENTS AT THE TISSUES

Tissue oxygen tensions vary considerably with metabolic activity. A resting tissue may have a PO_2 of about 40 mm Hg, while strenuous muscular activity can result in severe depletions which lower oxygen tension to less than 1 mm Hg. Since the arterial blood perfusing the tissues has an oxygen tension of about 100 mm Hg, diffusion is rapid with oxyhemoglobin unloading O_2 until depletion or equilibration occurs.

Metabolically active cells produce approximately 500 ml of CO_2 daily with PCO_2 increasing to 46–50 mm Hg. CO_2 diffuses rapidly into the red cells where the enzyme carbonic anhydrase catalyzes hydration to carbonic acid. The ionization of this weak acid is forced by the binding of hydrogen ions by reduced hemoglobin. This occurs as oxyhemoglobin is releasing oxygen.

$$H_2CO_3 + HbO_2^- \longrightarrow O_2 + HHb + HCO_3^-$$

Without this mechanism, solution of CO_2 would produce carbonic acid. Although this is a very weak acid, such large quantities could overwhelm buffer systems. Hemoglobin buffers carbonic acid, generating the 20 : 1 ratio of HCO_3^-/CO_2 and the slightly alkaline nature of the plasma.

Acid/Base Imbalance: Pulmonary Compensation

The bicarbonate/carbonic acid buffer system is the body's first line of defense against changes in blood pH, threatening acidosis or alkalosis. Acidosis is the more common threat and bicarbonate spent in buffering protons increases carbonic acid content. The danger is in overwhelming the system so that the capacity to buffer is impaired. The bicarbonate system is a good physiologic buffer because it is open-ended (i.e., carbonic acid is eliminated with ease as CO_2 by the lungs and bicarbonate is regenerated by the kidneys). The system is described by the Henderson-Hasselbalch equation which indicates that the normal plasma ratio of 20/1 (27 mEq/L HCO_3^-/1.35 mEq H_2CO_3) results in a blood pH of 7.4.

$$pH = pK + \log 20\ HCO_3^-/H_2CO_3$$
$$pH = 6.1 + 1.3 = 7.4$$

COMPENSATORY VENTILATION

The rate of pulmonary ventilation is mediated by central chemoreceptors located in the medulla near the origin of the ninth and tenth cranial nerves. These chemoreceptors are sensitive to the PCO_2 and the pH of the cerebrospinal fluid. In addition, peripheral chemoreceptors are located in the carotid and aortic bodies which contain afferent fibers to the respiratory center. The peripheral chemoreceptors are less sensitive to PCO_2, but this response becomes important in the presence of CNS depression due to drugs. Ventilation can also be regulated by a hypoxic response to low arterial PO_2 mediated peripherally through the carotid bodies. However, the hypoxic response does not occur until PO_2 drops to very low levels.

A normal rate of alveolar ventilation is sufficient to remove CO_2 produced by metabolism. In threatening acidosis, the PCO_2 increases. The respiratory center responds, accelerating the rate and depth of ventilation to remove excess carbonic acid. An increase of 10 mm Hg above normal PCO_2 will increase pulmonary ventilation fourfold. If alkalosis threatens, the PCO_2 decreases, the respiratory rate is slowed and CO_2 is retained, maintaining carbonic acid buffer capacity. Thus the 20/1 ratio is maintained, protecting the blood pH.

RESPIRATORY ACIDOSIS

Any disturbance of the rate of ventilation which leads to CO_2 retention can lead to respiratory acidosis. Depression of the respiratory center by drugs or anesthesia, obstruction or reduction of alveolar ventilation, by pulmonary diseases such as emphysema, pneumonia, or edema, paralysis of respiratory muscles, or diminished pulmonary circulation are typical clinical causes.

RESPIRATORY ALKALOSIS

Conditions which induce hyperventilation, such as fevers, CNS lesions, or hysteria can cause respiratory alkalosis. The condition can be self-induced by prolonged rapid, deep breathing. In respiratory alkalosis, CO_2 is blown off, depleting carbonic acid and increasing blood pH. A decrease in carbonic acid to 0.9 mEq, for example, would elevate blood pH to pH 7.6 if bicarbonate remained constant as is represented by the following:

$$\frac{HCO_3^-}{H_2CO_3}\ \frac{27\ mEq}{0.9\ mEq} = pH\ 7.6$$

The increase in pH is a result of decreased PCO_2. In the uncompensated condition there is low PCO_2, high pH, and slightly lowered bicarbonate. With renal compensation to eliminate bicarbonate, the pH approaches normal with a lowered bicarbonate concentration together with low PCO_2.

METABOLIC ACIDOSIS

Metabolic acidosis is caused by the overproduction of acid metabolites or the ingestion of acid. The primary event is depletion of bicarbonate in buffering excess acid.

$$HCO_3^- + H^+ \longrightarrow H_2CO_3$$

As bicarbonate is depleted, the carbonic acid and PCO_2 increase. A ratio of 10 HCO_3^-/0.5 H_2CO_3 would result in a normal blood pH of 7.4. However, to maintain buffer capacity bicarbonate must be regenerated. Clinically, diseases such as diabetes which produce ketoacids, toxemia, or starvation, overadministration of acids or acid salts, loss of alkaline fluids from prolonged diarrhea or fistular drainage, chronic dehydration in which chloride retention replaces bicarbonate, and chronic renal failure where bicarbonate is not conserved are typical causes.

METABOLIC ALKALOSIS

High bicarbonate levels and elevated blood pH characterize metabolic alkalosis which can be caused by ingestion of alkali or loss of acid. Overadministration of alkaline salts (lactates, bicarbonates, etc.) or persistent vomiting with loss of gastric acid are common clinical situations. The primary cause is bicarbonate retention. An increase in bicarbonate to 39 mEq, for example, would elevate blood pH to pH 7.6 if carbonic acid remained constant as is represented by the following:

$$\frac{HCO_3^-}{H_2CO_3} \frac{39\ mEq}{1.35\ mEq} = pH\ 7.6$$

Pulmonary compensation is rapid with decreased ventilation leading to CO_2 retention to protect blood pH. The reduction is usually in tidal volume, not in ventilatory rate. Often compensation is not complete because decreased tidal volume leads to hypoxia which influences increased tidal volume to counter the compensatory effect.

PART 4 _____

Renal Physiology

The kidneys are the prime regulators of the body in the important task of maintaining the constant composition of the body fluids. The kidneys selectively excrete and conserve essential water, electrolytes, sugars, and other metabolites. The kidneys regulate acid-base balance, excreting excess acid and synthesizing and reabsorbing bicarbonate. They regulate the extracellular osmolarity and fluid volume, using both endocrine and nonendocrine functions. In addition, the kidneys detoxify and excrete foreign compounds and passively excrete waste products, such as urea, uric acid, and creatinine. The hormonal function of the kidneys includes the production of erythropoietin (essential for red blood cell development), renin (trigger for the angiotensins), and in the transformation of vitamin D to the active hormone. They also play a role in gluconeogenesis, although the major organ involved in this process is the liver.

FUNCTIONAL ANATOMY

Anatomically, the longitudinal section of the kidney reveals an outer cortex, inner medulla, renal pelvis, and renal papilla. Most of the glomeruli, the filtration units, reside in the cortex. The renal pelvis is the expanded upper end of the ureter and the renal papillae are projections of the medulla into the lumen of a calyx.

The nephron is the functional unit of the kidney. There are approximately one million nephrons per kidney. The nephron begins in a tuft of capillaries called the glomerulus. Urine formation begins here by the separation of an essentially protein free filtrate from the blood perfusing the glomerular capillaries. The capillaries are unique as they lie between two arterioles, which permits fine adjustments of the pressure within the capillary bed. The glomerulus is enclosed in Bowman's capsule, which is an enlargement continuous with the lumen of the renal tubule and is comprised of specialized epithelial cells called podocytes.

The renal tubule is a long coiled structure divided into the proximal convoluted tubule, Henle's loop, and distal convoluted tubule. Groups of distal convoluted tubules empty into the collecting tubules, which form collecting ducts. These lead to papillary ducts which empty into the renal calyces.

The proximal convoluted tubule is a tortuous structure which functions in large scale movements of fluid and electrolytes and consists of cuboidal epithelium with a heavy brush border providing a large surface area. Many basal mitochondria provide energy for active transport.

Henle's loop commences with a descending limb and consists of thin descending, thin ascending, and thick ascending segments, each having a unique function. Cells in the ascending segments are impermeable to water, a characteristic essential for diluting urine. The ascending limb continues into the distal tubule. At this junction, the tubule comes into contact with the glomerulus in a region called the juxtaglomerular (JG) apparatus. Granular cells which produce renin and macula densa cells which function in control of renin secretion are found within the JG apparatus.

The distal convoluted tubule is important in the reabsorption of water and electrolytes. It has a cuboidal epithelium with little brush border and many mitochondria. The nephron as an individual unit ends here, since groups of distal convoluted tubules join and empty into collecting tubules.

The collecting tubules are also cuboidal with little brush border and few mitochondria. Here fine adjustments to urine concentration are made.

Nephron Types

Nephrons are classified by origin. Cortical (superficial) nephrons originate with the glomerulus just inside the capsule and have short Henle's loops that do not reach the medulla. Midcortical nephrons have glomeruli in the center of the cotex. Some have short Henle's loops which do not reach the medulla. Others have longer Henle's loops which extend partly into the medulla. The juxtamedullary nephrons have glomeruli on the border of the medulla and cortex and are of the long-loop type.

Blood Supply

The renal artery enters the kidney through the hilus and branches into interlobar arteries. At the medulla, they arch horizontally to form the arcuate arteries. Interlobular arteries pass outward through the cortex, giving rise to afferent arterioles which supply the glomerular capillary tufts. The glomerular capillary bed drains into an efferent arteriole, which supplies the capillary beds of the convoluted tubules, subsequently draining into the renal vein. The efferent aterioles derived from glomeruli close to the corticomedullary junction are an exception to this pathway. These become the vasa recta, straight vessels which descend into the medulla to follow the course of Henle's loops before returning to the cortex to drain into the renal vein.

The blood supply of a glomerulus usually supplies the same nephron. Peritubular capillaries surround the proximal and distal tubule of the same or adjacent nephrons and carry blood which has already been filtered by the glomerulus.

URINE FORMATION

The formation of urine involves ultrafiltration at the glomerulus, followed by selective reabsorption of water and solute, and selective tubular secretion of solute. The nephron functions passively in the collection of ultrafiltrate from the plasma. Reabsorption of solute from the tubuler lumen to the plasma is both active and passive, as is selective tubular secretion of solutes from the interstitial (peritubular) space into the lumen.

Glomerular Filtration

The afferent arteriole supplying the glomerulus is under high pressure, providing the hydrostatic pressure in the capillary tufts to drive filtration. Glomerular filtration produces an ultrafiltrate of essentially the same composition as blood plasma, but containing no protein.

Glomerular filtration involves passage of the plasma through the following barrier layers:

1. The capillary endothelium which is fenestrated with pores of sufficient size to prevent passage of cells but not proteins (700–1000 Å).
2. A basement membrane which is thick, trilaminar, and negatively charged, restrictive to large proteins and anions, but permeable to small proteins, such as albumin.
3. The epithelium of Bowman's capsule, where podocytes with interdigitating processes form filtration slits 70–1000 Å wide. Only very small proteins pass this barrier.

The filtration system is kept clean by mesangial cells, located between the endothelium and the basement membrane, which engulf particles stuck to the membrane.

FILTRATION FORCES

The hydrostatic pressure in the glomerular capillaries is high and can be held constant by arterioles on both sides of the capillary tuft. However, the oncotic pressure (colloidal osmotic pressure) is lower than normal in Bowman's interstital space because the glomerular capillaries are less permeable to protein than systemic capillaries. The oncotic pressure in the glomerular capillaries rises along the length of the capillary tuft, since protein is concentrated as fluid is removed.

The balance of hydrostatic and oncotic pressure determines filtration. For example, if the hydrostatic pressure in the glomerular capillary is 45 mm Hg and that in Bowman's space is 10 mm Hg, the net hydrostatic pressure, 35 mm Hg, will serve as a driving force toward Bowman's space. If the oncotic pressure in the glomerular capillary is 27 mm Hg and that in Bowman's space (normally protein free) is 0 mm Hg, the net opposing oncotic pressure, 27 mm Hg will draw fluid toward the capillary. The mean pressure (35 mm Hg net hydrostatic − 27 mm Hg net oncotic = 8 mm Hg) is a net hydrostatic force driving the filtrate into Bowman's space.

Filtration forces (q) may be described by the following equation:

$$q = K_f[(P_{GC} - P_{BS}) - (\pi_{GC} - \pi_{BS})]$$

In this equation, K_f is the filtration coefficient, which is proportional to the capillary area and permeability, P_{GC} is the hydrostatic pressure in the glomerular capillary, P_{BS} is the hydrostatic pressure in Bowman's space, and π_{GC} is the oncotic pressure in the glomerular capillary, opposing filtration. Normally, the oncotic pressure in Bowman's space (π_{BS}) is zero. In diseased states, if the oncotic presure in Bowman's space increases, it can reach an equilibrium point where the net mean pressure is zero and filtration will not occur.

GLOMERULAR FILTRATION RATE

The glomerular filtration rate (GFR) is the quantity of ultrafiltrate that passes per unit of time from the glomerulus into Bowman's space in all nephrons in both kidneys. Inulin, a small polysaccharide which is freely filterable, nontoxic, and not absorbed, secreted, or metabolized, is used to measure the GFR. Inulin is introduced into the blood, and the rate of urine production and the concentration of inulin excreted is measured. If urinary inulin output (Ui) is 125 mg/min and the flow volume (V) is 1 ml/min, and the plasma inulin concentration (Pi) is 1 mg/ml, then 125 ml of blood was filtered by the kidneys in 1 minute. The GFR is, therefore, 125 ml/minute.

$$GFR = \frac{Ui(mg/ml) \times V(ml/min)}{Pi(mg/ml)}$$

Normal GFR values are 125 ml/min for the male (normalized for 173 m^2 body surface area) and 110 ml/min for the female. GFR is lower for the young and elderly.

Factors affecting the GFR are glomerular capillary hydrostatic pressure, Bowman's space hydrostatic pressure, protein osmotic pressure, and the filtration coefficient. The capillary hydrostatic pressure is the most important variable and is largely determined by the resistance of the afferent arterioles. Intracapillary hydrostatic pressure increases in heart failure and is subject to change with systemic blood pressure as well as from drug and sympathetic nervous system influences. Bowman's space hydrostatic presure can be increased by obstruction of the ureter (e.g., kidney stones, edema, etc.) or by an increase in the protein osmotic pressure, which occurs in dehydration, starvation, tumors, etc. The filtration coefficient is influenced by changes in capillary permeability (acute glomerular nephritis increases permeability) as well as changes in the total area of the glomerular capillary bed. Area can be severely reduced by nephrectomy and destructive diseases.

RENAL CLEARANCE

Renal clearance (C, ml/min) measures the efficiency of the kidney to excrete a particular substance, and is the volume of plasma (ml) cleared of a substance (x) per unit of time (min). Clearance can also be described as the volume of plasma from which all of a substance appearing in the urine in 1 minute was derived. Clearance is described by the expression U × V/Px (urinary concentration × flow volume/plasma concentration).

Clearance will be equal to the GFR if a particular substance is not metabolized by the tubules, not secreted or reabsorbed by the tubules, not bound by plasma proteins, and is freely filterable. Inulin is such a substance. Therefore, Cin = GFR.

Comparison with the inulin clearance is used to determine the nature of the processes involved in the excretion of a substance. If clearance is lower than that of inulin, the substance must be reabsorbed from the tubule; if higher than inulin, the substance must be secreted.

Clinically, the creatinine clearance (Ccr) is frequently used to determine the GFR. Creatinine is an end product of muscle metabolism which is normaly added to the plasma at a constant rate. Ccr approximates the GFR as creatinine fits all the criteriea for clearance equivalent to GFR, except it is slightly secreted. Ccr should be slightly greater than insulin clearance and GFR. However, because methods of measurement detect other compounds than creatinine, clearance is calculated to be slightly less than inulin. Even though Ccr only approximates the GFR, it is widely used to measure kidney function.

Tubular Reabsorption

Most of the kidney's metabolic energy is spent in reabsorptive conservation of metabolites, a task of considerable magnitude. Tubular reabsorption involves the movement of a substance from the lumen of a tubule, across the epithelium, into the peritubular space, and back into the circulation via the peritubular capillaries. At a GFR of 125 ml/min, 180 L of water are filtered per day. Most is reabsorbed, with only 1–1.5 L of urine excreted. About 1.5 kg of salt are filtered daily, with only 2–3 g excreted. Urine contains only a little Na$^+$ and little or no bicarbonate. All glucose and amino acids are reabsorbed.

REABSORPTION RATE

The difference between the amount of a substance filtered and the amount that appears in the urine is the amount reabsorbed. The quantity excreted equals U (urinary concentration) × V (flow). The quantity filtered is called the filtered load (the amount of a substance presented to the tubules) and equals the plasma concentration PxGFR. The GFR is determined by Cin or Ccr and the rate of reabsorption (R) of a substance P is calculated as

$$R = (P_{[p]} \cdot GFR) - U_{[p]} \cdot V$$

The fractional excretion of a substance is determined from the amount per minute excreted and the amount per minute filtered and may be expressed as the following:

$$\frac{\text{Fractional}}{\text{excretion}} = \frac{\text{urine to plasma concentration of x}}{\text{urine to plasma concentration of inulin}}$$

The fractional excretion of Na^+ is one of the assessments for renal function.

TRANSPORT FACTORS

Reabsorption involves both passive and active transport of substances through several cell membranes. Passive transport moves a substance across a membrane in response to an electrial or chemical gradient. Energy is not directly involved. One substance may follow the gradient of another. Water, for example, follows sodium. Water movement is always passive as is transport of CO_2, NH_3, and urea.

The amount of a substance passively reabsorbed depends on the following:

1. Tubular permeability. The antidiuretic hormone (ADH), for example, influences collecting tubule permeability for water and urea.
2. Concentration and electrical gradients for the substance.
3. The rate of tubular fluid flow (V). If the flow increases there is less time for reabsorption.
4. The rate of blood flow in the peritubular capillaries. Increased rate of flow removes substances to maintain a concentration gradient. A fast blood flow rate favors reabsorption.

Active transport requires a transporter and energy input to move substances against concentration and electrical gradients. There are two types of transporters (i.e., those saturatable and those not saturatable at physiologic concentrations).

Glucose reabsorption is an example of saturatable transport. Glucose is reabsorbed only in the early proximal tubule and is dependent on sodium cotransport. Receptors for glucose and sodium are located on the lumenal side of the tubular cells. Sodium binding to the receptor increases the affinity of the receptor for glucose. Both glucose and sodium are translocated into the cell bound to the receptor. Once inside the cell, sodium is pumped into the peritubular space by the Na^+/K^+ ATPase pump and other Na^+ transporters. This prevents glucose rebinding to the cotransporter. Glucose is now passively transported into the peritubular space via a transporter on the basal membrane on the tubular cell. From the peritubular space glucose can diffuse into the peritubular capillaries.

TRANSPORT LIMITATION

A transport maximum (Tm) limits transport for a particular substance. At levels up to the Tm for glucose, for example, glucose reabsorption increases linearly as a function of plasma glucose concentrations. Normally, plasma glucose is far below the Tm and glucose does not appear in the urine. At levels above the Tm, glucose transporters are saturated so that glucose cannot be reabsorbed and it appears in the urine. The Tm for glucose is 375 mg/min for men. The renal threshold is the concentration at which plasma glucose first appears in the urine.

GLUCOSE TRANSPORT: DIABETES

In diabetes mellitus, plasma glucose levels become very high. The glucose transport mechanism becomes saturated and glucose spills into the urine. However, if the GFR is decreased (as in the elderly), less glucose is filtered per minute and all of the glucose that is filtered may be reabsorbed. Consequently, no glucose is spilled into the urine even though diabetes is present and blood glucose levels are high.

In the absence of diabetes, glucose may occur in the urine in conditions such as familial glycosuria, a genetic defect in which the Tm for glucose is lower than normal, so that glucose appears in the urine even at normal plasma levels.

GLUCOSE CLEARANCE

At low plasma glucose levels, all glucose is reabsorbed so that glucose clearance is zero. As glucose spills into the urine, the urinary glucose concentration increases. At very high glucose levels, the amount spilled into the urine will greatly exceed the amount reabsorbed.

If the Tm of a substance is very high (e.g., the Tm for glucose), the kidney has no role in the regulation of plasma levels. If the Tm of a substance is close to the normal plasma concentration (e.g., the Tm for phosphate), the kidneys regulate by excreting excess when the plasma levels increase slightly. If the Tm is fixed (e.g., glucose), the kidney has no role in the regulation of plasma levels. However, if the Tm is variable (e.g., the regulation of phosphate by parathyroid hormone), the kidney has a major role in regulating plasma levels.

AMINO ACID TRANSPORT

Similar to glucose, amino acid transport is active, occurs in the early proximal tubules, and is sodium dependent. Different carriers exist for each class of amino acids (i.e., basic, acidic, neutral, cystine, etc.). The Tm for amino acids is high enough to allow all amino acids to be reabsorbed.

Genetic disease affects amino acid transport. Fanconi's syndrome can cause infant death or severe disability and is associated with the inability to adequately transport certain amino acids, glucose, and phosphate. Cystinuria is due to failure to reabsorb cystine. Cystine has a low solubility so that kidney stones develop.

URIC ACID TRANSPORT

Uric acid transport is also similar to glucose transport. The kidney both reabsorbs and secretes uric acid. Increased plasma levels are usually caused by decreased tubular secretion, consequently, decreasing urinary excretion.

Na+ REABSORPTION AND EXCRETION

Sodium reabsorption involves a nonsaturable active transport system. Two-thirds of the Na^+Cl^- and H_2O filtered are reabsorbed by the proximal tubule. Na^+ is actively transported into the peritubular space from the lumen while H_2O and probably Cl^- passively follow the gradient generated by Na^+ transport.

The concentrations of the fluid reabsorbed, the fluid throughout the proximal tubule, and the plasma are equal. The resorbate (fluid absorbed) is isosmotic with respect to the proximal tubule fluid since Na^+ and H_2O are reabsorbed in the same proportion as is present in the lumen of the tubule. The resorbate is also isosmotic with respect to the plasma since the filtrate which enters the proximal tubule is simply filtered plasma. Thus, the total volume of fluid (a two-third decrease) changes in the proximal tubule.

The movement of Na^+ from the lumenal side of the proximal tubule to the peritubular side involves two different types of membranes with different electrical charges and concentration gradients of the ions involved on each side of the membrane (Fig. 8-9). The charge of the peritubular space is designated as 0 mV, with the electrical charges of other components measured with respect to this value. Movement of Na^+ opposes both electrical and concentration gradients and requires energy input. The active transport of Na^+ occurs only on the peritubular side of the proximal tubule. On the lumenal border, Na^+ entry into the cell occurs with the gradients and is probably by diffusion.

On the peritubular side, active transport involves two different Na^+ pumps. The Na^+/K^+ ATPase pump couples Na^+ transport out of the cell with K^+ entry. This pump is probably located on the lateral sides of the cell as well as on the cell's basal border. Other Na^+ pumps are present which do not couple Na^+ and K^+.

CHLORIDE REABSORPTION

Cl^- moves from concentrations of 108 mEq/L (lumenal), to 2 mEq/L (intracellular), to 103 mEq/L in the peritubular space. Overall, in a net sense, Cl^- is moving down a small concentration gradient as well as a small electrical gradient (-4 mV lumenal to 0 mV peritubular). No pumps for Cl^- have been found in the proximal tubules and Cl^- is postulated to move passively with Na^+. Na^+Cl^- may even act as a neutral entity when passing through tubular cell membranes.

	Lumen	Proximal Tubule Cells	Peritubular Space
Potential Difference	-4mV	-70mV	0mV
$[Na+]$	135mEq/L	20mEq/L	142mEq/L
$[Cl-]$	108mEq/L	2mEq/L	103mEq/L
$[K+]$	3.8mEq/L	150mEq/L	4mEq/L

Fig. 8-9. Electrochemical gradients of proximal tubule.

WATER MOVEMENT

Water moves in response to an osmotic gradient. Samples of fluid from the peritubular space, lumen of the early proximal tubule, and the plasma are isosmotic. The mechanism for generating the osmotic gradient involves Na^+ pumping out of the cell by active transport pumps located on the lateral borders of the tubular cells. This pumping concentrates Na^+ in the lateral intercellular space, establishing a local osmotic gradient. Water follows, accumulating with Na^+, and generating a hydrostatic force which causes channel flow between the cells and through the basement membrane into the peritubular space and capillaries. The high protein osmotic pressure and the decreased hydrostatic pressure of the blood in the peritubular capillaries favors movement of Na^+ and H_2O from the peritubular space into the peritubular capillaries. Although the tight junction between cells of the tubule at the lumenal side is leaky and allows some back movement of H_2O and Na^+, the mechanism is effective enough to reabsorb two-thirds of the filtered fluid volume. Of the 125 ml/min entering the tubule from Bowman's space, only 40 ml/min remains at the end of the proximal tubule.

ROLE OF HENLE'S LOOP

Transport of Na^+Cl^- out of the lumen and into the medullary space continues in the thick ascending portion of Henle's loop. The lumen in this segment is positive (due to removal of negative chloride ions) with respect to the peritubular space, a situation opposite that of the proximal tubule. In this area Cl^- is believed to be the actively transported ion with Na^+ following passively.

The ascending loop is impermeable to water and the fluid in the lumen becomes hyposmotic, since Na^+ pumping continues here. Approximately one half of the Na^+Cl^- entering this segment is removed, effectively diluting the developing urine. The ascending segment is, therefore, called the diluting segment.

THE DISTAL TUBULE

Fluid entering the distal tubule is hyposmotic and can remain so or can become isosmotic with plasma depending upon the total movement of water and Na^+ across the distal tubule. The distal tubule is less negative (-10 to -50 mV, depending on location) than the proximal tubule and the Na^+ concentration is lower, as approximately half is removed in Henle's loop. Movement of Na^+ across the lumenal border is by passive diffusion with active transport on the peritubular side. The distal tubules do not need to reabsorb bulk quantities of water and lateral intercellular channels do not exist here. Tight junctions between tubular cells are stronger. Hormonal control is exerted in the distal tubules and collecting ducts for further concentration of the developing urine.

RENAL REGULATION OF BLOOD VOLUME

Aldosterone

Aldosterone is a steroid hormone produced by the adrenal cortex in response to renin release by the juxtaglomerular apparatus. This hormone sets the level of Na^+ excretion to control blood volume. Aldosterone diffuses from the peritubular capillary into the peritubular space and is effective *only* from the peritubular side. On entering the tubular cell, aldosterone combines with a receptor found in the cytoplasm. The receptor-aldosterone complex can enter the nucleus and bind to the chromatin to stimulate synthesis of mRNA, which codes for the synthesis of aldosterone induced protein (AIP). AIP appears to act by either increasing the permeability of the lumenal membrane to Na^+ or by increasing Na^+ pumping activity on the peritubular side to increase Na^+ reabsorption. Two to three percent of the Na^+ remaining in the urine in the distal tubule is reabsorbed accompanied by water in the presence of aldosterone.

Cl^- movement in the distal tubule appears to be passive in a net sense. However, in some cases, such as severe salt deprivation, there is such a low Cl^- concentration in the lumen that a lumenal side pump is postulated.

Antidiuretic Hormone

Water movement is regulated by the antidiuretic hormone (ADH), a peptide hormone produced by the neurohypophysis in response to thirst. ADH acts on the peritubular side, combining with a receptor on the cell membrane to stimulate adenylate cyclase, increasing cAMP. cAMP influences phosphorylation of a lumenal membrane protein, increasing pore size and membrane permeability to water. Thus, ADH works against diuresis to produce a more concentrated urine and conserve water.

The Collecting Duct

The final volume and osmolarity of urine is determined by events in the collecting duct. The transtubular potential difference in the collecting duct is negative and Na^+ transport is active, with powerful Na^+ pumps capable of reducing the Na^+ level to essentially zero (99.99 percent can be removed). Cl^- passively follows Na^+. Water movement in the collecting ducts is under the control of ADH. Aldosterone influence is also exerted here.

Potassium Regulation

In the proximal tubule, K^+ concentrations are 3–8 mEq/L in the lumen, 150 mEq/L intracellularly, and 4 mEq/L in the peritubular space. Overall transport from 3.8–4 mEq/L requires active transport.

K^+ entry into the cell involves a lumenal membrane K^+ pump. The electrical gradient also favors movement into the cell. K^+ then diffuses passively into the peritubular space since the peritubular membrane is much more permeable to K^+ than the lumenal membrane. Some K^+ is pumped back into the cell by the Na^+/K^+ ATPase pump to maintain the intracellular K^+.

K^+ reabsorption in Henle's loop is vigorous and probably occurs in the thick ascending portion. Essentially all K^+ is reabsorbed in the proximal tubule and Henle's loop.

The distal tubule and collecting duct are responsible for K^+ balance since K^+ can be either reabsorbed or secreted in these areas. Reabsorption involves a K^+ pump on the lumenal side and passive diffusion into the peritubular space. If the body needs less K^+, secretion involves K^+ pumping into the cell on the peritubular side and passive diffusion into the lumen.

K^+ regulation is under the strictest control. An increase in plasma K^+ of 3–4 mEq/L can cause irreversible depolarization of muscle, nerve, and the heart (which remains in the contracted state). Death ensues quickly. A similar rise in plasma Na^+ (3–4 mEq/L) causes no discernible change.

Increased K^+ intake causes increased K^+ secretion by the distal tubule. Na^+ intake is also directly related to K^+ secretion; increased Na^+ intake increases K^+ secretion, with low Na^+ intake decreasing urinary K^+. In acidosis, high plasma H^+ causes K^+ and H^+ to exchange between the distal tubular cell and the peritubular space. The reduced intracellular K^+ results in reduced K^+ secretion. Aldosterone increases urinary K^+ by stimulating the secretory pathway, possibly by increasing Na^+/K^+ pumping activity. In addition, the water balance of the body affects K^+ secretion. In dehydration, intracellular water moves out into the plasma to maintain the blood volume. This increases intracellular K^+ concentration and enhances secretion.

Mechanism of Tubular Secretion

PASSIVE TRANSPORT: DIFFUSION TRAPPING

Tubular secretion involves movement of a substance from the peritubular capillary to the lumen of the renal tubule, an event opposite reabsorption. The secretory substance must be diffusable through the capillary wall, requiring it not be bound to plasma proteins. Once at the tubule cells, transport may be passive and require a transporter as the substance simply moves down electrochemical gradients.

Secretion may be facilitated by diffusion trapping mechanisms which operate to prevent back diffusion into the cell. The renal ammonium mechanism is an example. Ammonia, NH_3, is passively diffusable and is capable of binding a tubule proton to form the ammonium ion, $NH4^+$, which is not diffusable. Thus, ammonia nitrogen is trapped in the developing urine in a reaction which plays a role in the excretion of strong acid. Trapping is useful medically in cases of overdoses of drugs which are weak acids. An alkaline urine traps such drugs in their ionized form in the tubules.

ACTIVE TRANSPORT

Tm-limited active secretion occurs only in the proximal tubule. This mechanism results in the active removal of many drugs and foreign compounds, such as penicillin. Nonsaturatable active transport systems, such as those utilized by hydrogen ions, operate throughout the tubule.

RATE OF SECRETION

The rate of secretion (QS) can be calculated if the filtration rate (QF) and the rate of excretion (QE) for a substance is known. The amount excreted into the urine per minute equals the amount filtered at the glomerulus plus the amount transported into the tubule from the peritubular capillaries

$$QE = QF + QS$$

QE is calculated from the urine concentration $\times$ the urine flow rate; QF from the plasma concentration $\times$ GFR. For a secreted substance X, clearance X will be greater than the clearance of inulin if X is secreted in a net sense (i.e., CX will be greater than GFR). For a substance like K^+ which is both reabsorbed and secreted, only the net result can be calculated to determine if reabsorption or secretion predominate.

Renal Blood Flow Determination

α-Amino hippuric acid (PAH) is a compound isolated from horse urine, which is both secreted and excreted and is used to determine renal blood flow. Only a small amount of PAH is bound to plasma proteins so that the amount filtered per minute is a linear function of plasma concentration. The amount excreted is greater than the amount filtered. Therefore, PAH is also secreted.

The active transport mechansim for PAH is saturatable, with a Tm of about 80 mg/min. At low plasma PAH concentrations, almost all PAH is secreted from the proximal tubules. At higher plasma PAH concentrations, the amount secreted becomes less significant relative to the large amount filtered. Therefore, PAH clearance decreases as plasma concentration increases. At very low plasma PAH concentrations, the secretion mechanism is not saturated. Almost all PAH will be removed in one pass of blood through the kidney. Thus, PAH is very useful in determining renal blood flow (RBF), since flow of PAH will equal RBF.

Renal plasma flow (RPF) can be calculated if the concentrations of PAH in the renal artery (RA) and renal vein are known by using the Fick equation. If low concentrations of PAH are used for the determination, the PAH concentration in the renal vein is zero, since all PAH will be removed in one pass through the kidney. Therefore

$$RPF = \frac{U_{PAH} \cdot V}{RA_{PAH}}$$

Furthermore, since PAH is not acted upon by a tissue, the concentration in any artery will be the same as in any vein (except the renal vein where it is zero). A simple ventricular puncture gives the plasma concentration of PAH, simplifying the calculation to

$$RPF = \frac{U_{PAH} \cdot V}{Plasma_{PAH}}$$

The value derived is the approximate clearance of PAH as is represented by the following:

$$RPF_{PAH} \approx C_{PAH}$$

PAH is not totally removed in one renal pass because some blood bypasses the proximal tubule and is routed to the renal capsule, perirenal fat, etc. Therefore, clearance PAH actually measures the effective renal plasma flow (ERPF). About 90 percent of the total blood flow goes to the functional parts of the kidney, from which all of the plasma PAH is extracted. Effective renal blood flow (ERBF) is related to the hematocrit (45 percent of whole blood volume, whereas plasma is 55 percent of whole blood volume). Total renal blood flow can be determined using both extraction (0.90) and hematocrit (0.45) corrections as is represented by the following:

$$TRBF = \frac{C_{PAH}/0.9}{1 - 0.45}$$

The renal blood flow per minute averages about one fourth of the cardiac output. Clinically, substances similar to PAH which can be tagged with radioiodine are used for this test.

FILTRATION FRACTION

The filtration fraction (FF) is the percent of total renal plasma flow filtered at the glomerulus which appears in the tubule.

$$FF = \frac{GFR}{ERPF} = \frac{125 \text{ ml/min}}{660 \text{ ml/min}} = .19$$
(19 percent, normal adult value)

If the filtration fraction changes, the protein osmotic pressure of the blood in the peritubular capsule will also change and affect reabsorption of water and electrolytes.

AUTOREGULATION OF RENAL BLOOD FLOW

The renal blood flow and glomerular filtration rate must be precisely maintained and unaffected by variations in blood pressure, excitation, sleep, etc. There is a cyclic interdependence of renal and cardiovascular systems. RBF depends on adequate cardiac output, which depends on adequate venous return, which depends on the ability of the kidney to reabsorb water and electrolytes to maintain blood volume.

Autoregulation keeps RF and GFR constant over a wide arterial pressure range and is accomplished by adjustments in resistance (flow rate = pressure/resistance). Resistance is altered at the afferent and efferent arterioles, the renal arteriole tree, and the renal veins. Constriction of afferent and efferent arterioles is the most important mechanism (Fig. 8-10).

The autoregulatory mechanism is intrinsic to the kidney and does not depend solely on sympathetic innervation (nephrectomized or denervated kidney exhibits some autoregulation). The mechanism resides in the JG apparatus, which consists of specialized smooth muscle cells of the afferent arteriole at the junction with the distal tubule. Some cells of the efferent arteriole in the region of the macula densa may also have a role in autoregulation.

Two regulatory mechanisms have been postulated. The direct myogenic mechanism proposes that a change in renal artery resistance occurs in response to distension of the arterial wall. This is mediated by a change in the rate of renin secretion in the JG cell. The macula densa mechanism involves feedback from macula densa cells, with JG cells lining the arteriole acting as baroreceptors,

Afferent Constriction

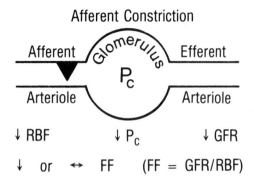

↓ RBF   ↓ P_c   ↓ GFR

↓ or ↔ FF   (FF = GFR/RBF)

Efferent Constriction

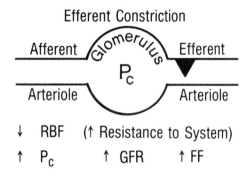

↓ RBF   (↑ Resistance to System)

↑ P_c   ↑ GFR   ↑ FF

Equal Constriction

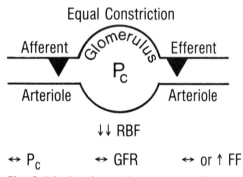

↓↓ RBF

↔ P_c   ↔ GFR   ↔ or ↑ FF

Fig. 8-10. Renal arteriole constrictive effects.

sensing pressure or stretch. JG cells respond by secreting renin, the catalyst of the angiotensin system.

Angiotensin II is a very potent vasoconstrictor and may have a negative feedback effect which prevents further renin secretion. Angiotensin II can assert a local effect by constricting renal arterioles, primarily the efferent arteriole. At high concentrations, it will constrict both efferent and afferent arterioles. Constriction of the efferent arteriole will raise the GFR. Angiotensin may also change the permeability of the glomerular capillaries.

THE CATECHOLAMINES

Epinephrine and norepinephrine directly constrict both afferent and efferent arterioles. At low concentrations, both constrict equally. However, at high concentrations afferent arterioles constrict preferentially, drastically reducing renal blood flow to shunt blood to other areas in the "fight or flight" response.

Direct innervation of both afferent and efferent arterioles by sympathetic fibers also causes constriction. Sympathetic nerve endings on the JG cells stimulate renin secretion as well. Mild sympathetic stimulation decreases RBF with no change in GFR. Rapid sympathetic firing decreases both RBF and GFR. (Congenital constriction of the renal artery results in systemic hypertension. Autoregulatory mechanisms may be overridden in renal pathology.)

Renal Oxygen Consumption

In most organs, including muscle, resting oxygen consumption remains fairly constant. As blood flow decreases, the AV difference rises proportionately. Kidney oxygen consumption per gram of tissue is greater than any other organ. Yet, the AV difference is the lowest. Basal renal oxygen consumption is approximately $100 \ \mu m \ O_2$ per 100 g kidney per minute. This is only one fifth of the total oxygen consumption of the normal kidney. Most of the oxygen consumed by the kidney is used to energize Na^+ reabsorption. As renal blood flow decreases from 700 to 200 ml/100 g/min, oxygen consumption decreases proportionately, with the AV difference remaining unchanged. Above the basal oxygen need, O_2 consumption is controlled by Na^+ reabsorption, which is related to GFR and to renal blood flow.

THE CONCENTRATION OF URINE

Limits of Concentration

The kidney can produce urine with a concentration range of one-sixth to four times that of plasma (50 mosm/kg to 1260 mosm/kg H_2O). A minimal amount of water is obligated for the excretion of solute which the kidney cannot reabsorb (600 mosm/day). This minimal amount of urine per day, called the obligatory water loss, is about 0.5 L per day. Urine cannot be concentrated further. The body can tolerate a water loss of up to 20 percent of total body weight. Survival time depends on how rapidly water is lost. A quick loss (hot, dry desert) can dehydrate in a day; a slower loss (cool, moist environment) can require several weeks.

Formation of Hypertonic Urine

At the cortex, the interstitium is isosmolar with the plasma (300 mosm/kg H_2O). At Henle's loops of juxtamedullary nephrons a concentration gradient is generated so that the interstitial regions of the outer and inner medulla become hypertonic. Interstitial concentration at the papillae is about 1200 mosm/kg H_2O. Therefore, water is withdrawn osmotically from the tubule by the higher solute concentration in the interstitium. The maximum amount of water that can be withdrawn would result in a maximum urine concentration equal to the concentration in the interstitium (1200 mosm/kg H_2O).

The concentration gradient in the interstitium develops a concentrated urine, with the presence of ADH required for withdrawal of H_2O. Henle's loops of the juxtamedullary nephrons generate the gradient, but because collecting ducts from all nephrons traverse this area, this mechanism concentrates urine outflow from all nephrons.

THE COUNTERCURRENT MECHANISM

The osmotic gradient is produced and maintained by the countercurrent mechanism. Countercurrent flow occurs when two fluids (or gases) move in opposite directions in two tubes in close proximity. Countercurrent flow helps regulate the temperature of the blood; arterial blood is cooled and venous blood is warmed by passive countercurrent heat exchange (Fig. 8-11). This effect can be enhanced by countercurrent multiplication, which uses active transfer in a limb of a countercurrent system to achieve a larger effect than that seen with passive exchange.

THE MEDULLARY UREA CYCLE: COUNTERCURRENT MULTIPLICATION

Countercurrent multiplication is used by the kidney to establish an osmotic gradient in the interstitium. The mechanism is cyclic. The first active transport step occurs in the thick ascending segment of Henle's loop. Here Cl^- is pumped; Na^+ follows. The thick ascending loop is impermeable to water and the transport of salt without water movement is the energy generating step. Moreover, the permeability to small molecules is low, so urea remains in the tubule. The permeabilities of Henle's loop, distal tubule, and collecting duct are the most important characteristics of the system. The loss of salt without water dilutes the developing urine to produce a hypotonic solution in the lumen of the thick ascending loop, which passes to the distal tubule.

The distal tubule is impermeable to urea and pumps Na^+ into the interstitium with Cl^- following (except when the tubular Cl^- is very low and active Cl^- pumping is thought to occur). Distal tubule permeability to water is dependent on the presence (permeable) or absence (impermeable) of ADH. ADH is effective in the distal third of the tubule. Water reabsorbed in the distal tubule goes into the cortex. The tubular fluid passes to the collecting duct.

The early collecting duct (outer medulla) is impermeable to urea. If ADH is present, the duct will be perme-

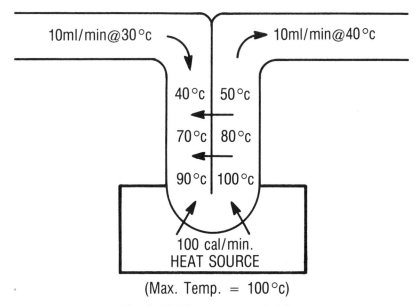

Fig. 8-11. Countercurrent principle.

able to water and the withdrawal of water will concentrate the remaining solutes. As the urine passes along the collecting duct into the inner medulla, the presence of ADH effects tubule permeability to both water and urea. Urea flows out into the medulla, adding to the salt already there from ascending loop transport to create an even greater osmotic gradient in the interstitium.

The urea in the interstitium can flow back into Henle's loop. If this occurs, the urea will travel back to the collecting duct and diffuse out again. The cyclic process resulting is called the medullary urea cycling. Urea trapped in this cycle plays a role in maintaining the concentration gradient. This role is important. In protein deficiency or starvation, for example, plasma urea falls and the ability of the kidney to concentrate urine is compromised to a maximum of 400–600 mosm/kg H_2O. This condition can be corrected by infusion of urea.

GRADIENT EFFECTS ON HENLE'S LOOP

The descending thin limb of the loop is permeable to water, with a low salt permeability. The fluid in the thin limb is in the environment of the urea and outer medullary concentration gradient. Thus, water is osmotically withdrawn, increasing the concentration of the remaining fluid. Enough water can be withdrawn here to produce a high concentration of Na^+Cl^- within the descending thin limb. At the bottom of Henle's loop, within the tubule, the osmolarity results from the high concentration of Na^+Cl^- with a contribution from urea. Outside the bottom of the loop, the interstitium osmolarity is contributed to by the high concentration of urea and a lesser concentration of NaCl. As the fluid enters the bottom of the loop, the permeability changes (i.e., the ascending limb is permeable to salt, but not to water). The high salt concentration at the bottom of the loop effectively primes the Na^+ or Cl^- pumps of the ascending limb. Thus, as fluid passes to the thick ascending limb, salt is again pumped out.

THE INTERSTITIUM CONCENTRATION GRADIENT

The following factors contribute to the gradient in the interstitium: (1) active transport of salt out of the thick ascending limb, (2) active transport of salt out of the late distal tubule and collecting duct, (3) withdrawal of urea out of the collecting duct, and (4) passive movement of salt out of the ascending limb (small contribution).

All of these contributions add up to a maximum concentration of 1200 mosm/kg H_2O in the inner medulla at the turn of Henle's loop, compared to a cortical concentration of 300 mosm/kg H_2O. The concentration of

urine depends on ADH and the permeability properties of the loop and tubule. The countercurrent mechanism produces a concentration gradient. Although the mechanism itself is found only with juxtamedullary nephrons, it concentrates all the urine because all collecting ducts pass through the medulla.

Renal Blood Flow: Water Reabsorption

Water withdrawn into the medulla must be reabsorbed into the circulation. However, straight, freely permeable capillaries in this area would upset the concentration gradient established by the nephrons. Therefore, the vasa recta capillaries are arranged in hairpin turns, utilizing countercurrent exchange for blood flow and the reabsorption of excess water. The capillaries arise from the efferent arteriole and are permeable to water, Na^+Cl^-, urea, etc., but not usually to proteins. There is a higher than normal protein osmotic pressure in these vessels. As the capillaries course from outer to inner medulla, the high Na^+Cl^- osmotic gradient is encountered. Water is withdrawn, Na^+Cl^- enters the vasa recta, and the protein concentration becomes even higher. Resistance in the capillaries increases and flow is impeded as the capillaries descend into the inner medulla. The capillaries then course back, meeting smaller and smaller osmotic gradients. Water flows back into the capillaries, diluting the proteins to decrease protein osmotic pressure. Salt leaves to the interstitium.

The osmotic lag helps to maintain the osmotic gradient despite capillary permeabilities, since it takes time for fluids to equilibrate on either side of the gradient. Therefore, at any given horizontal level on the descending side of the capillary, there is a greater concentration of solute outside than inside the capillary. This is reversed on the ascending side of the capillary. In descending, water leaves the capillary; in ascending, water enters. The loss of water from the descending capillary, when combined with the gain into the ascending loop gives a net gain of water equal to that lost from the collecting duct. In addition, the capillaries experience a net gain of Na^+Cl^-. However, neither addition is large enough to harm the interstitial concentration gradient.

Formation of Hypotonic Urine

The production of a hypotonic urine occurs as above except that ADH is low or absent so that water does not diffuse out of the distal tubule or collecting duct. With more water remaining in the collecting duct, the urea concentration is lower and medullary urea drops. Therefore, with hypotonic urine, medullary osmolarity is lower than for hypertonic urine production.

VARIATIONS IN URINE OSMOLARITY AND FLOW RATE

Urine osmolarity varies from 50 mosm/L to 1200 mosm/L (i.e., from 400 ml/day, the obligatory water loss to 2.5 L/day, the normal physiologic range). Normally urine is hypertonic, 500 mosm/L to 800 mosm/L (i.e., more concentrated than plasma). Hypotonic urine is unusual. The normal urine flow rate is 1 ml/min or 1.5 L/day.

EXCRETION OF UREA

Excretion of urea increases to a maximum value. Reabsorption of urea decreases as urine flow rate increases. When the urine flow rate is low (hypertonic urine), ADH levels are high and allow removal of urea from the distal portion of the collecting ducts. Urea clearance depends on the urine flow rate. The standard clearance is normally less than 2 ml/min.

DIURESIS

An increased urine flow rate above 2 ml/min can occur in conditions of decreased water reabsorption (water diuresis) or decreased salt reabsorption (osmotic diuresis). Water diuresis can be caused by the following:

1. Excessive fluid intake which dilutes plasma osmolarity, leading to decreased ADH production.
2. Lack of ADH (diabetes insipidus) in which the pituitary fails to elaborate ADH. Urine output can increase to 18–20 L per day in this condition. Certain drugs, such as alcohol, also suppress ADH production.
3. Nephrogenic diabetes insipidus in which the pituitary secretes normal amounts of ADH but the tubule cells do not respond.

Osmotic diuresis has two causes as is illustrated by the following:

1. Presentation to the kidney of a solute it cannot reabsorb. Mannitol is such a solute and is used clinically to induce diuresis. High glucose levels (diabetes mellitus) beyond the reabsorptive ability of the kidney also result in osmotic diuresis.
2. Drugs which inhibit reabsorption of ions. Drugs can act on the proximal tubule to inhibit Na^+ reabsorption, the thick ascending Henle's loop to inhibit Cl^- reabsorption, or the distal tubule, inhibiting Na^+. Some drugs

which inhibit reabsorption in the distal tubule also are antagonistic to aldosterone, further reducing Na^+ reabsorption.

PART 5

Acid Base Balance

Life could not exist without some mechanism for absorbing excess acid or base. The blood pH is alkaline and is maintained within the narrow normal range of about 7.37 to 7.42 that is essential to metabolic function. The buffer capacity of the blood was amply demonstrated by the physiologist Pitts who infused a dog with 156 ml of N HCL while adding the same amount of N HCL to 11 L of water, an amount equal to the dog's body fluid. The dog's blood pH dropped from 7.44 to 7.14. In contrast, the pH of the water dropped drastically from 7.0 to 1.8.

Buffers are chemical shock absorbers for H^+ and OH^- ions. Buffers defend as teams, resisting changes in pH to combat threats of acidosis or alkalosis. Acidosis is a condition in which blood pH is less than 7.37. If pH falls below 7.0, the CNS is suppressed, leading to coma and death. Alkalosis is a condition in which blood pH is greater than 7.42. If pH exceeds 7.8, tetany results, leading to death caused by tetany of the respiratory muscles. Acidosis is by far the more common threat, since essential protein, with its sulfur containing amino acids, constitutes an "acid-ash" diet, and acids are normal metabolic products. Vigorous exercise, for example, produces lactic acid.

ACID PRODUCTION

Between 13,000 and 20,000 mmole of CO_2 are produced daily by oxidative metabolism. This gas dissolves in the body fluids, hydrating to carbonic acid as shown by the following equation:

$$CO_2 + H_2O \rightleftharpoons H_2CO_3$$

Carbonic acid is called a volatile acid since it is excreted as CO_2 at the lungs.

Nonvolatile acid production consists of the daily production of 40–60 mmol of noncarbonic acid, chiefly sulfuric and phosphoric acids from the metabolism of amino acids and phospholipids.

BUFFER MECHANISMS

Bicarbonate/Carbonic Acid

Buffers defend as teams to resist changes in pH. The most effective buffers are weak acids and their conjugate bases. One member of the team binds H^+; the other donates H^+ to neutralize OH^-. The weaker the acid, the stronger the conjugate base. Carbonic acid is an extremely weak acid; HCO_3^-, its conjugate base is a good proton binder and is abundant in the body fluids. The bicarbonate/carbonic acid buffer system is the body's first line defense against threats to pH.

Conjugate base binds protons:

$$HCO_3^- + H^+ \longrightarrow H_2CO_3 \longrightarrow H_2O + CO_2 \uparrow \text{ (expired)}$$

Weak acid neutralizes base:

$$H_2CO_3 + OH^- \longrightarrow H_2O + HCO_3^-$$

Buffering is rapid and occurs extracellularly and intracellularly as the first line defense mechanism in acidosis or alkalosis. Buffering is an important, but temporary step, as the buffer is depleted and must be restored.

The second level response to the threat of acidosis or alkalosis is respiratory in which the lungs compensate by eliminating or retaining CO_2. The rate of respiration is altered, increasing in a very strong response if the blood is acidotic. If alkalosis threatens, respiration decreases somewhat (hypoxia must be avoided). This mechanism is not as rapid as buffering, but it is permanent and may be summarized by considering the bicarbonate reaction as

$$CO_2 + H_2O \longleftrightarrow H_2CO_3 \longleftrightarrow H^+ + HCO_3^-$$

If more CO_2 is exhaled, the reaction will shift to the left to decrease plasma H^+ concentration and compensate for acidosis. If CO_2 is retained, the reaction will shift to the right and plasma H^+ concentration increase to compensate for alkalosis.

The third level response to threats against pH occurs at the kidney, where excess H^+ is excreted and HCO_3^- is reabsorbed to compensate for acidosis. This shifts the bicarbonate reaction to the left so that more CO_2 is produced for elimination at the lungs. During alkalosis, when plasma H^+ decreases, the kidney reabsorbs less HCO_3^-, shifting the bicarbonate reaction to the right and increasing H^+ to compensate for the alkalosis. The kidney can also synthesize HCO_3^-.

THE HENDERSON-HASSELBALCH EQUATION

The bicarbonate/carbonic acid ratio is maintained in the plasma at 20 parts of bicarbonate to 1 part of carbonic acid. This ratio has been termed the alkaline (alkali) reserve and represents the base available for buffering acid. The Henderson-Hasselbalch equation describes buffer control of the blood and incorporates the pK (negative log of the ionization constant) of the weak acid as is represented by the following:

$$pH = pK + \log 20 \, (HCO_3^-/H_2CO_3)$$

Carbonic acid is in equilibrium with dissolved CO_2, which is measured clinically as the partial pressure of CO_2 (PCO_2), in mm Hg. A conversion factor of 0.03 mmol/L must be used to convert PCO_2 to dissolved CO_2. The dissolved CO_2 plus CO_2 in the gas phase represent total CO_2 concentration. At normal plasma levels, there are 24 mmol/L HCO_3^- and a normal PCO_2 of 40 mm Hg. The pK of the bicarbonate system is 6.1. Substituting normal values, the Henderson-Hasselbalch equation solves to equal 7.4, normal blood pH as is represented by the following:

$$pH = 6.1 + 1.3 = 7.4$$

The lungs and kidneys keep the ratio HCO_3^-/PCO_2 constant. Any change in either acid or base concentration is compensated by adjusting the ratio. The lungs adjust the H^+ concentration; the kidneys adjust the HCO_3^- concentration.

Auxiliary Buffer Systems

PLASMA AND TISSUE PROTEINS

Proteins contain basic amine and carboxylic acid groups. At physiologic pH, the amine groups are largely protonated (protein-NH_3^+), and behave as proton donors. The organic acid groups are largely dissociated as anions (protein-COO^-) and bind protons. Thus, they function as a buffer pair as represented by the following:

$$\text{basic protein-COO}^- + H^+ \longrightarrow \text{protein-COOH}$$

$$\text{acid protein-NH}_3^+ + OH^- \longrightarrow \text{protein-NH}_2 + H_2O$$

Plasma proteins bind about 0.11 mEq H^+/g protein. Blood contains 38.5 g protein/L so that total protein buffering capacity is about 4.25 mEq H^+/L.

HEMOGLOBIN

Oxyhemoglobin (HbO_2^-), the oxidized form, is a stronger acid than the reduced form, HHb. Reduced hemoglobin acts as a base to bind available protons.

$$HbO_2^- + H^+ \rightleftharpoons HHb + O_2$$

At the tissues, as oxygen is unloaded, hemoglobin binds protons from the dissociation of carbonic acid, forcing ionization to yield free HCO_3^-. The role of hemoglobin in the important task of generating the alkaline reserve is discussed with respiratory physiology. In addition, the free amine groups of hemoglobin (and other proteins) may bind with CO_2 to form carbamino compounds.

Hemoglobin is able to bind about 0.18 mEq H^+/g. Blood contains 150 g/L hemoglobin which is more effective than plasma proteins as a buffer.

PHOSPHATE BUFFERS

The presence of dibasic and monobasic phosphate anions provides an important intracellular buffer, with a minor role in plasma buffering. The phosphate anions are associated with Na^+ in the plasma and K^+ intracellularly. The anion pairs function as follows:

$$\text{conjugate base } HPO_4^{--} + H^+ \longrightarrow H_2PO_4^-$$

$$\text{weak acid } H_2PO_4^- + OH^- \longrightarrow HPO_4^{--} + H_2O$$

Intracellular buffers are important in chronic acidosis.

Reaction to Plasma Acid Load: Metabolic Acidosis

Metabolic acidosis is characterized by depletion of bicarbonate and lowering of blood pH. Clinically, causes of metabolic acidosis include (1) overproduction of acid metabolites by disease, toxemias, or starvation, (2) excessive administration of acids or acid salts (NH_4Cl) or

aspirin overdose, (3) excessive loss of alkaline fluids (prolonged diarrhea or fistula drainage), (4) renal acidosis in which kidney function is impaired and acid cannot be excreted nor bicarbonate regenerated, and (5) dehydration, due to chloride retention displacing bicarbonate.

The first reaction to threatening acidosis occurs within minutes. There is immediate buffering by the bicarbonate system. Respiration is stimulated as the CNS responds to increased H^+ and CO_2 is eliminated by the lungs. This system handles 12 percent of the total buffering.

The second reaction, also within minutes, is buffering by the plasma proteins, accounting for 1 percent of total buffer activity.

The third reaction also occurs quickly. H^+ diffuses into RBCs and is buffered by hemoglobin, phosphates, and intracellular bicarbonate. This accounts for 6–8 percent of total buffering.

The fourth reaction occurs in minutes to hours as H^+ crosses capillary walls into the interstitial compartment. Bicarbonate is the principal buffer in the interstitium, accounting for 30 percent of total buffering since there is four times more interstitial fluid than plasma. There is no protein buffering here, since proteins are restrained by the capillary membrane.

The fifth reaction occurs in several hours as H^+ diffuses into cells and is buffered by proteins in the tissues. H^+ enters the cell in a Na^+/K^+ exchange, increasing plasma K^+ and renal secretion of K^+. In chronic acidosis there can be a loss of K^+ due to this exchange. Much of this activity occurs in the bones and accounts for 51 percent of buffering.

One day after the acid load, blood pH returns to normal. However, only 25 percent of the acid has been eliminated. The remainder is sequestered and gradually eliminated by the kidneys. The kidney secretes H^+ slowly over several days. As HCO_3^- is consumed in buffering, the kidney replaces HCO_3^- by reabsorption and synthesis.

Reaction to Plasma Alkaline Load: Metabolic Alkalosis

Metabolic alkalosis is characterized by a large increase in bicarbonate and an elevated blood pH. Clinically, metabolic alkalosis is most commonly due to vomiting, with excessive loss of gastric juice or overadministration of a base forming salt, such as sodium bicarbonate or lactate.

Extracellular buffering accounts for 68 percent of the total. Respiration is depressed to retain carbonic acid (a limited effect due to hypoxia risk) and lactic acid is released from muscle and other cells. Bicarbonate enters the cells in exchange for Cl^-, while intracellular H^+ exits in exchange for Na^+ and K^+. Reabsorption of HCO_3^- by the kidney is decreased.

Differences in Buffering: Acidosis v Alkalosis

Respiratory compensation always occurs in acidosis, but not always in alkalosis. Lactic acid is involved in alkalosis as a compensatory mechanism but not in acidosis. Renal excretion of HCO_3^- in alkalosis is more rapid than excretion of H^+ in acidosis.

Respiratory Acid/Base Imbalance

When the lungs are the primary cause of acidosis (hypoventilation, emphysema, etc.), CO_2 retention results in increased H_2CO_3. Since H_2CO_3 cannot be buffered by HCO_3^-, all buffering is intracellular or by plasma proteins. CO_2 is permeable to the cell membrane and Na^+ and K^+ exchange with CO_2. CO_2 is then buffered by intracellular proteins. Buffering by hemoglobin in the RBC is important in this situation.

Respiratory acidosis and alkalosis are discussed further with respiratory physiology. Respiratory disturbances result in a more marked pH change as compared to metabolic disturbances, because HCO_3^- is lost. This situation requires renal compensation, a slower mechanism.

THE ROLE OF THE KIDNEY IN ACID BASE BALANCE

The kidneys function to regulate acid base balance by the excretion of H^+ and the reabsorption and synthesis of HCO_3^-.

Reabsorption of HCO_3^-

Bicarbonate is a threshold substance and most HCO_3^- is reabsorbed in the proximal tubule. In a threatening acidosis, HCO_3^- is depleted in buffering and will be in short supply. Effectively all HCO_3^- present will be reabsorbed in the proximal cells.

Since the lumenal membrane is impermeable to HCO_3^-, reabsorption is indirect. In the lumen HCO_3^- reacts with H^+ to form carbonic acid, which produces CO_2. CO_2 is membrane permeable and diffuses into the cell. In the tubular cell, CO_2 produced by metabolism as well as CO_2 entering from the lumen is hydrated to H_2CO_3 via carbonic anhydrase. The ionization of car-

bonic acid is forced by H^+ pumping into the lumen. Na^+ passively diffuses into the cell to replace secreted H^+. The HCO_3^- produced by ionization of intracellular carbonic acid diffuses across the permeable peritubular membrane accompanied by actively pumped Na^+. The net effect is reabsorbed $Na^+HCO_3^-$. Inhibition of carbonic anhydrase blocks sodium bicarbonate reabsorption, resulting in a large diuresis of $Na^+HCO_3^-$ and water.

The regulation of HCO_3^- reabsorption is controlled by (1) arterial PCO_2 (i.e., as plasma PCO_2 rises, CO_2 diffuses into the tubule cell to drive forward, via carbonic andrydrase, ionization of H_2CO_3 to HCO_3^- and H^+. Increased intracellular H^+ results in a greater H^+ secretion into the lumen, allowing more HCO_3^- to be reabsorbed); (2) plasma K^+ which influences HCO_3^- reabsorption in an inverse relationship related to K^+/H^+ exchange. Increased interstitial K^+ causes K^+ to enter the cell in exchange for intracellular H^+, decreasing HCO_3^- reabsorption and causing a more basic urine as the plasma becomes more acidic. If plasma K^+ is low (inadequate dietary K^+ or loss of K^+ in diarrhea), intracellular H^+ rises as K^+ falls, with increased HCO_3^- reabsorption; (3) plasma Cl^- (i.e., Cl^- and HCO_3^- are inversely related, mechanism unknown), and (4) adrenal steroids (i.e., HCO_3^- reabsorption is increased in Cushing's disease, a condition in which steroids are overproduced. In Addison's disease, steroid concentration falls, accompanied by decreased HCO_3^- reabsorption. This mechanism is related to the effect of steroids on K^+ flux. Steroids increase K^+ excretion, causing a fall in plasma K^+ which increases HCO_3^- reabsorption).

Excretion of HCO_3^-

In alkalosis when HCO_3^- concentration exceeds 28 mEq/L (the renal threshold), the kidney acts as a regulator of plasma HCO_3^-, and HCO_3^- is excreted.

Synthesis of HCO_3^-

EXCRETION OF WEAK ACID: TITRATABLE ACIDITY

The phosphate buffer is present in the plasma in a ratio 4:1 parts basic Na_2HPO_4/acidic NaH_2PO_4. Tubular activity in the regeneration of bicarbonate changes this ratio in the urine to 1:9 with the acid salt predominating. Weak acid anions, such as acetoacetate and β-hydroxybutyrate produced in diabetic acidosis, are also excreted by this mechanism as the undissociated acids. This scheme replaces bicarbonate lost in buffering. The Na^+/H^+ exchange in the distal tubules is influenced by aldosterone. The acid phosphate and organic acids produced in this manner are termed the titratable acidity and measure the extent to which bicarbonate has been depleted in buffering weak acids. Titratable acidity is determined by titrating the urine back to normal plasma pH 7.4 with standard alkali.

The mechanism involves the same metabolic scheme of carbonic anhydrase hydration of intracellular CO_2 and the removal of the ionization products of carbonic acid by H^+ pumping into the lumen and HCO_3^- diffusion into the peritubular interstitium. H^+ secreted into the lumen reacts with HPO_4^{--} or an organic acid anion and is excreted as the acid salt (NaH_2PO_4) or undissociated acid (Fig. 8-12).

EXCRETION OF STRONG ACID: THE RENAL AMMONIUM MECHANISM

The pH of the urine is normally between 5 and 7. Urine pH values lower than 4.5 are never found. Strong acids, such as HCl, produce pH values lower than this limit. In the presence of strong acid anions, such as sulfate from protein metabolism and chloride, a simple Na^+/H^+ exchange would produce sulfuric and hydrochloric acids with acidity levels harmful to renal tissue. Instead, the kidneys excrete strong acid anions as their ammonium salts.

Ammonia is produced within proximal and distal tubule cells and the collecting ducts by the deamination of glutamine and other amino acids rich in amine groups.

Ammonia diffuses into the lumen. Simultaneously, carbonic anhydrase activity via the previously summarized mechanism results in the pumping of H^+ into the lumen and the diffusion of HCO_3^- into the peritubular interstitium. Ammonia reacts with H^+ in the lumen to form the ammonium ion, NH_4^+ for the excretion of sulfates, chlorides, etc. as ammonium salts (Fig. 8-13).

Renal Pathology

In chronic renal disease, a loss of functioning renal mass occurs. As a result, renal ammonia production is decreased and the excretion of strong acid is compromised. However, H^+ may still be excreted via titratable acidity as long as H^+ pumping is sufficient and phosphate anions continue to be filtered in the remaining functional glomeruli. In renal tubule acidosis diseases, the kidney's ability to pump H^+ ions is a serious problem. Low plasma HCO_3^- results and if followed by high plasma Cl^-. If the proximal tubule cannot pump H^+, HCO_3^- is excreted, and plasma HCO_3^- and pH fall. The distal tubule can help to correct the low plasma pH level and is capable of building up a 1000:1 H^+ gradient. However, considerable HCO_3^- is still lost in the urine since the distal tubule is not as efficient as the proximal. Treatment involves the administration of HCO_3^-, resulting in a very basic urine.

When the distal tubule cannot pump H^+, the urine cannot be acidified below about pH 6.6. In this situation,

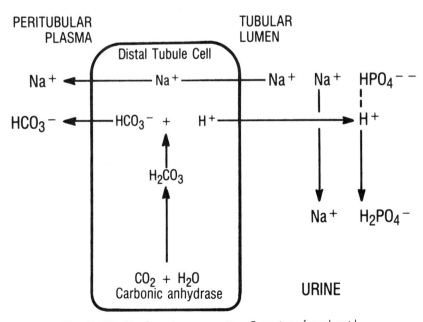

Fig. 8-12. Bicarbonate regeneration: Excretion of weak acid.

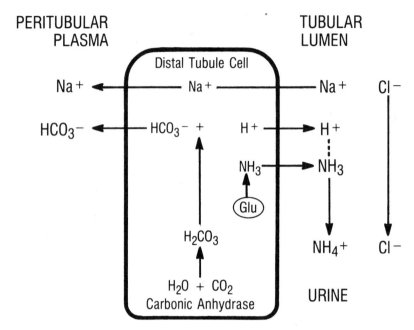

Fig. 8-13. Renal ammonium mechanism: Excretion of strong acid.

urine cannot be acidified and plasma pH will be acidic. This condition is also treated by administration of HCO_3^-, which is retained in this case at the proximal tubule.

WATER BALANCE

Normally, water distributes rapidly and uniformly throughout the fluid compartments. Water is gained by the body in fluid intake, in foods, as water of oxidation or "metabolic water." Water loss occurs chiefly in the urine. Appreciable loss also occurs via evaporation from the skin and lungs, either as insensible or sensible perspiration. The cardinal principle behind fluid balance is simply that new intake equals output.

Fluid Compartments of the Body

Water is the most abundant component of the body. The adult ranges between 50 to 70 percent water by weight. The percentage is dependent on the proportion of fat since fat excludes water. Almost one half of the body water is bound tightly by cellular proteins. Each cell is bathed by an interstitial (tissue) fluid, with transport from the environment performed by the circulatory system. Body fluid compartments and distribution of

total body water taken as 60 percent of body weight are as follows:

1. Intracellular fluid compartment (ICF), the fluid within the cells is 40 percent.
2. Extracellular compartment (ECF), the fluid outside the cells is 20 percent.
   Interstitial fluid is 16 percent.
   Plasma (vascular fluid) is 4 percent.

ELECTROLYTE COMPOSITION

In the extracellular fluid, Na^+ and Cl^- are the predominate cations, with small amounts of K^+, Mg^{++}, and Ca^{++} present. The predominant anions are Cl^- and HCO_3^-. Plasma contains a significant amount of protein anion which is absent in the interstitial fluid.

Intracellular fluid contains K^+ and Mg^{++} as the predominate cations, with a large amount of protein as well as phosphate and sufate anions.

Na^+ is the major osmotic species. The average cell membrane is an osmotic membrane, relatively impermeable to Na^+. The concentration of Na^+ in the plasma is regulated, in turn regulating the intracellular solutes in other compartments via water equilibrium. Water volume is regulated by the rate of Na^+ excretion, with osmolarity regulated by the rate of water absorption.

Regulation of Water Volume

Changes in blood pressure, venous pressure, and plasma osmolarity are regulatory signals directed to the hypothalamus via osmolar and vasoreceptors. Osmoreceptors, located in the hypothalamus, are sensitive to 1–2 percent changes in plasma osmolarity. In response to osmolarity increases, the hypothalamus increases ADH synthesis and secretion, thereby increasing water reabsorption to maintain fluid volume.

Two groups of vasoreceptors, low pressure venous receptors and the high pressure arterial receptors, influence fluid volume via the hypothalamus. Low pressure receptors are located in the left atrium of the heart and high pressure receptors are located in the carotid sinus and aortic arch. Vasoreceptors respond to increases in pressure and stretch, increasing the heart rate and relaying signals to the hypothalamus.

Volume and osmolarity act additively by way of these receptors. For example, a decrease in water intake causes a decrease in plasma volume, increasing plasma osmolarity to signal an increase in ADH release. The hypothalamus integrates signals with priority to plasma osmolarity (blood volume) until survival is affected. At this point, water volume takes priority.

FLUID SHIFTS

Fluid shifts are classified as (1) iso-osmotic in which both water and solute concentrations change proportionately, (2) hyperosmotic in which more water is lost than solutes, and (3) hypo-osmotic, in which more solutes are lost than water.

In extreme cases of iso-osmotic expansion, edema occurs as fluid moves into the interstitial space. Hypo-osmotic expansion may also be caused by ADH secreting tumors.

Regulatory Factors in NaCl Excretion

Normally, almost all Na^+ is reabsorbed with Cl^-. Some Na^+ is also reabsorbed in exchange for H^+ secreted by the tubules and a small amount is associated with K^+ secretion.

CHANGES IN THE GFR

Changes in the GFR affect Na^+ reabsorption and are commonly caused by (1) glomerular capillary pressure changes in which alterations in the systemic blood pressure are beyond renal autoregulatory control, (2) plasma protein osmotic (oncotic) pressure changes, (3) changes in sympathetic neural activity, and (4) changes in the renin-angiotension system.

Increases in the GFR present more Na^+ to the renal

tubules than can be absorbed in transit time. In addition, peritubular capillary protein osmotic pressure and peritubular capillary hydrostaic pressure are factors.

ADH RELEASE

Changes in ADH release are affected by plasma osmolarity (a direct relationship), blood pressure and blood volume (an inverse relationship), angiotensin II levels (a direct relationship), alcohol and caffeine, which act as diuretics to cause ADH secretion to cease, temperature (a direct relationship), and the sleep response, probably due to a drop in blood pressure since ADH secretion increases during sleep. Pain and emotional stress affect ADH unpredictably. Changes in ADH output and water absorption occur very rapidly, within minutes to hours. However, changes in sodium reabsorption can take days to readjust.

ALDOSTERONE OUTPUT

Aldosterone causes increased Na^+ reabsorption. The major regulator of aldosterone release is angiotensin II. At low levels, angiotensin II action is local, within the kidney. At higher levels, systemic effects cause an increase in peripheral vasoconstriction which increases blood pressure. This influences GFR increase and the filtration factor. Angiotensin II also influences the thirst mechanism.

The second factor which influences aldosterone output is the Na^+/K^+ balance. High Na^+ and K^+ levels directly effect the adrenal gland to increase aldosterone release; low levels of these cations inhibit aldosterone release.

BLOOD FLOW

Renal blood flow is redistributed in response to changes in plasma Na^+. If salt needs to be lost, more blood goes to the cortical nephrons. However, if salt needs to be conserved, more blood goes to the juxtamedullary nephrons.

In severe continued loss of water or salt, the kidney becomes helpless. For example, in response to water overload, aldosterone drops; if both Na^+ and water are lost, urine output peaks in 15 to 30 minutes after the plasma osmolarity is lowest. After 2 to 3 hours 1200 ml can be lost.

POTASSIUM EXCRETION

Most of the filtered K^+ is actively reabsorbed in the proximal tubules. K^+ may be secreted by the distal tubule cells. In this event, Na^+ is reabsorbed for excreted K^+.

PART 6 _____

Gastrointestinal System

The gastrointestinal tract is an open tube via which nutrients, minerals, vitamins, and water enter the body and complex molecules are broken down by the process of digestion to simple units for absorption into the lymph and blood. Undigested materials are excreted as feces.

Digestion begins in the mouth where starch is attacked by the salivary amylase (ptyalin). α-Amylase, the only important digestive enzyme in saliva, cleaves 1,4 glycosidic bonds. Amylase is optimally active at a neutral pH and is inactivated by high acid levels in the stomach. While the salivary amylase is capable of degrading starches to maltose, maltotrioses, and dextrins, the short period of activity in the mouth breaks only a few bonds in midchain. Thus, it is not essential for carbohydrate digestion.

Additional organic components of saliva are mucin, a glycoprotein which lubricates and aids in swallowing, and lysozyme, a bacteriocidal enzyme. Ionic components are those typical of extracellular fluid (Na^+, K^+, Cl^-, and HCO_3^-). HCO_3^- contributes to the pH of saliva, which ranges from $6.0-7.8$, depending on the flow rate. Small amounts of Ca^{++}, Mg^{++}, I^-, CNS^-, NO_3^-, urea, phosphates, and amino acids are present. Bacteria in the mouth convert nitrate to nitrite.

THE SALIVARY GLANDS

The main salivary glands, the parotid, submaxillary, and sublingual, are metabolically very active with a high O_2 consumption to provided energy for secretion. The acini structure exhibits mainly serous and mucous cells. The parotid gland (25 percent of total secretion) has only serous cells. The submaxillary gland (45 percent of total secretion) contains mainly serous cells; the sublingual (4 percent of total secretion) shows mainly mucous cells.

Secretions produced in acinar cells enter intercalated ducts which lead into intra- and extralobular ducts to the open gastrointestinal tract. The glands are innervated via sympathetic and parasympathetic fibers. Sympathetic stimulation is via the superior cervical ganglion, with norepinephrine release stimulating secretion. Parasympathetic postganglionic fibers release acetylcholine and affect a greater saliva production than sympathetic stim-ulation. The blood supply to the glands runs countercurrent to the flow of glandular secretion.

Mechanism of Salivary Secretion

Salivary secretion is similar to an ultrafiltrate of plasma, containing somewhat more HCO_3^-. The acinar cells actively secrete Na^+ (and possibly other ions), with water passively following. As fluid moves down the ducts, ions move in either direction and the net effect is removal of Na^+ and addition of K^+ to saliva. Since the ducts remove more ions than are added, the saliva is hypotonic. The composition varies with the efficiency of ion transport systems. At maximal flow, the saliva is richer in Na^+ with lower levels of K^+ than at basal flow rates.

Regulation of Salivary Secretion

The presence of food in the mouth (especially acidic foods) is a potent salivary stimulus. In addition, the sight, smell, and thought of food increase saliva production, primarily via parasympathetic stimulation. Fear and sleep inhibit secretion.

Parasympathetic stimulation stimulates a high volume of saliva, increasing cellular metabolism which results in the secretion of kallikrein into the blood. Kallikrein acts on a plasma protein to produce bradykinin, which dilates glandular blood vessels to increase flow. Increased blood flow is essential to sustain secretion. Parasympathetic stimulation also results in increased growth of the glands.

Stimulation of the sympathetic system results in a burst of salivary secretion due in part to contraction of the myoepithelial cells of the gland. This burst is accompanied by a transient vasoconstriction. Less saliva is produced via sympathetic stimulation than via parasympathetic stimulation.

There is no direct endocrine control of salivary secretion, except that mineralocorticoids increase Na^+ retention and K^+ output by the ducts. Thus, a high aldosterone level leads to a saliva which is low in Na^+ and high in K^+. The amount of secretion is not affected.

Drugs which are antagonists to acetylcholine and norepinephrine cause a dry mouth by interfering with normal nervous stimulation of salivation. Denervation of the glands or a regimen of low acid meals will cause the glands to atrophy due to lack of growth promoting action. If the sympathetic nerves to these glands are severed, their sensitivity to circulating epinephrine is greatly increased, a phenomenon called paralytic secretion.

Summary of Salivary Function

In summary, salivary secretion protects against acids and hot temperatures in the mouth, allows speech, lubricates food for easier swallowing, inhibits dental decay (due to HCO_3^- and Ca^{++}), and commences carbohydrate digestion. While the salivary glands are not absolutely necessary for digestion, they are essential for prevention of tooth decay.

GASTRIC SECRETION

Secretory Cell Types

Anatomically, the stomach is divided into the body or fundic region, the antrum or pyloric region, and the cardiac region. The stomach is lined with a thick mucous layer and surface mucosal cells which lie on top of the submucosa and muscle layers. Gastric glands containing several different types of secretory cells open into the mucous layer. In the fundic region, parietal (oxyntic) cells and mucous neck cells line the neck region of the glands and argentaffin cells and chief cells line their bases.

Surface mucous cells contain a large number of mucous granules on the lumenal side of the cell and secrete a glycoprotein mucus which serves to protect the underlying submucosa from stomach acid. Some of these cells are shed daily. The mucous neck cells also secrete protective mucus as well as a small amount of pepsinogen.

The chief (peptic) cells produce and secrete pepsinogen in response to appropriate stimuli. The zymogen (storage granules) for pepsinogen are the first to be secreted when the cell is stimulated. Cells are present only in the fundic region.

Parietal cells function to secrete acid and are present only in the fundic region.

Gastrin cells function to secrete the hormone gastrin into the blood. They contain secretory granules of gastrin predominately at the basal surface and microvilli with acid receptors. They are present only in the pyloric region.

MUCOSAL GROWTH AND REPLACEMENT

The gastric mucosa has a high turnover rate with a cell life of 1 to 2 days. Damaged glands can be replaced by surface mucosal cell differentiation into mucous neck cells, which can further differentiate into either parietal or chief cells. Both gastrin and growth hormone stimu-

late the growth of the gastric mucosa. The ability to replace mucosal cells is important in maintaining a protective barrier for the underlying cell layers.

Blood Supply

An extensive blood supply is necessary to produce large amounts of gastric secretions. Many anastomoses allow regions of the stomach to be tied off without preventing blood flow to other regions of the stomach. Gastric blood flow can be estimated by the clearance of a weak base from the blood. A weak base is unionized at physiologic pH, but ionizes once it diffuses into the highly acid stomach and cannot reenter the blood.

Innervation of the Stomach

Parasympathetic innervation is via vagal fibers to the secretory and endocrine cells via the myenteric and submucosal plexi. Stimulation increases gastric secretion.

Sympathetic innervation is also via the myenteric and submucosal plexi. The sympathetic system does not innervate the secretory cells of the stomach (some sympathetic innervation of intestinal secretory cells does occur). Sympathetic stimulation causes some vasoconstriction and is inhibitory to gastric secretion.

REFLEX SYSTEMS

In a peripheral reflex system, chemoreceptors and mechanoreceptors in the gastrointestinal tract send signals to the myenteric and submucosal plexi which are transmitted to gastric secretory and/or endocrine cells.

In an enterogastric reflex system, receptors in the intestine transmit signals to the celiac plexus which innervate the gastric blood vessels and muscles so that food in the intestine can effect activity in the stomach.

In an efferent system, mechanoreceptors and chemoreceptors can feed signals back to high centers of the brain in a long reflex arc involving vagal innervation of the stomach.

Composition of Gastric Secretion

PEPSIN

Pepsinogen (MW 42,000–43,000) is the inactive precursor to the proteolytic enzyme pepsin. The active enzyme is produced by the cleavage of a 29 amino acid inhibitory sequence from the N-terminus of pepsinogen. Activation occurs in the presence of acid or pepsin, itself.

Pepsin is only active in the acid pH range (1–4), with optimal activity at about pH 3. Pepsin is a nonspecific protease, with some preference to cleavage of bonds adjacent to internal hydrophobic amino acids.

Pepsinogen is released from chief cells in response to vagal (parasympathetic) stimulation and stomach acid or indirectly by gastrin (which influences acid release) and possibly secretin which is released from the duodenum in response to low pH. Pepsinogen is also produced by mucous neck cells.

INTRINSIC FACTOR

Intrinsic factor is a glycoprotein necessary for the uptake of vitamin B_{12} (cobalamin) and its precursors. In addition to intrinsic factor, transcobalamin II and the R protein are important in vitamin B_{12} metabolism. Transcobalamin II is necessary for transport in the blood and delivery to the cells. The R protein, located in the liver, has a high affinity for B_{12} and binds and stores the vitamin.

Intrinsic factor is synthesized and released by parietal (oxyntic) cells. Secretion is in response to vagal stimulation and gastrin. Lack of intrinsic factor leads to vitamin B_{12} deficiency.

OTHER CONSTITUENTS

Mucus is continuously produced by the active secretion and desquamation of surface mucosal cells. Secretion can be further induced by nervous stimulation and mechanical irritation.

A gastric lipase is present, but degrades only short chain fatty acids. Lysozyme degrades glycoproteins and bacterial cell walls, but does not digest the mucosal protective proteins. Urease, which hydrolyzes urea to ammonia, is only of importance in rare uremic conditions.

Bicarbonate is secreted by nonparietal mucous cells in a protective fluid with a neutral to alkaline pH. This fluid is trapped by mucus and the mixture of mucus, protein, and neutral fluid protects the underlying gastric cells against acid secretion.

The parietal cells are the source of acid secretion. Maximal stimulation can produce high H^+ concentrations (about 150 mmol).

Mechanism of Acid Secretion

The ability of the stomach to secrete acid is proportional to the number of parietal cells present. Events in the parietal cell involve active, coupled pumping of H^+ and Cl^- into the gastric juice. This activity results in a 1 : 1 ratio of H^+ and Cl^- and is accompanied by passive water transport.

The primary source of secreted H^+ appears to be from the ionization of water. The OH^- left behind is neutralized by the H^+ from the ionization of carbonic acid, produced by carbonic anhydrase activity on CO_2 and H_2O. The other product of carbonic acid ionization, HCO_3^- moves into the plasma.

The net effect of this mechanism is (1) H^+ moves into the gastric juice, (2) Cl^- moves from the plasma to the gastric juice and is replaced by HCO_3^- in a 1 : 1 exchange, (3) water loss results in an overall osmotic pressure rise, and (4) blood pH goes up as HCO_3^- replaces Cl^-, an event termed the postprandial alkaline tide.

The parietal cell is polarized with the serosal membrane positive, while the mucosal membrane is negative, mainly due to Cl^- pumping.

Phases of Gastric Secretion

The four phases of secretion are (1) the interdigestive phase in which no food is taken in and gastric secretion is minimal, (2) the cephalic phase in which food is in the mouth and gastric secretion increases to a substantial amount, (3) the gastric phase in which food enters the stomach and there is a substantial amount of secretion, and (4) the intestinal phase, in which food enters the intestine with a slight stimulation to slowing secretion.

Regulation of Acid Secretion

In the cephalic phase, acid secretion is caused by both direct innervation of the parietal cells by vagal release of acetylcholine and by innervation of gastric secreting G-cells in the antrum.

In the gastric phase, acid secretion is regulated by distension of the stomach. Response is via a short reflex arc in the submucosal plexus which releases acetylcholine onto parietal cells. A long reflex arc via the vagi also stimulates parietal cells. G-cells are also stimulated in the antrum. Amino acids and peptides from the meal also act directly on parietal cells to stimulate them and are able to stimulate antrum G-cells. In addition, Ca^{++} has some stimulatory effect.

In the intestinal phase, digested proteins act directly on intestinal G-cells to release gastrin and also act on intestinal endocrine glands to release enteroxyntin, an unidentified hormone with stimulatory effects on parietal cells.

The gastric mucosa has a high histamine content which has a potent stimulating effect on H^+ secretion, probably via cAMP. Two types of histamine receptors, H1 and H2, mediate parietal cell response. Blockage of

H1 receptors by antihistamines used to treat allergy has little effect on acid secretion. However, drugs that block H2 receptors, such as climetidine, are effective and are used to treat peptic ulcers.

Inhibition of Secretion

A pH of less than 3 in the antrum inhibits gastrin release. Entry of gastric contents into the duodenum causes inhibitory effects which decrease the amount of acid secretion. A low pH in the duodenum leads to release of the hormone secretin, which directly inhibits both gastric acid and gastrin release. A low pH in the duodenum also leads to a nervous reflex which inhibits acid secretion. In addition, when hyperosmotic solutions reach the duodenum, an unidentified "enterogastrone" is released which inhibits acid secretion. Fatty acids reaching the duodenum cause the release of (1) gastrin inhibitory peptide (GIP) which directly inhibits both gastric acid and gastrin secretion, (2) cholecystokinin (CCK) which leads to inhibition of gastric acid secretion only if gastrin is present, and (3) unidentified "enterogastrone."

Overall Acid Production

The production of acid is autoregulatory and is proportional to the buffering capacity of food in the stomach. Protein is the best buffer in food. Therefore, the total amount of H^+ secreted is proportional to the amount of protein consumed. Conditions such as gastric ulcer, gastritis, and gastric cancer decrease H^+ secretion. Emotional factors such as depression and fear decrease H^+ secretion while anger and anxiety cause an increase. Duodenal ulcers also increase both the rate and total amount of H^+ secretion. Men secrete more gastric H^+ than women.

Gastrin and vagal stimulation are the most important stimulators of acid secretion. The most important inhibitor is H^+ itself in the stomach.

Gastrin

Gastrin is a polypeptide hormone released by intestinal G-cells in two main circulating forms, gastrin 17 and gastrin 34, indicating the number of amino acids in the polypeptide chains. The two forms are equally potent and are present in equal molar concentrations. However, G-34 is longer lasting because of the increase in degradation time.

Physiologically, gastrin increases acid secretion by parietal cells. Gastrin also increases gastric mucosal blood flow. Trophically, gastrin acts on the gastrointestinal tract mucosa to stimulate growth of mucosal cells. The hormone also affects antral motility and causes closure of the lower esophageal sphincter.

At concentrations above physiologic levels, gastrin increases gallbladder contraction and intestinal motility as well as increasing enzyme and electrolyte secretion by the pancreas, liver, and intestine. Pharmacologic dosages also decrease intestinal absorption and gastric emptying and influence the release of insulin and glucagon.

STIMULANTS/INHIBITORS OF GASTRIN

Meat extracts, peptones, and amino acids act directly on the gastrin releasing G-cells. Other stimulants of gastrin secretion are histamine, caffeine, and alcohol.

The most potent physiologic inhibitor of gastrin secretion is acid which acts directly on the G-cells, with a probable action also via mucosal receptors. There is also duodenal inhibition of gastrin release. Other inhibitors include thiocyanate, carbonic anhydrase inhibitors, prostaglandins E1 and A, and H^+ receptor antagonists.

Gastric Absorption

Little absorption occurs in the stomach; short chain alcohols and short chain fatty acids are absorbed to some extent. Aspirin, a weak acid, is converted to the union-ized form in the stomach because of the low pH. This form is fat soluble and can diffuse into the gastric mucosa. At the neutral intracellular pH of the mucosal cell, aspirin becomes ionized again and diffuses into the blood. This can cause damage to the mucosal layer since it leads to histamine release and increases H^+ secretion. Hemorrhage and ulceration may result.

Summary: Gastric Function

The stomach functions to mix and break up the food bolus to a state called chyme, which is gradually released to the small intestine. Protein digestion begins in the stomach via pepsin degradation. Short chain fatty acids are digested and absorbed. H^+ secretion facilitates iron uptake, which is enhanced in the ferric (Fe^{+++}) form. The high acidity levels of the stomach function to kill bacteria. Gastric secretions also perform an important function in signaling the release of pancreatic enzymes.

Removal of the stomach is not life threatening with vitamin B_{12} therapy. Without therapy, B_{12} deficiency would develop some years later, since a 3 to 5 year supply of intrinsic factor is stored in the liver. However, the digestion and uptake of fat would be abnormal.

THE PANCREAS

Exocrine Function

The pancreas is an organ with both exocrine and endocrine functions. The exocrine function involves secretion of the digestive enzymes into the gastrointestinal tract. The acinar cells contain many storage granules for zymogens (proenzymes). They secrete most of the digestive enzymes and also a small amount of water, HCO_3^-, and Cl^-. Cholecystokinin (CCK or pancrozymin) is the primary stimulant for enzyme release. Gastrin at high concentrations and vagal stimulation also facilitate release of enzymes and pancreatic fluid. The hormones CCK and gastrin are secreted by the intestinal mucosa. The centroacinar cells and cells of the intercalated duct produce the bulk of pancreatic fluid which is rich in HCO_3^-.

Organic Components of Pancreatic Secretion

Trypsinogen (230 amino acids) is the inactive form of the protease trypsin. Conversion to the active enzyme occurs by cleavage of a 6 amino acid fragment from the *N*-terminus. Enterokinase, an enzyme secreted by the duodenal mucosa, activates trypsinogen and the presence of trypsin facilitates conversion of the proenzyme. Trypsin is a specific protease which cleaves peptide bonds on the carboxyl side of basic amino acids.

Chymotrypsinogen is the inactive precurosr of chymotrypsin, a specific protease which cleaves on the carboxyl side of aromatic amino acids. Conversion from the proenzyme is facilitated by the presence of trypsin.

Procarboxypeptidase A and B are inactive precursors of carboxypeptidase A and B which are converted to the active form by trypsin. Carboxypeptidase A cleaves individual amino acids from the carboxyl end of a peptide with preference for aromatic amino acids. Carboxypeptidase B functions in the same manner but prefers peptides with a basic amino acid at the carboxyl terminus.

Proelastase is converted to the active form, elastase, by trypsin and disgests the insoluble protein elastin.

Trypsin inhibitor (MW 10,000–12,000) plays an important role in protecting pancreatic cells from self-digestion as they contain large quantities of proteolytic enzymes. The inhibitor binds to and inactivates trypsin present in the acinar cells. The effects of trypsin inhibitor are overwhelmed quickly during active trypsin secretion.

The pancreatic amylase has the same specificity as the salivary α-amylase, cleaving 1–4 glycolytic bonds. The products are maltose, maltotriose, and 1–6 branched oligosaccharides.

Nucleases attack both ribonucleases and deoxyribonucleases.

At least four lipases are present in pancreatic juice. A lipase degrades long chain fatty acyl glycerides and one is specific for cholesterol esters. Both require the emulsifying action of the bile salts. Another lipase attacks short chain fatty acids and a fourth lipase is specific for lecithin and other phospholipids.

Dietary Trophic Effects

A diet high in proteins and/or fats results in an increase in the size of pancreatic cells and enzyme secretion. The pancreatic hormone CCK plays a role in the regulation of pancreatic growth.

The Pancreatic Fluid

The pancreatic enzymes have optimal activity around pH 7. The acid chyme arriving from the stomach is neutralized by the high HCO_3^- concentration of the alkaline pancreatic juice. The composition of pancreatic fluid depends on the rate of secretion. Maximal stimulation leads to maximal flow and results in a fluid high in HCO_3^- and low in Cl^-. Na^+ is the major cation. There is a 1:1 passive replacement of HCO_3^- by Cl^- as fluid passes down the duct. A high flow rate reduces exchange time.

The major driving force for HCO_3^- production is active Na^+ transport into the lumen of the duct. HCO_3^- and water follow passively. There is also active transport of H^+ into the plasma which is coupled to Na^+ movement from plasma into the cell. OH^- left behind within the cell combines with H_2CO_3 to yield HCO_3^-. CO_2 diffusing into the cell is converted to HCO_3^- by the action of carbonic anhydrase. HCO_3^- passively follows Na^+ into the lumen. Plasma CO_2 is the major source of HCO_3^-.

Stimulating Hormones for Pancreatic Secretion

Secretin elicits maximum response in effecting an increase in the volume of pancreatic fluid and the amount of HCO_3^-, but only results in a small increase in enzyme secretion. Low pH causes duodenal S-cells to release secretin.

CCK has the greatest effect on increasing enzyme secretion, with a small effect on increasing fluid volume and HCO_3^-. Amino acids, some peptides, and fats influence a small increase in secretin but a large increase in

CCK secretion. Secretin and CCK act synergistically to increase pancreatic secretory volume. Gastrin at very high levels has effects similar to CCK.

In summary, H^+ causes the release of secretin which stimulates an increase in flow of fluid and electrolytes in the pancreatic juice. Fat, peptides, and amino acids cause the release of CCK which stimulates an increase in pancreatic enzymes. Secretin and CCK are synergistic; one potentiates the action of the other.

CCK EFFECTS

CCK is a peptide hormone with the eight amino acid sequence at the carboxyl terminus required for activity. CCK peptides in the digestive tract are found mainly in the small intestine with some present in the colon. CCK peptides also occur in both the CNS and the peripheral nervous system, the pituitary, thyroid, and kidney. CCK-33 is found in small amounts in the cortex of brain, along with CCK-8 and CCK-4 which differ by amino acids at these positions. CCK-4 and gastrin-4 are the same compound.

In addition to effecting increased pancreatic enzyme secretion, CCK is a very potent stimulant for gallbladder contraction. CCK weakly stimulates fluid and electrolyte secretion from the liver and pancreas with synergistic action with secretin. CCK has a trophic effect on pancreatic growth, particularly of the acinar cells. The hormone reduces the rate of gastric emptying, which partially accounts for the slower gastric emptying after a high fat meal, since fat in the duodenum stimulates CCK release.

CCK is released mainly in the duodenum. Release is also effected in the remainder of the small intestine by certain amino acids and fats. Release is inhibited by trypsin and the bile acids. Response to the bile acids provides a regulatory mechanism for CCK release. CCK causes gallbladder contraction, resulting with the emptying of bile acids into the duodenum. The bile acids then inhibit more CCK release.

Pancreatic Enzyme Secretion

The mechanism of pancreatic enzyme secretion is postulated to occur by a hormone binding to a receptor in the cell membrane. This complex causes mobilization and release of the cell's normally sequestered Ca^{++} stores to stimulate enzyme secretion. Cyclic GMP may have a role in enzyme release, but apparently Ca^{++} is required.

Substances which stimulate enzyme secretion include acetylcholine, CCK, and gastrin.

BILE

Production and Secretion

Bile is continuously produced by the parenchymal cells of the liver and is secreted into the canaliculi where it enters the bile ducts. Duct cells contribute fluid and electrolytes to the bile whereas the bile salts and macromolecules are secreted predominantly by the hepatocytes.

Composition: The Bile Acids

Cholic, chenodeoxycholic, and lithocholic acid are the most important components of bile. Cholic acid is a cholesterol derivative produced by the liver. It is amphoteric with a nonpolar, steroid nucleus and polar hydroxyl groups occurring on carbons 3, 7, and 12 with a carboxyl group at the chain terminus. Cholic acid is a weak acid, with a pK_a of about 5. Conjugation of the amino acids taurine and glycine with cholic acid results in stronger acids. The bile salts are mainly Na^+ taurocholate (pK_a about 1.5) and Na^+ glycocholate (pK_a about 3).

Chenodeoxycholic acid is a derivative of cholic acid with one less hydroxyl group. The pKa is similar and it also conjugates with taurine and glycine to form bile salts.

The secondary bile acids, deoxycholic and lithocholic, are produced by the action of intestinal bacteria on cholic acid. Deoxycholic acid is absorbed from the intestine and is transported to the liver where it can conjugate with taurine and glycine to form functional bile acids. Lithocholic acid has limited polarity and on absorption is sulfonated by the liver for excretion via the intestine.

Other Bile Components

Cholesterol and lecithin are main constituents of bile. Bile also contains glycoproteins. Na^+, Cl^-, and HCO_3^- are predominate ions, with Na^+ also associated with bile acid anions.

Bilirubin is a degradation product of hemoglobin which is excreted in the bile. In the liver bilirubin is converted via a hepatic glucuronyl transferase into bilirubin glucuronide, the form in which it is excreted in the bile. In impaired liver function, the concentration of bilirubin, a yellow pigment, rises in the blood, leading to jaundice. The liver also excretes foreign substances as sulfate or glucuronide conjugates in the bile.

Bile Flow

Choleretics are substances which increase the rate of bile production and secretion. The bile acids themselves are important choleretics.

Bile acids can be newly synthesized or parenterally administered or recycled from the enterohepatic circulation. Increased bile salts from the latter source cause increased bile flow (the choleretic effect of bile salts).

Parenchymal as well as ductule cells secrete water and electrolytes. Secretin stimulates secretion from both cell types. Vagal stimulation also causes increased bile flow, an effect which can be blocked by anticholinergic drugs. Gastrin and CCK also affect bile flow but only at pharmacologic concentrations.

Enterohepatic Circulation of Bile Acids

Enterohepatic circulation of bile acids begins with bile secretion into the duodenum in response to a meal. In the terminal ileum the absorption of conjugated bile salts is an active process. Here salts enter the portal circulation for return to the liver where they induce more bile secretion and are resecreted themselves. Thus, bile salts are recycled during the course of a meal.

Deconjugated and unionized conjugated bile salts are passively absorbed in the small intestine. Bile salts which pass the active absorption site of the terminal ileum enter the colon where bacterial action splits off taurine and glycine. The hydroxyl groups are also removed resulting in the formation of the secondary bile acids, deoxycholic and lithocholic acids. Recycling of the bile acids is important since *de novo* synthesis by the liver would not produce enough bile for needs. *De novo* synthesis replenishes bile acids lost through excretion.

The Gallbladder

During the interdigestive phase, the sphincter of Oddi is closed and bile is stored and concentrated in the gallbladder. During a meal, the gallbladder is stimulated to contract by CCK and the vagal response to the presence of fat in the duodenum. Water, Na^+, and Cl^-, the principal electrolytes in bile, are removed in the gallbladder in the concentration process. Bile acids, cholesterol, lecithin, and other components remain. Although Na^+ decreases in quantity, Na^+ concentration actually increases in gallbladder bile because it is retained as the bile salt cation.

RELEASE OF CONCENTRATED BILE

In normal subjects, high concentrations of bile acids are found periodically in plasma in response to liquid meals. These particularly high levels are brought about by contractions of the gallbladder which release concentrated bile into the duodenum. Without a gallbladder, the large periodic changes are absent and the level of plasma bile acids is maintained at a fairly moderate level with only a slight increase in response to meals. If the bile acids cannot be absorbed properly, most will be lost. In this case, the first meal of the day induces the largest response, since *de novo* synthesis by the liver during sleep partially replenishes supply.

GALLSTONE FORMATION

Gallstones are formed by the precipitation of bile components, for example, cholesterol or the Ca^{++} salts of the bile acids. Stones of sufficient size can block the ducts.

INTESTINAL ABSORPTION

Transport Mechanisms

Absorption across the intestinal mucosa occurs by (1) Simple diffusion in which the solute either dissolves through the membrane or flows through membrane pores down its electrochemical gradient. No metabolic energy is required. (2) Facilitated diffusion which also occurs passively via the electrochemical gradient. No metabolic energy is required. (3) Active transport which occurs against the electrochemical gradient and involves a membrane carrier. Metabolic energy is required. (4) Exchange diffusion, in which one molecule runs down its electrochemical gradient while the other solute flows in the opposite direction against or with the electrochemical gradient. Metabolic energy is required. Carriers are usually located in the brush border membrane and may be temporarily or permanently missing in certain diseases.

Absorptive Surface and Cell Types

Undifferentiated secretory cells, located in the crypts and among the surface absorptive cells, secrete mucus which lubricates the chyme. Argentaffin and enterochromaffin cells are involved in endocrine function. They contain secretory granules for peptide hormones. Differentiated villous cells are histologically absorptive cells and are the most abundant cell type present.

Brunner's glands are mucous and enterokinase secreting glands located in the submucosa of the proximal small intestine. Regulation of the glands is both neural and hormonal. Mucous secretion protects this part of the intestine from the acid chyme released from the stomach.

Cell Components

The microvilli are lumenal membrane modifications which increase the surface area available for absorption. These processes contain the complex biological machinery of absorption (i.e., carriers and enzymes). The tight junctions are the closest approximation of two cell membranes, but are very leaky to water and small ions. The lateral intercellular space contains fluid recently transported. The glycocalyx is composed of glycoprotein adhering to the brush border and is the site of digestive enzymes.

Maturation of Cells

In maturing from the undifferentiated crypt cells to the surface absorptive cells, microvilli "grow" to increase surface area. Mitochondria increase to meet the increased metabolic requirement for absorption, with surface cells having a higher O_2 consumption. Cells lose their secretory granules since they are not needed for the cell's absorptive role. The cells become biologically more complicated, acquiring receptors and carriers. The cells also acquire a protein which increases the motility of the villi. Contraction of the villi mixes the unstirred surface layer in and around the glycocalyx, increasing absorptive efficiency.

Absorption of Water and Electrolytes

Water movement in the gastrointesinal tract responds to osmotic forces to maintain osmotic equilibrium with the plasma. Ingested fluids (2 L) and secretions (7 L) are almost totally reabsorbed daily in the intestines, with only 200 ml excreted in the stool.

Lumenal Na^+ and plasma Na^+ concentrations are approximately equal (140 mEq/L) with a large Na^+ flux occurring with water movement. Net Na^+ movement from lumen to plasma is against an electrical gradient since a potential difference of about 5 mV exists between the lumen (negative) and serosa (positive). Na^+ moves into the cell from the lumen along both electrical and chemical gradients (potential difference ~ -40 mV; intracellular Na^+ concentration ~ 15 mEq/L). Movement from the cell into the plasma occurs against the gradient and is assisted by a Na^+/K^+ ATPase pump located on the lateral intercellular membrane. Na^+ pumping produces a hyperosmolar solution in the lateral intercellular space to which water is osmotically drawn. Na^+ movement is, therefore, the primary event in water movement. Active transport of Na^+ also facilitates the absorption of glucose, amino acids, and other substances.

Chloride movement occurs against the electrochemical gradient from the lumen into the cell, but with the gradient from the cell to the plasma. Chloride can be actively reabsorbed in a 1 : 1 exchange with HCO_3^-, an important event in the neutralization of acid chyme.

K^+ movement occurs from the lumen into the cell against the concentration gradient, requiring active transport. At high enough K^+ levels in the lumen, movement can occur by simple diffusion. Na^+ movement via ATPase pumping is coupled to K^+ movement from the plasma into the cell.

Transport of Sugars

The end products of α-amylase digestion are dextrins (branched polymers of about eight glucose units), maltotrioses, and the disaccharide maltose. Oligosaccharidases located on the brush border of the mucosal cells, principally in the ileum, further degrade these to maltose.

Dissacharidases found in the lumen and on the glycocalyx of the brush border degrade sucrose, lactose, and maltose into their monomers (glucose, galactose, and fructose). Glucose and galactose are treated similarly by the intestine and share a common carrier. Absorption occurs against a gradient, assisted by very efficient, stereospecific, Na^+ dependent transporters which exhibit saturation kinetics. D-isomers are preferred. The transport mechanism appears to involve a brush border receptor for Na^+/glucose. Glucose moves into the cell via the Na^+/glucose carrier, but exits via a carrier that is not Na^+ dependent. Na^+ is removed via membrane ATPase pumping.

Fructose is transported by facilitated diffusion, with the intestine exhibiting a high transport capacity at high lumenal concentrations.

Protein and Amino Acid Transport

Both dietary protein and exogenous protein from saliva, gastric juices, pancreatic products, and desquamated cells of the intestinal mucosa are degraded in the gastrointestinal tract. Except for the first few days of life, intact proteins do not normally traverse the intestinal mucosa. Amino acids and small peptides are the degradation products absorbed.

Amino acids are actively transported by a system of stereospecific carriers which exhibit saturation kinetics. l-Amino acids are preferred. Transport of amino acids is augmented in the presence of Na^+. However, in the absence of Na^+, amino acids are still actively transported, although at diminished levels. Saturation kinetics are present with and without Na^+ for amino acid absorption, in contrast to sugar transport where there is essentially no sugar uptake without the presence of Na^+.

There are at least four transport mechanisms for

amino acids, some of which share carriers. Carriers transport structurally similar amino acids. The neutral amino acid system (glycine, alanine, etc.) exhibits Na^+ dependence. The basic amino acid system (lysine, arginine, etc.) is similar, but is independent of neutral amino acid transport and slower. The transport of cyclical proline and hydroxyproline occurs in a less distinct system which overlaps somewhat with neutral amino acid transport. Acidic amino acid transport (aspartic, glutamic, etc.) occurs via a separate system. Glutamic (GLU) and aspartic (ASP) acids are transaminated with pyruvic acid in the intestinal mucosa to form alanine. This modification lowers the mucosal concentration of GLU and ASP, maintaining a concentration gradient across the brush border favoring uptake of these amino acids.

Peptides are absorbed by a distinct mechanism involving a separate stereospecific carrier system from free amino acids. Peptides are hydrolyzed in the mucosa before entering the circulation.

Lipid Absorption

The bulk of lipid intake is in the form of water insoluble triglycerides, the simple dietary fats and oils. Ingested cholesterol esters present an absorptive problem because of their large size. Phospholipids must also be absorbed. In addition, the fat soluble vitamins (A, D, E, and K) are a small but important fraction of absorbed fats.

INTRALUMINAR PHASE

Ingested fat presents to the gut in large masses with a low surface area/mass ratio. Water insolubility presents a digestive challenge and requires emulsification by the action of the bile salts to break down a large mass of fat into smaller droplets, increasing the surface area. Lecithin and protein also act as emulsifying agents. Such agents have a nonpolar component which binds to the fat droplet and a polar component which interacts with water in a detergent action to solubilize the droplet.

The pancreatic lipase acts at the oil/water interface of the emulsion, catalyzing the hydrolysis of triglycerides into their constituent fatty acids and glycerol. Fatty acids appear as soaps in the alkaline, sodium rich intestinal fluid, aiding emulsification. Incomplete hydrolysis products, monoglycerides and some diglycerides, also appear.

Lipids tend to form micelles, a process aided by the bile salts. The bile acids and monoglycerides are key components of the micelle. Lecithin, cholesterol, fatty acids, and the fat soluble vitamins are also constituents. Components can move in and out of the micelle very rapidly. If the micelle is adjacent to the brush border, components can "jump" to the glycocalyx of the micro-

villi and then diffuse into the cell. The action of the bile salts is necessary for the absorption of phospholipids, cholesterol, and the fat soluble vitamins as well as triglyceride.

INTRACELLULAR PHASE

Fats are absorbed as fatty acids and glycerol, with some di- and triglyceride absorption also taking place. Phospholipids are broken down and absorbed as their constituent structures. Cholesterol may be esterified with fatty acids. The mucosal cells resynthesize triglycerides at the endoplasmic reticulum. In the golgi, lipids are packaged in chylomicrons, oil droplets enclosing triglycerides, phospholidpids, and cholesterol enclosed in a film of protein. The chylomicrons (about 0.3 μm) appear in the golgi vacuoles for extrusion by exocytosis from the basolateral cell membrane into the lymphatic system.

Medium chain fatty acids (8 – 12 carbons) are usually water soluble and diffuse from the lumen into the mucosal cell and into the portal venous system.

Dietary cholesterol represents about 1 g per day of total absorbed cholesterol. About 2 – 3 g of endogenous cholesterol from the bile and squamated cells is absorbed daily.

Iron Absorption

Dietary iron is absorbed as a complex with organic molecules. Iron containing hemoglobin and myoglobin enter the intestinal cells as intact molecules with their iron freed by the action of hemeoxidase and released into the intestinal lumen. Free iron (ferrous state-Fe^{++}) is actively transported on both mucosal and serosal sides of the intestinal cell. Iron is oxidized (ferric state-Fe^{+++}) in transit through the mucosal cell and reduced (Fe^{++}) at the vascular surface. Upon entering the blood, iron is again oxidized and combined with the B_1-globulin transferrin.

Iron from the lumen may be absorbed or excreted if not needed. Once in the mucosal cell, the iron can be absorbed into the blood or it can be stored in the cell and eventually lost when the cell is sloughed. In addition, there is a secretory pathway by which iron from the blood can be secreted into the cell.

The amount of iron present in the intestinal epithelium regulates iron uptake from the lumen. In the "iron deficient" state, mucosal cell iron stores have been depleted by body needs and the cell will accept more iron from the lumen. Essentially no iron will be lost via sloughing or as excreted iron. With "iron loading" the mucosa is less permeable to lumenal iron because intracellular iron is already high, resulting in an increase of unaccepted iron. In this case, a sloughed cell carries away a significant amount of iron. With iron loading, the secretory mechanism moving iron from the blood to the epithelial cell is also enhanced, while the rate that iron is transported to the blood is greatly diminished.

Calcium Absorption

Active transport of calcium into the mucosal cell takes place primarily in the duodenum if the lumenal concentration is about 5 mmol. Above 5 mmol, calcium diffuses into the cell and is actively transported out of the serosal side of the cell to the blood. Absorption is controlled by the active form of vitamin D (1,25 dihydroxy D_3) which is produced in the kidney. This metabolite induces the synthesis of a Ca^{++} binding protein in the mucosal cells. Production of 1,25 dihydroxy D_3 responds directly to plasma Ca^{++} levels, with response effective within a few hours.

Absorption of Water Soluble Vitamins

Several mechanisms of absorption appear to be utilized for different water soluble vitamins as is illustrated by the following:

1. A Na^+ dependent active transport mechanism involves active pumping into the cell and subsequent diffusion out the serosal side toward the blood. Vitamin C absorption is the best example.
2. Absorption and modification involves vitamin transport across the brush border into the cell where it is modified into another form, maintaining a low intracellular vitamin concentration to promote more absorption and prevent back diffusion out of the cell into the lumen. Some of the B-complex vitamins utilize this mechanism. Nicotinamide (NAD), for example, crosses the brush border by facilitated diffusion and is modified to NAD for absorption into the blood. Pyridoxine and thiamin are both modified intracellularly by phosphorylation.
3. Lumenal factor mediated absorption involves a factor F in the lumen which binds with the vitamin. This complex then crosses the brush border and breaks down before exiting the serosal side for net absorption into the blood. Vitamin B_{12} absorption is an example. B_{12} binds with a protein (R) in the stomach, which prevents the vitamin from being degraded by stomach acid, or being used by intestinal bacteria. Pancreatic proteases break down the R protein, releasing vitamin B_{12} which then binds to intrinsic factor (IF) to form a stable complex. In the ileum, this complex binds to a brush border and the vitamin component is taken into the cell.

GASTROINTESTINAL MOTILITY

Gastrointestinal motility is effected by the activity of the smooth muscle walls of the gastrointestinal tube, under neural and hormonal influence. Intestinal smooth muscle includes longitudinal and circular layers. Actin and myosin filaments interact via a modified sliding filament mechanism to produce long, slow, wormlike contractions. This mode of action differs drastically from the "spikes" of action potentials of striated muscle. Fibers are loosely arranged to allow for the smooth waves of peristalsis which are essential for proper digestion.

Segmented contractions are ringlike and occur at regular intervals, disappear, and are replaced by contractions in the segments previously relaxed. This action churns the chyme, presenting more surface area to the mucosal cells. The peristaltic wave is a circular contraction which occurs in response to stretch, forming behind the point of stimulation and moving to push chyme along the intestine toward the rectum.

Two types of electrical phenomenon are associated with gastrointestinal tract contractions. The slow waves of longitudinal smooth muscle depolarize caudally from the duodenum and result from a Na^+ dependent mechanism. No pressure changes in the gut are associated with slow waves. Action or "spike" potentials are a Ca^{++} dependent phenomenon which are of circular muscle origin and are associated with intraluminar pressure increases. Overall, slow waves provide the basic electrical rhythmic control of the gut and determine when spike potentials will occur. Spike potentials are the electrical equivalent of a muscle contraction. Peristalsis coordinates these events proximally to distally.

PART 7

Metabolism

ENDOCRINE INFLUENCE

The endocrine system is an internal communication system of ductless glands which utilizes hormones, chemical messengers released directly into the blood, to regulate metabolism. Organs well established as endocrine glands include the anterior and posterior pituitary, thyroid, parathyroids, adrenal cortex and medulla, ovaries, testes, islets of Langerhans in the pancreas, and various parts of the intestinal mucosa.

The nervous system is a rapid communications system which functions via action potentials to stimulate or inhibit specific target tissue and cells. In comparison, the endocrine system is a much slower communication mechanism, not as selective in the cells affected, but with more prolonged effects. The two systems are interrelated. For example, the hypothalamus, part of the CNS, produces and releases a number of hormones into the pituitary portal blood which travel a short distance to regulate the anterior pituitary. Hence, the nervous system affects an endocrine gland which regulates other endocrine glands in a very complex system. Hormones produced in the hypothalamus also travel down neurons to the posterior pituitary where they are stored within its nerve terminals. Nerve impulses from the CNS traveling down the spinal cord can regulate endocrine functions, such as the production and release of catecholamines by the adrenal medulla.

Characteristics of Hormones

Hormones are produced by a gland or neurosecretory cell, often stored where produced, and released into the blood in response to a specific stimulus. Release may be triggered by a nerve impulse or by a concentration change of the regulated metabolite in the blood perfusing the gland. When the hormone reaches its target cells, it modifies cell function to remove the stimulus that caused release of the hormone. Hormones often travel to distant target cells, but the distance may be short or even to adjacent cells.

Hormones are classified by their chemical structure. Amines include the thyroid hormones and catecholamines which retain the amino group of their precursor, tyrosine. Thyroid hormones are stored outside the cell, as thyroglobulin, and produced by iodination of the aromatic ring of tyrosine. Catcholamines are stored in secretory granules in the tissue where synthesized and produced by hydroxylation of the aromatic ring of tyrosine.

Steroids are derived from cholesterol, with synthesis involving hydroxylation and aromatization of the ring. Steroid hormones are stored as precursor cholesterol esters which are broken down on stimulation.

Protein hormones are produced from amino acids on the ribosomes of the endoplasmic reticulum. They are transported to the Golgi apparatus and stored in secretory vesicles. Synthesis of precursor hormones, such as proinsulin, involves additional amino acids which are cleaved to yield the active product. Small peptides and glycoproteins are also important classes of hormones.

Hormones regulate the biochemical processes of the body with effects that can be stimulatory, inhibitory, antagonistic, synergistic, or permissive. Production of a hormone occurs at a basal rate and may vary from that rate, with secretion subject to feedback regulation. When two hormones interact to control the same process, constant modulation exists. All hormones are rapidly lost by metabolic inactivation or excretion.

Pancreatic Hormones: Insulin

The pancreatic hormones are produced in the islets of Langerhans, highly vascularized cell clusters which represent 1–2 percent of the wet weight of the pancreas. Islet cells are innervated by adrenergic and cholinergic fibers of the autonomic nervous system. Specialized tight and gap junctions exist between islet cells which may enable islet cells to form a functional syncytium in which molecules from one cell influence hormonal secretion in adjacent cells.

Insulin is a polypeptide hormone (MW 6,000) produced by β-islet cells and consisting of A and B chains joined by two disulfide bridges. The hormone is synthesized as preproinsulin (MW 11,500), which is converted to proinsulin (MW 9,000) by cleavage of a 23 amino acid N-terminal fragment. Proinsulin contains the B chain at the N-terminus, followed by an intervening C peptide, followed by the A chain. Conversion to active insulin occurs by cleavage of the intervening C peptide by enzymes found in the granules of β-cells.

Insulin is an anabolic hormone released from pancreatic β cells in response to rising blood sugar levels and represents a series of firsts in protein chemistry. Insulin was the first protein hormone isolated in pure enough form for therapeutic use, the first to have amino acid sequence and tertiary structure determined, the first example of a prohormone, the first in the development of a radioimmunoassay, and the first produced by recombinant DNA.

CIRCULATION AND DEGRADATION OF INSULIN

Insulin circulates freely, with a basal peripheral concentration of about 400 pg/ml or 10 μU/ml (U = units). About 20–40 μg/h are produced by the pancreas to maintain the basal concentration. Insulin release is via the pancreatic vein to the portal vein where the concentration may be two to five times the peripheral concentration. Insulin concentration decreases during fasting and increases after meals. Insulin is rapidly cleared (t $\frac{1}{2}$ = 5–8 min), with the first pass through the liver clearing half the insulin produced. Degradation is by the action of insulin protease and glutathione transhydrogenase, which breaks disulfide bonds to inactive insulin in the liver. Some degradation also occurs in the kidneys.

C peptide, the insulin precursor, is produced in equimolar amounts with insulin and released to the circulation. C peptide has no known biological function but is used diagnostically to determine the endogenous rate of insulin synthesis in diabetics receiving insulin.

REGULATION OF INSULIN SECRETION

Primary Stimulus: Glucose. Blood glucose is the primary stimulator of insulin release. Action is via a feedback effect of the glucose level of blood perfusing the β-islet cells. Dose response shows little insulin released until the glucose concentration reaches 50–100 mg percent. At this point, insulin release is sigmoidal until glucose levels reach 250–300 mg percent, with the greatest response within the physiologic range, 90–150 mg percent.

Response to glucose stimulation is biphasic. An abrupt increase in blood glucose from 0–300 mg percent causes an initial spike of insulin release which may represent readily released secretory granules near the membrane or two pools of secretory granules, one released rapidly, the other more slowly. Sustained high glucose levels are characterized by an initial spike followed by drop off and a secondary insulin rise which is dependent on new insulin synthesis.

Insulin response to glucose differs by the route of administration. Intravenous glucose produces an abrupt rise in blood glucose but feeble insulin response. Intrajejunal glucose elicits a dramatic rise in insulin with little rise in blood glucose. The presence of glucose in the gut stimulates the gastrointestinal hormones, particularly gastric inhibitory peptide (GIP), which signals the islets cells to increase insulin in anticipation of the blood glucose load, an activity designed to prevent a dramatic rise in blood glucose.

Other Stimulators of Insulin Release. Additional stimulators of insulin include amino acids (arginine, leucine and others, since insulin is an anabolic hormone), intestinal hormones, primarily GIP, cAMP and its promotors which include β-adrenergic stimulating agents and theophylline which inhibits cAMP phosphodiesterase. Mannose, which is structurally similar to glucose, and sulfonylureas, oral hypoglycemic agents, also increase insulin secretion.

INHIBITORS OF INSULIN RELEASE

Insulin inhibitors include α-adrenergic stimulators and epinephrine, chemicals such as alloxan, which induces experimental diabetes, microtubule inhibitors which block vesicle transport, 2-deoxyglucose and mannoheptulose which interfere with glucose metabolism, and somatostatin.

MODE OF ACTION: INSULIN RECEPTOR

Insulin is bound by a specific receptor in target cell membranes which binds only insulin and analogs. The receptor is a glycoprotein complex of about 300,000–350,000 MW, with two α- and two β-subunits held together by disulfide bridges. The receptor exhibits protein kinase activity to phosphorylate one of its own subunits in response to binding insulin. Phosphorylation may be the initial signal generating cell response.

The receptor exhibits a negative cooperativity (i.e., the receptor affinity decreases as the number of receptors complexed with insulin increases). This may be a buffering mechanism to prevent the cell from responding to hyperinsulinemia. The receptor also exhibits down regulation (i.e., the number of receptors decreases in response to hyperinsulinemia). Obesity causes high blood insulin and a decreased number of receptors, whereas starvation increases the number of receptors.

The hormone and receptor are subsequently internalized (i.e., taken into the cell where insulin is degraded by lysosome). Intracellular insulin receptors have also been demonstrated on the nuclear membrane.

The effector system is unknown. However, insulin effects are rapid and are related to initial binding by the external membrane receptor. Glucose transport increases instantly and ion transport alters rapidly. Insulin also appears to play a role in the regulation of protein phosphatases, protein kinases, and enzyme phosphorylation. A second, unknown messenger may be involved, anaogous to, but not cAMP.

Secondary effects require time to develop. mRNA changes in response to insulin over hours to days and may be related to internalization or to internal receptors.

Glucagon

Glucagon, an antagonist to insulin, is secreted by the α-cells of the islets of Langerhans in response to lowered blood sugar levels. Glucagon stimulates glycogenolysis, mobilizing glucose. Glucagon also stimulates gluconeogenesis and lipolysis.

Glucagon is a single polypeptide chain of 29 amino acids (MW 3,500) and is synthesized with prepro- and proglucagon precursors. Glucagon circulates freely with a basal concentration of about 100 pg/ml. The hormone is rapidly cleared (t $\frac{1}{2}$ = 6 min), with 100–150 μg per day produced to maintain basal levels. Degradation takes place primarily in the liver with the kidney also participating.

REGULATION OF GLUCAGON SECRETION

Stimulators. The stimulators of glucagon release include amino acids, gastrointestinal hormones, primarily CCK and gastrin, β-adrenergic stimulators which increase cAMP, exercise, infection, and stress.

Inhibitors. The primary inhibitor of glucagon release is glucose, with lowered blood levels stimulating α-islet cells. The glucose effect is dependent on insulin. For glucose to inhibit glucagon, a basal level of insulin must be present. Release of somatostatin within the islet cells is also inhibitory to glucagon and is involved in overall hormone regulation.

MODE OF ACTION: GLUCAGON RECEPTOR

Glucagon binds to a receptor on the target cell membrane to initiate a cascade of reactions. Adenylate cyclase is activated to catalyze production of cAMP from ATP. cAMP then activates a cAMP dependent protein kinase which phosphorylates enzymes or membrane proteins to facilitate biological effects.

Somatostatin

Somatostatin, also known as the growth hormone release inhibiting hormone, inhibits both insulin and glucagon release and is produced in islet D cells. Somatostatin is a 14 amino acid peptide with an intrachain disulfide bridge. The hormone circulates in a 28 amino acid form which may be a precursor. Somatostatin is also found in the hypothalamus and inhibits the release of growth hormone from the anterior pituitary.

Blood Glucose Homeostasis

A constant blood glucose concentration is maintained by the interaction of insulin and glucagon. In the steady state condition, ingested glucose derived from dietary carbohydrate and endogenous glucose production are matched by glucose utilization. Endogenous glucose production takes place primarily in the liver when no ingested glucose is available, by the breakdown of liver glycogen stores (glycogenolysis) and by the conversion of amino acids, lactate, pyruvate, etc. into glucose in the process of gluconeogenesis. All tissues can utilize glucose. However, while some tissues, such as muscle and adipose, can utilize nonglucose substrates, glucose is essential for the brain.

Turnover of glucose persists and if input exceeds storage and utilization, hyperglycemia (diabetes) results. If utilization exceeds input, blood glucose concentration falls and hypoglycemia results. Since glucose is obligatory for the brain, hypoglycemia can be a CNS disaster, threatening life at blood concentrations below 20–30 mg percent.

Insulin has a major effect on endogenous glucose utilization, with glucagon and epinephrine the primary antagonists. Insulin acts by enhancing glucose transport into insulin sensitive tissues, muscle, adipose, etc. Insulin is not necessary for glucose entry into nervous tissue, liver, intestinal epithelium, red blood cells, and probably kidney tubule cells.

Inhibitors of glucose utilization are growth hormone (clinically elevated levels as seen in acromegaly produced type of diabetes) and adrenal glucocorticoids (clinically elevated levels as in Cushing's disease also produce a type of diabetes). The glucocorticoids elevate blood glucose levels by mobilizing amino acids and stimulating gluconeogenesis. Epinephrine, the fight or flight hormone, inhibits glucose utilization and is a powerful stimulus to glycogenolysis.

Hypoglycemia induced by infusing insulin elicits elevated growth hormone, cortisol, and catecholamine levels which bring about a recovery in blood glucose concentration. Without these hormones, hypoglycemia persists with slowed recovery.

INSULIN/GLUCAGON RATIO

The ratio of insulin to glucagon (I/G) is the important determinant of blood glucose concentration. After a large carbohydrate meal, as glucose is stored, the I/G ratio is high. In starvation, endogenous glucose production is turned on and the I/G ratio is low. The I/G ratio controls insulin and glucagon interaction and the blood glucose concentration.

The activity of alpha (glucagon secreting) and beta (insulin secreting) islet cells is coupled, with the perfusing blood glucose concentration determining which cell type is most stimulated. However, both cell types continuously produce and both hormones interact.

After a high carbohydrate meal, blood glucose is slightly elevated, stimulating insulin release by beta cells. Glucagon decreases with a shift in the I/G ratio favoring glucose utilization in muscle, adipose tissue, etc. In starvation, blood glucose concentration decreases slightly, with an insulin decrease and glucagon increase. The I/G ratio decrease favors glucose production, slowing utilization to insure a supply of glucose for the brain. In exercise, the muscles increase glucose utilization to supply energy needs (7–40 times basal amount). Glucagon increases, but insulin is unchanged, possibly decreasing slightly. The I/G decrease favors production of glucose to maintain constant blood glucose levels. After a high protein meal, amino acids stimulate both insulin and glucagon release. The I/G ratio remains constant, resulting in an unaltered blood glucose concentration.

Quantitative measurement of hormonal effects is difficult because of hormonal interrelation. Isotopic methods are utilized to measure glucose production and utilization. In such methods, somatostatin is infused to block insulin and glucagon release from the pancreas. Then, one hormone (insulin or glucagon) is infused to match the basal I/G ratio. Tracer determined glucose production, utilization, and concentration can then be measured.

GLUCOSE TOLERANCE TEST

The blood glucose concentration is diagnostic for diabetes mellitus. Glucose is administered orally (1.5 – 1.75 g/kg body weight) to the fasted subject. The blood sugar will immediately rise to abnormal levels, with recovery in 2 hours and a return to normal within 3 hours. The diabetic, when challenged with a glucose load, will exhibit a high fasting level and retain abnormal levels after three hours.

FUEL METABOLISM

Fuel Reserves

In starvation the fuel reserves of the body are sufficient to provide energy for metabolic requirements for 40 to 60 days. The important energy sources of the body are glucose, fatty acids, ketone bodies, and to a lesser extent, lactate, pyruvate, and amino acids. Four tissues are involved in the storage and redistribution of fuels as is illustrated by the following:

1. The adipose tissue is the primary fuel reserve of the body, storing fatty acids as triglycerides which appear in the adipocyte as oil droplets. The cell becomes one large lipid droplet with the nucleus and cytoplasm pushed to the periphery. Depot fat stores the highest potential energy in the least space, with triglyceride yielding 9 kcal/g on oxidation, compared to only 4 kcal/g for glycogen and protein. Triglyceride is abundant, representing a fuel reserve of over 110,000 kcal.

2. The liver is important because only liver glycogen can be broken down to yield free blood glucose. Liver glycogen represents short term fuel storage, capable of yielding only about 2,000 kcal, the equivalent of 1 day's energy requirement. The liver also possesses the enzymatic machinery for the production of glucose from amino acids and lactate (gluconeogenesis) and for the conversion of fatty acids to ketone bodies for fuel (ketogenesis).

3. Muscle has the capability of switching from one fuel type to another, depending on circumstances. Substrate requirements can increase dramatically (10–40 times) in exercise. Muscle represents about 40 percent of body weight and the largest store of protein which can provide amino acids for gluconeogenesis. About 6,000 g of muscle protein can yield 24,000 kcal, the caloric requirement for 10 days.

4. Brain tissue is important because its obligatory glucose requirement must be protected. Only in long term starvation does any adaptation occur.

Fuel Metabolism in Fasting

Normally 180 g of glucose per day, provided by liver glycogen and gluconeogenesis, are utilized primarily to support the nervous system. To provide the amino acid substrate for gluconeogenesis, 75 g of muscle protein are catabolized. In the fasting state, tissues such as heart, kidney, and muscle conserve glucose by switching their fuel source to fatty acids and ketone bodies. Fatty acids are mobilized from adipose tissue stores (160 g) to yield both fatty acids and glycerol (16 g) for gluconeogenesis. Fatty acids can be transported directly to heart, kidney, and muscle for utilization or can be transported to the liver for conversion to ketone bodies for release into the blood.

Long term starvation involves additional adaptive mechanisms. A major change occurs in the brain, which develops an ability to utilize ketone bodies to support energy needs, conserving glucose. The body reduces its need for glucose to a minimum. Liver glycogen has been long depleted and the only source of glucose is via gluconeogenesis. To conserve structural protein, only 20 g of muscle protein are now degraded to provide amino acids for gluconeogenesis, as opposed to 75 g in the short term fasting state.

Transitions in fuel utilization are dramatic during starvation. In the postabsorptive fed state, glucose contributes nearly all of the substrate for the brain as well as for other tissues. As starvation progresses, muscle tissue increases ketone utilization and the brain begins to utilize ketone bodies. After 2 to 3 weeks of starvation, fatty acids almost entirely support the energy needs of the body.

Adipose Tissue Metabolism

LIPOGENESIS

Adipose tissue takes up lipid from the chylomicrons and lipoproteins of the circulatory pool. A lipoprotein lipase located on the capillary endothelium converts triglycerides to glycerol and fatty acids which cross the adipocyte membrane. The activity of this enzyme increases in the fed state and decreases in the fasting state. In the cell, fatty acids are activated to acyl CoA intermediates for reesterification. Acetyl CoA units may be added or subtracted and the degree of saturation of dietary fatty acids may be altered by addition or removal of hydrogen. The pentose pathway is active in adipose tissue and generates the reducing equivalents (NADPH) for fatty acid biosynthesis. Resynthesis produces fat which is characteristic of the species and involves linkage of long chain fatty acids with α-glycerolphosphate, which arises from glucose metabolism in the adipocyte. Free glycerol is not a source of α-glycerolphosphate since the adipocyte lacks glycerokinase for this conversion. Free glycerol is released to the blood.

The reaction of α-glycerolphosphate with two activated fatty acid residues produces α-phosphatidic acid, which may link a third fatty acid to form triglyceride. Phospholipid synthesis occurs by a series of reactions in which α-phosphatidic acid is linked with choline, ethanolamine, or l-serine as the third component.

LYPOLYSIS

Fats are continuously being broken down (lipolysis), yielding free fatty acids which may be reesterified to netural fat, oxidized in the adipocyte for energy, or released to the circulation. Glycerol is released to the circulation and is an index of lipolysis.

Three distinct lipases cleave triglyceride sequentially to yield diglyceride, then monoglyceride, and finally glycerol and free fatty acid. The cleavage of the first fatty acid by a heavily regulated hormone sensitive lipase is the rate limiting step in lipolysis. Hormone sensitive lipase is the mobilizing lipase. The enzyme is more active when phosphorylated, a reaction requiring a cAMP dependent protein kinase. Dephosphorylation yields the more inactive form and is catalyzed by a phosphatase. Insulin favors dephosphorylation by either decreasing cAMP levels, by activating phosphodiesterase or by activating phosphoprotein phosphatase. This action damps triglyceride breakdown, favoring storage.

The adipose tissue is exquisitely sensitive to insulin. Insulin promotes lipogenesis, facilitating the transport of glucose across the cell membrane, essential to provide glycerol for triglyceride synthesis. Insulin increases lipoprotein lipase activity which provides fatty acids for transport into the adipocyte. The hormone damps lipolysis by influencing the inhibition of hormone sensitive lipase. Epinephrine and glucagon are insulin antagonists which promote lipolysis and the mobilization of depot lipid. Epinephrine acts by influencing an increase in hormone sensitive lipase activity.

Muscle Metabolism

Fuels metabolized to support muscle tissue are glucose, fatty acids, ketone bodies, lactate, and amino acids. Muscle shifts in substrate utilization occur primarily from glucose to fatty acids. Muscle metabolism differs with fiber type. White muscle is fast acting with few mitochondria and meets energy needs primarily through glycolysis. Pyruvate, the end product of anaerobic glycolysis, is reconverted to glucose in the liver via the Cori cycle. Red muscle has an abundance of mitochondria, is slower to contract, and utilizes glucose or fatty acids via the citrate cycle, with fatty acids the preferred substrate.

GLUCOSE TRANSPORT

Insulin responsive glucose transport into the cell is the rate limiting step in muscle metabolism of this substrate. Once in the cell, glucose is immediately phosphorylated to glucose-6-phosphate (G6P) via hexokinase. This effectively traps glucose in the cell, since the hexose esters are unable to diffuse (or be transported) out of the cell. Hexokinase is regulated by product inhibition. Inhibitors of glycolysis also inhibit hexokinase since break down of muscle glycogen yields G6P.

GLYCOGENESIS AND GLYCOGENOLYSIS

Storage of glucose as the polymer glycogen (glycogenesis) requires enormous energy input. G6P is rearranged to glucose-1-phosphate (G1P) and activated by the high energy nucleotide, uridine triphosphate (UTP) for attachment to the growing glycogen polymer. Breakdown of glycogen (glycogenolysis) requires cleavage of glucose units from the glycogen polymer by phosphorolysis, cleavage by phosphate. The enzyme phosphorylase is the catalyst and yields G1P as a product. Before entering other intracellular pathways, G1P is converted to G6P. Since glucose-6-phosphatase is absent in muscle, muscle glycogen is not a source of the blood sugar.

UTILIZATION OF GLUCOSE

Utilization of glucose requires conversion of G6P to lactate for anaerobic glycolysis or to acetyl CoA for aerobic metabolism via the citrate cycle. In this scheme, isomerase converts G6P to fructose-6-phosphate, with phosphofructokinase catalyzing conversion to fructose 1-6 diphosphate. ATP and citrate act as inhibitors of the phosphate diester reaction; AMP and inorganic phosphate act as activators.

Cleavage to the interconvertible trioses, dihydroxyacetone phosphate, and glyceraldehyde-3-phosphate, and rearrangement yields pyruvate. Pyruvate is reduced to lactate or is converted to acetyl CoA for entry into the citrate cycle. Pyruvate dehydrogenase catalyzes the latter reaction.

FATTY ACID UTILIZATION IN MUSCLE

Breakdown of plasma triglycerides by lipoprotein lipase allows fatty acids to enter the muscle cell. Fatty acids are activated to fatty acyl CoA. Transport into the mitochondrion requires combination with carnitine via the activity of fatty acyl carnitine transferase to form fatty acyl carnitine, the form in which fatty acids are transported across the mitochondrial membrane. Once in the mitochondrion, this complex is broken down to the activated fatty acid and carnitine. Fatty acyl CoA is broken down via β-oxidation to two carbon acetyl CoA fragments for entry into the citrate cycle.

The aerobic oxidation of nutrients and the release and transduction of their energy to regenerate ATP occurs in the process of cellular respiration. In the citrate cycle, nutrient carbon is eliminated as CO_2 and hydrogens and electrons are extracted and passed via a chain of respiratory enzymes to oxygen. Respiration is coupled to oxidative phosphorylation, a process which captures the energy released as electrons drop in electrical potential, and regenerates high energy phosphate.

In times of fatty acid abundance, muscle switches to utilization of fatty acids as the preferred substrate, increasing intracellular acetyl CoA. Acetyl CoA allosterically inhibits pyruvate dehydrogenase and activates pyruvate dehydrogenase kinase, leading to further inhibition. Citrate formed from the abundance of acetyl CoA enters the cytoplasm and inhibits phosphofructokinase to cause a build-up of G6P which inhibits hexokinase, sparing glucose utilization.

MUSCLE PROTEIN METABOLISM

In contrast with carbohydrate and fat, there is no specialized storage form for protein. Structural and functional muscle proteins must be catabolized to free amino acids into the circulation.

Synthesis of muscle proteins requires the uptake of amino acids from the blood by specific active membrane transport systems. Aminoacyl tRNAs are formed which polymerize on the ribosomes to form protein in reactions which include initiation, elongation of the amino acid chain, and termination; steps requiring both ATP and GTP. Catabolism of muscle protein utilizes lysosomes and soluble proteases. Free amino acids are released to the blood for redistribution.

Following a high protein meal, amino acids are taken up by muscle and converted to protein. During starva-

tion, muscle proteins are catabolized to provide energy via gluconeogenesis.

Regulation of Protein Synthesis/Degradation. Insulin is a key regulator of protein metabolism, causing an increase in protein synthesis within minutes. Insulin increases the translation of most mRNA by promoting the initiation step and inhibiting the rate of protein degradation. Amino acids, especially leucine, also stimulate protein synthesis at the initiation step of translation and inhibit protein catabolism. Growth hormone also stimulates protein synthesis. In contrast, glucocorticoids inhibit protein synthesis and stimulate degradation.

During the transition from the fed state to the starvation state, circulating insulin levels decrease, causing a decreased stimulation of protein synthesis as well as decreased inhibition of protein catabolism. The net result is a relative increase in protein degradation with release of free amino acids into the blood. Amino acids released from muscle during net proteolysis in the postabsorptive state are predominately alanine and glutamine (50-70 percent), although almost all amino acids are released to some extent. Alanine and glutamine constitute only 5-10 percent of the amino acids in muscle protein and must be synthesized *de novo* during negative nitrogen balance. Alanine released from muscle provides the key gluconeogenic substrate to the liver. Glutamine is primarily converted to alanine in the digestive tract. Alanine then enters the portal circulation and is cleared by the liver for utilization as a gluconeogenic substrate. In addition, glutamine can be metabolized by the kidney to release free ammonia, a deamination reaction which plays an important role in acid base balance.

The Glucose-Alanine Cycle

Glucose and alanine are related cyclically. Pyruvate arises primarily from the blood glucose, although other sources include muscle glycogen and glucogenic amino acids. Pyruvate may be transaminated to form alanine which serves as a transport vehicle for both carbon and nirogen (ammonia is toxic) from muscle to liver. The cycle has limitations. When alanine is formed from glucose intermediates and reused to form glucose, no net glucose is produced. Other gluconeogenic amino acids and glycerol must be utilized for a net positive glucose production.

THE LIVER: INTEGRATION OF METABOLIC EVENTS

The liver serves as the main integrator of metabolic events. Glucose can be converted to glycogen, or vice versa. Glucose can enter the glycolytic pathway to form pyruvate, which can be converted to acetyl CoA to make fatty acids, which are packaged into triglycerides and lipoproteins. The liver is the primary site of lipogenesis and most lipids are released into the blood as lipoproteins. Gluconeogenesis shares many common enzymes with glycolysis. Substrates include lactate and amino acids from muscle, glycerol from triglyceride metabolism in adipose tissue, and pyruvate. The liver is the only tissue with the capacity to form ketone bodies.

Carbohydrate Metabolism in the Liver

Glucose uptake by the liver is via a facilitated transport system which works constantly at full capacity and is not hormonally controlled. Glucose, therefore, equilibrates across the liver cell membrane in contrast to adipose and muscle tissues, in which uptake is hormonally controlled and there is virtually no free intracellular glucose. Liver contains glucokinase for phosphorylation of glucose to G6P. In contrast to muscle hexokinase, glucokinase is inducible, has a lower substrate affinity, and is not inhibited by its product, G6P. Only liver, kidney, and intestine have the enzyme glucose-6-phosphatase – absent in muscle – which is crucial to gluconeogenesis.

Liver Glycogen Metabolism

The depletion of liver glycogen during fasting is a rapid process. After 12 hours, most of the glycogen supply is gone. After 1 day, glycogen is almost totally depleted.

Glycogen synthesis and degradation are controlled by the activity of two key enzymes, glycogen synthetase and glycogen phosphorylase, which are under the control of a number of kinases. cAMP dependent protein kinase phosphorylates glycogen synthetase, rendering it inactive. It also phosphorylates and activates phosphorylase kinase which in turn phosphorylates and activates glycogen phosphorylase. The net effect is a relative cessation of glycogen synthesis and activation of its breakdown.

Glucagon exerts its most important action in the liver. Released in response to exercise or starvation, glucagon binds to hepatic receptors to activate adenylate cyclase, forming cAMP and initiating the cascade of events that mobilize glucose. Insulin has an antagonistic role to glucagon and influences the phosphorylation state of enzymes controlling glycogen synthesis.

Epinephrine activity is dependent upon the type of receptor on the liver cell membrane, which varies with nutritional states. When epinephrine interacts with a β-receptor, it activates adenylate cyclase (analogous to glucagon). Alpha receptor binding of epinephrine also causes glycogen breakdown. Ca^{++} is released and subsequently bound by calmodulin, which in turn activates a

different protein kinase. Five different protein kinases that phosphorylate glycogen synthetase on seven different sites are known. Insulin modifies only one of these sites, which differs from the site of phosphorylation by cAMP dependent protein kinase. This suggests that insulin does not act by interfering with cAMP dependent protein kinase.

The Gluconeogenic Pathway

The liver has a large capacity (150–300 g/day; 80 g/day after a 6 week fast) to synthesize glucose from endogenous substrates. During the postabsorptive state, greater than 90 percent of the glucose production is in the liver. During a long term fast, only about 55 percent of the glucose production occurs in the liver, with the rest contributed by the kidneys. Gluconeogenesis shares many of the same enzymes with glycolysis. However, three energy requiring steps of glycolysis are irreversible (i.e., the glucokinase, phosphofructokinase, and pyruvate kinase reactions). Four key enzymes are required to bypass these steps (i.e., pyruvate carboxylase, phosphoenolpyruvate carboxykinase, fructose diphosphatase, and glucose-6-phosphatase).

Amino acids are quantitatively the most important gluconeogenic substrate (50 percent), with alanine the most readily available. Pyruvate, lactate, and glycerol make up the difference. Gluconeogenesis is controlled hormonally and by substrate availability. Glucagon and insulin are key regulatory hormones. Glucagon is necessary to maintain the basal rate of gluconeogenesis in the postabsorptive state. Glucagon enhances the phosphorylation of pyruvate kinase, increasing its affinity for inhibitory allosteric regulators and permitting increased flux to glucose. Fructose 2-6 bisphosphate (F-2,6-P) is a key regulatory metabolite in the gluconeogenic pathway. Glucagon decreases the concentration of this metabolite, allowing flux in the direction of gluconeogenesis. Insulin increases the concentration of F-2,6-P, allowing glycolytic flux. The enzymes involved in the formation of this metabolite are also regulated by phosphorylation and affected by hormones. This represents yet another level of control in the cascade of regulation.

Lipogenesis in the Liver

In the liver, lipogenesis is dependent on the glycolytic pathway. When gluconeogenesis predominates, as during fasting and in diabetes, pyruvate kinase is inhibited, allowing substrates to enter the gluconeogenic pathway as pyruvate. When there is a high rate of free fatty acid delivery to the liver, oxidation to acetyl CoA inhibits pyruvate dehydrogenase and acts as a cofactor for pyruvate carboxylase. These events act to shuttle amino acid carbon via pyruvate to oxaloacetate, which leaves the mitochondrion and is converted to glucose via phosphoenol pyruvate in the cytoplasm. In gluconeogenesis, the glycolytic enzymes (glucokinase and phosphofructokinase) are relatively inactive, while fructose-1,6-diphosphatase and glucose-6-phosphatase are activated.

Lipogenesis occurs predominately in the fed state with the liver taking up dietary free fatty acids and glucose for conversion to triglycerides. Mitochondrial acetyl CoA levels drop. Pyruvate dehydrogenase inhibition is relieved, allowing formation of acetyl CoA and then citrate by reaction with oxaloacetate. Glucose entry activates glucokinase and phosphofructokinase to promote glycolysis. Glucokinase is enhanced by insulin, so that its concentration is increased in the fed state. Phosphofructokinase is activated allosterically by fructose-2,6-bisphosphate whose concentration is also elevated in the fed state. The pentose phosphate pathway is activated to provide reducing equivalents as NADPH for fatty acid synthesis. Phosphofructokinase is activated due to the high insulin/glucagon ratio in the fed state. These enzymes regulate the carbon flow to pyruvate which enters the mitochondria by conversion to oxaloacetate by pyruvate carboxylase.

Acetyl CoA condenses with oxaloacetate to form citrate which is transported out of the mitochondrion and converted back to acetyl CoA. This step is heavily regulated by acetyl CoA carboxylase (ACC), the rate limiting enzyme for fatty acid synthesis. Acetyl CoA units are linked via malonyl CoA into palmitic and other long chain fatty acids. Esterification to triglycerides is catalyzed by α-glycerolphosphate acetyltransferase, an enzyme activated in the fed state. Triglycerides are packaged with protein into very low density lipoproteins (VLDL) and released into the blood for transport to adipose tissue for storage.

The lipogenesis pathway is controlled chiefly by the availability of citrate and the activity of acetyl CoA carboxylase. A close correlation exists between the intracellular citrate concentration and the rate of lipogenesis. Glucagon slows lipogenesis with an associated fall in intracellular citrate. The addition of pyruvate dramatically increases citrate concentration. Glucagon, when added with pyruvate is less inhibitory. It appears that glucagon inhibits the flux of glucose to citrate via pyruvate kinase inhibition, inducing a significant increase in lipogenesis and citrate formation.

Acetyl CoA carboxylase exists in an inactive protomeric form and an active polymeric form. High citrate favors the polymeric, active form of ACC, while high fatty acyl CoA favors the inactive protomeric form. Phosphorylation is biased toward ACC inactivity. As long as citrate concentration is adequate, ACC activity will control the rate of lipogenesis.

Ketogenesis

The liver is the only organ which synthesizes ketone bodies. Fatty acids, primarily from adipose tissue, are ketone substrates. The major ketone bodies are β-hydroxybutyrate, which constitutes two-thirds of the blood ketones, and acetoacetate. Acetoacetate can undergo spontaneous decarboxylation to volatile acetone which can be detected in the breath in diabetic ketoacidosis.

The ketogenesis pathway is similar to that of muscle fatty acid oxidation. Fatty acids are activated to form fatty acyl CoA, which enters the mitochondrion via the carnitine transport mechanism. Fatty acyl CoA flux to triglyceride or ketone body is controlled by α-glycerolphosphate acyltransferase activity, which favors triglyceride formation, or carnitine acyltransferase I activity, which favors ketone body formation.

Once fatty acyl carnitine is in the mitochondrion, it is converted to fatty acyl CoA which undergoes β-oxidation, yielding acetyl CoA units. In the presence of β-ketoacylthiolase, two acetyl CoA molecules condense to form acetoacetyl CoA. Further manipulation to β-hydroxy β-methylglutaryl CoA (HMG CoA) permits cleavage to acetoacetate which is released into the blood.

β-hydroxybutyrate is formed by reduction of acetoacetate by NADH (from the β-oxidation of fatty acyl CoA) to acetyl CoA. Acetone results from the decarboxylation of acetoacetate.

REGULATION OF KETOGENESIS

Ketogenesis is limited by substrate availability and is influenced by any factor that controls the availability of fatty acids from adipose tissue. Control in the liver depends on the glucagon/insulin ration. Insulin primarily effects adipose tissue where it inhibits the breakdown of triglycerides. In the absence of insulin, there is an outpouring of fatty acids from adipose tissue to the liver. Glucagon stimulates ketogenesis in the liver.

The availability of carnitine is a regulator of ketogenesis. Malonyl CoA is a potent inhibitor of ketone body formation. High rates of lipigenesis result in increased levels of malonyl CoA which act to shut down ketogenesis. Conversely, when lipigenesis is inactive, inhibition of the carnitine system is removed. This permits fatty acids to enter liver mitochondria for conversion to ketone bodies.

PATHOLOGY OF KETOGENESIS

In diabetes, blood ketone body concentrations can reach acidotic levels. The flow of fatty acids to the liver as well as the activity of acylcarnitine transferase is increased in ketogenesis. Free fatty acids are mobilized rapidly from adipose tissue, with their metabolism in the liver channeled toward ketogenesis.

The advantages of ketone bodies as a fuel over glucose or fatty acids are two-fold as is illustrated by the following:

1. Ketone bodies are readily oxidizable substrates for tissues like muscle.
2. Fatty acids are water insoluble, unlike ketone bodies, so there is a limited capacity to transport fatty acids.

Ketogenesis is a normal physiologic process which only becomes a problem when acidosis results from an insulin deficiency, causing body ketone production to exceed utilization.

PART 8

Endocrine Controls

PITUITARY HORMONES

The pituitary or hypophysis is a community of glands, weighing about half a gram, and involved in the production of at least six hormones (Table 8-2). Located in the floor of the third ventricle within a pocket in the sphenoid bone, the pituitary consists of anterior and posterior lobes.

The Anterior Pituitary

The anterior lobe (adenohypophysis) arises from an outpocket of the oral cavity called Rathke's pouch. Five cell types are involved in the production of hormones. Only two cell types appear under light microscopy (i.e., acidophils, which elaborate prolactin and growth hormone, and basophils which produce the others). Anterior pituitary hormones are listed in Table 8-2.

Five cell types emerge using immunologic techniques involving antibodies to the various hormones. Luteinizing hormone (LH) and follicle stimulating hormone (FSH) are made within the same cell type. Growth hormone producing cells constitute the largest proportion of cells (30–40 percent), followed by cells producing adrenocorticotropic hormone (ACTH, 20 percent).

Table 8-2. Pituitary Hormones

Anterior Lobe - Adenohypophysis	
ACTH—Adrenocorticotropic hormone	
GH	—Growth hormone or Somatotropin (STH)
FSH	—Follicle stimulating hormone
LH	—Luteinizing hormone or Interstitial cell stimulating hormone (ICSH)
LTH	—Luteotropic hormone or Prolactin, luteotropin, mammotropin
TSH	—Thyroid stimulating hormone or thyrotropin
Intermediate Lobe - Pars Intermedia	
α-MSH	Melanocyte stimulating hormones or
β-MSH	Melanotropins
Posterior Lobe - Neurohypophysis	
ADH	—Vasopressin or antidiuretic hormone
Oxytocin	

HORMONE TYPES

Anterior pituitary hormones fall into three general categories (i.e., glycoproteins, somatomammotrophins, and corticotrophin related). FSH, LH, and thyrotropin (TSH) are glycoproteins of similar size and molecular weight, composed of alpha and beta subunits. These features are identical to those of chorionic gonadotrophin, a placental hormone. Specificity of action is determined by the beta subunit, which differs for each hormone of this type.

The somatomammotrophins include prolactin, growth hormone, and chorionic somatomammotrophin. These are similar single peptide chains, having two to three intrachain disulfide bridges and containing no carbohydrate. These hormones share homology in sequence resulting in overlapping effects.

The principal corticotrophin is ACTH, a small 39 amino acid hormone cleaved from a glycoprotein precursor. The first 24 amino acids in ACTH are preserved in all species and are required for full activity. The other 15 amino acids function only to slow the rate at which the hormone is degraded. The precursor molecule also contains sequences for melanocyte stimulating hormone (MSH), lipotropin, and the endorphins. Initial processing gives rise to an ACTH intermediate and lipotropin. Additional processing yields ACTH. The precursor exists in other parts of the brain and additional cleavage can yield other products. The endorphins, for example, contain the sequences for the enkephalins (opiate receptors).

Biosynthesis. The synthesis of pituitary hormones involves prohormones and is similar to that for insulin biosynthesis by pancreatic beta cells. All anterior pituitary cells secrete either protein or glycoprotein hormones from distinctive storage granules, which, on appropriate signal, discharge their contents by exocytosis. Since they receive no innervation from the hypothalamus, signals that control secretion are delivered by way of the hypophyseal portal system. All known stimulators and inhibitors of pituitary hormone release are peptides, with the possible exception of dopamine, which may be a prolactin inhibitory factor. Stimulus secretion coupling probably involves Ca^{++} with at least part of the response mediated by cyclic AMP.

GROWTH HORMONE

Growth hormone, an anterior pituitary somatomammotrophin, is a single chain polypeptide of 191 amino acids with two disulfide bridges forming structural loops. Growth hormone is synthesized as the prohormone by acidophilic cells of the anterior pituitary and is thought to circulate free in the blood.

Growth hormone affects virtually every tissue in the body, especially chondrocytes in bone growth. In almost all tissues growth hormone leads to an increase in mRNA and protein synthesis. In general, GH inhibits glucose uptake and causes insulin resistance in muscle and adipose tissue. While hormonal action in adipose, liver, and muscle is directly mediated, that in bone, heart, lung, and chondrocytes is affected via an intermediary regulator, somatomedin.

Role of Somatomedin. Somatomedin is produced by the liver in response to GH and is an important intermediary for body growth, while GH directly affects metabolism. A polypeptide (7,000 MW), somatomedin is similar in structure to proinsulin and can cross-react with insulin receptors, although it primarily acts via its own specific receptors. Two somatomedins are characterized (i.e., insulinlike growth factor I and insulinlike growth factor II).

Regulation of Growth Hormone Secretion. GH secretion is influenced by two hypothalamic hormones (i.e., somatostatin, which inhibits GH production and release, and growth hormone releasing hormone (GHRH), which increases GH). Somatomedin feedback to the hypothalamus decreases GH, and growth hormone itself exhibits feedback inhibition to the hypothalamus.

Factors that increase growth hormone secretion cause a decrease in energy metabolites and include a decrease in blood glucose, free fatty acids, and amino acids as well as exercise, stress, and REM sleep. Inhibitors of GH include increased blood glucose and free fatty acids.

GH Disorders. Clinically, deficiencies of GH caused by anterior pituitary tumors in early life will result in dwarfism. Deficiency in adulthood is generally compatible with life, but causes a hypoglycemic tendency. Excess of GH, usually caused by tumor, results in giantism if this occurs before the epiphyseal plates fuse. If GH excess occurs after epiphyseal fusion, acromegaly results, characterized by enlarged hands, feet, and protrusion of the jaw caused by increases in cartilage and soft tissue. GH excess can be treated by irradiation of anterior pituitary tumor cells or hypophysectomy.

The Posterior Pituitary

The posterior pituitary (neurohypophysis) is formed from a downpocket of the floor of the third ventricle and is continuous with the hypothalamus in this area. The posterior pituitary does not produce but rather stores hormones in nerve terminals.

The two hormones released from the hypothalamus and stored in the posterior pituitary are vasopression (ADH or antidiuretic hormone) and oxytocin. ADH and oxytocin are synthesized as prohormones in the hypothalamic supraoptic and paraventricular nuclei, respectively. The prohormone is cleaved to produce the hormone and a substance called neurophysin, which is also stored in the vesicles. Neurophysin may be important in the movement of the vesicle down the axon. Both ADH and oxytocin are small 9 amino acid peptides containing a disulfide bridge, with identical structures except at positions 3 and 8. Despite their similar structures, ADH and oxytocin have distinct actions.

OXYTOCIN

Oxytocin causes milk ejection and uterine contraction, with low pressor and antidiuretic activity. Oxytocin effects mammary gland myoepithelial cells, causing contraction to force milk into the ducts. It also activates smooth muscle uterine contractions and is widely used to induce labor.

VASOPRESSIN (ADH)

Vasopressin has a high pressor and antidiuretic activity and a lower uterine and milk ejection activity. Overlapping effects occur only with very high concentrations of the hormone. Vasopressin regulates plasma osmolality via sensitive receptors in the hypothalamus. A 1 percent change in osmolality can elicit a change in ADH secretion. As osmolality increases, ADH secretion increases. Blood volume regulation is via pressor receptors in the carotid sinus and aortic arch which sense pressure changes. Pressor receptors are also present in the low pressure systems such as the left atrium and central veins. These receptors produce negative feedback to decrease ADH. If blood volume drops, negative feedback impulses are decreased and ADH secretion increases.

HYPOTHALAMIC HORMONES

In addition to oxytocin and vasopressin, the hypothalamus produces at least seven hormones which regulate the release of hormones from the anterior pituitary.

The portal blood flow is the first indication of the functional relationship between the pituitary and the hypothalamus. Capillaries from the superior hypophyseal artery break up into a capilllary plexus in the area of the median eminence. Here portal vessels arise to form a capillary plexus surrounding anterior pituitary cells. A number of hormones released from nerve endings in the median eminence of the hypothalamus are carried to anterior pituitary cells by portal blood vessels via the pituitary stalk (Table 8-3).

Hypothalamic hormones are called releasing or inhibiting hormones, depending on their regulatory influence on anterior pituitary cells. There is some overlap involved in cell types. For example, thyrotropin releasing hormone (TRH) is a tripeptide with primary action on thyrotropin to stimulate release of TSH. However, TRH also effects prolactin and growth hormone in situations involving growth hormone secreting tumors. Hypothalamic hormones are found throughout the CNS, possibly acting as neurotransmitters.

Mode of Action

Anterior pituitary cells have membrane receptors for specific hypothalamic hormones. The binding of releasing or inhibiting hormones respectively influence production of cAMP by activation or inhibition of cAMP dependent protein kinase. Subsequent events lead to synthesis of anterior pituitary hormones.

Regulation

Target gland hormones can feed back at the level of the hypothalamus or the pituitary in a long loop mechanism to affect production of releasing factor or trophic hormone, respectively. Trophic hormone can also feed back (short loop) to the hypothalamus. Releasing factors themselves can influence their own production. It is proposed that retrograde flow within the portal vessels may carry releasing factors back to the hypothalamus from the anterior pituitary in an alter short loop feedback.

Feedback provides a diagnostistic tool. To determine the site of primary lesion in thyroid hormone deficiency, preparations of TSH and TRH serum can be used. If no increase in thyroid hormone occurs after giving TSH, the

Table 8-3. Hypothalamic Releasing Hormones

FSHRF	FSH	releasing hormone
GHRF	GH	releasing hormone
GHRIH	GH	release inhibiting hormone (Somatostatin)
LHRH	LH	releasing hormone
TRH	TSH	releasing hormone
CRF	ACTH	releasing factor (Corticotropin)
PIF	PIF	releasing factor
PRF	PR	releasing factor

lesion is at the level of the thyroid gland itself. However, if there is no increase in TSH after TRH administration, the lesion is at the level of the pituitary. If an increase in TSH alters TRH, then the lesion is at the level of the hypothalamus.

THYROID HORMONES

The thyroid is a follicular gland that produces iodine containing amino acid derivatives which regulate the normal level of metabolism in the tissues. In the active state, thyroid cells surround a colloid which is primarily thyroglobulin, a protein which binds tyrosine in peptide linkages, and is continuously secreted into the lumen of the follicle. The colloid acts as a reservoir to concentrate iodine for incorporation into tyrosine residues to form the active hormones, thyroxine (T_4) and 3,5,3′ triiodothyronine (T_3). When the gland is actively secreting, the cells take in colloid and degrade thyroglobulin to liberate active thyroid hormones. In the active state, growth of the gland is influenced by the TSH. In the inactive state, the cells atrophy and the amount of colloid increases.

Iodine Uptake by the Thyroid

The thyroid gland has considerable ability to concentrate and store iodine. The large pool of iodine in the gland is mainly in the colloid. The thyroid is able to transport iodide against an electrochemical gradient from the extrathyroidal inorganic iodide pool into the cell. T_4 and T_3 are secreted into the extrathyroidal organic iodide pool. The hormones are transported bound to plasma proteins.

Dietary iodine is normally ingested in excess of daily requirements (300 μg v 289 μg excreted). A small amount of extrathyroidal organic iodine is excreted in the feces. The remainder is recycled. Recycling occurs in extrathyroidal tissues which remove iodine from the thyroid hormones.

If iodine intake falls below necessary levels ($\sim 100\,\mu g$/ day), goiter develops. In this condition, thyroxine (T_4) and T_3 levels provide insufficient feedback to the pituitary to block the synthesis of TSH. Production of TSH increases with a trophic effect on the thyroid to produce a goiter.

Active Thyroid Hormones

Thyroxine (T_4) is the predominant hormone produced by the thyroid. The basic structure, called thyronine, consists of linked tyrosine residues, one of which is hydroxylated in the para position. Four iodine atoms are incorporated on the 3,5,3', and 5' positions of the two aromatic rings (Fig. 8-14).

3,5,3-Triiodothyronine (T_3) incorporates only three iodine atoms and lacks iodine at the 5' position. T_3 exhibits greater hormonal activity than T_4.

Monoiodotyrosine (MIT) and diiodotyrosine (DIT) are precursors of T_4 and T_3 and are present only to a small extent in the blood. The distribution of hormones in the thyroid is normally about 23 percent MIT, 33 percent DIT, 35 percent tryosine, and 7 percent T_3, with traces of related derivatives. Tyrosine and T_3 are the predominant forms secreted.

IODINATION: T_3 AND T_4 BIOSYNTHESIS

The plasma inorganic iodide concentration is fairly low. Active transport into the cell occurs via an iodide pump located on the capillary side of the thyroid cell. The thyroid cell secretes a peroxidase into the colloid which activates iodine for iodination of tyrosine in thyroglobulin to form MIT and DIT. Two DIT units or one DIT and one MIT are coupled to form T_4 and T_3, respectively. Thyroglobulin is a large protein with 10 times more T_4 than T_3 residues.

Under stimulation by TSH, colloid is taken back into the cell via pinocytosis, and thyroglobulin combines with lysosomes for degradation. Proteolysis yields the active hormones, T_4 and T_3 as well as MIT, DIT, and other constituent amino acids which may be recycled to make new thyroglobulin.

PLASMA PROTEIN BINDING

Thyroxine-binding globulin (TBG) has the highest affinity for T_4 and 60–70 percent of plasma thyroxine is bound to TBG. Thyroxine-binding prealbumin (TBPA) has less affinity for thyroxine, but is more abundant than TBG. About 10–20 percent of plasma thyroxine is bound to TBPA. Albumin has some affinity for thyroxine and a small percentage of plasma thyroxine is bound to albumin.

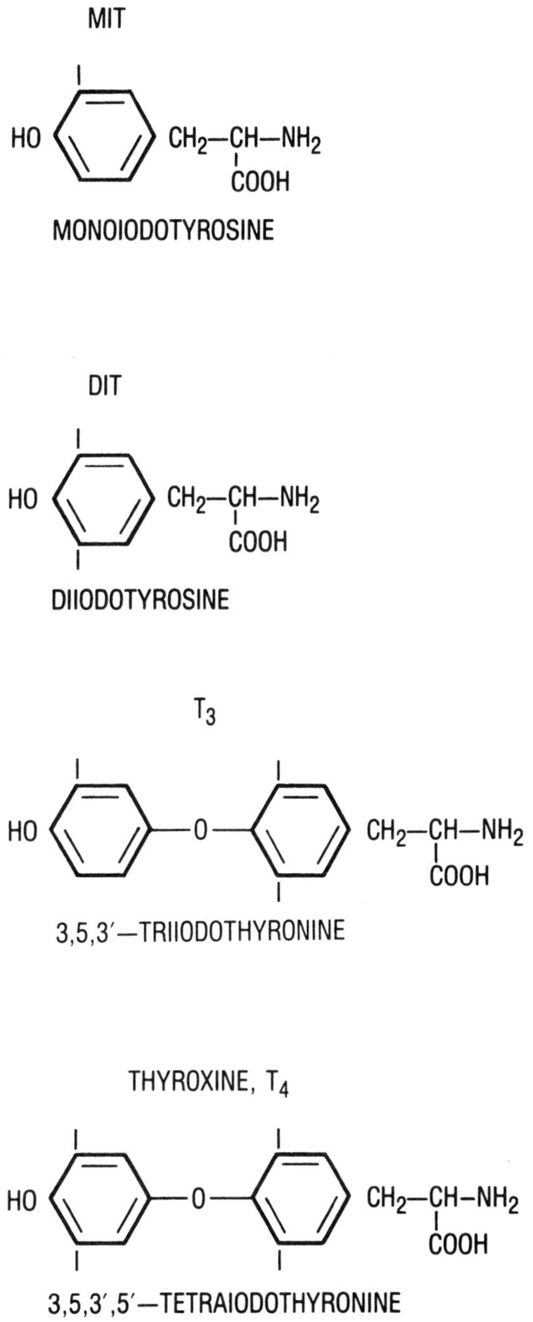

Fig. 8-14. Thyroid hormones.

A total of about 8 μg/dl of protein-bound thyroxine circulates in the plasma. In contrast, only about 0.003 μg/dl thyroxine is free. Free thyroxine is the form which provides feedback inhibition and is available for uptake in the tissues. Because thyroxine is tightly bound, the hormone has a long half-life (6.2 days v 1.0 days for T_3). T_3 concentration in the plasma is consistent with its shorter half-life as compared to T_4, while free T_3 concentration is closer to that of free T_4, also reflecting the lower affinity of T_3 for plasma binding proteins. About 80 percent of plasma T_3 is formed by the metabolism of T_4 to T_3 by extrathyroid tissues.

The amount of thyroxine binding proteins does not influence the concentration of free plasma thyroxine. If more protein is available to bind T_4, free T_4 concentration temporarily drops. This drop releases inhibition of TSH secretion until the T_4 level returns to normal.

Estrogen, along with other factors, can lead to an increase in thyroxine binding proteins. Androgens have the opposite effect, influencing their decrease. In both cases, free thyroxine concentrations remain normal.

In hyperthyroidism, feedback inhibition of thyroxine on TSH production is disturbed. More TSH is secreted, more thyroxine is secreted, and the free thyroxine concentration is increased, along with the total thyroxine concentration in the plasma. The level of thyroxine binding proteins remains normal.

In hypothyroidism, the thyroid does not respond to TSH, less thyroxine is made, and the free and total plasma levels of thyroxine decrease. Again, the level of thyroxine binding proteins is normal.

REGULATION OF SECRETION

TSH is a glycoprotein with alpha and beta subunits. Activity resides in the beta subunit. The hormone stimulates the thyroid gland to grow, take up iodine, and make and secrete thyroxine. T_4 and T_3 exert a negative feedback inhibition mainly at the level of the anterior pituitary. This limits TSH secretion, even though TRH is being produced in the hypothalamus. T_4 and T_3 have some inhibitory effect on the hypothalamus, reducing the output of TRH.

In animals subjected to cold for a long period of time, the higher brain centers signal the hypothalamus to release TRH and increase plasma levels of thyroxine. Thyroxine raises the basal metabolic rate (BMR), allowing for cold adaptation.

DEGRADATION

Degradation of thyroid hormones involves deiodination. The liver conjugates thyroxine to glucuronide for excretion in the bile. Some tissues, particularly the liver, can oxidatively deaminate or decarboxylate thyroxine for excretion.

Antithyroid Drugs

Antithyroid drugs interfere with the production of thyroxine. Thiocarbamides inhibit iodination and aminobenzenes (sulfonamides) block the iodide change to iodine. Anions, such as NO_3^-, block iodide uptake by either competing with I^- for the iodide pump or in some way inactivating it. The natural goitrogens and a large amount of iodide also inhibit thyroxine production.

Actions of Thyroxine

METABOLIC EFFECTS

Thyroxine exhibits a calorigenic effect, increasing the BMR and oxygen consumption in virtually all tissues. The brain, testes, and spleen are important exceptions which do not respond. Thyroxine increases the rate of protein degradation, and fatty acid and carbohydrate oxidation as well as enhancing carbohydrate absorption. Plasma cholesterol is decreased under the influence of thyroxine. The hormone also stimulates the CNS and potentiates the effects of catecholamines.

DEVELOPMENTAL EFFECTS

Thyroxine potentiates the effects of growth hormone in normal growth and skeletal bone development and is necessary for the development of the CNS and the myelination of nerves. Skeletal growth deficiency can be reversed by administration of thyroxine.

MECHANISM OF ACTION

Hormonal action is typical in that thyroxine binds to a receptor and goes to the nucleus to influence an increase in mRNA synthesis of specific proteins, possibly the membrane Na^+/K^+ ATPase since increased ATPase activity could account for the BMR increase. A direct effect on mitochondria causing uncoupling of respiration and oxidative phosphorylation has also been suggested as a mode of action.

Disorders of Thyroid Function

In children, hypothyroidism leads to cretinism in which the child becomes dwarfed and mentally retarded. In the adult, hypothyroidism is characterized by a low BMR, poor cold adaptation/tolerance, and slow mental processes, particularly speech. The condition in the adult is referred to as myxedema because of changes in glycoproteins in the skin. These undergo accelerated degradation in response to thyroxine, trapping water and leading to a puffiness in the skin and change in appearance. Carotenemia, a condition in which the skin yellows because of carotene build-up also occurs, since thyroid hormones are necessary for the conversion of carotene to vitamin A.

Hyperthyroidism leads to nervousness, weight loss,

intolerance of heat, and a high BMR. Hyperthyroidism can be caused by TSH secreting pituitary tumors and Graves' disease, a condition due to overproduction of an immunoglobulin (LATS) which binds to thyroid cell TSH receptors to stimulate the gland. Graves' disease is manifested by bulging eyes.

Hyperthyroidism may lead to heart failure because of the strain of chronic increased cardiac output influenced by thryoxine. Hyperthyroidism may also lead to liver failure, because the increased BMR depletes liver glycogen stores and disrupts normal metabolism.

ADRENAL HORMONES

The adrenal glands are located on the superior pole of each kidney. The inner adrenal medulla produces catecholamines, while the outer cortex produces steroids (i.e., glucocorticoids, mineralocorticoids, and sex hormones) that exert minor effects. Catecholamines and glucocorticoids interact in their effects. However, there is no important connection between the medulla and the cortex in terms of secretion.

THE ADRENAL CORTEX

The adrenal cortex can be divided into the zona glomerulosa, the outermost layer which secretes predominantly mineralocorticoids, the zona fasciculata, and the zona reticulata. The latter secrete glucocorticoids and some androgens. A fetal adrenal zone produces predominantly androgens which are used by the placenta as precursors for estrogen production. This zone is not present in the adult.

Trophic ACTH Effects

ACTH affects growth of the adrenal gland, in particular the zona fasciculata and the zona reticularis, which make up the bulk of the gland. When the stimulatory effect of ACTH is abolished by hypophysectomy, these two zones decrease in size and glucocorticoid production is diminished. The zona glomerulosa does not respond to the trophic effects of ACTH and is relatively unaffected by hypophysectomy.

GLUCOCORTIOCOIDS

The glucocorticoids and mineralocorticoids are structurally similar steroid hormones. All exhibit both glucocorticoid and mineralocorticoid activity.

Glucocorticoids primarily effect carbohydrate metabolism and include cortisol, corticosterone, and corti-

sone. Cortisol (hydrocortisone; 21-C steroid) is the predominant glucocorticoid secreted by the adrenal. Structurally, hydroxyl groups occupy positions 21, 11, and 17, with ketone groups on positions 3 and 20.

Corticosterone is secreted in much smaller amounts and differs structurally from cortisol in that it lacks a 17-α-hydroxyl group. Cortisone is formed from cortisol in the liver and has a ketone group instead of a hydroxyl group at the 11 position. It is not an important circulating steroid because it is metabolized further by the liver.

MINERALOCORTICOIDS

Mineralocorticoids primarily effect Na^+ retention and K^+ excretion. Aldosterone is the principle mineralocorticoid and is synthesized as the optically active D-isomer. Related to corticosterone, aldosterone has an aldehyde instead of a methyl group at position 28 so that the hemiacetyl form predominates.

Desoxycorticosterone is a precursor of corticosterone which exhibits weak mineralocorticoid acitivity and lacks the 11-hyroxyl group. The mineralocorticoid role of this hormone is minor, except when it is secreted in pathologic amounts.

Relative Activity. Cortisol is arbitrarily assigned a glucocorticoid activity of 1 and a mineralocorticoid activity of 1. Aldosterone has a mineralocorticoid activity that is 3,000 times greater than that of cortisol. Desoxycorticosterone has 30 times less mineralocorticoid acitivity than aldosterone.

Cortisol has the highest glucocorticoid activity, with cortisone and aldosterone exhibiting equal activity levels. In terms of actual secretion and presence in the blood, the mineralocorticoid activity comes from aldosterone and the glucocorticoid activity comes predominantly from cortisol, with a small contribution from corticosterone.

Synthetic Hormones

Synthetic corticosteroids include prednisolone, with a double bond in the 1 position of cortisol. Prednisolone is four times more active as a glucocorticoid than cortisol and does not exhibit mineralocorticoid activity. 9-Fluorocortisol is 10 times more active as a glucocorticoid and 100 times more active as a mineralocorticoid than cortisol. The derivative 9-fluoro-16-prednisolone (dexamethasone) is 25 times more active as a glucocorticoid but loses all mineralocorticoid activity. This is useful pharmacologically to promote pure glucocorticoidlike actions. High glucocorticoid activity is attributed to tight binding affinity for the cortisol receptor and a long half-life.

Biosynthesis of Adrenal Steroids

The adrenal synthesizes steroids from acetate or cholesterol precursors via the same reactions as ovarian and Leydig cells. Pregnenalone is synthesized from cholesterol and can be converted into progesterone or into 17-hydroxy progesterone.

Androgens and estrogens are produced in the zona fasciculata and the zona reticularis by the conversion of pregnenalone or progesterone. The predominant androgen secreted is dehydroepiandrosterone. Some androstene-dione is also secreted.

Very small amounts of estrogens are synthesized by the adrenal. Under normal circumstances, very little estradiol comes from the adrenal directly. However, some adrenal androgen is converted into estrogen by other tissues.

Cortisol and corticosterone synthesis involves the action of two enzyme systems on progesterone as precursor of corticosterone and 17-hydroxyprogesterone as a precursor of cortisol. The enzyme 21-hydroxylase converts the 21 methyl into a 21-hydroxyl group and 11-hydroxylase hydroxylates the 11 position. Both enzymes require NADPH and oxygen. The relative output of cortisol/corticosterone is 7 to 1 in favor of cortisol.

Mineralocorticoid production occurs in the outer zona glomerulosa. An enzyme system which hydroxylates corticosterone at the 18 position is present in significant amounts only in the zona glomerulosa. Subsequent dehydrogenation at the 18 position produces the aldehyde which is aldosterone. Both these reactions take place in the mitochondria. Aldosterone is formed in significant amounts only in the zona glomerulosa.

RELATIVE PLASMA CONCENTRATIONS

A very significant amount of adrenal cortical hormones are bound to plasma proteins, with total plasma concentrations including both free and bound proteins. The plasma concentration of cortisol is 25 times higher than that of corticosterone, and corticosterone is degraded more rapidly than cortisol.

Transcortin or cortisol-binding globulin (CBG) binds cortisol very tightly and corticosterone slightly less so. The binding capacity for cortisol is about 20 μg/100 ml, sufficient to bind most of the cortisol with only a small amount circulating free. Cortisol can bind to albumin, but the binding constant is much lower. Transcortin is synthesized in the liver and plasma levels are increased by estrogens and considerably elevated in pregnancy.

The half-life of cortisol is about 90 minutes, with slow uptake to the tissues because of tight transcortin binding.

The half-life of corticosterone is 50 minutes. Free and bound cortisol are interrelated by the equilibrium of binding. Plasma concentrations are about 0.5 μg/dl free cortisol to 13 μg/dl bound. Free cortisol is available for uptake, exerts hormonal action, and is degraded. Reduction of free cortisol feeds back to the pituitary, influencing the release of ACTH.

Plasma aldosterone is present in much smaller amounts than the glucocorticoids. However, these amounts are sufficient to produce sodium retaining effects. Aldosterone binds only to albumin and has a half-life of 20 minutes.

Deoxycorticosterone is present in approximately equal amounts to aldosterone, but is 30 times less active as a mineralocorticoid and contributes only a small effect on sodium retention, about 3 percent of the total.

The androgen, dehydroepiandrosterone, is present in substantial plasma concentrations compared to other cortical steroids.

HORMONE DEGRADATION

Degradation of adenal steroids occurs in the liver. The steps in cortisol degradation are typical and are initiated by reduction of the double bond of the A ring to a dihydro metabolite. Reduction of the 3 ketone group to a hydroxyl leads to a tetrahydro metabolite. Further reduction of the C-20 ketone gives corticolike derivatives and cleavage of the side chain produces 16-ketosteroids which have some androgenlike activity. "Tetrahydro" metabolites, corticolike derivatives and 17-ketosteroids are conjugated at the 3-hydroxyl position with glucuronide for excretion in the urine. The 11-hydroxyl group can be converted to a ketone to form cortisone, which is metabolized via the same reactions.

MODE AND REGULATION OF ACTION

Cortisol action is similar to that of other steroids and involves binding to a receptor and modification of mRNA synthesis in the nucleus. Regulation of cortisol secretion is predominantly under the control of ACTH. In addition to having a trophic effect on the adrenal cortex, ACTH binds to a receptor protein, leading to increased cAMP which stimulates a protein kinase, which phosphorylates an esterase. The esterase mobilizes stored cholesterol esters to free cholesterol. Enhanced uptake of cholesterol into the mitochondria and probably the stimulation of 20,22 lyase in response to cAMP result in increased production of progesterone. The availability of this substrate results in production of more cortisol.

Regulation of ACTH Secretion

The release of ACTH from the pituitary is subject to feedback inhibition by cortisol. Cortisol may also inhibit at the level of the hypothalamus. Reduction in cortisol levels releases inhibition to increase ACTH secretion, thus stimulating the adrenal cortex to produce more cortisol. ACTH release is stimulated by the release of corticotropin releasing hormone (CRH) from the hypothalamus.

Factors that influence the secretion of ACTH are generally related to stress and include toxins, trauma, infection, hypoglycemia, exercise, hemorrhage, pain, exposure to cold, emotional factors such as anxiety and apprehension, and sleep. In sleep, ACTH secretion follows the diurnal rhythm, with a major peak occurring early in the morning before wake up. These stimuli act directly to influence ACTH release via pathways which stimulate the hypothalamus.

There is good correlation between plasma ACTH and plasma glucocorticoid levels which supports the contention that ACTH regulates adrenal glucocorticoid secretion.

Metabolic Effects of Glucocorticoids

Glucocorticoids increase skeletal muscle protein breakdown, decrease glucose utilization, increase fatty acid release from adipose tissue, and increase liver gluconeogenesis. The increased release of amino acids can provide substrate for gluconeogenesis. Fatty acids provide an alternate fuel source to conserve glucose. Decreased uptake of glucose makes more glucose available for the heart and brain. These are extremely important physiologic reactions which are also modulated by other hormones such as glucagon and insulin.

PHARMACOLOGIC EFFECTS

Very high doses of glucocorticoids produce other effects of glucocorticoid excess. These include antiallergic effects caused by the inhibition of histamine release and anti-inflammatory effects.

HEMATOPOIETIC AND LYMPHOID EFFECTS

Glucocorticoids reduce the immune response. They inhibit lymphoid tissue by stimulating protein breakdown and decrease the number of circulating lymphocytes, eosinophils, etc. These effects could also contribute to anti-inflammatory effects. Glucocorticoids are required for normal erythropoiesis.

PSYCHONEURAL EFFECTS

Deficiencies in glucocorticoids lead to irritability, inability to concentrate, and other neurologic problems. The taste sensation is also greatly enhanced in deficiency. Glucocorticoid excess causes severe behavioral and emotional changes.

STRESS EFFECTS

Glucocorticoids enhance resistance to stress. In the absence of glucocorticoids, sensitivity to stress and noxious stimuli is greatly increased. A minor stress such as a toxic agent or an infection can be fatal in the absence of glucocorticoid secretion.

CARDIOVASCULAR EFFECTS

The glucocorticoids interact with catecholamines to exert cardiovascular effects. The catcholamines play an important role in maintaining vascular smooth muscle tone in the arteries, an effect which requires glucocorticoids. In excess, the mineralocorticoid activity exhibited by glucocorticoids influences some sodium retention.

OTHER ACTIONS

Excess amounts of glucocorticoids cause muscle tiring because of mobilization of muscle proteins. The calcium mobilizing effect leads to removal of calcium from bone and to bone weakness. In addition, connective tissue synthesis is reduced.

Glucocorticoids are needed for the excretion of a water load, with deficiency making water excretion extremely difficult. Glucocorticoids also act on the gastrointestinal tract to stimulate the secretion of a number of substances as well as on the respiratory system and the liver.

Mineralocorticoid Effects

Mineralocorticoids cause Na^+ retention and K^+ excretion by the kidney, salivary glands, sweat glands, and gastrointestinal tract. Secondarily to Na^+ retention, they increase plasma volume. In the long-term, kidney Na^+ retention escapes and the plasma volume increase ceases.

Adrenal insufficiency refers to the diminished ability of the zona glomerulosa to secrete aldosterone. This leads to a decrease in plasma Na^+ and an increase in plasma K^+. In primary hyperaldosteronism, excess aldosterone production effects some increase in plasma Na^+, with the effect ameliorated by the kidney escape phenomenon. In this condition, a substantial decrease occurs in plasma K^+ which leads to an increase in bicarbonate levels and metabolic alkalosis.

MODE OF ACTION

Aldosterone enters the cell and binds to a receptor which undergoes a conformational change in the cytoplasm. The receptor-aldosterone complex binds to the nucleus to turn on mRNA synthesis. Three different proteins have been hypothesized as the product of this genetic message (i.e., NADH isocitric dehydrogenase to increase metabolic activity with enhanced Na^+ uptake, membrane ATPase to increase Na^+ pumping, and permease in which a protein enhances Na^+ permeability). In any event, aldosterone binds to a receptor and activates Na^+ transport via the synthesis of a specific protein.

CONTROL OF SECRETION

Aldosterone secretion is controlled primarily by the renin-angiotensin system. Renin released from the kidney acts on angiotensinogen to form angiotensin I, which is converted to angiotensin II. Angiotensin II can act on the adrenal cortex to increase production and secretion of aldosterone. When aldosterone is secreted, there is an increase in Na^+ retention and water, which leads to an increase in the extracellular volume. This causes corresponding changes in blood pressure, which feeds back to reduce the secretion of renin. This feedback system tends to maintain normal plasma volume and normal Na^+ concentration.

Secretion of aldosterone is increased by angiotensin II, low plasma Na^+ levels, and high K^+ levels, the likely physiologic regulator. ACTH increases aldosterone transiently and in high doses and is only a minor factor in secretion. These factors, with the exception of Na^+, also increase cholesterol and pregnenalone in the zona glomerulosa.

There is a direct correlation between renin and aldosterone levels. High renin levels are associated with high aldosterone levels. This is related to posture, since more renin is released when standing.

Disorders of Adrenocortical Function

Complete loss of the adrenal gland either through surgery or disease is fatal without intervention. Both mineralocorticoids and glucocorticoids are lost. Aldosterone loss is most serious because the substantial Na^+ depletion and reduction in plasma volume lead to hypotension and shock. This is rapidly fatal unless mineralocorticoid is administered.

Replacement of only aldosterone without replacing glucocorticoids leads to a severe hypoglucocorticoidism. Effects are not as severe as aldosterone loss, but a spectrum of stresses may lead to a fatal collapse. With adequate food intake, the blood sugar is maintained. However, in the fasting condition, a fatal hypoglycemia develops because of the role of glucocorticoids in raising the blood sugar. Water excretion is difficult. Personality changes result, including the inability to concentrate. There is a lowering of the taste threshold, which is suppressed by glucocorticoids.

ADDISON'S DISEASE

In this condition, adrenal destruction is brought about by the autoimmune process or other means with a loss of both aldosterone and glucocorticoids. The syndrome develops slowly, with residual steroid production sufficient to maintain function for awhile. Most symptoms are due to absence of aldosterone (i.e., Na^+ loss, K^+ retention, dehydration, and hypotension). ACTH levels are greatly elevated, since there are no glucocorticoids to exert feedback inhibition of ACTH. ACTH in turn has little effect upon the diseased gland. Since ACTH has some MSH activity, prolonged exposure of high ACTH levels can lead to skin pigmentation.

CONN'S SYNDROME

Conn's syndrome leads to excess production of mineralocorticoids and is caused mainly by an aldosterone secreting tumor. Excess Na^+ retention leads to plasma volume increase and hypertension. K^+ depletion leads to muscle weakness and kidney damage. Metabolic alkalosis and a lowering of plasma Ca^{++} are secondary to the alkalosis.

CUSHING'S SYNDROME

Cushing's syndrome is caused by oversecretion of ACTH by pituitary microtumors or by excess releasing hormone. High ACTH levels increase glucocorticoid production but have no prolonged effect on aldosterone. Therefore, the manifestations of this disease are caused by the increased levels of glucocorticoids.

The disease can lead to severe mental aberrations, although for a short time a state of general euphoria may be experienced. Excess protein degradation leads to poor muscle development and wound healing. The mobilization of lipids from adipose tissue leads to a characteristic redistribution of fat to the abdomen and the back. Excess glucocorticoids cause elevated blood sugar and hyperglycemia which can lead to diabetes. Salt retention is caused by the mineralocorticoid activity of excess glucocorticoids. ACTH stimulates the production of excess 11-

deoxycorticosterone, which makes a large contribution to salt and water retention. This activity leads to K^+ depletion and hypertension.

ADRENOGENITAL SYNDROME

This abnormality is characterized by production of excess androgen and affects only females and boys before puberty. This syndrome can be caused by enzyme deficiency in the 21- or 11-hydroxylase which leads to low cortisol production. In this situation, more ACTH is produced since there is less feedback inhibition via cortisol and more steroid is made available to the pathway. Excess steroids will go from pregnenolone to the androgen producing pathway. Complete loss of the 11- or 21-hydroxylase leads to hypoglucocorticoidism and androgens as end products of steroid production. A partial enzyme deficiency leads to more or less normal amounts of glucocorticoids but excess androgens.

In the female, excess androgens lead to masculinization. This disorder can also occur through adrenal tumors that produce excess enzymes in the androgen biosynthetic pathway.

IATROGENIC HYPOGLUCOCORTICOIDISM

When high treatment levels of glucocorticoids act to suppress an inflammatory response over a long period, ACTH secretion from the pituitary is repressed by excess exogenous glucocorticoids. The adrenal gland zones producing glucocorticoids begin to atrophy from lack of ACTH. It takes several months for ACTH levels to reach normal after glucocorticoid treatment is stopped. Cortisol levels require an even longer period (6 months), since the first effect of ACTH is a trophic effect on the adrenal cortex.

THE ADRENAL MEDULLA

The adrenal medulla can be considered as displaced neural tissue since certain medullary enzymes and the catecholamines produced are also found in the sympathetic ganglia and the brain.

A significant fraction of the blood supply to the adrenal medulla is via the medullary artery. The cortical capillaries feed directly into the medulla. Blood from the cortex is very rich in the glucocorticoids secreted by cortical cells. This is important, since high levels of glucocorticoids are necessary for the induction of the enzyme essential for synthesis of epinephrine. Only 80 percent of the medullary cells stores epinephrine, with the remaining cells storing the precursor, norepinephrine. The difference between these cell types may simply be their

position relative to the medullary artery with its glucocorticoid rich blood supply. The medullary cells are innervated directly by preganglionic fibers of the splanchnic nerve. Stimulation of the nerve causes hormone release.

Catecholamine Hormones

Epinephrine and norepinephrine are both produced in the medulla. Epinephrine is the predominate hormone. The medulla is the only site of epinephrine synthesis so that the blood level (0.3 ng/ml) comes exclusively from this source. Norepinephrine is also found in the sympathetic system as a neurotransmitter. Blood levels of this hormone (0.2 ng/ml) come predominantly from nerve discharge, with only a small amount from the adrenal medulla. Epinephrine is the predominant hormone stored in the adrenal medulla.

BIOSYNTHESIS

The catecholamines are derivatives of the amino acids phenylalanine and tyrosine (Fig. 8-15). The introduction of a second hydroxyl group on the aromatic ring via tyrosine hydroxylase converts tyrosine to dopa (dihydroxyphenylalanine). Decarboxylation by the enzyme dopa decarboxylase yields dopamine, the first of three catecholamines. The activity of dopamine oxidase gives rise to norepinephrine. Methylation of norepinephrine by phenylethanolamine-N-methyl transferase converts to epinephrine.

Tyrosine hydroxylase and dopamine oxidase are found in brain, nerve endings, and the adrenal medulla. The phenylethanolamine-N-methyl transferase involved in the final conversion to epinephrine is found only in the adrenal medulla, the only source of epinephrine. All of the enzymes are cytoplasmic except dopamine oxidase which is found in the chromaffin granules. Therefore, the conversion of dopamine to norepinephrine involves dopamine transport into the chromaffin granules.

REGULATION OF SYNTHESIS

Catecholamine synthesis occurs under neural stimulation. Acute stimulation affects a rise in tyrosine hydroxylase (TH), the rate limiting enzyme in the synthetic pathway. TH is inhibited by catecholamine feedback. Chronic neural stimulation causes a rise in tyrosine hydroxylase and dopamine oxidase. ACTH also causes a rise in these enzymes. The effect is due directly to ACTH, not to ACTH's stimulation of glucocorticoid production. Glucocorticoids are needed for the induction of the N-methyl transferase.

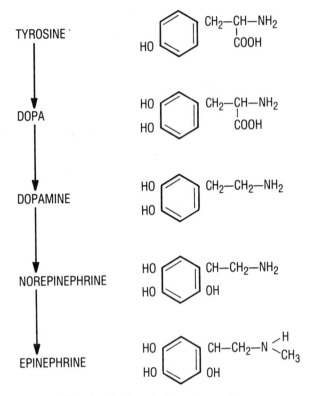

Fig. 8-15. Catecholamine biosynthesis.

CATECHOLAMINE STORAGE

Chromaffin granules contain large amounts of catecholamines and adenine nucleotides (especially ATP), substantial amounts of protein, and some Ca^{++}. The protein consists of some dopamine oxidase, but is primarily chromagranin A, necessary for storage of catecholamines and adenine nucleotides. Catecholamine transport into the granule takes place via a transporter which exchanges two protons for one single, positively charged catecholamine. The net effect is removal of one positive charge from the granule, with catecholamine transport driven by H^+ movement.

Reserpine blocks the catecholamine transporter and also the synthesis of norephinephrine. ATP is transported into the granules by a passive transporter protein. A final transport process removes two Na^+ in exchange for one Ca^{++}.

SECRETION

Secretion is controlled by neural stimulation via the splanchnic nerves. Stimuli to these nerves, such as pain, cold, anoxia, asphyxia, hypotension, hypoglycemia, severe exercise, or emotional stress, can lead to catecholamine secretion.

Chemical stimulants also influence secretion. The major chemical stimulant is acetylcholine, released during neural stimulation. Other stimulants include histamine, bradykinin (via angiotensin II), and glucagon.

Abnormal secretion can be caused by phenochromocytomas, tumors derived from the adrenal medulla which secrete norepinephrine indiscriminately without stimulation. Such tumors can be found in places other than the medulla.

The relative percentage of epinephrine and norepinephrine varies in different disorders. In asphyxia and hypoxia, the secretion of norepinephrine rises more than that of epinephrine. In hemorrhage, the increase is predominantly epinephrine, while the amount of norepinephrine is relatively unchanged from basal levels.

MECHANISM OF SECRETION

In the resting gland with catecholamine in the granules, Ca^{++} concentration in the cytosol is quite low. Secretion is initiated by acetylcholine released by preganglionic neurons which increases membrane permeability to Ca^{++}, allowing Ca^{++} to enter the cell. The granules are discharged via exocytosis in response to Ca^{++} exposure. When the stimulus is removed, Ca^{++} is bound, membrane permeability to Ca^{++} is diminished, and secretion decreases.

CATECHOLAMINE EFFECTS

Epinephrine is frequently called the fight or flight hormone. Under resting conditions the blood contains very little epinephrine. However, during excitement or stress, the adrenal medulla releases epinephrine and norepinephrine which exert potent physiologic effects—survival tactics to combat the emergency.

The release of catecholamine prepares the body for a crisis by stimulating cardiac output, diverting blood to muscle, mobilizing energy sources, and increasing the metabolic rate. The metabolic effects include increased glycogenolysis, lipolysis, and blood lactate, and decreased insulin release. There is a general calorigenic effect.

Catecholamine actions effect specific tissues as is illustrated by the following:

In the lung, dilation of bronchioles via epeinephrine causes increased ventilation which increases oxygen availability.

In the heart, catecholamines increase the force of contraction, the rate of metabolism, and the cardiac contractility.

In the blood vessels, the catecholamine effect is aided by vasoconstriction, which increases venous return and blood flow. Constriction of arteries to the skin and viscera causes elevated blood pressure. However, the arteries to the muscles are dilated, causing an increased blood flow to the muscles and the heart.

In the muscles, glycogenolysis increases available substrate and lactate.

In the liver, glycogenolysis increases to raise the blood glucose level and provide more fuel for the heart, muscle, and brain.

There are significant differences in the actions of epinephrine and norepinephrine. Epinephrine is more effective at inducing hyperglycemia; norepinephrine at increasing blood pressure. Cardiac output is increased by epinephrine. In the short-term, norepinephrine also increases cardiac output, but the long-term effect of this hormone is a reduction in cardiac output. Bradycardia may be produced reflexly in response to the increase in blood pressure and vasoconstriction.

In summary, in response to epinephrine, cardiac output and heart rate increase and total peripheral resistance decreases due to dilation of the vessels in skeletal muscle. Blood pressure increases. In response to norepinephrine, total peripheral resistance greatly increases, blood pressure substantially increases, and heart rate and cardiac output reflexly decrease.

MECHANISM OF ACTION

Receptors for catecholamines are separated into two categories. Alpha receptors are best stimulated by norepinephrine. Epinephrine is capable of stimulating both alpha and beta receptors. Beta receptors are further classified as $\beta 1$ receptors in the heart, while most other beta receptors are classified as $\beta 2$. Epinephrine and norepinephrine have about the same activity in alpha receptors, but epinephrine is much more effective in beta receptors.

In alpha receptors, binding appears to influence changes in Ca^{++} levels which mediate the effects. In beta receptors, the catecholamine binds and stimulates adenylate cyclase to increase cAMP production.

DEGRADATION

The main site of catecholamine catabolism is in the liver. Degradation involves transfer of a methyl group (catechol-o-methyl transferase, COMT) to a hydroxyl group of epinephrine or norepinephrine. Monoamine oxidase/aldehyde dehydrogenase (MO/AD) converts the amino group of catecholamines to an intermediate which can be methylated by COMT. The resultant metanephrine or normetanephrine is then conjugated to glucuronic acid and excreted.

Methyl transferase (COMT) is found in the liver and

kidney. Monamine oxidase is found only in the liver, kidney, salivary glands, and adrenergic nerve endings. Aldehyde dehydrogenase is found in all tissues. The uptake of catecholamines into tissues which can me-abolize them is of considerable importance in the control of their action parameters.

CALCIUM REGULATING HORMONES

Total body calcium averages aout 1,100 g, most of which is in the skeleton. The bone provides a reservoir for calcium regulation and is in a dynamic state of Ca^{++} flux. Under normal conditions, 0.5 g of Ca^{++} exchanges between the bone and extracellular fluid daily. There is some urinary excretion of calcium, but this is balanced by uptake of calcium from the gut. Normally, most of the dietary calcium is excreted in the feces.

Calcium Homeostasis

Plasma calcium is very tightly regulated and maintained at about 10 mg/dl. One half is in the free ionic state with most of the remaining calcium bound to plasma proteins. Maintenance of the free Ca^{++} level is important because of the role of Ca^{++} in blood clotting, muscle contraction, and nerve firing. Depressed calcium levels lead to uncontrolled firing of motor neurons, causing muscle spasms in a condition known as hypocalcemic tetany. Below 7 mg/dl, uncontrolled muscle contraction occurs and death from asphyxia can occur if spasm of the larynx becomes severe enough to obstruct the airway.

Calcium homeostasis involves three hormones and four tissues.

Parathyroid hormone (PTH), secreted by parathyroid cells, mobilizes Ca^{++} from bone.

Calcitonin, secreted by thyroid cells, inhibits Ca^{++} mobilization. Calcitonin is also produced in the thymus.

Active vitamin D_3 (1,25 dihydroxycholecalciferol) is produced by the kidney and affects Ca^{++} uptake in the gut. Vitamin D_3 is activated by hydroxylation of the 25 position in the liver and the 1 position in the kidney.

Hypocalcemic Tetany

Muscle spasms occur when plasma Ca^{++} falls significantly below 10 mg/dl. The tendency to tetany is dependent on plasma phosphate, magnesium, bicarbonate, and hydrogen ion concentrations. As free Ca^{++} rises, the tendency to hypocalcemic tetany decreases. Rising Mg^{++} levels decrease the tendency because Mg^{++} can replace Ca^{++}, releasing it from bound forms. Rising H^+ also influences the release of calcium from protein. Rising HCO_3^- and HPO_4^{--} increase the tendency because they both remove Ca^{++} from the plasma.

Calcium Uptake and Absorption

Both absorption and excretion of Ca^{++} occur in the gastrointestinal tract. Most of the ingested Ca^{++} is excreted. The amount of Ca^{++} absorbed balances the Ca^{++} urinary loss. The kidney conserves Ca^{++} so that only 2.5 mmol is lost in a filtered load of 250 mmol. The distribution of Ca^{++} in interstitial and extracellular fluids remains relatively constant.

The bone provides a very large reservoir of Ca^{++}, with about 100 mmol available for rapid exchange. The remainder, stable bone Ca^{++}, can only be mobilized very slowly. Normally, a small amount of Ca^{++} is deposited each day and an equal amount reabsorbed.

Three cell types influence Ca^{++} exchange in bone.

Osteoblasts are involved in bone synthesis and form a barrier defining an area of drastically different Ca^{++} concentration. These cells secrete collagen which forms a matrix for calcium phosphate deposition and secrete both acid and alkaline phosphatases. The phosphatases create an environment in which the solubility product is exceeded and calcium phosphates precipitate on the matrix.

Osteocytes develop from osteoblasts that become surrounded by bone. They have processes which connect them to osteoblasts and are able to mobilize and deposit Ca^{++} in the bone.

Osteoclasts are involved in the resorption of bone matrix. These cells secrete acid phosphatase and move Ca^{++} out of bone.

The resorption of Ca^{++} from bone (calcium mobilization) is stimulated by PTH, which is stimulated by low plasma Ca^{++} levels. Calcitonin stimulates increased deposition of Ca^{++} into bone and is stimulated by high plasma Ca^{++}.

Vitamin D_3

Dietary 7-dihydrocholesterol is a precursor of vitamin D_3. The ultraviolet wavelengths of sunlight energize the conversion of this precursor into vitamin D_3 (cholecalciferol). In the absence of sunlight, vitamin D_3 must be provided in the diet (cod liver oil is a source). The absence of vitamin D_3 leads to poor uptake of Ca^{++} from the gastrointestinal tract, leading to low plasma Ca^{++} and poor Ca^{++} deposition in bone. This condition causes rickets in children.

Vitamin D_3 is hydroxylated in the liver by 25-hydroxylase, and circulates to the kidney where it can be converted to 1,25 dihydrocholecalciferol, the active metabolite. The active form binds to an α-globulin for transport in the blood. A deficiency in 1-hydroxylase in the kidney will prevent D_3 conversion to the active form, leading to rickets in children and poor bone deposition in adults.

RENAL REGULATION OF VITAMIN D_3

Vitamin D_3 metabolism in the kidney is mediated by plasma Ca^{++} levels. High serum Ca^{++} levels lead to high production of inactive 24,25 dihydroxy D_3. Low plasma Ca^{++} levels lead to conversion to active 1,25 dihydroxy D_3 which promotes Ca^{++} uptake.

Regulation involves stimulation of PTH release by low plasma Ca^{++} levels. PTH directly affects the kidney, stimulating 1-hydroxylase which catalyzes conversion to the active 1,25 dihydroxy D_3 form. Low plasma phosphate levels also stimulate 1-hydroxylase. Increased calcium levels increase the formation of the inactive 24,25 dihydroxy D_3 derivative. 1,25 dihydroxy D_3 suppresses 1-hydroxylase and its own production via feedback inhibition and induces production of the inactive form.

MODE OF ACTION

The active vitamin affects intestinal calcium uptake. Intestinal absorption of calcium occurs via Ca^{++} stimulated ATPase, alkaline phosphatase, and Ca^{++} binding protein. Active 1,25 dihydroxy D_3 also influences increased phosphate absorption from the intestine.

Parathyroid Hormone

Parathyroid hormone (PTH) is a linear polypeptide secreted by parathyroid cells and consisting of 84 amino acid residues. Synthesis involves cleavage of the precursors preproPTH (115 amino acids) and proPTH (90 amino acids) to yield the active hormone. The hormone has a short half-life and is secreted into the blood where it can go to the bone, kidney, or liver where it can be cleaved to yield the N-terminal active fragment. The active fragment and PTH both circulate in the blood and act to increase plasma Ca^{++} and depress plasma phosphate.

REGULATION OF SECRETION

The secretory stimulus is provided by low plasma Ca^{++} levels which act directly on the parathyroid. PTH acts on bone to promote resorption of Ca^{++} and increases the formation of osteoclasts in the long-term. PTH acts on the kidney to enhance Ca^{++} retention and stimulate 1,25 dihyroxy D_3 which acts on the gut to increase Ca^{++} uptake. These actions mobilize Ca^{++} from bone and increase the plasma Ca^{++} level. The overall effect to raise plasma Ca^{++} is mediated by the ability of

PTH to increase cAMP levels at the target tissues (bone, kidney).

Parathyroidectomy will lead to death if PTH is not replaced, since adequate Ca^{++} levels are not maintained in the absence of this hormone.

Calcitonin

Calcitonin is a 32 amino acid peptide which inhibits bone resorption and is released from the parafollicular cells of the thyroid and also from the thymus.

PTH and calcitonin have antagonistic effects and act together to maintain plasma Ca^{++}. PTH is released in large amounts in response to low plasma Ca^{++} levels; calcitonin in response to high plasma Ca^{++}. PTH is the more important of the two, since calcitonin deficiency is very difficult to achieve. PTH and calcitonin affect all bone cells. PTH mobilizes bone calcium, while calcitonin inhibits this activity.

Glucocorticoids and Growth Hormone

Other hormonal influences include glucocorticoids and growth hormone. Glucocorticoids reduce Ca^{++} uptake in the intestine and increase bone degradation. The net effect is to lower plasma Ca^{++}. Growth hormone increases Ca^{++} uptake in the gut and increases urinary Ca^{++} excretion. The net effect is higher plasma Ca^{++}.

SEX HORMONES

The androgens and estrogens are steroid hormones normally secreted by both sexes that influence masculine and feminine characteristics. In the male, large amounts of androgens, principally testosterone, and small amounts of estrogens are secreted. In the female, estrogens predominate, but small amounts of androgens are also produced. The sex hormones, under the influence of the anterior pituitary gonadotropins, FSH and LH, develop and maintain sexuality and gametogenesis.

Male Hormones: The Androgens

The testes perform two important functions (i.e., the production of viable sperm and of the male hormone, testosterone). The seminiferous tubules, which make up the bulk of the testes are the site of sperm maturation. The interstitial (Leydig) cells, located in-between the seminiferous tubules, are the major site of testosterone production. Cholesterol, essential for testosterone synthesis, is stored as the ester in lipid droplets in the Leydig cells.

TESTOSTERONE

Testosterone is a 19 carbon steroid, hydroxylated at position 17, with a keto group at position 3, and a 4-5 double bond. Subtle differences in stereochemistry cause structurally similar steroids to exhibit different hormonal properties. Reduction of testosterone's double bond, for example, changes the 3-D structure to affect binding properties and yields the more active androgen, dihydrotestosterone (DHT).

Biosynthesis. The Leydig cells synthesize most of their endogenous cholesterol from acetyl CoA, with esterase activity freeing cholesterol from stored esters. The first step in testosterone biosynthesis is the conversion of cholesterol to pregnenolone, catalyzed by 20,22 lyase. Hydroxylation of the 17 position and side chain cleavage yield 17 ketosteroids which are converted to testosterone. In an alternate route, pregnenolone can be converted to progesterone, with 17-hydroxylase activity yielding androstene-3,17-dione, the immediate precursor of testosterone. Androstene-3,17-dione is an active steroid, but not as powerful as testosterone. These and other precursor molecules can be found in small amounts in the blood.

Control of Testosterone Secretion. Interstitial cell stimulating hormone (ICSH) increases testosterone production. This hormone is the same as luteinizing hormone (LH) in the female. LH is an anterior pituitary glycoprotein which stimulates testosterone by increasing cAMP concentration. cAMP stimulates esterase to free cholesterol and influences the conversion of cholesterol to pregnenolone via 20 – 22 lyase. LH is the most important factor in controlling androgen secretion to the blood. Prolactin potentiates the effect of LH on testosterone secretion.

FSH has a small effect on testosterone production, with a primary effect on stimulation of the seminiferous tubules. Increased blood flow also stimulates testosterone secretion, which moves out of cells by diffusion down a concentration gradient.

Prostaglandins may inhibit testosterone secretion, via small loop feedback.

SECRETION OF LH BY THE PITUITARY

Releasing factor from the hypothalamus stimulates release of LH (ICSH) from the pituitary, via a feedback loop activated by the LH level. LH release is pulsatile, occurring in bursts. An increase in the amplitude of the amount of LH release is mediated at the pituitary level. An increase in the frequency of release is mediated at the hypothalamic level.

Inhibitors of the system can either alter the magnitude or the frequency of release pulses. LH is inhibited by both high testosterone and high estrogen levels. The predominant effect of testosterone is to decrease the frequency of release via feedback on the hypothalmus. Estrogen decreases the amount of release via feedback to the pituitary.

TESTOSTERONE TRANSPORT AND DEGRADATION

Testosterone is transported bound to plasma proteins. Albumin binds about 40 percent, gonadosteroid binding globulin (GBG) another 40 percent, and other proteins about 16 percent. Only about 3 percent is free and represents hormone available for uptake and degradation in the tissues. In the female, nearly all of the small amount of testosterone produced is bound to GBG.

GBG is a glycoprotein (94,000 MW) with a high affinity for testosterone and estradiol. Tight binding by GBG and albumin enhances the release of testosterone from Leydig cells by effectively maintaining a low concentration of free testosterone in the blood. Synthesis of GBG (also called testosterone-estradiol binding globulin) is under feedback control by steroid hormones and is increased 10-fold by estrogen and 2-fold by testosterone.

Degradation of testosterone occurs mainly in the liver. The liver takes up either free or albumin bound testosterone. Degradation involves conversion to androstene-3,17-dione by reduction of the 3-keto group. Androgens are broken down into 17-keto steroid isomers, which are conjugated with glucuronic acid and excreted in the bile. The 17-keto steroid metabolites are active androgens, but not as active as testosterone.

TESTOSTERONE CONVERSIONS IN ACTIVE TISSUES

In target tissues, testosterone is converted into either of two active intermediates (i.e., DHT or estradiol). Conversion to DHT occurs via 5-reductase and is a major mediator of testosterone action. In some tissues, testosterone is converted to estradiol which mediates the effects of testosterone.

PLASMA ANDROGEN LEVELS

Androgen intermediates in the female are produced in the adrenals and ovaries. The primary site of production is the adrenal. Androstene-3,17-dione has some androgenlike effects and is higher in women.

In the male, testosterone is synthesized in the Leydig cells and secreted into the blood for conversion to the active metabolites, DHT and estradiol, in other cells. Androstene-3,17-dione and progesterone are also secreted by Leydig cells. Androstene-3,17-dione can be carried in the blood to other tissues and converted to estrone, which can enter the blood. Thus, steroid levels in the blood are regulated by their metabolism in other tissues.

ANDROGEN ACTIONS

Androgens stimulate spermatogenesis and are essential for viable sperm as well as embryonic differentiation of the male phenotype. The male hormones stimulate growth of external male genitalia and accessory sex glands such as the prostate and the seminal vesicles.

Androgens signal the development of male secondary sexual characteristics at puberty. They exhibit pronounced anabolic effects, influencing increased muscle mass and redistribution of body fat. Androgens lead to increased growth of long bone and epiphyseal plate closure. In the short-term, the effect is to increase growth; in the long-term, androgens reduce growth by epiphyseal closure.

CNS effects include increased libido and aggressive behavior. The hormone effects specific proteins in organs such as the liver and kidney which are androgen dependent.

MECHANISMS OF TESTOSTERONE ACTION

LH binds to the Leydig cell and causes release of testosterone. Testosterone binds to GBG and albumin in the blood, with about 3 percent free. Free testosterone is taken up into responsive tissues, such as skeletal muscle and kidneys, via a protein androgen receptor with a high affinity for testosterone. Testosterone and receptor enter the nucleus and turn on mRNA synthesis for specific new proteins.

In a second class of tissues, for example, prostate, free testosterone enters cells and is reduced by 5-reductase to DHT. DHT binds to a receptor protein and this complex effects nuclear mRNA. In a third class of tissues, the brain, for example, the effect of testosterone is mediated by estradiol. Estradiol binds to a specific and different cellular receptor to turn on appropirate mRNA.

FOLLICLE STIMULATING HORMONE

FSH, along with testosterone, is responsible for gametogenesis. The primary action of FSH is on Sertoli's cells, which extend the full thickness of the seminiferous epithelium and are the site of sperm maturation. FSH binds to receptors on Sertoli's cells, leading to an increase in cAMP, which leads to production of proteins which nourish and develop sperm. FSH also leads to an increase in the conversion of testosterone to estradiol which assists in the evolution of sperm. In addition, FSH increases the production of androgen binding protein (ABP) which carries testosterone to the sperm.

Female Hormones: Estrogens

THE OVARIAN CYCLE

At birth there are approximately two million ovarian follicles which are gradually lost through follicular atresia until about 400,000 remain at puberty. In the beginning of the ovarian cycle, about 20 follicles begin to grow, with the thecal layer and granulosa cells increasing. Most follicles regress; only one matures. The mature follicle contains a fluid filled antrum containing protein, carbohydrates, and steroid hormones. On maturing, the stigma of the mature follicle breaks with the expulsion of the ovum. After the release of the ovum, the follicle quickly fills with blood to become the corpus hemorrhagicum. The granulosa cells of the corpus hemorrhagicum then develop into the corpus luteum, a body of lipid containing cells which produce large amounts of steroids. The corpus luteum forms about 1 week after ovulation. If pregnancy does not occur, the corpus luteum regresses into the corpus albicans, and the cycle begins again. Menstruation occurs roughly midway between ovulations in the typical 28 day cycle.

Endocrine Influence. Initial follicular growth is stimulated by the FSH, which effects induction of more FSH receptors in the cells. At a certain state, the thecal layer begins producing estrogen. Locally, estrogens effect follicular growth. Blood estrogen levels also increase and other tissues are affected.

Close to ovulation estrogen levels increase rapidly and trigger the release of LH, which initiates ovulation. The granulosa cells, influenced by LH, then begin producing progesterone. Prolonged, elevated levels of estrogen and progesterone inhibit the release of FSH and LH from the pituitary. Unless pregnancy results, hormone levels decline and the corpus luteum regresses.

The ovarian cycle is divided into the follicular phase (follicle development) and the luteal phase (corpus luteum development). In the follicular phase, there is a high level of FSH and little estrogen and progesterone. FSH, enhanced by LH, stimulates the growth of the follicle. Eight days before ovulation, estradiol begins to increase with estrogen production in the maturing follicle. Estrogen causes a large surge in LH and a small surge in FSH.

In the luteal phase, after ovulation, the corpus luteum produces both estrogen and progesterone. During this period, basal body temperature is elevated due to the thermogenic properties of progesterone.

Effects of LH. Luteinizing hormone induces the production of progesterone. Locally this causes the production of proteolytic enzymes which weaken the follicular wall and change membrane permeability so that fluid enters the follicle, causing it to swell. The stigma breaks, the follicle ruptures, and the ovum is expelled.

CYCLIC CHANGES IN OTHER TISSUES

In the uterus, prior to ovulation, the endometrium is poorly developed. Under the influence of estrogen, the endometrial cells and glands proliferate. Glycogen is synthesized and stored. After ovulation, under the influence of estrogen and progesterone, the glands become more tortuous and begin secreting. If pregnancy does not occur, the estrogen and progesterone levels begin to fall and the spiral arteries contract.

Increased blood levels of estrogen and progesterone decrease FSH and LH; decreased levels stimulate FSH and LH. Ovarian estrogen and progesterone inhibit the production and release of FSH and LH by feedback inhibition of the pituitary and hypothalamus. With the appropriate rise in estrogen levels, the ventromedial arcuate nucleus of the hypothalamus releases LRF and FRF, leading to a large release in LH from the pituitary, producing ovulation. The mechanism is via feedback to the preoptic and suprachiasmatic nuclei. These paths represent both positive and negative feedback and are influenced by external stimuli, such as light, and higher neural centers. Lesions of the preoptic or suprachiasmatic nuclei block the facilitative feedback path so that only inhibition results. Therefore, LH surge and ovulation are abolished.

FEMALE REPRODUCTIVE LIFE

In the first 12 years, estrogen production is very low. At puberty more gonadotropin is released, causing some follicles to begin growing. Ovulation, however, does not occur because the estrogen rise is not rapid enough to cause the LH surge. The first few cycles are anovulatory. Years 13 to 45 represent the normal ovulatory cycle. The menopause occurs when all follicles have undergone follicular atresia (only about 400 are lost during the ovulatory years). The menopause occurs because gonadotropin cannot stimulate estrogen production. At menopause, with no estrogen response, there is no feedback inhibition and gonadotropin release skyrockets. Male gonadotropin levels remain constant after puberty.

ESTROGENS

The estrogens are 18 carbon steroids characterized by an aromatic A ring. Estradiol possesses beta hydroxyl groups at the 3 and 17 positions and is the most potent female hormone. Estradiol is in equilibrium with estrone, which has a 17 keto group and is less active. Hydroxylation of estrone in the 16 alpha position forms estriol which also has activity, but less than estradiol. Diethylstilbesterol and hexesterol are nonsteroid synthetics with estrogenlike properties.

Biosynthesis and Degradation. Testosterone and androstene-3,17-dione are intermediates in estrogen synthesis. Androgens are converted to estradiol by loss of a methyl group and aromatization of the A ring.

Most of the estradiol and other active estrogens released from the ovary are transported by albumin (60–70 percent). About 30 percent are carried on gonadotropin binding globulin (GBG), which has a higher affinity for testosterone. Even in the female, testosterone occupies most of the sites on the carrier. Only during the cycle peak and during pregnancy does estradiol binding approach that of testosterone for this carrier. Free estrogen represents 3–4 percent of the total and is readily available for uptake.

Degradation in the liver involves hydroxylation of the 16 position to form estriol which is excreted as a glucuronide or sulfate conjugate.

Estrogen Actions. Estrogens influence changes in follicle development and the uterine endometrium with the proliferative effects priming the glands for progesterone secretion. There is a trophic effect on the uterus, with an increase in uterine muscle activity. At puberty, the hormone increases the myometrium and overall uterine size. There is also a trophic effect on the breast.

Weak anabolic effects include increased growth in the long bones. Hormone stimulation of epiphyseal closure is more effective than that of the androgens which act through estrogen metabolites. There is also a weak effect on Na^+/water retention caused by interaction with adrenal corticoid receptors.

Estrogens effect a decrease in plasma cholesterol, an effect not well understood. Changes in skin texture and increased flow from sebaceous glands are also influenced by estrogens. The female secondary sexual characteristics are influenced. However, this effect is mainly caused by lack of androgens.

MECHANISM OF ACTION

The mechanism for estrogen action is the same as that of androgens and involves binding to an intracellular estrogen receptor which translocates to the nucleus to bind to specific chromatin sites, turning on mRNA.

Progestins

Progestins are hormones which influence a secretory endometrium suitable for ovum implantation. The progestins are a secretory product of four cell types (i.e., the adrenal cortex, the ovary, the Leydig cell, and the corpus luteum. Progesterone is the major physiologic progestin.

All of these cell types have the necessary enzymes for the biosynthesis of progesterone, 17-hydroxy progesterone, testosterone, 19-nortestosterone, and 17-β-estradiol. The cell type product depends on the relative enzyme amounts present in the biosynthetic pathway. Only the adrenal cortical cell has the 11,21 hydroxylases necessary to convert 17-hydroxy progesterone into cortisol, for example. In the ovary, 17-β-estradiol is the major product; in the testicular Leydig cell, testosterone; in the corpus luteum, progesterone, with 17-β-estradiol a minor product. The rate limiting step in all cases is the mitochondrial 20,22 lyase step and the localization of cholesterol esters.

PROGESTERONE

Progesterone is a C21 steroid which is an intermediate in steroid biosynthesis and the secretary product of the corpus luetum and the placenta. Progesterone is carried in the blood predominately bound to albumin. Some progesterone competes with cortisol for cortisol binding globulin, and some circulates free. Degradation of progesterone occurs in the liver where it is reduced to pregnanediol and excreted in the bile as pregnanediol glucuronide.

Actions of Progesterone. Progesterone has a role in ovulation and is involved in the cyclic changes of the endometrium, cervix, and vagina. The hormone stimulates growth of the lobules and alveoli in the breasts (estrogen stimulates growth of the ducts). Progesterone decreases the excitability of the myometrium, an action which opposes that of estrogen. It exhibits weak aldosteronelike effects on salt retention. A thermogenic effect increases the basal body temperature during the second half of the menstrual cycle.

Mechanism of Action. Progesterone, like estrogen and testosterone, binds to specific receptor molecules on the target cell membrane. The hormone/receptor complex then enters the nucleus and binds to nonhistone chromatin protein, turning on mRNA. The only difference between testosterone, estradiol, and progesterone in mechanism of action is that each has its own specific receptor and that testosterone action is dependent upon dihydrotestosterone in some tissues.

Fertilization and Pregnancy

The ovulated oocyte is picked up by the fimbrae of the fallopian tube and begins to travel toward the uterus. The cells of the fallopian tube provide the proper nutrient milieu and secretory products for maturation, requiring the influence of estrogen and progesterone.

Sperm travel, aided by uterine contractions, occurs at a greater rate than their independent swimming rate.

The life span of sperm is 24–76 hours; the ovum, about 24 hours. Fertilization occurs in the distal third of the fallopian tube. The fertilized ovum reaches the uterus at approximately the blastocyst stage in 3 days. During this time the uterus is preparing for the zygote by increasing glandular secretion, which requires progesterone and estrogen for cell growth.

Between day 5 and 6, implantation occurs. The cells surrunding the zygote fuse with the glycogen rich endometrium to form the placenta. The placenta is composed of maternal cells and fetal multinucleated cells and becomes a very active hormone producer.

PLACENTAL HORMONES

Human chorionic gonadotropin (hCG) is an important pregnancy hormone produced by the placenta. hCG is stucturally similar to LH and exhibits the physiologic effects of LH. The hormone functions in early pregnancy to maintain the corpus luteum and the production of progesterone. High levels of progesterone produced by the corpus luetum feed back to the pituitary to decrease LH secretion. At later stages of pregnancy, the level of hCG decreases and its role is less clear. It also stimulates the fetal testes to produce testosterone. The presence of hCG in the urine is used as a diagnostic indicator in many pregnancy tests.

Progesterone is also secreted by the placenta, but a lack of 17-hydroxylase prevents 17-hydroxy progesterone production. Progesterone concentration increases up until the time of delivery. In the early stages of pregnancy, the majority of the progesterone is secreted by the corpus luteum. However, at around 8 weeks of pregnancy, the placenta becomes the major producer. The corpus luteum is necessary in early pregnancy and is maintained throughout even though it atrophies somewhat after the fourth month.

Estrogen production by the placenta requires a source of androgens since the 17-hydroxy progesterone intermediate is not available. The fetal adrenals supply most of the androgens, with maternal and placental contributions. The fetal pregnenolone-16-hydroxydehydroepiandosterone pathway provides androgens in sulfate form. These are desulfated to enter the placenta by a sulfatase on the fetal placental barrier.

Human chorionic somatotropin, hCS, (also called human placental lactogen or chorionic growth hormone prolactin) is a protein synthesized by the placenta in large quantities, approximately 1 g per day near term. hCS effects an increase in lipolysis and gluconeogenesis, while decreasing glucose uptake in activity similar to that of growth hormone. The hormone can cause diabetic symptoms in some pregnant women. hCS has a significant effect on nitrogen and calcium retention, a prolactinlike effect on the breast, and increases erythropoiesis and aldosterone excretion. hCS is used clinically for placental monitoring.

Chorionic thyrotropin is a placental hormone similar to TSH which stimulates the production of thyroid hormones.

PITUITARY SECRETION DURING PREGNANCY

Secretion of ACTH, TSH, and GH increases during pregnancy, while secretion of FSH and LH decreases because of feedback inhibition from high levels of estrogen and progesterone.

Parturition (Delivery)

Estrogen increases myometrium excitability, while progesterone decreases excitability. The ratio of estrogen/progesterone increases during pregnancy, resulting in an increase in myometrial muscle excitability. Relaxin is a small polypeptide hormone produced by the ovary which may relax pelvic ligaments. Oxytocin is released from the posterior pituitary in response to stimulation of neurons by signals from cervical stimulation and sucking. Oxytocin causes milk release and enhances labor. Many nonhormonal factors come into play at the time of delivery with local mechanical reflexes clearly very important.

Lactation

The major hormones involved in lactation are estrogen, which influences development of the mammary ducts in the postpubertal stage, progesterone, which stimulates the development of secretory lobules and alveoli, and prolactin and placental lactogen, which are involved in the synthesis of precursors for initial milk production. Oxytocin is needed for continued milk production. Growth hormones, insulin, and corticosteroids play minor roles.

PROLACTIN

Prolactin has a trophic effect on the breast, stimulating milk production. Prolactin, placental lactogen, and growth hormone all have similar structures and actions. Prolactin inhibitory factor (PIF), secreted by the hypothalamus, controls the secretion of prolactin. Estrogen stimulates prolactin secretion by inhibiting the release of PIF. Therefore, prolactin increases with the increase in estrogen levels during pregnancy. Suckling also inhibits PIF and thereby increases prolactin production. Suckling also maintains milk production by causing the release of oxytocin which is necessary for the ejection of milk by stimulating the myoepithelial cells of the breast lobules. The secretion of prolactin is episodic in its amounts during a 24 hour period.

POSTPARTUM EFFECTS

Estrogen and progesterone levels fall enormously after delivery, with 6 to 8 weeks elapsing before normal ovarian cycles are reestablished. This length of time is extended by suckling.

Contraception. Many methods of contraception are based on the prevention of the surge of LH that causes ovulation. Estrogens and progesterone can prevent the LH surge. Most oral contraceptives are mixtures of estrogens and progesterones, even though either one can perform this function alone. They function by inhibiting the release of gonadotropin releasing factors (FSHRH, LHRH) which results in a lack of follicle development and an absence of ovulation. The levels of estrogen and progesterone can be manipulated so that the normal menstrual cycle can be maintained.

STEROIDS IN DEVELOPMENT AND DIFFERENTIATION

The Sexual Phenotype: Sex Chromosomes

The human cell contains 46 chromosomes, 22 autosomic pairs and 2 sex chromosomes. Male cells with a diploid number of chromosomes contain an X and a Y chromosome; females carry only X chromosomes. The Y chromosome contains a gene that codes for the production of testes; two X chromosomes are needed for proper ovary development. Therefore, the zygote inheriting the XY combination is male; the XX zygote is female. Only one X chromosome is active, the other is inactivated and becomes a Barr body, visible near the nuclear membrane in various cell types or as a chromatin "drumstick" in the nuclei of 1–15 percent of the polymorphonuclear leukocytes in females. The basic gonadol embryonic plan is inherently female. In the positive sense, the sex determinant is coded on the Y chromosome.

Gonadal Sex: The XY Antigen

In the early embryonic stage, the gonads are indifferent. At 6 weeks in the male, the testes start to develop. At 9 weeks in the female, the same gonadal structure develops into ovaries. Evidence points to the HY antigen as organizing indifferent gonads into testes.

The HY antigen is a membrane glycoprotein which is the testes determining gene product. Normally, the gene controlling the expression of this protein is on the Y chromosome. The HY antigen is the director of differentiation of the heterogametic gonad.

GENITAL SEX

By the 7th week of development, the embryo exhibits both male and female primordial genital ducts. In the female, the müllerian ducts differentiate into the uterus and fallopian tubes. In the male, the wolffian ducts develop into the vas deferens, epididymis, seminiferous tubules, and ejaculatory ducts. In the developing female, the wolffian ducts regress; in the developing male, the müllerian ducts regress.

In the male, testicular hormones lead to normal development of the male internal genitalia. Testosterone and its metabolites are responsible for the continued growth and differentiation of the wolffian ducts. Testosterone causes seminal vesicle, epididymis, and vas deferens development and is also important in the development of external genitalia. The testes also produce müllerian regression factor (MRF), a protein which leads to regression of the müllerian tubes.

In the normal female, the gonads develop into ovaries. Hormones are not necessary for the development of the müllerian tubes into the uterus and fallopian tubes. The wolffian tubes regress with the development of the external female genitalia.

If the gonads are removed from the bipotential male or female zygote, both internal and external development is female. The XY male develops both external and internal genitalia under the influence of testosterone. If the gonads are castrated, treatment with testosterone causes development of the wolffian ducts and external genitalia in the male pattern.

The same primordial structure that develops into the penis with androgens develops into the clitoris without such exposure. The development of the female structure is not hormone dependent, therefore.

In summary, in the male, the presence of the Y chromosome leads to HY antigen production, which informs a bipotential gonad to form the embryonic testes. The testes produce testosterone, which influences the development of male internal and external genitalia and MRF which blocks development of female internal genitalia. At puberty testosterone causes male secondary sexual characteristics.

In the female, a biopotential gonad develops into embryonic ovaries in the absence of HY antigen. In the absence of androgens, the female develops normal internal and external genitalia.

Testosterone v Dihydrotestosterone

The enzyme 5-reductase is found in later embryonic development in the seminal vesicles but is absent in the epididymis. It appears that testosterone causes these structures to differentiate. The scrotum, penis, and prostate have considerable amounts of 5-reductase at the time of development and dihydrotestosterone appears responsible for their development.

Chromosomal Disorders

A developmental disorder in which the XX female is exposed to androgens during embryonic development can cause the external genitalia to become male. Androgen secreting adrenal tumors or drug administration can also lead to this condition.

In the male, developmental disorders include testicular feminization in which there are no androgen receptors, 5-reductase inactivity, and MRF inactivity, which allows both wolffian and müllerian ducts to develop.

Testicular feminization is a rare inherited condition in which XY phenotypes have testes, but neither müllerian nor wolffian ducts develop. The external genitalia look female and normal female development continues at puberty with substantial breast development. Even though the testes produce large amounts of testosterone in this condition, as well as MRF, male development does not occur because testosterone is converted to estrogens. This disorder is an X-linked recessive disorder in which the receptor for androgen is missing or will not bind androgen. The result is a phenotype female with abdominal testes. The disorder is not responsive to testosterone or dihydrotestosterone since there is a receptor deficiency.

Action of Testosterone on the Neonatal Brain

Testosterone secreted from the fetal testes acts on the neonatal brain to inactivate the cyclic gonadotropin release center needed for ovulation in females. The action is mediated by conversion of testosterone to estrogen in the appropriate brain cells.

Hormonal Activity at Puberty

At puberty there is a change in the plasma testosterone levels in males and in plasma estradiol levels in females. These changes are mediated by a resetting of the feedback mechanism controlling the release of the pituitary gonadotropins which influence the production of steroid hormones by the gonads. The larger amounts of gonadotropin released influence the production of larger amounts of steroids.

Levels of FSH and LH also Increase During Puberty

Abnormal development can result in an earlier than normal precocious puberty in which both gonadotropin and steroid levels are changed to adultlike levels. Precocious pseudopuberty is caused by steroid hormone production increases without increases in gonadotropin levels. There is no spermatogenesis or ovarian development in this condition which can be caused by androgen secreting tumors. Male characteristics occur if androgens are produced in substantial amounts.

REFERENCES

Berne RM, Levy MN: Physiology. 1st ed. CV Mosby Co., St. Louis, 1983

Davenport HW: Physiology of the Digestive Tract. 5th Ed. Year Book Medical Publishers, Chicago, 1982

Ganong WF: Review of Medical Physiology. 11th Ed. Lang Medical Publishers, Los Altos, 1983

Rushmer RF: Cardiovascular Dynamics. 4th Ed. Saunders, Philadelphia, 1976

Valtin H: Renal Function: Metabolism Preserving Fluid and Solute Balance in Health 2nd Ed. Little, Brown, and Co., Boston, 1983

West JB: Respiratory Physiology — The Essentials. 2nd Ed. Williams & Wilkins, Baltimore, 1979

MULTIPLE CHOICE QUESTIONS

Choose the one best answer to each question.

1. At normal blood glucose concentrations, cellular entry of glucose across the cell membrane occurs via the following process:
   A. Osmosis
   B. Simple diffusion
   C. Active transport
   D. Facilitated diffusion
   E. None of the above

2. Conductance of the nerve impulse without loss of voltage can best be explained by the accompanying event:
   A. Depolarization of the cell membrane
   B. Decreased K^+ conductance
   C. Increased K^+ conductance
   D. Decreased Na^+ conductance
   E. Increased Na^+ conductance

3. Conductance at the skeletal neuromuscular junction involves increased ion permeability in the mus-

cle cell membrane caused by release of neurotransmitter at the nerve ending. Substances involved are:
A. Norepinephrine, K^+, Cl^-
B. Norepinephrine, Na^+, K^+
C. Acetylcholine, Na^+, Mg^{++}
D. Acetylcholine, Na^+, K^+
E. Acetylcholine, Ca^{++}

4. In muscle, excitation/contraction coupling does not require:
A. Transverse tubule membrane depolarization
B. Actin-myosin cross linkages
C. Sequestering of Ca^{++} by the sarcoplasmic reticulum
D. ATP
E. Binding of Ca^{++} by troponin C

5. The normal pacemaker activity of the heart which dictates the rhythm of the cardiac cycle resides in:
A. The bundle of His
B. The AV (atrioventricular) node
C. The Purkinje fibers
D. The SA (sinoatrial) node
E. All of the above

6. In the conventions representing electrocardiogram waves:
A. The R wave indicates atrial depolarization
B. The S wave indicates atrial depolarization
C. The P wave indicates ventricular depolarization
D. The T wave indicates ventricular repolarization
E. None of the above

7. Closure of the aortic valve in the normal cardiac cycle is followed by:
A. Mitral valve opening prior to atrial depolarization
B. Ventricular depolarization prior to AV nodal depolarization
C. Ventricular depolarization prior to mitral valve closure
D. Rising ventricular pressure
E. None of the above

8. Stroke volume is increased by:
A. Digitalis
B. Lowering of systemic blood pressure
C. Increased venous return
D. Sympathetic cardiac stimulation
E. All of the above

9. The total lung capacity is equal to:
A. Vital capacity + dead space
B. Vital capacity + functional residual capacity
C. Vital capacity + residual volume
D. Tidal volume + expiratory residual volume
E. Approximately 3 liters

10. Physiologic shunting:
A. Increases in pulmonary edema
B. Normally represents 2 – 5 percent of cardiac output
C. Is contributed by bronchial arteries
D. Is contributed in part by coronary veins
E. All of the above

11. Glomerular filtration rate measurement requires a substance which is filtered but not absorbed, secreted, or metabolized, such as:
A. Fructose
B. Creatinine
C. Inulin
D. PAH (para-aminohippuric acid)
E. None of the above

12. In passing through the kidneys, filtered glucose is reabsorbed in the following:
A. Henle's loop (ascending limb)
B. Henle's loop (descending limb)
C. Proximal convoluted tubule
D. Distal convoluted tubule
E. Collecting duct

13. Renal hydrogen ion excretion occurs via the following mechanism:
A. Excretion with bicarbonates via carbonic anhydrase
B. Excretion with chlorides
C. Excretion with sulfates
D. Excretion as ammonium salts
E. All of the above

14. The primary cause of metabolic acidosis is:
A. Bicarbonate excess
B. Bicarbonate deficiency
C. CO_2 excess
D. CO_2 deficiency
E. None of the above

Choose the correct answers to each of the following questions, indicating:

A   if 1, 2, and 3 are correct
B   if 1 and 3 are correct
C   if 2 and 4 are correct
D   if 1, 2, 3, and 4 are correct

15. Gastric acid secretion is stimulated by the following:
    1. Alcohol
    2. Secretin
    3. Glucocorticoids
    4. Enterogastrone

16. The exocrine function of the pancreas includes release of substances which promote:
    1. Lipid breakdown
    2. Carbohydrate breakdown
    3. Protein breakdown
    4. Neutralization of acid chyme

17. Bile salts promote lipid absorption by:
    1. Reduction of surface tension
    2. Emulsification of fat
    3. Stimulation of reesterification within mucosal cells
    4. Micelle formation

18. Insulin increases glucose uptake in the following tissues:
    1. Adipose
    2. Skeletal muscle
    3. Uterine
    4. Intestinal mucosa

19. Glucagon promotes the following effects:
    1. Increase in glycogenolysis in the liver
    2. Decrease in gluconeogenesis
    3. Glycosuria when liver glycogen is exhausted
    4. Hypoglycemia

20. Effects of thyroxine include:
    1. Increased rate of oxygen consumption
    2. Increased rate of protein synthesis
    3. Increased calorigenesis
    4. None of the above

21. The following disorders are accompanied by high levels of parathyroid hormone:
    1. Parathyroid hyperplasia
    2. Parathyroid adenoma
    3. Pseudoparathyroidism
    4. Chronic renal failure

22. Hormones produced by the adrenal cortex include:
    1. Sex hormones
    2. Glucocorticoids
    3. Mineralocorticoids
    4. Glucagon

23. Aldosterone secretion is stimulated by the following:
    1. Renin-angiotensin system
    2. ACTH
    3. Low plasma Na^+
    4. High plasma Na^+

24. Hormones involved in the control of calcium homeostasis include:
    1. Calcitonin
    2. Vitamin D_3
    3. Parathyroid hormone
    4. Insulin

25. Following ovulation, the corpus luteum normally secretes:
    1. Luteinizing hormone
    2. Estrogen
    3. Growth hormone
    4. Progesterone

Answers

1 D	2 E	3 D	4 C	5 D
6 D	7 A	8 E	9 C	10 E
11 C	12 C	13 D	14 B	15 B
16 D	17 D	18 A	19 B	20 A
21 D	22 A	23 A	24 A	25 C

Section 2

Clinical Sciences

9

Internal Medicine

John W. Burnside

CARDIOVASCULAR DISEASE

Cardiovascular disease is a major cause of morbidity and mortality in the United States. Slightly more than 50 percent of all deaths are attributable to cardiovascular disease. Approximately 15 percent of the adult population suffer from hypertension. Congenital heart disease occurs in 0.5 to 1.0 percent of all live births. Rheumatic heart disease, although much less frequent in recent years, still accounts for 15,000 deaths a year and affects over 100,000 children and 1.6 million adults.

Coronary, cerebrovascular, and hypertensive diseases all increase in prevalence with age. Hypertension is present in 8 percent of the population under age 45, usually asymptomatic. Over age 65, 44 percent of women and 35 percent of men have hypertension. Symptomatic or detectable coronary artery disease is present in 6 percent of men aged 45 to 64 and in 5 percent of men over 65. Women, seemingly protected from coronary disease during ovarian functioning, have an incidence of coronary disease of only 3 percent prior to 65 but this increases to 8 percent in the over 65 age group.

Recent data released by the Department of Health and Human Services of the United States government indicate that the incidence of death from cardiovascular disease is declining. Although it is difficult to ascertain the reason or reasons for this decline, current thinking is that it is the result of more aggressive identification and treatment of hypertension. Additionally the elucidation of risk factors and the general public education of these risks may have resulted in some behavioral changes responsible for the diminishing death rate.

General Considerations in Heart Disease

A rational approach to the definition of heart disease requires discipline and clarity of thought. The New York Heart Association suggests that the following elements be considered in order to render a complete diagnosis.

1. Etiology: Is the disease congenital, rheumatic, hypertensive, or arteriosclerotic?
2. Anatomy: What anatomical or functional unit of the heart is involved?
3. Physiology: Are there findings of abnormal rhythms, congestive failure, or ischemia?
4. Disability: What is the individual functional level?

The New York Heart Association further defines the disability level as follows:

Class I: No symptoms on ordinary activity.
Class II: Symptoms occur on ordinary activity.
Class III: Symptoms occur on less than ordinary activity.
Class IV: Symptoms present at rest.

One significant advantage of this system of classification is that it is defined according to the life standards of the individual being assessed.

The response of the cardiovascular system to disease is limited. The signs and symptoms share commonalities regardless of the etiology. The end result of most cardiac insults is either pain, arrhythmia, or heart failure.

PAIN

Pain is the hallmark of most coronary artery diseases and most inflammations of the pericardium. It is usually recognized as originating from the heart but occasionally is referred to more remote sites such as the epigastrium, jaw, or arm.

ARRHYTHMIAS

Arrhythmias, when symptomatic, are usually described as palpitations or flutterings in the chest. Most any form of heart disease may be associated with arrhythmias as can many noncardiac diseases such as hyperthyroidism, pulmonary disease, and altered metabolic states.

HEART FAILURE

Heart failure may be the end result of almost any variety of heart disease. The physiologic definition of congestive heart failure is an elevated end diastolic pressure of the ventricle. This represents the earliest attempt by the system to compensate for an inadequate cardiac output once the mechanisms of increased stroke volume and faster heart rate have been unsuccessful in meeting the needs. The increased end diastolic pressure increases the stretch on the myofibrils and increases contractility (Starling's law).

Three main hemodynamic changes lead to the major signs and symptoms of congestive heart failure. The first is a decreased cardiac output or at least inadequate output for the need; occasionally the output is increased over normal but it is still inadequate for the need, so-called high output failure. The second is an increased left atrial pressure reflecting the increased ventricular end diastolic pressure. This leads to pulmonary venous hypertension with lung congestion. When acute and severe, this congestion leads to the transudation of fluid into the alveoli with marked dyspnea (i.e., acute pulmonary edema). A similar change occurs in the right atrium with the production of systemic venous hypertension. A similar transudation of fluid may occur in the lower extremities producing pitting edema of the legs. As the pressure increases the fluid accumulation may occur in the peritoneal cavity, and the visceral organs will become congested with blood. Because the organs, especially the kidneys, perceive inadequate perfusion, hormonal events are called into play to increase the blood volume. Aldosterone, the most potent of these mediators, causes the retention of salt and water which further aggravates the edematous state.

The symptomatic representation of congestive heart failure is usually a combination of fatigue and dyspnea (both exertional and paroxysmal nocturnal dyspnea). Further the patient will note nocturia and ankle swelling. The signs of congestive failure include, tachycardia, elevated jugular venous pressure, basilar pulmonary rales, third heart sounds, and occasionally liver enlargement and pitting edema of the lower extremities or of the sacrum if the patient has been at bed rest.

The therapy of heart failure must first be directed to reversing any potentially reversible etiology (e.g., hyperthryoidism, fluid overload, uncompensated hypertension, etc.). Basic therapeutic measures may include the use of oxygen to maximize delivery to tissues, reduction of the congested state through the use of sodium restriction in the diet, and the use of diuretic agents. Thiazide diuretics are mostly used. The more potent loop diuretics, furosemide or ethacrynic acid, are sometimes required. With either of these careful attention to maintainence of adequate serum potassium levels is mandatory. Spironolactone, which specifically inhibits the effects of aldosterone, may promote the necessary diuresis without the loss of potassium.

The reduction of the volume overloaded state is known as preload reduction. Further enhancement of cardiac output occurs with afterload reduction. Many vasodilator drugs are useful here especially the vasoactive antihypertensives. The major thrust of treatment however remains with the improvement of myocardial performance. This is best accomplished by the use of digitalis preparations or other inotropic agents. Although the precise mechanism of the action of digitalis is still subject to study, the end result is enhanced contractility of the myocardium. Digitalis has a narrow therapeutic index and toxicity is common. This may take the form of gastrointestinal disturbance, altered visual acuity, and actual cardiotoxicity with the production of potentially fatal arrhthymias. Laboratory assays of the serum concentration of digitalis permits easy monitoring of the adequacy of the dose.

Congenital Heart Disease

The etiologies of congenital heart disease are not completely understood. They represent a complicated combination and interplay of environment and heredity. Overall the incidence of congenital heart disease is greater in males than females. Environmental teratogens include infectious agents such as the rubella virus which causes an increased incidence of patent ductus arteriosus and pulmonary stenosis, and the drug thalidomide which was responsible for multiple congenital defects. It is likely that other infectious and chemical agents are responsible for some congenital heart diseases. Other probable factors include the age of the mother, chromosomal abnormalities, altitude during fetal life, and prematurity.

A useful classification of congenital heart disease is as follows:

1. Abnormal systemic pulmonary communications
   Left to right shunt — acyanotic
   Right to left shunt — cyanotic
      Decreased pulmonary vascularity
      Increased pulmonary vascularity
2. Without shunts
3. Cardiac malposition

ATRIAL SEPTAL DEFECT

Communication from one atrium to the other may occur at three levels. The sinus venosa defect allows the superior vena cava to empty into both atria at once, the ostium secundum defect occurs at midatrial levels and the ostium primum or endocardial cushion defect is a low defect which may also involve the ventricles and tricuspid valves.

The ostium secundum defect is the most common congenital heart lesion of children and young adults. Initially, there is a left to right shunt owing to the slightly higher pressure in the left atrium. At this point the condition is acyanotic. The major defect is pulmonary flooding and the increased flow is often evident on the chest x-ray. The clinical findings include a systolic pulmonary flow murmur and fixed splitting of the second heart sound. If the shunt is large enough, the right ventricle will hypertrophy and the pressure in the pulmonary circuit will rise. When the pulmonary vascular resistance rises, the backup pressure will reach the right atrium and the shunt may reverse leading to cyanosis. At this point the lesion is no longer surgically correctable.

The less common primum defect is more difficult to correct surgically. The findings are more variable since the defect may also permit left to right shunting at the ventricular level and the malformed mitral and or tricuspid valves may permit regurgitation into the atria.

VENTRICULAR SEPTAL DEFECT

This defect although usually small in size produces dramatic findings of systolic murmur and frequently a thrill felt over the precordium. The high pressure of the left ventricle may allow a large left to right shunt with marked increase in pulmonary vascularity. The shunt may decrease as the right ventricle achieves systemic pressures but the shunt very rarely reverses in the absence of other defects. Both ventricles will hypertrophy and this will be evident on the electrocardiogram and

chest x-ray. The treatment is surgical although a number of these will close spontaneously prior to adult life.

PATENT DUCTUS ARTERIOSUS

This is the second or third most common congenital defect. It is more common in women, and rubella during pregnancy is a clear etiologic agent. This lesion is the persistence of a structure utilized during fetal existence. Generally, the ductus closes within the first week of life. The ductus originates just beyond the bifurcation of the main pulmonary artery and joins the aorta just distal to the left subclavian artery.

The expected result of this communication is a left to right shunt since the pressure gradient is such. The amount of the shunt is determined by the size of the ductus and the difference between the systemic and pulmonary vascular resistance.

If the shunt is large, heart failure may occur early in life. Smaller shunts may be consistent with asymptomatic existence. The physical findings are quite characteristic with a machinerylike continuous murmur. A thrill is often felt. A diastolic filling rumble reflects the increased volume of blood returning to the left ventricle from the engorged pulmonary circuit.

Ligation of the ductus is the definitive treatment and was the earliest cardiac congenital surgery performed. In certain circumstances of prematurity, the patent ductus can be closed pharmacologically with the use of prostaglandin inhibitors such as indomethacin.

EISENMENGER'S SYNDROME

The three lesions just described, atrial septal defect, ventricular septal defect, and patent ductus arteriosus may develop the Eisenmenger's syndrome. The increased flow through the pulmonary circuit may lead to an increased vascular resistance. As this resistance increases the pressure in the pulmonary artery rises and hence the pressure in the right ventricle and atrium rises. If these pressures become as high as those on the left side of the heart the shunt will cease or become bidirectional. Occasionally the pressures on the right side will exceed those on the systemic side and a reversal of the shunt will occur with the development of cyanosis.

VENTRICULAR SEPTAL DEFECT WITH PULMONARY STENOSIS (TETRALOGY OF FALLOT)

There is a great variability in the clinical expression of this lesion. Usually this is a cyanotic congenital heart disease. Severe pulmonary stenosis forces a right to left shunt through the ventricular septal defect. There is also usually right ventricular hypertrophy and some overriding of the aorta to complete the tetrad. The pulmonary obstruction is progressive so that while initially acyanotic the lesion eventually produces cyanosis.

Additional abnormalities which may be present include a right sided aortic arch, persistent left superior vena cava, incomplete pulmonary valve, and an abnormal origin of the left anterior descending coronary artery.

The clinical picture is of cyanosis appearing early in life. Dyspnea is common and patients frequently squat to relieve it. Episodes of syncope secondary to hypoxia may occur. Clubbing of the fingers and toes is common. A systolic murmur from the pulmonary valve will be heard. If the obstruction is not severe the murmur will be loud. Treatment is primarily surgical.

TRANSPOSITION OF THE GREAT VESSELS

This cyanotic disease is the result of abnormal division of the aorta and pulmonary artery. If complete this is incompatable with life since the two circuits are then independent. Most patients have an associated atrial septal defect which allows mixing and life. Others will have either a ventricular septal defect or a patent ductus arteriosus.

The disease is more prevalent in males and in offspring of diabetic mothers. The children so affected usually grow poorly and are dyspneic and cyanotic. Seventy-five percent will die by 6 months of age and very few survive to adult years. Surgical correction is difficult. The most successful approach is to redirect the venous inflow to the atria.

COARCTATION OF THE AORTA

This is a very common defect. The usual coarctation of the aorta occurs at the locus of the ligamentum arteriosus (the residual of the ductus arteriosus). It occurs in 1 of every 2,000 people and is much more common in men than women. If it occurs in a woman the diagnosis of Turner's syndrome should be suspected.

Every young man with hypertension should be checked for a coarctation. They typically demonstate hypertension when measured in the arms but will have low pressures in the legs. The mechanism of hypertension is probably renal in that the kidneys perceived reduced perfusion pressure and elaborate renin.

Many patients are asymptomatic while others will complain of headaches, nosebleeds, and claudication of the legs. A murmur is common and the collateral circulation may be audible over the posterior ribs. The left ventricle is usually hyperdynamic and may be hypertrophied. Patients are at risk for bacterial endocarditis, cerebral hemorrhage from associated cerebral artery aneurysms or heart failure. Treatment is surgical. The ideal age to repair this defect is around puberty.

PULMONARY STENOSIS

The obstruction is usually valvular but may be sub- or supravalvular in site. Right ventricular hypertrophy will result. The symptoms are fatigue, dyspnea, and occasionally syncope.

DEXTROCARDIA

When the cardiac apex lies in the right chest together with situs inversus (i.e., complete reversal of all organs) there are generally no significant problems. When, however, the heart is reversed alone or when the heart is right but all other organs are reversed, multiple other congenital anomalies should be anticipated.

Valvular Heart Disease

Rheumatic fever is declining in incidence yet it remains the single most common etiology of acquired valvular heart disease. Valvular heart disease may also be the result of ischemic, infective, and degenerative processes involving the valves or their support structures:

MITRAL VALVE DISEASE

The mitral valve is the most commonly affected valve as the result of rheumatic heart disease. The valve may be affected during the period of acute carditis, and return to normal only to represent profound symptoms later in life as the progressive scarring occurs.

Mitral stenosis occurs in 40 percent of patients with rheumatic heart disease and is most common in women. The usual age at onset of symptoms is 35 to 45 years. The valve leaflets become thickened and the commissures fuse. The chordae tendinae thicken, fuse, and foreshorten. These changes reduce the cross section of the mitral valve orifice. This produces a large pressure gradient across the valve. The pressure in the right atrium increases and the atrium dilates. The elevated pressure head is further back transmitted into the pulmonary venous circuit. If substantial back pressure exists the alveoli may leak fluid causing pulmonary edema. Over a long period of time, this pressure is further transmitted to the right side of the heart with the production of right ventricular hypertrophy.

Symptomatically, the patient with mitral stenosis complains first of fatigue, later of dyspnea, and occasionally of hemoptysis and palpitations. The examination frequently shows atrial fibrillation from the distended atrium, a loud first heart sound, an opening snap caused by the late opening of the mitral valve just after the second heart sound, and a diastolic rumble heard at the apex and axilla.

Mitral regurgitation is also a common result of rheumatic heart disease. This lesion also occurs when the chordae or papillary muscles are diseased. The chordae may be congenitally lax as in the click syndrome. This disease is usually detected in the younger patient and when symptomatic may produce atypical chest pain or palpitations. It may accompany Marfan's syndrome. The chordae also may rupture as a result of bacterial endocarditis. The papillary muscles are the end point of coronary circulation. They may be acutely dysfunctional during ischemia causing transient mitral regurgitation. The entire papillary muscle may infarct and rupture causing acute and severe regurgitation.

When the mitral valve is incompetent similar changes occur as in mitral stenosis. Differently, however the left ventricular volume increases since much is wasted in the backward ejection. The ventricle enlarges and may fail. The examination also differs in that the left ventricle will be easily palpable, the murmur is holosystolic, and there may be a diastolic filling rumble as the regurgitated volume falls back into the left ventricle.

Some older patients have calcification of the mitral valve annulus. This distorts the mitral orifice causing the leaflets to drop over the heavy calcification. A combination of mitral stenosis and regurgitation may result. The patient may have relatively loud murmurs but is usually asymptomatic. They are at risk for bacterial endocarditis.

AORTIC VALVE DISEASE

Aortic valve stenosis may accompany mitral valve disease following rheumatic fever. When the aortic valve alone is stenotic, the etiology is more likely to be calcific. A bicuspid aortic valve is particularly prone to calcification in older years. An accompaniment to arterioslcerosis may also be calcification in the sinuses of Valsalva leading to stenosis of the valve. Whatever the etiology, the left ventricle faced with obstruction must increase the pressure head in order to eject blood. This results in hypertrophy of the ventricle. Symptomatically, patients with aortic stenosis will have chest painlike angina, exertional syncope, and finally failure of the ventricle. The examination will show a hypertrophied ventricle, a diamond shaped systolic ejection murmur at the base of the heart with radiation to the neck, slow low volume pulses, and a small pulse pressure.

Idiopathic hypertrophic subaortic stenosis is not a true valvular stenosis. It may be genetic in origin. Anatomically this disorder is characterized by an asymmetrically thickened interventricular septum. As the ventricle ejects the hypertrophied septum partially obstructs outflow. The left ventricular impulse is accentuated and the systolic murmur is more localized with little radiation to the neck. A fourth heart sound is heard. The murmur is louder if the ventricle ejects faster or if the ventricular volume is less as after a Valsalva maneuver or the administration of amyl nitrate.

Aortic regurgitation may also be seen in rheumatic heart disease. It may also be the result of endocarditis of a bicuspid valve, syphilis with dilatation of the aortic root, or following aortic dissection. The left ventricle both enlarges and hypertrophies since the cardiac output must be increased markedly. The symptoms are of congestive heart failure, fatigue, and sometimes chest pain. The ventricle is easily felt and the characteristic diastolic blowing murmur is loudest over the upper left parasternal border. The pulses are dramatically accentuated and the pulse pressure is very large.

Bacterial Endocarditis

Two conditions are usually required for the development of bacterial endocarditis. First, there must be an episode of bacteremia. This may occur with "dirty" surgery such as rectal or genitourinary surgery or dental procedures, the use of intravenous illicit drugs or during an episode of sepsis from some other primarily affected organ systems (e.g., cholecystitis, pneumonia, or diverticulitis). Second, bacterial endocarditis is enhanced when the heart valves are somehow abnormal. This situation obtains in the presence of rheumatic heart disease or congenital heart disease.

Bacterial endocarditis is traditionally separated into acute and subacute although the distinctions are not very sharp. The difference is usually determined by the offending organism. When bacteria or fungi gain access to the blood stream and attach to a heart valve, they colonize and form vegetations. The local effect is to destroy and alter the normal anatomy of the valve usually rendering it incompetent. The valve or chordae may rupture or perforate or become aneurysmal. Acute bacterial endocarditis is most often caused by *Staphylococcus aureus* and the damage may be sudden and explosive demanding immediate surgery for life preservation. Subacute endocarditis is the more usual presentation.

The patient will complain of malaise, intermittent fever, arthralgia, and muscle pain. The physical findings are those of the cardiac lesion as well as the embolic and vasculitis sequelae of the heart lesion. The mitral and aortic valves are the most commonly involved. Right sided lesions, when they occur, are most common in intravenous substance abusers. In addition to the regurgitant murmurs, the patient may have splenomegaly and petechiae in the conjunctiva or the digits, particularly under the finger or toe nails. The latter may well be a form or vasculitis rather than emboli. Emboli to the kidneys can also be detected by the presence of blood in the urine. Emboli to the fundi appear as white-centered hemorrhages called Roth spots.

Positive blood cultures in the presence of the above constitutes the diagnosis. The organism may be bacterial or fungal and appropriate culture medium is necessary. Antibiotic sensitivities based on the in vitro tests of the recovered organism are required. Patients frequently are mildly anemic and have an elevated sedimentation rate, leukocytosis, and hematuria. Multiple cultures should be taken if the diagnosis is suspected.

Appropriate treatment consists of organism specific antibiotics parenterally administered, support of failing cardiac function, and occasionally emergency valve replacement.

Cardiovascular Syphilis

Syphilis and all of the complications of that disease have been declining in incidence in the United States. When the treponemes attack the vascular system, they produce a vasculitis with a particular predilection for the vasavasorum. Many of these nutrient arteries are located in the aorta and great trunk vessels. The resulting damage leads to aneurysm formation of the ascending aorta, dilatation of the aortic root with aortic insufficiency, and compromise of the coronary artery ostia. The disease is most common in men in their 40s and 50s.

Coronary Heart Disease

Although declining in incidence, coronary heart disease is a major cause of death in all industrialized countries. Most of the nearly 500,000 deaths annually in the United States occur suddenly before any medical intervention is possible. The advent of the specialized coronary care units, closed chest cardiac massage, and rapid response emergency teams in the field caused a significant drop in mortality. The major hope of a further reduction in deaths is in the recognition and interdiction of the many risk factors.

The Framingham Study and other large scale epidemiologic studies identified several risk factors. Age is a factor. Prior to menopause women have a lower incidence of coronary disease but subsequently catch up after menopause. Hypertension, cigarette smoking, hypercholesterolemia, obesity, diabetes mellitus, sedentary life style, and a Type A personality have all been implicated as risk factors. A family history of premature coronary disease increases the risk implicating genetic factors

as well. Recent evidence suggests that a high density lipoprotein (HDL) may be protective.

Pathologically, the basis of the disease is atherosclerosis. Many years pass from the origin of the process to the development of symptoms. The process includes the development of smooth muscle proliferation in the intima, aggregation of platelets, the deposition of a variety of lipids, and finally compromise of the lumen. The occlusive event may be a clot, a hemorrhage into a plaque, or just an expansion of the plaque.

Clinically, coronary heart disease takes several recognizable forms. Angina pectoris, myocardial infarction, arrhthymias with occasional sudden death, and ischemic cardiomyopathy.

ANGINA PECTORIS

The myocardium even at rest consumes large quantities of oxygen. The extraction of oxygen is nearly maximal at all times. Cardiac pain is caused by inadequate oxygen delivery to the muscle. It, therefore, almost always indicates an inadequate flow, assuming a normal amount of hemoglobin and a normal hemoglobin oxygen unloading capability (severe anemia and carbon monoxide poisoning would be examples of exceptions). The volume of blood carried by the coronaries is dependent on the degree of dilatation of the coronaries, the heart rate, ejection volume, and left ventricular wall tension. The wall tension is in turn dependent on the diameter of the left ventricle and pressure within the ventricle. When the coronary flow is less than that required for the oxygen needs, myocardial ischemia occurs. If brief and reversed the syndrome of pain is called angina. If sustained, irreversible myocardial damage results.

The responsiveness of the coronary arteries themselves is quite important. When oxygen demand increases, normal coronaries will dilate to permit increased flow. Stiff atherosclerotic vessels are incapable of doing this. Also, it has been recently recognized that abnormal spasm of coronaries which are otherwise normal may produce angina. This is called Prinzmetal's angina and should be suspected in the younger patient, especially women, with elevated ST segments on the electrocardiogram during pain.

Clinically, the patient will report an oppressive heaviness of the chest during exertion. This is particularly likely during walking up an incline or in the cold weather. The patient may clench a fist over the sternum when describing the discomfort. It may radiate to the left arm or jaw and may be accompanied by a sense of doom. It may be misinterpreted as indigestion or gas pains and is sometimes associated with nausea, vomiting, or sweating. It dissipates with rest or following a nitroglycerin tablet. Many patients know exactly how much exertion will bring on an attack. Three to 5 percent of patients with angina will die each year.

There are few findings during an attack. The patient may appear distressed and there may be signs of transient left ventricular failure with the development of a diastolic gallop, reversed splitting of the second heart sound, and a soft murmur of mitral regurgitation. During an attack, the electrocardiogram will show ST segment depression in excess of 0.1 mV whereas in the absence of pain the tracting may be normal.

Exercise stress testing is a method of producing diagnostic symptoms and electrocardiographic changes under controlled circumstances. The most popular current method is to exercise the patient until 85–90 percent of the maximal predicted heart rate for that age group is attained. Continuous monitoring by the electrocardiogram and of pulse blood pressure and patient's symptoms are required.

Stress testing allows a functional assessment. Coronary arteriography allows an anatomical assessment. In skilled laboratories the morbidity and mortality of the test is low (0.1 percent mortality). The major arteries are visualized and the degree of luminal narrowing can be determined. The test is used to assess patients with (1) persistent symptoms in spite of maximum medical therapy, (2) as a diagnostic measure when the nature of the pain is unclear and/or the stress test is equivocal, (3) for evaluation of graft patency, and (4) for those patients with strongly positive stress tests or those about to have valvular surgery.

Treatment of angina may be medical or surgical. The first step in medical management is to lessen the influence of other factors on either oxygen demand or availability. Hypertension, cigarette smoking, correction of anemia, and weight reduction may all be salutory. Three classes of drugs are used specifically for angina (i.e., nitrates, β-blockers and calcium channel blockers).

Nitroglycerin is the treatment of choice for the acute attack. Given sublingually, it will abort the pain within 3 to 5 minutes. It is effective by causing vasodilatation both of the coronary arteries and peripheral veins and arteriolar beds. The ventricular wall tension may be lessened, further enhancing myocardial blood flow. The drug is also available for intravenous use in the emergency room or coronary care unit and in a long acting form for prevention of attacks.

Propranalol was the first β-adrenergic blocker used in the United States. All of the β-blockers slow the heart rate, reduce the blood pressure, and reduce the left ventricular contractility thereby improving coronary flow. These agents combined with nitrate treatment can be very effective in reducing or ablating angina. They probably interfere with the natural history of coronary disease although some controversy still exists.

Calcium channel blocking agents are the most recent additions to the treatment of angina. They are potent vasodilators and have a negative ionotropic action on the myocardium.

Coronary artery surgery consists of bypassing areas of narrowing or obstruction through the grafting of venous limbs from the aorta to the coronary artery distal to the lesion. Not everyone agrees on the complete indications for this procedure. It should be performed on patients with significant obstructions of the main left coronary artery and should not be performed on patients with diffuse distal vascular disease. In other circumstances many factors contribute to the decision such as the patient's inclinations, surgical expertize, adequacy of medical management, and other complicating medical illnesses. The mortality in experienced hands is 1–2 percent, graft patency is 80 percent, and at one year, 50 percent of the patients become asymptomatic.

CARDIOMYOPATHIES

A group of diseases which are characterized by myocardial dysfunction and failure but which are not caused by any of the common entities such as valvular, congenital, or coronary artery disease are called cardiomyopathies. They are divided into primary diseases of the myocardium and secondary cardiomyopathies.

Secondary Cardiomyopathies. This group includes certain metabolic, neurologic, and immunologic diseases and are rare. Diseases associated with cardiomyopathies including the following:

1. Amyoloidosis
2. Friedreich's ataxia
3. Glycogen storage disease
4. Hemochromotosis
5. Hurler's syndrome
6. Lupus erythematosis
7. Muscular dystrophy
8. Myotonia dystrophica
9. Polyarteritis nodosa
10. Sarcoidosis
11. Scleroderma

Primary Cardiomyopathies. These diseases are divided according to their clinical characteristics since etiologies are unknown.

Hypertrophic cardiomyopathies share the feature of ventricular hypertrophy which may be diffuse or asymmetric involving especially the interventricular septum. It is probably an autosomal dominantly inherited genetic disease. When the septal hypertrophy is dominant the disease is called idiopathic hypertrophic subaortic stenosis (IHSS). The symptoms are much like aortic stenosis. The findings include a fourth heart sound and a systolic murmur which will increase with the Valsalva maneuver. Treatment consists of drugs which slow the rate of cardiac ejection such as β-blockers, or in some surgical resection of part of the septum.

Congestive cardiomyopathies are characterized by massive cardiac enlargement and dilatation with signs and symptoms of congestive heart failure. The causes are probably multiple and may include remote viral myocarditis and toxins such as alcohol and antineoplastic drugs. Treatment is supportive and symptomatic. Arterial dilators, digitalis, diuretics, and anticoagulants to reduce the incidence of both intraventricular thrombosis and peripheral thrombophlebitis are recommended.

Obliterative cardiomyopathy is rare and is characterized by a stiff myocardium, valvular abnormalities and heart failure. It may selectively involve one or the other ventricles with obliteration of the cavity. Endomyocardial fibroelastosis is the most common type in the United States and is often seen in the pediatric age group.

Restrictive cardiomyopathy is also rare and presents with a picture similar to constrictive pericarditis with impaired ventricular filling.

PERICARDIAL DISEASES

The pericardium, like other serosal membranes, may be the focus of inflammation and subsequent fibrosis and scarring. As a result of inflammation it may produce excessive fluid impeding the filling of the heart. It is also an occasional focus for the deposit of metastatic cancer cells.

Acute pericarditis may be caused by injury, infection (viral, bacterial, or fungal), immune diseases, underlying myocardial infarction, or malignant disease. Pain in the chest aggravated or relieved by a change in position is the cardinal symptom. A pericardial friction rub is the cardinal finding. The rub is typically three phased, superficial sounding, and likened to the sound of wet leather being rubbed.

Pericardial effusion is almost always present with pericarditis. The fluid may be serous, serosanguinous, or frankly bloody. When the effusion is large the friction rub may disappear as the grating surfaces are separated.

Pericardial tamponade results when the effusion is of such magnitude that it impedes the filling of the ventricles. This is clinically more apparent on the right side of the heart. The neck veins will be distended and increase in distention with inspiration (i.e., the reverse of the normal situation). Similarly, the systolic pressure will drop during inspiration as the tensing of the pericardium further impedes ejection from the left ventricle (e.g., pulsus paradoxus).

Constrictive pericarditis is caused by severe scarring of the pericardium and may be the end result of pericarditis. The findings are similar to pericardial tamponade except that the cardiac size will be normal or only slightly enlarged. The most common discovered cause is tuberculosis but most have no known etiology. Mild disease may be treated medically, severe disease requires surgery.

Hypertension

Hypertension is the most common cardiovascular disease in the United States, responsible for 250,000 deaths annually from the complications of stroke, heart attack, and kidney failure. It affects between 20 and 60 million citizens. Although blood pressure should be considered a continuum (the lower the better) epidemiologic studies use levels of 140/90 and greater as the cutoff point.

The vast majority of patients (95 percent) have essential hypertension. There is no specific identifiable cause. Pathophysiologically, the early finding is of increased cardiac output and later a fall in output with a rise in peripheral resistance.

Early hypertension is usually asymptomatic and discovered during an examination for some other reason. With long standing or severe disease, the patient may complain of headache, usually occipital and worse in the morning, epistaxis, angina, congestive heart failure, or cerebrovascular symptoms of dizziness or blackouts. The review with the patient must include family history, use of drugs, diet, smoking, exercise, and weight.

Secondary hypertension, although present in only a few individuals, is searched for since some are completely correctable. Secondary hypertension is associated with a variety of primary diseases as is illustrated by the following:

1. Renal disease: Glomerular, polycystic, diabetic, traumatic, renin producing tumors, drug nephritis
2. Renal artery stenosis: Fibromuscular or atherosclerotic
3. Adrenal disease: Cortical or medullary, aldosteronism, Cushing's syndrome, pheochromocytoma
4. Drug-induced: Estrogens, corticosteroids, sympathetic stimulants
5. Coarctation of the aorta
6. Toxemia of pregnancy
7. Central nervous system disease: Increased intracranial pressure

The renin-angiotensin system operates in many patients with both primary and secondary hypertension. Renin is secreted by the kidney. It acts enzymatically on angiotensinogen in plasma releasing angiotensin I which is subsequently converted to the vasoactive angiotensin II. Angiotensin II is a very potent vasoconstrictor. It also stimulates the secretion of aldosterone which enhances the retention of sodium from the kidney thereby increasing blood volume. Unanswered yet is why this normal homeostatic mechanism should be disturbed in hypertensive patients.

Treatment of hypertension reduces the morbidity and mortality of the disease. Drugs either singularly or in combination designed to approach different facets of the pathophysiology provide the major approach to primary and some secondary hypertensives.

Drugs used in hypertension include the following:

1. Diuretics: Chloruretic (thiazide), loop (furosemide), and potassium sparing (spironolactone)
2. β-Adrenergic receptor blocking agents: Propranolol
3. α-Receptor blockers: Phenoxybenzamine
4. Vasodilators: Hydralazine, diazoxide
5. Central active: Reserpine, methyldopa, clonidine
6. Autonomic blockers: Guanethidine

COR PULMONALE

Hypertension of the lesser circuit is the hallmark of cor pulmonale. It is always the result of a pulmonary abnormality rather than primary disease of the right ventricle. The increased pressures in the pulmonary vascularity cause enlargement and hypertrophy of the right ventricle. The most common pulmonary disease leading to cor pulmonale is chronic obstructive lung disease. Other causes include diffuse interstitial disease of the lungs, primary disease of the pulmonary arterioles leading to increased resistance, neuromuscular diseases of pulmonary mechanics such as kyphoscoliosis or amyotrophic lateral sclerosis, central nervous system disease with low pulmonary drive, and chronic high altitude sickness.

The symptoms are those of right ventricular failure and dyspnea. Peripheral fluid accumulation is common, ascites from hepatic congestion may be part of the picture. The physical findings are of right ventricular disease with a palpable enlarged right ventricle, elevated neck veins, hepatomegaly, and edema. The chest x-ray will show right ventricular enlargement and may show underlying pulmonary disease if that is etiologic. The electrocardiogram provides confirmatory evidence.

ATHEROSCLEROSIS

Atherosclerosis is a disease of arteries, spotty in distribution, increasing in prevalence with age and with clinical manifestations which are determined by the site of the plaques. There is no diagnostic blood test for the disease. Its presence is inferred by the various clinical syndromes which it causes. Coronary heart disease is the most reliable marker for the presence of atherosclerosis as is intermittent claudication. Cerebrovascular accidents are less reliable markers since these events may also be caused by hemorrhage or thrombosis.

Although the cause of atherosclerosis is unknown, epidemiologic evidence points strongly to hyperlipemia and hypertension as contributing agents to its acceleration. Treatment is best focused on these two elements to afford prevention of the lesions since there is no convincing evidence that once established that plaques can be made to resolve.

The two major lipids of clinical importance are cholesterol and triglycerides. These are variously combined with phospholipids for transport and handling. These combinations are called lipoproteins of which there are four major classes. Key lipoproteins are the high density and low density lipoproteins (HDL and LDL respectively). The incidence of ischemic heart disease appears to be directly related to the level of LDL and inversely correlated with HDL.

Treatment of hyperlipidemia depends on the type detected. Dietary management is important for all and may require attention to saturated fats and carbohydrates. Drugs used influence either the production of lipids or decrease the pool through gastrointestinal binding.

Peripheral Vascular Disease

Aneruysms are classifed by etiology and location. They most commonly affect the aorta and its major branches but may occur anywhere in the arterial tree. Aneurysms may be congenital, inherited, or acquired.

Congenital aneurysms are one cause of cerebrovascular accidents resulting from their rupture. The event is usually experienced by a relatively young patient presenting with severe headache and the presence of blood in the cerebrospinal fluid. Inherited diseases predisposing to aneurysms include polycystic kidney disease with a high association of aneurysms, Marfan's syndrome which includes medial cystic necrosis of the arteries with the development of dissecting aneurysms of the aorta, and homocystinuria which has similar vascular lesions. Acquired aneurysms are most often the result of atherosclerosis involving the thoracic or abdominal aorta. Under these circumstances, the saccular dilations are at risk for rupture and are best treated surgically by replacement. Dissecting aneurysms may be treated surgically with replacement of the affected vasculature or decompression of the dissection or medically by decreasing the rapidity (shear strength) of left ventricular ejection.

Another category of acquired aneurysms is infectious

disease. Syphilis affects the aorta through direct invasion of the adventitia by the treponemes which obliterate the vasavasorum. The subsequent dilation results in aneurysm formation, aortic dilatation with aortic regurgitation, and compromise of the coronary ostia. Many bacteria may, in addition, spread from bacterial endocarditis, injury, or surgery to invade arteries at various locations and produce mycotic aneurysms. Treatment is surgical.

Vasculitis is a process characterized by inflammation of blood vessels which results in rupture or occlusion of the vessel with a resultant clinical picture determined by the vessel involved. There are hindreds of conditions which are either the cause of vasculitis or are associated with vasculitis. Classifications are confusing and only partially helpful clinically. It is perhaps best to consider some broad categories and vessel size until we understand the etiologies better.

Hypersensitivity vasculitis includes polyarteritis nodosa and allergic angiitis and granulomatosis. These separate categories present with vasculitis as the major clinical feature. Both are probably immunologic in origin. Polyarteritis is thought to result from the deposition of immune complexes in the vessel wall and allergic angiitis is frequently associated with severe asthma. The former rarely involves the lung. Both require biopsy for diagnosis and respond to combinations of corticosteroids and cytotoxic drugs.

Wegener's granulomatosis is a distinct pathologic entity with a predilection for the upper and lower respiratory tract and kidney. Giant cell arteritis has a predilection for large elastic arteries of the aortic arch and large immediate muscular branches. Takayasu's arteritis involves similar sized vessels but usually results in occlusions of the affected arteries.

Many infectious agents involve blood vessels and lead to vasculitis. This is particularly true of the fungal agents and treponemes.

Vasculitis may be a part of a more systemic disease. Rheumatoid arthritis and systemic lupus erythematosis are such examples. The disease here is thought to be the result of immune complex deposition in the vessels.

Thrombophlebitis is a common disorder usually involving veins of the lower extremity. The usual clinical presentation consists of pain, redness, and swelling. When the disease involves deep veins of the leg especially those proximal to the knee, a very great risk of embolic events exists. Risk factors for thrombophlebitis include varicose veins, congestive failure, muscular paresis, and obesity. When thrombophlebitis involves other veins or is recurrent, the clinician should consider the possibility of an occult neoplasm especially a mucin secreting adenocarcinoma.

PULMONARY DISEASES

Normal Pulmonary Function and Testing

The prime function of the lungs is to exchange gas providing oxygen and disposing of carbon dioxide. There also exist some metablic functions of the lung including the conversion of some hormones and surveillance against invasion by foreign substances.

To accomplish these functions, the lung provides a complicated mechanism which is mechanical and biochemical. Maximum exposure of air to the capillary network is afforded by the unique structure of the lung.

The assessment of pulmonary function best begins with a test of the adequacy of this gas exchange. Arterial blood gases provide the marker of the major function and are an important measurement in any patient with pulmonary disease. Measurement of the PO_2, PCO_2, and pH provide information unavailable by any other technique. Hypoxia and hypercapnia exist in varying combinations and provide valuable clues as to the nature of the pulmonary disorder. Hypoxia has many root causes. Hypercapnia always indicates alveolar hypoventilation. The diffusion of carbon dioxide across the alveolar capillary membrane occurs seven times as fast as the diffusion of oxygen. For this reason, it can be concluded that the patient with an elevated carbon dioxide level must have inadequate exposure of ambient air to the alveolar space. Hypoxia on the other hand may be present because of small changes in the ventilation perfusion ratio, because of thickening of the exchange membrane, and because of inadequate oxygen carrying capacity of the blood, etc.

The other major measurement of pulmonary function consists of an evaluation of the flow of air. Pulmonary function tests measure both the flows and volumes of air exchanged.

The volumes in the lungs are divided into the following:

1. Total lung capacity
2. Residual volume (that which is left after complete expiration)
3. Tidal volume (the volume of air exchanged in a breath at rest)
4. Inspiratory reserve (the amount in excess of the tidal volume which can be inspired in a deep breath)
5. Expiratory reserve (the amount in excess of the tidal volume which can be expired with maximum effort)
6. Dead space (the volume of air contained in nongas exchanging space such as the trachea)
7. Vital capacity (the difference between the total lung capacity and the residual volume)

To further refine our understanding of pulmonary function, we examine the flow rates of all except the residual volume. We measure the amount of air moved as a function of time. The usual flow measurements consist of (1) FVC, the forced vital capacity or the amount of air moved with maximum expiration following maximum inspiration, (2) FEV_1, the volume of air moved in the first second of a forced expiration following a forced inspiration, (3) FEV_3, the same measurement at 3 seconds, and (4) $FEV_{25-75\%}$, a measurement of the slope of the line between 25 percent and 75 percent of the FVC, a helpful measurement of obstruction of small airways.

Many pulmonary diseases are divided into obstructive or restrictive abnormalities. Restrictive lung diseases share the major characteristic of reduced volumes of the lung. On the other hand, the common denominator of obstructive lung disease is a diminution of flow rates.

Obstructive Lung Disease

The diseases listed below share an increase in total lung capacity. As a result, these patients will display findings of increased anteroposterior diameters of the chest, flat diaphragms on radiographic examination, and dyspnea. Usually, the increase in capacity of the lung is an increase in nonfunctional volume, either dead space or residual volume.

CHRONIC BRONCHITIS

Chronic bronchitis is diagnosed by the history. A patient who relates the production of sputum daily for at least 3 months for 2 consecutive years has chronic bronchitis. The most common etiologic agent is cigarette smoke although other irritants including chronic low grade infection may be operative. Pathologically the bronchi show hyperplasia of the muscular and mucous secreting apparatus. Obstruction to air flow comes late in the pathology of the disease. Such patients, when symptomatic will show diminished flow rates and increased total lung capacity. They will complain of cough with sputum production easy fatiguability, frequent infections of the respiratory tract, and dyspnea. Blood gases will show carbon dioxide retention and hypoxia in the advanced state and the right heart may fail.

BRONCHIECTASIS

Bronchiectasis is a form of chronic bronchitis. It is defined as a fixed dilatation of bronchi associated with chronic inflammation. This form of chronic bronchitis often has its origin in childhood either as a result of a congenital abnormality of the bronchi or as a result of childhood pneumonia which leaves permanent damage to some bronchi. There is a frequent association of chronic sinusitis and this may indicate some basic defect in the respiratory tract surveillance against infection. The disease may be focal in location affecting just one lung or lobe. The diagnosis frequently requires bronchograms to define the abnormal saccular anatomy. Treatment may require surgical resection of the affected lobe.

CYSTIC FIBROSIS

Cystic fibrosis is a systemic disorder which produces obstructive lung disease by virtue of abnormal mucous production. The thick mucous plugs airways and predisposes to infection, bronchiectasis, and cor pulmonale.

EMPHYSEMA

Unlike chronic bronchitis which is a clinical diagnosis, emphysema is diagnosed pathologically. The pattern is that of destruction of alveolar walls with subsequent enlargement of air spaces, but fewer of them. The basic mechanism is unknown. Several pathologic patterns can be identified but they bare little correlation to potential etiologies or clinical syndromes. The result of all forms is a loss of total gas exchanging area and lung compliance. Obstruction to airflow results from the collapse of small airways during expiration. The patient with emphysema is more likely to have hypoxia without hypercapnia than the patient with chronic bronchitis. Sputum production may also be less but dyspnea and fatigue will be common.

ASTHMA

Asthma is a very common variety of obstructive lung disease affecting between 2 and 6 percent of the American population. It is a disease of complex and probably multiple etiologies. It is characterized by hyper-reactive airways which under appropriate stimuli will constrict and obstruct flow. An important part of asthma is that it is reversible.

A third of the patients with asthma have a clear atopic basis for the disease, in another third allergy is an important component, and the remainder have no identifiable hypersensitivity state. The inciting agent in asthma may be allergic, infectious, toxic, or emotional. In the majority of patients the appropriate question is not which one but how much of each is playing a role.

Clinically, the patient with asthma reports episodes of dyspnea and wheezing between which times he/she may be well. The disease often has its onset in childhood with a secondary peak appearance after age 40. Blood counts often show eosinophilia, pulmonary function tests show obstruction, and blood gases may show hypoxia and, when quite severe, hypercapnia.

Treatment consists of avoidance of known precipitating agents. During attacks the use of β-adrenergic agonists such as epinephrine and more recently available selective β-2-agonists are quite effective. Similarly, sympathetic amines such as ephedrine and terbutaline may be effective in treating the acute attack or as prophylaxis. Theophylline, administered orally, is an effective first line drug for prophylaxis or treatment of the acute attack. Corticosteroids either systemically or in an inhaled variety are effective but their use is reserved for those refractory to other modes of treatment.

The drug treatment of asthma is designed either to interfere with the chemical mediators of the disease or to block the reactions of those mediators. Histamine from mast cells, slow reacting substance of anaphylaxis (SRS-A), platelet activating factor, eosinophilic chemotactic factor, and prostoglandins are a few of the mediators. The common reactive pathway consists of smooth muscular contraction of the airways, increased resistance to expiratory flow, hyperinflation, and hypersecretion of bronchial mucus.

Restrictive Lung Diseases

Restrictive lung diseases, whatever their cause, have the common attribute of reduced lung volumes rather than interference with flow rates. These diseases affect either the interstitium of the lung, the peripheral alveoli, or the mechanical apparatus of respiration. Lungs with restrictive disease are often stiff and lack compliance.

The etiologies are diverse. Severe remote infectious disease may result in scarring of the interstitium. Metastatic malignancy diffusely infiltrating the lymphatics of the lung will show a restrictive pattern. Many toxins will similarly affect the lung such as mustard gas, uremia, hypercalcemia, paraquat, silica, asbestos, berrylium, and coal dust. Drugs have been implicated such as antineoplastic agents, sulfa compounds such as furadantin, and others. Late radiation scarring will also produce pulmonary fibrosis and restrictive diseases. Immunologic diseases are sometimes associated with restrictive lung disease (e.g., hypersensitivity pneumonitis, Goodpasture's syndrome with antibodies to pulmonary basement membrane antigen, Wegener's syndrome which is probably a primary vascular insult, systemic lupus erythematosis, and scleroderma).

Occasionally the process has no identifiable origin and is called diffuse interstitial fibrosis. Other disorders of unknown origin include pulmonary alveolar proteinosis which is characterized by the extensive weeping of proteinacious material, desquamative interstitial pneumonitis in which the alveoli are filled with shed pneu-

mocytes, and indiopathic pulmonary hemosiderosis a disease of iron deficiency anemia and the deposition of large quantities of hemosiderin and iron in the alveolar walls.

Anything which interferes with the mechanics of respiration will appear as a restrictive process. Poliomyelitis, amyotrophic lateral sclerosis, and other neuropathic disorders are in this category. Severe kyphoscoliosis is often associated with restrictive lung disease which may be the result of the mechanical deformity or may be another manifestation of abnormal connective tissue.

Clinically, patients with restrictive lung disease complain of dyspnea but infrequently have a productive cough. They will generally have more severe hypoxia rather than hypercapnia. They are usually thin, do not have barrel chests, and they work hard to breath.

Treatment begins with an attempt to define the basic process. This demands a very careful history with an emphasis on exposures and other diseases, involves appropriate blood work which may include a test for precipitating antigens, and may extend to a lung biopsy for pathologic examination. Unfortunately, by the time many patients become symptomatic and present for evaluation the process has extended to nondiagnostic diffuse interstitial scarring. Long term oxygen therapy is often of value in the late phases.

Pulmonary Embolism

Embolism to the lung most commonly is by a clot. Other substances can be implicated under some circumstances. Fat emboli are seen following trauma and long bone fractures, amniotic fluid in the partuient patient, air under many circumstances, and foreign material in the intravenous drug abuser.

Pulmonary thromboembolism constitutes the largest problem of this disease both because of the numbers and the high mortality. Autopsy data suggest that emboli may be found in 20 to 60 percent of patients so examined. Probably 35 percent of patients who have unrecognized pulmonary emboli will die of the disorder. Our diagnostic accuracy may be as low as 50 percent.

Factors which predispose to the development of venous thrombosis include congestive heart failure, chronic venous insufficiency, trauma with soft tissue injury, surgery, paralysis, the use of birth control pills, and prolonged immobilization. Under these circumstances a clot will form usually in the lower extremity or pelvis. The condition most often is a phlebothrombosis rather than thrombophlebitis with little attendant inflammation and therefore frequently with few clinical findings.

The clot breaks free with motion, straining at stool, or manipulation, and floats freely until it lodges in the pulmonary arterial tree. The larger the embolic load the more proximal the obstruction and the more serious the initial threat to life.

A complicated sequence of events ensues. The obstruction to flow elevates the pulmonary artery pressure. There is probably a release of vasoactive substances causing vasoconstriction with a further increase in pressure. Bronchospasm may be added. There now exists an imbalance between ventilation and perfusion with resultant hypoxia. If the lung is not normal, the clot may eventuate in infarction of the pulmonary tissue.

The classical clinical picture is of a patient who suddenly becomes breathless. He may experience a substernal chest heaviness, wheezing, and marked anxiety. The findings include dyspnea, tachycardia, bronchospasm, and an accentuated pulmonic closure sound. Often however the picture is not classical and may be only confusion in an elderly patient or unexplained hypoxia. If the process proceeds to infarction of the lung, the clinician will note the presence of fever, a pleuritic rub, and perhaps hemoptysis.

The diagnosis is treacherous. The chest x-ray may be normal. Hypoperfusion, plump pulmonary artery trunks, or, in the case of infarction, an infiltrate may be seen. The electrocardiogram may show right heart strain, right bundle branch block, or atrial arrythmias. Blood gases invariably show hypoxia usually without carbon dioxide retention.

Radioisotope scanning of the lung will show perfusion defects while the ventilation scan will show normal air flow. This is most helpful in the presence of a normal x-ray. Pulmonary angiography may be required to yield a definitive diagnosis. Most patients will be shown by venography to have disease of the deep veins of the lower leg or thigh.

The treatment of choice is anticoagulation with heparin during the acute episode followed by long term anticoagulation as long as the predisposing condition exists. Also of value in some circumstances is the use of thrombolytic therapy with streptokinase of urokinase. Surgical interruption of the inferior vena cava is a last resort measure.

Infectious Disease of the Lungs

Normal defense mechanisms of the lungs include the filter mechanics dictated by the size of the airways. Particulate matter will reach the alveoli only if it is 10 μm or smaller. Ciliary action clears most matter. The lung is rich in macrophages which ingest much foreign material including infectious agents. Also important is the secretion of IgA which has sterilizing qualities. The lung may become infected when any of these mechanisms are defective or when the patient has any other debilitating disease.

PNEUMONIA

Pneumonia accounts for perhaps 10 percent of admissions to acute care hospitals. Pneumonia should first be distinguished by the site of origin. Community acquired pneumonia is usually caused by *Streptococcus* pneumoniae or by mycoplasma. *Klebsiella* or *Staphylococcus* organisms may be acquired in the community as well but are usually seen in the compromised host. *Staphylococcus* and gram-negative pneumonia are more commonly the result of hospital acquired infections. Aspiration of gastric contents is another common source of pneumonia. Beginning as a chemical pneumonitis because of the acid burn of the lung, this process frequently becomes superinfected with other organisms.

Streptococcus pneumoniae commonly presents with shaking chills, fever, and cough with sputum production. Hypoxia and pleurisy may be present. Mycoplasma, usually seen in younger adults, is less dramatic with a lower fever, less sputum production, and a more indolent course. *Legionella* pneumonia was identified after a 1976 epidemic in Philadelphia, is caused by a fastidious organism, and is characterized by fever, chills, a nonproductive cough, severe debility, and multilobe consolidation. It has a 15 percent mortality rate.

The diagnosis is established by the clinical findings of rales, rhonchi, or signs of consolidation, together with a chest x-ray showing either lobar consolidation with *Streptococcus* pneumoniae or bronchopneumonia with mycobacterium or staphylococcus. Sputum should be examined for white cells and Gram stained for predominant organisms. Sputum and blood cultures will confirm the offending organism and lead to the selection of the appropriate antibiotics. Oxygen and other supportive measures are required.

PULMONARY TUBERCULOSIS

Mycobacteria are slow growing organisms prevalent throughout history. The spread is primarily by droplet inhalation. The primary infection is the result of the organisms causing a mild lower lobe pneumonia. They are ingested by macrophages, transported to hilar lymph nodes, and encapsulated but usually not destroyed.

After approximately 6 weeks the host develops cell-mediated immunity and the skin test with purified protein derivative (PPD) becomes positive. Under the appropriate circumstances diabetes, debility, steroid use, etc. later develops and the disease reactivates. The granuloma liquefy, break down, and produce upper lobe pneumonia with cavitation, cough, sputum, night sweats, and inanition.

Hematogenous spread of the tubercle bacillus may lead to metastatic infections in the bone or kidneys. Bovine tuberculosis is transmitted by contaminated milk, and when infectious to humans usually causes disease in the lymphatics of the small intestine, especially Peyer's patches of the terminal ileum.

Drug therapy for tuberculosis is quite effective. Because of the slow growth of the organisms treatment must continue for many months to a year. Cavitary tuberculosis requires two drug treatments. The drugs of choice are isoniazid and ethambutol. Secondary drugs used for resistant organisms or in patients intolerate of the primary drugs.

LUNG ABSCESS AND EMPYEMA

Lung abscess usually follows a necrotizing pneumonia. *Staphylococcus* or anarobic gram-negative organisms frequently set the stage. The cavity left by the necrosis of lung tissue is partially filled with bacteria, white cells, and debris. When in communication with a major bronchus, heavy foul sputum production results.

An empyema is said to exist when infected fluid is found in the pleural space. This too is most often the result of an antecedent pneumonia which spreads infection to adjacent pleural spaces but may also be the result of a penetrating wound of the chest with the introduction of bacteria. The pleural fluid will be exudative (high protein content and contain white cells) and will show bacteria.

The diagnosis of a lung abscess is usually made by a chest x-ray which shows a cavity with an air fluid level. An empyema will show as a pleural effusion on a chest x-ray. Bacteriologic examination of material from the abscess or from a thorocentesis with empyema is mandatory. Treatment requires antibiotics specific for the offending organisms and may also require surgery (i.e., either pleural drainage with an empyema or resection of a lung abscess).

Cancer of the Lung

Cancer of the lung is of tremendous epidemiologic importance. More than 100,000 people die annually of this disease. It accounts for 21 percent of all cancers in men and 5.8 percent of all cancers in women. It is rising in frequency in women. The peak incidence is in the sixth decade of life and the 5 year survival from diagnosis is only 8 percent.

Many etiologic factors may be implicated. Cigarette smoking is clearly the major offender. Exposure to radon gas, arsenic, nickle, iron oxides, chromium, and asbestos all have been shown to be associated with an increased incidence of cancer of the lungs. With asbestos the increased incidence is seen in those who also smoke. There

are four basic histologic types of cancer which behave differently.

Squamous cell carcinoma accounts for 40 percent of lung cancer. It is usually found near the hilum arising from a major bronchus. It has the best prognosis since it usually is diagnosed before distant metastases are present.

Adenocarcinoma accounts for 15 percent of lung cancers. This disease more often is found in the periphery of the lung and may be associated with scars of the lung. It is less strongly associated with cigarette smoking.

Small cell anaplastic carcinoma accounts for 25 percent of lung cancers. It is the most aggressive of lung tumors and is almost always metastatic at the time of diagnosis with deposits found in bone marrow, brain, and or liver. Untreated, it has a less than 6 month survival rate.

Large cell anaplastic carcinoma is intermediate in aggression. It may actually consist of several varieties of cancer. It usually is seen near the mediastinum.

The symptomatic representation of these tumors can be divided into local and distant effects. Cough, sputum production, hemoptysis, and pain locally are common. Adjacent structure involvement may lead to pericarditis, esophageal obstruction, superior vena caval obstruction, or Pancoast's syndrome of involvement of the brachial plexus. Distant effects can result from metastases such as seizures, bone pain, or liver dysfunction. Some peculiar nonmetastatic effects are seen with some of these tumors. Hypertrophic pulmonary osteoarthropathy is a syndrome of clubbing and periosteal hypertrophy of long bones which can be painful in the arms and legs. These tumors may also secrete hormones (polypeptide hormones) leading to Cushing's, hyperparathyroidism or inappropriate antidiuretic, syndrome.

The diagnosis is made by biopsy of primary or metastatic lesions. Treatment is guided by the cell type and the extent of the disease. If localized and squamous, surgical resection is recommended. Small cell anaplastic is a nonsurgical disease since it is so frequently metastatic. It responds very rapidly to radiation and multiple drug treatment but equally quickly will relapse. Survival can usually be extended to at least 1 year and in a few cases many years. Oncologists believe that this disease may be curable with multiple drug regimens.

GASTROINTESTINAL DISEASES

Esophageal Diseases

The major function of the esophagus is to transport food and liquid from the mouth to the stomach. Disorders of the esophagus influence either the delivery to the stomach or permit the reflux of material from the stomach to the esophagus or above.

Symptomatically, the most important complaint of esophageal disease is dysphagia. It is important to ascertain if the dysphagia is for solids, liquids, or both. Dysphagia for liquids alone most often indicates disease of the pharynx of a neurologic origin since it is much more difficult to form a bolus of liquid than solids in the pharynx. Mechanical obstruction presents early with solid dysphagia and later with liquid dysphagia. Pain is the second most important symptom. Frequently the pain is with swallowing but may occur independently and be confused with angina pectoris, pleurisy, or gallbladder disease.

GASTROESOPHAGEAL REFLUX AND ESOPHAGITIS

When gastric contents are permitted to come in contact with the esophagus, the patient will complain of heartburn. The esophagus is not designed to withstand the assault of gastric acid and pepsin, and will react with inflammation. The usual mechanism is an incompetent lower esophageal sphincter which fails as a one way valve. This may be the result of an hiatus hernia, neuromuscular disease, or scleroderma. An hiatus hernia is a defect in the diaphragm which allows a portion of the stomach to slide into the thoracic cavity. The additional support to the esophageal sphincter is not present and it becomes incompetent. Hiatus hernia is almost always seen in obese patients who complain of heartburn after eating and particularly when lying down after meals. The treatment of esophagitis is both mechanical and chemical. Antacids, H-2 blockers, elevation of the head of the bed, and occasionally surgery to correct a hernia have all been used with success.

DIFFUSE ESOPHAGEAL SPASM

This episodic disease plagues patients in the midlife years. Pain may be intense, occasionally related to hot or cold food but frequently coming on without association with active swallowing. It is a disorder of esophageal motility with intense simultaneous repetitive contractions of the esophagus. It is diagnosed by esophageal manometry during an acute attack. It is frequently confused with coronary artery pain. Treatment with smooth muscle relaxants such as nitroglycerin is helpful.

ACHALASIA

Achalasia is uncommon and the cause is unknown. In this disorder, the esophagus loses peristalsis altogether. In addition, the lower esophageal sphincter fails to relax

and allow free transit of food to the stomach. The result is that the esophagus becomes markedly dilated. The patient will complain of chest discomfort, regurgitation of undigested food, and weight loss. A barium swallow shows an enormously distended esophagus terminating in a beaklike small orifice to the stomach. The condition predisposes to carcinoma of the esophagus. It is treated surgically by dilatation of myotomy.

ESOPHAGEAL CARCINOMA

This disease occurs in older men and is more common in some groups and populations than others (high incidence in Japan). Some predisposing factors include, alcoholism, achalasia, and lye burns of the esophagus. Most are squamous cell carcinomas and the remainder adenocarcinomas. Some of the latter undoubtedly arise from the stomach near the esophagus. Only half of these are operable at the time of diagnosis and the 5 year survival is a disappointing 5 percent.

Gastric Diseases

CANCER OF THE STOMACH

Worldwide, cancer of the stomach is very important. In the United States it is less prevalent than in Japan and the incidence appears to be declining. This cancer is treacherous since symptoms are frequently minimal until late in the disease. Also, the spread of this tumor is centrifugal with involvement of lymph nodes in several different chains unlike cancer of the colon.

Eighty percent of gastric cancers are adenocarcinomas. The remainder are lymphomas, leimyosarcomas, and rarely carcinoid type tumors.

The etiology is unknown although there is a mild genetic predisposition. Patients with atrophic gastric mucosa are at risk for this cancer especially those with pernicious anemia in whom the incidence of cancer of the stomach is 6 percent.

The diagnosis is suspected by x-rays showing ulcerlike lesions especially in the antrum or lesser curvature of the stomach. Biopsy through an endoscope confirms the suspicion. Treatment for cure is surgery. Paliation may be obtained with the use of chemotherapy.

GASTRITIS

Acute erosive gastritis is an important cause of upper gastrointestinal bleeding. It may occur with no known etiologic features or may be the result of aspirin use, alcohol ingestion, acute stress such as body burns or trauma, or ingestion of toxic substances.

The patient presents with either hematemesis or melena frequently without pain. The diagnosis is established by endoscopy since barium studies will be normal as the ulceration is very shallow. Usually a self-limited disease, bleeding may be treated with iced gastric lavage. Once bleeding ceases, treatment with antacids is recommended.

MISCELLANEOUS GASTRIC DISORDERS

Acute gastric dilatation may be a life threatening event. It may occur as a result of diabetic acidosis, total body casting, pneumonia, or the inappropriate use of anticholinergics.

The Mallory-Weiss syndrome consists of gastric hemorrhage following a tear of the mucosa at the gastroesophageal junction following prolonged retching.

Bezoars of the stomach are concretions of ingested nondigestible material such as hair. They may obstruct the stomach and are usually seen in patients with a psychiatric disturbance.

Acid Peptic Diseases

Upper gastrointestinal ulcers share similar symptoms and all are related to the penetration of the normal protective barriers of the mucosa by acid and digestive enzymes. Eighty percent of such ulcers occur in the proximal portion of the duodenum and most of the rest occur in the stomach. Probably 10 percent of the population has ulcer disease at some time in their life.

Many factors bear on the development of ulcers. There is probably always an element of gastric hypersecretion of acid. There are genetic factors (more common in Type O blood type), vagal influences, and some neuropsychiatric influences. Gastric hypersecretion is most marked in patients with the Z-E syndrome of hypergastrinemia secondary to a gastrin secreting tumor(s) of the pancreas. Glucocorticoids are also important. Ulcers are more common in Cushing's disease or with the exogenous use of steroids and are very rare in patients with Addison's disease. Ulcers are more common in patients with hypercalcemia or hyperparathyroidism.

The symptom complex is characteristic and consists of midepigastric pain relieved by food or antacids. Typically the pain begins 2 to 2½ hours following meals. Patients relate a burning, gnawing, or hungerlike discomfort. Often the pain wakes the patient from sleep in the early morning hours. Other patients report no symptoms and may not present until there is perforation or bleeding.

The diagnosis is made with x-rays and/or endoscopy. The treatment for perforation is surgery. Medical treatment currently has vastly reduced the need for gastrectomy. Antacids, rest, dietary changes, and most importantly, the judicious use of H-2 blockers such as cimetidine usually result in complete amelioration of symptoms. The disease is frequently recurrent over months and years with peak symptomatic periods in the spring and fall.

Small Intestine Diseases

GENERAL PRESENTATIONS

The symptomatic presentations of small intestine diseases are those related to motility disturbance, pain, bleeding, or malabsorption. Ileus, obstruction and diarrhea indicate motility problems. Pain from the small intestine usually presents about the umbilicus and frequently comes in peristalic waves, more frequent in periodicity, the higher the pathology in the tract. Bleeding beyond the Treitz ligament appears as melena, and above the ligament as hematemesis. Malabsorption merits additional discussion.

MALABSORPTION

Several categories of mechanisms result in malabsorption. Inadequate digestion of food is seen postgastrectomy in some patients. Another major cause is inadequate pancreatic lipase as seen in chronic pancreatitis, cystic fibrosis, pancreatic carcinoma, and the ulcerogenic pancreatic tumors of the Z-E syndrome.

Diminished bile salts lead to malabsorption. Hepatobiliary disease with either diminished production of bile salts or inadequate delivery to the gut is the most common cause. Bacterial overgrowth in the small bowel secondary to stasis, as seen in blind loops, scleroderma, and fistulas, will result in bile salt deficiency. Bile salt pools may be depleted if there is disease of the terminal ileum which is responsible for the reabsorption of bile.

The gut absorptive surface is diminished with resection of long portions of the bowel or with the development of fistulas which allow food to bypass absorptive surfaces.

Lymphatic obstruction as seen in bowel lymphoma, intestinal lymphagiectasis, and Whipple's disease results in malabsorption.

Vascular diseases leading to malabsorption may be arterial or venous. Arterial insufficiency for any reason will impede absorption and digestion. Venous hypertension as in congestive heart failure and constrictive pericarditis similarly can lead to malabsorption.

Malabsorption is prominent in diseases of the mucosa

itself. Inflammatory or infiltrative diseases such as amyloid and regional enteritis characteristically show findings of malabsorption. Biochemical deficiencies of the mucosa are seen in nontropical sprue (gluten induced enteropathy) and enzyme deficiencies of which disaccharidase deficiency is the prototype.

Endocrine disease may include malabsorption as part of the clinical picture. Hyper- or hypothyroidism, Addison's disease, diabetes mellitus, and carcinoid tumors are examples.

Clinically, malabsorption has weight loss as the hallmark. There are frequently recognized changes in the stool with increased bulk, flatulence, and frequency. Hypoproteinemia, vitamin deficiencies, and low grade anemia are all common. Other findings will be related to the causative disease.

REGIONAL ENTERITIS

Regional enteritis, also called Crohn's disease is a chronic illness of the gut of unknown cause. It appears more frequently in caucasions than blacks and slightly more frequently in Ashkenazi Jews.

The disease most commonly involves the distal ileum but any portion of the gut from the esophagus to rectum can be involved. Pathologically, regional enteritis involves the entire thickness of the gut wall which distinguishes it from ulcerative colitis, a mucosal disease. Characteristically, the disease involves portions of the bowel with intervening areas remaining quite normal. These skipped areas are important diagnostically on x-ray. The process begins with inflammation and over time progresses to stricture with a high propensity to adhere to adjacent structures and the development of fistulas.

Treatment is supportive for the complications. Surgery should be reserved for those with clear indications. Drug therapy with salicylazosulfapyridine (Azulfadine) may afford long term control. Corticosteroids are useful for acute inflammatory events but not for stricture. Occasionally immunosuppressive treatment with azathioprine proves helpful.

VASCULAR DISEASES

The bowel is fed from the celiac axis and the superior and inferior mesenteric arteries. The former two supply primarily the small intestine.

Acute ischemia of the small bowel occurs with occlusion of either the celiac axis (rare) or of the superior mesenteric artery. Emboli from the heart should be suspected in the patient with congestive heart failure, mitral stenosis, or documented arrhythmias especially atrial fibrillation. Thrombosis of the vessels are seen in atherosclerotic disease. Such patients may report prodromes of intestinal angina.

Intestinal angina is a clinical syndrome caused by mesenteric vascular insufficiency. Patients complain of abdominal pain shortly after eating, and experience weight loss either because they eat less or have malabsorption.

Vasculitis of the bowel usually occurs as part of a systemic vasculitis. Periarteritis nodosa, systemic lupus erythematosis, and allergic vasculitis (Henoch-Schönlein purpura) are examples. Large vessel disease leads to infarctions and small vessel disease to bleeding.

APPENDICITIS

This disease seen most often in the first two decades of life, is a clinically diagnosed illness. Appendicitis is a disease of no more than 5 days. The onset is with anorexia followed by dull pain about the umbilicus which migrates to the right lower quadrant. Nausea and vomiting, seen in about 50 percent of cases occurs after pain. Tenderness is always elicited somewhere but varies according to the location of the appendix (right or left side, retrocecal, or high in the right upper quadrant). Low grade fever and an elevated white blood cell count together with this history should prompt surgical intervention. Perforation hightens mortality rates especially at the extremes of life.

Diseases of the Colon and Rectum

Patients with disorders of the colon and rectum will present with pain, change in bowel habits or bleeding from the rectum. The pain of lower bowel disease frequently refers to the lower quadrants. Diarrhea or constipation must be interpreted in light of the patients established lifelong patterns of elimination. Bleeding from the colon will be maroon colored stools or bright red blood noted on the stool, mixed with the stool, on the paper, or in the bowel.

MEGACOLON

A dilated colon may be congenital or acquired. The most common congenital form is aganglionic megacolon also called Hirschprung's disease. An absence of ganglionic cells in a small portion of the colon prohibits that portion from relaxing normally and results in proximal dilatation sometimes of massive proportions. Treatment is surgical resection of the aganglionic segment.

Similar ganglionic dysfunction can result from trypanosomiasis infection. Occasionally, megacolon is a manifestation of psychiatric disease. It may also complicate ulcerative colitis.

DIVERTICULOSIS

Diverticula of the colon are hernias of the mucosa through the muscular layers. They increase in incidence with age. When symptomatic, they cause either bleeding or pain and fever from localized infection.

IRRITABLE COLON SYNDROME

This syndrome manifests as pain and alternating diarrhea and constipation. The etiology is unknown but it is thought to be an exaggerated colonic reaction to psycholgical stress.

ULCERATIVE COLITIS

This inflammatory disease of the colon has no known etiology. Unlike granulomatous disease, ulcerative colitis is usually confined to the colon and rectum, and is almost exclusively a mucosal disease such that fistulas and abscesses are less frequent. The disease follows a variable course from mild ulcerative proctitis to life threatening pancolonic disease. The major symptom is bloody diarrhea often with systemic complaints of fever and weight loss.

The diagnosis is established by sigmoidoscopy which reveals friable mucosa which bleeds easily. Barium studies demonstrate the extent of the colon involved. Complications include perforation, toxic megacolon, serious hemorrhage, malnutrition, liver disease, and occasionally arthritis.

Therapy includes nutritional support sometimes including hyperalimentation with bowel rest. Corticosteroids may be required for acute episodes either parenterally or as steroid enemas. Sulfsalazine (Azulfadine) is useful as a maintenance drug. Experience with immunosupressants indicates they may be salutory. Toxic megacolon may demand emergency colectomy. Some specialists recommend total colectomy for long standing disease because of the increased incidence of carcinoma in such patients.

The major differential diagnostic considerations are ischemic colitis, granulomatous colitis, and amebiasis of the colon.

TUMORS OF THE COLON

Polyps of the colon are common, usually are benign, and usually are located in the rectosigmoid region. The most common is the adenomatous polyp which is benign, frequently grows on a stalk, and may bleed.

Villous adenomas are usually more sessile, broad based, and composed of delicate fronds some of which will show atypia or frank neoplasia in 50 percent of cases. Rarely, villous adenomas cause severe watery diarrhea. They should be removed surgically.

Cancer of the colon is most often adenocarcinoma. Most (75 percent) occur in the rectosigmoid and 15 percent are found in the cecum. The earliest finding of these tumors is microscopic bleeding into the stool. The diagnosis is established by sigmoidoscopy and or barium enema and the treatment is surgery.

Hepatobiliary Diseases

HEPATITIS

Generically, hepatitis is the term for inflammation of the liver. It may be the result of infection, toxin exposure, drugs, or alcohol.

Infectious hepatitis is the result of viral invasion of the hepatocytes. Three types of viruses have been implicated, hepatitis A or infectious hepatitis, hepatitis B or serum hepatitis and non A non B hepatitis which is seen post-transfusionally.

Hepatitis A, infectious hepatitis, is transmitted by the fecal oral route and is epidemic in nature. The incubation period is 10 to 50 days, has little prodrome, is characterized by jaundice, anorexia, low grade fever, and mild abdominal pain. Rarely does one become a carrier of hepatitis A. Immunoglobulin prophylaxis is recommended for immediate contacts of hepatitis A.

Hepatitis B is transmitted by blood or blood products and contaminated needles. Incubation is longer ranging from 40 to 180 days and there may be a prodrome of myalgias, arthralgias, or urticaria. Hepatitis B may exist as a carrier state with few symptoms.

Either type may be fulminant leading to death. Hepatitis B however is the only one which may lead to chronic persistent hepatitis (relatively benign carrier state) or chronic active hepatitis (relatively serious which may lead to cirrhosis and death).

Hepatitis B is reliably diagnosed serologically by the demonstration of hepatitis B surface antigen.

CIRRHOSIS

Cirrhosis is end stage fibrosis of the liver which may be the result of any prolonged hepatic insult. Most commonly the insult is alcoholism, but it may also result form chronic active hepatitis, hemochromotosis, some drugs, or idiopathically. The usual sequence leading to cirrhosis is first fatty metamorphosis then progressive scarring bridging portal triads and finally such significant cell drop out that function is markedly reduced. The scarring impedes blood flow and leads to hypertension of the portal circuit. This backup pressure causes the spleen to enlarge and may lead to esophageal varices and bleeding. The functional loss prohibits normal detoxification with NH_3 buildup, normal conjugation with jaundice, and normal synthesis with bleeding. The abnormalities of ammonia metabolism are probably responsible for the hepatic encephalopathy accompanying end stage liver disease.

Alcoholic cirrhosis, the most common variety is related to the amount and duration of alcohol abuse. The precise mechanism is in dispute. Although nutritional deprivation is common, there is also an element of direct alcohol toxicity. This toxicity seems to vary from individual to individual. The earliest change is fatty infiltration during which time the patient may be asymptomatic, and hepatomegaly may be the only finding. Subsequently, the fat is replaced with scar, the liver shrinks in size, and complaints of cirrhosis emerge. A frequent physical finding in the midstage in men is the development of hyperestrinemia. Body hair diminishes, breast enlargement occurs together with testicular atrophy, a female escutcheon, spider angiomata, and a diminished libido. The alcoholic may also experience alcoholic hepatitis with a tender liver, fever, leukocytosis, and transiently disordered liver function. Improvement in survival only attends abstinence from alcohol.

Hemochromotosis is a metabolic form of cirrhosis. The disease may be inherited as an autosomal dominant with varying penetrance. Alternatively, it can result from iron overload in other conditions such as thalassemia or from conditions requiring frequent lifelong transfusions. In addition to affecting the liver, the iron overload in hemochromotosis affects other organs, most notably the pancreas, thyroid and adrenals, and heart. The iron precipitates and there is intense fibrotic reaction in all these organs. The liver scars to a micronodular cirrhosis and biopsy will show the characteristic iron deposition. The symptom complex of hemochromotosis includes those of cirrhosis as mentioned above. In addition the skin is pigmented, diabetes or hypothryoidism from scarring of those organs may appear, and cardiac arrhythmias are common. Phlebotomy is the treatment of choice. It may be required as often as weekly for several years in order to adequately deplete the excessive stores of iron.

Wilson's disease, another metabolic form of cirrhosis is related to disordered copper metabolism. It appears that the liver is unable to adequately excrete copper. The accumulation leads to cirrhosis. The nervous system is also affected with tremors, ataxia, and changes in mentation. Treatment is with chelation of the copper by penicillamine.

Biliary cirrhosis is characterized by chronic intrahepatic cholestasis. The primary variety has no known etiology but is probably immunologic. More common in women, this disease usually appears between age 40 and 55 and at first appears as obstructive jaundice. Biopsy shows intense bile duct proliferation and dilatation with fibrosis and occasionally granulomas. It progresses to cirrhosis with necrosis of hepatocytes especially around portal areas. Portal hypertension, variceal bleeding, ascites, and malabsorption characterize end stage disease. Treatment is unsatisfactory.

GALLSTONES

This common disorder is found in 10 percent of the population and probably near 30 percent of those over 65 years of age. Most are asymptomatic.

Two types of stones are recognized. Most (95 percent) are cholesterol stones and the remainder are pigment stones. Cholesterol stones are caused by the precipitation of cholesterol which occurs when the concentration of cholesterol in relation to bile acids and lecithin is high. Pigment stones are the result of a high bile pigment as a result of hemolysis of blood.

Acute cholecystitis occurs usually when a stone becomes lodged in the cystic or common bile duct. Pain, nausea, vomiting, and fever result. The pain is usually constant, not periastalic, and is referred to the right upper quadrant. Chronic cholecystitis has variable manifestations. Although frequently found in those who are obese, female, multiparous and with a positive family history, the oft stated intolerance to fatty foods is probably not as accurate as once thought.

The diagnosis is established by cholecystograms or ultrasound studies. If asymptomatic, gallstones should be left alone unless the patient is a diabetic. Infection and gangrene is more common in such patients and can be rapidly fatal.

Pancreatic Diseases

PANCREATIC CARCINOMA

Pancreatic cancer is the third most common gastrointestinal malignancy. It is more common in men, smokers, and alcoholics. Adenocarcinoma is the most common pathologic type. Seventy percent occur in the head of the pancreas. Typical symptoms include back pain, weight loss, and frequently depression. If the lesion obstructs the common duct, jaundice and a palpable gallbladder may be present. This treacherous malignancy is often incurable by the time the diagnosis is established. Only 25 percent are resectable and the 5 year survival is only 1 percent.

The diagnosis is established by upper gastrointestinal x-rays, ultrasound, or CT scan of the abdomen.

PANCREATITIS

Acute pancreatitis manifests as severe abdominal pain, nausea, and vomiting. It is the result of alcoholism, trauma, gallstone obstruction of the pancreatic duct, some drugs, and some viral infections (mumps). The patient will be quite ill as a result of the edema of the pancreas with occasional hemorrhage and autolysis of the gland. Patients are treated with intravenous fluids, nasogastric suction, and, if indicated, antibiotics.

Chronic pancreatitis results from alcoholism, biliary tract disease, cystic fibrosis, hyperparathyroidism, hyperlipemia, or idiopathic reasons. It may be represented as chronic low grade abdominal pain or punctuated episodes of pain. Pancreatic insufficiency results with malabsorption, weight loss and sometimes diabetes mellitus. The diagnosis is suggested by the finding of pancreatic calcifications or retrograde endoscopic cholecystopancreatography. Treatment is with supplemental pancreatic enzymes, attention to the offending agent, and insulin if required.

A pancreatic pseudocyst may result from either acute or chronic pancreatitis. This saclike accumulation of serum and pancreatic fluid can reach very large size. It may be palpable and the cause of persistent pain. Treatment is surgical.

NEUROLOGIC DISEASES

Dementia

Dementia is characterized by a gradual loss of higher intellectual function. Motor loss occurs only very late in the disease. Remote memory is disproportionately preserved when compared to recent memory. The process most commonly accompanies advanced years but occasionally has its onset in the late 40s or 50s.

Alzheimer's disease is the most common cause of dementia (50 percent). This progressive cerebral degeneration has no known cause. There may be early slight lateralization of the findings but these do not persist. The diagnosis can only be made with pathologic assurance with the appearance of neurofibrillary tangles and plaques. There is no specific treatment.

Fifteen percent of dementias are the result of diffuse cerebrovascular disease. In both cerebrovascular disease and Alzheimer's, computerized axial tomography will show diffuse cerebral atrophy which is nondiagnostic.

Perhaps fifteen percent of dementias are the result of other diagnosable disorders. Low pressure hydrocephalus is a rare cause but important because it is treatable. This condition may be suggested by the appearance of incontinence and difficulty walking. The CT scan will

show atrophy but little space between the cortex and the calvarium. Alcoholism, vitamin deficiencies (B_1, B_6, and B_{12}), myxedema, and syphilis are other etiologies to consider.

Huntington's chorea is a rare dominantly inherited form of dementia. The onset is in the fourth or fifth decade. Distinguishing features include the appearance of choreiform motions followed by depression and profound dementia leading to death.

Lower Motor Neuron Diseases

Lesions anywhere in the lower motor neuron lead to wasting, weakness, and loss of reflexes. Fasciculations are common if the lesion is close to the spinal cord and not present in lesions of the very distal nerve.

Amyotrophic lateral sclerosis is a rare form of lower and upper motor neuron diseases. The features are those of wasting, weakness, and fasciculations. Pyramidal tract findings are also prominent. The disease is fatal usually within 7 years of diagnosis. The cause and treatment are unknown.

Progressive muscular atrophy is a slowly progressive lower motor neuron disease involving predominantly the arms and legs. Long survival is common but no treatment has been found to influence the disorder.

Peripheral Nerve Lesions

Disorders of the peripheral nerves may be single or multiple. Single nerve lesions are called neuropathies and multiple nerve involvements are called either mononeuritis multiplex involving multiple disparate nerves or polyneuropathy which is a symmetrical nerve involvement. Mononeuritis multiplex often accompanies systemic disorders with vasculitis such as systemic lupus erythematosis or rheumatoid arthritis. The most common cause of polyneuropathy is diabetes mellitus where the involvement is particularly likely to involve sensory nerves.

Many major distal nerves may be subject to entrapment between bone and fascial sheath. The most common is carpal tunnel syndrome where the median nerve is trapped in the carpal tunnel producing wasting of the thenar eminence and weakness of the interosseus muscles of the first three fingers.

Guillain-Barré Syndrome

Also called acute infective polyneuritis, the Guillain-Barré syndrome most often follows an upper respiratory tract infection. It may also appear after immunization for other viral diseases or idiopathically. The paralysis is usually ascending first involving the lower extremities then progressing to involve the upper extremities and the muscles of respiration. The latter involvement may lead to the need for mechanical ventilation. Cranial nerves may become involved. Recovery usually occurs but may be prolonged taking up to 6 months. The only known treatment is supportive awaiting resolution.

Neuromuscular Junction

The arrival of an impulse at the neuromuscular junction causes the release of acetylcholine which transmits the impulse chemically to receptors on the motor endplate. Many drugs act on this junction either to promote the effects of acetylcholine or block its effects.

Myasthenia gravis most commonly affects women in midlife. The most common clinical feature is fatiguability of muscle with repetitive use. The first muscle affected will vary and may be the lids, the pharynx, or small muscle units of the hands. They may develop lid droop, diplopia, or profound weakness of the hands. There is no wasting and no fasciculations. With rest, motor strength improves. The electromyogram is diagnostic. The diagnosis can also be suggested by a positive response to neostigmine which is an anticholinesterase drug. By inhibiting cholinesterase the effects of the reduced amount of acetylcholine are enhanced and the weakness will disappear. The disease is thought probably to be the effects of an immunologic disorder. There is a known incidence of thymoma and some patients will achieve complete remission with thymectomy. Treatment otherwise is with the use of long acting cholinesterase inhibitors.

The myasthenic syndrome, also called the Eaton-Lambert syndrome, is so called since it somewhat mimics myasthenia gravis. The patient will complain of fatigue but on examination the weakness will be found to affect predominantly proximal limb girdle muscles, and improves with exercise as opposed to classic myasthenia. The importance of recognizing this disease is because it usually presages the clinical manifestations of carcinoma of the lung.

Muscular Dystrophies

The muscular dystrophies are divided according to the clinical manifestations and mode of inheritance.

Duchenne dystrophy is a sex-linked recessive disorder appearing in childhood. The major early finding is proximal muscle weakness. Pseudohypertrophy of the muscles is secondary to enlargement of individual fibers which is apparent pathologically. The condition, which is untreatable, is slowly progressive leading to wheelchair existence and frequently respiratory complications as the chest support becomes involved.

Facioscapulohumeral dystrophy is inherited as an autosomal dominant and therefore affects both males and females. Girdle muscle weakness, usually pectoral, appears in adolescence and progresses slowly. In many the disease is consistent with a relatively normal life-style with little progression to other muscles.

Myotonic disorders are characterized by the inability to relax muscles following voluntary contraction. Dystrophia myotonica appears in adolescence or later. It is dominantly inherited and when fully blown shows myotonia, frontal baldness, cataracts, and testicular atrophy. Myotonia congenita appears at birth as widespread myotonia frequently with hypertrophy of muscles.

Parkinson's Disease

This disease of the basal ganglia may be the result of remote encephalitis (especially the influenza infections suffered by many in 1918). Biochemically, it is characterized by the degeneration of the dopaminergic pathways of the globus pallidus and substantia nigra. The clinical picture is of rigidity, bradykinesia, and resting tremor. The rigidity has a cogwheeling feeling to motion by the examiner, facial expression is lost, the patient shows a shuffling gait with trouble negotiating turns, and a tendency to topple forward (festination). The tremor is characteristic, most noted in the hands as a "pill rolling" seven per second tremor which disappears with intention. Treatment aimed at restoring dopamine levels in the brain has assisted many patients. The levo form of dopa, the immediate precursor of dopamine, will cross the blood brain barrier and is effective in many patients. A dopamine agonist, bromocryptine, and the antiviral agent, amantidine, have also been found useful.

Infectious Diseases

Acute pyogenic meningitis is the result of bacterial invasion either hematogenously from a remote site or by direct extension from a nearby locus such as a sinus or middle ear. Host deficiencies are important predisposing factors. Many organisms may cause bacterial meningitis but the clinical picture is similar. The patient will exhibit fever, headache, and vomiting. There will be signs of meningeal irritation, epilepsy, common in children, and coma may occur. The diagnosis is established by examination of the cerebrospinal fluid which will show a leukocytosis and elevated protein and depressed glucose levels. The specific organism may be suggested by Gram stain but cultures are required for definitive identification and sensitivity testing.

Syphilis and tuberculosis are the most common causes of chronic pyogenic meningitis. The symptoms are less dramatic and may include headache, malaise, confusion, vomiting, and somnolence. Fever is usually low grade. Examination of the cerebrospinal fluid may show increased pressure, lymphocytosis, and increased protein and depressed glucose levels. The tubercle bacillus may be slow growing and delay the diagnosis. A positive test for reagin indicates the likelihood of syphilis.

Viral infections rarely are contained to just the meninges. Meningoencephalitis is more common and the disease is not rare. Many viral agents may produce infection of the central nervous system. Most are benign and self-limiting with headache, meningism, low grade fever, photophobia, and malaise. The cerebrospinal fluid will show predominantly lymphocytes; the protein is normal and the glucose is also normal.

A few viral infections are more devastating. Herpes simplex may cause an acute necrotizing encephalitis with death. The findings relate to the predilection for this virus to affect the temporal lobes. A tumor like mass may be seen on scans of the brain. Treatment with cytosine arabinoside has met with variable success but is the only available therapy. Rabies virus will infect the brain following a bite by an infected animal. The virus tracks up peripheral nerves and untreated leads to death. Pharyngeal spasm, a common symptom, leads to the term "hydrophobia." Untreated, the disease is invariably fatal.

Subacute sclerosing panencephalitis, progressive multifocal leukoencephalopathy, and Jakob-Creutzfeldt disease are all thought to be the result of viral infections.

Seizures

Seizures are the result of a disorderly discharge of neurons in the central nervous system. The onset and terminus are abrupt and the symptomatology findings relate to the area(s) involved with the discharge. Seizures are divided into partial and generalized.

Partial seizures are simple or complex. Simple seizures result from a localized contained discharge. The seizure may consist of motor, sensory, or autonomic symptoms or combinations. Focal jerks, posturing, and speech arrest are common symptoms. Sensory complaints may consist of hallucinations, odors, and tastes or labyrinthian changes. Complex partial seizures, also called psychomotor or temporal lobe seizures, present with an aura of cognitive, affective, or psychomotor symptoms. There is frequently an alteration of consciousness. The attack resolves gradually with confusion or drowsiness.

There are several types of generalized seizures. Petit mal seizures are very brief, have no aura, and few aftereffects. These brief "spells" are often accompanied by automatisms such as lip smacking, clonic jerks, or changes in postural tone. Grand mal seizures may begin with localized jerks and spread to total body jerking (Jack-

sonian march) or may be bilateral and total from the outset. There is sudden loss of consciousness followed by a tonic contraction of all muscles with apnea then followed by the clonic jerking motion of all major motor units. Incontinence of urine and stool may occur. The clonic phase lasts for minutes or longer (status epilepticus). The patient wakes slowly with a postictal state of coma lightening to somnolence to lethargy to sleep.

With any variety of epilepsy it is important to investigate any organic lesion which may be responsible such as tumor, abscess, scar, or metabolic abnormality. The electroencephalogram may be diagnostic even in the seizure free period and may localize a lesion.

CEREBROVASCULAR DISEASE

Intracranial Hemorrhage

Extradural hemorrhage is almost always the result of a severe blow to the head. The middle meningeal artery is subject to tear with fractures across the temple. Since this is arterial bleeding the syndrome appears rapidly. The blow usually causes unconsciousness following which there may be a lucid interval with the progression to coma again in hours. Hemiplegia with fixed dilated pupils is usually found. This represents a surgical emergency.

Subdural hemorrhage also usually follows an injury but the trauma may be much milder and more remote in time such that the patient may not even recall the event. Here the bleeding is venous and the progression slower. Signs will depend on the location with headaches, seizures, personality changes, or focal motor deficits being common. Subdural hematomas may be treated surgically or conservatively depending on the clinical severity.

Subarachnoid hemorrhage is most often the result of a ruptured aneurysm of the circle of Willis. When this congenital sacular aneurysm ruptures the clinical syndrome abruptly presents. Usually, the patient complains of a severe headache with nausea and vomiting. Meningism and a bloody cerebrospinal fluid strongly suggest the diagnosis. This is a disorder of young to middle aged adults. Surgical ligation of the aneurysm or its supply is occasionally required.

Intracerebral hemorrhage is seen in patients with long standing hypertension. The perforating arteries off of the circle of Willis are the ones which most commonly rupture. Bleeding therefore is most common in the internal capsule, thalamus, and upper brain stem. The presentation is abrupt with severe deficits and poor prognosis. The hemorrhage may rupture into the ventricle.

Cerebrovascular Ischemia

Transient ischemic attacks last less than 24 hours. They are generally associated with atherosclerotic vascular disease. Thirty percent of patients with transient ischemic attacks will complete a stroke within a year. When cerebral vessels are compromised the patient will show contralateral long tract signs. If the vertebrobasilar system is involved the symptoms are ataxia, dizziness, nausea, and vomiting.

Cerebral thrombosis results when a compromised vessel becomes completely occluded by in situ thrombosis. The development of the stroke is slower than an embolus. The findings are of contralateral paresis and aphasia if the dominant hemisphere is involved. The most common predisposing disease is atherosclerosis but occasionally other blood vessel diseases may lead to thrombosis such as arteritis from infectious or immunologic diseases.

Cerebral embolus causes abrupt disruption of function. The findings relate to the vessel involved but most often these are branches of the internal carotid artery. The two most common sites of origin are the heart and the carotid bifurcation. Patients may dislodge a clot from a mural thrombus of the left ventricle following a myocardial infarction or from the left atrium as a result of mitral valve disease. Cardiac arrhythmias predispose to such emboli. Atherosclerotic plaques of the carotid bifurcation may slough and embolize. If some of this debris flows into the retinal artery the patient will have a characteristic transient blindness (i.e., amaurosis fugax). Rarely an air embolus will follow cardiac surgery. Clot or air may also rarely cross a patent foramen ovale or atrial septal defect and embolize to the brain.

Intracranial Tumors

Tumors may arise from a variety of brain tissues. Meningiomas are benign and arise from the meninges. Gliomas which have variable malignant potential arise from glial cells. The pituitary and pineal are two other common sources. Primary tumors of the brain do not metastasize and are classified as malignant or benign by their invasiveness of the surrounding normal brain. The findings vary according to location. Frontal lobe tumors may have few findings until they are very large. Personality disorders and dementia are common. Conversely, tumors of the posterior fossa become symptomatic early since there is little room for silent expansion. Such patients usually have severe headaches because of early hydrocephalus. The brain is a common site for metastatic disease. Breast and lung cancers lead the list.

Demyelinating Diseases

Multiple sclerosis is a demyelinating disorder characterized by randomly distributed plaques throughout the central white matter. The plaques tend to evolve and resolve yielding waxing and waning clinical findings. Changes in cerebellar pathways are common and produce nystagmus, ataxia, and dysarthria. The cord may be involved with pyramidal and posterior column findings but peripheral nerves are not involved. Incontinence is an important diagnostic clue. The disease is most often seen between ages 20 and 40 and is more common in women than men. The cause is most likely immunologic. Cerebrospinal immunoglobulins may be characteristically altered. There is no satisfactory treatment although patients may have very long survivals.

Progressive multifocal leukoencephalopathy has a patchy demyelinization but the lesions do not tend to resolve as in multiple sclerosis. It is diffuse and asymmetric involving the cerebral hemispheres. Hemiplegia, hemianopsia, aphasia, or dysarthria are common complaints. The cerebrospinal fluid is normal. It is very likely caused by a slow virus. The disease is almost always seen in the face of altered immunity in patients with leukemia, lymphoma, or carcinomatosis.

Subacute sclerosing panencephalitis is a progressive fatal disease of children and adolescents. The insidious onset progresses to death within a year. The cerebrum is widely involved. The disease is thought to be caused by the measles virus.

HEMATOLOGIC DISEASES

Disorders of Erythrocytes

ANEMIAS — DEFICIENCIES OF PRODUCTION

Anemias may be characterized as deficiencies of red cell or hemoglobin production or shortened red cell survival.

The major deficiency states include iron, vitamin B_{12}, and folic acid deficiencies. Symptomatically, all of the anemias present with varying degrees of lassitude, fatigue, and weakness. Other symptoms may point to a specific deficiency and the symptoms of all are tempered by both the severity of the anemia and the rapidity of its occurrence.

Iron deficiency is the most common cause of anemia. It is characterized as a microcytic hypochromic anemia with low serum iron, increased iron binding capacity, and diminished iron stores in the marrow. It is imperative to identify the reason for the iron deficiency which may be secondary to blood loss, poor dietary intake, or excessive iron loss. Treatment is replacement with iron either orally or parenterally.

Megaloblastic anemias are usually the result of vitamin B_{12} or folic acid deficiency. The red cell membrane production is abnormal but hemoglobin synthesis is normal. The result is fewer cells which are large and packed with hemoglobin. Vitamin B_{12} deficiency occurs in pernicious anemia which is an inherited disorder of the production of stomach intrinsic factor such that vitamin B_{12} cannot be absorbed properly. Other causes of vitamin B_{12} deficiency include small bowel disorders which prevent absorption such as total stomach resection or disease of the terminal ileum where vitamin B_{12} is absorbed. In addition to the anemia, patients with vitamin B_{12} deficiency are at hazard for the development of subacute combined degeneration of the spinal cord. With this condition, patients will complain of paresthesias and will be found to have deficient proprioception and vibratory sensation in the lower extremities.

Folic acid deficiency will produce the same findings in the peripheral blood smear of megaloblastic anemia, but patients do not develop the neurologic consequences. Folic acid deficiency is seen in dietary inadequacy, alcoholism, pregnancy, and as a result of some drugs, notably phenytoin, used for seizure control.

Treatment of either folic acid or vitamin B_{12} deficiency is replacement of the vitamin orally or parenterally.

The anemia of chronic disease is very common and probably represents a failure of the stem cells of the marrow. The red cells are usually normochromic and normocytic. Iron levels will be low as will the iron binding capacity, and the marrow will show normal to increased amounts of iron. The anemia is usually not severe and the treatment of the anemia is the treatment of the underlying chronic disease.

Aplastic anemia results from partial or complete failure of the stem cell of the marrow. It is frequently accompanied by failure of other cellular elements. Half are of unknown cause and the remainder are found to be the result of toxins, chemicals, drugs, or radiation. A few result from other diseases such as miliary tuberculosis, viral hepatitis, or pancreatitis.

ANEMIAS — (SHORTENED SURVIVAL)

The normal life span of the red cell is 120 days. Under a variety of circumstances this survival may be shortened. The marrow will respond by increased production. If the magnitude of the loss exceeds the marrow's ability to compensate, anemia will become apparent.

Hemolytic anemias are the result of premature destruction of red cells and may be congenital or acquired.

Hereditary spherocytosis is a dominantly inherited disorder in which the red cell membrane is abnormal and the cells become spherical and are destroyed by the reticuloendothelial system. Patients with this disease have anemia, splenomegaly, and may be jaundiced because of the increased bilirubin load and may develop pigment gallstones. Splenectomy provides excellent symptomatic control.

Sickle cell anemia is a disease of blacks characterized by an abnormal hemoglobin. Hemoglobin S deforms in the presence of low oxygen tension and the red cells assume bizarre sickle shapes. The manifestations of the illness include the symptoms of chronic anemia punctuated by crises of pain in the back extremities and abdomen. The homozygote is much more severely affected than the heterozygote. No treatment other than symptomatic relief is available.

Thallasemia, also an inherited disorder, appears mostly in patients of Mediterranean descent. Patients with this disease continue to produce fetal hemoglobin rather than graduate to the production of normal adult forms of hemoglobin. Here too the homozygote has a much more severe disease and may die in childhood. Splenectomy is sometimes symptomatically helpful.

Autoimmune hemolytic anemias consist of a variety of disorders in which antibodies against some part of the red cell cause premature destruction of the cells. The condition is seen in a variety of other diseases. The antibodies are divided in the cold and warm varieties. Cold antibodies are those demonstrated best at temperatures under 37°C. These cold antibodies occur in infectious mononucleosis, myocoplasma infections, or spontaneously. The warm antibodies are more often associated with lymphomas, leukemias, collagen vascular diseases, or spontaneously. Treatment with steroids is usually helpful.

Blood loss from any source is, or course a common cause of diminished survival. The loss may be gastrointestinal, renal, endometrial, or pulmonary.

Polycythemia

Polycythemia is an absolute elevation of the hemoglobin level in the blood. It must be differentiated from apparent polycythemia secondary to dehydration. It is divided into primary polycythemia and secondary causes.

Polycythemia vera is a primary increase in the production of hemoglobin from stem cells of the marrow. It may also affect the other cellular elements such that leukocytosis and thrombocytosis are also seen. The patient will have symptoms of sludging with headaches, visual disturbances, lassitude, and fatigue. Most will have spenomegaly. The disease is chronic and may eventuate in myelofibrosis or leukemia. Phlebotomy affords symptomatic relief but no other treatment is curative.

Secondary polycythemia may be seen in states of poor oxygenation or secondary to increased production of erythropoietin. Pulmonary disease, cyanotic congenital heart disease, and the presence of abnormal hemoglobins with high tenacity for oxygen will all result in a secondary increase in hemoglobin production. A few diseases of the kidney may result in increased erythropoetin.

Disorders of White Blood Cells

ACUTE LEUKEMIAS

Leukemias are neoplastic diseases of one of the blood forming elements. They are classified according to the cell type of origin and the degree of differentiation of the malignant cell. Thus acute leukemias are those with very primitive cells and those that tend to be more aggressive. All leukemias untreated are fatal.

There are two major forms of acute leukemia, acute lymphoblastic leukemia and acute nonlymphoblastic leukemia. They are so divided because of similarities in distribution and clinical behavior. The nonlymphoblastic leukemias may be further divided by cell of origin such as myelocytic, monocytic, myelomonocytic, and erythroleukemia, a rare leukemia of red cell origin. Often the distinction is difficult since the immaturity of the cells makes clear identification impossible. Acute nonlymphoblastic leukemias are also referred to as acute myelogenous leukemias.

The signs and symptoms of both types are somewhat similar. Marrow failure leads to anemia, bleeding diathesis with concomitant malaise, and fatigue. Fever because of susceptibility to infection or fever *de nova* is common. Tissue infiltration by leukemic cells may provoke central nervous system disease, hepatic dysfunction, hypersplenism, vascular infarctions, and bone and joint pain.

The diagnosis is suggested by the findings of high white blood cell counts and the presence of blast cells in the peripheral blood. Bone marrow examinations show packed marrow with a dominance of the immature elements.

The etiolgoy of the acute leukemias is unknown. There is evidence implicating virus causation, radiation injury, and spontaneous chromosomal damage.

Treatment of the acute leukemias is varible. Acute lymphoblastic leukemia tends to be a disease of children and has a good prognosis when aggressively treated with combination chemotherapy and sometimes radiation therapy. Remission rates of 90 percent are expected. Drugs used include corticosteroids, vina-alkaloids, methotrexate, alkylating agents, asparaginase, and others. Effective treatment is more difficult when this disease appears in adults.

The acute myelogenous leukemias appear more often in adults and have a worse prognosis. Fewer drugs have been shown to be helpful. Cytosine arabinoside and antracycline antibiotics such as daunorubicin are marginally effective. Chemotherapeutic agents are further limited in all acute leukemias because of the low therapeutic index, the marked susceptibility to infection, and the damage to normal marrow cells incurred.

CHRONIC LEUKEMIA

The chronic leukemias tend to appear in later life and are characterized by more mature cells appearing in the blood. The course tends to be more indolent and may extend for years.

Chronic lymphocytic leukemia is characterized by the appearance in the blood of normal mature appearing lymphocytes in great numbers. Symptoms are usually mild and the disease is often found by happenstance. The patient may complain of fatigue and malaise and may note some lymphadenopathy. The cells tend to infiltrate various reticuloendothelial structures such as nodes, the spleen, and liver. Such patients are at risk for pneumococcal infections and thromboembolic events. Treatment is held until the patient is symptomatic or until infiltration of marrow or organs begins to produce complications especially of profound anemia or thrombocytopenia. Prednisone and chlorambucil are the most often used drugs. Occassionally radiation therapy is used for massive or troublesome splenomegaly.

Chronic myelogenous leukemia is a disease of myeloid elements. It is more aggressive than chronic lymphocytic leukemia and after a period of time, this disease usually progresses to acute leukemia and death. Fatigue, sweating, dyspepsia, weight loss, and pain or dragging feelings in the left upper quadrant may prompt the patient to seek attention. Splenomegaly is usual but lymphadenopathy is not. The peripheral smear and bone marrow confirm the diagnosis. The Philadelphia chromosome (a deletion of the long arm of a number 22 chromosome) is found in 85 percent of marrow preparations. Drug treatment of this disorder is constantly evolving and as yet it is unsatisfactory for prolonging life beyond 3 to 5 years.

LYMPHOMAS

Lymphomas are a diverse spectrum of malignant diseases originated in lymphoid tissue usually of nodes. They are arbitrarily separated into Hodgkin's disease and the non-Hodgkin's lymphomas. The etiology of the lymphomas is unknown although there is strong evidence implicating the Epstein-Barr virus in the genesis of the rare Burkitt's lymphoma first described in African children.

The diagnosis and classification of the lymphoma requires evaluation of tissue. The types are defined by cellular characteristics and the extent of the disease is graded according to location of the disease and associated symptoms. Classifications of the lymphomas are still in flux.

Hodgkin's disease is a lymphoma which usually appears in young adults as painless nodal enlargement. The nodes will be rubbery and matted and appear in typical node areas of the neck, axilla, and groin. Occasionally they will first be detected on a routine chest x-ray. Other patients may appear with fever of unexplained origin, weight loss, anorexia, or night sweats. Generalized severe pruritus may be the original complaint.

The disease, untreated, pursues a relentless course terminating in death in months to few years. Late complications include hematologic abnormalities, infections, and obstruction of node draining areas.

Node biopsies reveal pathologic changes including the typical Reed-Sternberg giant cell. Further characterization of the cell pattern allows additional classification.

Hodgkin's and other lymphomas are staged as follows:

Stage I: Involvement of a single node bearing region.
Stage II: Involvement of two or more node regions contiguous and on the same side of the diaphragm.
Stage III: Involvement of two or more node regions on both sides of the diaphragm.
Stage IV: Multiple or disseminated foci of involvement including extralymphatic tissue.

Each stage is further given an A or B classification according to the presence or absence of systemic symptoms such as fever, night sweats, or weight loss.

Treatment of Hodgkin's disease has changed and progressed in recent years. Radiation and chemotherapy now afford significant increases in life expectancy and a much greater chance for cure. At least half of patients with Hodgkin's disease can expect long term survival and probably cure.

Non-Hodgkin's lymphomas are a diverse group of malignancies of lymphoid tissue with variable manifestations. Diffuse histiocytic lymphoma is the most common and is sometimes called reticulum cell sarcoma.

Such patients present with localized but rapidly progressive nodal enlargement. This may appear in nontypical node areas such as the gastrointestinal tract, Waldeyer's ring in the pharynx, the bone, thryoid, or testes. Any visceral organ may subsequently become involved and signs and symptoms will be appropriate to the area diseased.

The role and parameters of radiation therapy and chemotherapy in this group of diseases is less well defined than in Hodgkin's disease. Aggressive staging and combination therapy still affords a 50 percent response rate.

Platelet Disorders

THROMBOCYTOPENIA

A platelet count of less than 100,000/cc is generally considered to be thrombocytopenia. Although there is a general association between the level of depression of the platelet count and the complication of bleeding, it is important to remember that both numbers and individual function are important. Thus counts of 15,000 normal platelets may not result in bleeding but higher counts of abnormal platelets will yield bleeding.

Patients with quantitative or qualitative disorders of platelets will present with bleeding usually of the skin as manifested by petechiae and purpura, or of mucous membranes of the mouth, rectum, or vagina. Low platelet counts result either from defective production from the marrow or increased destruction.

Inhibition of platelet production is frequently the result of drug administration. Marrow replacement is by foreign elements or as part of myelofibrosis, as aplastic anemia of any cuase, or as a deficiency of thrombopoietin, the hormone which stimulates platelet production. The maturation of platelets may be inhibited by vitamin deficiencies such as vitamin B_{12} or folic acid or rare inherited disorders.

Accelerated destruction of platelets may occur from a variety of mechanisms. The most common is antibody mediated destruction. The antibodies may be directed against the platelet as in idiopathic thrombocytopenic purpura or systemic lupus erythematosis, or the leukemias or the platelet may be an innocent bystander. In the latter category, antibodies nonspecifically attach to the platelets which are then filtered out by the reticuloendothelial system. Many drugs precipitate these reactions. Platelets may also be subject to early destruction through consumption in a process of vasculitis or splenomegaly for any cause such as in portal hypertension where the enlarged spleen may indiscriminantly destroy platelets or other blood elements.

Idiopathic thrombocytopenic purpura deserves special mention. The chief findings of this disease are bleeding into the skin and into hollow viscera. It may be a fulminant acute disorder or may be chronic and long standing. The platelets are normal but decreased in number. The blood smear will show large platelets, a sign of immaturity. Platelet antibodies can usually be demonstrated with difficulty. Treatment with steroids, splenectomy, and immunosuppressants have been met with variable success. Plasmapheresis has shown effectiveness in preliminary studies.

THROMBOCYTHEMIA

Thrombocythemia is arbitrarily defined as a sustained elevation of platelets to more than 800,000/cc. Transient elevations of platelets will occur after hemorrhage or splenectomy. Patients with true thrombocythemia are at risk for both spontaneous bleeding and clotting. The disorder may accompany polycythemia vera.

Bleeding Disorders

Abnormal bleeding may result from disorders of blood vessel integrity, clotting factors or platelets. The pattern and location of the bleeding may provide a clue to the origin. Laboratory tests of value include the bleeding time, platelet count measurement of the prothrombin time, partial thromboplastin time, and measurement of the specific clotting proteins.

VASCULAR BLEEDING

Bleeding which is the result of vascular disease is usually not extensive, usually mucosal or skin in location, and usually associated with some systemic illness.

Infectious diseases such as rickettsial infections, fungal infections, and meningococcemia set up a vasculitis. The presentation, in addition to the signs and symptoms of the infection, include petechiae which are palpable and purpura of skin and mucous membranes.

Many drug reactions can present with vasculitis and bleeding. Penicillin and the sulfonamides are the most common offenders. A peculiar form of allergic vasculitis is called Henoch-Schönlein purpura. This disease, usually seen in children following an infection or drug reaction, presents with a purpuric rash, arthralgias, hematuria, and occult bleeding in the stools. It is usually self-limited and resolves without treatment.

Scurvy causes vascular bleeding through disorder collagen growth as a result of the vitamin C deficiency.

Hereditary hemorrhagic telangiectasia is an inherited disease of blood vessels. Multiple dilated capillaries and arterioles develop progressively with age. Bleeding may develop in the lungs, gastrointestinal tract, kidneys, or skin. No specific treatment is available.

COAGULATION DEFECTS

Bleeding as the result of a coagulation defect is usually seen as an inherited condition and is usually the result of a single clotting deficiency.

Classic hemophilia is a sex-linked recessive disease which therefore is seen almost exclusively in males and is transmitted by females. The deficiency of Factor VIII is variable in intensity and the bleeding reflects this. Those with 25 percent or more of the factor may be little troubled. Since the platelet function is normal, patients with hemophilia will form a platelet plug which will hold immmediate bleeding but subsequent to the injury extensive bleeding may then occur. For the same reason, skin and mucous membrane bleeding is uncommon. Rather, deep tissue bleeding is the rule. A special problem is hemarthrosis which when repeated may cripple the patient and reqrue aggressive surgery to correct. The diagnosis is established with the family history and the demonstration of depressed levels of Factor VIII. Treatment is with replacement of the factor either as fresh plasma or usually as cryoprecipitate.

Von Willebrand's disease is inherited as an autosomal dominant and combines moderate Factor VIII deficiency with a defect in platelet aggregation. Since platelets are involved, bleeding will come from skin and mucous membranes. Treatment with Factor VIII will help those severely affected.

Factor IX, Christmas factor, deficiency is inherited and appears much as does classic hemophilia. Treatment is with Factor IX concentrates

Factor XI deficiency causes signs and symptoms similar to mild to moderate hemophilia. It is treated with fresh frozen plasma.

Vitamin K deficiency will yield an acquired bleeding disease. Vitamin K is a fat soluble vitamin. Deficiency of this vitamin most commonly occurs with biliary tract obstruction which prevents absorption of the vitamin. Malabsorption for other reasons may result in vitamin K deficiency as well. Without the vitamin the liver is unable to manufacture prothrombin. Bleeding may occur anywhere but joint bleeding is rare. The prothrombin time will be prolonged and treatment with parenteral vitamin K will reverse the disorder promptly.

Disseminated intravascular coagulation (DIC) merits special mention. This complex disorder may follow many different insults. Shock, burns, septicemia, anaphylaxis, and neoplasms have all been described as antecedents. The suggested mechanism involves diffuse small vessel clotting with the subsequent utilization of all clotting factors and platelets which then permits uncontrolled bleeding. Laboratory studies will show diminished platelets, low levels of fibrinogen, prolonged prothrombin times, and the presence in the blood of fibrin split products. The first step in therapy requires attention to the insulting event. Heparin is needed to prevent the ongoing consumption of clotting factors and replacement of the factors may be required to control bleeding.

SPLENIC DISORDERS

Splenomegaly occurs as the result of increased pressure in the splenic vein as in portal hypertension or because of infiltration of the organ by hematopoietic cells or diseases of reticuloendothelial cells.

Hypersplenism results when an enlarged spleen becomes overactive in its screening function. Red cells, platelets or white cells may be prematurely destroyed either as a group or singly. The peripheral smear shows early cells in circulation (reticulocytes), immature white cells, or large young platelets. If the disorder is primary splenectomy may be effective otherwise treatment is directed to the underlying disease.

Splenic infarctions are common. Clot from the heart or valves lodges in the splenic circulation. Acute left upper quadrant pain may be the only symptom.

Hyposplenism results from congenital absence of the spleen, surgery, or autoinfarction splenectomy. Patients without a spleen function normally but seem to be more susceptible to infections with *Streptococcus* pneumonia. Prophylactic immunization is indicated.

RENAL DISEASES

Glomerular Diseases

Glomerular diseases present with variable manifestations. Hypertension and the nephrotic syndrome are common as are less specific complaints of malaise, fatigue, and weight loss. The patient may note smokey urine, present with uremia or massive edema. The urine in patients with glomerular disease typically will show protein loss and may show red cells and importantly, red cell casts. The latter almost always indicates glomerular disease.

The nephrotic syndrome most often is the result of a glomerular abnormality. Characteristically, there is the loss of more than 2 g of protein a day. The resultant hypoalbuminemia lead to decreased oncotic pressure and the development of significant edema without findings of congestive heart failure. Nephrosis results from intrinsic renal disease affecting the glomerulus, systemic diseases in which the glomerulus is an innocent bystander, and systemic diseases which result in increased

renal vein pressure such as constrictive pericarditis or severe right heart failure.

GLOMERULONEPHRITIS

Several pathologic events result in inflammatory dysfunction of the glomerulus. The filtering mechanism of the glomerulus can be damaged if the membrane is clogged with the immune complexes. The prototype here is poststreptococcal glomerulonephritis, especially streptococcal pharyngitis or dermatitis. This mechanism is also implicated in systemic lupus erythematosis, polyarteritis nodosa, Wegener's granulomatosis, some malignancies, and in the allergic glomerulonephritis of subacute bacterial endocarditis.

The basement membrane may, alternatively, be subject to direct antibody reaction as in Goodpasture's syndrome of pulmonary hemorrhage and glomerulonephritis. In this disease, antibodies which react with pulmonary tissue also react with the basement membrane of the glomerulus.

The glomerulus may also be injured by the deposition of fibrin in its loops. Many Type I allergic reactions may lead to such a state with interference with glomerular function.

Systemic diseases affect the glomerulus. The classic example is diabetes mellitus. Diabetic nephropathy shows characteristic changes in the glomerulus with resultant insufficiency and azotemia. Similarly, amyloid deposits will affect the kidney and commonly result in significant proteinuria and large kidneys from the infiltrative process.

The gold standard of diagnostic methods is a renal biopsy. The diseases are classified by the location and distribution of the glomerular lesions. Thin sections and often electronmicroscopic sections are required. Immunoflourescent staining may also indicate the pathogenic mechanisms.

Treatment is directed at the offending mechanism and often requires the use of corticosteroids or immunosuppressant drugs.

Vascular Diseases

Nephrosclerosis is the most common disease of a vascular nature which affects the kidneys. This disease presents pathologically as intimal proliferation of medium and large sized arterioles of the kidney. It is usually, but not always, associated with long standing hypertension. The clinical presentation is not very specific, often no more telling than mild to severe azotemia detected on laboratory screening.

An acute vasculitis of the kidneys accompanies malignant hypertension and is a cause of death in patients with progressive systemic sclerosis (scleroderma).

Arterial occlusion of the kidney most commonly occurs following embolic episodes from the heart. Rarely in situ thrombosis occurs at an area of stenosis. The patient complains of acute pain in the flank, fever, and shows hematuria and sometimes hypertension.

Renal vein thrombosis results from renal cell carcinoma or extension of phlebothrombosis of the inferior vena cava. The patient complains of pain and shows both proteinuria and hematuria. The prognosis is poor.

Tubular Diseases

The primary function of the renal tubules is to acidify and concentrate the urine. Disorders of tubules, then are suggested by the presence of urine which is neutral in pH and which fails to concentrate above a specific gravity of 1.01.

Acute tubular necrosis is a form or acute renal failure in which the tubules are primarily affected. The syndrome is common and has many causes. Drug toxicities are a common cause with antimicrobials, iodine (from contrast materials), and organic solvents such as carbon tetrachloride. Acute tubular necrosis may also follow crush injuries in which the kidney is called to filter large amounts of debris from rhabdomyolysis. Probably the most common cause however is shock from hemorrhage resulting in inadequate renal perfusion for a period of time.

Several mechanisms may be involved in the pathogenesis of acute tubular necrosis. Renal vasoconstriction, plugging of tubules with inspissated debris, and a back diffusion of ultrafiltrate through damaged membranes are often alluded to as causes. Clinically, the syndrome occurs from hours to days after the event. Although a fall in urine output is common, the syndrome may begin with normal or even increased urine flow. The urine however will be dilute and unacidified; early in the course of the disease the urine often shows desquamated tubular cells and red blood cells (rarely casts of red cells). Further, the urine will contain large amounts of sodium which will help to distinguish this from acute glomerular disease. Treatment consists of close control of fluid and electrolyte supplementation and a careful prophylaxis for infection which is the most common cause of death. Recovery will occur in about 70 percent of patients with uncomplicated disease. Dialysis is not usually needed.

RENAL TUBULAR ACIDOSIS

A distinctive variety of renal tubular disease is renal tubular acidosis (RTA). The disease is said to exist whenever the patient is found to have a metabolic acidosis as a result of the loss of sodium bicarbonate from the kidney.

Classic or distal (type I) renal tubular acidosis is severe, presents usually in childhood, and causes severe acidosis. The urine remains alkalotic even in the presence of severe acidosis. Growth retardation, rickets, and osteomalacia may be the initial complaints. It is usually caused as an autosomal dominant inherited disease but may also be the accompaniment of drug toxicity (amphotericin, gentamicin), immune disorders (Sjögren's disease, systemic lupus erythematosus SLE), or hyperparathyroidism. The laboratory shows acidosis with a normal anion gap. There will be renal wasting of sodium and potassium as well. Hypercalciuria is a constant feature and may declare itself as renal stones or nephrocalcinosis on x-ray. Treatment is directed at the underlying disorder if it can be identified and with the replacement of bicarbonate if it cannot.

Another variety of renal tubular acidosis is proximal (type II) RTA. In this disorder the defect is in acidification in the proximal tubule. Generally, less severe, the urine will become acid when metabolic acidosis occurs since the distal tubule can compensate somewhat. The disorder can be an accompaniment of amyloidosis, multiple myeloma, medullary cystic disease, or drug reactions (cadmium, lead, outdated tetracyclines). Treatment may require massive doses of alkali and potassium replacement.

Interstitial Disease

Renal outflow obstruction is responsible for about half of the cases of interstitial nephropathy. The obstruction is distal to the collecting system and may be anywhere downstream. Probably the most common cause is prostatic enlargement. Other causes include urethral strictures from trauma, infection, or congenital narrowing. Bilateral ureteral obstruction may result from retroperitoneal fibrosis which is idiopathic, the result of radiation, or rarely from drugs (Sansert) or from encroachment by enlarged nodes of malignant disease. The urinary tract proximal to the obstruction dilates and eventually the back pressure reduces glomerular filtration. The interstitium at first is edematous and eventually fibrotic. Gradual azotemia results often with few symptoms until the late stages of the disease. Infection often superimposes on the obstruction and may be the presenting complaint. With relief of obstruction a surprising degree of recovery often ensues.

Toxic nephropathies are another variety of interstitial disease. Heavy metal poisoning with mercury or arsenic or lead may result in interstitial nephropathy. Drugs are sometimes implicated. The most carefully researched is an entity known as analgesic associated nephropathy. Although circumstantial, the evidence strongly implicates long term heavy ingestion of phenacetin as etiologic. Patients, usually adult women with a long history of headache or other pain syndromes, present with insidiously developing complaints of gastrointestinal distress, fatigue, or hypertension. They may have episodes of acute pain when tips of papillae are sloughed and passed. Treatment is withdrawal of the agent.

Another category of interstitial disease is allergic nephropathy as a reaction to drugs or some toxins. The biopsy will show diffuse infiltration with chronic inflammatory cells and occasionally eosinophils. Nephrosis often accompanies this disease with or without oliguria and azotemia. Interstitial nephropathy is also seen with chronic hyperuricemia and sometimes for no known reason.

Infectious Diseases

Urinary tract infections are extremely common. It is important to discern if the infection is confined to the bladder or extends to the renal parenchyma. Infections are frequently asymptomatic and are an important cause of chronic renal failure. Females predominate and predisposing features include diabetes mellitus, obstruction to flow, or instrumentation.

Cystitis presents with frequency, urgency, burning, and small volume voiding. Systemic symptoms are mild. The urine shows white cells and bacteriuria but no white blood cell casts.

Pyelonephritis is infection of the kidney and usually is acquired in a retrograde fashion from below. In acute disease, the patient is ill with high fever, flank pain, and often dysuriia. In addition to bacteriuria the urine shows white blood cell casts. Therapy requires appropriate antibiotics, fluid replacement, and attention to any inciting disease such as diabetes or obstruction to flow such as a stone, prostatic enlargement, or tumor. Chronic pyelonephritis represents a significant cause of renal failure, may be asymptomatic and show only chronic pyuria. Sterile pyuria should alert the clinician to the possibility of renal tuberculosis.

NEPRHOLITHIASIS

Stones have many sources. When they pass through the ureter the symptom complex is characteristic. The pain is severe, colicky, and tends to move as the stone moves. First felt in the flank it later moves to the lower quadrant and then to the groin or testicle. The urine shows hematuria and mild proteinuria. Stones may be calcium as in hyperparathryoidism, oxalate as in hyperoxaluria, uric acid from hyperuricosuria (radiolucent), or mixed from a chronic nidus of infection.

Treatment is expectant since most stones will pass spontaneously with the assistance of fluid loading and analgesics. Occasionally retrograde removal or laparotomy is necessary. Associated infection must be specifically treated.

Polycystic Renal Disease

This is the most common congenital disorder of the kidneys. This autosomal dominant disease is thought to be a fetal failure of cortical medullary match-up. Cysts develop which gradually enlarge eventually causing renal enlargement, bleeding, pain, and infection. Symptoms may not appear until the fourth or fifth decade.

Renal Cell Cancer

The incidence of this cancer rises sharply after age 40 and although comprising less than 1 percent of malignancies it frequently presents with unusual features. Patients with renal cell cancers may present with fever, polycythemia, unexplained leukocytosis, hypercalcemia from ectopic parathyroid hormone production, or nonmetastatic liver function abnormalities. The tumor has a propensity to invade and occlude the renal vein and inferior vena cava. Primary treatment is surgical. Chemotherapy is palliative.

FLUID, ELECTROLYTES, AND ACID BASE DISORDERS

The osmolality of the extracellular fluid is maintained within very narrow limits. Normally, the serum osmolality is 280 mosm/L. The homeostatic mechanisms consist of thirst and the action of the antidiuretic hormone (ADH) from the posterior pituitary. The most common threat is hyperosmolality which is combatted by an increase in thirst and the secretion of ADH which promotes renal fluid retention.

Hyponatremia accompanies hypo-osmolality and usually results from the stronger drive to maintain volume status. Thus, following severe fluid loss the body will sacrifice osmolality in order to maintain volume. A deficiency of ADH, or cortisol and mineralocorticoids or of thyroid will also result in hyponatremia. Hyponatremia can also result from fluid excess as in psychogenic water drinking or the inappropriate secretion of ADH (SIADH). The loss of sodium through sweat, diarrhea, vomiting, or diuretics with free access of water also results in a low sodium concentration.

Hypernatremia, on the other hand, will result from free water loss as in the absence of ADH or following an osmotic diuresis such as severe hyperglycemia. Burns, hyperventilation with fever, osmotic diarrhea, and the absence of thirst also yield hypernatremia.

Potassium exists predominantly within cells. Serum potassium levels will fall with diuretic use where it is exchanged for sodium in the renal tubule. In alkalotic states, hydrogen ion will exit cells and potassium will replace it. A check of urine potassium tells if the hypokalemia is the result of renal potassium loss when the concentration in the urine exceeds 40 mEq/L. Complications of hypokalemia predominantly involve neuromuscular and cardiac activity. Patients will complain of muscle cramps and weakness and may be found to have cardiac arrhythmias.

Potassium excess results when the ion is shifted out of cells as in acidosis. Hyperkalemia also occurs with hemolysis of red cells, rhabdomyolysis, and the use of aldosterone antagonists such as spironolactone. Hyperkalemia interferes with cardiac excitation first showing as peaked T waves later producing heart block and standstill.

The pH of arterial blood is carefully maintained at 7.4 through a delicate balance of renal and pulmonary determined homeostasis. The usual metabolic threat is acidosis. Both acidosis and alkalosis is countered by buffers of bicarbonate carbonic acid, phosphates, and proteins.

Metabolic acidosis is defined as an acid pH and a depressed level of bicarbonate. The normal acid load of metabolism is buffer by the bicarbonate system and excreted by the kidney which in the process regenerates the bicarbonate. Acid loads of diabetic ketoacidosis, lactic acidosis, or the ingestion of acid overwhelm the system and result in metabolic acidosis. The compensatory mechanisms include the elaboration of additional bicarbonate by the kidney and hyperventilation which blows off CO_2. The kidney will attempt additional unloading of acid through the use of phosphate buffers and ammonia. Some of the additional acid may be converted by the liver to bicarbonate.

Metabolic alkalosis is defined by an elevated pH and an excess of bicarbonate. It may result from gastrointestinal or renal loss of H^+ ion, the intracellular shift of H^+ ion as in hypokalemia, alkali ingestion, or a high renal threshold for bicarbonate. The latter will be seen in potassium depletion, hypercalcemia, and chloride depletion with hypovolemia. The most common clinical cause of metabolic acidosis is the use of diuretics. Compensatory mechanisms include the involvement of tissue buffers, the renal loss of bicarbonate, and perhaps a small contribution from hypoventilation to retain CO_2.

Respiratory acidosis is defined by an elevated CO_2 concentration and acidosis. This always implies alveolar hypoventilation. Since carbon dioxide is so readily diffusible, retention can only come about if a large number of alveoli are not ventilated. It most commonly occurs from chronic lung disease but may also come about as the result of central nervous system disease, airway obstruction, or pneumothorax. Compensation depends on the renal generation and retention of additional bicarbonate. This takes 3 to 5 days in the acute state.

Respiratory alkalosis is defined by an elevated pH and a low carbon dioxide. It results from hyperventilation which may be psychogenic or may be induced by some drugs or central nervous system diseases. It is compensated for by additional renal excretion of bicarbonate.

ENDOCRINE DISEASES

Most endocrine diseases are the result of too little or too much of a given hormone. The disturbance may result from an abnormality of the specific gland itself or a disturbance of its servomechanism (i.e., positive and negative feedback controls). Rarely the disturbance is the result of an abnormal hormone, target organ unresponsiveness (pseudohypoparathyroidism), target organ overresponsiveness (virilizing syndrome), or interfering substances.

Because of their systemic influences, endocrine diseases share many common symptoms such as weakness, fatigue, menstural changes, weight changes, impotence, hypertension, or abnormal growth patterns.

Hypothalamus

Neurosecretory cells here stimulate the pituitary with releasing hormones such as thyroid releasing hormone (TRH), luteinizing hormone releasing hormone, (LHRH), and somatostatin which inhibits the release of growth hormone. TRH has the additional effect of stimulating prolactin release.

Pituitary (Adenohypophysis)

Originating from Rathke's pouch, these specialized cells provide master control for several glands. Tumors of this region may release uninhibited amounts of growth hormone leading to giantism or acromegaly. Other tumors may not release any hormones but will cause destruction of the normal cells leading to panhypopituitarism with insufficiency of growth hormone, adrenocorticotropic hormone (ACTH), luteinizing hormone (LH), and follicle stimulating hormone (FSH). Tumors here will also cause bitemporal loss of vision because of the proximity to the optic nerves. Tumors of the pituitary are either microadenomas of secretory cells or neoplasms of the original pouch (craniopharyngiomas). The anterior pituitary may also be destroyed by infarction following a postpartum hemorrhage (Sheehan's syndrome).

Pituitary (Neurohypophysis)

Cells here are of neural crest origin and are known to produce vasopressin or antidiuretic hormone. This hormone responds to changes in osmotic pressure in the serum. When the pressure rises, the hormone is released and effects the tubules of the kidney to conserve water.

Loss of this hormone leads to diabetes insipidus with a profound diuresis, dehydration, hypertonicity, and collapse if the deficiency is complete. Partial deficiency is more common. This may be effectively treated with sulfonylureas which increase the effectiveness of the hormone. In complete deficiency the patient requires replacement by vasopressin either insufflated or injected.

The syndrome of inappropriate antidiuretic hormone (SIADH) is fairly common. Many tumors, especially of the lung, secrete this hormone. The sustained release of the hormone causes water retention, hyponatremia, and hypo-osmolality. This may lead to seizures. The condition is diagnosed by finding urine which is inappropriately concentrated when compared with the osmolarity of the serum. Other conditions which may lead to SIADH include pulmonary diseases such as tuberculosis, some drugs and head trauma or brain disease such as meningitis. It is treated by water restriction.

Thyroid Diseases

Hypothyroidism is the result of an absolute or relative deficiency of thyroid hormone. It may be the result of inadequate amounts of thyroid releasing hormone from the pituitary (secondary hypothyroidism) or primary disease of the gland itself. Primary hypothyroidism is usually associated with a large gland while secondary hypothyroidism is not.

Whatever the cause, the symptoms are those of a hypometabolic state. Fatigue, lassitude, weight change, thickening of the skin, deepening of the voice, constipation, slow relaxing reflexes, puffy myxedematous skin, and frequently the loss of the lateral third of the eyebrows.

Causes of primary failure include deficiency of iodine, congenital abnormalities of the synthesis of the thyroid hormone, inflammation of the gland (acute thyroiditis or chronic Hashimoto's thyroiditis), or following surgery or radiation of the gland.

The diagnosis is established by finding low levels of thyroid hormone. Primary versus secondary is determined by the level of the thyroid stimulating hormone (TSH).

Hyperthyroidism is most commonly the result of Graves' disease. This disease consists of hyperthyroidism, goiter, and ophthalmopathy. The gland is diffusely and symmetrically enlarged and proptosis is evident. The patient will complain of nervousness, irritability, fatigue, heat intolerance, and frequently oligomenorrhea, palpitations, sweating, and tremor. It is a disease of women (7:1) and may be immunologic in origin.

A toxic nodular goiter may produce hyperthyroidism. Autonomous nodules pour out thyroid hormone which does not respond to control by TSH.

The diagnosis is established by finding high levels of thyroid hormone, occasionally high levels of tri-iodinated thyroid hormone, and very high uptake by radioactive scanning of the gland.

The hyperthyroid gland may be treated by extirpation, radioactive iodine administration, or the use of antithyroid drugs which interfere with the production of the hormone. β-Blockers may assist in the acute phases to reduce the hyperadrenergic state.

Thyroid Cancer

The most common thyroid cancer is a papillary carcinoma. This slow indolent cancer spreads most commonly to regional nodes, is common in younger age groups, and is consistent with a long survival when treated surgically and with thyroid replacement.

Follicular carcinoma is less common, spreads hematogenously and frequently is active enough to take up radioactive iodine which when given in large doses may be therapeutic.

Anaplastic cancers of the thyroid are extremely aggressive, more common in the elderly, and usually fatal.

Adrenal Cortex

Cushing's syndrome is the term for unmodulated excretion of corticosteroids from the adrenal. The original disease was described as a result of a pituitary adenoma with hypersecretion of ACTH. Currently the syndrome name is applied to any condition resulting in hypersecretion.

Cushing's syndrome may arise from an adrenal adenoma, unilateral or bilateral. Adrenal cancers may be endocrinologically active and tumors of other tissues may result in high levels of ACTH with resultant hypersecretion.

Whatever the etiology, the patient with Cushing's syndrome develops centripetal obesity, fatigue, muscle weakness, hirsutism, moon facies, a buffalo hump over the upper thoracic spine, ecchkymoses, and pigmented striae.

The diagnosis rests on the finding of elevated levels of cortisol which are unmodulated. This is determined by showing no reduction in levels following the exogenous administration of cortisone. Measurement of ACTH levels permits the determination of primary v secondary hypercortisism. Treatment for adrenal adenomas is surgery which may be effective as well for nonmetastatic carcinoma.

Hyperaldosteronism results when an offending adenoma secretes this hormone. Seventy-five percent of these cases are the result of unilateral adenomas of the adrenal. The patient presents with mild hypertension, a low potassium and an elevated serum bicarbonate. In spite of the salt and water retaining properties of aldosterone, these patients do not show edema. The diagnosis is suggested by the finding of elevated levels of aldosterone when corrected for the sodium balance. The treatment of choice is surgery although some patients are well controlled with the use of aldosterone antagonists.

Addison's disease is the inadequate production of corticosteroids from the adrenal. The most common cause of such destruction of the adrenals is an autoimmune process. In this context other autoimmune disease may also be present such as pernicious anemia and Hashimoto's thyroiditis. In earlier years, tuberculous destruction of the adrenals was common.

The patient with Addison's disease complains of fatigue, weight loss, nausea, and vomiting. Because of the very high levels of ACTH, they will be hyperpigmented. The deficient release of aldosterone leads to hypotension and hyperkalemia. A low cortisol level which does not increase with the infusion of ACTH suggests the diagnosis. It is treated with replacement of corticosteroids.

Pheochromocytoma is a rare lesion of the adrenal medulla. The overproduction of epinephrine or norepinephrine leads to sustained or paroxysmal hypertension. It is an important cause of reversible hypertension and although rare needs to be considered in all hypertensive patients. Fifty percent of pheochromocytomas are located in the adrenal and 6 percent are malignant. In addition to hypertension, patients complain of sweats, episodes of pallor with nausea, and abdominal pain. Patients may be hypoglycemic. The measurement of catecholamines in the urine together with CT scanning will usually establish the diagnosis. The nonadrenal pheochromocytomas may be located anywhere that neural crest cells are located.

Treatment of pheochromocytoma is preferentially surgery when the lesion can be extirpated. α-Blockade with dibenzyline and β-blockade with any of several such agents may prove symptomatically helpful.

Parathyroid Diseases

The parathyroid glands which are four in number and located behind the thyroid are responsible for the release of parathyroid hormone. The hormone responds to the level of ionized calcium in the plasma which provides a negative feedback.

Parathyroid hormone acts to increase the renal excretion of phosphorus, and increase the level of calcium in the blood by increasing gastrointestinal absorption and encouraging activity by osteoclasts to release calcium from the bone.

These glands also secrete calcitonin which comes from the parafollicular cells. This hormone opposes the action of parathyroid hormone but its role is probably minor.

The unopposed secretion of parathyroid hormone results in hyperparathyroidism. The elevated calcium and depressed phosphorus levels are accompanied by the clinical syndrome of fatigue, lassitude, weakness, apathy and depression often with pruritus, arrhythmias, renal stones, and osteoporosis. The disease is more common in women and is most often the result of a single adenoma.

The diagnosis is established by the finding of elevated calcium, depressed phosphorus, and elevated parathyroid hormone levels. The treatment of the hypercalcemia may be a medical emergency if the level is quite high. Large volumes of fluids with a forced diuresis is effective. Mithramycin therapy paralyzes osteoclastic activity and lowers calcium. The definitive step is surgery.

Diabetes Mellitus

Diabetes mellitus is a relative or absolute deficiency of insulin. This hormone, secreted by the β-cells of the pancreas responds to the level of blood sugar. It is opposed by glucagon which serves to increase the level of glucose.

The normal action of insulin is to facilitate the passage of glucose across the cell membrane and enhance the synthesis of glycogen, the uptake of amino acids, and lipogenesis. If the cellular supply of glucose is deficient, glucagon secretion increases blood glucose.

An important concept in the understanding of diabetes has been developed (i.e., insulin receptors located on cells provide a binding point for insulin and are critical for insulin to be active). Diabetes may result from inadequate secretion of insulin from the pancreas or by a reduction in the number of functioning receptor sites on cells.

Type I diabetes is insulin requiring diabetes previously called juvenile diabetes, while type II diabetes is noninsulin dependent. Type I usually onsets in childhood or young adult years, occurs suddenly, requires insulin therapy, and is prone to develop ketoacidosis. Type II is often asymptomatic, onsets in the 40s, has low likelihood of ketoacidosis, and has a strong hereditary predilection.

Insulin levels may be quite high in type II diabetes in the presence of insulin resistance. Insulin binding sites may be deficient in number or may be occupied by anti-insulin binding site antibodies. Levels of insulin are low in type I diabetes and in the forms of diabetes related to known diseases of the pancreas such as chronic pancreatitis or postpancreatectomy.

The complications of diabetes are legion. The vascular complications involve both large and small vessels. Large vessels develop premature atherosclerosis. The small vessel microangiopathy is characterized by thickening of the basement membrane and proliferation of small vessels. When this occurs in the eye as retinopathy the result is microaneurysm formation with hemorrhages and exudates and blindness. Diabetic nephropathy is the vascular disease of the kidneys. The glomeruli show marked thickening of the basement membranes and the patient develops hypertension and renal failure.

The nervous system is subject to important complications. Most common is a sensory neuropathy. Stocking glove paresthesias are common in the adult. Cranial nerve palsies may appear and may be the initial manifestation of diabetes. The vascular disease may affect the vasa nervorum with resultant infarction of a nerve producing diabetic amyotrophy, a painful sometimes motor deficiency which is unilateral.

Diabetic ketoacidosis is a life threatening complication. The lack of insulin allows marked hyperglycemia. This promotes an osmotic diuresis and dehydration. The cells sense starvation of glucose and resort to the use of lipids for energy. Lipolysis frees fatty acids for the liver which converts these to ketones such as β-hydroxybutyrate and acetoacetate. The more effective use of the free fatty acids requires small amounts of insulin. The ketones are acidic and the blood pH subsequently falls.

Hyperosmolar nonketotic coma may be seen in the older patient. It is presumed that small amounts of insulin are present in these circumstances and the acidosis is thereby avoided. Coma results from the very high glucose levels and dehydration which produce a hyperosmolar state.

The treatment of type I diabetes and diabetic ketoacidosis requires insulin. In ketoacidosis the dehydration must be corrected. Constant infusion of insulin is gaining favor as the modality to correct ketoacidosis. Potassium loss is also prevalent and must be corrected. Once the ketoacidosis is corrected, the patient needs education, dietary instruction, and a program of insulin injections which meets his/her requirements.

Type II diabetes frequently responds to dietary control. When this is inadequate oral hypoglycemic agents may be used. Most of these are sulfonylurea derivatives. There is some evidence that these drugs may accelerate atherosclerosis.

Gonadal Disorders

Klinefelter's syndrome is an inherited disorder in which there is duplication of the X chromosome in phenotypical males. The XXY complement results in a hypergonadotropic hypogonadism. It occurs in approximately 1 in 500 male births and is therefore quite common. Patients so afflicted have small firm sclerotic testes

and present with arrested pubertal development. They may appear quite eunuchoid or have fairly normal appearance because of the variable penetrance of the disorder. Gynecomastia, absence of facial or body hair, and a female escutcheon are the most blatant expressions of the disorder.

Infection (bilateral mumps orchitis) or trauma may also result in hypergonadotropic hypogonadism. Because the seminiferous tubules are primarily affected in mumps, sperm production is depressed. Testosterone loss is usually less marked.

Hypogonadotropic hypogonadism is of course the result of deficient pituitary drive to the testes. One peculiar variety is the Kallmanns' syndrome of anosmia and hypogonadism which occurs independently of other pituitary deficiencies. Any disorder of the pituitary may result in hypogonadotropism such as tumor or infarction. If prepubertal, the result is eunuchism, if postpubertal, ammenorrhea and impotence results.

Primary ammenorrhea is the absence of spontaneous menarche by age 16. Primary disorders causing this syndrome include Turner's syndrome XO, gonadal dysgenesis of XX or XY karyotypes or true hemaphroditism, and the polycystic ovary syndrome. Patients with Turner's syndrome have associated body habitus abnormalities of webbed neck and high carying angle of the arms together with the absence of the Barr body in the buccal smear. Patients with testicular feminization are unresponsive to normal testosterone and as a consequence develop into phenotypical females but have no uterus and therefore are ammenorrheic. Primary ammenorrhea will of course occur with prebuteral pituitary ablation of LH and FSH from tumors.

Secondary ammenorrhea presents a more difficult differential diagnosis. The diagnosis of pregnancy must of course be excluded. In the United States a very common cause is anorexia nervosa, a psychiatric disorder of profound weight loss and abnormal hypothalamic (pituitary) control mechanisms. Vigorous prolonged exercise may also predispose to secondary ammenorrhea as in marathon runners. The mechanism is unclear. Finally, premature menopause may account for secondary ammenorrhea. Usual menopause occurs in the fifth decade but in some much earlier. In these patients the syndrome is accompanied by profound elevations of gonadotropins while in the others levels are depressed.

Polycystic ovarian disease is a form of secondary ammenorrhea which is preceded by a period of oligomenorrhea. Associated findings include a variable amount of hirsutism, acne, and obesity. LH is elevated, FSH is depressed, and production rates of testosterone are characteristically elevated. Infertility is common and may be related to failure to release ova from the gonad. The capsule of the ovary becomes thickened in this disorder.

Neoplasms of the Reproductive Tract

Prostatic carcinoma follows only lung cancer in prevalence. It is strikingly a disease of advanced years with 90 percent of cases appearing after age 60. Most have metastases at the time of diagnosis. The favored site of metastases is bone and in such cases an elevated acid phosphatase is helpful although there are about 10 percent false positives and false negatives with this test. The bone metastases are usually osteoblastic and readily evident on plain films. Radical prostatectomy in the absence of metastases offers the chance of cure. This is sometimes accompanied by extensive pelvic lymphadenectomy. Once metastatic, palliation is possible through the use of hormonal manipulation designed to reduce the levels or effect of testosterone. Ochiectomy or the administration of exogenous estrogens are equally effective. No advantage is gained by using both measures.

Testicular cancer, on the other hand has a high cure rate even when metastatic. The peak incidence is in the 20s to 30s although the incidence is low (1 percent of male cancers). These are tumors of germ cells. These pluripotential cells may then manifest as tumors of most any variety. Broadly, they are divided into seminoma and nonseminoma. Nonseminoma tumors may appear as teratomas with a variety of cell elements, embryonal cell carcinoma or undifferentiated cancer. Half are seminomas for which radiation therapy is highly effective even with metastases. Localized disease of course is best treated with orchiectomy. Nonseminomas require more aggressive combinations of treatment. Helpful parameters to follow in this disease are levels of α-fetoprotein, or human chorionic gonadotropin either, or both, which may be elaborated by the tumor and can serve as a marker of progression or recurrence. Multiple chemotherapeutic agents together with surgery and radiation affords cure in 75 percent of patients with nonseminomas. The only known predisposing feature of testicular cancer is cryptorchism which increases the risk by 30 to 40 fold.

Cervical cancer has had a marked reduction in mortality owing to the widespread use of the Pap smear for early detection. Predisposing factors include early onset of sexual activity, early pregnancy, type II herpes virus, and multiple sexual partners. Squamous dysplasia occurs first followed by carcinoma in situ and later frank squamous cell cancer which will metastasize first to local nodes and later widely. Conization of the cervix or hysterectomy is the treatment of choice for localized disease. More extensive involvement requires a more radical form of surgery or radiation. Extensive disease responds only partially to multiple chemotherapies.

Ovarian cancer is less common but appears to be increasing in frequency. Most tumors are epithelial in origin; only 3 to 4 percent are germ cell in origin. The disease is characteristically silent until widespread or very large. Often, the presenting finding is of a large pelvic mass since cystic developments are common. Surgery is recommended for almost all patients even when the disease has spilled into the peritoneum. There is evidence that removal of large tumor mass allows more effective treatment with chemotheapy. Cure is possible and increased survival common with multiple chemotherapies.

Endometrial cancer is more common. Associations with obesity, hypertension, and diabetes are well known as is the association with polycystic ovarian disease. Exogenous estrogens may predispose to endometrial cancer while combinations of estrogen and progesterone may be protective. Vaginal bleeding is the most common early symptom. The early diagnosis is best obtained through curettage of the endometrium. Surgery, radiation, and chemotherapy are all used depending on the stage of the disease.

INFECTIOUS DISEASES

Infectious diseases are the purview of every practicing physician regardless of the discipline. The spectrum of offending organisms and clinical pictures varies widely and great strides are continually made in improving diagnosis and therapy with substantial reductions of morbidity and mortality (Table 9-1).

Most infectious processes involve a reservoir, a vector, and a host. Many times each is separate but one organism may be any of the two or all three. The organisms responsible for causing disease vary in infectivity and virulence. Some agents are extremely infectious such as

Table 9-1. The Diverse Nature of Infecting Agents

Agent	Size (μm)	Extracellular
Virus	0.1	No
Mycoplasma	0.25	Yes
Chlamydia	0.3	No
Rickettsia	0.45	No
Bacteria	1.0	Yes
Actinomyces	1.0	Yes
Fungus	4.0	Yes
Protozoa	40.0	Yes
Helminths	1.0	Yes

chicken pox while others lack ease of transmission such as leprosy and tuberculosis.

The virulence of an organism is a function of the invader itself and the condition of the host being attacked. Rabies is highly virulent in even the healthiest host. The immunosuppressed host may be a fatal victim of an otherwise low virulence infectant.

Virulence of the organism is related to its ability to invade tissue, a property which is facilitated by enzymes and protective coatings such as the antiphagocytic coatings of some bacteria. Further damaging effects occur as a result of toxins elaborated by the organism. These diffusable exotoxins cause effects remote from the site of infection. Similarly, virulence may be facilitated by the hosts own response to infection. The classic example here is reactivation tuberculosis where the damage is as much a result of the host sensitization as it is of the mycobacterium itself.

The human organisms resistance relates to the integrity of skin and mucous membranes, the ability to phagocytose invaders, the ability to elaborate humoral antibodies, and the ability to mobilize cellular immunity of thymus origin. Burns, neutropenia, chemotherapy for cancer, steroids, and general debility will interfere with these mechanisms.

Viral Diseases

Viruses are small obligate intracellular organisms which contain either RNA or DNA wrapped in a capsid. They capture the cell's synthetic ability and force replication and subsequent release of new infective particles. Antibiotics are ineffective. Infected cells may produce interferon, a nonspecific substance which aids cellular resistance to invasion. Humoral immunity generally results from viral infections.

The herpes viruses cause a variety of diseases. Herpes I is responsible for cold sores and keratitis. Herpes II causes genital herpes. Both types tend to remain dormant within cells and recur at irregular intervals. With depressed immunity they may disseminate to widespread skin or central nervous system disease.

Varicella is also a herpes virus and is responsible for chickenpox in children and herpes zoster in the adult. Chickenpox has an incubation of about 2 weeks following which there is the development of a rash which becomes vesicular within a day. The lesions come in crops and the disease is usually mild. Zoster is a disease of adults. The virus resides in a sensory nerve root and causes intense pain and vesicles in a dermatomal distribution.

Cytomegalovirus leads to a serious disease in children. They become systemically ill frequently with jaundice and fever. It may also result in chorioretinitis and neurologic damage.

EB virus most often is the cause of infectious mononucleosis in young adults. A prodrome of sore throat and fever develops into a full blown systemic illness with malaise, fatigue, myalgias, occasional nausea and vomiting, and lymphadenopathy. Laboratory studies will show atypical lymphocytes, heterophile antibodies which will agglutinate sheep red blood cells, and sometimes abnormal liver function tests. The disease is self-limiting. Steroids are occasionally necessary if splenomegaly is significant. This virus has also been implicated as the cause of Burkitt's lymphoma in Africa and elsewhere.

Influenza virus is an RNA virus and tends to appear in cycles. It is notorius for changing its antigenic qualities in subtle ways which allow hosts to be reinfected. The incubation period for disease is a few days following which fever appears abruptly together with chills, malaise, myalgias, and dry cough. The duration is about a week with complete resolution although a secondary pneumonia may complicate the disease. Killed virus vaccines are recommended annually for those strains most likely to appear.

Mumps virus affects predominantly children. The syndrome of parotitis and low grade fever appears 18 days after exposure. Occasionally the infection involves the testis or pancreas and may cause sterility. With pancreatitis or parotitis the serum amylase is elevated. The disease is mild.

Measles is an exanthematous disease of children. Contagion is by respiratory droplets and appears with an incubation period of about 2 weeks. Initial coryza fever conjunctivitis and photophobia develops into a diffuse rash 4 days later. The disease is contagious before the rash appears and it can be a serious illness. Koplik spots are pathognomonic and are recognized as small red spots usually on the buccal or larial mucosa of the mouth.

Rabies is a viral disease transmitted to man by animal saliva. The disease exists endemically in many animal populations in the United States and the most common contacts which pass rabies to man are racoon, skunks, bats, and foxes. The disease is almost uniformly fatal.

Following a bite by a rabid animal, the patient first notes paresthesias at the site. As the virus ascends the nerve root, progressive increase in motor tone results with tetanic contractions followed by flaccid paralysis and death. The term hydrophobia relates to the tetanic contractions of the pharynx which result with attempts to swallow.

The diagnosis can be ascertained by a positive fluorescent rabies antibody (FRA) test applied to biopsied tissue. The only treatment is prophylaxis. An initial injection of rabies immune globulin is followed by serial injections of human diploid cell rabies vaccine.

The enterovirus group consists of the polio virus, coxsackie group, and ECHO virus. They are frequent causes of gastroenteritis with diarrhea and vomiting which is self-limiting.

Polio virus, following the gastroenteritis, may develop into a rapidly ascending paralysis involving motor and cranial nerves. The trivalent oral polio vaccine, which is a live virus, has been responsible for a markedly reduced incidence of polio in the United States.

Coxsackie A virus causes herpangina which is a painful ulcerative disease of the mouth. Small erythematous papules which may ulcerate and which are located anywhere on the buccal mucosa suggest the diagnosis. Coxsackie B virus causes pleurodynia. This form of pleurisy is most often seen in the summer and early fall months. Pleural effusion is rare and the disease lasts about a week. This virus can also cause myocarditis with pain, arrythmias, occasional congestive heart failure, and rarely long term cardiomyopathy.

Chlamydia, Mycoplasma, and Rickettsia

Chlamydia is an obligate intracellular organism which has both RNA and DNA, a cell wall, and is susceptible to antibiotics. *Chlamydia psittaci* cause psittacosis, a respiratory infection transmitted by birds, and *Chlamydia trachomitis* causes trachoma, a leading cause of blindness, and nongonococcal urethritis. It can be diagnosed by a complement fixation test and is treated with tetracycline, erythromycin, or sulfa drugs.

Mycoplasma is a fastidious organism which will grow in a cell free extract with difficulty. The organism possesses no cell wall. It causes primary atypical pneumonia (PAP) in young adults. The syndrome consists of mild fever, cough, and an infiltrate on chest x-ray. Half of the patients develop cold agglutinins which help in the diagnosis. The clinical course may be shortened with the use of tetracycline. A complement fixation test helps establish the diagnosis.

Rickettsia organisms are intracellular and usually cause a vasculitis. The most important disease caused by the *Rickettsia* is Rocky Mountain spotted fever. Transmitted by ticks, the responsible rickettsia lead to a syndrome of rash involving first the palms and soles. The rash spreads centrally and is followed by fever, headache, myalgias, abdominal pain, and occasionally disseminated intravascular coagulation. The diagnosis is supported by the finding of nonspecific antibodies which will agglutinate proteus bacteria type OX-2 and OX-19 (Weil-Felix reaction). A complement fixation test is

more definitive but may not be positive until late in the disease. Tetracycline and chloramphenicol are effective antibiotics.

Bacterial Disease

Bacteria possess DNA and ribosomes together with a well defined cell wall but still have no defined nucleus. They divide by binary fission. Some bacteria can form spores (clostridia) which provide a dormant state.

Bacteria are classified according to shape (i.e., cocci, bacilli, or pleomorphic), and by staining characteristics (i.e., gram-positive, gram-negative, or acid fast). Further classification includes oxygen requirements (i.e., aerobic, microaerophilic, or anaerobic).

Pneumococci (*Streptococcus pneumoniae*) are gram-positive cocci. They have a protective polysaccharide capsule which resists phagocytosis. This same capsule prevents the organism from being destructive to tissue and impedes its ability to spread rapidly throughout tissue. It is the most common cause of adult pneumonia which is a lobar variety and presents with fever, chills, cough, and sputum production. Pneumococci are an important cause of meningitis in the adult and also may be a cause of septicemia. Rarely the organism will infect a joint or the middle ear. The organism is routinely sensitive to penicillin and grows readily in the diagnostic laboratory. An extract of the capsular polysaccharides is available as a vaccine. The vaccine affords 80 percent protection and is best used in the elderly, those with chronic lung disease, after splenectomy, and for immunosuppressed patients.

Staphylococci cause great human misery. These gram-positive cocci vary in virulence from the near saprophytic. *Staphylococcus epidermidis* to the aggressive *Staphylococcus aureus*. They produce their effects through the immediate invasion of tissue and the elaboration of potent exotoxins. A common manifestation is furuncles and boils especially in diabetic patients. They cause cellulitis, bacteremia, endocarditis, destructive bronchopneumonia, metastatic abscesses, osteomyelitis, septic arthritis, and food poisoning. The latter is through the elaboration of exotoxin, in contaminated food, producing profound diarrhea and vomiting when ingested. Staphylococci are an important form of hospital acquired infections. Some are sensitive to penicillin but the more dangerous varieties elaborate penicillinase and some are resistant to semisynthetic penicillins. Therapy is best directed by the results of sensitivity testing in the laboratory.

Streptococci are gram-positive cocci which grow in chains in the laboratory. They produce a variety of diseases related to their ability to spread rapidly in tissues, which is facilitated by their elaboration of enzymes such as streptokinase. Further, they can precipitate dangerous host reactions as in rheumatic heart disease and glomerulonephritis.

Viridans and Group D streptococci are important agents in subacute bacterial endocarditis. The bacteria form a nidus on previously damaged heart valves and slowly produce progressive destruction of the valve (most often the aortic or mitral valve). The disease may be indolent, producing malaise, low grade fever, night sweats, and weight loss. The finding of splenomegaly, murmur, fever, and splinter hemorrhages under the nails or in the conjunctiva suggest the diagnosis. The organism is susceptible to penicillin which must be given from 4 to 6 weeks parenterally.

Group B streptococcus causes neonatal sepsis and meningitis. Group A streptococcus is the usual cause of tonsillitis and may lead to scarlet fever, rheumatic fever, or glomerulonephritis. Streptococcal infections of the skin may be in the form of erysipelas or impetigo. Erysipelas is a toxic disease of abrupt onset. A small area of cellulitis may produce a very sick patient with high fever and toxicity. Impetigo, a more indolent disease of children, demonstrates chronic nodular lesions of the skin which may be pruritic and are contagious.

Rheumatic fever occurs 1 to 5 weeks after a streptococcal pharyngitis. It does not occur after skin infection. The hallmarks of acute rheumatic fever include signs of carditis, migratory polyarthritis, chorea (St. Vitus' dance), subcutaneous nodules, and erythema marginatum. The latter is a painless evanescent, macular, faintly red rash which looks like smoke rings. The disease is probably caused by the cross-reactivity of antibodies directed against the streptococcus which affects myocardial tissue. The acute disease is treated with aspirin and rarely requires corticosteroids. Long-standing disease may cause valvular lesions requiring surgical repair.

Acute poststreptococcal glomerulonephritis follows either skin or throat infection. Two weeks after the episode the patient develops hypertension, fluid retention with edema, and a typical urine sediment of glomerulonephritis. Most patients recover completely.

Neisseria are gram-positive, lancet-shaped diplococci. Gonorrhea, meningitis, and gonococcemia are the major manifestations of infection. Gonorrhea is a venereal disease. In the male the disease produces a urethritis with pain on urination and a discharge. Women may be asymptomatic. During menses, the organism can migrate from the cervix up the fallopian tubes and produce an abscess and sterility.

Neisseria meningitis affects young adults frequently in the military or schools. A fulminant bacteremia associated with the meningitis can be fatal. The patient shows evidence of disseminated intravascular coagulation, skin rash of petechiae and purpura, and may suffer adrenal hemorrhage and collapse. It has a 20 percent mortality.

A milder form of gonococcemia can follow gonorrhea. Skin lesions will be evident and the organism then has a predilection for joints, especially the small joints of the hands and feet.

The neisseria is a fastidious organism and difficult to grow in the laboratory. It is treated with penicillin. Prophylaxis for those who contact a patient with meningitis interestingly is ineffective with penicillin. Rifampin is the drug of choice.

Salmonella, Shigella, and Cholera

Salmonella are gram-negative bacilli with a reservoir in fowl, turtles, and poultry products. The usual gastrointestinal salmonellosis (*S enteritidis*) appears within 24 hours of ingestion and consists of fever, abdominal pain, and diarrhea. A stool smear will show white blood cells and the organism is readily cultured. If seriously ill, patients can be treated with chloramphenicol. Most require no antibiotics.

Salmonella typhi causes typhoid fever a somewhat more serious illness. Man is the primary resevoir and it is spread by fecal contact. An incubation period of 10 days results in the development of fever, headache, abdominal pain, and usually, constipation. The patient will demonstrate abdominal tenderness, splenomegaly, bradycardia, and a faint erythematous trunkal rash. The liver may also be enlarged and abnormal liver function tests may be found. The organisms can be cultured from the blood, urine, and stool. The disease may be fatal. Treatment with ampicillin or chloramphenicol is recommended. Some patients will develop a carrier state. A common resevoir for such carriers is the gallbladder which is already diseased with chronic cholecystitis or stones.

Shigella is a gram-negative bacillus which directly invades the intestinal mucosa. Man is the resevoir and the disease favors children and travelers. Fever, abdominal pain, and watery diarrhea appears after a 2 to 3 day incubation period. The stool shows blood and mucus and will be culture positive. The disease is usually self-limited but may require antibiotic treatment with ampicillin.

Cholera is caused by *Vibrio cholera* a gram-negative rod. The severe watery diarrhea results from the elaboration of a potent enterotoxin by the organisms. This toxin causes a profuse weeping from the mucosa. The organism is water borne. Treatment, to be successful, must include attention to replacement of the large volumes of water and electrolytes lost. The organism is sensitive to tetracycline.

PLAGUE AND TULAREMIA

Yersinia pestis, a gram-negative bacillis, is responsible for plague. Transmitted by fleas from animal reservoirs, plague affecting the lungs is highly contagious. In addition to this pneumonic plague, the organism may also localize to lymph nodes which become enlarged, tender, and may drain as "bubos" as bubonic plague. Septicemia may also be found and the disease has a case fatality rate of 20 percent. Streptomycin is the drug of choice.

Francisella turalensis causes tularemia. The disease follows direct contact with infected rodents or rabbits. A skin ulcer appears with regional lymphadenopathy and fever. The organism is sensitive to streptomycin.

ENTEROBACTERIA

This group of gram-negative organisms inhabit the normal lower bowel. They are important causes of hospital acquired infections in debilitated hosts. Organisms of the genera *Proteus, Klebsiella, Escherichia,* and *Citrobacter* are the major organisms. *E coli* is the most common cause of urinary tract infections and also causes diarrhea and neonatal meningitis. *Klebsiella* causes pneumonia especially in alcoholics and those with chronic lung disease. This group of bacteria have variable sensitivities to antibiotics and sensitivity testing is required. Those which stalk hospitals are notorious for having acquired antibiotic resistance. The aminoglycosides, cephalosporins, and ampicillin are the most commonly used agents.

HEMOPHILUS

This pleomorphic gram-negative bacillus causes childhood otitis media, meningitis, and pneumonia. Treatment is with ampicillin or chloramphenicol.

ANAEROBES

The anaerobic bacilli are exquisitely sensitive to oxygen and will not grow in its presence. Special culture techniques are required. They make up the predominant organisms in the normal bowel. Most infectious are endogenous (i.e., they are carried in the patient and become pathogenic under appropriate circumstances). They are common causes of abdominal, pelvic, or wound abscesses. Some form gas which may be seen on x-rays. The pus is usually foul smelling and cultures will identify the offending anaerobe. Treatment requires the correct antibiotic and surgical drainage. The bacteria may also yield septicemia.

CLOSTRIDIA

Clostridia form spores and are gram-positive bacilli. The soil is their resevoir and they produce disease usually by contamination of wounds. The local infection is minor. The major manifestations of illness come from the elaboration of a potent neurotoxin with strychnine-like properties. After a few days of incubation, *Clostridium* tetanus elaborates enough toxin to cause spasm with trismus of the mouth and jaw and eventual respiratory paralysis. Tetanus has a 50 percent mortality. It is treated by local drainage of the abscess followed by hyperimmune globulin. Prophylaxis is maintained by tetanus immunization which is effective for 10 years.

Clostridium botulinum causes disease solely by toxin effects ingested with contaminated foods. The toxin inhibits the release of acetylcholine from the myoneural junction. Diplopia and dysphagia are the earliest symptoms which occur within 24 hours of ingestion followed by a symmetrical descending paralysis with fever and confusion. Treatment includes support of respiration and equine antitoxin.

Clostridium perfringens causes gas gangrene. The organism resides in the gut and vagina as well as the soil and will contaminate wounds favoring anaerobic conditions. Enzyme production destroys surrounding tissue. Patients with this condition are quite ill and show high fever and severe local wound pain. Treatment is with surgical debridement and penicillin.

Clostridium difficile is an opportunistic organism which is the agent responsible for pseudomembranous colitis after antibiotic usage. The toxin elaborated causes a diffuse diarrhea and colonic weeping of mucus and fluids.

DIPTHERIA

Corynebacterium diphtheriae are gram-positive aerobic bacilli which make a cytotoxic toxin. Diphtheria is a disease of children and is spread by respiratory droplets. After a 2 to 4 day incubation period, the patient complains of fever, sore throat, and dysphagia. Findings include local lymphadenopathy and the characteristic dirty gray membrane in the posterior pharynx. The heart and central nervous system may become involved with myocarditis or cranial nerve palsies. The organism requires special media to grow. Prevention with immunization has reduced this disease to a rarity. Treatment is with penicillin or erythromycin.

SPIROCHETES

These highly motile organisms do not stain well and are best seen by dark field microscopy. *Treponema* pallidum causes syphilis, Borellia causes relapsing fever, *Leptospira interrogans* causes leptospirosis and another spirochete has now been implicated in the tick borne disease Lyme arthritis.

Syphilis is a venereal disease with many clinical manifestations. The primary lesion is the chancre appearing on the penis or cervix or mouth. This ulcer is painless, indurated, and will disappear in about a month. In another month to 6 weeks, secondary syphilis appears as a dermatologic condition with macules on the palms and soles or as soft papules in the perineum called condyloma lata. A low grade fever and lymphadenopathy are also present. The disease then becomes latent for a period of months to years. Tertiary syphilis affects predominantly the cardiovascular and neurologic systems. The aortitis which may occur results from the obliterative endarteritis of the vasa vasorum. Neurosyphilis may cause general paresis, tabes dorsalis, or neuropathies. The diagnosis can be made by dark field examination of genital chancres. Four weeks after the chancre the patient will have a positive reagin test. This nonspecific test should be followed by a test for fluorescent treponema antibody (FTA). The organisms are sensitive to penicillin.

MYCOBACTERIA

These are fastidious slow growing bacilli. Mycobacterium tuberculosis produces a destructive immune reaction in the host. The primary infection is contracted by respiratory droplets. A local infection in lower lobe alveoli is usually asymptomatic. The organisms drain to regional hilar lymph nodes, are engulfed by histiocytes, and result in a granuloma which may calcify. At this point the patient diplays delayed hypersensitivity as manifest by a positive skin test to purified protein derivative (PPD). After a variable period of time the local nodes may casease, break down, and release organisms. This time the infection is worse because of the cytotoxic effects of the immunity. Classically disease now involves the upper lobes of the lung and may disseminate hematogenously to the bone, brain, kidneys, or elsewhere. This secondary or reactivation tuberculosis is more likely to occur in the debilitated patient with diabetes or immunosuppressed patient with steroids or lymphoma. The diagnosis is made by culture which may take several weeks to grow. Because of organism resistance, sensitivi-

ties are important. Two drugs are recommended for the same reason. Isoniazid plus ethambutol or isoniazid plus rifampin are recommended.

ASPERGILLOSIS

This ubiquitous saprophyte produces three distinct syndromes in man. The fugus may form a fugus ball in a preexisting lung cavity, may cause a hemorrhagic necrotizing pneumonia in the immunocompromised host, or may produce a hypersensitivity bronchitis. The diagnosis is made by examination of the sputum and culture. Treatment is with amphotericin B.

CANDIDA

Candida albicans is a microscopic yeast found normally in the gut, vagina, or mouth. Infection, when it occurs, is generally of the skin or mucous membranes. Thrush, a common pharyngeal infection, is suggested by the finding of white patches over erythematous patches. More severe infection involves the skin in some endocrinopathies or patients with deficiencies of cell-mediated immunity. The organism is easily cultured and may be found in the blood. Topical treatment with oral nystatin or systemic therapy with amphotericin B or 5-fluorocytosine is effective.

CRYPTOCOCCUS

Cyrptococcus neoformans is a yeast found predominantly in pigeon droppings and is an unusual cause of disease. Patients who become infected are usually suffering from other diseases which impair their immunity such as lymphoma or the administration of steroids. It may produce a mild pneumonia or a life threatening meningitis. The latter can be indolent and is diagnosed by examination of the cerebrospinal fluid with india ink to highlight the organism and culture. Cryptococcal antigen can also be detected in the blood and cerebrospinal fluid. Treatment of choice is amphotericin B or 5 fluorocytosine.

HISTOPLASMOSIS

This fungus is endemic in the Ohio and Mississippi river valleys in the soil and in bird excreta. The organism is inhaled and produces a tuberculosislike illness. If it disseminates it may be rapidly fatal with a serious interstitial pneumonia and adrenal hemorrhage and insufficiency. Cultures of blood, sputum, lymph nodes, or bone marrow may yield the organisms. Treatment is with amphotericin B.

MALARIA

Malaria is a parasitic disease found in the tropics spread by mosquitoes. Fever, chills, headaches, and myalgias predominate. The disease saw an increase in the United States with returning veterans of the Vietnam war. *Plasmodium vivax* is the most common variety. *Plasmodium falciparum* is the most serious. Both may be relapsing and can be visualized on blood smears. Prophylaxis is best achieved with the use of chloroquine.

AMEBIASIS

Entamoeba histolytica lives as a trophozoite or cyst. The trophozoite penetrates the intestinal mucosa following ingestion and produces a diarrhea or colitis picture. Cysts are passed in the stool. The disease may extend to the formation of liver abscesses. It is treated with metronidazole.

GIARDIA

This flagellate is an infectant of the upper gastrointestinal tract and usually produces mild flatulence and variable bowel habits. It is diagnosed by a duodenal aspirate and treated with metronidazole.

RHEUMATIC DISEASES

Approximately 30 million Americans suffer from rheumatic diseases. There are perhaps 60 different varieties of the illness. They are syndromes of pain, stiffness, muscle weakness, and signs and symptoms of inflammation. Few are of known etiology and most are defined by the joints involved, age, sex, serologic markers, x-rays, and associated conditions.

Rheumatoid Arthritis

This disease of unknown etiology appears to be immunologically mediated. The trigger insult is unknown and may be infectious. As a result of this insult, a reaction which is continuous and self-sustaining occurs with prolonged damage to the target organ (e.g., the synovial lining of joints).

The disease predominantly affects women with a peak incidence in the 40s although both sexes and all ages may present with the disease. There is no single diagnostic test for rheumatoid arthritis. It is rather a syndrome of symptoms and signs.

Symptomatically, the patient complains of polyarthralgias involving symmetrical joints frequently in the hands, wrists, knees, hips, elbows, and shoulders. The spine is usually spared and the temporomandibular joints are involved in this disease but in few others. Morning stiffness, malaise, muscle weakness, weight loss, and occasional low grade fever may also be complaints.

The examination shows fusiform swelling of the small joints of the fingers and the synovial thickening of other involved joints with or without fluid, warmth, and signs of ligamentous laxity about the involved joints.

Laboratory studies generally show a mild anemia of chronic disease, an elevated sedimentation rate, and the presence of rheumatoid factor. Rheumatoid factor is an IgM antibody against IgG and, while not diagnostic for the disease, is strongly suggestive.

Early x-ray changes are those of osteoporosis around inflamed joints. Later changes include erosions, loss of cartilage space, and subluxation. The synovial fluid when examined has an elevated white count, poor viscosity, and may show rhagocytes (white blood cells with dense deposits of IgM-IgG complexes).

Treatment in addition to rest, nutrition, and physical therapy includes a variety of drugs. Aspirin in therapeutic doses is the first drug of choice. Parenteral gold is a remittive agent successful in perhaps 65 percent of patients. Nonsteroidal anti-inflammatory agents are frequently helpful in controlling pain and inflammation. Steroids are widely used but carry grave side effects. Penicillamine is also useful and may reduce the titer of rheumatoid factor. This is particularly important in patients who develop the vasculitis of rheumatoid arthritis.

Ankylosing Spondylitis

Unlike rheumatoid arthritis, anklylosing spondylitis affects men more than women. It usually appears in the second or third decade as low back pain.

This illness affects predominantly the axial skeleton beginning with the sacroiliac joints and moving up the apophyseal joints of the spine to the neck. It finally results in complete fusion of the spine. The pathogenesis is unknown. There is a high proportion of patients (90 percent) with the HLA-B27 phenotype. This tissue marker is present in only 6 percent of the general population. It is suggested that it indicates an unusual predilection for the immunologic reaction which causes the disease.

Symptomatically, the onset is insidious with low back pain and malaise. The pain progresses up the spine with progressive limitation of motion. As it begins to affect the posterior articulation of the ribs, respiratory effort is increased and restrictive lung disease appears.

There is no single diagnostic test. The rheumatoid factor will be negative, the sedimentation rate elevated, and the x-rays characteristic.

Treatment must include vigorous physical therapy so that fusion, when it occurs, is in the most advantageous position. Nonsteroidal anti-inflammatory agents (e.g., indomethacin and tolmetin) are quite useful in this disease. They provide good pain relief and may delay the onset of fusion.

Psoriatic Arthritis

This disease also has a high incidence of HLA-B27 positivity. It occurs in association with psoriatic skin disease. It affects the small distal interphalangeal joints of the fingers and toes and the apophyseal joints of the spine.

The patient will complain of pain, redness, and stiffness. The examination shows sausage shaped swelling of the digits affected and limitation of spine movement if it is involved. The skin shows psoriatic plaques and pitting of the finger and toe nails. X-rays may show characteristic erosions of distal joints. Treatment is difficult and requires attention to both the arthritis and skin disease. Aspirin, nonsteroidals, steroids, and occasionally methotrexate have been used.

Reiter's Syndrome

Reiter's is a syndrome of polyarthritis, conjunctivitis, and urethritis. A fourth component of mucosal ulcerations may also be seen. The pathogenesis is unknown but probably results from an infectious illness and a subsequent reaction to it. The disease has been known to follow chlamydia, yersinia, and shigella infections. HLA-B27 positivity is seen in this disease as well but somewhat less than in ankylosing spondylitis (85 percent).

The disease may be confused with gonococcal arthritis. It is seen most often in young men. Various parts or combinations of the triad may be seen at any one point in time. Treatment is symptomatic. Joint destruction is rare and the disease is usually not lifelong.

Systemic Lupus Erythematosis

This is a chronic disease immunologically mediated of unknown cause with many manifestations. It affects women eight times more than men.

The disease affects small blood vessels and serosal surfaces. The clinical manifestations may include any combination of the following:

1. Nondeforming polyarthralgias
2. Alopecia
3. Characteristic facial rash
4. Pleurisy
5. Neurologic complaints and findings
6. Nephritis
7. Fever, weight loss, and malaise
8. Photosensitivity
9. Raynaud's phenomenon

This impressive list indicates the variable clinical picture which may result.

Patients with this disease characteristically have antibodies against nuclear material of their own cells (i.e., antinuclear antibodies, ANA).

Antibodies to nuclear material show different patterns depending on the protein material of the antibody. The fluorescent pattern may be speckled (relatively nonspecific), homogenous (most suspicious for SLE), peripheral, or nucleolar. More specific tests show antibodies against specific components of the cell. The one most closely allied with systemic lupus erythematosis is anti-double stranded DNA antibody. Both the direct reaction of antigen and antibody and the deposition of complexes formed by this reaction are thought to contribute to the clinical signs and symptoms.

Ninety percent of patients with lupus will show antinuclear antibodies but not everyone with the antibodies has lupus. They are also seen in patients with progressive systemic sclerosis, some with rheumatoid arthritis, and also as a function of age.

Other autoantibodies occur in this disease and may show as autoimmune hemolytic anemia, idiopathic thrombocytopenia, or leukopenia. Complex deposition is the cause of the renal disease of lupus. A characteristic picture of complex deposition is recognized on kidney biopsies examined under electron microscopy.

Therapy consists of aspirin, antimalarials, corticosteroids, immunosupressants, and cytotoxics. Nephritis demands the most aggressive treatment.

Progressive Systemic Sclerosis

Progressive systemic sclerosis or scleroderma is a disease of unknown cause characterized by an excessive accumulation of collagen and evidence of small vessel vasculitis. It is four times more common in women and generally begins in midlife.

Initially, patients will complain of Raynaud's phenomenon of cold induced vasospasm of the hands. They will relate that their hands become chalky white with a sharp border to normal skin. Subsequently, the color change is to purple and then red with rewarming which is painful. The next manifestation is fusiform swelling of the digits much like early rheumatoid arthritis. Next, the skin becomes tight, loses definition and becomes hidebound. Ulcers of the digits may appear with necrosis and autoamputation. Multiple skin telangiectases are frequently seen.

Visceral components include dysphagia from disorder esophageal motility, small bowel dilatation and dysfunction, cardiac sclerosis, pulmonary interstitial sclerosis, and fatal renal vasculitis.

Most patients have ANA, usually of the speckled variety, an elvated sedimentation rate, and a few other specific laboratory findings. Some recent evidence suggests that 50 percent of patients with progressive systemic sclerosis will have anticentromere antibodies.

Treatment is difficult and largely ineffective.

Polymyositis

Polymyositis is an inflammatory disease of striated muscle. It may be associated with a skin rash in which case it is called dermatomyositis. The rash appears on the face, neck, and upper arms and is a purplish dusky macular eruption with some tissue edema.

The muscle disease is most profound in proximal muscles where it produces weakness atrophy and some pain. The disease affects women more than men (2:1) and occurs with a peak in childhood and a second peak in mid- to late life. When it occurs in late life it may be a marker to an occult malignancy (8–9 percent).

The diagnosis is supported by the clinical findings together with an elevated sedimentation rate and high levels of muscle enzymes (CPK, SGOT, or aldolase), electromyograms showing sustained fibrillations and a muscle biopsy showing an active round cell, inflammatory infiltrate with loss of muscle fibers.

Treatment with corticosteroids is effective usually in childhood. The adult variety may require methotrexate treatment if steroids fail.

Polymyalgia Rheumatica

This disease is a syndrome characterized by pain in the shoulder and pelvic girdles together with systemic symptoms of fever, anorexia, weight loss, and lassitude. It is a disease of later life usually seen in persons over 50 years of age. The laboratory tests are nonspecific and include very high sedimentation rates, anemia or chronic disease, normal muscle enzymes, and muscle biopsies. The response to corticosteroids is dramatic and may be diagnostically helpful. Steroids are required because of the high incidence of association with giant cell arteritis which if untreated may lead to blindness or infarctions of any of the territories supplied by the aortic arch vessels.

Crystal Joint Diseases

Uric acid, calcium pyrophosphate dihydrate, and hydroxyapatite may all cause acute arthritis secondary to crystals in the joint space. The supposed mchanism includes the deposition of crystals which are phagocytosed by white cells with the resultant release of proteolytic enzymes from the white cells producing acute inflammation.

Gout is a monoarticular or pauciarticular disease caused by the deposition of uric acid crystals in the synovial space. The most commonly affected joint is the first metatarsal phalangeal joint but other joints may be affected. The patient complains of the acute onset of severe pain and swelling of the joint. Examination shows all the signs of inflammation and the diagnosis is established by the demonstration of uric acid crystals in the synovial fluid. These crystals are needle shaped and strongly negatively birefringent under polarized light.

Patients with hyperuricemia may be overproducers of uric acid (80 percent) or underexcreters of uric acid (20 percent) because of a primary renal defect in the handling of uric acid. Overproducers may be so on a genetic basis or because of another disease with rapid protein turnover such as psoriasis or myeloproliferative disorders. The disease seems to be facilitated by the presence of testosterone and inhibited by the presence of estrogen since it does not appear in men till after puberty and does not appear in women until after menopause.

The acute attack of gout can be treated by the administration of colchicine (orally or parenterally) or phenylbutazone. The production of uric acid can be retarded by the use of allopurinol which is a xanthine oxidase inhibitor and is therefore a prophylactic drug. Uric acid excretion can be facilitated by the use of probenecid which inhibits the reabsorption of uric acid by the renal tubule. The latter drug must be used with caution in the overproducer since the patient is then at risk for the development of renal stones.

Pseudogout is so named because of its clinical similarity to gout. The offending crystal is calcium pyrophosphate dihydrate. The disease is also prominent in men in middle age as is gout. Weight bearing joints are favored as is the shoulder. There is a strong association with chondrocalcinosis which may be apparent on x-rays. The diagnosis is established by the finding of weakly positively birefringent crystals of rhomboid shape in synovial fluid. Associated diseases include gout, hyperparathyroidism, hemochromotosis, and diabetes mellitus. Treatment with butazolidin is effective. No prophylactic measures are known.

Inflammatory osteoarthritis is a variant of osteoarthritis (vida infra) characterized by a history of symptoms suggestive of rheumatoid arthritis with pain, swelling, and redness of joints but with clinical findings of osteoarthritis. The disease is caused by the shedding of hydroxyapatite crystals from eburnated joints into the synovial space with the same crystal inflammation as gout or pseudogout. Patients generally have an elevated sedimentation rate and aggressive osteoarthritis. Treatment with anti-inflammatory drugs is indicated.

Osteoarthritis

This is the most common variety of arthritis. It has both environmental and genetic features. It is seen in virtually everyone with aging but is most prominent in families especially among women.

Osteoarthritis is also the final pathway of joint injury and so will be seen late in the course of rheumatoid arthritis or other joint diseases. The disease has a predilection for the joints of the hands and the weight bearing joints especially the spine, hips, and knees. The process is multifaceted and includes the loss of joint cartilage, injury to the underlying bone, and remodeling with overgrowth of bone about the affected joints. It is usually seen in multiple joints of a given patient but may occur in a single joint which has been the subject of previous injury such as trauma, aseptic necrosis, or congenital dislocation. A particular variety of the osteoarthritis is seen in the Charcot joint which is a joint denervated by a central nervous system disorder such as lues, sryngomyelia, or diabetic neuropathy. Under these conditions the failure to feel pain permits continued injury to go unnoticed and result in severe osteoarthritis.

The usual patient will show changes in the distal interphalangeal joints (Heberden's nodes), limitation of motion about the spine particularly the cervical spine, bony enlargement of the knees, and limitation of motion of the hips. Severe spine disease may present with signs and symptoms of nerve root entrapments of the cervical or lumbosacral spine.

There are no diagnostic laboratory tests. X-rays show the typical changes of loss of joint space, compression osteosclerosis, and bony overgrowth.

Treatment is largely symptomatic with physical therapy, weight control, and analgesics.

Low Back Pain

There is no single cause of low back pain but because of the magnitude of this complaint it deserves special mention. Disorders which result in low back pain include muscle strain, anklyosing spondylitis, osteoarthritis, spondylolysis, spinal stenosis, superior articular facet syndrome, and malingering. A careful history and physical and radiologic evaluation will usually reveal the etiology.

ALLERGY AND IMMUNOLOGY

The major components of the immunologic system include lymphocytes, phagocytes, complement, and immunoglobulins. The immunologic phenomenon consists of exposure to an antigen followed by the reaction of reexposure.

Lymphocytes are divided into T- and B-cells. T-cells derive from the thymus and are responsible for cellular immunity. Subclasses of T-cells are designated as helper, suppressor, and killer cells. B-cells respond to antigenic stimulus by producing immunoglobulins. B-cells are so called because of their concentration in the bursa of birds. No single similar locus is found in man.

Immunoglobulins are classified by molecular weight and other characteristics. IgG is the largest component of immunoglobulins (75 percent). These immunoglobulins fix complement, cross the placenta, and usually follow an infectious process. IgM, a large size immunoglobulin, is the first immunoglobulin to appear following an infection. IgM also fixes complement. IgA accounts for about 10 percent of the immunoglobulins. IgA is found abundantly in secretions of the bronchi, upper airways, and gut. They are thought to coat virus and bacteria as a surface protection. IgD is found in only trace amounts. IgE, also called reagin, participates mainly in allergic reactions during which it activates mast cells to release their enzymes.

Immunologic reactions in health and disease are classified according to the timing of the reaction and the participants in the reaction.

Type I Reactions

This is an immediate reaction. IgE participates in response to a sensitizing antigen by promoting the release of histamine from mast cells, involving the slow reacting substance of anaphylaxis (SRS-A), and causing local or systemic vasodilatation. The simplest reaction is allergic rhinitis and the most complex is anaphylaxis with vascular collapse and death. Asthma affects about 5 percent of the population and the clinical manifestations are heavily dependent on type I reactions. Urticaria and angioedema are other type I reactions.

Type II Reactions

Type II reactions are cytotoxic to cells. This type involves IgG or IgM immunoglobulins which together with complement promote phagocytosis by histiocytes.

Examples of type II reactions include immune hemolytic anemias, idiopathic thrombocytopenic purpura, and acute graft reactions in transplant recipients.

Type III Reactions

A type III reaction is the result of complexes of antigen and antibody which are trapped in tissue and promote injury by their presence. Usually, these complexes localize within vessels and cause a vasculitis, the symptoms and signs of which are dependent on the organ affected. The nephritis of systemic lupus erythematosis, the arthus reaction, and serum sickness are examples. Many forms of vasculitis are probably the result of this complex deposition phenomenon but have not yet been identified as such. Serum sickness is the prototype reaction. After acute exposure to foreign serum protein, the body responds by developing antibodies. These antibodies, over a 2 week period, appear and complex with the offending antigen. The complexes are then sifted out in various reticuloendothelial locations where local reactions can occur. Fever, lymphadenopathy, skin rash, and arthralgias are the dominant symptoms.

Type IV Reactions

Type IV reactions are cell-mediated and involve T-cells and macrophages. Complement and antibody is not involved. Sensitized T-cells, when exposed to their marker antigen, react with local tissue injury. Delayed hypersensitivity as with a positive skin test for PPD is the classic example. Contact dermatitis is another example of Type IV reaction.

It is important to remember that drug reactions may be of any of these type reactions.

Immunodeficiency Syndromes

B-cell deficiency, either in numbers or effectiveness, may be acquired or congenital. The major manifestation is recurrent infectious diseases with bacteria.

T-cell deficiency results in a propensity to develop intracellular parasites and opportunistic infections with fungi, pneumocystis, cryptococcus, tuberculosis, and many viruses.

SKIN DISEASES

A full discourse of dermatologic diseases is not possible in the scope of this text. Selected, are topics of either great significance because of frequency or because of their implications such as cutaneous signs of internal disease.

Classification of Dermatologic Diseases

Many of the dermatologic diagnoses are established by the appearance, location, and duration of the lesions. A careful description of skin lesions provides the index from which the clinician can find the appropriate diagnosis. A few of the descriptives are the following:

Macule: A nonpalpable lesion in the plane of the skin identifiable by its color
Papule: An elevated lesion
Nodule: A palpable skin lesion extending below the plane of the skin
Tumor: A large palpable lesion usually greater than 5 cm both above and below the skin
Plaque: A large palpable lesion with a surface area in excess of depth; they may be a coalescence of papules
Vesicles and Bullae: Elevated lesions containing fluid; a bulla is larger than a vesicle
Pustule: A raised lesion containing pus
Scale: The accumulation of epidermal debris

A careful description of the distribution is also important. Lesions may be prominent in the palms and soles as in secondary syphilis, trunkal as in pityriasis rosea, confined to a dermatome as in herpes zoster, or total body as in exfoliative dermatitis.

Psoriasis

Psoriasis is a chronic skin condition characterized by scaling papules and plaques which may involve any area of the body. The lesions are preferential to the extensor surfaces especially over the elbows and knees. The scalp and nail beds are also frequently involved. The disease may occur at any age with no sex predominance. The etiology is unknown. Pathophysiologically, there is remarkable rapidity of skin growth in the involved patches. This rapid turnover explains the heaped up scaling skin and the rapid protein turnover accounts for the elevated uric acid often found in these patients. The disease affects more than one million Americans. Occasionally, the lesions assume a pustular form. The pustules are sterile and the lesions can be localized especially to hands and feet or generalized. Rarely, exfoliative dermatitis results with a generalized skin shedding and erythema. In either disseminated pustular psoriasis or exfoliative erythroderma, mortality is signficant. The open skin permits septicemia and there is loss of temperature control and loss of fluids and electrolytes.

Psoriasis is treated but not cured. The safest modality is ultraviolet light. Patients often report improvement during the summer months. This paliative result from ultraviolet light has been extended to photochemotherapy or the combination of light and chemicals. Topical tars or steroids together with light or the oral administration of psoralen, which localizes in the skin, is followed by ultraviolet light.

Pityriasis Rosea

The history is very important in the diagnosis of this disease. The patient will report the appearance of a single macule called the "herald" patch. This is followed in a few days by the appearance of a diffuse maculopapular rash involving the trunk but sparing the face. The lesions are pale coppery in color and often have small scales. There are few symptoms and the disease is self-limited, disappearing in about 6 weeks.

Lichen Planus

Lichen planus is a papulosquamous disorder which is usually localized with a preference for the lumbar region, anterior lower legs, wrists, ankles, genitalia, and mucous membranes. The lesions are geographic, violaceous, and flattopped often coalescing into plaques. A lacelike pattern of white lines may be apparent on the surface called Wickham's striae. These are particularly helpful in mouth lesions. The etiology is unknown and the treatment is unsatisfactory.

Phemphigus Vulgaris

The group of phemphigus diseases are bullous diseases and are associated with autoantibodies. These diseases are very serious in terms of morbidity and mortality. Phemphigus vulgaris is the prototype and is seen in men and women between age 40 and 60. The bullae may appear anywhere often beginning in the mouth. When they rupture there are ulcers which weep and become secondarily infected. Untreated, the illness is fatal in a little more than a year. Pathologically, the splitting of the skin layers occurs within the epidermis. Treatment requires high doses of corticosteroids and occasionally immunosuppressants.

Phemphigoid is less aggressive, appears like phemphigus, occurs in older patients, and may remit spontaneously. In this disease, the split is between the epidermis and dermis, the bullae are tougher and heal more rapidly.

Dermatitis Herpetiformis

This disorder usually presents with intense pruritus and excoriated papules or vesicles in a distribution over the buttocks, shoulders, elbows, and knees. There is der-

moepidermal separation with microabscesses. There is diffuse deposition of immunoglobulins, especially IgA.

The disease appears most frequently in men in the later years of life. It has an interesting association with celiac disease or nontropical sprue. Treatment with dapsone is very effective.

Erythema Multiforme

This is an important illness for the company that it keeps. It is related most often to an antigen-antibody reaction often following a viral illness or the administration of drugs. It occurs between age 10 and 40. It is an acute inflammatory disease involving the skin, mucous membranes, and occasionally internal organs. The lesions are variable macular, papular, vesicular, and bullous. A characteristic pattern is the iris lesion of a serpiginous circle with central clearing. They most often appear on the face, neck, forearms, and legs. There is variability in the clinical expression of the disease ranging from a mild eruption which is self-limiting to a severe life threatening disease involving the total body.

The most severe form is called Stevens-Johnson syndrome. It begins over a few days to 2 weeks with fever, malaise, and sore throat. It rapidly progresses to an abrupt appearance of bullae all over the body and mucous membranes. The bullae rupture, become ulcerated, and weep. The mortality is 10 percent. Treatment is with corticosteroids and supportive care.

Erythema Nodosum

This too is an inflammatory disease of the skin. It is characterized by the appearance of red painful nodules on the anterior lower legs and occasionally arms. It is a systemic reaction to a number of infectious or inflammatory diseases. The patient will report a very painful spot which only later becomes brightly erythematous and nodular. The lesions resolve much as a bruise. It is most often seen in association with a streptococcal pharyngitis, tuberculosis, and sarcoidosis. Other infectious diseases may be associated. It occurs most often in women in their early years. It may last several weeks and the treatment is directed at the underlying illness.

Malignant Tumors of the Skin

Basal cell carcinomas of the skin are the most common and the least malignant of the skin cancers. They arise from the basal layer of cells in the epidermis. Ultraviolet exposure increases the risk of basal cell cancers and hence they are more frequent in sun exposed areas and rare in darkly pigmented people. A well advanced basal cell has a pearly rolled edge with a depressed shiny center. Treatment with surgery or radiation is curative.

Epidermoid or squamous cell cancers of the skin are more aggressive. Ultraviolet light, radiation, arsenicals and tars, chronic trauma, or ulceration are frequent predisposing causes. Squamous cell cancers account for about 10 percent of all skin cancers. They are less papular than the basal cell cancers and they tend to ulcerate and invade deeper structures although they rarely metastasize. Surgery and radiation are therapies of choice.

Malignant melanomas account for about 5 percent of skin tumors and are the most aggressive variety. It originates from melanocytes. This tumor is increasing in frequency, has no sex predilection and is much more frequent in whites than blacks. The tumor may appear anywhere on the body but prefers sun exposed areas. Four types of malignant melanoma are recognized.

Lentigo maligna is a pigmented macule usually seen on the face of the elderly. It varies considerably in appearance and changes with time. As it becomes more aggressive it will invade deeper structures. The treatment is simple excision.

The superficial spreading melanoma is the most common form of the disease. It is slightly elevated irregular in shape and variable in color. The individual lesion may have shades of red white and black. (This combination of colors is an important clue to all melanomas.) With time the lesion becomes more nodular.

Nodular melanomas are the most treacherous. They are the quickest growing and metastasize early and widely.

Acrolentiginous melanomas is similar in appearance to a pigmented nevus but is very aggressive. It curiously has a tendency to appear on the hands, feet, oral mucous membranes, and genitalia of blacks and orientals.

A careful histologic examination of melanomas provides prognostic information. The depth of invasion of the skin is classified from level I to level V. At level I the cancer is confined to the epidermis and at level V it has invaded subcutaneous fat.

The primary treatment of melanomas is surgical excision with a wide margin. If metastatic, chemotherapy is added. There may be a very long latent period between the primary and the appearance of metastases (as long as 30 years).

Kaposi's hemorrhagic sarcoma has become an important skin cancer. It has recently been associated with a high degree to the autoimmune deficiency syndrome (AIDS) seen in homosexual men, hemophiliacs, and some drug abusers. The disease appears on the feet and hands first as dark red to purple nodular lesions. Visceral involvement especially the gastrointestinal tract commonly follows. The lesions are very radiosensitive.

Mycosis fungoides occurs in the skin and is a variety of lymphoma. It is a somewhat indolent disease with a natural history of up to 10 years between appearance and death. The initial lesions are papulosquamous usually quite pruritic. Next, plaques appear which are palpable, and finally frank tumor masses are apparent. The lesions almost always have a striking but variable color and prefer the trunk although almost the entire skin may become involved. Chemotherapy is directed by the stage of involvement and distribution of the lesions. Since the disease is always multifocal surgery has limited usefulness.

Dermatitis

Several inflammatory diseases of skin are noteworthy. Contact dermatitis is an inflammatory state secondary to contact with an irritant or allergen. With irritants anyone will react given enough exposure but allergic reactions are patient specific. Since they are of the delayed hypersensitivity variety, the reaction to allergens will take several days to weeks to become manifest. When the reaction is acute the lesions will be intensely pruritic and inflamed. Blisters and ulcers with weeping and secondary infection may occur. More chronic reactions may be lichenified, excoriated, and crusted. The location of the lesions of course depends on the area of contact.

Atopic dermatitis may appear at virtually any age and is also mediated by immune mechanisms. These lesions which are usually weeping and inflamed appear characteristically on the buttock, face, scalp, neck, and palms. Older lesions become lichenified and favor the flexor surfaces such as the popliteal fossa and antecubital space. A specific allergen cannot usually be identified but a strong personal and family history of atopy is common. Treatment with topical corticosteroids and oral antihistamines is salutory.

Acne vulgaris is an inflammatory disease of the pilosebaceous apparatus and is most commonly seen in young men and women. The lesions erupt on the face, neck, back, upper arms, and chest. The skin in affected individuals is often oily. The cause is unknown although hormones often play a role. The rise in testosterone with puberty, the association with the use of birth control pills, and the frequent exacerbation just prior to menses point to this fact. Some drugs such as phenytoin, bromides, and iodides may also precipitate the lesions. When extensive and markedly inflamed, acne lesions will scar and disfigure. Topical benzoyl peroxide, sulfur, and salicylic acid are all used with variable success. Vitamin A (Retin A) or tetracylcine are used orally.

Acne rosacea unlike vulgaris is a disease of old age. There is inflammation with telangiectases, erythema, and pustules over the face especially the nose. When severe, there is marked hypertrophy of the sebaceous glands leading to deforming rhinophyma (the bulbous nose). Alcoholism predisposes to acne rosacea.

Cutaneous Signs of Internal Malignancy

Acanthosis nigricans is a curious lesion which may be benign or associated with an internal malignancy. The disease is recognized as a velvety palpable dark colored eruption in the axillae, folds of the neck, and groin. The lesions produce no symptoms. The cancers with which it keeps company are generally of the gastrointestinal tract. When benign, it may be seen in patients with diabetes mellitus, especially those with insulin resistance or simply with obesity.

Dermatomyositis appearing in the patient over 50 should prompt a search for malignancy. This disease shows a characteristic malar or butterfly erythema. The lids are usually edematous and similar lesions may be seen on the extensor surfaces of the fingers. Telangiectasis of the nail bed are helpful findings in this disease and systemic lupus erythematosis. The myositis component when present combines pain and weakness of proximal motor units. Muscle enzymes are markedly elevated in the serum. Treatment is directed to the underlying malignancy.

REFERENCES

Thorn, Adams, Braunwald, Isselbacher, Petersdorf (eds): Harrison's Principles of Internal Medicine. 8th Ed. McGraw Hill Co., New York, 1977
  The sections on cardiovascular diseases and infectious diseases are particularly well written.
Beeson, McDermott, Wyngaarden (eds): Cecil: Textbook of Medicine. 15th Ed. WB Saunders Co., Philadelphia, 1979
  Generally a very well written text. The pulmonary section is recommended.
Stein (ed): Internal Medicine. Little Brown Co., Boston, 1983
  This text flows nicely and contains many little pearls. The endocrinology section is quite lucid.
Kaye, Rose (eds): Fundamentals of Internal Medicine. CV Mosby, St. Louis, 1983
  The section on neoplasia is well organized and presented. Other sections are quite variable.

MULTIPLE CHOICE QUESTIONS

1. Although many patients with hypertension are termed "idiopathic" remediable causes of hypertension should be searched for by history, physical examination, and appropriate laboratory screens. A patient has the following electrolytes reported: Sodium 146 mEq/L, potassium 2.8 mEq/L, and bicarbonate of 38 mEq/L. He is taking no medications. Appropriate workup should be instituted for which of the following?
   A. Coarctation of the aorta
   B. Cushing's disease
   C. Thyrotoxicosis
   D. Primary aldosteronism
   E. Pheochromocytoma

2. A 20-year-old woman is referred for evaluation of a heart murmur. She states that a heart murmur has been heard as long as she can remember. Presently, she has no symptoms and is referred for assessment of possible organic heart disease. Her physical findings are confined to the upper left sternal border where a grade 3/6 systolic ejection murmur is heard. The second heart sound is abnormal with fixed splitting. A chest x-ray is reported as evidence for increased pulmonary blood flow. The patient is not cyanotic. The most likely diagnosis is:
   A. Tetralogy of fallot
   B. Congenital aortic stenosis
   C. Atrial septal defect
   D. Pulmonary insufficiency
   E. Innocent murmur of childhood

3. A patient with aortic stenosis has been followed for several years and is asymptomatic. At your next evaluation in the office, which of the following would be an indication for cardiac catheterization?
   A. Angina, and/or heart failure, and/or syncope
   B. Angina pectoris
   C. Congestive heart failure
   D. Increased intensity of the murmur
   E. Ventricular premature beats

4. A 60-year-old man is admitted to the hospital with a diagnosis of chronic pulmonary disease with acute decompensation. The diagnosis is established most definitively by which one of the following tests?
   A. Minute volume of ventilation
   B. Expiratory flow rate
   C. Arterial blood gases
   D. Ventilatory response to carbon dioxide

5. Which statement is correct regarding the management of patients with bronchgenic carcinoma?
   A. Hypercalcemia essentially eliminates the chances for a surgical cure
   B. Hyponatremia is most frequently due to bilateral metastatic adrenal destruction

C. A liver scan may well show metastases even when the physical examination and liver function tests are normal

D. Lesions most likely to be cured by resection are those of nonoat cell variety, located in the periphery, and less than 2 cc in diameter

6. Which one of the following is the least likely complication of granulomatous (Crohn's disease) enteritis?
   A. Bowel obstruction
   B. Bowel fistulization
   C. Gastrointestinal bleeding
   D. Free perforation with generalized peritonitis
   E. Abscess formation

For the next five questions answer as follows:

A   if the question is associated with A only
B   if the question is associated with B only
C   if the question is associated with both A and B
D   if the question is associated with neither A nor B

7. Pain may cause
   A. Coronary artery dilatation
   B. Excretion of catecholamines which can cause an increase in heart rate, cardiac output, and heart work.
   C. Both
   D. Neither

8. In the syndrome of inappropriate antidiuretic hormone, life threatening cerebral dysfunction may require rapid restitution of the serum sodium.
   A. Water deprivation may be too slow.
   B. Hypertonic saline is not efficacious
   C. Both
   D. Neither

9. Gastroesophageal reflux may occur
   A. With hiatal hernia
   B. Without hiatal hernia
   C. Both
   D. Neither

10. In regard to the measurement of thyroid antibodies
    A. A high titer is useful in the diagnosis of hyperthyroidism due to Hashimoto's thyroiditis
    B. They are of limited value in the initial diagnosis of hyperthyroidism as antibodies are also found in a small percentage of normal people as well as in patients with other, nontoxic, thyroid disorders
    C. Both
    D. Neither

11. Nodular deposits of immunoglobulins are deposited on the basement membrane of the glomerulus in
    A. Systemic lupus erythematosis
    B. Poststreptococcal glomerulonephritis
    C. Both
    D. Neither

Pick the best answer.

12. Patients with severe chronic renal failure may not be expected to have the following manifestation
    A. Peripheral neuropathy
    B. Severe thrombocytopenia
    C. Hyperphosphatemia
    D. Anemia
    E. Nausea and vomiting

13. Which of the following have not been associated with the mononucleosis syndrome?
    A. EB virus
    B. Cytomegalovirus
    C. Herpes simplex
    D. *Toxoplasma gondii*
    E. Coxsackie virus

14. A 50-year-old man with chronic obstructive lung disease is admitted with fever, shaking chills, and cough. The chest x-ray shows a lobar pneumonia. The most likely bacteria causing this illness is:
    A. *Streptococcus* pneumoniae
    B. Pseudomonas
    C. *E coli*
    D. Mycobacterium
    E. *Streptococcus viridans*

15. In congenital spherocytosis:
    A. Hemoglobin electrophoresis usually establishes the diagnosis
    B. The defect is inherited as a sex-linked trait.
    C. It may result in chronic hemolytic anemia
    D. It characteristically causes hemolytic anemia following exposure to certain drugs.
    E. The red cells have decreased osmotic fragility

16. Which of the following may not be a manifestation of systemic lupus erythematosis?
    A. Positive antinuclear antibody
    B. Raynaud's phenomenon
    C. A false positive treponema inhibition test for syphilis
    D. Pleuritis/pericarditis
    E. Facial erythema

For the next five questions use the following key:

    A. If 1, 2, and 3 are correct
    B. If 1 and 3 are correct
    C. If 2 and 4 are correct
    D. If if only 4 is correct
    E. If all statements are correct

17. Osteomalacia is associated with
    1. Malabsorption syndrome
    2. Normal or low serum calcium
    3. Depressed serum phosphate
    4. Normal serum alkaline phosphatase

18. A palpable mass in the renal area may be produced by
    1. Neoplasm
    2. Perinephric abscess
    3. Polycystic kidneys
    4. Hydronephrosis

19. Myasthenia gravis
    1. Is a chronic disease with a tendency to remission and relapse
    2. Involves impairment of conduction at the myoneural junction which is temporarily relieved by cholinesterase inhibitors such as physostigmine and neostigmine
    3. Occurs most commonly between the ages of 20 and 50
    4. Affects men more frequently than women

20. Multifocal atrial tachycardia
    1. Is often caused by digitalis toxicity
    2. Is seen in older patients and commonly in those with chronic lung disease
    3. Has a p–r interval which is constant beat to beat
    4. Has a high mortality rate

21. Erythema nodosum may accompany
    1. Streptococcal infections
    2. Chronic lymphocytic leukemia
    3. Sarcoidosis
    4. Malaria

Answers to Multiple Choice Questions

1 D	**2** C	**3** A	**4** C	**5** D
6 D	**7** B	**8** C	**9** C	**10** C
11 C	**12** B	**13** C	**14** A	**15** C
16 C	**17** A	**18** D	**19** A	**20** C
21 B				

10

Obstetrics and Gynecology

Charles W. Whitney, John J. Botti, and Rodrigue Mortel

PART 1 _____

Obstetrics

Obstetrics and gynecology is the field of medicine that deals with parturition and aims to reduce to a strict minimum maternal and infant mortality and morbidity.

The maternal mortality rate is defined as death during pregnancy or as a result of pregnancy complications. In 1982, maternal mortality in the U.S. was 8.9 per 100,000 live births. The major causes of maternal death are hemorrhage, toxemia of pregnancy, and infection. Recently, with improvement in maternal death rates from the major causes, there has been a relative increased mortality frequency from thromboembolism, anesthesia, and cardiac disease. Advanced maternal age, high parity, and socioeconomic disadvantage are associated with increased maternal mortality and morbidity.

Infant mortality rate is the number of infant deaths under 1 year of age per 1,000 live births. In 1980, United States infant mortality was 12.5 per 1,000 live births. The perinatal mortality rate is comprised of fetal and neonatal mortality rates. The perinatal mortality rate in the United States in 1980 was 16.8 per 1,000 total births, evenly divided between fetal mortality and neonatal mortality. Historical improvement of infant and perina-

tal mortality is related to the improved general health of the population, better maternal nutrition, decreased out-of-hospital births, and improved medical care of the preterm infant. The incidence of birth defects and mental retardation parallels that of perinatal mortality. Both are influenced by the rate of premature births. A major concern in obstetric medicine is the prevention of premature birth, which occurs in approximately 5 percent of all pregnancies but which is associated with 85 percent of perinatal mortality.

MATERNAL PHYSIOLOGY

Nutritional Needs

Size at birth and later development are related to maternal weight gain. The National Research Council recommends an average weight gain of 24 pounds during pregnancy. Ideal weight gain should be a function of prepregnancy weight and ideal body weight-versus-height and age. A daily increase of approximately 300 kilocalories, including an increase of approximately 30 g of protein, should satisfy the nutritional needs of most pregnant women. Pregnant adolescents, especially those less than 14 years of age whose own growth is incomplete, require between 2,400 and 2,700 kcal per day, including 1.3 to 1.7 g/kg protein per day.

Two dietary items frequently in short supply during the course of pregnancy are iron and folic acid. The total iron required in pregnancy is about 1.5 g incorporated into an increase in red cell mass and fetal blood formation. Without supplementation during pregnancy, maternal serum iron concentration, hematocrit, and percent transferrin saturation decrease. In response, serum iron binding capacity and gut iron absorption increase. Oral iron supplementation will benefit these patients and is recommended for all pregnant women regardless of initial hemoglobin concentration at the time of conception. Due to absorptive limitations, the amount of iron needed to fulfill maternal and fetal needs is approximately 60 mg of elemental iron or approximately 300 mg of iron sulfate per day.

Folic acid is required for rapid cellular metabolism and growth. Daily requirements amount to 1 mg. Other essential nutrients usually found in the diet include calcium, iodide, and fluoride. Recommended daily allowances for pregnancy nutrition are shown in Table 10-1.

Circulation

Blood volume increases up to 40 percent; there is a 25 percent increase in red blood cell (RBC) volume but an approximately 50 percent increase in plasma volume. There is an increase in reticulocyte count and in the amounts of hemoglobin-F found in the maternal circulation. Because of the differential expansion of plasma and RBC volumes, hemoglobin concentration decreases from a non-pregnant average of 13.3 g/100 ml to 12.1 g/100 ml in the third trimester. Total protein concentration is reduced for the same reason. Venous pressure is increased in the lower extremities in response to compression of the vena cava by the gravid uterus. This increase is most often noted with the patient in the supine position; in the lateral recumbent position, the pressure effect is minimized.

Cardiac output increases by a maximum of approximately 1.5 L between the 28th and 32nd week. The major portion of the increase in cardiac output is distributed to the uterus; a smaller fractional increase goes to the kidneys. A 15 percent increase each in pulse rate and in stroke volume account for the increase in cardiac output. Because of the hemodynamic changes, cardiac murmurs may become new but non-pathologic findings during pregnancy. During labor, contractions of the uterus may cause an increase in cardiac output by a further 30 percent with modest rises in blood pressure. This may be further increased during the second stage of labor, but is minimized by the lateral recumbent position.

Maternal blood pressure decreases during early pregnancy, with a greater reduction in diastolic blood pressure contributing to a widening of pulse pressure. Establishment of a low resistance placental circulation

Table 10-1. Recommended Dietary Allowances

| | Nonpregnant females | | | | | |
	11–14 yr[a]	15–18 yr[b]	19–22 yr[c]	23–50 yr[d]	Pregnancy	Lactation
Energy, kcal	2400	2100	2100	2000	+300	+500
Protein, g	44	48	46	46	+30	+20
Vitamin A, IU	4000	4000	4000	4000	5000	6000
Vitamin D, IU	400	400	400		400	400
Vitamin E, IU	12	12	12	12	15	15
Ascorbic acid, mg	45	45	45	45	60	80
Folacin, μg	400	400	400	400	800	600
Niacin mg	16	14	14	13	+2	+4
Riboflavin, mg	1.3	1.4	1.4	1.2	+0.3	+0.5
Thiamine, mg	1.2	1.1	1.1	1.0	+0.3	+0.3
Vitamin B_6, mg	1.6	2.0	2.0	2.0	2.5	2.5
Vitamin B_{12}, μg	3	3	3	3	4	4
Calcium, mg	1200	1200	800	800	1200	1200
Phosphorus, mg	1200	1200	800	800	1200	1200
Iodine, μg	115	115	100	100	125	150
Iron, mg	18	18	18	18	d	18
Magnesium, mg	300	300	300	300	450	450
Zinc, mg	15	15	15	15	20	25

[a] Weight, 44 kg (97 lb); height, 155 cm (62 in).
[b] Weight, 54 kg (119 lb); height, 162 cm (65 in).
[c] Weight, 58 kg (128 lb); height, 162 cm (65 in).
[d] The increased requirements of pregnancy cannot usually be met by ordinary diets; therefore, the use of supplemental iron is recommended.
Source: Food & Nutrition Board: Nutrition in Maternal Health Care.

appears to play a role in the changes in blood pressure and cardiac output. During labor, blood pressure may increase 15 to 30 torr with a contraction, but returns to normal values postpartum. Circulation time does not change during pregnancy and electrocardiographic findings are consistent with left axis deviation, a function of diaphragm elevation during pregnancy.

Pulmonary Function

Tidal volume increases during pregnancy, in part through decreases in inspiratory reserve capacity and in expiratory reserve. There is no change in vital capacity. Pulmonary airway resistance decreases and conductance increases. The respiratory rate increases by 20 percent during pregnancy and, with increased tidal volume, leads to an increase in minute volume and alveolar ventilation. The net increase in oxygen consumption and in decreased partial pressure of carbon dioxide is mediated directly on the respiratory center by progesterone. Thus, the sensation of dyspnea is common during pregnancy. Pulmonary function reverts to the nonpregnant state within 24 hours after birth.

Gastrointestinal Function

Nausea and vomiting is common during early pregnancy, secondary to hormonal effects on gastrointestinal and metabolic functions. Esophageal reflux is common and hiatus hernia may become clinically evident. The large and small intestines are displaced into the upper abdomen by the pregnant uterus. The appendix is displaced to the mid or upper right quadrant and may cause confusion in diagnosis of the acute abdomen during pregnancy. The motility of the gastrointestinal tract is reduced with an increase in gastric emptying time and in intestinal transit time. Constipation occurs in association with these changes. Similar changes in gall bladder motility, along with metabolic changes, are associated with an increased incidence of cholelithiasis and cholecystitis. The hemorrhoidal veins enlarge and become symptomatic because of increased venous pressure and constipation. With the onset of labor, gastric motility effectively ceases and it should be assumed that all patients in labor have a full stomach when considering anesthetics and airway integrity.

Liver function is unchanged during pregnancy. Carbohydrate metabolism is blunted by several pregnancy hormones that interfere with the peripheral utilization of glucose but which also increase free fatty acid concentrations. Pancreatic insulin secretion increases in response. If this hyper-insulinemic response is insufficient, chemical diabetes may become manifest during pregnancy.

Renal System

Hormonally mediated smooth muscle relaxation during pregnancy contributes to hydroureter and dilation of the renal calyces. Another cause is the compression of the ureter against the pelvic brim by expansion of the uterus during pregnancy. Increased urinary stasis results, with increased risk of asymptomatic bacteruria and pyelonephritis during pregnancy. Three to 6 percent of pregnant women have asyptomatic bacteruria. About one-third of these women, if untreated, will have pyelonephritis during pregnancy. A diagnosis of pyelonephritis is an indication for radiographic investigation of the renal collecting system after pregnancy.

Renal function is most efficient with the patient in the left lateral recumbent position. Renal plasma flow increases by approximately 50 percent early in the second trimester. Glomerular filtration rate increases by a similar amount. These changes are probably mediated by estrogen and progesterone. Sodium handling by the kidney is increased. The renin-angiotensin system responds to increased clearance by activation of aldosterone for sodium retention. The net effect is a 6 L expansion in total body water which correlates well with the increase in venous capacity stimulated by progesterone effects on vascular smooth muscle. An increase in angiotensin-II activity is offset by a decrease in vascular smooth muscle tone during pregnancy. Angiotensin-II resistance is diminished in preeclampsia.

Increased glomerular filtration rates result in decreased concentrations of blood urea nitrogen (BUN), creatinine, and uric acid. Under pathologic circumstances such as preeclampsia, the appearance of apparently normal BUN and creatinine concentrations is an early suggestion of renal impairment.

Postpartum, renal plasma flow decreases quickly and diuresis occurs between the second and fifth postpartum day.

Hematologic System

With good pre-pregnancy nutrition and health, early pregnancy hemoglobin/hematocrit should change little during pregnancy if supplemental iron is given. Red blood cell morphology is unchanged in normal pregnancy. There is a slight increase in white blood cell concentration with normal ranges to 15,000/mm^3 and with a normal differential count. Platelet concentrations are unchanged during normal pregnancy. Plasma protein fractions change in the following fashion: there is a decrease in albumin and γ-globulin while α- and β-globulins increase. A small decrease in total protein per liter of plasma occurs. Serum fibrinogen concentration is increased 40 to 50 percent during pregnancy, up to 600 mg/dl. Because of these changes in fibrinogen concentration, there is an increase in the erythrocyte sedimentation rate during pregnancy. Factors VII, VIII, IX, and X are increased during pregnancy as well. There is some suggestion that these changes represent a hypercoagulable state in pregnancy as venous thrombosis and pulmonary embolism are more frequent. These changes revert to non-pregnant levels rapidly after birth.

Neurologic System

Increases in fluid accumulation in the peripheral nervous system during pregnancy are associated with increased headache, chorea graviderum, and carpal tunnel syndrome. Peripheral compression is relatively common because of the aforementioned changes. Growth of the gravid uterus with compression in the pelvic region and lordotic changes in the spinal column contribute to pelvic nerve root compression, and sciatica can be a vexing problem during pregnancy.

Reproductive Function

Maternal reproductive adaptation to pregnancy includes an increase in uterine mass from approximately 70 g in the nonpregnant state to between 1.2 and 2 kg at term. Uterine blood flow increases 10-fold, to 650 ml/min at term, but flow per 100 g uterus is unchanged. These changes are stimulated chiefly by the action of estrogen and possibly by progesterone. In growing, the uterus displaces abdominal contents laterally and superiorly and the uterus dextrorotates, probably from the location of the rectosigmoid in the left lower pelvis. Uterine contractility gradually increases throughout pregnancy.

During pregnancy, there is a pronounced softening and cyanosis of the cervix associated with hormonal and vascular changes. There is increased vascularity and edema of the entire cervix. The cervix contains a small amount of smooth muscle but is comprised mainly of connective tissue. Change in the character of this connective tissue near term is associated with ripening and softening of the cervix in preparation for labor and delivery. Many of these late pregnancy changes appear to be due to prostaglandin activation of cervical collagenases.

The main function of one of the ovaries during pregnancy is to maintain the corpus luteum during the time of implantation until placental hormones are sufficiently elaborated to support the products of conception. The amount of progesterone produced by the corpus luteum of pregnancy decreases between the sixth and eighth week after the last menstrual period. Relaxin is a protein hormone also secreted by the corpus luteum during human pregnancy. The specific role of relaxin is obscure at this time.

The vagina also undergoes loosening of the connective tissue and hypertrophy of the smooth muscle cells which result in an increase in the length of the vaginal walls in preparation for eventual delivery.

During pregnancy, major changes in breast tissue include hypertrophy of the mammary alveoli with glandular differentiation. There is an increase in breast weight under these conditions and, after the first few months, colostrum can be expressed from the nipples by gentle massage.

Endocrine Changes

The pituitary enlarges during pregnancy. There is an increase in prolactin secretion and a decrease in follicle-stimulating hormone (FSH) and luteinizing hormone (LH) secretion. Blood supply to the pituitary gland appears to be critical during pregnancy. Severe postpartum maternal hemorrhage has been associated with postpartum infarction of the pituitary gland (Sheehan's syndrome), resulting in hypopituitarism. The pituitary gland appears not to be necessary for successful pregnancy if the patient is maintained on replacement therapy with thyroid, corticosteroid, and antidiuretic hormones. There is a gradual increase in the secretion of oxytocin throughout pregnancy. Oxytocin does not appear to be essential for the onset of successful labor. Adrenocorticotropic (ACTH) hormone activity does not appear to be increased.

Thyroid activity is increased during pregnancy with an estrogen-induced increase in thyroid binding globulin. A human chorionic thyrotropin has been isolated from the placenta and may also have an effect on increased thyroid activity. Basal metabolic rate is increased approximately 25 percent during pregnancy with an increase in total thyroxine and a decrease in resin uptake of thyroid hormone. The free thyroid index remains unchanged during pregnancy, as does the clinically euthyroid state. Adrenocortical activity is increased along with corticosteroid binding globulin in pregnancy. Free cortisol concentrations in the plasma remain unchanged.

Estrogen and progesterone play important roles in the physiologic changes in pregnancy and in early endocrine maintenance of the conceptus. Estradiol 17-B is the estrogen produced in highest concentration by the ovary before pregnancy and is essential for ovulation, fertilization and implantation. The placenta, however, is the chief source of estrogens during pregnancy. Instead of estradiol, the estrogen most actively produced is estriol, whose precursor is 16 hydroxyepiandrostenedione sulphate (16-OH-DHEAS), produced chiefly by the fetus.

The placenta is incapable of producing estrogens de novo and is reliant upon both maternal and fetal precursors. The major source of estriol precursor is the fetal zone of the fetal adrenal cortex. Estriol is conjugated in maternal liver to estriol glucuronide, which is excreted in maternal urine. Estriol concentrations in maternal plasma or urine are used to assess feto-placental function.

Progesterone is produced by the placenta without need for major precursors. Progesterone from the corpus luteum functions to prepare the endometrium for blastocyst implantation. Progesterone also decreases spontaneous uterine activity and inhibits uterine response to oxytocic hormones. By 12 weeks gestation, the placenta is the major source of progesterone secretion.

The onset of labor may be associated with changes in the metabolism of progesterone by fetal membranes, which renders lysosomes unstable and results in the release of phospholipase A2. This, in turn, increases the availability of arachidonic acid for conversion to prostaglandins.

Three major protein hormones are synthesized by the placenta. They are human chorionic gonadotropin (HCG), human placental lactogen (HPL) and human chorionic thyrotropin (HCT). HCT does not appear to be as important as HCG and HLP in pregnancy activity except in molar pregnancy. HCG is a glycoprotein, containing alpha and beta subunits. The alpha subunit appears to be similar, but not identical, to subunits of FSH and LH, as well as thyrotropin. The beta subunit is specific for human chorionic gonadotropin and has become the basis for sensitive tests of early pregnancy or of gonadotropin secreting tumors. HCG is produced in the syncytiotrophoblast. HCG in plasma and urine are highest at about 60 days gestation. Serum levels peak around 100,000 milli-international units per mililiter (mIU/ml), then decrease by 90 percent at term. Peak values of HCG in the urine range from 20,000 to 100,000 mIU/day and decrease to approximately 20 percent of these values later in pregnancy. Most commercial urine pregnancy tests detect HCG at 1,500 to 3,000 mIU/ml. Radioimmunoassay of urine can detect HCG as low as 50 mIU/ml. Pure beta HCG can be detected as low as 5 mIU/ml in plasma. Beta HCG detection of pregnancy is dependent upon laboratory standards but results in excess of 50 mIU/ml are generally diagnostic and may be found as early as 8 days after fertilization.

HPL is a single chain polypeptide similar to human growth hormone. HPL has several activities in human pregnancy. It appears to play a role in maintaining the corpus luteum in early pregnancy, but its main activity appears to be related to its growth hormone-like and metabolic effects. HPL is associated with mobilization of fat stores in the mother and an increase in circulating free fatty acids. Maternal insulin resistance may be partly due to placental lactogen. The reduced sensitivity to plasma insulin in response to a standard glucose load is HPL-mediated. It is postulated that the role of HPL is to spare protein and glucose for fetal consumption while free fatty acids become available for maternal fuel needs. HPL also appears to be necessary for lactogenic response in pregnancy. HPL has been shown to stimulate breast development and casein synthesis, and is found in much larger concentrations in the mother compared with the fetus, suggesting a maternal function for the hormone. Because of rapid clearance, circulating HPL is 1 to 5 mg/ml and is directly proportional to the amount of placental tissue present. HPL has been used as a measure of fetal and placental well-being but because of a large range of normal values with gestation, it has not achieved popularity as a critical screen.

Lactation requires contributions by progesterone, estrogen, prolactin, thyroxine, cortisol, and insulin in addition to placental lactogen. Together, they stimulate growth and development of the milk-secreting apparatus. The increased levels of estrogen and progesterone during pregnancy appear to interfere with the lactogenic stimulus. Plasma prolactin is essential in lactation; although plasma levels decrease after pregnancy, the act of suckling triggers a rise in prolactin concentration. Oxytocin also plays a role; contraction of the myoepithelial cells is stimulated by oxytocin release (let-down factor).

During pregnancy, colostrum is secreted by the breast. It contains more protein and minerals but less sugar and fat than mature milk. Mature milk contains immunoglobulin G (IgG), proteins, lactose, water, and fat. Of the proteins, casein is in highest concentration. The nutrients are synthesized in the alveolar secretory cells, utilizing circulating plasma precursors. Human milk is a poor source of vitamin B_{12} and iron.

FETO-PLACENTAL PHYSIOLOGY

Immunology of Pregnancy

Only half of the fetal complement of genetic material is maternally derived. As an allograft, it should be immunologically rejected. Successful completion of pregnancy has been explained by the following hypotheses: the fetus is antigenically immature, the uterus is an immunologically privileged site, the fetus and mother are separated by a physical barrier, or the state of maternal immunological competence is modified during pregnancy. However, both the placenta and the fetus possess immunologic antigenicity early in pregnancy. Moreover, the uterus has vascular and lymphatic drainage, and does not appear to be immunologically privileged as are several other areas of the body. Extrauterine sites of continued pregnancy also argue against this theory. Generalized immunosuppression in the pregnant female has not been demonstrated. Maternal lymphocytes have been repeatedly shown to react against foreign antigens, although reduction of T-cell activity and depressed lymphocyte transformation have been noted. A blocking antibody has been postulated that protects the fetus from circulating sensitized T-cells. The increase in corticosteroid hormones during pregnancy may also play a role in modifying the immunologic response.

The separation of the mother and fetus by the placenta may provide protection by imposing limitations in the number of immunologically competent cells transferred to the fetus. A fibrinoid-like layer of the trophoblast consisting of a mucopolysaccharide rich in hyaluronic and sialic acids may prevent the trophoblast from expressing its antigenicity. Maternal tolerance cannot be explained by a single factor but may be considered a complex mechanism influenced by several of the previously mentioned factors.

Placental Exchange

A major function of the placenta is to transfer oxygen and nutrients from the mother to the fetus, and waste products from fetus to mother. The substances are transferred across the placenta by simple diffusion across a gradient (blood gases and electrolytes), facilitated diffusion (carbohydrates), active transport (amino acids, iron), bulk flow, and pinocytosis (proteins, hormones). Distribution of drugs to the fetus is dependent upon molecular weight of the drug, variations in maternal and fetal pH, ionized and unionized concentrations, metabolism and excretion of the drug by mother and fetus. Bacteria and viruses traverse the placenta by different mechanisms. Viruses obtain entrance to the fetal circulation very rapidly, while bacteria may actually have to infect the placenta prior to transport to the fetus. Protozoans and malignant diseases are, with few exceptions, barred from further access to the fetus by the placenta.

Placental Development

In the primitive blastodermic vesicle, a single layer of ectoderm differentiates into trophoblasts which invade the decidua of the endometrium. Maternal blood vessels are tapped and form large lacunae that are soon filled with maternal blood. The trophoblastic proliferation forms a large complex of channels that become the intervillous space and primary villous stalks. Blood vessels develop from cytotrophoblast in the stalks. By the 17th day, a placental circulation is established. The trophoblast differentiates into cytotrophoblast cells and an outer syncitiotrophoblast. The combined trophoblast attached to the decidua basalis of the uterus comprise the chorionic plate which defines the implantation site of the placenta (Fig. 10-1). The decidua overlying the ovum and separating it from the rest of the uterine cavity is called the decidua capsularis. The remainder of the uterus is lined by the decidua vera. The decidua vera and decidua basalis are composed of three layers, the zona compacta, the zona spongiosa, and the zona basalis. The first two form the zona functionalis of the chorion. The zona basalis remains after delivery and gives rise to a new endometrium. As the invading trophoblast meets the decidua, a zone of fibrinoid degeneration (Nitabuch's layer), is formed. When this layer is absent, abnormal invasion of the myometrium may occur as in placenta accreta.

The villi that meet with the decidua basalis form the chorion frondosum, the fetal component of the placenta. As the placenta grows and ages, the underlying stroma of the placenta becomes denser and the cells become more tightly packed. The syncitium thins, there is an increase in the number of capillaries from the fetus to the villi, and the capillary-villus distance is reduced. The syncitiotrophoblast is a source of placental steroids. The cytotrophoblast does not synthesize placental hormones.

The circulation of the mature placenta has derivations from both the mother and the developing fetus. Blood enters the maternal intervillous space directly through branches of the uterine artery. The force of maternal blood pressure is approximately 70 torr at the tips of the spiral arteries. The spurt of arterial blood diffuses rapidly and peripherally through the space, is collected in uterine veins, and continues to the internal hypogastric veins for return to the maternal heart. A small fraction drains through the ovarian veins. Uterine blood flow is affected by uterine contractions, venous blood flow being cut off prior to arterial inflow. Approximately 80 percent of uterine blood flow is directed to the intervillous space during pregnancy. Increases in the size of the placenta and fetus are associated with increases in uterine blood flow, as in multiple gestation. Chronic vascular disease, severe malnutrition, heavy cigarette use, renal insufficiency, and decreased plasma volume are associated with decreases in uterine blood flow and retarded development of the fetus and placenta.

The fetal placental circulation consists of umbilical arterial flow branching into progressively smaller vessels and villous capillaries. The maternal and fetal circulations are separated only by thin capillary-syncitiotrophoblast. The fetal placental veins gradually unite to form the single umbilical vein of the fetus. There is no evidence of local or humoral control of the fetal placental circulation.

Maternal-fetal gas exchange involves maternal and

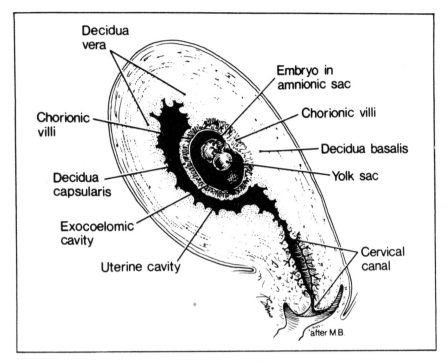

Fig. 10-1. Chorion frondosum and chorion laeve of early pregnancy. Three portions of the decidua (basalis, capsularis, and parietalis, or vera) are also illustrated. (Pritchard JA, McDonald PC: Williams Obstetrics, 16th ed. Appleton-Century-Crofts, New York, 1980.)

fetal red blood cells as well as blood flow and limiting membranes in the intervillous space. Fetal red blood cells contain hemoglobin F or fetal hemoglobin that manifests a greater affinity for oxygen than adult hemoglobin at physiologic pH and PCO_2. The hemoglobin content of fetal blood is substantially higher than that of the mother so that oxygen capacity per ml is increased. The partial pressure of oxygen in umbilical venous blood is probably not greater than 45 torr but is sufficient to meet the metabolic needs of the fetus. Partial pressure of carbon dioxide in umbilical venous blood before labor is ordinarily 40 to 45 torr with a pH range of 7.30 to 7.38. The fetus has only limited ability to increase its respiratory exchange area during times of metabolic stress, so that buffering systems are important for maintenance of homeostasis.

Water exchange between the products of conception and the mother is very large at term, approaching 4 L per hour. The largest proportion moves across the placenta. Net exchange, however, is small. With fetal or placental disease, amniotic fluid volume may be reduced (renal agenesis) or increased (duodenal atresia, anencephaly). The normal volume of amniotic fluid at term is approximately 1 L. Volumes in excess of 2 L are referred to as polyhydramnios. Twenty-five to 30 percent of patients with polyhydramnios have evidence of fetal congenital abnormalities.

Early Development of the Embryo

After fertilization, the zygote, containing the combined genetic material of its parents, travels down the fallopian tube toward implantation in the endometrium (Fig. 10-2). The zygote undergoes cleavage from a one-cell to a multicellular mass between 36 hours and $4\frac{1}{2}$ days after fertilization. By this time, a blastocyst with an inner cell mass has been formed. Implantation occurs 6 to 8 days after fertilization. The trophoblast develops from that portion of the blastocyst that does not contain the inner cell mass. The inner cell mass differentiates into the embryonic disc, containing ectoderm and an underlying layer of endoderm. Between the embryonic disc and trophoblast, small cells develop that will become the amnion and amniotic cavity. At 9 to 12 days, syncitiotrophoblast develops. By 12 days, the embryo is approxiately 1 mm in diameter. Cells within the amniotic cavity form the body stalk which later develops into the umbilical cord. The endoderm eventually forms the yolk sac and the gut. Cellular proliferation of the embryonic disc proceeds along an axis that becomes the mesoderm of the primitive streak. Thus, three germ layers give rise to various organs of the body. The ectoderm develops into the nervous system, the epidermis, and such derivatives as the lens of the eye and hair. The endoderm develops into the lining of the gastrointestinal tract and

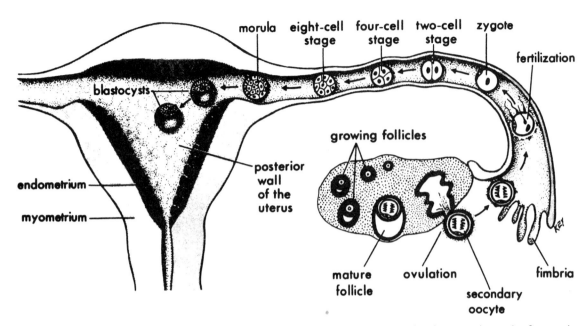

Fig. 10-2. Diagrammatic summary of the ovarian cycle, fertilization, and human development during the first week. Developmental stage 1 begins with fertilization and ends when the zygote forms. Stage 2 (days 2 to 3) comprises the early stages of cleavage (from 2 to about 16 cells or the morula). Stage 3 (days 4 to 5) consists of the free unattached blastocyst. Stage 4 (days 5 to 6) is represented by the blastocyst attaching to the center of the posterior wall of the uterus, the usual site of implantation. (Moore: The Developing Human, 2nd ed. WB Saunders, Philadelphia, 1977.)

derivative organs (liver, pancreas, thyroid). The dermis, skeleton, connective tissue, vascular and urogenital systems, and most skeletal and smooth muscle arise from the mesoderm.

In the third postfertilization week (fifth week of gestation), the primitive streak differentiates into cephalic and caudal ends. As the yolk sac enlarges, the body stalk becomes defined and a narrow endodermal diverticulum called the allantois becomes visible. Embryologically, the notocord is developed as an extension of the primitive streak and becomes the early supporting structure during embryonic life. Subsequent development of the primitive streak is directed at development of the head. A neural groove develops as folds on either side of the neural plate and the mesoderm becomes divided into discrete blocks called somites. Those cephalad form the occipital region of the head, while those in the midportion are associated with development of the spinal cord. The rapid growth of the embryonic head slows down after the fourth week; by the seventh week, the neck is visible and the embryo can be identified as having a human habitus.

From fertilization to 8 weeks of pregnancy, the developing form is called an embryo. During this time, major organ system formation occurs. After 8 weeks it is referred to as a fetus. Differentiation of previously formed organs and growth are the major elements of this portion of intrauterine life.

By the end of the fourth week, the embryo measures between 4 and 5 mm in length, the heart and pericardium are prominent, and arm and leg buds are present. By the end of the sixth week, the embryo measures approximately 24 mm in length and the head is still quite large compared to the trunk. Fingers and toes are present and the external ears are already formed. By the beginning of fetal life, the embryo measures nearly 40 mm in length. Few new major structures are formed thereafter. When the uterus has become palpable above the symphysis pubis, at 12 weeks, ossification centers have appeared in most bones and the external genitalia begin to differentiate into male or female sex. The phenotypic sex of the fetus can be determined by approximately 16 weeks of gestational age. Other differentiating factors seen with increasing gestation include the following: 20 weeks—fetal weight equals 300 g; 24 weeks—fetal weight approximately 650 g, eyelids fused; 28 weeks—fetal weight approximately 1,000 to 1,200 g, vernix caseosa is present, fetal eyelids open, fetal respiratory activity and purposeful neurologic activity present.

The bones of the fetal head differentiate early into a protective covering for the brain. They consist of the frontal, parietal, and occipital bones. They are approximated by membranous spaces called sutures. The enclosed membranous space, the anterior and posterior fontanelles, also provide landmarks during labor. Other cephalic areas become sensory structures.

The fetal circulation undergoes multiple changes during embryologic life. Fundamental differences between fetal and adult circulations exist because of the specialized function of the placenta and umbilical cord. The single umbilical vein carries oxygenated blood from the placenta, ascends to the liver and divides, with a small portion of umbilical blood flow supplying the hepatic veins. The major portion continues to the portal sinus where a fetal vessel, the ductus venosus, traverses the liver to enter directly into the inferior vena cava. Blood flow into the fetal heart contains both oxygenated blood from the ductus venosus and less oxygenated blood from the inferior vena cava. The upper inferior vena cava contains blood whose oxygen content is higher than that of the superior vena cava and the aorta.

Several anatomic changes are seen in the fetal heart. The foramen ovale is an opening in the right atrium directly off the inferior vena cava, which allows oxygenated blood deflected by another structure, the crista dividens, to flow into the left atrium. Most of the less oxygenated blood from the superior vena cava enters directly into the right ventricle. This arrangement permits delivery of more highly oxygenated blood to the left ventricle than if complete admixture had occurred in the right atrium. The oxygenated blood of the left ventricle perfuses the heart and brain first. About two-thirds of the less oxygenated blood in the right ventricle is shunted through the ductus arteriosus into the descending aorta and the remainder goes to the lungs. Because of the shunts just described, both ventricles of the fetal heart work in parallel rather than in series. High pulmonary vascular resistance accounts for low blood flow in the fetal pulmonary circuit and maintains the gradient for shunting of oxygenated blood to the heart and brain.

After birth, the umbilical vessels, the ductus arteriosus, the foramen ovale, and the ductus venosus normally constrict or collapse. These effects are mediated through decreased regional prostaglandin elaboration, necessary for maintenance of some fetal circulatory shunts.

The volume of fetal blood at term is approximately 80 ml/kg. When combined with the content of placental blood, the total fetal placental blood volume at term is approximately 125 ml/kg of fetus. Seventy-five percent of total hemoglobin at term is hemoglobin F. This proportion decreases in the first 12 months after birth.

Vitamin K-dependent coagulation factors usually decrease after birth and may lead to newborn hemorrhage. Platelet counts, total plasma protein and plasma albumin are similar to concentrations found in the adult. IgG is present in approximately the same concentration in maternal and cord sera but IgA and IgM are considerably lower in cord sera.

The urinary system of the fetus undergoes numerous developmental changes before definitive development of the kidney and collecting system. Two primitive urinary systems, the pronephros and mesonephros, precede the development of the adult metanephros. Impaired development of the urinary system can occur as a result of embryologic failure of one of the two primitive systems. The fetus continues to secrete wastes through the umbilical circulation. Hourly urine production by the fetus gradually increases throughout pregnancy and may be used as a marker of fetal renal integrity. Obstruction of the urinary collecting system in the fetus may be associated with damage to the ureters and kidneys.

One of the most important features of fetal development is maturation of the fetal lung. The survival of the infant born prematurely is most often dependent upon the degree of respiratory maturation. Anatomically, terminal bronchioles and alveoli are present in the fetal lung between 24 and 26 weeks of gestation. The ability of these structures to inflate and remain inflated is dependent upon a surface active protein, surfactant. The principal component of surfactant is dipalmitoyl lecithin, formed in the lamellar bodies of type II pneumocytes in the lung.

The digestive system is active as early as the eleventh week of gestation. Fetal swallowing is a factor in the amount of amniotic fluid present in later pregnancy. Newborns with tracheo-esophageal fistula or duodenal atresia often present in pregnancy with polyhydramnios. Meconium is undigested debris from swallowed amniotic fluid as well as products of secretion and excretion by the gastrointestinal tract that may be excreted by the fetus in hypoxic situations.

The fetal liver has limited capacity for converting free bilirubin to its conjugated derivative. During fetal life, unconjugated bilirubin may be transported across the placenta to be processed by the mother. The fetal pancreas secretes insulin as early as 12 weeks of pregnancy. Fetal growth is probably determined partly by the action of insulin on maternally supplied glucose. Glucagon has been identified at 8 weeks of gestation but this does not seem to be an important regulatory hormone during fetal life.

The fetal pituitary gland synthesizes and stores virtually all the primary hormones and appears to be capable of secreting these hormones early in gestation. Thyroid stimulating hormone appears early and the thyroid concentrates iodide by 11 weeks of pregnancy. The fetus appears to be dependent on its own thyroid functions. Fetal parathormone is also present in the first trimester. Newborns of mothers with hyperparathyroidism may have hypocalcemia at birth which suggests fetal regulatory mechanisms are present early.

The fetal adrenal gland is much larger in relation to total body size than that of the adult. The fetal zone of the cortex contributes precursors for placental estrogen biosynthesis. The adrenal is responsive to fetal ACTH release and utilizes progesterone and cholesterol for endogenous corticoid synthesis and steroidogenesis. The fetal adrenal also synthesizes aldosterone and catecholamines.

Fetal testosterone is developed by the fetal testis as early as 10 weeks gestation. The capacity for steroidogenesis by the ovary of the female fetus is absent before the development of primary follicles in the second half of gestation.

The development of the fetal nervous system begins early in the embryo. The forebrain is separated from the midbrain and hindbrain by 4 weeks gestation. Neural cells lining the neural tube differentiate into neuroblasts and spongioblasts; the former become mature neurons while the latter become supporting glial cells which invest the neurons. The glial cells continue to proliferate through life. The neurons form the gray matter of the brain while the marginal layers of the neurons, the axons, along with the glial cells, form the white matter. The brain further subdivides into five major regions that eventually become the cerebral hemispheres, the thalamus and hypothalamus, the midbrain, the cerebellum and pons, and the medulla. The pituitary gland develops as an evagination of the floor of the midbrain region.

Thymus-dependent lymphocytes appear during the first trimester and the thymus continues to grow, reaching its maximum size shortly before birth. Immunologic tissue appears in the spleen at approximately 20 weeks; maximum bone marrow activity is attained by 30 weeks gestation. Lymphocytes produced from the marrow eventually become the source of circulating immunoglobulins. Elements of the complement system are also evident by the end of the first trimester. IgG is produced by the fetus but the major fetal immunoglobulin is IgM.

Sexual Differentiation of the Fetus

Genetic sex is established at the time of fertilization by assignment of an XX (female) or XY (male) sex chromosome pair. An abnormal number of sex chromosomes (XO, XXY, XYY, XXX, etc.), is associated with biochemical and functional disorders of sexual differentiation. The gonad is a toti-potential organ that has the capability of differentiating either into a biochemically male or female organ. Gonadal sex is determined by the action of a locus on the Y chromosome to bring about differentiation of the primitive gonad as a testis. The absence of the H-Y antigen for male differentiation will allow the gonad to continue development as an ovary. Phenotypic sex differentiation will ultimately be dependent on fetoplacental hormones. Absence of male hormones or end-organ unresponsiveness to testosterone

will cause development of a phenotypic female. The male fetal testis elaborates mullerian duct inhibitory factor, which causes mullerian duct (uterine tube and vagina) regression, and testosterone, which stimulates development of the wolffian ducts (seminal vesicles, vas deferens, epididymis). Dihydrotestosterone causes virilization of the external genitalia, at approximately 6 weeks gestation with Leydig cell differentiation. Absence of this enzyme or of androgen receptor proteins generally results in failure of end-organ differentiation and a phenotypic female. The germ cells of the male and female are derived from the primitive yolk sac and migrate to the gonadal tissue during the fifth week of embryonic life. Primitive spermatogonia will become spermatozoa during puberty under the influence of testosterone. In the female, the germ cells enter meiotic prophase at the end of the first trimester; primordial, then graffian follicles will appear during the second half of pregnancy. Ovarian estrogen formation starts with the appearance of the follicles.

Sexual differentiation in the brain occurs in the hypothalamus, depending upon the type and concentration of sex hormones that are present at hypothalamic receptor sites during fetal development.

GENETICS

Basic Concepts

The normal chromosome complement in humans consists of 46 chromosomes, including 44 autosomes and 2 sex chromosomes, XY or XX. Chromosomes are found in 23 homologous pairs derived equally from maternal and paternal sources. There are seven groups of chromosomes (A to G) based on morphologic characteristics. X and Y chromosomes are not placed in these groups. Pairs of chromosomes arranged into groups according to size and morphology comprise the karyotype. Chromosomal abnormalities are alterations in either structure or number. These abnormalities occur generally during cell division.

Mitosis or somatic cell division is a process of maintaining genetic constancy within an organism when growth and development occur (Fig. 10-3). The result of mitosis is two identical daughter cells. Mitosis is divided into five stages; interphase, prophase, metaphase, anaphase, and telophase.

Interphase is also known as the resting stage. The diploid number (2N = 46) of chromosomes is maintained. Chromosomal material, however, is replicated during this stage so that the amount of DNA is doubled.

Prophase consists of condensation of chromatic material into doubled chromosomes with a common centro-

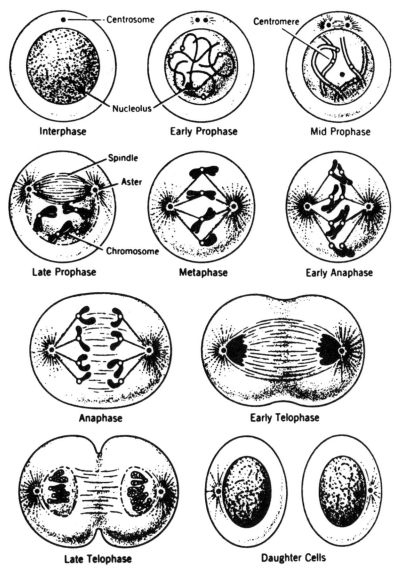

Fig. 10-3. Mitosis in an animal cell with four chromosomes. (From Gardner: Principles of Genetics. 4th Ed. Wiley, New York, 1972.)

mere. The centromere is a point of attachment of the sister chromatids on the mitotic spindle and determines the movements of chromosomes during cell division. Prophase ends as the chromosomes migrate toward the center of the nucleus.

Metaphase is the alignment along the equatorial plane of paired chromatids and attachment to the spindle fiber by the centromes, which doubles and splits longitudinally.

During anaphase, the spindle fibers migrate away from the equatorial plane toward the poles of the cell accompanied by separation of the centromere and movement of the separated chromatids to opposite poles.

In telophase, the new chromosomes continue to their respective poles. Two clusters of chromosomes are again seen. The cell contracts at the equator and separation of the cytoplasm occurs into two identical cells. The nuclear membrane and nuclei reform and the chromosomes attenuate. During this stage, the diploid number is still 2N, but the DNA content has been reduced to its normal complement.

Meiosis is a process by which the diploid number of chromosomes (2N) is reduced to a haploid (N = 23) number (Fig. 10-4). Meiosis occurs only in germ cells. Meiosis allows for genetic variation through random assortment and disjunction of homologous chromosomes. Each of the meiotic divisions have the same five stages as

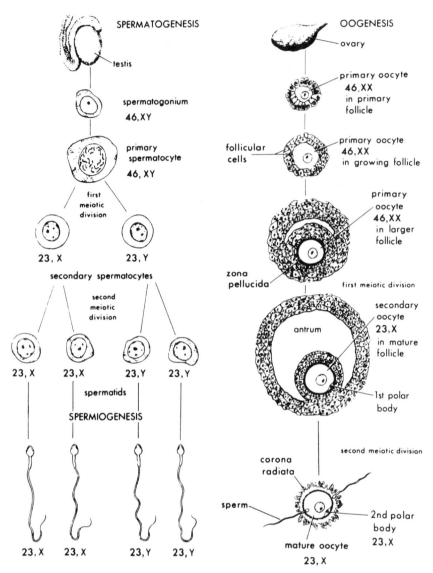

Fig. 10-4. Drawings comparing spermatogenesis and oogenesis. The chromosome complement of the germ cells is shown at each stage. The number designates the total number of chromosomes, including the sex chromosome(s) shown after the comma. Note that (1) following the two meiotic divisions, the diploid number of chromosomes, 46, is reduced to the haploid number, 23; (2) four sperms form from one primary spermactocyte, whereas ony one mature oocyte (ovum) results from maturation of a primary oocyte; and (3) the cytoplasm is conserved during oogenesis to form one large cell, the mature oocyte (ovum). (Moore KL: The Developing Human. WB Saunders, Philadelphia, 1977.)

mitosis. The processes differ in that meiosis involves two divisions with only one replication of genetic material. In the first stage each chromosome replicates but pairs with its homologue. Each pair lines up along the equatorial plane. By random assortment, these homologues segregate during the first phase resulting in two clusters of randomly paired chromosomes at opposite ends of the cell. The chromosome number has been reduced by one-half (reduction division). The second division is similar to mitosis in that individual chromosomes align themselves along the equatorial plate with division of the centromeres and movement of the chromosomes to opposite poles. As a result of this division, the haploid number is maintained with half the normal complement of DNA of a somatic cell. The daughter cells of the second division are generally identical (except for crossover recombination), unlike those in the first division.

In the male, meiosis of the spermatocyte leads to the formation of four mature spermatozoa; in the female, meiosis in the oogonia leads to the formation of one mature egg and two inactive polar bodies.

There is a delicate balance in the amount and kind of chromosome material compatible with normal human development. Changes in the number of chromosomes, in amount of chromosomal material, or in structural relationships lead to abnormal karyotypes that may be pathologic. Multiples of the haploid number of germ cells is known as polyploidy. This is manifested in somatic cells as triploidy (3N = 69) or tetraploidy (4N = 92). An aberration of individual chromosome number (N = 44, 45, 47, 48, etc.) is called aneuploidy. The presence of three homologous chromosomes in a cell is referred to as trisomy (e.g., 47 XY, 21$^+$) the absence of one of a pair of homologous chromosomes is termed monosomy (e.g., 45, XO). The mechanisms leading to abnormalities of chromosome number are listed below.

1. Nondisjunction; during meiosis, failure of chromosomes to sort themselves in equal numbers into daughter cells. One daughter cell receives one chromosome too many and the other receives one too few. Absence of chromosome material is probably more disruptive than excess material. Nondisjunction at later cell division may result in myxoploidy or mosaicism, in which a population of normal and trisomic or monosomic cells co-exist in a single individual. Clinical nondisjunction syndromes include Down's syndrome (trisomy 21), Edward's syndrome (trisomy 18), and Patau's syndrome (trisomy 13).

Trisomy 21 is the most common trisomy, occurring in approximately 1 per 600 live births. Pure nondisjunction is casual in 95 percent of the cases, the remainder caused by translocation or mosaicism. The newborn has a characteristic appearance with upward slanting eyes, epicanthal folds, dermatoglyphic changes, and various levels of mental retardation with, in some instances, cardiac and gastrointestinal complications. Down's syndrome infants may live well into adulthood. Other aneuploid syndromes are lethal early in life. The incidence of Down's syndrome in women age 30 is about 0.6 per 1,000 births and increases gradually to approximately 20 to 50 per 1,000 in mothers at age 45. Nondisjunction appears to be a phenomena related to maternal age but not to paternal age.

Monosomy of autosomes almost always causes early intrauterine demise of the conceptus.

Nondisjunction of sex chromosomes is clinically important but may be compatible with a productive life. Klinefelter's syndrome (47 XXY) is found in 2 per 1,000 live births. This syndrome is associated with sterility, mental subnormality, and alterations in the male habitus. Turner's syndrome, (45 XO) is a phenotypic female compatible with life although often found in spontaneous abortions. Among the malformations noted in

Turner's syndrome are infantile genitalia, short stature, sterility, and ovarian agenesis. This syndrome occurs in 1 per 2,500 live births. Triple XXX females, approximately 1 per 1,600 live births, are apparently normal individuals but may be associated with mental retardation and infertility.

2. Translocation is the transfer of a segment of chromosomal material to another chromosome leading to an imbalance of material in each daughter cell. Two nonhomologous chromosomes may simultaneously break near their ends and join with each other to form a single chromosome such as a D/G translocation. If no genetic material is lost in cell division, a balanced translocation exists and the person is usually clinically unaffected and capable of reproduction. Whether the offspring will be affected depends on the amount of genetic material transferred in reduction division. The risk that a balanced translocation carrier will have an affected child is greater than that of a normal individual. It is, however, independent of maternal age.

3. Deletion is loss of chromosome material following a break in the chromosome arm, resulting in loss of material or partial monosomy. The most well known clinical syndrome related to deletion is termed cri-du-chat, which is a partial monosomy for the number 5 chromosome. These infants have severe mental retardation and most die early in childhood.

Genes are portions of DNA molecules whose function is to direct the synthesis of specific polypeptides. The polypeptides, in turn, may be involved in the production of enzymes. Under normal circumstances, as DNA replicates, an exact reproduction of second generation DNA occurs, insuring the correct transcription of genetic information to daughter cells. Genotype refers to an individual's genetic constitution and the phenotype to the physical expression of genes. An allele is the alternative form of a gene. Homozygous refers to identical genetic allele pairing. Heterozygous indicates the presence of different genetic forms or alleles at similar gene sites or loci of homologous chromosomes. Alleles interact to determine phenotypic traits. When two different alleles are paired, the trait of only one of the alleles is phenotypically expressed (dominant trait) and the individual is said to be a carrier of a recessive allele or trait. There may be variation in the phenotypic expression of a dominant allele (variable expressivity).

Inheritance patterns in human genetic expressivity are in the following patterns:

1. Autosomal dominant

    The phenotypic expression appears in every generation.

    Half the children of an affected person on the average will have the trait.

The trait is not transmitted by unaffected persons to their children.

Male and female are equally likely to transmit or have the trait.

2. Autosomal recessive

The trait most commonly appears only in siblings and not in their parents or offspring.

One-fourth of the sibs of the affected person on the average are affected.

Males and females are equally likely to be affected.

The parents of the affected person may be consanguineous.

3. X-linked recessive

The incidence of the trait is higher in males than in females.

The trait is passed through all the daughters of an affected man to half of the daughters' sons.

The trait is not transmitted from father to son.

4. X-linked dominant

The trait is transmitted from affected males to all their daughters and none of their sons.

An affected female is heterozygous; she will transmit the condition to half her children.

Affected homozygous females will transmit the trait to all of their children.

Affected females are twice as common as affected males and express their condition in a milder form.

Single gene disorders often manifest as inborn errors of metabolism. These result from a metabolic block caused by the deficiency or absence of a single enzyme. There are many rare neonatal and childhood diseases associated with this type of inheritance and a description of them is beyond the scope of this discussion. In general, autosomal recessive inheritance is the most common underlying factor.

Multigenic disorders involve the environmentally influenced interactions of a number of different gene pairs. They are common conditions and include hypertension, diabetes, and peptic ulcer. In the newborn, neural tube closure defects and possibly certain types of heart disease are associated with multifactorial inheritance.

Counseling

About 10 percent of all conceptions are chromosomally abnormal, but a large number abort before viability. Approximately 60 percent of spontaneous first and early second trimester abortions are due to chromosomal abnormalities. Patients who have had a spontaneous abortion associated with chromosomal abnormality have a greater risk than the normal population for a second chromosomally abnormal abortion in future pregnancies. Nevertheless, only a small proportion of mothers having multiple abortions have balanced chromosomal translocations so that markers of future pregnancy risk are not common. The overall risk of chromosome abnormalities at birth is 1.1 per 1,000. Single gene disorders are probably higher than the 1 percent risk that has historically been quoted. The most common of these disorders include Tay-Sachs disease, a disorder of lipid metabolism, inherited as an autosomal recessive disorder, in some descendants of Eastern European Jews; the hemoglobinopathies, including sickle cell disease and thalassemia, representing structural protein abnormalities; deficiencies in protein membrane transport, including α-1 antitrypsin deficiency which is manifested as cystic fibrosis, affecting about 1 in 1,600 newborns.

Because of the impact of these diseases on quality of life and cost to society, recognition of parents at risk is an important part of appropriate care. Documentation of family history, including first-degree (parents, siblings, and subsequent offspring) and second-degree relatives (grandparents, aunts and uncles and half sibs) provides a comprehensive assessment of the gene pool risk for an affected offspring. A complete reproductive history, age at the time of diagnosis, and present status of an affected person are important. Previous pregnancy loss may be a clue to future potentially affected offspring. The second part of the family history consists of asking specific questions to elicit a history of inherited disorders amenable to diagnosis or prevention. This screening history should be carried out before conception and updated between pregnancies.

Laboratory tests useful in prenatal screening include: maternal serum alpha-feto protein (5 to 7 percent false positive); ultrasound for evaluating structural abnormalities of the fetus in utero, as well as for amniocentesis; amniocentesis as the primary means of evaluation during pregnancy, for karyotype and alpha-fetoprotein analysis; specific metabolic tests of amniotic fluid, if available, when a discernible disorder is known to be prevalent within the family; and fetoscopy with sampling of fetal blood for several disorders, limited to a few centers. Prenatal counseling may include consideration of adoption or artificial insemination by an individual from an unaffected gene pool to decrease the risk of abnormal offspring.

Specific patients for whom these tests may be important include mothers age 35 years or more, parents of a previous trisomic infant, known translocation carrier state in one of the parents, history of X-linked disorders, previous child affected by a metabolic disease amenable to antenatal diagnosis, and patients with a prior history of an infant affected by spina bifida, anencephaly, or hydrocephalus.

PRENATAL CARE

The objectives of prenatal care include recognition and treatment of diseases present in the mother or fetus, pregnancy education of the family, provision of psychologic, financial, and social service support for the patient, and provision of nutritional and activity guidelines during pregnancy.

Identification of the high-risk patient is basic to good obstetric care. Between one-third and one-half of patients who subsequently develop serious problems during pregnancy may be recognized during the first prenatal visit. Age less than 16 years or greater than 35 years, malnutrition, and low socioeconomic background are risk factors. A pregnancy history that suggests increased risk includes previous abortion or premature delivery, previous bleeding disorders during pregnancy, history of cesarean section, erythroblastosis, and a gravidity greater than five. Present pregnancy risks include anemia, diabetes, hypertension, renal or other medical diseases, bleeding during pregnancy, malpresentation, deficient prenatal care, and erythroblastosis. Nevertheless, at least 50 percent of maternal complications occur in patients classified as low-risk during their first prenatal visit. When risk indices are used to assess the likelihood of perinatal complications, excellent outcomes are seen in low-risk groups while high-risk groups have increasing perinatal mortality with increasing risk assessment scores. Intrapartum factors may cause a change in risk.

Development of a risk index requires a careful history and physical examination, including age, date of last menstrual period, and complete menstrual history. Use of contraception before conception is important. With menstrual cycles approximating 26 to 30 days, a calculation of an estimated date of confinement is possible based on Naegele's rule of counting 280 days from the first day of the last menstrual period or, from a practical standpoint, by subtracting 3 calendar months and adding 7 days to the first day of the last normal menstrual period. Ovulation usually occurs approximately 14 days before the next anticipated menstrual period. If a patient has a 35-day cycle, an extra 7 days should be added to Naegel's rule, if calculating from the date of the last menstrual period. The history should also include year of occurrence, duration, and problems with each previous pregnancy. Length and conduct of labor and complications during labor and delivery also should be documented. Mode of delivery, type of anesthesia used and the condition of the infant at birth complete the history of labor and delivery. Postpartum complications, including infection and postpartum bleeding, should not be ignored. A history of pregnancy hypertension may be of importance for future pregnancy if underlying benign essential hypertension is present.

Symptoms of pregnancy that might interfere with daily health, prepregnancy planning, and wish to continue pregnancy should be recorded. General and pelvic examinations should be performed on all pregnant patients. The pelvic examination should confirm the diagnosis and time of gestation, provide an estimation of the capacity of the pelvis, and discover any abnormalities that mitigate against conducting normal pregnancy, labor, and delivery.

Diagnostic signs, symptoms, and tests for pregnancy may be subdivided into positive, probable, and presumptive. Positive determinants of pregnancy are the establishment of a fetal heart rate, distinct from the mother's; determination of fetal activity by the examiner; and sonographic or radiographic diagnosis of intrauterine gestation.

Probable signs of pregnancy include increasing size of the maternal abdomen; changes in uterine size, shape, and consistency; changes in cervical shape and consistency, and Braxton-Hicks contractions, balottement, outlining of the fetus, and positive biochemical tests for pregnancy.

Presumptive signs of pregnancy include amenorrhea, changes in the breasts, vaginal discoloration, abdominal striae, nausea and vomiting, fatigue, urinary disturbances, and maternal perception of fetal activity.

Fetal heart rate may be determined by auscultation at 17 to 20 weeks of gestation. By Doppler ultrasound, fetal heart sounds may be heard as early as 8 to 9 weeks of gestation. Fetal activity may be felt by the examiner after 20 weeks of gestation and sonographic diagnosis of intrauterine gestation may occur as early as 5 weeks after the last menstrual period. Radiographic diagnosis is largely historical since ultrasound appears to have less potential adverse effect on the fetus. Ultrasound has become an important dimension of obstetrics because of its capability to determine gestational age, diagnose multiple gestation, to contribute to the diagnosis of ectopic pregnancy, and to discover fetal abnormalities.

Among the probable signs of pregnancy, changes in the uterus are most characteristic. Hegar's sign, a softening of the cervical isthmus, occurs at 6 to 8 weeks of pregnancy. Chadwick's sign is cyanosis of the cervix. By 12 weeks, the uterus has grown to the top of the symphysis pubis. By 20 weeks, the uterus is at the umbilicus. From 16 to 36 weeks, the growth of the uterus is approximately 1 cm per week, when using MacDonald's measurement of the distance between the symphysis pubis and the top of the fundus.

Any of the probable signs of pregnancy may be in error. The use of biochemical pregnancy test to diagnose pregnancy depends on the sensitivity of the test for chorionic gonadotropin as well as its specificity against other hormones that have a biochemical structure similar to

HCG. LH possesses a subunit structure similar to HCG. An elevated LH may cause many pregnancy tests to react, giving a false positive result. This interference may be seen in commercial immunoassays and in the radio-receptor assay. However, the beta subunit for HCG is specific only for HCG and does not cross-react with LH. The patient may have positive beta HCG levels when pregnancy is not present, as in neoplastic diseases with HCG-like substances secreted by the tumor. Home pregnancy tests rely upon immunoassay methods that are relatively sensitive but nonspecific, contributing to a higher false positive rate. Almost all the urine immuno-chemistry tests are obscured by proteinuria, giving false positive results.

A positive pregnancy test does not rule out extrauterine pregnancy or fetal death since placental hormone production may continue even after a missed abortion.

The differential diagnosis for patients with presumptive signs of pregnancy includes amenorrhea and/or galactorrhea secondary either to stress, medication, or pituitary tumor, pseudocyesis, and ovarian failure with secondary amenorrhea and increased LH hormone secretion.

THE PELVIS IN PREGNANCY

Because of the shape of the pelvis, it is difficult to delineate specific structures in relationship to the eventual presenting part of the fetus. Therefore, the pelvis has been described as having four imaginary planes: the plane of the pelvic inlet, the plane of the pelvic outlet, the plane of greatest pelvic dimensions, and the plane of least pelvic dimensions or midpelvis. At the plane of the pelvic inlet, the configuration of the pelvis is usually round or gynecoid. Obstetrically important diameters of the pelvic inlet include the anterior-posterior diameter, the shortest distance between the sacral promentory and the symphysis pubis, designated the obstetric conjugate. Normally, the obstetric conjugate measures at least 10 cm. The transverse diameter represents the greatest distance between the pelvic sidewalls at the level of the pelvic inlet (average, 13.5 cm). The oblique diameters of the inlet average 13 cm. The obstetric conjugate cannot be measured directly. For clinical purposes, the diagonal conjugate, which extends from the lower symphysis pubis to the sacral prominence, may be measured. The diagonal conjugate should measure at least 11.5 cm. The pelvic outlet consists of three important diameters: the anterior-posterior, or the lower margin of the symphysis pubis to the tip of the sacrum (11.5 cm); the transverse diameter between the inner edges of the ischial tuberosities (10 cm); and the posterior sagittal diameter, or the tip of the sacrum to the right-angled intersection between the ischial tuberosities (7.5 cm). The interspinous diameter represents the smallest diameter of the mid pelvis and should measure at least 10 cm. The anterior-posterior diameter at the level of the ischial spines measures at least 11.5 cm.

The outlet of the pelvis can be measured in the transverse diameter from the innermost aspect of the ischial tuberosities. Measurements greater than 8 cm are considered normal. The angle of the subpubic arch should measure at least 90°.

The support of the bony pelvis, which is comprised of the sacrum, the coccyx, and the innominate bones, consists of both fibro-cartilage and ligaments of the two pelvic rami anteriorly and of the sacroiliac joints posteriorly.

Clinical measurements are obtained to assess the pelvic passage during labor. X-Ray pelvimetry has been used in sizing the bony pelvis but should be used only in few clinical circumstances. These include previous injury or disease affecting the bony pelvis and breech presentation at term. Pelvic dimensions change with increasing gestation because of ligamentous relaxation.

Pelvic Shapes

There are four general pelvic shapes or types: (1) Gynecoid—characteristically well-rounded segments with a slightly oval or round configuration throughout. Sidewalls are straight and the spines are not prominent. This type is found in approximately one-half of women. (2) Android—a short posterior inlet, converging pelvic sidewalls, prominent ischial spines, and narrowed subpubic arch. Approximately one-third of women have some form of android pelvis. (3) Anthropoid—the anterior-posterior diameter of the inlet is greater than transverse diameter with a large sacrosciatic notch and convergent sidewalls. The anthropoid pelvis is generally deeper than other types. (4) Platypelloid—flattened with a short anterior-posterior and wide transverse diameter. The sacrum is usually curved and rotated backward so that the pelvis is shallow. This type of pelvis is uncommon, occurring in less than 3 percent of women.

Most pelves are intermediate or of mixed type rather than one of the four pure types. When other potential problems are factored, android pelves are most often associated with complicated labor and delivery and gynecoid pelves least often.

Symptoms of Early Pregnancy and Therapy

Pregnancy should be considered a normal physiologic state. General health care ideally begins before pregnancy to ascertain diseases and developmental abnormalities, appropriate nutrition, and basic exercise characteristics. There are several problems common to normal pregnancy. One of the most common symptoms of early pregnancy is nausea and/or vomiting. The exact cause is not clear but is assumed to be associated with changes in circulating pregnancy hormones. Psychological components may be involved in some patients. Occurrence is common in the morning or when the stomach is empty. Management consists of more frequent feedings and the use of easily digestible carbohydrates.

Backache occurs in many pregnant women. It is associated with fatigue and excessive activity. Ligamentous changes in the pelvis, the increasing size of the gravid uterus and descent of the fetal presenting part into the pelvis contribute to pressure in the lower back and sciatic pain. Management consists of rest, the use of a maternity girdle, and referral to an orthopedic specialist if the problem persists or worsens.

Headache is largely treated symptomatically. Most decrease in severity and may disappear by midpregnancy. In later pregnancy, headache may be a symptom of more serious disease, especially preeclampsia.

Varicosities are exaggerated by pregnancy because of progesterone effects on smooth muscle. Rest, elevation of the lower extremities, and the use of waist-high support hose may be beneficial when symptoms are present. Surgical correction is not advised during pregnancy. Varicosities of the hemorrhoidal veins also appear during pregnancy, due to the obstruction of venous return by the pregnant uterus. Swelling may be relieved by use of topical anesthetics and stool softeners.

Constipation is due to decreased transit through the large intestine. This problem may be counterbalanced by having the patient increase water intake in addition to more frequent use of high-fiber foods. Stool softeners may also be used.

Heartburn is caused by reflux of gastric contents into the lower esophagus, due to compression and displacement of the stomach by the uterus and by hormonal changes on gastric motility. Relief may be obtained by the use of antacid preparations and frequent, small meals. Other symptoms include the normal increase of urinary frequency, fatigue and insomnia, and leukorrhea during pregnancy.

Patient counselling during early prenatal visits is important in the optimal care of pregnancy. A patient may engage in physical activity during pregnancy to the extent that she has engaged in similar activity prior to pregnancy, but she may need to modify that activity during pregnancy. Nonweight-bearing exercise presents the least amount of stress during pregnancy, but moderate exercise, with periodic modification and consideration of other environmental factors, is probably appropriate. Activities that may contribute to injury of the mother or

of the conceptus and potentially hypoxic situations should be avoided. This also applies to physical labor. Adequate rest periods should be provided during the working day. Patients with previous complications of pregnancy that may be recurrent should minimize work and exercise.

Coital activity may be continued during pregnancy unless there is a history of previous perinatal loss or present bleeding, threatened premature labor, premature rupture of fetal membranes, or patient discomfort. It has not been conclusively determined that maternal orgasm is associated with harm to the fetus.

Patients may bathe throughout pregnancy using either showers or tub baths. Douching should be avoided.

Smoking during pregnancy should be avoided. If pregnancy is planned, prepregnancy curtailment of smoking is best. Infants of smoking mothers are smaller than those of nonsmoking mothers and perinatal mortality and morbidity are increased. The incidence of bleeding disorders in pregnancy are also increased when the mother has previously smoked. Cigarette smoke contains over 2,000 chemicals, including carbon monoxide, which functionally inactivates fetal and maternal hemoglobin, and nicotine, which causes vasoconstriction of the uterine arteries. Smoking women also tend to have a reduced caloric intake.

Counseling mothers related to alcohol ingestion during pregnancy is difficult. Fetal alcohol syndrome, which consists of pre- and postnatal growth retardation, typical craniofacial abnormalities, and impaired motor and developmental function in later life, has been noted in newborns of mothers who consumed excessive amounts of alcohol during pregnancy. The syndrome has not been found in women who have consumed less than the equivalent of one mixed drink per day, but abstinence is the only absolutely safe course to insure no fetal effects.

Chronic use by the expectant mother of hard drugs is potentially harmful to the fetus. Poor fetal growth is common and acute maternal drug withdrawal may be hazardous for the fetus.

Routine dental care may be given during pregnancy. Hypnotic anesthetics are not recommended in the dentist's office because of potential maternal and fetal hypoxia.

Laboratory screening during the first office visit should consist of hemoglobin or hematocrit, clean catch urinalysis and screen for bacteria, blood type and Rh antibody screen, pap smear of the cervix, serology, and, unless the patient is known to have had acquired immunity, a rubella titer. In high-risk groups, cervical cultures for gonococcus and herpes simplex virus and serologic hepatitis B screening are recommended.

Subsequent visits should be monthly until 32 weeks and then more frequently thereafter. At each visit, uterine height is measured and the fetal heart rate should be assessed after the twentieth week. Fetal position is determined by Leopold's maneuvers. The patient's blood pressure and urinalysis are recorded at each office visit. The presence of glucose in the urine is not a sensitive indicator for glucose intolerance. During subsequent visits, patients should be questioned about quantity and quality of fetal activity and whether other problems have developed since previous visits. If the patient develops high-risk signs, she may require the services of a medical care team consisting of the obstetrician, other physicians, a dietician, nurse, and social worker.

Tests of Fetal Status

ESTRIOL

The measurement of estriol is the primary biochemical test for fetal well-being during pregnancy. Estriol is an estrogen formed in large quantities by the fetoplacental unit during pregnancy. Its precursor, fetal dehydroepiandrosterone sulfate (DHEA-S) is hydroxylated by the fetal liver and aromatized in the placenta to estriol. The amount of estriol in the maternal urine and plasma rises progressively through pregnancy. Profiles of urine conjugated estriol and serum conjugated and un-conjugated estriol have been determined for normal pregnancy. Single measurements of either urinary or serum estriol are not sufficient to reflect the status of the fetoplacental unit. A 40 percent decrease from previous 3-day means of serum or urine estriols is of significance in assessing fetal well-being. Plasma unconjugated estriol may be a more sensitive indicator of the fetoplacental unit without addressing maternal metabolism. Decreasing values have been associated with fetal jeopardy in several pregnancy disorders.

Other biochemical assays of fetal well-being include human placental lctogen in maternal plasma, DHEA-S, and measurements of progesterone levels or their metabolites. None of these biochemical tests offer any advantage over estriol assays and are infrequently employed.

Major biophysical tests of fetal well-being consist of the nonstress test (NST) and the contraction stress test (CST) or oxytocin challenge test (OCT). The NST is based on the premise that with fetal activity, an acceleration of fetal cardiac rate will occur. Fetal heart rate is recorded electronically while the mother marks fetal movement on the monitor. The test is generally considered normal when two accelerations of at least 15 beats per minute above baseline heart rate are recorded for at least 15 seconds. The test is considered to be as reliable as the oxytocin challenge test in verifying fetal well-being. Absence of accelerations and of activity may be asso-

ciated with physiologic sleep in the fetus (30 to 60 minute cycles); this may account for the low incidence of positive oxytocin challenge tests when a nonreactive nonstress test is recorded.

The contraction stress test or oxytocin challenge test has become a standard for evaluating the fetus during the third trimester when fetal jeopardy is suspected. Electronic recording of fetal heart rate is performed in conjunction with uterine activity, identified by a tocographic transducer. Baseline uterine activity and fetal heart rate are recorded for 15 to 30 minutes. If three spontaneous uterine contractions, each lasting at least 30 seconds, are detected in a 10-minute segment, the criteria for contraction stress test are fulfilled and the fetal cardiac response to contractions is evaluated. In the absence of uterine activity and abnormalities of fetal heart rate, an intravenous oxytocin infusion is started at 0.5 ml/min and increased at 15-minute intervals until three contractions in 10 minutes is recorded. A finding of persistent late decelerations of the fetal heart rate is defined as a positive or abnormal OCT. A negative test shows no late decelerations of the fetal heart rate under similar circumstances. A suspicious test shows irregular late decelerations or other nonperiodic changes in fetal heart rate. Hyperstimulation and uterine contractions more frequent than every 2 minutes, or lasting longer than 90 seconds, negate the validity of a positive test. Oxytocin challenge tests are unsatisfactory if a poor recording is obtained. A normal test is generally reassuring that fetal condition will not deteriorate within a week. False negative tests are found in approximately 0.5 percent of all tests. False positive tests are more common. Sixty percent of inductions after positive contraction stress tests show no signs of fetal distress or neonatal complications.

Fetal movement is frequent during the second half of pregnancy. Thus, a profile of normal daily fetal movement counts has been used as an indicator of fetal health. A persistent 50 percent or greater decrease in fetal movement is abnormal and requires more sophisticated testing.

Amniocentesis is used in late pregnancy to determine fetal lung maturity, to diagnose intraamniotic infection in patients at risk, and to indirectly assess elevated amniotic fluid bilirubin in rhesus isoimmunization. Chromosomal analysis may also be performed. Fetoscopy is a technique employed to observe the fetus for gross abnormalities and to obtain fetal blood for analysis. This method of fetal examination has been used during the second trimester to diagnose classic hemophilia, sickle cell disease, and beta thalassemia. Fetoscopy should be considered a research tool only. The use of radiography, amniography, and amnioscopy are used less frequently for pregnancy diagnosis because of newer technology, especially ultrasonography.

Ultrasonography can study fetal motion and fetal urination as well as to survey fetal anatomy, placental localization, and changes in amniotic fluid volume. Ultrasonography may be subdivided into B-scan, which provides a static cross-sectional picture allowing identification of size, shape, and location of a structure; real time, which documents movements of structures in a two dimensional plane; and M-mode, to study the fetal heart for abnormalities of structure or activity.

Parturition

Labor is a process by which the uterus expels the products of conception after at least 20 weeks gestation. Normal labor is characterized by periodic uterine contractions that produce gradual cervical effacement, dilatation and descent of the fetal presenting part. Uterine contractions usually occur at intervals of less than 10 minutes and become more frequent with advancing labor. Labor is divided into three stages: onset of labor to complete dilatation of the cervix, complete dilatation to birth of the fetus, and birth of the fetus to delivery of the placenta.

What initiates human labor is not entirely clear, but it appears that the fetus, the placenta, and the uterus have contributory roles. At the cellular level, prostaglandins are produced from fetal membranes through phospholipase A-2 action on arachidonic acid precursors. The prostaglandins mediate free calcium release in the myometrium and changes in cervical connective tissue. In concert, these lead to an increase in effective uterine contractions. There is evidence that some prostaglandin activity also occurs in the decidua vera of the endomyometrium.

Fetal cortisol pathways are more active at term and may be involved in phospholipase A-2 activation. The contribution of maternal oxytocin to labor initiation appears to be very small. The fetus is also a source of oxytocin which gradually increases at the time of parturition. The gradual stretch of uterine fibers during pregnancy appears to make them more susceptible to prostaglandin-induced changes in intracellular calcium. The changing relationship of progesterone and estrogen concentrations in late pregnancy probably contribute to increasing uterine myofibril electrical activity. When these activities are in concert, uterine contractions become more frequent and stronger. In patients with twins or polyhydramnios, labor often begins prematurely because the volume of the uterus is increased and smooth muscle fibers are stretched disproportionately. Changes in placental integrity such as found in placenta previa, abruption, and preeclampsia are associated with earlier activation of parturition events. Anencephaly, with poorly developed fetal endocrinologic pathways, is often associated with prolonged pregnancy.

Normal Labor

Changes in uterine contraction frequency and intensity distinguishes true labor from false labor, in which uterine contractions are characterized by irregularity and brevity. The mucous plug that filled the cervical canal during pregnancy is discharged as "show," frequently near the onset of labor. Contraction frequency may be infrequent in early labor but increases to every $2\frac{1}{2}$ to 3 minutes by the active phase of labor. Intensity increases from approximately 40 torr to greater than 75 torr during the same time period. Under normal circumstances, baseline uterine tone is 10 to 15 torr. Generally, a relaxation phase of at least 60 seconds is noted between contractions.

The propagation of uterine contractions normally occurs from pacemakers in the fundus near the uterotubal junction. When this fundal dominance is inhibited by pacemakers elsewhere in the uterus, incoordinate activity may result, manifested in several labor disorders. Mechanical stretching of the cervix, known as the Ferguson reflex, may enhance uterine activity in labor.

In labor, the uterus differentiates into an upper segment which actively contracts and a lower segment, the thinned out isthmus of the nonpregnant uterus which dilates in response to the activity of the superior segment. With contractions, the upper segment contracts, retracts, and expels the fetus through the greatly expanded, thinned out fibromuscular tube of the lower segment. The myometrial cells of the upper segment become relatively fixed at a shorter length and the upper segment becomes progressively thickened during labor. Muscular fibers in the lower segment stretch and become thinner during labor, forming a physiologic retraction ring.

Effacement of the cervix is the shortening of the cervical canal from a structure of approximately 2 cm in length to one in which the canal is virtually an orifice with paper-thin edges. Muscular fibers in the vicinity of the internal os are pulled upward into the lower uterine segment shortly before and during labor. The work of labor is related to the resistance offered by the cervix to dilatation. In the second stage of labor, the resistance may be exerted by the muscles of the pelvic floor. For the fetal head to pass through the cervix at term, the cervical canal must dilate to a diameter of about 10 cm. With each contraction, the hydrostatic action of the amniotic sac or the presenting part helps to dilate the cervical canal.

The pattern of cervical dilatation during normal labor is in the shape of a sigmoid curve (Fig. 10-5). Two phases of cervical dilatation have been defined, the latent phase

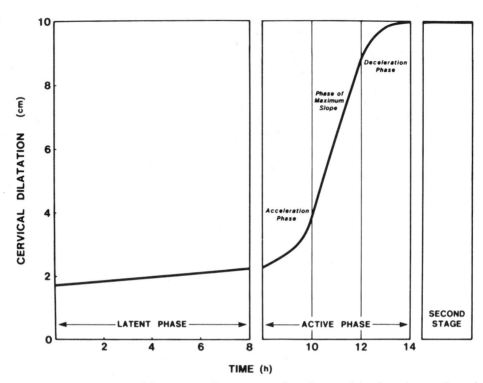

Fig. 10-5. Composite of the average dilatation curve for nulliparous labor based on analysis of the data derived from the patterns traced by a large, nearly consecutive series of gravidas. The first stage is divided into a relatively flat latent phase and rapidly progressive active phase. The active phase has three identifiable component parts — an acceleration phase, a linear phase of maximum slope, and a deceleration phase. (Friedman: Labor: Clinical Evaluation and Management, 2nd ed. Appleton, New York, 1978.)

and the active phase. The latent phase is a variable phase of uterine work until the cervix is dilated approximately 3 to 4 cm. Thereafter, more rapid changes in the cervix occur; this is referred to as the active phase. The active phase may be further subdivided into an acceleration phase, a phase of maximum slope, when the most rapid changes occur, and the deceleration phase. Nulligravidas and multiparous patients have different lengths of the latent and active phases. Prolongation of the latent phase has little bearing on the subsequent course of labor but characteristics of the active phase are generally predictive of the outcome of labor. The pattern of descent plays an important role in defining the prognosis of labor. In many nulliparous patients, engagement of the fetal head into the pelvis occurs prior to labor and further descent does not occur until active labor. In multiparous patients and in nulliparous patients without previous engagement, descent often occurs during the first stage of labor. Active descent usually takes place after cervical dilatation has progressed for some time. Once descent has started, it normally continues until the fetal presenting part reaches the pelvic floor. Should this not occur, there is often a discrepancy in the relationship of the fetal presenting part to the pelvic floor.

Spontaneous rupture of the membranes most often occurs during the active phase of labor. Once dilatation is complete, intraabdominal pressure by the mother contributes to expulsion of the fetus. Several changes occur in the tone of vagina and pelvic floor during the second stage of labor to help propel the fetus toward delivery.

The third stage of labor includes placental separation which occurs as the result of a decrease in uterine volume and subsequent buckling of the placenta. In general, the placenta will be spontaneously expelled from the uterus and artificial removal of the placenta should be reserved for instances of postpartum hemorrhage.

Presentation of the Fetus in Labor

Generally, the fetus presents in labor in longitudinal lie, and most often with vertex foremost within the birth canal. This is referred to as a vertex presentation. Uncommonly, the fetus may present in a transverse lie or an oblique lie, in which the fetal axis is in a non-parallel plane with the maternal long axis. Longitudinal lies are present in over 99 percent of labors at term. Other longitudinal presentations beside vertex include breech, face, and brow presentations. Ordinarily, the head is flexed sharply with the chin on the thorax forming the vertex or occiput presentation. If the neck is sharply extended, the face presents first (< 1 percent). Brow presentation is an unstable presentation and generally will convert either to a vertex or a face presentation.

If the fetus presents by the breech (4 percent), the thighs may be flexed with the legs extended over the anterior surface of the body. This is referred to as frank breech presentation. A complete breech occurs when the knee and hip joints are flexed and an incomplete breech or footling breech occurs when both the hip and knee of one or both legs is extended.

Once fetal presentation and lie have been determined, position (left, right, or direct) of the presenting part is determined. Most commonly, the vertex, or occiput presents first. Consequently, the fetus may present in a right or left occiput position. The third component of position is whether the presenting part is anterior, transverse, or posterior. Most commonly, the fetus presents as an occiput anterior or transverse in either right or left position.

Diagnosis of presentation and position of the fetus may be performed by Leopold's maneuvers. Additionally, vaginal examination should give information about cervical effacement and dilatation, presentation and position of the presenting part, and integrity of the fetal membranes. Measurements of the relative dimensions of the fetal presenting part and the pelvic cavity are performed. During labor, the head will adapt to the diameters of the pelvis by several maneuvers and by molding. The maneuvers, commonly referred to as cardinal movements, include engagement, descent, flexion, internal rotation, extension, external rotation, and expulsion. Several of these mechanisms occur simultaneously in labor; the shape of the fetal head changes or is molded to allow for passage through the lower pelvis. The passage of the greatest transverse diameter of the fetal head through the pelvic inlet is designated "engagement." The fetal head tends to accommodate to the transverse axis of the pelvic inlet and the sagittal suture generally lies midway between the symphysis and the sacral promontory. Deflection of the sagittal suture outside of this plane is referred to as "asynclitism." Moderate degrees of asynclitism occur in normal labor.

When the head flexes, its presenting diameter changes from a larger occipitofrontal diameter to a shorter suboccipitobregmatic diameter. With delivery, the head externally rotates back or restitutes to the prelabor position.

A fetus who presents in an engaged occiput anterior position should deliver vaginally under normal obstetric circumstances. If a fetus continues labor in a occiput posterior or transverse position, these deviations

from normal presentations may cause obstetric difficulties.

Conduct of Normal Labor and Delivery

Identification of labor includes the differentiation of true from false labor. True labor generally occurs at regular intervals which gradually shorten, with gradual increase in contraction intensity. There is discomfort in lower back and abdomen with cervical dilatation. This type of labor is not stopped by sedation. False labor usually is controlled by sedation with little change in the cervix. Once labor is diagnosed, the condition of the mother and her fetus should be ascertained through history and physical examination. Frequency and intensity of uterine contractions are noted along with the degree of maternal discomfort. Heart rate, presentation, and size of the fetus are evaluated abdominally. Fetal heart rate should be checked at the end of a contraction to identify potentially pathologic tachycardia, bradycardia, or decrease from baseline heart rate.

Unless there has been heavy vaginal bleeding, a vaginal examination may be performed under aseptic conditins. Membrane status and the condition of the cervix including softness, effacement, dilatation, and location should be assessed.

Station refers to the relationship of the presenting part to the ischial spines of the maternal pelvis. The ischial spines are considered at zero station. If the presenting part is above the ischial spines, it is considered (in centimeter intervals), at a minus station, below the ischial spines at a positive station. Clinical pelvimetry, the measurement of the relationship of the presenting part to the sacrum, pelvic sidewalls, and the subpubic arch, should be performed to determine the feasibility of vaginal delivery.

Detection of ruptured membranes is important in the examination of the patient who may be in labor. Patients should be admitted for evaluation if they have fluid leakage or ruptured amniotic membranes. Membrane rupture may be the first sign of labor. Unusually, the umbilical cord may prolapse after rupture of membranes. Prolonged rupture of fetal membranes may result in infection of the fetal membranes, or chorioamnionitis, threatening both mother and fetus.

Spontaneous rupture of membranes may be documented by visualization of free flowing fluid from the cervix, arborization of amniotic fluid on a dried glass slide (fern test), or by documentation of alkaline pH of amniotic fluid on nitrazine paper. Urine can also show an alkaline pH, making this test less reliable.

If a patient is in labor or has ruptured membranes, several laboratory studies should be performed. Serum hemoglobin, blood type and antibody screen and urinalysis for protein should be performed. Maternal vital signs should be repeated periodically, including blood pressure, pulse, respiratory rate, and temperature. Use of enemas and perineal shaving should be individualized to patient needs and few clinical circumstances.

Fetal heart rate and uterine activity should be accurately recorded during labor. During the first stage of labor, fetal heart rate should be recorded immediately after a contraction, at 15-minute intervals. In the second stage, evaluation should be at 5-minute intervals. Uterine activity is palpated at similar intervals; vaginal examination should be performed as infrequently as possible. Patients may be reexamined if contractions become more uncomfortable, if the patient desires medication, if there are abnormal decelerations, marked decreases in fetal heart rate, if there is an increase in vaginal bleeding, or if the patient has a sense of rectal pressure and feels the need to push. Vaginal examination should always be performed immediately after rupture of membranes to rule out cord prolapse.

The average first stage of labor in nulliparous women is approximately 8 hours and in parous women about 5 hours. The second stage is approximately 50 to 60 minutes in nulliparous women and 20 to 30 minutes in multiparous patients. The third stage is completed in approximately 5 to 10 minutes. Variations are common but prolongation of any of these stages may represent clinical problems.

Dysfunctional labor occurs in several clinical forms. Prolonged latent phase is defined as continued contractions longer than 20 hours without cervical dilatation greater than 3 to 4 cm in nulliparous patients and longer than 14 hours in multiparous patients. Prolonged latent phase is frequently associated with excessive analgesia. The differential diagnosis includes false labor (20 percent). Prolonged latent phase is treated by sedation or by intravenous oxytocin. Sedation is usually followed by active phase labor. Contractions may cease, leading to a diagnosis of false labor.

Protracted active phase occurs when the rate of cervical dilatation is less than 1.2 cm per hour in nulliparous patients and less than 1.5 cm per hour in multiparous patients. Protracted descent is less than 1 cm per hour in nulliparous patients and less than 3 cm per hour in multiparous patients. Average dilatation is approximately 3 cm per hour in active phase. Protraction disorders are associated with cephalopelvic disproportion or excessive sedation or anesthesia. Oxytocics should be used cautiously to ameliorate the disorder. Cesarean section may be indicated for lack of progress or deterioration of maternal or fetal condition.

Secondary arrest of dilatation and descent occur when there is absence of dilatation or descent for 2 hours during the active phase of labor, once descent has started. This disorder is also associated with cephalopelvic disproportion but may also be due to conduction anesthesia or dysfunctional labor. If the patient does not have clinical cephalopelvic disproportion, treatment by oxytocin stimulation is frequently helpful.

Precipitate labor occurs when there is unusually rapid progress of cervical dilatation, greater than 5 cm per hour in nulliparous patients and greater than 10 cm per hour in multiparous patients. This disorder is more frequent in multiparous patients and is associated with trauma and fetal asphyxia. Carefully controlled delivery should minimize some of these problems.

Fetal monitoring addresses the response of the fetus to changes in uterine blood flow during labor. Normal fetal heart rate should range between 120 and 160 beats per minute. Baseline fetal heart rate should be ascertained immediately after contractions. Relative bradycardia exists with a fetal heart rate of 100 to 120 beats per minute and relative tachycardia may be defined as a fetal heart rate of between 160 to 180 beats per minute. These findings, if transient, are rarely associated with problems. Fetal heart rates of greater than 180 beats per minute or less than 100 beats per minute are often associated with abnormalities of fetal oxygenation. If these changes are auscultated, electronic fetal monitoring is warranted. Electronic fetal monitoring can ascertain fetal heart rate variability, which is the beat-to-beat variation in baseline heart rate due to intact central nervous system control mechanisms. Variability of between 6 to 10 beats per minute is reassuring if obtained by an internal fetal heart rate electrode. External electronic monitoring is not as accurate in determining variability. Fetal heart rate responses to uterine contractions, known as periodic changes, are important determinants of fetal well-being in labor. Accelerations of fetal heart rate or mild decelerations in phase with uterine contractions, are reassuring when associated with good beat-to-beat variability. Variable decelerations are changes in fetal heart rate of variable onset, variable rates of deceleration, and of variable duration. They are usually in phase with uterine contractions. Infrequent variable decelerations are not associated with fetal hypoxia, but if persistent and prolonged, they may indicate impaired uteroplacental exchange. Decelerations starting later in a uterine contraction and continuing after the contraction has ceased indicate fetal hypoxia. If persistent, further evaluation or management of these late decelerations is required including the possibility of emergency delivery.

Nonperiodic fetal heart rate changes include both accelerations and decelerations not associated with uterine contractions. Accelerations may be associated with fetal activity and are reassuring. Decelerations unassociated with uterine activity may be due to changes in fetal position. They indicate cord compression, sometimes associated with decreased amounts of amniotic fluid, and may be a sign of fetal distress if persistent.

Other signs of potential fetal distress in labor include the passage of meconium, prolonged bradycardia less than 100 beats per minute, and tachycardia greater than 180 beats per minute.

When possible, the biophysical diagnosis of fetal distress should be confirmed by biochemical tests. Fetal scalp pH sampling will detect fetal acidemia. If maternal acid-base balance is normal, fetal pH ≥ 7.25 is considered normal. A scalp pH of < 7.20 indicates fetal acidemia and correlates with other signs of fetal distress and neonatal depression. A scalp pH between these two values requires immediate retesting.

Management of fetal distress includes maternal position change, oxygen administration, decreasing uterine activity, correction of maternal hypotension if present, examination for cord prolapse and labor progress, and operative delivery if other methods do not improve fetal status.

During labor, maternal position is important in maintaining uterine blood flow. The sitting position or lateral recumbent position, if comfortable for the patient, is ideal. The supine position is associated with hypotension because blood return from the lower extremities is impeded by the gravid uterus. Maternal hypotension and fetal bradycardia have been noted with the supine hypotension syndrome.

Amniotomy should be performed for clinical indications only. These include obstetrically indicated induction or augmentation of labor when amniotomy may be helpful, inadequate external evaluation of fetal heart rate response to uterine activity, and increased maternal bleeding in labor or abruption.

The second stage of labor is often heralded by slowing of the fetal heart rate with fetal head compression. Prompt recovery of fetal heart rate is usually seen under these circumstances. The mother experiences an urge to push and constant attendance and coaching of maternal efforts is important. The second stage may be shortened appreciably by appropriate coaching and maternal position.

In the delivery room, the attendant should gown and glove in an aseptic fashion and the patient should be prepped for delivery. Episiotomy is a surgical incision of the perineum for delivery of the fetal head. This procedure may be helpful for primigravid patients to decrease the potential for fetal head trauma from constant pushing against the intact perineum. Episiotomy reduces the frequency of lacerations and heals better. Protection of the pelvic floor is increased by performance of a modified Ritgen maneuver, which displaces some of the pressure of the fetal head away from the perineal body and toward the vaginal orifice.

Once the fetal head is delivered, immediate suctioning of the mouth and nasopharanyx is performed and the face is wiped dry. Approximately 25 percent of infants will present with a loose nuchal cord which may be reduced before full delivery. After delivery, the cord is clamped and the newborn is examined.

The third stage of labor, separation and delivery of the placenta, is manifested by four signs; (1) the uterus becomes firm and globular; (2) a sudden gush of blood; (3) the uterus rises in the abdomen as the placenta is delivered into the lower uterine segment; and (4) the umbilical cord elongates. These signs occur without the need for traction by the operator and manual removal is warranted only if there is excessive vaginal bleeding, or if placental separation has not occurred within a reasonable amount of time (30 minutes). The delivered placenta should be inspected to determine whether any portions are retained in the uterus. After delivery, the uterus should be examined for evidence of atony and injury. Massage of the postpartum uterus often increases uterine tone. The cervix, vaginal walls, and episiotomy site should be inspected for evidence of injury and should be repaired. Oxytocics may be used to increase uterine tone and decrease bleeding. When uterine atony is present, as shown by a soft uterus and increased vaginal bleeding, intravenous oxytocin in dilute solution should be used. Oxytocin should not be administered as an intravenous bolus. Ergot alkaloids, including ergonovine, have also been used to decrease postpartum bleeding but may increase blood pressure, and should be limited to patients who are not hypertensive. Vaginal and intramuscular prostaglandins are also used to decrease uterine atony.

Vaginal lacerations may result from delivery and include the following; First degree — simple tears of perineal skin or vaginal mucosa; Second degree — the tearing of the muscle and fascia of the perineal body; Third degree — tearing of the anal sphincter muscle; Fourth degree — disruption of the rectal mucosa. Recognition and proper repair of third and fourth degree lacerations is essential to prevent fecal incontinence and recto-vaginal fistula formation.

Labor Induction

The elective induction of labor has been associated with several problems, including iatrogenic prematurity and operative delivery. Induction of labor may be indicated for several medical or obstetric problems. A partial list includes premature rupture of fetal membranes at term, medical or obstetric conditions threatening the health of the fetus (diabetes mellitus, preeclampsia, small for gestational age infants near term), and prolonged pregnancy.

The inducibility of the cervix may be assessed by using the Bishop's score of labor inducibility (Table 10-2). The more favorable the inducibility score, the more likely is normal labor to ensue. Oxytocin is the best agent for inducing labor, when given intravenously in dilute solution by a constant infusion pump. Sublingual and intravenous drip oxytocin have also been used but cannot be controlled so well as an infusion pump. Uterine sensitivity to oxytocin increases throughout pregnancy and hypertonic uterine contractions may be caused by indiscriminate administration of oxytocin. Amniotomy has been used to initiate labor but has the disadvantage of requiring a very ripe cervix and of contributing to complications if the fetal head is not descended into the pelvis. Prolapse of the umbilical cord and fetal bleeding from vasa previa may result from amniotomy. Intravenous prostaglandins have been used for labor induction but are not more effective than oxytocin. Intravaginal prostaglandins are efficacious in stimulating labor in patients with intrauterine fetal demise in the second trimester. In lower dosage, they may ripen the cervix for successful induction in high risk patients.

Uterine activity in labor may be hypotonic, hypertonic, or incoordinate, depending on the frequency of contractions and the relaxation phase between contractions. Hypotonic contractions or secondary inertia are noted late in the active phase and respond well to oxytocin. Hypertonic uterine contractions may be seen with precipitate labor or in protracted active phase disorders. With the latter, poor labor progression continues despite an increase in uterine activity. The primary method of management for this disorder is sedation. Incoordinate uterine activity is manifested by frequent, irregular contractions of variable duration and is manifested by a lack of labor progress; this problem too may be managed by sedation.

Table 10-2. Bishop Scoring of Inducibility of Labor

	Score			
Factor	0	1	2	3
Dilatation, cm	Closed	1–2	3–4	5 or more
Effacement, %	0–30	40–50	60–70	80 or more
Station	−3	−2	−1.0	+1, +2
Consistency	Firm	Medium	Soft	
Position	Posterior	Mid	Anterior	

(From Romney, et al. (eds): Gynecology and Obstetrics. The Health Care of Women, 2nd Ed. McGraw-Hill, New York, 1981.)

Analgesia and Anesthesia

When considering analgesia and anesthesia during labor and delivery, the following principles should be observed. (1) The consideration of the safety of two patients. Oversedation of the fetus may contribute to poor neonatal cardiorespiratory response. (2) The medication used should not interfere with the progress of labor and delivery. (3) Any woman in labor should be considered to have a full stomach because of the absence of gastric emptying during labor. (4) Analgesia-anesthesia should be used in an environment of patient education and proper psychological management. (5) Delivery of a pain relief system should not interfere with oxygen transfer to the mother or fetus. (6) Use of analgesia or anesthesia during labor and delivery requires supervision of oxygenation and vital signs.

Analgesia-anesthesia may be considered in terms of levels of care. More invasive and extensive management may be necessary with increased labor progress or with complications of labor. Most patients benefit from early pregnancy information about the course of labor. Psychoprophylactic methods or Lamaze classes are helpful in educating patients to the realities of pain in labor and to patient relaxation techniques. When these techniques are insufficient for labor management, the attendant may consider the following agents:

(1) Sedation-analgesia with narcotic analgesics. These agents may be given intramuscularly or intravenously. When given by the intravenous route, they are more predictable in their action and clearance. Meperidine and alphaprodine are the most frequently used agents. Given in small intravenous doses, these drugs are cleared from the maternal and fetal circulations within 1.5 to 2 hours and may be given with some time predictability prior to delivery. Morphine sulfate is a less attractive agent because of its more profound central nervous system depressant action on the neonate. Ataractics (promethazine, hydroxyzine) add to the analgesia effect and relax the patient. Barbiturates have been used for similar purposes. When narcotics are used for labor and delivery, a narcotic antagonist should be available for the possibility of a maternal reaction or neonatal depression.

(2) Paracervical block. Local anesthetic is injected near sensory ganglia located in the lateral cervix. The local anesthesia prevents sensory transmission from a T 10–T 12, L1 distribution and intrauterine discomfort is usually obliterated. Complications from this method include transient fetal bradycardia and direct injection into the uterine circulation or into the fetus. Fetal distress and fetal death have been recorded in the rare situation of direct fetal injection. Generally, a short-acting local anesthetic should be used.

(3) Regional anesthesia. Epidural anesthesia is an ex-

cellent means of pain relief. Its use requires adequate knowledge of neuroanatomy and potential complications of use during pregnancy. Epidural anesthesia is usually provided through a catheter inserted into one of the lumbar interspaces. Onset of action is dependent on the type of local anesthesia used but usually starts within 10 minutes of injection. Epidural anesthesia may also be sympatholytic. Therefore, the patient should be pretreated with intravenous fluids to minimize the effects of sequestering blood volume in the capacitance vessels of the lower extremities. Circulating levels of local anesthesia are usually small and direct fetal effects are generally not a problem. Epidural anesthesia rarely affects the progress of labor and ultimately, the type of delivery, but when used appropriately, this method should not interfere with normal labor and delivery.

Anesthesia for delivery is determined by neuroanatomical areas. The lower pelvic region is served by sensory fibers from the S 2 – S 4 region. The simplest method of anesthesia for delivery is a local anesthetic injected for episiotomy. Infiltration of the pudendal canal near the ischial spines blocks sensory fibers throughout the lower vagina and perineum and is referred to as a pudendal block. This method has a 90 percent success rate in experienced hands. Side-effects include the development of a hematoma when the pudendal artery or vein is inadvertently injured. A pudendal block is usually insufficient anesthesia for forceps delivery.

Regional methods of anesthesia are excellent for delivery and include subarachnoid block and epidural anesthesia. Subarachnoid block or spinal anesthesia is similar to epidural anesthesia in the neuroanatomic region involved. The advantages of spinal anesthesia include rapid onset of action and relative ease of administration. Complications of spinal anesthesia include hypotension with insufficient vascular volume, central nervous system stimulation with inadvertant injection of anesthetic into intravascular spaces, and total spinal anesthesia when the drug affects higher neural segments. Postpartum headache occurs in 5 to 10 percent of patients and transient bladder dysfunction has been described. Infection is rare. Spinal and epidural anesthesia should be used with caution and appropriate monitoring, if at all, under circumstances of severe late pregnancy bleeding or hypertension.

The use of general anesthesia requires knowledge of respiratory tract anatomy since artificial ventilation and tracheal intubation are required. The onset of action of a general anesthetic, when used in conjunction with a short-acting barbiturate or a muscle relaxant may be quite rapid and appropriate for emergency deliveries. A patient should be considered to have a full stomach with the potential for aspiration (Mendelsohn's syndrome). General anesthesia is a central nervous system depressant and may cause uterine relaxation when certain halogenated anesthetics are used. This effect may be helpful during difficult delivery but may also be of potential risk when requiring uterine hemostasis. When general anesthesia is used for delivery, high concentrations of inspired oxygen are beneficial. The use of clear antacids or cimetidine has been recommended prior to intubation to diminish the incidence of aspiration syndromes.

OPERATIVE DELIVERY

When maternal efforts to complete the second stage of labor fail or if other complications of labor jeopardize the fetus or mother, operative intervention may be necessary. The most commonly used procedures are forceps delivery, vacuum extraction, and cesarean delivery.

Forceps are paired, interlocking blades, designed to facilitate safe delivery of the fetal head through the maternal pelvis. Forceps are indicated only after engagement of the vertex into the pelvis. Low forceps consists of application when the fetal head is in the occiput anterior or posterior position on the pelvic floor. Midforceps refers to procedures performed when the fetal head has not yet rotated to occiput anterior or posterior or has not reached the pelvic floor. Any rotational forceps delivery of the engaged vertex is a midforceps operation. High forceps is application to the unengaged head, a dangerous and obsolete practice. Some forceps are specifically designed for traction while other designs facilitate rotation of the fetal head.

Forceps may be used to shorten second stage labor. Several complications of the second stage, especially fetal distress, hemorrhage, and regional anesthesia effects, may be indications for forceps delivery. Prerequisites for forceps delivery are complete cervical dilation, engagement of the fetal head, favorable position of the fetus, and pelvic dimensions that permit vaginal delivery. In the case of breech delivery, forceps application to the aftercoming fetal head prevents neck hyperextension and neurologic injury.

Vacuum extraction is used under similar circumstances as are forceps. Newer designs of the suction cup for application to the fetal vertex facilitate its use and have minimized complications associated with earlier designs. Vacuum extraction usually augments maternal expulsive efforts when the fetus is in occiput anterior position. It is less helpful when regional anesthesia prevents maternal pushing. The method is associated with a low incidence of birth trauma.

Cesarean delivery is usually indicated for cephalopelvic disproportion but may also be indicated for a variety of maternal and fetal disorders, including fetal distress, prolapsed umbilical cord, some breech presentations, unstable third trimester bleeding disorders, and previous cesarean section. Up to 20 percent of term pregnancies end in cesarean deliveries. Morbidity and mortality are more frequent with cesarean delivery; anesthesia complications, infection, and hemorrhage are the most frequently associated factors.

Cesarean delivery is usually made through a transverse incision in the lower uterine segment to minimize the risk of future rupture. A trial of labor and vaginal delivery after previous cesarean delivery may be considered provided the patient has not had a classical cesarean scar and pelvic dimensions are adequate. If the fetus presents with a transverse lie or with an anterior placenta previa, a vertical or classical incision may be necessary. The risk of uterine rupture in future pregnancy is 0.2 to 0.5 percent. Fetal loss is approximately 50 percent if rupture occurs.

Postpartum Hemorrhage

The loss of more than 600 ml blood at delivery occurs in four percent of parturients. Postpartum hemorrhage is the primary cause of maternal deaths in the United States. Uterine atony is the most common form of this disorder. Predisposing causes include overdistension of the uterus because of a large fetus, multiple pregnancy, and polyhydramnios. High parity, prolonged labor, rapid delivery, general anesthesia, retained uterine fragments, vaginal and cervical lacerations, and coagulopathies are also associated with postpartum hemorrhage. Management consists of uterine massage, intravenous oxytocic infusion, and transfusion and curettage when placental fragments remain. Uterine packing is generally contraindicated.

Puerperium

The puerperium is the period from delivery until the return of the reproductive organs to a normal, nonpregnant state, approximately 6 to 8 weeks. After delivery, the uterus continues to contract and assumes a position midway between the umbilicus and symphysis pubis. The cervical os closes within days. Since most postpartum problems occur in the first few hours after birth, maternal vital signs, uterine size and tone, and character of vaginal bleeding should be checked frequently for several hours and the patient should not be oversedated. Early puerperal complications include infection, bleeding, eclampsia, and venous thrombosis.

Uterine discharge, or lochia gradually changes from a blood-mixed lochia rubra to a more watery lochia serosa during the first postpartum week. During the next 2 to 3 weeks, lochia alba consisting of leukocytes and epithetical cells is seen in most nonlactating women, and menses often recur between 6 to 8 weeks postpartum. Continued lactation may delay ovulation and menses indefinitely but should not be considered as adequate contraception.

Ambulation should start immediately postpartum as protection against venous thrombosis. Diet should emphasize antenatal considerations for protein and calories, especially in the nursing mother. Mild analgesics may be used for puerperal pain without depressing the infant if the mother is lactating.

Lactation is usually started by the fourth postpartum day in response to withdrawal of pregnancy hormones and postpartum neurohypohyseal release of prolactin and oxytocin. Oxytocin release is further stimulated by suckling.

Breast-feeding may start immediately after delivery with a gradual increase from 3 to 10 minutes feeding per breast as colostrum gives way to a greater supply of mature milk. Gentle washing of the nipples after feeding is sufficient to prevent nipple cracking and infection. Breast feeding with neonatal vitamin supplementation is sufficient nutrition for the first half year if infant growth has been normal.

Suppression of lactation may be desired postpartum and is best accomplished by tight binding of the breasts with a bra or binder, ice to the axilla, and analgesics. Bromocryptine, a prolactin antagonist, may also be used but causes nausea and vomiting in 10 percent of patients.

Complications of the late puerperium include endomyometritis, urinary tract infection, hemorrhage due to subinvolution of the placental site, mastitis, venous thrombosis, and postpartum depression. Postpartum infection is signified by temperature of at least 38°C, documented on at least 2 of the first 10 days postpartum, exclusive of the first 24 hours.

Endomyometritis is commonly due to normal bacterial inhabitants of the genital tract: coliforms, aerobic and anerobic streptococcus, and staphylococcus. This disorder is more commonly associated with prolonged labor, operative delivery, multiple vaginal exams, hemorrhage, and debilitation. Diagnosis is made by findings of fever, uterine tenderness, and abnormal or foul-smelling lochia. Leukocytosis may be present and lochial or endometrial cultures are often positive but contamination by normal vaginal flora is common. Management consists of broad-spectrum parenteral antibiotics, bedrest, fluids, and analgesia. Persistence of the infection may lead to pelvic cellulitis or pelvic thrombophelebitis. The latter is often associated with bacteriodes fragilis infection and responds to appropriate antibiotics and intravenous heparin.

Urinary tract infections are more frequent during the puerperium because of delivery trauma, frequent catheterization, indwelling catheters from cesarean delivery, and hypotonia of the bladder. Urinary tract infections usually manifest on the first or second postpartum day, endomyometritis is clinically apparent usually after the second day. Diagnosis is made by urinalysis and culture of urine from women with complaints of dysuria or retention. Coliforms are the most common pathogens and treatment consists of oral or systemic antibiotics, rest, and increased fluid intake.

Mastitis or breast infection is most often unilateral and may cause engorgement, fever, and pain. Abscess formation occasionally occurs. The offending organism frequently is staphylococcus aureus that enters nipple fissures from the neonate's oronasopharynx. Prevention consists of good personal hygiene and elimination of virulent organisms from nursery personnel. Management includes isolation of suspected infants, culture of maternal milk, and a 10-day course of appropriate antibiotics. Breast feeding may continue as treatment is started. Rarely, abscess formation requires incision and drainage.

Venous thrombosis is more frequent postpartum than during pregnancy. Trauma at delivery, stasis of lower extremity blood flow, and coagulation changes postpartum contribute to the increased frequency. Deep venous thrombosis is associated with an increased risk of pulmonary embolus. Anticoagulant therapy is necessary; heparin, given intravenously as 5,000 to 10,000 units at 4 to 5 hour intervals, or at 800 to 1000 units per hour by infusion pump, is the cornerstone of therapy. Therapy is continued with sodium warfarin after approximately 1 week of IV heparin therapy. Pulmonary embolism may be suspected because of patient dyspnea, chest pain, tachypnea, tachycardia, or apprehension, with abnormal pulmonary or cardiac exams. Diagnosis is made by arterial blood gases and either ventilation-perfusion scans or pulmonary angiography. Treatment consists of systemic anticoagulation and oxygen therapy. Persistence of the problem may require surgical intervention in the form of vena caval ligation.

DISORDERS OF THE FETUS

The fetus may be adversely affected by the following categories of disorders: immunologic-erythroblastosis fetalis, abnormal fetal growth, asphyxia, infection, and developmental abnormalities.

Erythroblastosis is a hematologic disease unique to the fetus. The affected fetus is most often the product of a Rh-negative mother and a Rh-positive, ABO-compatible father. If the fetus is Rh-positive (autosomal dominant), fetal cells entering the maternal circulation stimulate an antibody response. Maternal IgG antibodies can also cross the placenta with relative ease and continue to attack RBCs of the fetus. Isoimmunization may also occur if the mother has irregular antibodies (Kell, Duffy, Kidd, etc.). Destruction of the antibody-fetal cell complex occurs in the fetal spleen. If severe enough, fetal anemia, hypoproteinemia, and ultimately heart failure result.

Fifteen percent of women are Rh-negative. Because of Rh-compatible paternity, and immunologic and placental circulatory reasons, 2 percent of Rh isoimmunization occurs during pregnancy. Most occurrences result from delivery and are evident by the subsequent pregnancy. Therefore, all pregnant women should have a Rh antibody screen during the first prenatal visit. If Rh-negative, the patient is at risk to become sensitized during pregnancy or delivery. The antibody screen should be repeated at 28 weeks. If negative, the patient is a candidate for antepartum prophylaxis with Rh-immune globulin (RHIG). Generally this is sufficient to prevent isoimmunization before labor. If the screen remains negative, the patient is then a candidate for Rho(D) immune globulin prophylaxis at delivery.

With a positive screen, Rh antibody titers are performed. If a previous infant was erythroblastotic or the titer is increasing, amniocentesis is necessary. The timing of amniocentesis depends on history and should start at least by 26 weeks of pregnancy. Laboratory analysis consists of spectrophotometric analysis of amniotic fluid at 450 nanometers, compared to normal or baseline readings (delta O.D. 450). The delta O.D. 450 is plotted against gestational age based on a nomogram devised by Liley. Depending on the gestational age and the absorption of amniotic fluid, the fetus may be mildly, moderately, or severely affected (Zones I to III). Repeat amniocentesis establishes a trend of bilirubin pigment production. The frequency of amniocentesis depends on the severity of fetal condition. If severe fetal involvement is determined to be present, management consists either of delivery of the fetus if lung maturity is assured or intrauterine fetal transfusion. This procedure may be repeated periodically until fetal lung maturity is present. Further management as a neonate is less risky. With mild or moderate isoimmunization (Zones I, II) periodic examination of the amniotic fluid determines the safety of continuing pregnancy. It is prudent to deliver these pregnancies with a mature L/S ratio, usually between 37 and 39 weeks gestation.

Erythroblastosis fetalis may be prevented by giving RHIG to non-sensitized Rh-negative women within 72 hours after delivery. RHIG, 300 μl, is sufficient to neutralize 30 ml of fetal blood or 15 ml of fetal RBCs in maternal circulation. With abruption, placenta previa, traumatic delivery, or manual removal of the placenta, a quantitative test of fetal RBCs in the maternal circulation determines the proper dose of RHIG to be given (Kleihauer-Betke test).

Abnormal fetal growth consists of either small for gestational age (SGA) or large for gestational age (LGA) infants. Small for gestational age infants are found in both premature and term pregnancies. Their perinatal mortality is approximately 10 times that of pregnancies with normal fetal growth. SGA infants are associated with first pregnancies, advanced maternal age, teenage pregnancy, multiple gestation, pregnancy-induced hypertension, congenital infections, and chromosomal abnormalities. Placental pathology is a relatively uncommon cause of growth retardation.

When intrauterine growth retardation is suspected, management starts with confirmation of gestational age and the size of the infant by ultrasonic examinations. Amniocentesis may be used to assess fetal lung maturity when fetal growth is impaired. Assessment also includes nonstress or oxytocin challenge tests. The incidence of fetal distress and asphyxia during labor and delivery is increased in SGA infants. Therefore, electronic fetal monitoring is essential in management.

LGA infants include infants who show an increase in all body proportions, and infants of diabetic mothers who have more body fat leading to an increased weight-to-length ratio. LGA infants have a significantly higher mortality rate than appropriately grown infants. Much of the increased mortality is attributed to problems at the time of delivery. The incidence of cephalopelvic disproportion is increased and may lead to asphyxia or birth trauma. At delivery, shoulder dystocia may be a problem. LGA infants are at increased risk for head injury and peripheral nerve palsy. The large infant of the diabetic mother is prone to hyperviscosity and venous thrombosis.

Perinatal asphyxia is a function of the duration of oxygen deprivation and the availability of glucose for anaerobic metabolism. If the length or frequency of contractions in labor is excessive, fetoplacental reserves decrease and hypoxia results. Maternal contributions to fetal circulatory compromise include supine hypotension syndrome, hypotension following conduction anesthesia, and hypertensive or vascular disease before labor. The use of oxytocin challenge tests or non-stress tests may predict potential fetal compromise before the onset of labor. Management of fetal asphyxia includes reduction of uterine contractility or increasing maternal arterial PO_2 during labor. If a favorable response is not obtained, operative delivery should be expedited.

Maternal infections that affect the fetus include the following. (1) Viral infections: rubella, cytomegalovirus, and herpes simplex virus. The first two are systemic infections which are more devastating if acquired early in pregnancy. Herpes simplex virus is usually acquired when a fetus passes through an infected birth canal. Fetal problems encountered from rubella include congenital

heart disease, cataracts, hearing loss, and mental retardation. Cytomegalovirus is associated with fetal death, severe brain damage, hearing and visual loss, and learning disabilities. Herpes simplex infections very often are associated with death or brain damage. (2) Protozoan infections: toxoplasmosis. This infection is acquired from a protozoan that is present in uncooked meat and in cat feces. Fetal infection may include early pregnancy loss, chorioretinitis, hydrocephalus, and anemia. Long-term effects in infants who survive include central nervous system damage. Previous infection protects the mother and the fetus from acquiring the disease. (3) Syphilis: Every pregnant mother should have a screen for syphilis antibodies early in the pregnancy. A confirming test of a positve screen is an indication for antibiotic therapy. Neonatal effects of syphilis include systemic infection, central nervous system disease, and various skeletal disorders.

Group B streptococcal disease has become an important focus of perinatal infection. It is generally acquired via the maternal birth canal and may be associated with premature onset of labor or premature rupture of membranes. The disease may manifest as severe pneumonia which often leads to perinatal death. Because *Streptococcus agalactiae* is a frequent inhabitant of the maternal birth canal, and neonatal disease is distinctly uncommon, screening cultures are not helpful in asymptomatic patients. Patients with a history of having had a neonate with group B streptococcal disease should be carefully assessed for the possibility of prophylactic treatment during labor.

Listeria infections have also been associated with premature onset of labor, rupture of the membranes, and early pregnancy loss.

NEWBORN ADAPTATION

The major changes in the adjustment to extrauterine life are conversion to an adult circulation by closure of several fetal cardiac shunts, air expansion of the fluid-filled lung for oxygen exchange, increased neural input from the environment, increased gastrointestinal absorption of nutrients, and increased use of fat stores to maintain a neutral thermal environment.

These adjustments may be interfered with by perinatal asphyxia, congenital or acquired disorders, or by systemic pharmacologic poisoning that interferes with central nervous system control in the neonatal environment. Neonatal support may be necessary under these circumstances.

Indications for resuscitation include absence of breathing or hyperventilation, a heart rate less than 100 beats per minute, sluggish neonatal response, and evidence of acute or prolonged intrauterine insults (e.g., infant of diabetic mother, growth retardation).

Resuscitation consists of ventilation, circulation, temperature stabilization, glucose regulation, and hydration.

Ventilation is improved by suctioning the nasopharynx and mouth and by oxygen, given by intermittent positive pressure. Temperature stability is maximized by drying the newborn's skin and radiant heat. Intravenous glucose and hydration may be necessary to maintain circulation and energy requirements.

NEWBORN DISORDERS

Intrauterine asphyxia may contribute to acidosis at birth, especially in cases of neonatal respiratory distress syndrome, congenital heart disease, and other congenital abnormalities. Management includes support of circulation, administration of oxygen and judicious use of sodium bicarbonate. Respiratory acidosis is usually treated with respiratory support only. Persistent metabolic acidosis is a common sign of an inborn error of metabolism.

Blood glucose levels less than 30 mg/100 ml blood indicate a need for glucose replacement. Hypoglycemia is common in small and large for gestational age infants, as well as in newborns with post-maturity syndrome, asphyxia, or infection. At least 100 ml/kg per day of 10 percent dextrose solution is used to maintain blood concentrations of at least 40 mg/dl. Hypocalcemia may be found in association with asphyxia, intrauterine growth retardation, prematurity, and neonatal hypoglycemia. Parathormone resistance is thought to play a role in this problem. Ionized, nonprotein bound calcium (60 percent of total newborn calcium) is the active component of serum calcium. Intravenous calcium is indicated with neonatal seizures, central nervous system irritability, and hypocalcemia in prematurity, with physiologic serum calcium as the goal. Hypomagnesemia may be found in conjunction with hypocalcemia. Magnesium replacement is similar to calcium therapy, both in indication and in dose.

Hyperbilirubinemia, a by-product of heme metabolism in the newborn, is due to either increased production — most often from hemolysis-isoimmunization, or decreased excretion — most often due to slow onset of conjugation. Therapy depends on appropriate diagnosis and includes correction of the cause, exchange transfusion, and phototherapy.

Respiratory disease is the leading cause of neonatal death in newborns, especially in prematures. Among the disorders are pulmonary hypoplasia and agenesis, mediastinal tumors and cysts, diaphragmatic hernia, and airway obstruction. However, hyaline membrane disease is the most prevalent disorder. Variants of hyaline membrane disease include transient tachypnea and congenital pneumonia. Aspiration syndromes, spontaneous pneumothorax, and persistent fetal circulation are sometimes encountered in cases of perinatal asphyxia. Respiratory distress is commonly associated with asphyxia, hypothermia, infection, hypoglycemia, and acidosis. Respiratory distress may be the first sign of congenital heart disease.

In the most common forms of hyaline membrane disease (HMD), stability of the alveoli and resistance to expiratory collapse are decreased by the absence or decreased production of surfactant. This surface tension-lowering phospholipid contains lecithin and sphingomyelin in concentrations that may be measured in amniotic fluid to determine fetal lung maturity (L/S ratio). When the L/S ratio is immature, the infant presents with tachypnea, retractions, nasal flaring, cyanosis, and expiratory grunting. Reticulogranular radiologic changes are characteristic. Laboratory findings include decreased pH and PO_2, and increased PCO_2. HMD is treated by oxygen, assisted ventilation, temperature and volume support, energy regulation, and hydration. Antibiotics and bicarbonate therapy may be helpful in selected cases. Most infants who survive early HMD, if unassociated with infection or congenital abnormalities, go on to recovery. Complications of the disease include intraventricular hemorrhage, pneumothorax, retrolental fibroplasia with oxygen therapy, and bronchopulmonary dysplasia.

Transient tachypnea may be clinically indistinguishable from HMD but has a more benign course. Congenital and acquired pneumonias may have a course similar to HMD and may complicate treatment of HMD. Meconium aspiration is a complication of perinatal asphyxiation manifested by clinical and radiologic evidence of air trapping and emphysema. Respiratory support is necessary. Prevention is the most effective therapy. When meconium staining is recognized in labor, attention should be given to emptying the oral and nasal cavities of secretions at delivery. Laryngoscopy and tracheal suctioning may be necessary. Persistance of fetal circulation is the continued shunting of substantial quantities of hypo-oxygenated blood away from the lungs of the neonate. This disease is associated with intrapartum asphyxia but is uncommon. Assisted ventilation and pulmonary vasodilators may help to correct this disorder.

Infection in the newborn is infrequent but devastating. Septicemia, meningitis and pneumonia in the neonatal period have mortality rates as high as 50 percent. When instrumentaion is used, the limited ability of the newborn to mount an immunologic response is associated with increased infection. Prolonged and premature rupture of fetal membranes, prolonged labor, and traumatic delivery also predispose to infection. The source of neonatal infection is often ascending vaginal flora that may include transplacentally acquired organisms. Viral infections are usually acquired transplacentally although herpes simplex is acquired during delivery.

Infection may be manifested by altered neonatal response, including lethargy, irritability and poor feeding. Gastrointestinal and respiratory function are impaired and jaundice is also notable with neonatal infection. Laboratory tests suggesting neonatal infection include leukopenia or leukocytosis, hypoglycemia, thrombocytopenia and anemia, hyperbilirubinemia, and electrolyte disorders. Chest x-rays and Gram's stains of gastric aspirate material may be diagnostic for pneumonia or generalized septicemia. Blood cultures, examination of urine, and lumbar puncture for cerebrospinal fluid evaluation complete the exam. Antibiotic treatment, temperature support, attention to perfusion status, and ventilatory support are essential to good outcome.

DISEASES SPECIFIC TO PREGNANCY

Abortion

Spontaneous abortion is loss of the products of conception through natural causes before viability, which extends to 20 weeks of gestation or a fetal weight of 500 g in many states. Approximately 15 percent of all recognized pregnancies terminate in spontaneous abortion, although the true incidence is probably higher. Approximately 60 percent of spontaneous abortions result from nonrecurrent chromosomal abnormalities. The role of radiation, anesthesia, inorganic agents, and immune response remains unclear. Congenital anomalies of the uterus are probably not associated with first trimester abortions but can precipitate abortions in the second trimester or premature delivery.

The process of spontaneous abortion may be subdivided into the following categories. (1) Threatened abortion: pregnancy with vaginal bleeding, with or without cramps, and with a closed cervix. Approximately one-third of all pregnant patients will have first trimester bleeding and fifty percent of these will abort. In the remainder, there appears to be an increase in prematurity, placenta previa, abruption, and congenital anomalies. The differential diagnosis is missed abortion and can be ruled out by the use of ultrasound scanning to determine the viability of the embryo. Management is expectant and education is important to reduce anxiety. Diminished activity may be appropriate for several days. (2) Incomplete abortion: the products of conception have been incompletely expelled. Excessive bleeding may result and infection is a potential complication. Therapy usually consists of evacuation of the uterus by vacuum aspiration or sharp curettage. (3) Inevitable abortion: tissue has not been passed but the cervix is dilated in the presence of pain and bleeding. Treatment is the same as for incomplete abortion. (4) Complete abortion: the products of conception have been totally expelled, the uterus is empty and contracted. Infrequently, curettage may be performed. (5) Missed abortion: embryonic death has been present without expulsion. The uterus usually decreases in size or remains unchanged. After several weeks, coagulation defects may occur because of hypofibrinogenemia. Once missed abortion is recognized, expectant management may be considered but curettage may be required to complete the abortion.

The risk of subsequent abortion is approximately 15 percent. The risk increases gradually if more than one previous abortion has occurred. In general, miscarriage does not jeopardize a patient's chances of having children in the future.

Incompetent cervix occurs in approximately 1 in 500 pregnancies and is a cause of second trimester abortion. The internal os of the cervix dilates spontaneously and silently and a history of painless dilatation with previous pregnancy is characteristic. Incompetent cervix is managed by cervical cerclage. If this procedure is successful, pregnancy may be continued with the cerclage in place until term. The suture is then cut and labor is allowed to progress. Cerclage should be performed when the risk of spontaneous abortion is decreased after the first trimester.

Ectopic pregnancy is the implantation of a fertilized ovum outside the endometrial cavity. Ninety-eight percent of ectopic pregnancies occur in the fallopian tube, most often in the ampullary portion. Tubal pregnancy is serious because of maternal bleeding and accounts for 10 percent of maternal deaths each year. Tubal pregnancies occur in approximately 1 to 2 percent of pregnancies. The condition is more common in patients with a history of pelvic inflammatory disease, tubal sterilization, tuboplasty, and endometriosis. Higher maternal age and gravidity are also associated with increased incidence of tubal pregnancy. IUD use has been associated with ectopic pregnancy. Many tubal pregnancies rupture, causing severe abdominal hemorrhage. Pain, amenorrhea, and irregular vaginal bleeding are present in 80 percent of cases. Manifestations of the problem may include shoulder pain, syncope, hypotension, and tachycardia. Vaginal exam usually reveals a fullness or tenderness in the adnexea or cul-de-sac. Diagnosis is often made by culdocentesis. Positive results consist of nonclotting blood or bloody fluid and mandates surgical exploration. Standard pregnancy tests are not diagnostic. However, laboratory assessment of quantitative beta HCG may be helpful in differentiating uterine from ectopic pregnancy. The finding of an empty uterus by ultrasonographic examination in conjunction with positive beta HCG is also diagnostic.

Management of tubal pregnancy is surgical; salpingectomy of the affected site is usually necessary. However, salpingostomy may be performed to preserve potential fertility. Nevertheless, the chances of a repeat tubal pregnancy are significantly increased.

Treatment of ovarian pregnancy is salpingo-oophorectomy. Cervical pregnancy can be life threatening because of the profuse hemorrhage that occurs. Its treatment may include a requirement for hysterectomy. Ectopic pregnancies may implant in the broad ligament, pelvic wall, intestine, mesentary or omentum. If successful reimplantation occurs, pregnancy may progress to viability as an abdominal pregnancy. Delivery is accomplished by laparotomy and careful ligation of the umbilical cord. The placenta should not be detached.

Multiple Pregnancy

Twin pregnancy is the most common form of multiple gestation, occurring in approximately 1 in 85 pregnancies. Monozygotic or identical twins occur once in approximately 250 pregnancies. The development of dizygotic or nonidentical twins is influenced by several factors including race, genetics, maternal age and parity, and administration of ovulation-inducing drugs. Monozygotic pregnancies are independent of these factors. Monozygotic twins, unlike dizygotic twins, result from fertilization of one ovum and share virtually all the genetic material under normal circumstances. Monozygotic twins may occur anywhere from separation at the two cell stage up to separation after the primitive streak has developed. In the latter, the development of conjoined twins is likely.

Twin gestation is important for both maternal and fetal reasons. Maternal complications with twin gestation include preeclampsia, anemia, hemorrhage, and intrapartum complications. For the fetus, perinatal mortality is two to three times greater than in singleton pregnancies, primarily because of prematurity, prolapse of the umbilical cord, and asphyxia. The frequency of SGA infants is increased with multiple pregnancy. Large differences in size between twins suggests the presence of a twin transfusion syndrome. This results from anastomoses between the placental circulations of each twin. Classically, one twin is smaller with chronic intrauterine underperfusion and malnutrition. The larger twin is polycythemic and may be hydropic as well.

Multiple gestation should be suspected whenever the pregnant uterus is too large for gestation. The presence of excessive amniotic fluid or the palpation of numerous small parts or more than one head should also suggest the diagnosis. However, 25 percent of multiple gestations are not diagnosed until after the delivery of the first fetus. Early diagnosis of twin gestation can be made by ultrasonography or radiography.

Management of multiple pregnancies should include frequent prenatal examinations to detect maternal and fetal complications. Patients will require iron supplementation to minimize the chances of maternal anemia. Patients should be educated about the early signs of premature labor and the potential benefit of increased bedrest to fetal growth. Serial ultrasound is helpful in determining whether intrauterine growth retardation is present. Since twin gestation is associated with an increased risk of congenital fetal abnormalities, ultrasound may be helpful in early diagnosis of such problems. If abnormalities of fetal growth are detected, fetal nonstress tests are appropriate in the third trimester.

The management of twin labor is important because of several potential problems. Dysfunctional labor is more frequent in multiple pregnancy as is premature labor. The latter may be treated with tocolytic agents and bed-rest. Fetal presentation is important in management. Delivery of the first twin is usually vaginal, although some types of breech presentation, especially with a fetus less than 1,500 g, may be more appropriately delivered by cesarean section. Other indications for cesarean section are the same as with singleton presentations. Delivery of the second twin will depend on fetal presentation. If delivery can be effected in less than 20 minutes after delivery of the first twin with a healthy monitored fetus, the second fetus may be delivered by internal podalic version and breech extraction or by guiding the fetal head into the pelvis for vertex delivery. If the second twin presents as transverse or oblique lie, cannot be guided into the pelvis, or if fetal distress occurs, general anesthesia should be administered and cesarean section may be necessary. Following delivery of the twins and removal of the placenta, oxytocin should be given intravenously to enhance contraction and prevent postpartum hemorrhage.

DISORDERS OF PLACENTA AND MEMBRANES

The latent period between rupture of membranes or amniorrhexis and onset of labor required for the definition of premature rupture of membranes (PROM) is most often quoted at 1 hour. The duration of the latent period is greater in preterm gestation than in term pregnancies. Labor begins spontaneously after 72 hours in only 70 percent of preterm pregnancies. At gestational ages of less than 32 weeks, perinatal mortality from hyaline membrane disease is so high that delaying delivery may improve fetal survival without significantly increasing the incidence of chorioamnionitis and maternal or fetal infection. Diagnosis of premature rupture of membranes is important in determining the further management of a pregnancy remote from term. In considering the heightened possibility of preterm delivery, betamethasone therapy reduces the risk of hyaline membrane disease and does not, in most studies, appear to be associated with an increase in chorioamnionitis. The immaturity of other organ systems argues against the indiscriminate delivery of preterm pregnancies after premature rupture of membranes, unless infection or other fetal or maternal complications suggest a more expedient course. Conservative management of premature rupture of membranes remote from term still remains potentially hazardous to mother and fetus. The risk of sepsis for both is of real concern.

Premature rupture of membranes is also associated with a higher incidence of fetal malpresentation. The abdominal delivery of smaller infants under these circumstances is associated with a higher maternal infection risk. Antibiotic prophylaxis is recommended.

Generally, premature membrane rupture at term should be expeditiously delivered, if necessary, with augmentation by oxytocin.

Placental Abruption

Placental abruption, or premature separation of the normally implanted placenta, is detachment from the uterine wall at any time between the twentieth week of pregnancy and the end of labor. Eighty-five to ninety percent are mild to moderate, but the remainder are associated with a maternal mortality rate as high as 10 percent. Mortality is related to hemorrhagic shock, renal failure, and pituitary insufficiency. When managed aggressively with blood and fluid replacement and expeditious delivery, maternal mortality is almost nonexistent. Abruption is complete if the placenta is totally detached from the uterine wall, or partial if a portion still remains in connection with the uterus. Abruption may or may not be associated with vaginal bleeding. A concealed abruption occurs when blood does not appear externally but is retained between the placenta and the uterus. Concealed abruption is associated with a higher maternal and fetal morbidity and mortality. Marginal sinus rupture is limited placental separation at the margin and is often associated with normal outcome.

Placental abruption is seen in 1 to 2 percent of deliveries. Approximately 50 percent of placental separations occur before the onset of labor. Fetal compromise occurs in 25 percent of cases. Fetal hypoxia and death are dependent upon the amount and duration of placental separation, maternal hypertension and hypovolemic shock. With complete placental abruption, fetal mortality rate approaches 100 percent.

Factors associated with placental abruption include acute and chronic hypertension, sudden decompression of the uterus, occlusion of the inferior vena cava, older maternal age, high parity, and cigarette use. The role of infection in abruptio placenta has not been defined. Half the patients with abruption have underlying hyertensive diseases. Women with previous placental abruption are more likely to develop the same complication in subsequent pregnancies.

The pathophysiology of abruption includes degeneration of the decidua basalis associated with acute degenerative arteriolitis. In severe abruption, the entire uterine musculature may contain extravasated blood. This is characteristically referred to as a Couvelaire uterus.

A major complication of abruptio placenta is disseminated intravascular coagulopathy (DIC). This disorder is caused by an abnormal activation of the coagulation cascade, especially by decidual thromboplastin. The continued consumption of fibrinogen, coupled with the increasing production of plasmin from plasminogen, contributes to incoagubility of the circulation and rapid, abnormal bleeding.

The classical symptoms of abruption are vaginal bleeding with uterine tenderness and increased uterine tone. The mother often becomes hypotensive with the intensity of shock directly related to maternal blood loss. Differential diagnosis includes placenta previa, rupture of the uterus, torsion of the uterus, ruptured uterine varices, and acute surgical conditions causing abdominal pain. Mild abruption may initially present with painless vaginal bleeding. Diagnostic ultrasound is often helpful in differentiating between abruptio placenta and placent previa.

Management includes restoration of an effective circulation by intravenous administration of fluids and blood. In situations where the fetus is still alive and potentially viable, delivery, usually by cesarean section, should follow stabilization of maternal circulation. Maternal hemorrhagic shock should be treated with enough blood and balanced salt solution to maintain a hematocrit of at least 30 percent and a urinary output of at least 30 ml/hr. Measurement of central venous pressure may be helpful in monitoring replacement fluids. The use of fresh frozen plasma, cryoprecipitate and platelet transfusions will correct circulating deficits of these agents.

Artificial rupture of fetal membranes will tend to minimize hemorrhage and also reduce the extent of DIC. The fetus should be directly monitored and delivery expedited.

Complications of severe abruptio placenta include renal failure and pituitary necrosis.

Placenta Previa

Placenta previa complicates 0.3 to 0.5 percent of all pregnancies. It consists of abnormal implantation of the placenta in the lower uterine segment with partial or complete covering of the cervical os. Diagnosis depends upon finding placental tissue in the cervical os either before or during labor. A previa may be described as complete, partial, or low-lying. The latter is not actually a previa, but an implantation of the lower uterine segment. Placenta previa is associated with multifetal gestation, eccentric insertion of the umbilical cord in the placenta, previous cesarean section, previous placenta previa and maternal smoking.

Hemorrhage is caused by partial separation of the uterus from the placenta and increasing uterine irritability or contractions. The lower uterine segment cannot contract in the face of placental separation and painless vaginal bleeding results. The earlier in pregnancy the bleeding is noted, the more extensive is the placenta previa. Subsequent episodes of bleeding after the first episode are often more hazardous to maternal health.

Diagnosis is made by localization of the placenta by ultrasonography.

Abnormal fetal presentation is more frequent with placent previa, occurring in as many as 20 percent of all cases. Vaginal examination for diagnosing placenta previa is only occasionally necessary, and is never permissible unless the patient is in an operating room and preparations have been made for immediate cesarean section should torrential hemorrhage occur from the examination. Management of placenta previa depends upon gestational age and fetal maturity.

Placenta accreta is abnormal adherence of placenta to myometrium due to absence of decidua between the trophoblast and myometrium. Placenta increta involves a more extensive invasion of the myometrium, and placenta percreta is penetration through the full thickness of the myometrium and cerosa. Placenta accreta is rare but often occurs in conjunction with placenta previa. Hysterectomy may be required to control the bleeding. Mortality rates as high as 6 percent have been recorded, even with hysterectomy, due to excessive blood loss and delay in therapy.

Polyhydramnios is amniotic fluid in excess of 2,000 ml. Normal amniotic fluid volume is approximately 1 L in the late third trimester with a gradual small reduction in volume later in pregnancy. The diagnosis of polyhydramnios may be confirmed by ultrasound. Polyhydramnios is increased in maternal diabetes mellitus, preeclampsia and hypertension, anemia, and pyelo-

nephritis. Fetal associations with polyhydramnios include congenital anomalies (25 to 30 percent), multiple gestation, Rh sensitization, and placental chorioangiomas.

Management of polyhydramnios consists of evaluating the condition of the fetus and the mother and testing for specific causes of the underlying problem. The use of ultrasound, fetal heart rate monitoring, selected amniography and Rh antibody titers should be considered.

Since the risk of premature labor and malpresentation is increased, further management includes bed-rest in the lateral recumbent position and prevention or treatment of premature labor. In severe cases, amniocentesis has been performed to remove excess fluid with varying results. The mother is at increased risk for postpartum hemorrhage and cesarean section because of malpresentation or cord prolapse.

Oligohydramnios is the depletion or absence of amniotic fluid. Oligohydramnios is seen in prolonged pregnancy and in women with chronic amniotic fluid leakage. It has also been found in conjunction with fetal renal abnormalities, especially renal agenesis or Potter's syndrome. Intrauterine growth retardation is a prominent feature with oligohydramnios. The diagnosis is made by physical examination and ultrasound. Further evaluation for fetal well-being by fetal nonstress tests or oxytocin challenge tests is appropriate. Management in labor is dependent upon knowledge of underlying fetal abnormalities, if any, and fetal response to the stress of labor. Cesarean section is often required because of fetal distress due to cord compression and decreased uteroplacental reserve.

Disorders of the Uterus

Rupture of the uterus is an infrequent occurrence (1 in 2,000 deliveries) but is associated with occasional maternal mortality and a fetal mortality of up to 50 percent. Rupture of the unscarred uterus before the onset of labor is extremely rare. Uterine anomalies such as bicornuate uterus and placental abnormalities are associated with spontaneous rupture. Grand multiparity, neglected cephalopelvic disproportion, hydrocephalus, and tumors obstructing the birth canal have also been described with spontaneous rupture. Induction or stimulation of labor in patients with these problems should be avoided.

Previous uterine surgery, including classical cesarean section, myomectomy, or uterine plastic procedures increase the risk of uterine scar rupture with subsequent pregnancy. However, the use of low segment transverse cesarean section has rarely been associated with subsequent uterine rupture and maternal or fetal mortality. Previous classical cesarean section is a contraindication to labor with subsequent pregnancy. In several institutions, with appropriate conditions, vaginal delivery following previous low segment transverse cesarean section may be justified. Traumatic rupture of the uterus is a rare occurrence, previously associated with improper and excessive management of abnormal presentations and manual removal of the placenta. Uterine rupture may also occur following the use of oxytocic agents.

Clinically, the patient complains of pain, cessation of uterine contractions, and bleeding and shock are common findings. If the patient is undelivered, there may be greater ease in palpating fetal parts. Hematuria may be part of the clinical picture. Management includes immediate correction of hypovelemia followed by surgery to correct the problem. Hysterectomy is often required although hemostatis has been obtained with bilateral hypogastric artery litigation.

Inversion of the uterus occurs with forceful management of the third stage of labor when strong fundal pressure or traction on the umbilical cord is performed before placental separation. Inversion is a rare occurrence but may be life threatening. Incomplete inversion occurs when the uterine fundus is inverted but has not descended beyond the cervix and complete inversion is passage of the fundus through the cervix. The patient may present with bleeding and shock. Management consists of treating the shock and correcting the inversion. The latter often requires a surgical approach under general anesthesia for uterine relaxation. After replacement is complete, oxytocic agents should be administered to prevent recurrence of the inversion.

Hypertensive States of Pregnancy

Previously described as pregnancy toxemias, the pregnancy-associated hypertensive states include the following.

1. Mild disorders
   A. gestational edema
   B. gestational proteinuria
   C. gestational hypertension
2. Acute disorders
   A. preeclampsia — eclampsia
   B. chronic hypertension with superimposed preeclampsia or eclampsia
3. Chronic hypertensive disease of whatever cause
4. Unclassified hypertensive disorders with insufficient information to classify the hypertensive state.

Edema is the accumulation of fluid with weight gain of 5 pounds or more in 1 week. In spite of gross weight gain and edema, most patients in this category have normal pregnancies and offspring.

Gestational proteinuria is the presence of proteinuria in the absence of hypertension or edema, renal infection, or renal vascular disease during pregnancy. Mild gestational proteinuria alone does not affect the fetus.

Gestational hypertension is the development of an increase in systolic blood pressure of 30 torr or diastolic blood pressure of 15 torr during pregnancy or within the first 24 hours postpartum in previously normotensive women, unassociated with proteinuria or edema. Gestational hypertensive patients often have a family history of hypertension and many later develop essential hypertension.

Preeclampsia is the development of hypertension with proteinuria, edema, or both after the twentieth week of gestation. It may develop earlier with gestational trophoblastic disease. Progression of preeclampsia without proper treatment results in eclamptic convulsions.

Preeclampsia is characteristically a disease of the indigent primagravida who has received little or no prenatal care. There are many exceptions to this characterization. Succeeding pregnancies usually are not marked by preeclampsia-eclampsia, leading to a number of theories about the etiology of this disease. Preeclampsia is considered severe with any one of the following signs or symptoms: (1) blood pressure greater than 16 torr systolic, or 110 torr diastolic on at least two occasions at least 6 hours apart, with the patient resting in bed; (2) proteinuria of 5 grams or more in 24 hours; (3) oliguria (less than 500 ml/24 hours); (4) cerebral or visual disturbances; (5) epigastric pain; (6) pulmonary edema/cyanosis; (7) thrombocytopenia (less than $100,000/mm^3$); and (8) severe intrauterine growth retardation.

Eclampsia is still one of the frequent causes of maternal death with a mortality rate of 3 to 5 percent. Fetal mortality is between 17 and 20 percent.

Placental ischemia is a characteristic of this disease. Immunologic and antibody reactions between maternal and fetal tissues and the vasoconstrictive activity of disordered prostaglandin activity have been suggested as causes of the disease.

The pathophysiology of the disease involves generalized vasospasm that can be evaluated clinically by physical exam. Increased peripheral resistance is associated with the onset of hypertension. Vascular sensitivity to pressor substances such as angiotensin II, norepinephrine, and vasopressin is increased. Sodium retention has been noted in preeclampsia and there is a marked reduction in size of the vascular compartment as plasma escapes into the interstitial space, causing edema. Central venous pressure is low.

As a result, there is decreased circulation to vital organs, especially the brain, liver, kidney, and placenta. Cerebral resistance is measurably increased and decreased oxygenation of the brain resulting from vasospasm produces cerebral irritability and eventually seizures if unmanaged. Metabolic dysfunction of kidney and liver are noted in patients with severe preeclampsia and decreased perfusion of the placenta is characterized by small, infarcted placentas and SGA infants.

Renal blood flow, glomerular filtration rate, and uric acid clearance are all decreased with preeclampsia. Renin substrate, the renin activating system, and angiotension II are augmented to a lesser degree in preeclamptic patients than in patients without the disease.

Management of the preeclamptic patient includes evaluation of the clinical severity of maternal disease and insuring the well-being of the fetus. Milder cases of preeclampsia are managed by continuing pregnancy until fetal maturity is achieved. However, with severe, unremitting disease, delivery is the treatment of choice because of catastrophic risks to both mother and fetus. Combined clinical observation and laboratory tests are useful in judging the clinical status of preeclamptic patients. They should include (1) vital signs, blood pressure, and pulse. (2) Volume input and output; decreased urinary output is an ominous sign. (3) Daily weight; continued weight gain, especially after bed-rest, indicates unrelenting fluid retention. (4) Measurement of deep tendon reflexes to monitor central irritability. (5) Observation for impending symptoms including headaches, scotomata, epigastric pain. (6) Fetal evaluation including amniocentesis for L/S ratio, fetal monitoring, and serial sonography for fetal growth. Laboratory studies should include 24-hour urine protein, urinalysis and culture, blood urea nitrogen and serum creatinine, serum uric acid, platelet count, and liver enzyme studies if the patient has severe preeclampsia.

The guidelines of preeclampsia management during pregnancy include the following. The only definitive treatment is delivery of the fetus and placenta. Bed-rest with observation must be an integral part of conservative management. Treatment must take into account the severity of the preeclampsia balanced against the viability of the infant.

Treatment includes anticonvulsant therapy with magnesium sulfate when the preeclamptic patient is in labor. Therapy may be instituted prior to labor, but if required, serious thought should be given to the delivery of the fetus. Magnesium sulfate depresses activity at the interneuronal and myoneuronal junctions, and there is some evidence for a central effect. An intravenous loading dose (4 to 6 g) should be slowly given, followed by a maintenance dose of approximately 1 to 2 g per hour via infusion pump. Medication may also be given intramuscularly. Excessive plasma concentration is evidenced by decreased respirations or the disappearance of reflexes. Intravenous calcium gluconate reverses the effect of the magnesium sulfate.

An airway should be maintained and oxygen therapy should be administered during management of eclamptic patients. With eclampsia, delivery should be undertaken once the patient's condition has been stabilized on anticonvulsant therapy. Approximately 20 to 30 percent of patients do not respond to oxytocin induction and require cesarean section. The fetus should be monitored for evidence of decreased uteroplacental reserve; if fetal distress is present, operative delivery is indicated.

After delivery, severely preeclamptic or eclamptic patients must be observed carefully. Anticonvulsant therapy should be maintained until evidence of decreased peripheral vascular resistance has occurred, manifested by a decrease in blood pressure and diuresis, usually during the first 24 hours postpartum.

Patients with essential hypertension may not gain excessive edema weight as seen with preeclampsia. Intrauterine growth retardation and fetal demise are serious risks in this group of patients. Placental abruption is also more likely to occur. Antihypertensive medication is an integral part of management in pregnancy complicated by essential hypertension. Oral alpha-methyl-dopa is a good first-line drug to maintain diastolic blood pressure less than 90 torr. In severe superimposed preeclampsia, the use of intravenous apresoline may be required to treat a hypertensive emergency. Blood pressure should be lowered so as not to contribute to maternal hypotension which may threaten circulation to the placenta and fetus. Monitoring of fetal well-being during pregnancy in these patients is an absolute necessity.

DISEASE COMPLICATING PREGNANCY

Diseases that occur outside of pregnancy may occur during pregnancy and those diseases that are more common to reproductive age women are relatively common during pregnancy as well. The physiologic changes of pregnancy may mask some of the normal signs and symptoms of several of these diseases. What may appear to be normal physiologic manifestations for the nonpregnant state may be an abnormal response for a patient who is pregnant. These general guidelines should be remembered in patients who have a significant medical history and who become pregnant.

Disorders of the Cardiovascular System

The signs and symptoms of organic heart disease must be differentiated from normal manifestations. Cardiac murmurs, cardiomegaly and pedal edema are normally found in pregnancy. Clinical evaluation of the cardiovascular system is, thus, very important in the pregnant patient. Certain laboratory procedures may confirm the presence of pulmonary congestion or changes in pressure and circulation time. Anemia is to be avoided in pregnant patients with underlying cardiovascular disease.

The most significant basis for determining prognosis of the cardiac patient in pregnancy is functional capacity. The functional criteria established by the New York Heart Association are a valuable index; Class I — cardiac disorder without limitation of physical activity; Class II — slight to moderate limitation of physical activity; Class III — marked limitation of physical activity so that less than ordinary activity causes discomfort; Class IV — severely impaired physical activity and significant discomfort at rest. Patients in classes I and II have an excellent prognosis in pregnancy and require little more than routine care. Patients in the other classes have a higher incidence of complications and require special supervision. Historically, fetal loss with maternal cardiac disease has been high, ranging between 30 to 50 percent. More recent preventative care and proper management of maternal vascular complications has been associated with a marked improvement in prenatal survival.

Older gravidas with a history of cardiac decompensation are at most risk for maternal morbidity and mortality. Myocarditis, atrial fibrillation, severe anemia and hypertension magnify maternal hazards. The mortality rate of pregnant patients with severe cardiac complications has been as high as 20 percent. With modern medical management and counseling, however, the risk of maternal mortality should be close to nonexistent.

Disorders of the cardiovascular system may be divided into congenital and acquired diseases. Presently, maternal congenital heart disease is the most frequent pregnancy cardiac disease since rheumatic heart disease has decreased in frequency.

The diagnosis of congenital cardiac defects may be made for the first time when a patient appears for obstetric care. If the patient is asymptomatic without a history of cardiac difficulties, further studies may be deferred until after the pregnancy. Patients with severe congenital heart disease usually do not maintain physical conditioning consistent with successful reproduction. Of the maternal congenital cardiac defects in pregnancy, only Eisenmenger's syndrome is associated with unacceptable maternal mortality, approximately 25 percent. Of the more frequently found congenital abnormalities, patent ductus arteriosis, atrial septal defect, corrected coarctation of the aorta and small ventricular septal defects account for approximately 80 percent. As a rule, these patients do not have major cardiovascular complications during pregnancy as long as cardiac disability prior to pregnancy was minimal.

Patients with uncorrected major congenital abnormalities such as Tetralogy of Fallot, coarctation of the aorta, and pulmonary stenosis have increased complications during pregnancy with a higher maternal mortality. These patients benefit from counseling and prepregnancy corrective surgery.

Coronary artery disease is extremely uncommon in women of child-bearing age. Cardiac arrhythmias are as common as in the nonpregnant population of the same reproductive age. Management is the same. Premature cardiac beats are a common finding during pregnancy and are almost never associated with underlying organic heart disease. As long as maternal circulation is not affected by arrhythmias, the fetus does not seem to be at increased risk. Management includes proper diet and attention to normal blood volume, removal from undue physical stress, and attention to appropriate weight gain. Antibacterial prophylaxis during labor and delivery is important in these patients.

Cardinal principles in labor management with cardiac disease are pain relief, avoidance of hypotension, adequate oxygenation of mother and fetus, and maintenance in the left lateral recumbent position. Oxytocin may be used as necessary. It is advisble to shorten the second stage of labor by forceps delivery once the fetus presents in a position that will not cause harm to either the fetus or the mother. Regional anesthesia is probably the best technique for managing a pregnant cardiac patient as long as care is taken to avoid hypotension. Management of the puerperium is important because maternal heart may be under greater stress with the rapid mobilization of fluids into the cardiovascular system.

Venous thrombosis is relatively common in pregnancy. It is associated with hormonally mediated stasis of venous circulation in the lower extremities and with increasing coagulability of maternal blood. Thrombophlebitis may be superficial or in the deeper veins. If superficial, usually the only treatment is circulatory support with an elastic bandage and administration of analgesics. Rarely is heparin necessary for treatment. The use of anti-inflammatory agents is problematic because of the potential risk of premature closure of the fetal ductus arteriosis.

Diagnosis of deep vein thrombosis is difficult to establish but the hazards are greater. Pulmonary embolus is a direct complication and should be prevented by early and aggressive management of the underlying disease. Patients may be symptomatic with fever, leg pain, unilateral edema, and tenderness to palpation of affected veins. Management consists of anticoagulation with intravenous heparin, which does not cross the placenta. Therefore, it is an ideal agent to use during pregnancy. The use of a continuous intravenous infusion after initial loading allows for uniform maintenance of activated partial thromboplastin time at approximately $1\frac{1}{2}$ to 2 times normal. If long-term therapy is required because of the length of pregnancy, heparin is still preferable to coumarin derivatives and has been given in daily subcutaneous doses.

Pulmonary embolism does not occur often but maternal mortality is sufficiently high enough to make it an important disease during pregnancy. Diagnosis may be made by abnormal arterial blood gases and electrocardiographic evidence of heart strain. Arteriographic demonstration of occluded pulmonary artery branchs or ventilation perfusion scans of the lung are diagnostic. Treatment consists of the administration of parenteral fluids and oxygen, anticoagulation, and surgery if the previous mentioned methods are unsuccessful. In patients with pelvic thrombophlebitis and recurrent pulmonary emboli, inferior vena cava ligation is indicated.

Disorders of the Respiratory System

The incidence of tuberculosis is uncommon in pregnancy. There does not appear to be a specific effect of tuberculosis on pregnancy. Opinion is divided whether the altered immunologic state of pregnancy allows tuberculosis to become more active during or shortly after pregnancy. Management of active tuberculosis continues to be combined chemotherapy. Obstetric care should not be altered by the diagnosis of tuberculosis. Conduct of labor and delivery are based upon obstetric considerations. Choice of anesthesia may be individualized and the presence of active pulmonary tuberculosis must be made known to the anesthesiologist. Combined chemotherapy should include isoniazid. Streptomycin may be ototoxic for the fetus but the benetfit/risk ratio may require its use. Resistance to certain drugs should be a caution for a patient to become pregnant since control of the disease process might be unreliable.

Bronchiectasis, sarcoidosis, respiratory tract allergies and cystic fibrosis are distinctly rare complications during pregnancy. With the exception of cystic fibrosis, they should not interfere with the normal conduct of pregnancy. Management may be difficult in patients who have asthma or pneumonia during pregnancy because of decreased respiratory reserves.

Disorders of the Urinary Tract

Disorders of the urinary tract are important during pregnancy because of anatomic changes associated with pregnancy. Bacteruria is defined as the presence of 100,000 bacteria/ml of urine obtained from a midstream voided specimen, found in 5 to 7 percent of pregnant women. Eighty percent of positive cultures are due to gram negative bacteria. Bacteruria is important since over 30 percent of women with this finding who are untreated ultimately develop pyelonephritis during pregnancy. Pyelonephritis is found in less than 3 percent of women who are treated for asmyptomatic bacteria.

There appears to be a relationship between urinary tract infections and fetal welfare. There is an increased rate of prematurity with pyelonephritis and possibly with asymptomatic bacteria. Management of bacteruria consists of 2 weeks of active antibiotic therapy to which the organism is sensitive. Tetracycline and chloramphenicol are contraindicated during pregnancy. Sulfonamides should be used with caution after the beginning of the third trimester because of displacement of bilirubin from fetal carrier proteins.

Cystitis may occur during or shortly after labor related to trauma to the base of the bladder and instrumentation with catheters. Postpartum bacteruria is approximately 2 to 4 percent. Pyelonephritis, on the other hand, is a serious complication that may occur at any time during pregnancy. It is more common in primagravidas and is often preceded by asymptomatic bacteria or cystitis. The problem may be related to anatomic and hormonal changes in pregnancy contributing to stasis of the ureters and physiologic hydroureter. Pyelonephritis usually presents with urgency, frequency, and dysuria. Pain, and tenderness, chills, and high fever are often found in conjunction with pyelonephritis. Diagnosis is made by urinalysis and culture. Treatment should include hospitalization, bed-rest, hydration, and parenteral administration of a broad spectrum antibiotic. Persistent pyelonephritis may contribute to renal disease and it is incumbent to reevaluate maternal urine after treatment for an urinary tract infection during pregnancy.

Urinary tract calculi are not common but, when present, contribute to infection, pain, renal damage, and premature labor. Renal stones often are lodged at the ureteropelvic junction. A patient may present with colicky pain radiating down the ureter and into the groin with urgency, frequency, and hematuria. These symptoms remit with passage of the calculus. Diagnosis is by ultrasonographic evaluation of renal stones, or the use of an intravenous pyelogram. Bed-rest and hydration are important parts of management; surgical management of renal stones is usually not necessary during pregnancy and most patients will pass the stone with proper analgesia and hydration support. If the stone does not pass, the use of indwelling ureteral catheters or stents have helped in the maintenance of pregnancy to fetal maturity.

Acute glomerulonephritis is a rare complication of pregnancy with urinary protein, casts, and urethrocytes. Blood pressure may be elevated. Once the diagnosis is established the patient should be at bed-rest with a low-salt diet. A course of antibiotic therapy should be administered and anti-hypertensive agents used as necessary. With early treatment, the patient usually experiences a diuresis with a normal blood pressure and reduction in albuminuria and hematuria. Pregnancy will then tend to proceed normally to term. With treatment delays there is an increased risk of abortion, stillbirth, and premature labor. Approximately 5 percent of patients with acute glomerulonephritis fail to respond to treatment and progress to renal failure. Management of these patients is by hemodialysis, although some people have suggested that therapeutic abortion may help. Patients with chronic glomerulonephritis may develop superimposed preeclampsia and an increased risk of perinatal mortality. Renal function in these patients should be determined periodically during pregnancy and an increase in maternal bed-rest should be helpful. How long pregnancy should be continued is a function of fetal monitoring in the third trimester.

The nephrotic syndrome is characterized by massive proteiniuria, lipiduria, hypoalbuminemia, and hypercholesterolemia with massive edema. An immunologic basis for this problem has been postulated but not proven. Management depends upon accurate diagnosis and renal biopsy may be necessary. Management consists of bed-rest, and a high-protein, low-salt diet. Baseline laboratory studies of renal function and fetal wellbeing should be continued with hospitalization. Cortico-steroids may be effective in decreasing protein loss by the kidneys and may have the added benefit of increasing fetal lung maturity.

Acute renal failure is the decrease in urine excretion to less than 500 ml in 24 hours. The primary etiology in pregnancy is hemorrhage leading to maternal hypovolemia and hypotension. Septic shock or infection and severe preeclampsia and eclampsia as well as disseminated intravascular coagulation have been associated with acute renal failure. The primary sign of renal failure is decreased urine output. Progressive deterioration may be accompanied by increases in neuromuscular irritability, acidosis, and convulsions. Early diagnosis and institution of appropriate therapy are associated with a return to near normal renal function. Management consists of hourly evaluation of urine output and adequate fluid and blood replacement. Stimulation of urine excretion with the use of intravenous diuretics may be helpful in reversing a trend toward renal failure. Infections should be treated appropriately with antibiotics and preeclamptic conditions that contribute to tubular necrosis should be managed conservatively. DIC must be managed aggressively with appropriate plasma factors to prevent durther deterioration of the kidney and other organs.

Congenital anomalies of the urinary tract are often discovered during pregnancy and are more common if they are maternal uterine anomalies. In the case of polycystic kidney disease, it may be proper to recommend early completion of family by patients because of the chronic and progressive nature of the disease. Pregnancy is possible after renal transplantation but the consideration of other systemic diseases in association with trans-plantation care should be taken into account before advising a patient to undertake or avoid pregnancy.

Hematologic Disorders in Pregnancy

The most common hematologic disorders during pregnancy include iron deficiency anemia, folic acid anemia, and the hemoglobinopathies. Iron deficiency anemia is present when maternal hemoglobin values are below 10 g/100 ml. A blood smear will show varying degrees of hypochromia, microcytosis, and anisocytosis. Total serum iron binding capacity is normally elevated in pregnancy but the iron content is abnormal if less than 15 percent of total iron binding capacity. Management consists of therapeutic doses of ferrous sulfate or its equivalent in elemental iron. This amounts to approximately 600 to 900 mg/day of the sulfate salt or 1,200 to 1,800 mg of ferrous gluconate salt. A maximum reticulocyte count should be expected within 5 to 10 days with a gradual increase in hemoglobin concentration over the next 2 to 3 months.

Megaloblastic anemia of pregnancy is related to folic acid deficiency and very rarely from vitamin B_{12} deficiency. Patients should respond to oral folic acid, 1 mg daily. Clinical responses may take up to 2 to 6 weeks. Prophylactic administration of folic acid 1 mg/day orally should be prescribed as routine in pregnancy. Aplastic anemia and hemolytic anemia are rare complications during pregnancy. Their management is similar to management outside of pregnancy. Sickle-cell disease or hemoglobin-SS disease is an inherited autosomal dominant disorder of hemoglobin structure that contributes to sickling under circumstances of decreased oxygen tension. Once sickling occurs, blood flow is impaired by multiple intracapillary thromboses and RBCs may be removed from the circulation by phagocytes. Women with sickle-cell disease have reduced fertility potential and have a higher incidence of abortion, stillbirths, neonatal death, and premature labor. Fetal wastage is approximately 35 percent. Patients with sickle trait or hemoglobin AS disease have normal fertility. They may be subject to a higher incidence of urinary tract infections, but there is no increased incidence of abortion, stillbirths, prematurity, or newborn infant problems. Maternal death from sickle-cell disease is as high as 10 percent when patients are not adequately cared for. Management consists of proper hydration, oxygenation, and exchange transfusions in circumstances of crises. In some centers, the use of prophylactic exchange transfusion to maintain a minimal level of maternal hemoglobin appars to be associated with an increase in perinatal survival and a decrease in maternal morbidity. Iron therapy should not be increased in these patients.

The thalassemias have a varied response in pregnancy.

Patients with homozygous beta thalassemia present with severe anemia, and have difficulty in maintaining health into the reproductive years. Pregnancy has not been reported in these patients. Heterozygous thalassemia minor is not as serious a condition although chronic hemolytic anemia may be present. Patients with thalassemia trait have normal fertility and pregnancy. Folic acid supplementation is important in these patients.

Immunologic thrombocytopenic purpura (ITP) is characterized by purpuric skin lesions, easy bruising, and hemorrhages from orifices associated with the reduction in the number of blood platelets. The disease is frequent in young, reproductive age females in both acute and chronic forms. Thrombocytopenia may also occur in relationship to drug ingestion, exposure to noxious substances, allergies, recent viral infections, toxemia of pregnancy, and other diseases. The patient's peripheral platelet count is often less than $100,000/mm^3$ with a prolonged bleeding time and normal clotting time. Plasma clotting factors and cell counts are otherwise normal. ITP antibodies may cross the placenta and are associated with transient thrombocytopenic purpura in infants born to mothers with the disease. There is increased risk of perinatal morbidity and mortality when the mother presents with ITP in pregnancy. If the mother has not been appropriately treated and is thrombocytopenic, the risk of hemorrhage and hematoma formation during delivery or surgery is increased. Splenectomy or steroid therapy may normalize maternal platelet counts.

Life-threatening bleeding is a potential complication in the fetus or newborn of a patient with ITP. Management of the fetus during pregnancy is the same, whether the patient has had a splenectomy or is receiving corticosteroid therapy. Platelet antibody (IgG) can cross the placenta and the fetal spleen is capable of removing antibody coated platelets, increasing the risk of perinatal thrombocytopenia. Maternal and fetal platelet counts do not necessarily coincide so that direct assessment of fetal hemostasis is by a scalp sample for quantitative platelet count. If the fetal platelet count is greater than $50,000/mm^3$, vaginal delivery may proceed. If the platelet count is less than $50,000/mm^3$, then careful cesarean delivery is indicated.

The factor deficiency that is of most clinical importance is von Willibrand's disease, a disorder of factor VIII concentration with abnormalities of platelet function. Postpartum hemorrhage is the most common occurrence during pregnancy and is treated by the infusion of cryoprecipitate.

The most common acquired bleeding disorder is disseminated intravascular coagulation. Activation of the fibrinolytic system results in circulating fibrin split products that act as anticoagulants. This is seen frequently with amniotic fluid embolism, septic abortion, hydatidiform mole, missed abortion, and toxemia of pregnancy. Management consists of replacement of coagulation factors by fresh frozen plasma or cryoprecipitate.

Disorders of the Endocrine System

DIABETES MELLITUS

During pregnancy, maternal carbohydrate metabolism undergoes major alterations. Glucose is the primary energy requirement for the human fetus. The mother transfers some of her energy requirements to the oxidation of fats due to interference of glucose-insulin relationships by human placental lactogen and placental insulinase. This allows glucose to become available for the fetus. To maintain homeostasis in the face of insulin antagonism and enhanced degradation, maternal pancreatic beta cells increase insulin production. Maternal insulin activity increases with pregnancy. Minor deficiencies of insulin production become overt under these circumstances. With a glucose load, maternal insulin response may be overstressed, resulting in hyperglycemia during pregnancy.

Maternal diabetes during pregnancy is classified according to duration of disease and time of onset as well as underlying organ complications (Table 10-3).

Several disorders are associated with the natural history of diabetes, including retinopathy, neuropathy, and nephropathy. Diabetes complicating pregnancy occurs in almost 2 percent of all gestations. Some patients have not been diagnosed prior to gestation, some have adult

Table 10-3. Classification of Diabetes in Pregnancy

Class	Description
A	Gestational diabetes with normal fasting plasma glucose and postprandial plasma glucose < 120 mg/100 ml
B_1	Gestational diabetes with fasting hyperglycemia and/or postprandial plasma glucose > 120 mg/100 ml
B_2	Overt diabetes, onset after age 20, and duration less than 10 years
C	Overt diabetes, onset before age 20, or duration 10 to 20 years
D	Overt diabetes, duration more than 20 years or onset before age 10, benign retinopathy
E^a	Calcified pelvic vessels
F	Nephropathy (proteinuria, azotemia)
R	Malignant (proliferative) retinopathy (retinitis proliferans)

Modified from White, P: Pregnancy and diabetes. In Marbel A, White P, Bradley RF, and Krall LP (eds.): Joslin's Diabetes Mellitus. 11th ed. Lea & Febiger, Philadelphia, 1971.

[a] This classification is generally not employed in current practice.

onset diabetes, and the remainder have juvenile-onset insulin-dependent diabetes.

Insulin requirements usually increase during gestation and decrease markedly after delivery. The use of oral hypoglycemics is not warranted during pregnancy because of potential effects on fetal pancreatic activity. Preeclampsia and pyelonephritis are more frequent with diabetic pregnancy. Several problems associated with diabetes may become accelerated during pregnancy, especially retinopathy. Postpartum condition does not differ markedly from preconceptional condition, however. Maternal mortality is less than 1 percent.

Diabetes does exert a deleterious influence on pregnancy. Polyhydramnios is present more frequently in diabetic pregnancies and may be associated with premature labor. Preeclampsia is more frequent with increased risk of perinatal mortality and morbidity. Perinatal mortality is approximately 1 to 3 percent with proper care and attention to maternal glucose control. Otherwise, rates as high as 15 to 20 percent have been recorded. Mortality is due to prematurity, maternal ketoacidosis, preeclampsia, and poor uteroplacental function. Infants of diabetic mothers have a threefold increase in the incidence of major congenital abnormalities. The risk of anomalies increases with the severity of maternal diabetes. Diabetic ketoacidosis is frequently lethal for the fetus. Macrosomia or the LGA infant is a frequent complication. The excessive weight of the newborn under these circumstances is probably related to overutilization of glucose in utero. Intrauterine growth retardation, although uncommon in diabetic pregnancy, is seen more frequently in classes D to R and is associated with reduced utero-placental circulation. Fetal beta cell response is excessive, due to exposure to maternal hyperglycemia. The hypersecretion of insulin does not stop at birth and hypoglycemia is a potentially severe problem in the neonatal period.

The principles of diabetic management in pregnancy include diagnosis, preferably prepregnancy, with careful evaluation and classification of the diabetic woman; meticulous management of diabetes throughout pregnancy, labor, and delivery; delivery at an optimal time for fetal survival; and immediate and intensive neonatal observation and care of the baby.

Recent information suggests the benefit of strict prepregnancy control of diabetes in reducing the incidence of congenital abnormalities. Although this requires confirmation, strict diabetic control appears to help maternal well-being as well. Management includes dietary control in all classes, and insulin treatment in classes B through R. The prescribed diet is based on ideal body weight of the patient and ranges between 1,800–2,500 kcal daily. This approximates to 30 to 35 kcal/kg, 25 to 30 percent for each of three meals with the remainder to

be taken as a bed-time snack. The goal of such therapy is to maintain fasting plasma glucose less than 105 mg percent and 2-hour postprandial glucose less than 140 mg percent. For insulin-dependent diabetes, plasma glucose concentrations should be the same although some investigators have suggested even lower peak plasma glucose after eating. Because of individualized requirements based on diet, activity, and metabolism of glucose with exogenous insulin, the use of daily blood glucose monitoring has become the mainstay of patient management during pregnancy complicated by insulin-dependent diabetes. Self-determined blood glucose concentrations three to four times a day determine the changing requirement for insulin during pregnancy.

Insulin management for class B to R diabetes usually requires a short and medium- to long-acting insulin given together twice daily to cover prandial glucose surges. Optimal management minimizes postprandial fluctuations in blood glucose as a response to dietary intake.

Periodic evaluation of fetal growth, maternal blood pressure, renal function, and neurologic and opthalmalogic changes during pregnancy are performed on all insulin-dependent diabetics. Insulin requirements increase progressively in most pregnant patients. Exogenous insulin given to the mother does not appear to cross the placenta or affect the fetus.

In the third trimester, non-stress fetal monitoring is performed at least weekly to assess fetal well-being. In pregnancies where strict maintenance of euglycemia has been documented, these patients may be allowed to continue to term with a better chance of vaginal delivery. If prognostically bad signs are evident during pregnancy (pyelonephritis, maternal hypertension, ketoacidosis, or patient noncompliance) more aggressive management of pregnancy should be pursued with early hospitalization of the patient and delivery with evidence of fetal lung maturity. Under these circumstances, operative delivery is more likely. Biochemical monitoring by maternal urinary estriol excretion or serum unconjugated estriols has also been used to monitor the integrity of the feto-placental unit. In diabetic pregnancy, timing of fetal lung maturity appears to be delayed. Obstetric management may also require induction of labor with intravenous oxytocin and maintenance of euglycemia by insulin pump and glucose infusion. Failed attempts at vaginal delivery within a reasonable interval are an indication for cesarean delivery.

THYROID DISORDERS

In pregnancy, estrogen-induced increases in thyroid binding globulin are accompanied by increased production of thyroxine to maintain normal plasma binding concentrations. The concentration of free thyroxine in plasma is unchanged. The proportional number of free sites on thyroid binding globulin are unchanged during pregnancy but the total number of sites is increased. Consequently, resin T3 uptake is decreased during pregnancy. The basal metabolic rate of the mother increases progressively throughout pregnancy but this is a reflection of the sum of maternal and fetal metabolic activities.

Severe hyperthyroidism antidating pregnancy is associated with amenorrhea and infertility. With proper management before pregnancy, a patient with hyperthyroidism may become pregnant. Thyrotoxicosis is to be avoided during pregnancy because of the increased frequency of abortion, premature labor and preeclampsia. Hyperthyroidism appears to have little affect on the course of pregnancy. Adequate control is associated with a good outcome. Pregnancy does not appear to change the course of hyperthyroidism. Some patients with hyperthyroidism have remissions during pregnancy, possibly as a result of increased binding to thyroglobulin. Also, the immunologic basis of some states of hyperthyroidism may be diminished during pregnancy.

Iodine and antithyroid drugs readily cross the placenta. Human fetal thyroid tissue avidly accumulates iodine at the end of the first trimester. Consequently, the use of radioactive iodine for maternal diagnosis or therapy is contraindicated during pregnancy. Thyroid-stimulating hormone does not appear to cross the placenta and thyroxine crosses with difficulty. Transient neonatal hyperthyroidism is associated with long-acting thyroid stimulator activity on the fetal-thyroid. Management with anti-thyroid medication effects on the fetus include transient or more long-term neonatal hypothyroidism.

Management is based on maintaining maternal euthyroidism at the lowest dose of antithyroid medication to protect the fetus. In mild cases, no treatment may be required. Treatment may also be decreased later in pregnancy. The antithyroid drugs currently in use for treating hyperthyroidism are carbimazole, methylthiouracil, and propylthiouracil. Excessive exposure of these drugs to the fetus may result in congenital goiter, fetal hypothyroidism, and mental retardation. These drugs are also excreted in breast milk. Propylthiouracil is most commonly used, with treatment of 100 to 200 mg three times daily until the euthyroid state is reached. Thereafter, the dose may be reduced with further control. Surgical management of thyrotoxicosis should be reserved for hyperthyroidism unresponsive to medical therapy. After thyroidectomy, thyroid hormone substitution may be necessary to avoid the risk of maternal hypothyroidism.

Hypothyroidism is infrequently encountered during pregnancy and is associated with increased rates of infertility. Euthyroid control is obtained with thyroid replacement therapy.

Hyperparathyroidism is distinctly unusual in pregnancy. Parathyroid disease results from solitary or multiple adenomas, hyperplasia, or carcinoma. There is excessive secretion of parathormone, serum calcium is elevated, and urine calcium is increased. Most affected patients have calcium and phosphate renal stones. The symptoms of muscular weakness, psychosis, hypophosphatemia, and decreased bone density may also be present in secondary hyperparathyroidism, which occurs with chronic renal insufficiency. Treatment for primary hyperparathyroidism is surgical. Postoperative treatment includes vitamin D and calcium therapy.

Hypoparathyroidism is equally rare and is often secondary to surgery. The most frequent manifestation is hypocalcemic tetany. This disorder is controlled by supplying adequate amounts of calcium along with vitamin D.

Pituitary disorders are rarely found during pregnancy. Prolactin secreting adenoma is a problem during pregnancy because of continued stimulation and growth. Generally, patients with untreated prolactin secreting adenomas should be counseled to have medical or surgical management prior to conception. Hypopituitarism, which may have been related to a previous pituitary necrosis during pregnancy, is associated with infertility unless adequate replacement therapy is available. With successful conception, replacement of other pituitary hormones should insure normal outcome for pregnancy.

Cushing's syndrome is rarely seen in pregnancy. The disease results from adrenocortical hyperfunction secondary to hyperplasia, adenoma, or carcinoma of the adrenal gland, or to increased pituitary secretion of ACTH. Rarely, pregnancy may occur in the course of the disease. Treatment may include bilateral adrenalectomy or pituitary radiation. Replacement therapy is necessary after surgery. Infants born to mothers with untreated Cushing's syndrome may have adrenal insufficiency and require immediate treatment at birth.

The adrenogenital syndrome is the overproduction of androgens by the fetal adrenal cortex and is usually an inborn error of metabolism. One of several enzyme deficiencies is associated with a specific clinical presentation of one or more of the following: virilization of females, salt loss, premature isosexual development, hypertension, and hypokalemia. Many of these do not become clinical problems for the fetus until after delivery. The syndrome may not appear until puberty or later in life. Patients have become pregnant with this syndrome and hormonal replacement therapy with cortisone or surgical correction are usually successful.

Primary aldosteronism is a rare condition during pregnancy with hypertension, hypokalemia, and normal renal function. Administration of spironolactone will be helpful in management but surgery may be required, especially if a tumor of the adrenal cortex is present.

Adrenal hormone deficiencies are extremely uncommon and are treated by replacement of gluco- and mineralocorticoids. Maternal and fetal mortality from pheochromocytoma are quite high during pregnancy and early diagnosis should be followed by surgical management. Operative management includes the use of anerergic blocking agents.

Ovarian disorders are relatively common during pregnancy. Differential diagnosis includes corpus luteum cyst, and benign and malignant tumors. Diagnosis may be difficult in pregnancy because of the size of the gravid uterus. Abortion and hemorrhage are common complications of ovarian neoplasms during pregnancy. Surgical exploration is indicated for all persistent adnexal masses by early second trimester. Adult cystic teratomas make up 25 to 40 percent of all ovarian masses; one-third are cystadenomas with potential for malignant transformation. These uterine cysts are found as exaggerated ovarian response to excessive gonadotropin stimulation. They are frequently associated with gestational trophoblastic disease, but may be found in patients with twin gestation.

The optimal time for surgical intervention for ovarian tumors is in the second trimester. Ovarian lesions found to be borderline malignancies should allow the obstetrician to be conservative and maintain pregnancy. The chance of a more aggressive malignancy should be discussed with the patient before surgery to determine whether or not to maintain pregnancy.

Connective tissue disorders are more common among women and therefore are not rare during pregnancy. The most important of these is systemic lupus erythematosus (SLE), a collagen disease with variable clinical manifestations. The characteristic findings of skin rash, arthritis, renal damage, anemia, leukopenia and thrombocytopenia may be present during pregnancy. If renal disease is present, the likelihood of superimposed preeclampsia is increased. Pregnancy does not appear to alter the course of SLE. The major effects of SLE on pregnancy are increases in fetal wastage, preeclampsia, intrauterine growth retardation, and complete fetal heart block. Management consists of careful assessment of maternal control during pregnancy, including periodic assessment of components of the complement system, and anti-DNA. Decreases in complement components are often harbingers of worsening disease. Increases in daily corticosteroid dosage appear to be of benefit in maintaining maternal health.

The course of rheumatoid arthritis is usually improved during pregnancy although treatment may be maintained without using nonsteroidal antiinflamma-tory agents. However, in patients who have severe disability because of the underlying disease, management of labor and delivery may be modified.

Scleroderma is rarely seen with pregnancy but there appears to be an increased pregnancy wastage, including spontaneous abortion, premature labor, and impaired uteroplacental function. Periarteritis nodosum is equally rare and is associated with increased maternal mortality. Because of the risk of dissecting aneurysm, especially associated with changes in cardiac output, Marfan's syndrome may be lethal during pregnancy. Management of pregnancy includes evaluation for hypertensive changes and abnormalities of fetal growth as well as active management of labor and delivery.

Disorders of the gastrointestinal system during pregnancy include viral hepatitis, acute fatty liver, recurrent jaundice of pregnancy, cholestatis, and cirrhosis. None of these disorders are found with any frequency in pregnancy. Fetal wastage may be high, from early abortion or premature labor. Hepatitis B is important when hepatitis B surface antigen is persistent in the mother without development of hepatitis B antibody. The risk of neonatal infection is increased in contact with the mother. Consequently, the use of hepatitis B immune globulin is recommended at the time of delivery with later administration of hepatitis B vaccine for infant protection.

Acute fatty liver presents with severe jaundice, epigastric pain, and vomiting, frequently accompanied by stillbirth, usually in the last trimester of pregnancy. The biochemical profile is compatible with acute liver failure. The etiology of the condition is unclear. Treatment is supportive and mortality is high. Cholestasis is a condition characterized by jaundice and pruritus, due to deposition of bile salts under maternal skin. The syndrome is limited to pregnancy and to the use of oral contraceptives. Pregnancy cholestasis increases the risk of maternal postpartum hemorrhage, prematurity, and fetal distress. Treatment should include careful assessment of fetal well-being. Patients with cirrhosis may consider pregnancy when there is no evidence of portal hypertension or severely deteriorated liver function. Patients with previous porta caval shunts may also be considered as potential candidates for pregnancy.

Cholecystitis and cholelithiasis are common during pregnancy because of changes in circulating estrogens, hypercholesterolemia, and biliary hypotonia. Right upper quandrant pain with radiation is characteristic of the disease although the differential diagnosis includes hepatic disease, pyelonephritis, and renal stones. Diagnosis is made by ultrasonography and acute management consists of administration of appropriate intravenous fluids with antispasmodics, analgesics, and in some cases antibiotics. Most patients improve with this regimen. Surgery is best avoided during pregnancy but may be necessary when more conservative therapy fails.

Acute pancreatitis presents with the same clinical picture in pregnancy as in the nongravid state. Onset is characterized by severe upper abdominal pain and vomiting. Fever, distension, and decreased bowel sounds may be present. Diagnosis is based on a high index of suspicion and elevated serum amylase concentrations. Serum lipase increases more slowly but tends to remain elevated longer. Since the concentration of these enzymes may be elevated in other acute abdominal conditions, x-ray examination of the abdomen may often reveal a sentinel loop pattern of ileus. Treatment consists of complete rest for the pancreas. This includes intravenous fluids, nasogastric suction, anticholinergic medication, and antibiotics to control associated infection. Other volume expanders, including blood, plasma, or serum albumin, may be necessary. Because of large changes in plasma volume, urine output should be monitored.

Peptic ulcer is distinctly uncommon during pregnancy and treatment is generally the same as in the nonpregnant state.

Appendicitis is the acute surgical condition most frequently encountered during pregnancy. There is an increase in maternal and fetal mortality and morbidity, usually associated with delay in diagnosis and treatment. The displacement of the appendix from its position in the right lower quadrant, increasing pregnancy gastrointestinal symptoms, and physiologic leukocytosis of pregnancy are associated with delayed diagnosis. The classical signs of peritoneal irritation noted with appendicitis may not be present during pregnancy. Diagnosis rests upon a high index of suspicion and careful attention to history. Differential diagnosis include urinary tract disease, adnexal pathology, and degeneration of uterine leiomyomata. Exploratory laparatomy is necessary for diagnosis and should not be delayed because the patient is pregnant. Generally, removal of the appendix is indicated and abdominal or cul-de-sac drainage may be required if leakage has occurred into the abdominal cavity. Cesarean section should not be attempted at the time of appendiceal disease.

Regional enteritis does not appear to affect the outcome of pregnancy nor is the course of ileitis affected by pregnancy if inactive at the time of conception. The course is likely to be severe when it presents for the first time during pregnancy. Exacerbation occurs after delivery in up to 50 percent of affected patients. Management is generally symptomatic and supportive but may include surgical intervention. Pregnancy may actually be associated with worsening ulcerative colitis. Medical management ought to be tried first and should include dietary manipulation, rest, and sedation, and possibly corticosteroids or antiinflammatory medications. The latter should be considered carefully in light of potential fetal complications. Surgery may be unavoidable but colectomy should be delayed, if possible, until after delivery.

Other causes of intestinal obstruction are distinctly rare during pregnancy but should be taken into account in the differential diagnosis of gastrointestinal complications.

Disorders of the neuromuscular system generally include epilepsy, peripheral neuropathies, carpel tunnel syndrome, and intracranial disorders.

The effect of pregnancy on epilepsy is not entirely clear; some patients have an increase in seizure frequency during pregnancy and others a decrease. Uncontrolled epilepsy may have a deleterious effect on pregnancy. Abortion and premature labor are not usually the result of seizures but there is some suggestion that there is an increase in congenital disorders among offspring. The use of phenytoin (Dilantin) has also been associated with a neonatal syndrome of facial dysmorphism, intrauterine growth retardation, and later developmental delay and mental retardation. Approximately 10 percent of newborns exposed to Dilantin in utero have this syndrome.

Nevertheless, anticonvulsant therapy should be followed into pregnancy because of the risks to both mother and fetus of increasing seizures. Changes in maternal absorption and metabolism mandate periodic measurement of serum Dilantin concentrations. Careful adjustment is necessary to decrease seizure frequency. Supplementary folic acid should be given in a dose necessary for normal pregnancy requirements only, as increasing doses of this medication compete with Dilantin for receptor sites.

Peripheral neuropathies usually affect the lower extremities due to hormonally mediated and structural changes in the lower back, and increasing pressure of the gravid uterus on peripheral nerve trunks. Bed-rest and management to increase tone of the lower back and abdominal muscles may benefit this spectrum of disorders. Carpal tunnel syndrome or compression of the median nerve is relatively common during pregnancy. Management includes splinting of the hand, the use of corticosteroids, and in some cases, surgical release of the nerve from the compressing ligament of the wrist.

Intracranial vascular disorders include subarachnoid hemorrhage, cerebral thrombosis, and arteriovenous malformations. The first disorder is most often associated with rupture of a congenital aneurysm. Management of these disorders is the same as in the nonpregnant state. They are associated with an increase in maternal mortality. Multiple sclerosis, brain tumors, and myasthenia gravis are extremely uncommon during pregnancy and their course is not affected by pregnancy.

Disorders of the skin include pruritus of pregnancy or prurigo gestationis, herpes gestationis, impetigo herpetiformis, and persistent urticarial plaques and papules. Of these, herpes gestationis is associated with an increased risk of fetal wastage and is probably associated with an altered immunologic environment. Impetigo herpetiformis threatens fetal well-being and may be potentially fatal to the mother. Persistent urticarial plaques and papules also appear to have an immunologic basis. The treatment of all these disorders is with systemic corticosteroids.

Various cancers are important during pregnancy because of their increased association in women of reproductive age. The treatment required for cancer may jeopardize the fetus or impair the mother's ability to care for her child.

Carcinoma of the breast and carcinoma of the cervix are the most frequent malignancies seen during pregnancy although melanoma, leukemia, and malignancies of the gastrointestinal tract and central nervous system may also be present. The finding of a breast mass during pregnancy is somewhat more difficult because of changes in breast tissue. Mammography and excisional biopsy are necessary to make a diagnosis. Once breast carcinoma is diagnosed, appropriate therapy should be undertaken. For the most part, modified radical mastectomy is still the treatment of choice in this country, although some advocate the use of simple mastectomy followed by radiation therapy to contiguous regions of the chest and axilla. Five-year survival rates for pregnant women with normal axillary nodes is the same as that of nonpregnant women. Therapeutic abortion is generally not recommended, even with the use of chemotherapy.

Carcinoma of the cervix ranges from carcinoma in situ to more invasive cancer. In the former, periodic evaluation during pregnancy with diagnostic and therapeutic cone biopsy of the cervix may be warranted, depending on the extent of the lesion by colposcopy and directed biopsy. Invasive carcinoma requires radical treatment by either extended hysterectomy or radiotherapy, both of which are incompatible with maintenance of pregnancy. The timing of diagnosis in pregnancy in terms of potential fetal viability is important. In no case of invasive carcinoma should a patient be allowed to deliver vaginally.

INFECTION

Multiple factors are important in gynecologic and obstetric infection. Socioeconomic background, impaired immunologic response, and diminished host defense mechanisms have been associated with complications in management of infectious disease. The microbiology of the genital tract is important in considering infection. Several bacterial organisms native to the reproductive tract may become pathogens under certain circumstances. In other cases, the offending organism is definitely exogenous. This has led to critical investigations of sexual transmission as well as the establishment of strict aseptic technique during obstetric and surgical procedures. Reduction of infectious morbidity and mortality, especially in obstetrics, from these changes was present before the availability of antibiotics for clinical practice.

Changes in vaginal flora in individuals and between population groups may be a function of socioeconomic and sexual practices. Because of these findings, it is difficult to describe normal and pathogenic vaginal flora in women. Many of the organisms in the vagina are capable of causing serious infectious disease when host defense mechanisms are altered. Better information about this has remained incomplete until recently because of difficulties in isolation and identification of certain microorganisms. Accurate identification depends on rapid transport to the laboratory and the use of appropriate media. With careful culturing techniques, anaerobic bacteria, mycoplasma, certain viruses, yeast, and protozoa have been encountered with greater frequency than previously. Under normal circumstances, the uterus has several mechanisms for protecting itself against bacteria that manage to survive the antibacterial effects of cervical mucus and enter the uterine cavity. The use of foreign bodies, such as intrauterine devices, or the breakdown of other physiologic barriers, may cause this protective milieu to be breeched.

Infections of the female generative tract may be subdivided into more localized infections of the vagina and urinary tract and systemic infections including the kidneys, the uterus, fallopian tubes, and ovaries.

Acute Localized Infections

Neisseria gonorrhoeae has been the most important pathogen in the nonpregnant female. Gonorrhea exists in epidemic proportions in the United States. These infections are usually not life-threatening, but because of salpingo-oophoritis, with resultant tubal occlusion or pelvic abscess formation, infertility may be a long-term residual effect. *Neisseria gonorrhoeae* may cause local infection including symptomatic vulvovaginitis in premenstrual or postmenopausal women, urinary tract symptoms, and abnormal uterine bleeding. Only a small fraction of women of child-bearing age exposed to *neisseria gonorrhoeae* will develop symptomatic salpingo-oophoritis.

Vaginitis is one of the most common complaints of

patients seen in daily office practice. Infections include *Gardnerella vaginitis (hemophilus vaginalis)* vaginitis, an asymptomatic, localized infection that may not cause vaginal discomfort but, because of its offensive odor and discharge, comes to the physician's attention. Several medications have been used to eradicate this pathogen but metronidazole appears to be the most effective.

The fungus *Candida albicans* is frequently a cause of vaginal infections in sexually active women. Candidiasis may be a complication of systemic antibiotic infection for infection elsewhere in the body. Pregnancy and uncontrolled diabetes have also been associated with an increased frequency of candida vaginitis. There is some evidence that oral contraceptive ingestion may increase candida infections. Diagnosis is made by the clinical appearance of a curd-like white discharge in a patient with vulvar pruritus and inflamed vulva. The presence of mycelia in a potassium hydroxide wet mount preparation of vaginal secretions or the growth of candida on Sabouraud's medium confirms the clinical suspicion of candida vaginitis. A number of antifungal agents are effective in treatment. The protozoan *Trichomonas vaginalis* is also a cause of vulvovaginitis. It causes itching, burning, and malodorous discharge. Red, punctate lesions may be seen on an inflamed cervix, giving it a strawberry-like appearance. The presence of motile trichomonads in a wet mount preparation of vaginal secretions is diagnostic. Metronidazole is the agent of choice against this infection. When reinfection occurs, both sexual partners should be treated.

Infection of the paraurethral (Skene's) and vaginal (Bartholin's) glands may cause acute symptoms. *Neisseria gonorrhoeae* is often a pathogen, but in many cultures, a mixed flora is found. Because of inflammation, flow of glandular secretions may be stopped, causing soft tissue infection with abscess formation. Antibiotics may be helpful in preventing the spread of soft tissue inflammation but care requires establishment of operative drainage to maintain flow of secretions and prevent reinfection.

Viruses are responsible for some localized female genital urinary tract problems. Herpes simplex virus (HSV) is the most important because of its clinical spectrum and its association with potential problems in childbearing. The diagnosis of HSV vulvovaginitis is made clinically by seeing inflamed, ulcerated small lesions of the vulva, vaginal introitus, and cervix in conjunction with moderate to severe discomfort. Primary HSV infection may be associated with urinary retention and fever. There is no cure for the disease but the use of acyclovir has been associated with improvement in the course of primary infection.

Condyloma acuminatum will also cause symptomatic problems as well as vaginal outlet obstruction. Manage-

ment of venereal warts consists of either short exposure to podophyllin or cryotherapy.

Lymphogranuloma venereum is a disease process caused by *Chlamydia trachomatis*. The disease is manifested by progressive formation of draining sinuses, perirectal and isheorectal abscesses, and eventual stricture or edema of the labia and clitoris. Chlamydia is susceptible to tetracycline and clindamycin. Early treatment can result in cure and prevention of disfiguring lesions.

Chancroid is a debilitating infection of the lower genital tract caused by the gram-negative bacillus. *Hemophilus ducreyi*. This disease is most often seen in tropical climates. The genital infection progresses to painful vaginal lesions and infected inguinal nodes with suppuration and drainage. The organism is sensitive to both sulfa drugs and tetracycline.

Granuloma inguinale results from infection by the bacteria *Calymmatobacterium granulomatis*. With this infection, ulceration, granulation, and extensive fibrosis of the vulvar region may occur. The organisms are sensitive to tetracycline.

Treponema pallidum is the bacillus that causes syphilis. The primary route of infection is sexual. The primary lesion or chancre is found as a painless ulcer of the labia or cervix. The untreated primary lesion may heal spontaneously within 3 to 9 weeks after exposure. Unless the patient seeks medical attention, however, the disease will go undiagnosed and untreated.

Urinary Tract Infections

Urinary tract infections are the most frequent infections in women. Heterosexual activity may play a role in asymptomatic bacteriuria. Colonization of the vaginal canal with potentially pathogenic bacteria because of sexual activity or poor hygiene leads to an increased risk of urinary tract infection.

A carefully collected clean voided midstream urine with more than 100,000 bacteria/ml is 80 percent diagnostic of bacteruria. The majority of organisms responsible for urinary tract infection are gram-negative enteric organisms. The predominant pathogen is *Escherichia coli*. Systemic antibiotics that are concentrated in the urinary tract are the treatment of choice for urinary tract infections with appropriate sensitivity. Cultures should be obtained 2 days after therapy is started and again a week after therapy is completed to be certain that the infection has been cured. Patients with symptoms limited to the lower urinary tract are treated for 3 to 10 days with oral agents. In patients with clinical evidence of pyelonephritis, parenteral antibiotics should be started for a 10 to 14 day course of therapy. Recurrence of infection indicates further evaluation by urologic and radiologic procedures to determine whether abnormalities of the urinary tract exist.

Systemic infections that affect the reproductive system, in order of importance, are gonorrhea, syphilis, and tuberculosis. Gonorrhea may have local manifestations, as previously described. In many cases, this infection may be asymptomatic. Pharyngeal gonococcal disease has been described also and is probably associated with orogenital contact. Because of the asymptomatic nature of local gonorrhea, it is important to screen certain high-risk populations by culturing the cervical canal during routine exams. Thayer-Martin media will be approximately 90 percent accurate. Routine cultures of the rectum and urethra in high-risk populations will increase the yield of diagnosis.

If localized gonorrhea is untreated or inadequately treated, the disease may spread by direct extension from the endocervical canal to the endometrial cavity, fallopian tubes, and peritoneal cavity. This is more likely at menstruation when the endocervical canal becomes dilated and the mucus plug disintegrates. The organism quickly spreads by direct extension to the mucosal lining of the fallopian tube. The antitoxin produced by the gonococcus causes an inflammatory reaction at the site of contact with eventual tissue destruction and tubal scarring. Virulence of the organism, tissue resistance, and availability of treatment are decisive factors in the arrest or progression of disease at this stage. With progression of disease, the tubes eventually become thickened and occluded. Extensive damage occurs to the tube and the muscularis and serosa become involved with severe infections. As a result, the patient has an increased potential for ectopic pregnancy, infertility, and chronic disease.

Patients may present with lower quadrant pain, elevated temperature, and nausea and vomiting. Abdominal distention and muscular guarding may be apparent with examination. Untreated or poorly treated endosalpingitis may form large abscesses involving both the fallopian tube and the ovary (tuboovarian abscess). The treatment of local gonococcal disease and systemic disease are initially the same. For most patients, Neisseria gonorrhea is exquisitely sensitive to penicillin. Effective treatment is obtained with administration of 4.8 million units of procaine penicillin G in divided doses at one visit. Probenecid 1 g given orally 30 minutes prior to antibiotic injection prevents rapid excretion of the penicillin and permits high blood levels of the antibiotic. Initial therapy should be followed by oral ampicillin 500 mg 4 times/day for 10 days or, if the patient is penicillin-sensitive, she should receive tetracyline hydrochloride 1.5 g initially followed by 0.5 g, 4 times/day for 10 days. Spectinomycin, 2 g intramuscularly should be restricted to treatment of penicillinase-producing organisms or to recurrent disease. In pregnancy, if a patient is allergic to

penicillin, erythromycin 0.5 g 4 times/day for 7 days is the treatment of choice. For subacute salpingitis, hospitalization is indicated if the patient is febrile, dehydrated, if she has leukocytosis, or reliability of follow-up is questionable. Higher antibiotic dosages may be required for systemic disease (Fitzhugh-Curtis Syndrome). Parenteral penicillin in dosages of 10 to 20 million units per day in divided doses should be instituted. Because gram-negative organisms and anaerobic bacteria have been associated with gonococcal disease, addition of an aminoglycoside and clindamycin may be indicated. Complications such as bacteremia, arthritis, endocarditis, etc. must be individualized for management. If there is question of potential surgery, the patient should not be fed. Bed-rest in a semi-Fowler's position may help to localize an abscess in the cul-de-sac area and allow for incision and drainage. Once the patient has had endosalpingitis, certain restrictions are appropriate for the future. In these patients, the intrauterine device is contraindicated.

The systemic manifestations of syphilis start approximately 2 months after exposure. Although syphilis is systemic within 24 hours of primary infection, primary disease may clinically disappear within 3 to 9 weeks of exposure. Secondary syphilis begins with complaints of malaise, headache, and anorexia. A generalized skin rash with lesions on the mucus membranes make this stage highly contagious and characteristic for diagnosis. Tertiary syphilis begins when secondary syphilis resolves spontaneously or is inadequately treated. It may manifest by ulcerative lesions of the skin known as gummas. These lesions may appear within 1 to 10 years following initial exposure. Complications of syphilis appear approximately 8 to 10 years following initial contact. They include effects on almost all organ systems. Syphilis of more than 1 year's duration requires more extensive therapy than primary syphilis.

Specific tests for syphilis include the following serologic tests:

1. Nontreponemal tests; VDRL, RPR. These tests are determinations of nonspecific antibodies against certain antigens of the treponeme. They are standard screening tests and become reactive within 2 weeks after the appearance of a primary lesion or 4 to 5 weeks following initial infection. Titers rise rapidly thereafter. A titer of 1 : 8 or less may signify either a false positive reaction or the presence of disease. Titers of 1 : 32 or greater signify the pressure of the disease. The reported titer is not an indication of the infectiousness of the disease. Clinical data obtained from the patient are necessary to interpret test results.

2. Treponemal tests: When nontreponemal screening tests are positive, a confirmatory test may be necessary. The most commonly used test is the fluorescent treponemal antibody-absorption (FTA-ABS) test. It is the

most sensitive clinical test to diagnose all stages of syphilis. False positive reactions do occur but are infrequent. False positive reactions are usually associated with disorders of serum proteins. Patient information is still necessary in formulating a diagnosis and plan. The VDRL is usually employed for followup examination after treatment. Repeat testing should be done monthly for 6 months and then less frequently. The tests will become negative and remain so with adequate treatment. Patients with a positive titer after 12 months of treatment should have a lumbar puncture for cerebrospinal fluid evaluation. If syphilis has been present for several years before diagnosis and treatment, serology may remain positive.

3. Dark field examination of sera permits an absolute and immediate diagnosis of syphilis. This test is inaccessible to most physicians but may be appropriate to confirm disease in borderline cases.

4. Biopsy may be appropriate when dark field examination is not available.

Treatment of syphilis depends on the stage of the disease. For primary or secondary syphilis, a single intramuscular injection of 2.4 million units of benzathine penicillin G is curative in the majority of cases. An alternative schedule is procaine penicillin G 600,000 units intramuscularly daily for 8 to 10 days, or procaine penicillin G with 2 percent aluminum monosterate 2.4 million units IM followed by an additional 1.2 million units in each of 2 subsequent injections 3 days apart. Patient reliability may be important in deciding the course of treatment. With patients who have penicillin allergy, tetracycline hydrochloride 0.5 g 4 times/day for 15 days or erythromycin 0.5 g 4 times/day for 15 days is appropriate.

Syphilis of more than 1 year's duration (latent, intermediate, cardiovascular, late benign, neurosyphilis) should be treated with benzathine penicillin G 7.2 million units total, given in 2.4 million unit doses weekly for three weeks. An alternative choice would be to increase procaine penicillin G to 9 million units, given in 600,000 unit doses intramuscularly on a daily basis for 15 days. Treatment with erythromycin or tetracycline should be for at least 30 days. Treatment should be carried out in conjunction with followup serologic testing.

Tuberculosis is uncommonly a cause of reproductive tract infection or abnormalities. It is a major cause of infertility elsewhere, but is distinctly uncommon in the United States. If conception is successful, pregnancy loss is still a potential problem.

Other systemic infections that may have a bearing on reproductive health include surgical gastrointestinal diseases such as appendicitis, diverticulitis, and bowel injury. Suppurative complications of these diseases and subsequent formation of fibrous adhesions may anatom-

ically obstruct passage of the egg from the ovary to the tube where fertilization usually takes place. Septic or criminal abortion used to be a major cause of maternal morbidity and mortality and subsequent infertility. With the advent of more liberal standards for therapeutic abortion, this particular problem has become increasingly infrequent in clinical obstetric and gynecologic medicine. Postoperative infections of the urogenital tract also contribute to female morbidity, mortality, and subsequent infertility. Manipulation of the vaginal canal during surgery in the premenopausal woman is especially important because of the continuous reservoir of potential pathogens in this organ. Attempts at eradicating all organisms in the vagina prior to surgery meet with failure so that the use of prophylactic antibiotics during vaginal surgery is appropriate.

Pelvic and systemic infections are still potential problems after gynecologic surgery and have been the impetus for careful aseptic technique by surgeons and the use of prophylactic antibiotics during major surgery. Other sources of postoperative infection are the urinary and respiratory tracts. Proper postoperative management should include maintenance of high arterial PO_2 and lung aeration through coughing and deep breathing. Under these circumstances, pneumonia and atelectasis are minimized. In the urinary tract, persistence of indwelling urinary catheters contributes to an increased risk of bladder or kidney infection. Therefore, it is appropriate to remove these catheters as soon as the patient is able to void without complications. The development of a closed collecting system for urinary drainage has decreased the incidence of invasion by bacteria. In some cases antibiotic prophylaxis may be appropriate.

When a febrile response is observed in the postoperative period, and the respiratory and urinary tracts do not seem to be offending areas, more systemic manifestations may be further documented by a positive blood culture. The chance of finding the most likely causative organism in postoperative infection outside of the urine and sputum is in cultures from active pockets of infection such as the wound in drainage from an operative site or from the blood stream. Bacteremia is an early sign of a potentially devastating septicemia. Acquisition of a blood culture involves aseptic treatment of sites for venipuncture and aerobic and anaerobic bacteria culturing.

In general, postoperative wound and pelvic infections are associated with surgery in a contaminated operative field, the use of instruments and materials that, as foreign bodies, tend to support bacterial growth, poor hemostasis at the operative site, and active intercurrent infection. Age at surgery may be important because of host factors, but an intriguing difference is noted with vaginal surgery. Premenopausal women tend to have higher rates of infection than postmenopausal women after vaginal surgery. The reasons for this are not clear but probably involve hormonal and local circulation differences.

Antibiotic therapy for infection will depend upon the causative organisms, the site of infection, patient susceptibility to side effects of the antibiotic, host renal and hepatic function for metabolism of the drug, the potential development of bacterial resistance in the use of certain agents, and route of administration of agents. With pregnant patients, effects of certain agents on fetal growth and development should be taken into account. Localized or regionalized infections may be initially treated with a single agent if the organism is known to be susceptible and the infection is not immediately life-threatening. In obstetric and gynecologic medicine, the enteric gram-negative pathogens have often been primary organisms of infection and therefore are susceptible to broad spectrum penicillins such as ampicillin as well as to the aminoglycoside agents. The prevalence of mixed infections or purely anaerobic type infections have made the use of clindamycin and metronidazole an integral part of overall management for gynecologic infection. Therefore, when gynecologic infection exists without knowledge of the offending organism, it has become appropriate to use broad spectrum medications that cover several pathogens and patients often receive a combination of a penicillin, aminoglycoside, and a chemotherapeutic agent whose chief activity is against anerobic bacteria. Newer cepahlosporins and penicillins have become available that may provide broad coverage for several organisms that are resistant pathogens in the genital tract.

PART 2

Gynecology

ANATOMY

The female reproductive system can be conveniently divided into the internal and the external genitalia. The internal genitalia includes the uterus, the fallopian tubes and the ovaries. The external genitalia consists of the vulva and vagina.

External Genitalia

The vulva is made up of the mons, the paired labia minora and majora, and the midline clitoris, urethra, vaginal orifice, and the perineal body. The mons is a hair

covered mound of adipose tissue overriding the pubic symphysis. The pared labia majora are two skin covered adipose tissues that lie longitudinally along the lateral vulva. Medial to the labia majora lie the labia minora. These two folds of tissue arise near the clitoris and descend approximately two-thirds of the way to the perineum. The skin overlying the labia minora is devoid of hair but does contain many sebaceous glands. The clitoris is a midline erectile organ about 6 to 8 mm in diameter. The erectile tissue of the clitoris is composed of two corpura cavernosa. The urethra is a tubular structure arising from the bladder base and extending to the visible external urethral meatus. It is lined by a stratified transitional epithelium near the bladder, gradually changing to a stratified squamous eptihelium externally. Inferior to the meatus are the orifices of the pararetheral or Skene's glands. The majority of the vulvar blood supply is derived from the internal pudendal artery, a branch of the hypogastric or internal iliac artery. The venous drainage follows a similar course. The lymphatic drainage of the vulva is in a superior direction towards the mons. The major lymphatic chains being the superficial inguinal lymph nodes which drain to the femoral nodes and then via the node of Cloquet to the pelvic nodes.

The vagina is a tubular structure lined by squamous epithelium and surrounded by an inner circular and an outer muscular layer. It extends from the vulva horizontally to the uterine end for a distance of 9 to 10 cm. The uterine end widens into the fornices of the vagina into which the ectocervix protrudes. The vagina receives its blood supply via the vaginal artery, a branch of the hypogastric and from branches of the uterine and internal pudendal arteries. The venous efflux follows veins of the same names. The vaginal lymphatic drainage is similar to that of the vulva in the lower half and to that of the cervix in the upper half. The vagina is bounded anteriorly by the bladder. The upper third anteriorly is in close approximation to the bladder trigone and the intravesicle portions of the ureter course along the anterior vaginal wall. The vagina is bounded posteriorly by the rectum save for the upper third in the region of the posterior vaginal fornix. At the posterior fornix, the vagina is covered above by parietal peritoneum and it is through this area that the peritoneal cavity can be entered using the procedures called culdocentesis and colpotomy.

Internal Genitalia

The uterus is comprised of the cervix and uterine fundus. The cervix has an intravaginal portion surrounded by the anterior and posterior vaginal fornices and laterally by the two lateral vaginal fornices. The intravaginal portion is covered by squamous epithelium similar to that of the vagina. This epithelium extends to the external cervical os where it merges with the epithelium of the endocervix. The endocervical epithelium is a racemose mucus secreting columnar epithelium that extends upward approximately 2 cm. along the endocervical canal to the internal cervical os. The cervical stroma is composed of spindle cells. The internal os marks the transition from the endocervix to the uterine cavity. The cervical blood supply arises from branches of the uterine and vaginal arteries. The cervical lymphatic drainage occurs in a step wise predictable manner to the parametrial, obturator, iliac, and finally the paraaortic nodes.

The uterus is a pear shaped muscular organ lined by an epithelium that varies histologically depending upon its hormonal milieu to be described later. This lining or endometrium covers a conical shaped cavity. The uterus is usually situated at a right angle to the long axis of the vagina but it may be rotated posteriorly or retroverted. It also may flex upon itself anteriorly or posteriorly, a condition termed anteflexion or retroflexion. The upper portion of the fundus is dome like in shape and is marked laterally by the cornua where each fallopian tube attaches. The uterine wall is made up of smooth muscle cells that freely interlace. The uterus is covered by parietal peritoneum which reflected off the posterior surface on to the rectum at the cul-de-sac of Douglas. The peritoneum anteriorily is reflected on to the bladder. The lateral peritoneum is reflected on to the pelvic side walls as the broad ligaments, the upper portion of which includes the fallopian tubes. The lower portion of the broad ligament is thickened and contains connective tissue. This is the cardinal ligament. The uterosacral ligaments are thickened connective tissue structures that arise from the posterior wall of the uterus and extend posteriorly around the rectum to insert onto the sacral promontory. The paired round ligaments arise from the anterior aspect of the uterine fundus and pass to the internal inguinal ring. From the ring, they traverse the inguinal canal to fuse with the connective tissue of the groin. The uterine blood supply comes from the uterine arteries which are branches of the anterior division of the hypogastric artery.

The fallopian tubes are paired muscular tubes that insert into the uterine cornua. The tubes are covered by peritoneum. They have a muscular coat arranged in an inner circular and an outer longitudinal layer. The epithelium is folded becoming more so as the distal end or fimbria of the tube is approached. The tubes are divided into four portions. The interstitial or intramural portion penetrates the myometrium and enters the endometrial cavity. The isthmus is the name given to the portion of the tube near the uterus. The ampulla is a larger diameter middle portion and finally the fimbria is the distal end. The tubes serve as a conduit for the ova to reach the uterine cavity. The blood supply comes from branches of the ovarian and uterine arteries.

The ovaries are paired structures that are roughly almond shaped and white in color. They are attached to the posterior leaf of the broad ligament at the hilum of the ovary through which the ovarian blood supply passes. The ovary is covered by a mesothelial layer that is given the name germinal epthelium. Beneath the epithelium is the ovarian stroma a portion of which is thickened and termed the tunica albuginea. The stroma is composed of spindle cells. The stroma and the epithelium constitute the ovarian cortex. The follicular elements or germ cells are contained in the ovarian stroma. The histology of the follicles and their changes will be described subsequently. The central portion of the ovary is termed the medulla.

Pelvic Support

The genitalia are supported by the perineum which is made up of the pelvic and urogenital diaphragms. The pelvic diaphragm is composed mainly of the levator ani muscles and some contribution of the coccygeous muscles. The levator ani muscles arise from the pubic rami, the ischial spines, and the obturator internus fascia. These paired muscles meet in the midline at the median raphee which extends to the coccyx. The pelvic diaphragm is pierced by the rectum, vagina, and urethra. The urogenital diaphragm lies superficial to the pelvic diaphragm in the area bounded by the pubic symphysis and the ischial tuberosities.

EMBRYOLOGIC ANATOMY

Genetic sex is determined at conception. Those X-bearing ova that are fertilized by an X-bearing sperm are endowed with a female genetic sex, whereas those receiving a Y-bearing chromosome become male. Following determination of genetic sex, three stages of sexual development occur, gondal, internal genital, and external genital. Double X-bearing germ cells proliferate in the ectoderm of the yolk sac. By 6 weeks of development they must have migrated to the developing gonad for complete development to occur. This bipotential gonad will differentiate into an ovary if the germ cells that arrive are of female genetic sex. The germ cells settle into the gondal cortex and lead to development of an ovary by 11 to 12 weeks of fetal life with a complement of approximately 6 to 7 million ova.

The route of development of the interior genitalia is determined by the hormonal milieu in which it is found. All embryos possess the primordia of either male or female internal genitalia. The Wolffian ducts, mesonephric ductal structures, in the presence of testosterone and Mullerian inhibiting factor (MIF) proliferate into mesonephric structures such as the vas deferens, seminal vesicles, and epididymis. In the presence of estrogens and the absence of müllerian inhibiting factor the müllerian or paramesonephric ducts proliferate into the uterus, tubes, cervix, and perhaps the upper vagina by 8 to 16 weeks of pregnancy. The Mullerian ducts begin as invaginations of the coelomic epithelium. The cranial end remains open into the pelvic cavity as the ostia of the fallopian tubes at their fimbriated end. The distal end of each paramesonephric duct rotates across the midline and fuses with its counterpart from the other side to form the uterus and cervix. Remnants of the wolffian duct may persist as the epoophoron, paraoophoron, and Gartner's duct cysts along the vagina and cervix.

Development of the external genitalia is determined by the presence or absence of male sex steroid hormones, namely, androgens. If the gonad is XX and its secretion does not contain significant quantities of androgens the bipotential anlage proceeds along female lines. The genital tubercle becomes the clitoris, the genital folds, the labia minora and the genital swellings the labia majora. This occurs during the second trimester of pregnancy. The solid caudal end of the müllerian ducts reach the urogenital sinus at 9 weeks of development at the vaginal plate. At 5 months of development the plate is canalizing as the vagina. The most caudal end develops with the external genitalia as the vestibule or opening of the vagina.

Congenital anomalies that do not result in the ambiguity of the external genitalia are not usually discovered until puberty when pain, and amenorrhea occur or later when repeated pregnancy wastage has been explored. These defects are divided into failures of canalization (i.e., imperforated hymen, vaginal septa, and vaginal absence); failure of the development of Mullerian Ductal derivatives (i.e., absence of the uterus, tubes, or vagina), or fusion defects (i.e., arcuate uteri, septate uterus or bicornuate uteri, or uterine didelphys). An imperforate hymen presents as primary amenorrhea, with cyclic cramps and pain. The blocked efflux of menstrual flow may cause a hematocolpos. There is no association with urinary tract defects as seen in the other Mullerian defects. Transverse vaginal septa are usually incomplete and found only when dyspareunia or hemorrhage secondary to delivery occurs. Septa are seen with increased frequency in patients exposed to diethylstilbestrol in utero. Vaginal absence may be an isolated finding but is usually found in association with an absent uterus.

Complete absence of the Mullerian duct derivatives, uterus, tubes and vagina usually presents as primary amenorrhea, sterility, and inability to achieve intercourse. Workup of the urinary tract is indicated because these women will be found to have renal defects in approximately 50 percent of the cases. Treatment is the creation of an artificial vagina. This is usually successful for coitus but these patients remain sterile. Phenotypic females with congential absence of the vagina may have female or male karyotypes. The phenotypic and karyotypic females with uterine absence will be sterile and will present with primary amenorrhea. Those with male karyotype have testicular feminization in which there is absence of response to the normal circulating male levels of testosterone. These individuals should have bilateral gonadectomy as there is a 25 percent incidence of malignant tumors developing in these gonads. This is followed by estrogen replacement.

Unicornuate uteri may be accompanied by rudimentary uterine horns or ductal remnants. If there is a functioning endometrium in the rudimentary horn, there may be cyclical pain and an enlarging pelvic or paravaginal mass. Treatment is surgical excision of the rudimentary horn. There is a high association with urinary tract abnormalities. Fusion defects may be slight presenting only as a dimple on the uterine fundus. Midline uterine septa are associated with repeated pregnancy wastage in the first and second trimesters. Treatment is excision of the septum. Bicornuate uteri have two endometrial cavities communicating with a single normal appearing cervix. These patients have an increased chance of pregnancy wastage in the second trimester. Uterine didelphys is a complete duplication of the uterus, cervix with or without duplication of the vagina.

Once the female genitalia have developed in utero, there is little change save for some somatic growth until puberty. The first indication of puberty is the growth spurt manifested mainly by an increase in height. The breast bud then usually develops though the two may be reversed. Pubarche or sexual hair growth is in response to adrenal androgens and occurs about 2 years prior to axillary hair growth. Menarche or the appearance of menses is the last event in a sequence of changes that is termed puberty. The first 12 to 18 months of menses are usually anovulatory and are therefore irregular and may be occasionally heavy. The mean age in the United States of menarche is 12.8 years with a range of 9 to 18 years of age.

ENDOCRINOLOGY

The ultimate control of reproduction resides in the brain and hypothalamus by virtue of their release of releasing factors. Conceptually, it is useful to consider that there are two centers of control. A tonic center and a cyclic center. The tonic center is located in the medial basal hypothalamus and controls the basal secretion of gonadotropin releasing factor (GNRH). This center is under negative feedback control by circulating estrogens. The cyclic center is located in the anterior hypothalmus near the preoptic area. It is under positive estrogen feedback and is responsible for the midcycle surge of gonadotropins. GNRH is a decapeptide of known amino acid sequence. GNRH is delivered to the anterior pituitary via the hypothalamic pituitary portal axis. GNRH once released stimulates the pituitary to release the gonadotropins LH and FSH. These glycloproteins can be measured by radio-amino assays. Each gonadotropin is made of two chains, an alpha and a beta. The alpha chains are the same for both the pituitary gonadotropins and the HCG secreted by the placenta during pregnancy. The beta chain of each is distinct and gives each gonadotropin its unique identity and biologic effect.

In the female, FSH is responsible for follicular growth in the ovary. FSH also stimulates the follicles to produce estrogen. Circulating levels of FSH vary with the menstrual cycle between 8 and 15 MIU/ml save for the time of ovulation when levels greater than 20 MIU/ml may be found. Postmenopausally levels greater than 100 MIU/ml are frequently found.

LH is the major gonadotropin responsible for ovulation. Under positive feedback stimulus of estrogen which rises in response to FSH at ovulation, the level of LH is high at approximately 80 MIU/ml as compared to the normal levels of 10 to 20 MIU/ml. Approximately 24 hours after the LH surge, the ovary releases a single ovum, ovulation. Human chorionic gonadotropin, HCG, is secreted by the placenta during pregnancy and rarely by ovarian tumors. It is also a glycoprotein that has the same alpha subunit as does FSH and LH. The beta subunit gives its specificity and unique identity. The cell of origin is the syncytiotrophoblastic cell of the placenta. Blood levels peak at 50 to 100 IU/ml at 60 days of pregnancy and then gradually decline. Following delivery, there is a sharp decrease usually being completed at 2 weeks postpartum. Its major physiologic role is to maintain the corpus luteum of early pregnancy until the placental production of estrogen and progesterone is well established. It is the HCG that is measured in most pregnancy tests whether they are biologic, immunologic or using radioimmunoassay.

Steroid Hormones

All the biologically active steroid hormones are of similar basic structure. They differ mainly in the number of carbon atoms. The C21 steroids are corticoids and progestins, the C19s are androgens and the C18 steroids are the estrogens. A simplified schema for the metabolism of the steroids is shown in Figure 10-6.

Estrogens

Estrogens are the classic female hormones. The major circulating estrogen is Estradiol or E_2. It is this steroid that is responsible for the female effects, increase in size of gential tissues and breast, and proliferation of the vaginal epithelium and the endometrium. Estrogens also cause changes in several circulating blood proteins namely, globulins secreted by the liver. Thyroxine binding globulin (TBG), transcortin (CBG), and sex steroid binding globulin (SBG) are increased by estrogens. Estrogens also have other metabolic effects on salt and water metabolism, and calcium metabolism. Given postmenopausally, estrogens alleviate some of the effects of osteoporosis. Estrogens also have different effects on the various lipoprotein fractions.

Estrogens are secreted by the ovary with a small contribution from the adrenal and peripheral sources. During pregnancy, the placenta becomes a major source of estrogen mainly estriol E_3. Estrogen levels fluctuate with the menstrual cycle as shown. (Fig. 10-7). Blood levels of

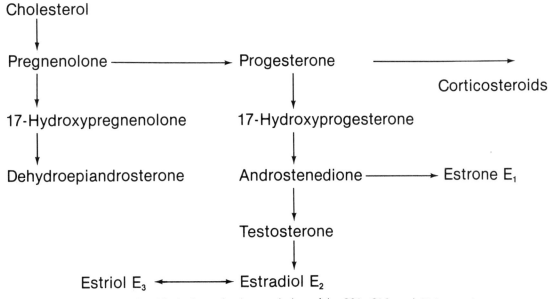

Fig. 10-6. Simplified schema for the metabolism of the C21, C19, and C18 steroids.

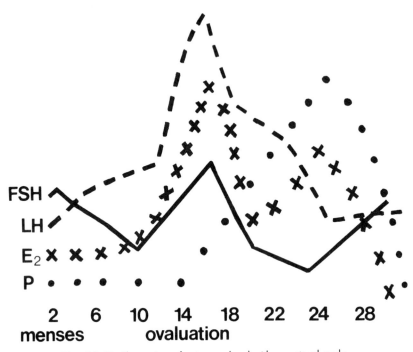

FSH LH	40	32	24	16	8	mIU/ml
E$_2$	500	400	300	200	100	pg/ml
Progesterone	10	8	6	4	2	ng/ml

Fig. 10-7. Fluctuation of estrogen level with menstrual cycle.

estradiol range from 40 to 100 pg/ml during the early proliferative phase of the menstrual cycle, peak at 300 to 400 pg/ml at mid cycle or ovulation and decline to 200 to 300 pg during the luteal phase. The second major circulating estrogen is estrone. Where 85 to 90 percent of circulating of estradiol is the result of direct ovarian secretion, only 70 to 80 percent of estrone is derived from the ovary. The remainder comes from the peripheral conversion of adrenal androgens, mainly androstenedione. Approximately 1 percent of androstenedione is converted to estrone. This occurs in the peripheral adipose tissue. This accounts for 20 to 40 μg per day of estrone. The percentage conversion to estrone increases with age and with the percentage of body fat. Estrogens can be measured in the serum by radioimmunoassay and as urinary metabolites by the same techniques.

Progesterone

Progesterone causes the endometrium to differentiate. Progesterone is secreted throughout the menstrual cycle but the greatest amount is present during the luteal phase or after ovulation and formation of the corpus luteum. Progesterone causes the endometrium to differentiate from a proliferative phase to a secretory pattern with the appearance of increased glands and glandular secretion.

The endocervical mucus becomes thick and viscous under the influence of protesterone. Systemically, progesterone causes an increase in basal body temperature of approximately ½ to 1°F. Progesterone is naturietic, stimulates respiration, and generally causes relaxation of smooth muscle including that of the uterus.

Metabolites of progesterone can be measured in the urine, the major one being pregnanediol. Levels range from 1 mg/24 hours during the follicular phase to a 3 to 6 mg/day at the peak of the luteal phase. Blood progesterone levels follow a similar pattern. During the follicular phase, levels are less than 1 ng/ml rising to a peak of greater than 10 ng/ml at the midluteal phase. Progesterone is secreted predominantly by the corpus luteum, a fact which explains the low follicular levels and the much higher midluteal levels. This midluteal rise in progesterone is presumptive evidence of ovulation though the only definitive proof of that is pregnancy.

Steroid Receptors

All of the biologically active steroids exert their effects by the mediation of intracellular receptor proteins. The steroid diffuses through the cell membrane by passive diffusion. Intracytoplasmically they bind to receptor proteins. The steroid hormone receptor protein complex then translocates to the nucleus where binding to DNA occurs. The steroid then induces RNA synthesis and ultimately protein synthesis. The synthesized proteins translate the biological effects of the steroids. Estrogen induces the production of its own receptor and the receptor for progesterone. Progesterone conversely reduces the synthesis of both estrogen and progesterone receptors. This is one mechanism that controls steroid action.

Androgens

The normal ovary also secretes androgens in small amounts with the highest levels occuring at midcycle. Ovarian androgens arise from the ovarian stromal cells. Of the circulating androgens in the female, testosterone is the most androgenic. Approximately 20 percent comes from direct ovarian secretion and approximately 35 percent from secretion by the adrenal gland. The remainder comes from the peripheral conversion of androstenedione and dehydroepiandrosterone to testosterone.

Ovarian Cycle

The above described protein and steroidal hormones interact in a dynamic way with the positive and negative feedback relationships involving the hypothalmus, pituitary, the ovaries, and the endometrium. The menstrual cycle can be divided into three phases: the follicular, the ovulatory, and the luteal phases when speaking of the ovary, and the proliferative and secretory phases respectively when speaking of the endometrium. Shortly prior to menses, FSH levels begin to rise. This is secondary to falling estradiol levels by a negative feedback mechanism in the hypothalmus. FSH stimulates follicles within the ovary to begin to grow. The mechanism by which the follicle destined to ovulate during any one cycle is selected is unknown. As the follicle grows and matures, estradiol levels begin to rise. Steroidogenesis in the ovaries is predominantly dependent upon LH stimulation, but FSH contributes in that FSH increases the number of LH receptors and therefore increases LH action. As ovulation approaches, FSH levels begin to fall, secondary to the negative feedback effects of increasing estradiol levels. Concurrent with the rising estradiol levels, the endometrium is undergoing proliferation. Hence the proliferative phase of the menstrual cycle. The endometrium becomes thicker. The endometrial epithelium including that of the glands becomes taller and the cells become columnar. Mitotic figures are seen in the glands and stroma.

At midcycle, a surge of estradiol from the developing follicle occurs. Those follicles stimulated by FSH but not destined to ovulate become atretic and regress. The estradiol surge stimulates a positive feedback mechanism acting via the cyclic center of the hypothalmus which causes an outpouring of pituitary LH and to a lesser degree of FSH. Approximately 24 hours after the LH surge, ovulation or the release of the egg from the ovary occurs. The exact mechanism of ovulation is unknown, but increased intrafollicular pressure is not responsible. The LH surge also induces luteinization of the follicle. The granulosa cells enlarge and capillaries penetrate the follicle. Concurrent with the luteinization of the follicle, progesterone secretion increases in such a way that at midluteal phase, serum progesterone levels greater than 3 ng/ml occur. Concurrent with the rise in progesterone levels, there is a change in the endometrium from a proliferative to a secretory endometrium. The first change seen is the appearance of subnuclear vacuoles. The endometrial glands become tortuous. The stroma becomes thicker and more vascular.

The activity of the corpus luteum peaks at day 8 past ovulation. The life span of the corpus luteum is limited to 14 days if pregnancy does not intervene. The mechanism of this limited life span is unclear. As the activity of the corpus luteum declines, progesterone levels in the serum fall. Estradiol levels that displayed a secondary rise after ovulation also begin to fall. The nadir levels of both hormones being reached just prior to the next menses. With the decline of hormone levels, the endometrium begins to regress—the late luteal or secretory phase. The endometrial stromal cells enlarge, a decidual change, and the stroma becomes edematous. Ultimately the hormonal support of the endometrium is gone and the endometrium sloughs—menses. The basal layer of the endometrium does not slough but remains to regenerate the endometrium for the next cycle. When pregnancy supervenes, placental trophoblastic secretion of HCG maintains the corpus luteum. HCG appears at the peak of the corpus luteum function, 9 to 13 days post ovulation. HCG maintains steroidogenesis in the corpus luteum until 9 to 10 weeks of gestation at which time placental steroidogenesis is well-established.

SIGNS AND SYMPTOMS

Gynecologic Examination

As in all areas of medicine, gynecologic examination begins with a careful and thorough history. Details unique to the gynecologic history include the menstrual and pregnancy history. The timing, duration, and amount of menstrual bleeding should be elicited. The dates of the last two menstrual periods are obtained. A history of any change in the frequency, length, and/or amount of bleeding should be obtained, particularly the absence of expected bleeding or increased bleeding. Details of the previous pregnancies including spontaneous abortions should be obtained. Details of contraceptive practices are recorded. Any associated symptom needs to be explored. Pain, if present, should be described in terms of severity, location, radiation, onset, time course, and aggravating and relieving factors. Any associated gastrointestinal or urinary symptom should be elicited. A thorough history in terms of review of systems, past history, and social history should not be minimized because the patient is seeking gynecologic evaluation.

Physical examination again begins with sound general examination principles. Vital signs are recorded. A thorough general examination is done. Gynecologic physical examination begins with the patient being suitably robed in a comfortable position in the presence of a chaperone. The dorsal lithotomy position usually is most comfortable for both the patient and the physician. The external genitalia are first inspected and then palpated. The vulva is a skin covered organ and any other dermatologic disorder may be present on the vulva. Any lesion noted is described in terms of location, size, extension to other structures, pain, and tenderness. The urethra should be milked so that any discharge from the Skene's and paraurethral glands that is noted can be cultured.

A lubricated and warmed speculum is then inserted and the cervix visualized. Any lesion on the cervix is noted as to the location, size, color, and bleeding. The Papanicolaou smear is then obtained. A swab is twirled in the endocrvix and the swab then placed on a microscopic slide and immediately fixed. The ectocervix or the region of the transformation zone is scraped with a spatula and also immediately placed upon a slide and fixed. In the post menopausal patient, a posterior vaginal fornix sample is obtained and treated as above. The slides are labeled and an appropriate history of the patient including menstrual status, hormone administration, and any other pertinent physical or historical findings are submitted to the cytopathologist. As the speculum is being removed, the vaginal walls are noted for discharge or lesions. In patients who were DES-exposed in utero, separate Pap smears should be obtained from each vaginal wall.

The bimanual exam is then undertaken. The vaginal wall should be palpated particularly in the DES exposed offspring. The cervix is palpated. The uterine fundus is palpated and notation made of size, location, shape, and tenderness. The adnexal areas are then palpated and again with care to note tenderness, size, shape, mobility, and/or nodularity. Asking the patient to cough would reveal any weakness in the vaginal structures. Also a spurt of urine from the urethra may indicate urinary stress incontinence. A bulge appearing at the vaginal apex between the uterosacral ligaments may indicate an internal hernia or enterocele. This may contain small bowel. The uterus may also descend down the vaginal barrel indicating uterine descensus. Both levators are then separated which may reveal a rectocele. The rectovaginal examination is a routine part of any gynecologic examination. This allows for confirmation of the vaginal findings, and in addition, supplies information about the parametria and uterosacral ligaments. Any tenderness or nodularity in these areas is noted. A stool guaiac is indicated with the rectal examination. All the above findings are recorded in the patient's chart including normal findings.

Pain

Pain of gynecologic origin may be acute or chronic. Acute pelvic pain may be due to gynecologic or nongynecologic causes. In addition, those conditions requiring operative intervention must be separated quickly from those that do not. The principles of evaluation of pain of pelvic origin are the same as those for the evaluation of pain of nonpelvic origin.

Pain of sudden onset may be due to perforation of a hollow viscus such as rupture of a tubal pregnancy. With obstruction or inflammation of a hollow viscus, the pain is more slow in onset and reaches a peak after an interval of several hours. Things to consider are intestinal obstruction, appendicitis, or salpingitis. Colicky or crampy pelvic pain is secondary to the muscular contractions of the hollow organ such as intestine, uterus, or appendix. Pregnancy symptoms with a tender unilateral adnexal mass suggests ectopic pregnancy. Bilateral pelvic pain with fever and cervical motion tenderness is usually seen with acute pelvic inflammatory disease. High fever and elevated white blood counts suggest tubal ovarian abscess.

Nongynecologic pain of pelvic origin includes appendicitis, diverticulitis, and intestinal or ureteral obstruction. Appendicitis presents with epigastric pain followed by anorexia, nausea, and vomiting. In a few hours the pain localizes to the right lower quadrant. There will be right lower abdominal tenderness, fever, and leukocytosis. The presentation can be atypical. When pregnancy is associated with acute appendicitis, the pain's location may be atypical because of the gravid uterus, the cecum, and the appendix rise out of the pelvis. Left lower quadrant pain associated with a history of irritable bowel symptoms, fever, leukocytosis, and constipation suggests acute diverticulitis. Intestinal obstruction of any cause is seen with nausea, vomiting, colicky abdominal pain, and distention. The more proximal in the GI tract that the obstruction occurs, the quicker the vomiting will be seen. The more distal the obstruction, the greater the abdominal distention. The patient will usually have high pitched bowel sounds. Ureteral obstruction presents with flank pain radiating to the groin and pelvis. The pain may be very severe. The most common causation is a ureteral calculus.

Chronic pelvic pain may be due to pelvic tumors, chronic inflammatory disease, pelvic congestion, and other causes. Uterine fibroids present with pelvic achiness or heaviness. Pressure on the rectum or bladder can cause symptoms referrable to these organs. Severe pain is unusual unless infarction has occurred. Large ovarian tumors, unless they undergo torsion, are usually asymptomatic. Patients with a history of acute pelvic inflammation can go on to a chronic disabling pelvic pain syndrome. This may be due to pelvic adhesions, or distention of the fallopian tubes with pus or fluid, pyrosalpinx, or hydrosalpinx. Pelvic congestion syndrome occurs predominantly in women of the 40 to 50 age group and is characterized by pelvic discomfort prior to menstruation.

Dysmenorrhea

Cyclical pelvic pain with menstruation is termed dysmenorrhea. This colicky pain occurs with ovulatory cycles and typically begins after the onset of menses. It is mainly due to the release of prostaglandins which causes uterine smooth muscle contraction. Increased prostaglandin levels had been observed in the menstrual fluid of patients with dysmenorrhea. The pain begins with the menstrual period or just prior to same, but typically peaks during early menstruation. On pelvic exam, no abnormalities are appreciated that could suggest organic pathology such as endometriosis. Combination oral contraceptive pills have been shown to be of benefit in patients with primary dysmenorrhea. They work by decreasing bleeding and tissue slough. Also they have been shown to decrease prostaglandin levels in the endometrium. With increased understanding of the role of prostaglandins in dysmenorrhea, prostaglandin synthesis inhibitors have been used as treatment. Indomethacin, mefenamic acid, ibuprofen, and other antiprostaglandin agents have been shown to decrease dysmenorrhea. In patients who do not respond to prostaglandin inhibitors or oral contraceptives, laparoscopy should be considered to rule out organic pathology.

Premenstrual Syndrome

Premenstrual syndrome is an entity with protean manifestations. To be truly classified as the premenstrual syndrome symptoms must occur within 7 days prior to menses. Symptoms include mood changes, irritability, emotional instability, changes in libido, appetite changes, breast changes, headache, generalized aches and pains, nausea or vomiting, abdominal bloating, and weight gain and/or edema. The incidence tends to increase with increasing age. Several mechanisms are postulated including dietary deficiencies such as zinc and B_6, estrogen and progesterone changes, prolactin alterations, and psychiatric causes. Prostaglandins have also been implicated. Supportive evidence is obtained in that primary dysmenorrhea frequently accompanies the premenstrual syndrome. Due to the many theories of causation, there are many proposed treatments. Bloating and edema can be treated with mild diuretics. Because prolactin has been implicated, studies using bromergocryptine have been undertaken and a definite effect was seen for mastalgia but not for the other symptoms. Pyridoxine and high-protein diets, have been tried also. The observation that the premenstrual syndrome is associated with ovulatory cycles has prompted the use of oral contraceptives. Prostaglandin inhibitors have also been used with some success. Recently, progesterone by injection, suppository, or orally active analogues have been used with some success. In general, no specific single treatment is effective for all patients but treatment must be individualized using any of the above methods.

Amenorrhea

Amenorrhea is the absence of expected vaginal bleeding. Traditionally amenorrhea was divided into primary, failure to institute menstruation, versus secondary, failure to reestablish expected bleeding pattern after 6 months of its absence. A system is outlined that will allow for the evaluation of amenorrhea of any cause. The workup should be instituted for the following criteria: absence of menstruation by age 14 coupled with the absence of secondary sexual characteristics, absence of menstruation by age 16 with secondary sexual characteristics, or absence of menstruation for 6 months or a length of time greater than three normal cycle lengths. In any woman of reproductive age with amenorrhea, pregnancy must be first ruled out. This can be accomplished by pelvic examination and pregnancy testing.

A serum prolactin level is first obtained. If this is elevated, the patient should be evaluated as in the outline on galactorrhea. If the prolactin level is normal, no further workup for this etiology is needed. Then the adequacy of the circulating estrogen and the completeness of the outflow test is assessed by progesterone challenge. Progesterone in oil (200 mg IM) or oral medroxyprogesterone acetate 10 mg for 5 days by mouth is given. A positive result is the appearance within 2 to 7 days of vaginal bleeding. If this occurs, a diagnosis of anovulation is established. There are consequences of anovulation: the first is the difficulty this may cause in establishing pregnancy when desired. The second is that without ovulation, there is no progesterone-induced differentiation and sloughing of the endometrium. Therefore, the endometrium is continually exposed to an estrogenic stimulus to proliferate. This can lead to endometrial hyperplasia and possibly endometrial carcinoma. If the patient is anovulatory and does not desire pregnancy, the patient should be treated with progesterone as outlined above, every 3 months to induce withdrawal bleeding and differentiation of the endometrium. The 3-month interval will allow for the spontaneous resumption of ovulation to become apparent. If the patient is anovulatory and desires pregnancy, ovulation can be induced by the procedure outlined below.

If no bleeding occurs in response to exogenous progesterone the patient should be given estrogen usually in the form of Premarin 2.5 mg by mouth daily for 21 days. During the last 5 days of the estrogen administration, progesterone is also given as outlined above. Two results can occur. Vaginal bleeding may or may not occur. If there is no vaginal bleeding, an abnormality in the outflow tract may be suspected that needs to be evaluated such as absence of an endometrium, congenital anomalies, or endometrial trauma (i.e., Asherman's syndrome). Asherman's syndrome is destruction of the endometrium secondary due to previous intrauterine scarring usually by curettage. If pelvic examination reveals a normal uterus, obstruction to the outflow tract may be due to such abnormality as vaginal septa. If there is no palpable uterus, there may be congenital absence of the Mullerian structures or testicular feminization. This situation can be elucidated by obtaining a karyotype. The patient with a congenital absence will have a normal karyotype whereas the patient with testicular feminization will have a XY karyotype. These patients have testes rather than ovaries. These gonads should be removed because of the high incidence of malignancy.

The patient that experiences vaginal bleeding after estrogen and progesterone administration should have gonadotropin assays obtained. There are two possibilities. The gonadotropins, FSH and LH, will be high or normal. If the gonadotropins are high, the diagnosis of ovarian failure is established. In those patients with normal gonadotropins, the diagnosis of CNS and/or pituitary disorder is established.

Patients with high gonadotropins should also have a karyotype. As 45 XO karyotype indicates Turner's syndrome. Most of these patients have short stature, webbed neck, shield chest, increased carrying angle of the arm, cardiac and renal abnormalities, and hypergonadotrophic amenorrhea. These patients are treated with hormonal replacement, estrogen and progesterone. Patients with hormonal failure may have mosaicism with chromosomes of different cell lines in the same individual.

Again, the patient with a Y chromosome in the mosaic should have gonadectomy. Gonadel agenesis or complete failure of the gonads to form is a syndrome of unknown cause. These patients are treated with hormonal replacement. The resistant ovarian syndrome includes patients with elevated gonadotropins and ovarian follicles in the ovary. These patients need ovarian biopsy to document the diagnosis. A subgroup of patients with the resistant ovarian syndrome are those in premature menopause. The average age of menopause in the United States is 52 years, but in some patients ovarian function ceases much earlier, between 30 and 38 years of age.

Those patients with low gonadotropins have defects in the pituitary and/or the CNS or hypothalamus. A patient with low gonadotropin should have skull films, prolactin assays if not done previously, and visual field examinations coupled with polytomography of the sella turcica. The purpose of this workup is to rule out a pituitary tumor. Patients who are found to have a pituitary tumor, usually a benign adenoma, should have a neurosurgical consultation. The tumors can be removed surgically, radiated, or treated with drugs likely to lower prolactin levels if elevated. If the workup for a pituitary tumor is negative, the patient can be suspected to have hypothalamic amenorrhea. This can be the result of stressful life situations, a surprisingly common cause of amenorrhea. Weight changes can also induce amenorrhea by a hypothalamic mechanism. A particularly severe case is that of anorexia nervosa. These patients display profound weight loss secondary to dieting, amenorrhea, and a variety of endocrine and psychiatric abnormalities. The reinstitution of proper diet and weight gain will cause menses to return. A rare cause of amenorrhea is hypogonadotropism and anosmia. These patients respond to the induction of ovulation. Finally, postpill amenorrhea or amenorrhea occurring after cessation of the oral contraceptive pills is amenorrhea persisting greater than 6 months after the discontinuation of the pills. The general incidence is less than 1 percent. These patients are evaluated as would be any patient with amenorrhea.

Anovulation

Anovulation can be discovered during the workup of amenorrhea but anovulation can be associated with other complaints such as excess or dysfunctional bleeding, infertility, hirsutism, and with the polycystic ovarian syndrome. This syndrome, given eponym Stein-Leventhall syndrome, includes anovulation manifested as amenorrhea or irregular heavy bleeding, hirsutism, and relative obesity with palpably enlarged ovaries. Usually the ovaries are large and are covered by a thick white capsule. Histologically the ovaries display numerous follicles and a dense stroma. The current thinking is that these ovaries are the result of chronic anovulation and not the cause. Treatment depends upon the patient's wishes. Those patients who desire pregnancy can have ovulation induced. Those patients not desirous of pregnancy and who have amenorrhea or oligomenorrhea are treated with periodic progestational withdrawal. Hirsutism is evaluated and treated as below. Patients desirous of absolute contraception need to be critically evaluated for proper contraceptive methods.

Abnormal Bleeding Patterns

Before abnormal bleeding patterns can be discussed, normal bleeding patterns must be defined. Most normal women of reproductive age display reproduceable bleeding in terms of timing and duration. The patterns though different from woman to woman are usually the same in any given individual though changes from the norm are frequent. First menses usually occurs around age 13 with a range of 9 to 18 years. The average interval for ovulatory cycles is 29 plus or minus 2 days with a normal range of 24 to 44 days. The mean duration of flow is 5 days plus or minus 2 days and relatively constant for any one individual. Average blood loss ranges from 30 to 100 ml. Average age of cessation of menses is approximately age 52 with a range of 35 to 55. Any deviation from these means deserves evaluation. Vaginal bleeding that occurs in the premenarchal or more correctly in a patient prior to the expected age of menarche is termed premenarchal bleeding. This needs to be evaluated in the context of the individual particularly with attention of the presence or absence of other secondary sexual characteristics. If other secondary sexual characteristics are present, a source of estrogen can be presumed. This can be either ovarian or exogenous. History will elucidate exogenous estrogen use. Ovarian sources can be secondary to estrogen-producing tumors. Therefore these patients deserve a thorough pelvic examination. Ovarian estrogen can also be the result of gonadotropin stimulation of the ovary.

Premenarchal vaginal bleeding without secondary sexual characteristics is usually due to local causes. Foreign bodies may be found. Infections such as pinworms, β-hemolytic streptococcus, staphylococcus, or E coli may be found secondary to fecal contamination or from other sites of infection. Cultures for *Neisseria gonorrhea* should also be obtained. A positive result should raise a suspicion of sexual assault or child abuse. In the 2 to 6 age group, a prolapsed urethra should be sought. A rare but deadly cause of vaginal bleeding in the premenarchal child is sarcoma botryoides (rhabdomyosarcoma). This extremely malignant tumor presents as polypoid masses arising from the cervix or upper vagina.

Heavy bleeding during the reproductive years has numerous causes including leiomyomata, polyps, adenomyosis, dysfunctional uterine bleeding, and always the suspicion of carcinoma. Sub-mucus fibroids present with cyclic bleeding that is initially normal and then becomes heavier. At dilatation and curettage, a defect may be felt on the uterine wall. Endometrial polyps present with bleeding that consists of spotting following a normal period. Polyps may be found on dilatation and curettage or visualized by hysteroscopy. Adenomyosis presents with a heavy bleeding accompanied by dysmenorrhea in a tender, symmetrically enlarged uterus. Blood dyscrasias should also be considered. Intrauterine contraceptive device users frequently report heavier menstrual bleeding. Dysfunctional uterine bleeding is excess bleeding that has no demonstrable, organic cause. This bleeding is the result of chronic anovulation for the most part. These patients have infrequent but heavy bleeding. Due to the persistent estrogen stimulation of the endometrium and the failure of progesterone secretion to differentiate the endometrium, the endometrium becomes thickened. It eventually overgrows the ability of the circulating estrogens to support it and heavy bleeding ensues. This diagnosis rests on the failure to demonstrate an organic cause and histologic confirmation of proliferative or hyperplastic endometrium on biopsy or dilatation and curettage. The treatment is similar to that of anovulation as outlined previously. This type of bleeding is frequently seen in the peri-menopausal age group. It should be remembered that with any heavy bleeding in a woman of reproductive age, pregnancy and its complications must be thought of and ruled out.

Any vaginal bleeding occurring in a patient who has ceased normal cyclical menstrual function for greater than 6 months and who are more than 45 years of age, is a cause for concern. In the group of postmenopausal patients, the first duty of the physician is to rule out malignancy. Malignancy of the cervix, ovary, vagina, or vulva can also present with postmenopausal vaginal bleeding but endometrial cancer is the most common malignant cause. In actuality, the most common cause of postmenopausal vaginal bleeding is atrophic change in the cervix, vagina, or the endometrium. This does not allow the clinician to avoid the workup for malignancy. These patients deserve examination under anesthesia and fractional dilatation and curettage.

Bleeding that occurs between what otherwise would be normal cyclic bleeding is termed intermenstrual bleeding. Spotting that occurs at midcycle around the expected time of ovulation is a relatively frequent occurrence. This is due to the midcycle drop in estrogen levels. Premenstrual staining may be due to an inadequate luteal phase. Bleeding that has no relationship to the menstrual cycles raises the suspicion of malignancy, particularly cervical carcinoma. These patients also have contact bleeding or bleeding after intercourse or after examination.

Discharge

Discharge from the vagina and genital pruritus are among the most common complaints that bring patients to their gynecologist. These symptoms can occur concurrently or separately and they have a variety of causes. There is a normal amount of vaginal discharge secondary to secretions of the Bartholin Skene's and aprocrine glands of the vulva, from the vaginal mucosa, and the cervix. These white semisolid secretions usually have a pH of 3.8 to 4.2 and are usually odorless. Microscopic examination of the discharge reveals clumps of epithelial cells without leukocytes.

Monilial vaginitis is secondary to the fungus *Candida albicans* and is perhaps the most common cause of abnormal discharge. It can occur in an otherwise normal woman but tends to be associated with pregnancy, antibiotic use, and perhaps with the use of oral contraceptives. Diabetics are particularly prone to this infection. The discharge is cheezy white and associated with intense pruritus. Mycelia can be seen when a drop of the discharge is placed on a microscopic slide and covered with a 10 percent potassium hydroxide (KOH) solution. The KOH dissolves the epithelial cells. Cultures can confirm the diagnosis. Local antifungal agents such as Nystatin, Miconidazole, or Clotrimazole are usually effective. Alkaline douches may be helpful as the organism needs an acid environment to flourish. Gentian violet staining may be of value in recalcitrant cases.

Trichomonas vaginalis, a parasite, causes a greenish, malodorous discharge that is typically worse at the time of menstruation. The cervix and vagina display a strawberry-red inflammation. The motile parasite can be identified by the beating of its very active flagella when a drop of discharge is mixed with saline and observed under a microscope slide. Treatment involves oral Metronidazole. Vinegar douches help give symptomatic relief. The male partner must be strongly urged to seek consultation and be treated concurrently. Failure to do so will inevitably result in reinfection.

Nonspecific vaginitis as it was termed in the past is caused by the bacterial organism, Gardenerella. This disease presents with malodorous vaginal discharge usually without associated pruritus. The pH of the discharge is 5.0 to 5.5 This diagnosis can be confirmed by the findings of clue cells on a wet prep as is done for the diagnosis of *Trichomonas*. No trichomonads are seen. A clue cell is a superficial cell with short bacilli clustered around its edges. Treatment again must stress concurrent treatment of the male partner. Oral antibiotics with gram-negative coverage are needed such as Metronidazole or Ampicillin.

Atrophic vaginitis is a disease of the postmenopausal patient or the patient who has lost ovarian function. With the loss of estrogen the vaginal mucosa becomes thin and transluscent. It is easily secondarily infected by bacteria. Intravaginal estrogen cream usually results in prompt relief. This can be given daily for relief and then one to two times per week.

Disorders of Pelvic Support

Pelvic relaxation is a generic term that may be applied to a variety of defects including cystocele, rectocele, enterocoele, and uterine prolapse. Uterine prolapse is the descent of the uterus along with axis of the vagina. There may be various degrees of descent from slight to complete prolapse of the uterus out of the introitus. The prolapsed uterus is subject to trauma and may become irritated leading to bleeding. Symptoms of genital relaxation tend to worsen as the day progresses as gravity further pulls down the pelvic structures. Treatment of uterine prolapse usually involves surgery. Hysterectomy, coupled with repair of the anterior and posterior vaginal walls is usually needed. Patients occasionally may be treated with culpoclesis in which the anterior and posterior vaginal walls are approximated. The patient who cannot tolerate surgery may be fitted with a pessary.

Cystocele is a bulging and weakness of the anterior vaginal wall. Symptoms are those of a pressure sensation or urinary complaints. Urinary complaints are usually incomplete emptying of the bladder with a feeling of needing to void again after a short interval from previous voiding. Secondary infection may lead to dysuria and urgency. Treatment is again surgical, usually with repair of the anterior vaginal wall.

Rectocele is a bulging of the posterior vaginal wall with the large bowel presenting in the defect. The patient may have a pressure sensation, constipation, and the not infrequently seen symptom of needing to place a finger in the vagina to complete evacuation of the rectum. Treatment is again surgical. The vaginal mucosa is removed from the rectum. The levator ani muscles are then approximated across the midline with repair of the vaginal mucosa.

Enterocoele is a true vaginal hernia with a peritoneal lined sac bulging into the posterior upper vagina. The sac may contain small bowel. Enterocoeles are frequently found with other pelvic relaxations and after previous vaginal surgery. Treatment is surgical and includes the principles of hernia repair as done elsewhere. The sac must be excised and the normal anatomy reestablished.

Posthysterectomy vaginal vault prolapse presents with bulging of the anterior and posterior walls to the introitus. Treatment is surgical with many different procedures described.

URINARY INCONTINENCE

Urinary incontinence is the involuntary loss of urine via the urethra that is socially unacceptable to the patient. If such loss occurs following coughing, sneezing, straining, or any other measure that increases intraabdominal pressure, it is termed stress incontinence and is usually associated with some anatomical defect. Urgency incontinence is the inability to hold urine once the urge to void is first felt. This suggests urinary tract infection, inflammation of the bladder base, and occasionally detrussor dysenergia. Detrussor dysenergia more commonly presents as the sudden loss or urine without urgency and without any straining. Overflow incontinence is the dribbling of urine that occurs with large atonic bladders or large cystoceles.

Normal voiding or micturation is dependent on a highly organized sequence of events. As the normal bladder fills and dilates, a sensation of the need to void is felt. These nerve impulses travel to the spinal cord and then upward to the motor cortex. The normal individual is able to inhibit the efferent arc and prevent voiding. If voiding is desired, voluntary impulses are transmitted via the pudendal nerves causing relaxation of the pelvic diaphragm. This allows the bladder neck to descend. The abdominal muscles are flexed which slightly increases the intraabdominal pressure. The detrussor or the smooth muscle of the bladder then contracts causing the bladder to empty.

STRESS INCONTINENCE

Stress incontinence of urine is usually associated with some anatomic defect that allows intra-abdominal pressure to be transmitted directly to the bladder. Concurrently there may be descent of the bladder base and proximal urethra such that intra-abdominal pressure is not transmitted to the urethra. Conditions that increase intra-abdominal pressure, such as obesity, chronic coughing secondary to pulmonary problems, and heavy lifting, exacerbate the anatomical defects and can cause incontinence. The patient with incontinence with these factors should be suspected to have an anatomic defect. Stress incontinence is frequently associated with previous vaginal surgery. The demonstration of loss of urine via the urethra with measures that increase intra-abdominal pressure is necessary to make the diagnosis. This may be accomplished in the lithotomy position though occasionally such loss can be demonstrated only when the patient stands. A variety of other techniques have been championed including x-ray studies of the bladder and urethra, the Marshall test, cystometric studies, and recording of intravesicle and intravaginal pressures. It is important that other causes of incontinence be ruled out before any operative intervention is planned. Urine cultures are obtained to rule out infections. Any infection found should be treated, as this will frequently cause the incontinence to become less aggravated. Cystometric studies may demonstrate uninhibited bladder contractions, detrussor dysenergia. Cystoscopic studies rule out inflammation of the bladder. A variety of operative procedures for the correction of stress incontinence have been devised. The majority involve restoring the bladder base and proximal urethra to an intra-abdominal position where they are subject to increased intraabdominal pressure. The success rate for most procedures is 80 percent. Some patients have a great deal of relief by the use of Kegel's exercises, which strengthen the muscles of the pelvic diaphragm. These are accomplished by the patient alternately starting and stopping her urinary stream.

DETRUSSOR DYSENERGIA

Detrussor dysenergia is increasingly being recognized as a cause of urinary incontinence. These patients display sudden involuntary loss of urine usually without stress or urgency. The bladder will empty completely in these patients. Cystometric studies where bladder pressures are recorded may help confirm the diagnosis. Treatment includes using parasympathetic drugs that prevent involuntary bladder contractions.

OVERFLOW INCONTINENCE

Overflow incontinence secondary to large cystoceles will be helped by operative repair. Overflow incontinence secondary to neurological defects will not. The diagnosis of overflow incontinence is confirmed by the finding of a large volume of urine remaining in the bladder after voiding (i.e., a large residual urine volume).

URETHRAL DIVERTICULA

Urethral diverticula are an uncommon cause of urinary incontinence. They may serve as a source of recurring urinary tract infections. These are frequently palpated under the urethra and small amounts of urine can be expressed. The patient complains of dribbling a small amount of urine after voiding. Urethroscopy may demonstrate the defect. Treatment is surgical excision.

FISTULA

The continued passage of urine by the vagina should raise the suspicion of a urinary fistula such as a vesicovaginal or an ureterovaginal fistula. These frequently occur after pelvic surgery or childbirth. A variety of simple techniques will help elucidate the diagnosis. After placement of a colored solution such as methylene blue in the bladder, the dye will appear in the vagina if a vesicovaginal fistula is present. Treatment for a vesicovaginal fistula is surgical repair by a variety of techniques. If leakage of dye does not occur with methylene blue placed in the bladder, one should suspect a ureterovaginal fistula. This can be diagnosed by giving a systemic dye that is secreted by the kidney such as indigo carmine. After 20 to 30 minutes, blue dye will appear in the vagina. This confirms the diagnosis of a ureterovaginal fistula. An intravenous pyelogram is done to document the site of leakage and to rule out concurrent obstruction. Treatment is again, surgical correction via a variety of techniques.

Pelvic Masses

Masses in the pelvis may arise from any of the structures in the pelvis, the reproductive organs, uterus, tubes, ovaries, the urinary tract, and the gastrointestinal tract. Masses that present with other associated findings are described elsewhere. The differential diagnosis of the asymptomatic pelvis mass is described. Ovarian masses are among the most common pelvic masses. Ovarian masses may be functional, inflammatory, or neoplastic. The workup of an ovarian mass depends upon the status of the patient in terms of reproductive age. In women of reproductive age, functional masses are the most common. These functional masses are either follicular cyst or corpus luteum cysts. These cysts are usually asymptomatic but large ones may present with feelings of pelvic discomfort. Follicular cysts are abnormal enlargements of the follicle. The normal follicle seldom becomes greater than 3 cm in size. Any follicle larger is termed a follicular cyst. These cysts are usually 6 to 8 cm in size but some may reach 20 cm. These cysts are usually unilateral. They develop during the reproductive years secondary to stimulation of the ovary by gonadotropins. The natural history is that they tend to regress over time usually within 2 to 3 months. Therefore, a woman of reproductive age with an asymptomatic ovarian cyst may be followed for 2 to 3 months. If the cysts regress, no further workup is indicated. If the cysts persist, the patient must have histologic diagnosis of this mass. Some physicians advocate placing the patient on oral contraceptive pills for what is felt to be a functional cyst. The rationale is that this will suppress gonadotropins and

decrease stimulation of the ovary and may cause the cyst to regress quicker.

Corpus luteum cysts are unilateral cysts of 6 to 8 cm in diameter. They result after ovulation with excess bleeding into the cavity. They are more apt to be symptomatic than follicular cysts. By definition, they can only occur in ovulatory women, and tend to regress in 2 to 3 months. Rupture with intraperitoneal bleeding can occur. Because of these above findings, guidelines for the management of unilateral cysts in women of reproductive age are as follows: if the cyst is unilateral and less than 6 to 8 cm in diameter, the patient may be followed for 2 to 3 normal cycles as would be done for what is felt to be follicular cyst. The remainder of the management is unchanged. Fixed, solid, bilateral, or symptomatic masses need prompt investigation. Any pelvic mass greater than 6 to 8 cm in diameter also deserves prompt investigation. This investigation is in the form of laparotomy with removal of the mass and immediate frozen section to rule out a malignant process. Premenarchal patients with abdominal masses also deserve immediate exploration as there is a high incidence of malignant germ cell tumors in this age group. Postmenopausal patients with adnexal masses also deserve immediate exploration because of the high chance that there may be an epithelial malignancy of the ovary. Indeed, if one palpates what would be a normal sized ovary for a woman of reproductive age in a woman of postmenopausal age, the patient should be immediately explored. The normal postmenopausal ovary is not palpable. It becomes palpable only when there is an abnormal enlargement. This is the so-called postmenopausal palpable ovarian syndrome, (PMPO). These ovaries harbor a high incidence of neoplasia. Endometriomas are masses that develop secondary to pelvic endometriosis. These masses are usually found in a background of pelvic pain and dysmenorrhea but may be asymptomatic. They are usually fixed and tender. Paraovarian cysts are found between the leaves of the broad ligament and are usually between 5 and 8 cm in diameter. They arise from the remnants of the mesonephric ducts and tubules.

Tubal causes of pelvic masses may be due to inflammatory processes (i.e., pyosalpinx, hydrosalpinx, and neoplastic lesions, both benign and malignant). Ectopic pregnancy may present as a mass but there is usually a history of menstrual irregularity and pelvic pain. The uterus may also give rise to pelvic masses that most common being uterine leiomyomata or fibroids. The gastrointestinal tract can give rise to pelvic masses. Fecal material in the large bowel can be misinterpreted as a pelvic mass. Examination of the patient after an enema will clarify this situation. Gaseous distention of the cecum may present as a right-sided pelvic mass. Repeated examination will reveal the effervescent nature of these masses. Diverticula of the sigmoid can cause left-sided pelvic masses. Barium enema will clarify this situation. A firm posterior nonmobile mass may represent a pelvic kidney. An intravenous pyelogram will elucidate this. Appendiceal abscesses should be considered in a patient with a history of symptoms of acute appendicitis with fever and an elevated white blood cell count. These masses can also be asymptomatic. Another pitfall in the workup of pelvic masses is an overdistended bladder. Voiding prior to the pelvic examination will help prevent this. If there is still a question, the bladder can be emptied via catheterization.

Hirsutism

Hirsutism is the growth of hair in excess amounts in areas that are not normally associated with the female phenotype. Scalp, leg, pubic, and axillary hair are considered normal. Whereas breast, facial, or abdominal hair is not. Hair does not grow continuously but in a cyclic fashion. There is an anagen phase during which the hair grows actively. This phase is of different lengths for different areas of the body. A catagen phase of rapid involution follows and the hair is shed. The hair shaft then enters a quiet phase of telogen during which there is no growth. Sexual hair is that hair that responds to sex steroids, particularly androgens. Androgens cause hair growth in length and diameter. Estrogenic effects on sexual hair are essentially the opposite causing finer, lighter, and slower growing hair. It must be remembered that there is a racial distribution of hair growth with Caucasians having greater hair growth than Orientals. Also within groups there are familial dispositions to the amount of hair in any one individual.

The main cause of continuous hair growth is excess androgen levels, primarily testosterone. The first step in the workup of hirsutism is a 24-hour urinary assay for 17-ketosteroids. The goal here is to rule out adrenal causes of excess androgen secretion. If the 17-ketosteroids are less than 20 mg for 24 hours, the diagnosis of persistent anovulation and excess production of androgen from the ovarian stroma or end organ hypersensitivity to a normal level of androgens is established. These patients, if they are desirous of pregnancy, can have ovulation induced. Those who do not desire pregnancy can be treated with oral contraceptives. These regimes both interrupt the steady state of ovarian androgen production by decreasing LH stimulation of the ovary. These treatments will decrease further hair growth. Hair that is already present will have to be removed by electrolysis or other means. Patients with normal 17-ketosteroids who are ovulatory have end organ hypersensitivity of the hair follicle to androgens. These patients can usually be successfully treated with oral contraceptives. Patients with

elevated 17-ketosteroids and signs of Cushing syndrome need to be screened by giving Dexamethasone at night and checking the morning cortisol level. Failure to suppress indicates that further workup is needed. Patients without signs of Cushing syndrome are given 5 days of suppression and the 17-ketosteroids levels are rechecked. If there is no suppression, the patient needs to be evaluated for adrenal neoplasia. Suppression to a level of less than 4 mg per 24 hours suggests adrenal hyperplasia whereas to 5 to 10 mg per 24 hours indicates the patient is anovulatory. The 17-ketosteroids determinations may be replaced by blood levels of dehydroepiandrosterone (DS). Patients with adrenal hyperplasia are treated with continuous glucocorticoids. Those with persistent anovulation are treated as above. Serum testosterone levels may be normal in patients with hirsutism. Androgens decrease the sex steroid binding globulin levels and the total testosterone level may be normal but the free level is elevated. An absolute level of greater than 2 mg per ml suggests an ovarian androgen producing tumor. In addition, patients with rapidly progressive hirsutism and signs of virilization such as clitoromegaly, deep voice, should be evaluated for androgen-producing tumors. In patients with a normal pelvic examination, it may be necessary to do venous catheterization studies of the ovarian and adrenal veins to locate the source of excess androgen. Computerized actual tomographic scanning of the adrenals may be helpful.

Galactorrhea

Galactorrhea is the appearance of mammary secretion of a milky fluid that is inappropriate in timing. Secretion that is bloody or other than white or clear should suggest local breast disease and the patient needs careful breast examination. Full development and function of the breast depends upon a variety of hormones and their interactions including insulin, cortisol, thyroxine, and growth hormone. In the evaluation of galactorrhea, prolactin level is of central importance. Prolactin is released by the pituitary gland and is under a tonic inhibition by prolactin inhibiting factor (PIF) that is transported from the hypothalamus via the portal axis to the pituitary. Prolactin stimulates the breast to produce milk. PIF secretion is controlled by a variety of factors. Estrogen decreases PIF, therefore estrogen-containing birth control pills can cause galactorrhea. Breast stimulation via suckling or foreplay can decrease PIF as can any defect in the afferent sensory arc such as herpes zoster of the chest wall or cranial/spinal lesions. Many drugs including opiates, tycyclic anti-depressants alpha-methyldopamine, and in particular the phenothiazines decrease PIF and therefore increase prolactin secretion. The most worrisome source of elevated prolactin is a pituitary adenoma. These benign tumors cause significant effects in addition to the secretion of the prolactin. By pressure effect, they can cause changes in other pituitary hormones. Enlargement can also lead to compression of the optic chiasma with visual and neurologic symptoms. The first step in the evaluation of galactorrhea is the measurement of the serum prolactin level. Normally the level is less than 10 ng/ml. During pregnancy, levels greater than 200 ng/ml are seen. Nearly all patients with galactorrhea will have prolactin levels in excess of 20 ng/ml and levels greater than 50 ng/ml are strongly suggestive of a tumor. All patients with galactorrhea deserve a CT scan of the sellae turcica. This will usually demonstrate a tumor if it is present. If a tumor is found, there are a variety of treatment options including the pituitary radiation, surgical removal, and drug therapy. Patients without an abnormality of the sellae turcica can be treated with the medications. Patients whose galactorrhea is secondary to other medications seldom have prolactin levels above 50 ng/ml. Withdrawal of the offending agents will usually abate the galactorrhea. Patients with elevated prolactin levels and no tumor may be treated medically. Many medications have been used including DOPA and pyridoxine. Bromoergocryptine is a specific inhibitor of prolactin secretion. It will cause a decrease in serum prolactin levels relatively promptly and most patients respond within 2 to 3 months. In patients who are anovulatory and have galactorrhea, bromoergocryptine is the drug of choice for inducing ovulation and it is very successful. Bromoergocryptine has also been used to treat pituitary tumors and some tumors have regressed.

Infertility

Infertility or the relative inability to achieve pregnancy is defined as absence of any pregnancy after 1 year of unprotected intercourse. Infertility is due to a variety of causes both male and female. In 40 percent of the cases the male factor is deficient, and in 60 percent the female factor is deficient including failure of ovulation 10 to 15 percent, tubal pathology 20 to 30 percent, cervical factors 5 percent, and 10 to 20 percent of the patients are infertile for unknown reasons. There are great advantages to interviewing both partners in the couple seeking advice for the evaluation of infertility. It allows for correlation of historical facts and an explanation of the studies necessary for an infertility workup. The first step is the evaluation of the male partner. This is done by means of a semen analysis. A normal semen analysis has a volume of 2 to 3 cc with a sperm count of greater than 20 million per cc. Pregnancies have occurred with lesser sperm counts but the percentage drops with further decreases in the count. At least half the spermatozoa should be motile and 60 percent should be normal forms. Ab-

normalities of the semen analysis deserve referral to a urologist who is interested in male infertility. Following the attainment of a normal semen analysis a postcoital test is done. This test is done around the time of expected ovulation as determined by basal body temperature charts. Basal body temperature charts help to time all infertility tests and also confirm that the patient is ovulatory. Following ovulation there is a $\frac{1}{2}$ to 1 °F increase in basal body temperature secondary to corpus luteum secretion of progesterone. The temperature should be obtained daily upon awakening. A flat basal body temperature is indicative of anovulation. Forty-eight hours prior to the expected rise in basal body temperature as determined from earlier basal body temperature charts intercourse is prescribed. Within a few hours of intercourse cervical mucus is removed. If ovulation has occurred the cervical mucus should be clear and watery and should display spinnbarkeit or the ability to be stretched a great distance. The mucus should be looked at microscopically to determine the presence and motility of sperm. Greater than five motile sperm per high power microscopic field is considered adequate for pregnancy to occur. The mucus when dried should also display a fernlike pattern microscopically. If the mucus is thick, opaque, and viscous, timing of the test may be wrong. But if on repeated tests the same results are found, a diagnosis of hostile cervical mucus is made. Such poor quality cervical mucus can be treated with midcycle estrogen replacement. Cervical mucus of good quality that repeatedly displays dead sperm is a vexing problem. Sophisticated tests for sperm allergy may be needed.

For pregnancy to occur, sperm must be transported to and fertilize the egg. The fertilized ovum is then transported to the endometrial cavity. For this to occur the fallopian tubes must be patent. A history of pelvic inflammatory disease, ruptured appendix, previous pelvic surgery, endometriosis, should all suggest tubal pathology. Tubal patency can be assessed by infusing CO_2 gas transcervically and listening over the lower abdomen for the sound of gas bubbling. Most feel that hysterosalpingography (HSG) has replaced the CO_2 or Rubin test. This x-ray procedure is performed 2 to 6 days after a normal menstrual period. A radioopaque dye is instilled transvertically into the uterine cavity. The relative merits of oil-based and water-based x-rayed media are debated. The dye should freely spill into the peritoneal cavity. HSG has the added advantage of showing uterine defects. If tubal blockage is shown, a variety of operative procedures are available for repair. The next step is endometrial biopsy performed 2 to 3 days prior to the expected menstrual period. From the histology (i.e., examination of the endometrial sample), additional confirmation of ovulation can be obtained as evidenced by typical postovulatory endometrial changes. It is also possible to date the endometrium as to its point of the menstrual cycle. An endometrial biopsy that is dated greater than 2 days behind the expected cycle date as determined by the subsequent menstrual period is termed an inadequate luteal phase. These patients typically have a luteal phase of less than 10 days as opposed to the normal 14 days. Replacement with progesterone may aid these patients. Endometrial biopsy may also show other unsuspected endometrial pathology such as tuberculosis or chronic endometritis. Patients who are anovulatory by history, basal body temperature chart, and endometrial biopsy are candidates for induction of ovulation. Patients with anovulation and elevated prolactin levels may benefit from Bromoergocryptine. Patients who are anovulatory with normal gonadotropins and estrogens are considered candidates for clomiphene therapy. Clomiphene is a nonsteroidal antiestrogenic compound that is bound by the hypothalmus preventing the binding of estrogen to the same sites. The hypothalamus cannot perceive the circulating estrogen due to the competitive binding of clomiphene and therefore releases gonadotropins. The levels of FSH and LH rise with clomiphene administration. This stimulates follicular growth. Clomiphene is given for 5 days beginning on the fifth day after the onset of menstrual period. Basal body temperature charts are taken to determine if ovulation occurs. The dose can be escalated if ovulation does not occur. The patient must be followed closely as Clomiphene can cause ovarian enlargement. Other side-effects include flushing, nausea, vomiting, headaches, and visual symptoms. Multiple pregnancies have occurred but these are mostly twins. The overall success rate in terms of induction of ovulation is 70 percent and the pregnancy rate is 40 percent. Patients who are deficient in gonadotropins are candidates for human menopausal gonadatropin therapy. This therapy requires specialized care and expertise to monitor. Patients who are normal by all the other tests are candidates for laparoscopy. This oprative technique allows visualization of the pelvic organs. Transcervical injection of a colored dye will afford another confirmation of tubal patency. Twenty percent of women will have previously unsuspected pathology of the pelvic organs including endometriosis, pelvic adhesions, and old pelvic inflammatory disease. A variety of surgical techniques are available to correct these defects. Finally, 10 to 20 percent of couples who have no discernible or treatable cause for their infertility, should be counselled for adoption.

Venereal Disease

Classically, the common venereal diseases were considered to be syphilis and gonorrhea. The list of diseases that are transmitted sexually has increased such that they are now designated sexually transmitted diseases and include, in addition to the above, condyloma, chan-

croid, granuloma inguinale, lymphogranuloma venereum, herpes, Gardernerella, trachoma, and pelvic inflammatory disease. Syphilis, gonorrhea, herpes simplex, and pelvic inflammatory disease will be discussed in this section.

GONORRHEA

Gonorrhea is caused by Neisseirra gonorrhea, a gramnegative intracellular diplococcus. Direct physical contact is needed for infection to occur. The organism can infect the urethra, vulva, vagina, Bartholin's glands, cervix, fallopian tubes, anus, pharynx, and can even be disseminated. Three to 21 days following exposure, local redness and swelling occur at the site of contact. Disease may be localized forming a purulent exudate or become disseminated. Urethral involvement may cause symptoms of urinary tract infection. Palpation of the urethra can cause purulent material to be expressed from the Skene's glands. The vulva and vagina are uncommon sites of primary infection except in premenarchal and postmenopausal patients when there are low levels of circulating estrogen. The exception is the Bartholin gland that can become infected forming a Bartholin's abscess. Treatment of this consists of marsupialization coupled with antibiotics. The endocervix is a very common site of gonococcal infection and also serves as a conduit for the organism to spread upward to the uterus and tubes. The cervix may be reddened with a profuse, irritating discharge. Rectal infection may lead to perirectal abscess formation. Pharyngeal infection presents like streptococcal pharyngitis with a reddened pharynx and occasionally a purulent exudate. Detection of gonorrhea begins with a history of exposure including the possibility of rectal or oral infection. Definitive diagnosis rests on culturing the organisms. The site to be cultured is swabbed. The swabs are then plated in a Thayer-Martin media and immediately placed in a 5 percent CO_2 atmosphere or a candle jar. For the treatment of local gonorrhea, penicillin remains the drug of choice. Doses of 2,400,000 units of aqueous penicillin G given intramuscularly in each buttock are felt to be adequate for cervical, rectal, or pharyngeal gonorrhea. This is followed by oral pennicillin or tetracycline for 10 days. Penicillinase-producing gonorrhea are an increasing problem. These can be found by test of cure cultures from the same site that the original cultures were obtained. Patients with penicillinase-producing gonorrhea may be treated with spectinomycin or cefoxitin.

Undiagnosed or untreated gonococcal infection of the lower genital tract can spread to the upper genital tract. This occurs particularly at the time of menstruation when the endometrial cavity harbors a great deal of necrotic tissue and blood. From the endometrial cavity, the organisms quickly spread to the mucosa of the fallopian tubes. The tubes become inflamed and fill with exudate that may spill into the peritoneal cavity causing pelvic peritoneal irritation and possibly spread to the upper abdomen. Symptomatically the patients will complain of pain in both lower quadrants, occasionally nausea, vomiting, and fever. On examination, exudate may be seen arising from the endocervical canal. The uterus is usually tender on exam and particularly with motion of the cervix. The adnexa will be tender to palpation. Patients will display fever and leukocytosis. It is extremely important to recognize salpingitis because if left untreated, the tubes can become permanently scarred leading to chronic pelvic pain, infertility, and an increased risk of ectopic pregnancy. Uncomplicated gonococcal salpingitis can be treated with penicillin as outlined above. But only 50 percent of salpingitis is due to gonococcus. A variety of other pathogens are now known to be included. The equation, salpingitis equals gonococcal infection is no longer true. Nongonococcal salpingitis may be a primary infection or secondary to suprainfection after the gonococcus has caused tubal damage. A variety of aerobic and anaerobic organisms are now known to be associated with pelvic inflammatory disease including Eschereria, bacteroides species, and aerobic and anaerobic streptococci. *Chlamydia trachomatis* is being increasingly recognized as a possible pathogen. Also users of intrauterine devices are now known to have an increased risk for the development of nongonococcal salpingitis. Patients with salpingitis in whom the diagnosis of gonococcal disease cannot be made immediately can be treated with penicillin as for gonococcal salpingitis. Increasingly, it is becoming apparent that there are many patients who may benefit from intravenous broad spectrum antibiotics that are effective also against the gonococcus. Also with the increasing knowledge of the role of anaerobic bacteria, anaerobic coverage is suggested. Patients who respond to such intravenous therapy may develop less tubal scarring. Patients who do not respond to intravenous antibiotics should be considered for operative intervention.

SYPHILIS

Syphilis is caused by an anaerobic spirochete, *Treponema pallidum.* Syphilis can gain access to the body via moist, mucus membranes and is then disseminated by the blood stream. The incubation time for the spirochete is 10 to 60 days. Usually within 2 to 3 weeks a chancre develops at the site of exposure. The chancre is an ulcerated, indurated, lesion of the vulva, vagina, cervix, or oral cavity that is painless. If undetected, the chancre will heal in 3 to 9 weeks. A few months later, signs of secondary syphilis may appear with malaise, headache, and a generalized rash with a predilection for the palms of the

hands and the soles of the feet. If untreated, secondary syphilis goes on to tertiary syphilis with varied and widespread manifestations involving several organ systems.

The diagnosis of syphilis rests on the dark field examination and serologic tests. Material from the lesion is obtained by denuding the base so that serum is expressed. The serum is then quickly touched with a glass slide and a cover-slip placed over it. The slide is then immediately viewed under a dark field microscope. Treponemas will appear as a tightly coiled organism that rotates on its long axis and can flex on its long axis. Serologic tests for syphilis are divided into nonTreponemal tests for the presence of nonspecific antibodies (Venereal Disease Research Laboratories, serologic test for syphilis, rapid plasma reagin) and treponemal tests, which are specific for Treponemal antibodies (FTA, FTA-ABS). The nontreponemal tests are relatively inexpensive and become positive in 1 to 2 weeks subsequent to the appearance of lesions and 4 to 5 weeks subsequent to contact. A rising titer indicates disease. The titer does not give information about the infectious status of the patients. These tests will revert to a negative approximately 12 months after therapy but may remain positive. False positive tests may be biologically false positives. Biologic false positive tests can be due to collagen vascular diseases, measles, drug abuse, pregnancy, and aging. The specific Treponema serologic tests are very specific and have few false positives. These tests can be used to clarify the situation of the weekly positive nonTreponemal test. The test can also be used to confirm the diagnosis when there is strong clinical suspicion but a negative nonTreponemal test. As many as one-half of the patients with latent syphilis may be negative with the nonTreponemal serologic test. Biopsies of lesions are not that helpful in making the diagnosis of syphilis, but may be necessary to rule out coexistent malignancy.

Pencillin remains the mainstay in treatment of syphilis. Primary and secondary syphilis can be treated by Benzanthine penicillin 2,400,000 units in one dose or procaine penicillin 600,000 IM daily for 8 to 10 days. Erythromycin or tetracycline can be used for patients allergic to penicillin. Latent or neurosyphilis is treated with Benzanthine penicillin 2,400,000 units IM weekly for 3 weeks or aqueous penicillin 600,000 units IM for 15 days. The patient must be followed after treatment by serologic testing. A rising titer indicates reinfection and the patient must be retreated.

HERPES SIMPLEX

Herpes simplex is a viral infection of the genital tract which has become the second most common sexually transmitted disease. This virus produces a variety of symptoms involving the mouth, skin, and urogenital tract. Most genital tract infections are caused by herpes simplex type II whereas type I infections commonly involve the mouth and the face though both can be found at the opposite location. The virus causes a primary infection, then goes latent in the dorsal sensory root ganglia. Many causes of reactivation have been proposed including stress, temperature changes, fever, drugs, sunlight, and menses. Primary genital disease begins with malaise, headache, and fever. This occurs 2 to 20 days after contact. Pain, tenderness, and pruritus of the contact area quickly follows. Multiple raised vesicles appear on the vulva, vagina, and cervix. The vesicles rupture, leaving 1 to 3 mm shallow, painful ulcers with a slight surrounding erythema. The lesions persist for 1 to 3 weeks. The virus becomes latent and antibodies develop against the viral antigens. After the latent period which is extremely variable, the virus can reactivate and cause vesicles that follow a similar course. The generalized symptoms are less severe with reinfection, and the total course of the illness is shorter. The diagnosis of herpes is made by finding of typical lesions. Cytologic studies obtained from the lesions will how multinucleated cells. A rise in antibody titer from acute and convalescent phase sera will confirm primary infection. The virus can also be grown in tissue culture. Material is obtained by aspirating the vesicles. Treatment of herpes remains a frustrating topic for both patient and physician. Symptomatic relief can be obtained by analgesics, topical anesthetics, sitz baths, and antibiotics to prevent superimposed infection. Recently Acyclovir has been shown to decrease virus shedding and shorten the course of primary infection when applied topically. The patient should be counseled that they are infectious and can transmit the disease particularly when lesions are present.

CONDYLOMA ACCUMINATA

Condyloma accuminata are caused by a papovavirus that clinically presents as a cauliflower-like squamous papilloma of the vulva, vagina, or cervix. Flat lesions of the cervix that present only when an abnormal Pap smear is being evaluated by a colposcopy have recently been described. The finding of koilocytic atypia in cervical biopsies is also felt to be secondary to condyloma infection. One to 3 months after sexual contact, lesions may be found. Lesions range in size from a few millimeters to many centimeters. A variety of treatments are available including Podophyllin, electrocautery, cryosurgery, laser cautery, and surgical excision. Podophyllin 25 percent in benzoin is applied to the lesion and removed after 4 to 6 hours. Podophyllin is used for vulvar lesions. Vaginal lesions are best treated by electrocautery, laser, or surgical excision. Cervical lesions can be treated with cryosurgery. Large lesions are best excised. Lesions that are not typical condyloma accuminata should be biopsied as condyloma lata are manifestations of secondary syphilis.

PUBIC LICE

Pediculosist pubis (pubic lice) and scabies are parasitic infections that can be transmitted sexually and nonsexually. Diagnosis is made by finding the parasites on the vulvar skin. Both are treated by gamma benzene hydrochloride or benzoyl benzoate.

VULVAR DISEASE

Vulvar Infections

The vulva being a skin covered structure is susceptible to most generalized dermatologic diseases. A variety of infections are often seen in the vulva including herpes and condyloma as previously described. Another viral disease that is frequently observed on the vulva is molluscum contagiosum, which is caused by a pox virus. It presents as multiple umbilicated papules up to 1 cm in size occasionally with pruritus. They are treated by expressing each lesion and applying a caustic agent to the cavity so formed. They can also be curetted with a dermal curette.

Behçet's syndrome is an unknown disorder in the United States characterized by genital and oral ulcerations and ocular inflammation. The etiology may be viral or autoimmune. Small vesicles appear on the genitals and in the mouth. They ulcerate and leave a cavity covered by gray tissue. Healing leads to fibrosis and scarring with pain and dyspareunia being the result. Ocular lesions begin as an inflammation that progresses to iridocyclitis. Behçet's syndrome is treated by systemic corticosteroids.

The vulva is susceptible to fungal infections other than candida. Tinea curus is caused by dermatophytic fungi. It causes a reddened lesion with sharp margins. The patient presents with complaints of vulvar pruritus. Scrapings of the lesion will reveal filamentous forms on potassium hydroxide prep. The lesion is treated with topical clotrimazole. Tinea vesicolor may occur elsewhere on the body and it is usually asymptomatic. It is also treated by clotrimazole.

Granulomatous Diseases of the Vulva

The vulva is the site of granulomatous diseases that are infectious in origin. The lesions are more common in tropical countries. Chancroid is caused by *Hemophilius ducreyi.* Three to 5 days following contact, a papule appears that quickly breaks down into an ulcerated lesion with a reddened swollen border. The ulcer itself becomes painful in contrast to a chancre and it is malodorous. The regional lymph nodes become suppurated. The diagnosis can be confirmed by finding short gram-negative bacilli on gram stain and by culturing on blood agar. Tetracycline and sulpha compounds are effective treatments. Lymphopathia venereum or lymphogranulomo venereum (LGV) is caused by a chlamydial organism that is difficult to culture. One to 4 weeks after contact, the patient develops nonspecific symptoms of malaise, headache, and fever. The inguinal lymph nodes become swollen and painful. This is more common in females who develop enlargement of the perianal and perirectal nodes. Obstruction of lymphatic channels can cause elephantiasis of the vulva. The vulva can ulcerate and anal and rectal strictures can occur. The diagnosis can be confirmed by the Frei test. LGV is treated with Tetracycline and sulpha drugs. Extensive lesions may have to be surgically excised.

Granuloma inguinale is caused by Donovania granulomatis. Eight to 12 weeks following contact a papule forms that quickly ulcerates. The initial ulcers are painless. Secondary infection leads to scarring fibrosis and lymphatic obstruction. Biopsy of the lesion's edge will show intracytoplasmic Donovan bodies. Granuloma inguinale is treated with tetracycline.

White Vulvar Lesions

White lesions of the vulva have a variety of causes. The two underying mechanisms are loss of pigmentation and hyperkeratosis. The possibilities range from benign lesions to premalignant lesions and frankly malignant processes. The workup of white vulvar lesions rests on biopsy and histologic examinations. Vulvar biopsies are easily accomplished by using dermal punch biopsy instruments. After infiltrating the area with local anesthesia, the biopsy is taken by rotating the punch into the lesion. The resulting defect can be cauterized or sutured. Guidance as to where to obtain the biopsy material can be obtained by colposcopy of the vulva or toluidine blue staining. Toluidine blue is a nuclear stain and areas with increased nuclear activity will stain blue. Vitiligo is depigmentation that is usually due to chronic irritation of the vulva.

Vulvar Tumors

A variety of cystic tumors can arise from the vulva. Epidermal inclusion cysts are found most commonly in the labia majora. They are filled with a cheezy keratinatious material, or sebaceous cyst. They are usually asymptomatic and require no treatment unless they are symptomatic. Hidradenoma is a lesion arising from the vulvar sweat glands. These lesions of the labia majora are usually 1 cm in size. They are treated with surgical excision. Fox-Fordyce disease is very rare. Patients complain of pruritus and small papules arising from sweat glands. The axilla may also be involved. Birth control pills give symptomatic relief. Syringoma are small asymptomatic or pruritic papules seen beneath the vulvar skin. Mucus cysts of the vulva arise from the epithelium of the urogenital sinus. These cysts are usually small and asymptomatic. Large symptomatic cysts may need to be excised.

The Bartholin glands open into the vestibule by a ductal system. When the ducts become obstructed, cysts of the glands ensue. Gonorrheal infection of the glands is a frequent cause of Bartholin's duct abscesses. These abscesses present as very painful and tender enlargements of the gland. The area overlying the gland is reddened and edematous. The mass is tender and fluctuant to palpation. They range is size from 2 to 6 cm in diameter. If not drained, they will usually rupture within 72 hours. Local heat may hasten drainage. Treatment of Bartholin's abscesses involve marsupialization of the duct. Noninfected cysts of the Bartholin's gland may be the sequelae of earlier infection, insipated mucus, trauma, and congenital defects. Noninfected cysts that are large may cause discomfort. If so, they are opened into the cyst wall, and epithelium is sutured to the skin to also marsupialize the cyst and allow for further drainage. A Bartholin's gland abscess occurring in a postmenopausal patient should be highly suspect for harboring an adenocarcinoma. These patients should have the gland excised. There are many benign lesions of the vulva. Acrochordon is a benign fibroepithelial polyp. It is commonly referred to as a skin tag. There is no malignant potential. Pigmented nevi of the vulva may be raised or flat. Their significance lies in the fact that they may represent a starting point for vulvar melanoma. Therefore pigmented lesions and junctional nevi should be excised particularly when they are discovered during pregnancy.

Vulvar Dystrophies

The term vulvar dystrophy has replaced a previously used and confusing variety of terms that have both clinical and pathological connotations. The vulvar dystrophies include lichen sclerosis, hyperplastic dystrophy with and without atypia, and mixed vulvar dystrophy with and without atypia. All classes of dystrophy may present with similar appearing lesions and the same lesion may appear different in the same patient in different areas. The diagnosis rests on knowing the histology of the lesion. All the vulvar dystrophies cause the patient to complain of vulvar pruritus. The vulvar pruritus causes vulvar scratching and excoriation that can worsen the lesion and lead to superinfection.

Lichen sclerosis et atrophicus though thought to be predominantly a vulvar disease can be found elsewhere on the body. Vulvar locations include the labia, perineal area, and clitoris. Lichen sclerosis begins as a white, maculopapular lesion. On occasion, the lesion can involve the entire vulva. The vulvar tissue particularly the clitoris and labia atrophy and shrink. The shrinkage may be so severe as to cause the introitus to become stenotic. The clinical term kraurosis vulvae is used to describe this condition. On biopsy, atrophy of the epithelium with hyperkeratosis is noted. Underneath there is a thick collagen layer and chronic inflammatory cells. This lesion is not a precancerous entity. Locally applied testosterone gives marked relief of pruritus and results of thickening and softening of the vulvar skin. This needs to be coupled with local hygenic measures. The vulvar skin should be kept dry. Underwear should be cotton to allow moisture to evaporate. Use of a hair dryer to dry the vulva rather than towel will prevent excoiation. No deodorants, perfumes or douches should be used. Mild soaps are used for washing.

Hyperplastic dystrophies may be reddened or white, elevated or flat. The patients also complain of pruritus. Histologically, the lesions have hyperkeratosis, acanthosis, and irregular thickening of the horny layer. There is an underlying inflammation of the dermis made up of lymphocytes and plasma cells. It is important that presence or absence of atypia is noted on histologic examination because lesions without atypia have minimal malignant potential whereas those with atypia have a definite increased incidence of subsequent vulvar malignancy. Atypia is defined as variations in nuclear size and shape, and hyperchromasia. Increased mitotic activity begins in the more basal layers and progresses toward the surface as the lesion progresses. If there is full thickness epithelial atypia, the diagnosis of carcinoma in situ of the vulva is made. Treatment includes local measures described above. Relief of pruritus will allow healing. This can be accomplished by local application of steroid creams and antipruritic agents. Healing will usually occur. Despite signs of improvement, the patient should be followed frequently with liberal use of biopsy to document resolution and more importantly to rule out progression particularly in patients with atypia. Patients with mixed dystrophy both hyperplastic and lichen's sclerosis can be treated with alternating corticosteroid and testosterone locally.

Carcinoma in situ of the vulva is being increasingly recognized in younger and younger women. It appears to be a different lesion in younger patients as opposed to older individuals. In young women, CIS of the vulva may be pruritic but is more commonly asymptomatic. The lesion may be white, red, flat, thickened, and some appear as condylomatous lesions or papules. It tends to be multifocal in the young patient. Diagnosis rests on the liberal use of biopsy and histologic review. A variety of treatment options have been considered, including only following well documented lesions. Radical vulvar operations are no longer indicated for the young patient. Lesions may be locally excised or laser cauterized. Topical 5-FU also has been used with success. Frequently in the young patient, lesions will spontaneously regress. In the older, postmenopausal patient, vulvar CIS tends to be unifocal and has a greater tendency to progress to invasion. These patients should have a more extensive resection and a simple vulvectomy is advocated by many. Approximately 30 percent of patients with vulvar CIS will have had previous preinvasive or invasive lesion of the cervix or concomitant lesion of the cervix or will develop subsequently preinvasive or invasive lesions of the cervix.

Vulvar Carcinoma

Carcinoma of the vulva is the fourth most common gynecologic cancer but accounts for less than 1 percent of all female cancers. The vast majority are squamous cell carcinomas. This is a disease of the postmenopausal patient with a mean age at diagnosis of 65 years. These women tend to be overweight, hypertensive, diabetic, and nulliparous, though none of these are hard and fast. Fifteen percent of women with squamous carcinoma of the vulva have an antecedent, simultaneous, or subsequent CIS or invasive disease of the cervix. The vulva is readily accessible for inspection but frequently the interval from patient presentation to her physician to diagnosis is very long. Even longer is the time from onset of symptoms to consultation with a physician. In one out of three patients, this interval is greater than 12 months. Patients complain of pruritus, mass, ulcerations, bleeding, or dysuria secondary to urine passing over the lesion. Obstruction of the inguinal lymph nodes by tumor may cause lymphedema of the lower extremities. The lesion may arise in any part of the vulva but the labia majora, labia minora, and clitoris are the most common. The lesions are usually unifocal but kissing lesions on each labia are also seen. The lesion can be ulcerated, exophytic, or infiltrative. Size ranges from less than 1 cm to cancers encompassing the entire vulva. There can be extension to the pubic bone, anus, vagina, urethra, rectum, and bladder. Diagnosis is obtained by biopsy of the lesion. Vulvar squamous carcinoma progresses by local extension and by lymph node dissemination. The lymphatics of the vulva drain into the inguinal nodes superficial and deep then via the node of Cloquet to the deep pelvic nodes.

Once the diagnosis is made, the patient's tumor needs to be staged. Staging includes clinical assessment of the vulva, and extension to local structures, and evaluation of the regional lymph nodes. Cystoscopy and proctosigmoidoscopy will bring out bladder or rectal involvement. A simplified staging system follows. Stage I lesions are those cases of less than 2 cm in diameter confined to the vulva with nonpalpable nodes or palpable nodes that are not suspicious of cancer. Stage II lesions are greater than 2 cm in diameter with nonpalpable nodes or palpable nodes that are not suspicious of cancer. Stage III lesions are lesions of any size with the extension into the urethra, vagina, or anus or lesions with palpable nodes that are suspicious of harboring tumor metastasis. Stage IV lesions are lesions of any size with bladder, rectal involvement, tumors fixed to bone, fixed ulcerated nodes, or distant metastasis. This staging though clinical in nature, has been shown to predict survival. The overall survival for stage I lesions is greater than 90 percent. With stage IV lesions, the 5-year survival is only 15 percent. Within any stage lesions, patients whose inguinal nodes are shown to be histologically negative, have a much higher survival than those with positive inguinal nodes. The mainstay of the treatment of vulvar cancer has been and remains the radical vulvectomy coupled with an inguinal lymphadenectomy. Despite the fact that the disease occurs in the postmenopausal age groups, the patients do very well with what is essentially a superficial operation. The major complications are wound breakdown and vascular events such as thrombophlebitis, pulmonary embolism, and lymphedema. Patients who are found to have positive groin nodes can have their pelvic nodes treated by excision or radiotherapy. Recurrent lesions are treated by wide local excision.

Vulvar Melanomas

The second most common vulvar cancer is vulvar melanoma. These lesions occur predominantly in the peri- and postmenopausal patients. They may arise from a preexisting nevus. Patients complain of pruritus, enlargement of a previously known mole or nevus, or by bleeding. The majority are found on the labia minora and clitoris. The lesions can be raised, flat, or ulcerated. The lesions are usually brown or black but amelanotic melanomas also occur on the vulva. Vulvar melanoma does not display the predictable behavior of squamous cell carcinoma of the vulvar. Small lesions can metastasize quickly. The major determinant of survival appears to be the level of invasion of the dermis as has been shown for melanomas elsewhere in the body. The deeper the invasion, the worse is the prognosis. Nearly one-half of patients will have groin metastases at diagnosis. Treatment is radical vulvectomy with inguinal lym-

phadenectomy. The vulvar respond poorly to radiation therapy. Chemotherapy has not been shown to be helpful for vulvar melanomas.

Basal Cell Carcinoma of the Vulva

Basal cell carcinoma of the vulva, like basal cell carcinoma found elsewhere, are usually locally invasive and do not metastasize. These lesions are found on the labia majora and are seldom greater than 2 cm in diameter. Treatment is wide local excision.

Vulvar Paget's Disease

Paget's disease of the vulva occurs in postmenopausal women who complain of pruritus. The lesion is reddened, well demarcated, and occasionally whitened and ulcerated. Extension to the anus is common. Treatment is vulvectomy as the lesion is multifocal and frequently extensive histologic changes are found beyond clinically visible lesions. Also in 20 percent of the cases, there is an underlying invasive adenocarcinoma arising in sweat glands. These patients should be treated by radical vulvectomy. This disease has a great propensity for local recurrence.

Other Vulvar Malignancies

Vulvar adenocarcinomas usually occur in the Bartholin's gland. The patients present with a mass in the region of Bartholin's gland. The disease also tends to be more advanced at diagnosis than is epidermoid carcinoma of the vulvar. The recommended treatment is radical vulvectomy with inguinal lymphadenectomy. Vulvar sarcomas are very rare lesions that tend to be locally aggressive. Verrucous carcinoma is a rare tumor that appears as a condylomatous lesion of the vulva. This lesion should not be radiated as this may allow the lesion to take on a more aggressive behavior. Treatment is radical vulvectomy.

VAGINA

Viral, bacterial, and fungal diseases of the vagina have been previously described. Many of the rare diseases that can involve the vagina have also been previously described with the vulvar diseases. Atrophic vaginitis does need further discussion. With the withdrawal of estrogens at menopause, the vaginal epithelium becomes thin and appears pale with areas of petechiae. The thin mucosa is easily traumatized and secondarily infected. The patient will complain of discharge, pruritus, burning, and tenderness. Dyspareunia is particularly distressing to the patient. Bleeding if present, will be in the form of staining or spotting. This discharge is thin and watery with a pH of greater than 6.5. A Pap smear taken from the vaginal side walls will show a pattern of estrogen deficiency. Treatment with intravaginal estrogen cream usually gives prompt relief.

Vaginal Cystic Tumors

Vaginal cysts may be mesonephric, paramesonephric, and urogenital sinus in origin. Gartner's duct cysts arise from the remnants of the Wolffian ducts (mesonephric ducts). They occur along the lateral wall of the vagina. Paramesonephric cysts are derived from the remnants of the paramesonephric Mullerian epthelium. They can occur anywhere in the vagina. Mucus cysts have origin from the epithelium of the urogenital sinus. They occur in the vestibule near the clitoris and hymenal ring. Most of these cysts are small, less than 2 cm in diameter, and are asymptomatic. Larger ones may need to be removed if pain or dyspareunia occurs.

Vaginal adenosis is a condition in which columnar epithelium similar to that of the endocervix occurs in ectopic locations such as the vagina. This is usually the result of in utero DES exposure.

Vaginal Intraepithelial Neoplasia

Vaginal intraepithelial neoplasia (VIN) is the vaginal counterpart of cervical intraepithelial neoplasia. The vaginal epithelium displays changes that range from mild dysplasia to CIS. There is no invasion of the submucosal tissues. Vaginal intraepithelial neoplasia is by itself a rare lesion occurring in 1 to 3 percent of patients. Forty percent of the patients will have had prior CIS of the cervix or vulva, and 15 percent will present with concomitant lesions of these organs. Predisposing factors include previous radiation therapy, immunosuppression, and the field carcinogenesis theory. The field carcinogenesis theory states that all the lower genital tract tissues, cervix, vagina, and the vulva are susceptible to the same stimulus and react with the same process. VIN is found in the upper third of the vagina in nearly 90 percent of the cases. In posthysterectomy patients, the common site of abnormalities are the 3 and 9 o'clock positions in the vaginal cuff where two small tunnels may exist. Intraepithelial neoplasia is most commonly discovered when an abnormal Pap smear is being evaluated. Patients who have had a hysterectomy for in situ or invasive cervical cancer should continue to have frequent Pap smears so that the neoplasms of the vagina can be found. Intraepithelial lesions of the vagina are usually white appearing and sharply demarcated. Diagnosis rests on obtaining a biopsy of the lesion for histologic confirmation. Lugol

staining of the vagina may aid in locating the lesion. The vaginal epthelium is glycogenated and will stain dark brown when iodine solutions (Lugol's solution) is applied. Any area that is nonglycongenated because of ulceration, neoplasia, trauma, or infection will not take up the stain. This is the so-called Schiller's test. Nonstaining areas will direct the physician to the area that needs to be biopsied. Colposcopy can also be used as described subsequently. In general, vaginal intraepithelial neoplastic lesions will be white with areas of punctation. Biopsy is mandatory so that areas of invasion can be ruled out. Treatment options for VIN include surgical excision, local destructive techniques, and local application of chemotherapeutic agents. Radiation therapy is not recommended as it will cause shortening of the vagina, dyspareunia, and ovarian failure. Unifocal lesions can be surgically excised or destroyed locally with lasers or electrocautery. In a posthysterectomy patient, the upper vagina can be excised (upper vaginectomy). Multifocal lesions may require total vaginectomy with reconstruction of the vagina. Topical application of 5-FU has been used with minimal success. In an occasional postmenopausal patient, application of estrogen creams may lead to regression of the lesion.

Vaginal Carcinoma

Primary invasive carcinoma of the vagina is a rare lesion comprising 1 to 2 percent of all gynecologic cancers. Lesions that involve the cervix and vagina are categorized as cervical cancers, and lesions that involve the vagina and vulva are classified as vulvar cancers. The predominant histologic type is squamous cell carcinomas though adenocarcinomas, sarcomas, and melanomas do occur. Patients' age range from 35 to 70 years with the average age being 62 years. The true etiology is unknown but the same epidemiologic factors that are associated with cervical cancer are also found in vaginal cancer. In addition, prior radiation therapy has been implicated.

Patients usually present with vaginal discharge, frequently bloody. Irregular bleeding or postmenopausal vaginal bleeding are also frequent. Urinary symptoms can occur particularly when the anterior vaginal wall is involved. The lesions are readily apparent on speculum exam and a diagnosis can be confirmed by biopsy. Vaginal cancers spread by direct extension and by lymph node dissemination. Upper vaginal lesions metastasize to the pelvic nodes and lower vaginal lesions to the inguinal and femoral nodes. Once the diagnosis is made, studies are done to stage the patient's disease. The following studies are indicated: examination under anesthesia, chest x-ray, intravenous pyelogram, barium enema, cystoscopy, and proctosigmoidoscopy. The staging of vaginal carcinoma is as follows:

Stage I — the carcinoma is limited to the vaginal wall.

Stage II — the carcinoma involves the subvaginal tissues but has not extended onto the pelvic side wall.

Stage III — the carcinoma has extended to the pelvic side wall.

Stage IV — the carcinoma has extended beyond the true pelvis or has involved the mucosa of the bladder or rectum.

Stage IVA — spread to adjacent organs

Stage IVB — spread to distant organs.

Radiation therapy remains the mainstay in the treatment of vaginal carcinoma. This is a combination of external whole pelvis radiotherapy to treat the pelvic nodes and intracavitary brachytherapy. The external radiation field should encompass the pelvic nodes and the vaginal tube to a point 2 cm below the lesion. This will also shrink a large bulky tumor. Radium or cesium sources are then placed in the vagina to deliver a high dose directly to the lesion. Small Stage I lesions occupying the upper vagina may be treated with radical surgery to include pelvic lymphadenectomy. The overall 5-year survival rate approaches 50 percent with Stage I and II lesions approaching 80 to 90 percent.

Vaginal Adenocarcinoma

Until about 10 years ago, primary vaginal adenocarcinoma was a very rare lesion and indeed a biopsy of adenocarcinoma from the vagina triggered a search for a site of primary disease. The primary vaginal adenocarcinomas that were described were in elderly women. Now vaginal adenocarcinoma is seen in young women. This is felt to be secondary to in utero diethylstilbesterol (DES) exposure. In the 1940s and 1950s, DES was given during pregnancy for many high-risk conditions. In the early 1970s it became apparent that there was an increased incidence of adenocarcinomas of the vagina and cervix in these in utero-exposed offspring. The carcinoma was of a uniform histologic type, a clear-cell adenocarcinoma. These patients range in age from 7 to 30 years. The presenting symptoms were abnormal vaginal bleeding and discharge with a great many cases discovered when asymptomatic. These lesions may involve the cervix and vagina with the predominance of cases arising in the upper vaginal wall anteriorly. The carcinoma was almost universally associated with adenosis. Adenosis is the finding of endocervical-type epithelium in ectopic locations such as the ectocervix and vagina. These lesions are benign. Indeed, vaginal adenosis is a much

more common finding in DES-exposed offspring than is adenocarcinoma. Therapy of clear-cell carcinoma of the vagina is not standardized but both surgery and radiation therapy have been employed. Lymph node metastases are relatively high and metastases to the lung are more common than with squamous-cell carcinoma of the vagina. Recurrences after therapy are relatively high with most occurring within 3 years of therapy. Sites of recurrence are the pelvis (greater than 50 percent), lungs, and supraclavicular nodes.

Other Changes Related to in Utero DES Exposure

In addition to adenocarcinoma and adenosis, other changes are associated with in utero DES exposure. Transverse vaginal ridges, abnormal cervical shapes (cocks comb cervix), cervical eversions, vaginal hoods, and pseudopolyps. One or more of these abnormalities are seen in 60 percent of the patients with in utero DES exposure. The development of clear-cell carcinoma from areas of adenosis has not been definitely established. Nonetheless, these patients warrant close observation. DES-exposed offspring should have a gynecological examination beginning at menarche or earlier if symptoms of unusual discharge or bleeding occur. The entire cervix and vagina should be inspected and palpated. Cytologic samples are obtained from the cervix and vaginal walls. Lugol's staining and colposcopy may aid in localizing lesions. On colposcopic examination, areas of adenosis will appear red and granular. The lesions are confirmed to be adenosis by biopsy. Once the diagnosis is confirmed, no therapy is needed. The natural history of adenosis is that it will gradually be transformed into mature squamous epithelium over time.

Vaginal Melanoma

Vaginal melanomas are very rare lesions. These lesions occur predominantly in post-menopausal women who present with vaginal discharge or bleeding. It occurs most frequently on the anterior vaginal wall. The lesions may be fungating or ulcerative and are usually black or brown. Treatment is radical surgery. Radiation therapy and chemotherapy are not effective. Overall survival is very poor.

Vaginal Sarcomas

Vaginal leiomyosarcomas and fibrosarcomas have been reported. The most common vaginal sarcoma though is sarcoma botryoides. This is a rhabdomyosarcoma that involves the vagina and/or cervix. It occurs in infants and young children who present with large grape-like vaginal masses that cause bleeding and discharge. Chemotherapy has recently become the primary treatment. Surgery is used only to resect lesions that persist following aggressive chemotherapy.

CERVIX

The cervix can be involved with a variety of acute infections. Viral infections include herpes and condyloma. Bacterial infections include gonorrhea, Gardenerella, and syphilis. The common vaginal infections of Candida and Trichomonas can involve the cervix. Chronic cervicitis is found histologically in the cervices of 90 to 95 percent of women. This is asymptomatic and of little consequence.

Cervical polyps arise from the endocervical canal and range in size from a few millimeters to greater than 3 cm. Most are asymptomatic but patients may complain of menorrhagia or discharge. Treatment is surgical removal by ligating the pedicle. The cervix can also harbor leiomyomas, hemangiomas, and endometriomas.

Cervical Intraepithelial Neoplasia

During the past few years, a great deal of knowlege about the origin, natural history, diagnosis, and treatment of preinvasive lesions of the uterine cervix has emerged. The exact etiologic agents involved in the initiation and promotion of these changes are unkown. However, several epidemiologic points have been associated. Cervical squamous preinvasive and invasive lesions do not develop in the absence of sexual intercourse. Young age at first coitus, multiple sexual partners, and lower socioeconomic status are all associated with an increased incidence. Histones in the sperm heads have been implicated. Herpes simplex type II viral infections have also been epidemiologically associated and by the findings of increased antibody titers in patients with cervical neoplasia. Also viral proteins and DNA have been identified in cervical neoplastic lesions. Similar data is also found for human papilloma virus. Several lesions that were in the past termed dysplasia of the cervix have now been shown to represent flat condyloma virus infection. These lesions are white appearing under colposcopy with areas of mosaic and punctation. Histologically they display thickened epithelium with cytoplasmic vacuolization. These lesions are evaluated and treated similarly to preinvasive lesions of the uterine cervix. Studies indicate that cervical neoplasia is a spectrum of disease from mild changes to invasive carcinoma and that it is a deviation from a normal dynamic process. This process occurs in the transformation zone. The transformation zone is the area of the cervix that was initially covered by columnar epithelium. Through a process termed squamous metaplasia, the columnar endocervical-like epithelium is converted to mature squamous epithelium. Squamous metaplasia is most active in utero, during puberty, and during pregnancy. Nearly 70 percent of females have columnar epithelium on the ectocervix at birth. If while this process of squamous metaplasia is active, particularly around puberty, the patient is exposed to the supposed carcinogen associated with intercourse (histones, viruses, etc.) it is conceivable that the process could be directed along an abnormal path to dysplasia rather than along the normal path to mature squamous epithelium. Dysplastic changes have been graded from mild, moderate, to severe dysplasia depending upon the thickness of the epithelium that is abnormal. When the entire thickness of the epithelium is abnormal, it is termed carcinoma in situ (CIS). Recently these designations have been termed cervical intraepithelial neoplasia (CIN) I (mild dysplasia) when the lower third of the epithelium is abnormal, CIN II (moderate dysplasia) when the lower two-thirds of the epithelium is involved and CIN III (severe dysplasia, CIS) when the entire or nearly the entire epithelium shows abnormalities. The abnormalities one sees are hyperchromasia, increased nuclear cytoplasmic ratio, and nuclear atypia. The mainstay for the detection of CIN is the Papanicolaou smear. With properly obtained smears, the diagnostic accuracy approaches 90 percent. The Pap smear is obtained by sampling the endocervix and the transformation zone. The smears are prepared as previously described. Any sexually active woman should have a yearly Pap smear. Certain low-risk groups may need less frequent sampling. Unfortunately despite its proven value, some studies indicate that nearly 50 percent of women have never had even one screening Pap smear. The Pap smear is the best method for the detection of abnormalities of the cervical epithelium. Further studies are indicated to completely evaluate the disease. The workup of the abnormal Pap is outlined below. The workup of the abnormal Pap smear does not cease until histologic diagnosis that explains the abnormality seen on the Pap smear is obtained (Fig. 10-8). The utilization of the above algorhythm reduces the need for conization of the cervix by 80 percent. Cone biopsy of the cervix was the main technique utilized in the past. Colposcopy and directed biopsies allow for the diagnosis using less hazardous and expensive techniques. This is particularly important now that cervical neoplasia is being seen in younger and younger women many of whom have not completed their childbearing desires. The first step is to re-examine the patient. If a gross cervical lesion is seen, it is biopsied immediately. If invasive disease is found, the patient undergoes staging and definitive therapy as outlined below. If no gross lesion is seen, colposcopy and

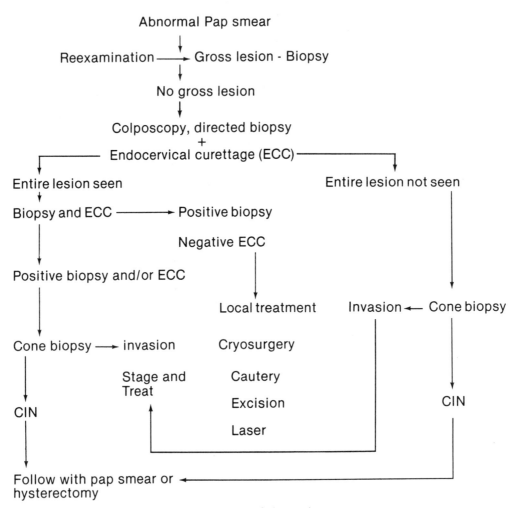

Fig. 10-8. Workup of abnormal Pap smear.

directed biopsy are undertaken. Colposcopy is the visualization of the cervix under magnification of 8 to 40 times. Care is taken to visualize the transformation zone. One percent acetic acid is placed on the cervix to dry out the mucous and bring out abnormal areas. These abnormal areas appear white. Within the white area (white epithelium) there may be small red dots (punctation), red vessels that divide the white epithelium into small plaques (mosaic), or atypical vessels. These are the areas that need to be biopsied. In addition to cervical biopsy, an endocervical curettage is recommended. Endocervical curettage (ECC) involves scraping the endocervix with a small curette and submitting the specimen so obtained separately for pathologic review. The ECC will bring out abnormalities of the endocervix that cannot be seen by the colposcope. If the entire lesion is seen and the ECC is negative, the patient can be treated without further workup as outlined below. If the entire lesion is not seen, a condition termed "unsatisfactory colposcopy" or if the ECC is positive for dysplasia, the patient should

undergo diagnostic conization. The histologic review of the cone biopsy specimen will determine the need for further therapy. If at any time during the sequence, invasive carcinoma is found, the workup ceases and the patient is staged and treated for invasive disease. A variety of local destructive techniques are available to treat preinvasive lesions of the cervix if the entire lesion is seen and the ECC is negative. These include local excision, cryosurgery, electrocautery, laser ablation, and conization of the cervix.

Local excision may be accomplished in the office or in the operating room. Because of possible bleeding and the difficulty of the technique, local excision is not frequently used. Electrocautery uses an electrically heated probe to destroy the cervical epithelium. The probe burns off the transformation zone and ablates the abnormal area. The area then heals with normal squamous epithelium. Perhaps the most frequently utilized technique is cryosurgery. This involves placing a refrigerated probe against the cervix. The cervical tissue freezes and the tissue undergoes necrosis and sloughing. This office technique is very effective and carries only the mild side-effect of mild cramping during the procedure and a great deal of discharge subsequently. The overall success rate as judged by subsequent Pap smears approaches 90 percent. Some investigators do not advocate using cryosurgery for CIN Grade III lesions because of a higher failure rate. They recommend conization for this group of patients. Carbon dioxide lasers have been used recently to destroy the transformation zone. This technique is more expensive but gives results similar to those of cryosurgery. It does have the advantage of a faster healing phase. Complications are bleeding that occurs approximately in 1 percent of patients.

Conization of the cervix has two indications for diagnosis and as therapy. The diagnostic indication for cone biopsy are unsatisfactory colposcopy, positive endocervical curettage, or biopsy that shows questionable invasion or microinvasion.

In many patients what was done originally as a diagnostic cone biopsy may be considered therapeutic if noninvasion is noted, the patient is desirous of further childbearing, and the margins of the cone are histologically free of disease. Complications of cone biopsy are immediate and delayed. Immediate complications include hemorrhage, perforation, and the risk of anesthesia and expensive hospitalization. Delayed complications include bleeding at 10 to 14 days, subsequent servical stenosis, infertility, and cervical incompetence. The latter three tend to be related to the extent of the cone biopsy. Larger biopsies carry a greater risk for these complications. A controversial area is in the patient with CIN III on cone biopsy or directed biopsy. Some authors advocate the cone biopsy as therapy and others advocate hysterectomy. The rate for recurrent CIN is about twice that seen with hysterectomy for those patients treated by cone biopsy alone. The rate of subsequent invasive cancers is about equal. The choice of therapy appears to rest upon the patient's need and desire to retain childbearing capacity.

Invasive Cervical Carcinoma

Invasive carcinoma of the cervix is the sixth most common invasive cancer in women overall with approximately 16,000 new cases annually and over 7,000 deaths in the United States. It is a disease of the parous women with a peak age incidence of 45 to 55 years though it is being seen in younger women. Abnormal vaginal bleeding is present in nearly 90 percent of the patients. Postcoital bleeding and vaginal disharge are also common. Some are discovered during the workup of an abnormal Pap smear. Pain and urinary symptoms are relatively late symptoms and suggest advanced disease.

Over 90 percent are squamous carcinomas. Other types include adenocarcinomas, (5 percent) and a variety of others including melanomas and sarcomas. Squamous carcinoma is a relatively predictable disease in terms of mechanism of spread. It spreads locally from the cervix into the vagina, parametrium, bladder, and rectum. It also disseminates via lymphatics again in a predictable, stepwise manner to the parametrial nodes, obturator nodes, iliac nodes, and then to the para-aortic lymph nodes. The lesion may be fungating forming large polypoid lesions. The lesions may be ulcerated involving the cervix and upper vagina. Other lesions may not be visible but present as a stony, hard cervix. The diagnosis can readily be obtained by biopsy.

Once the diagnosis is obtained, the patient undergoes a staging workup. This includes examination under anesthesia to detect parametrial and vaginal extension, cytoscopy, proctoscopy, barium enema, intravenous pyelogram, and chest x-ray. The staging criteria are as follows:

Stage I—lesions confined to the cervix
Stage IA—microinvasions
Stage IB—all other Stage I lesions
Stage II—lesions involving the parametrium but not to the pelvic side wall and/or the upper vagina
Stage IIA—upper two-thirds of the vagina
Stage IIB—parametrial involvement
Stage III—lesions involving the parametrium to the pelvic side wall and/or the lower third of the vagina
Stage IIIA—lower third of the vagina
Stage IIIB—pelvic side wall involvement
Stage IV—extension to the bladder or rectum confirmed histologically or distant metastasis
Stage IVA—bladder or rectal involvement
Stage IVB—distant metastases

Microinvasion is defined as a lesion that has less than 3 mm of invasion below the basement membrane, no vascular channel involvement, and no confluence of tongues of invasive tissue. The finding of hydronephrosis or a nonfunctioning kidney that cannot be explained otherwise is sufficient to allot a case to stage III-B. Other findings such as laparotomy findings or other x-ray studies are not sufficient to change a patient's stage of disease. The incidence of positive nodes in both the pelvis and para-aortic area and survival vary with the stage of the disease as outlined in Table 10-4.

Radiation therapy and radical pelvic surgery are both effective in the treatment of cervical carcinoma. The choice of therapy depends upon the condition of the patient, expertise of the physician caring for the patient,

Table 10-4. Incidence and Survival of Positive Nodes in the Pelvis and Para-aortic Areas

	Positive Pelvic Nodes (%)	Positive Para-aortic Nodes(%)	Survival (%)
I.	15	8	90
II.	30	15	75
III.	45	20–25	45
IV.	—	—	15

and the extent of the disease. Stage IA lesions can be treated with simple hysterectomy with a very high success rate. Patients with Stage IB or IIA lesions can be treated with either radiation therapy or radical hysterectomy with pelvic and para-aortic lymphadenectomy. The overall success rate for both techniques is approximately 90 percent. Radical hysterectomy involves removal of the uterus, parametrium, and upper vagina. Pelvic lymphadenectomy consists of clearing all large pelvic vessels of lymph nodes bearing tissue. Advantages of surgical therapy include preservation of ovarian and vaginal function. Complications of radical surgery include bleeding, pelvic infection, damage to the urinary tract (i.e., vesicovaginal or ureterovaginal fistula and neurogenic bladder). These complications are immediate and surgically correctable. Radiation therapy offers the advantage of being applicable to all patients even those who are not surgical candidates. Complications of radiation therapy are either early or late. Early complications include nausea, diarrhea, and skin changes. Late complications are due to necrosis and scarring secondary to the endarteritis that radiation therapy causes and include fistula, rectovaginal and vesicovaginal, bowel obstruction (usually the terminal ileum), and radiation cystitis and/or proctitis. These complications are difficult to manage. Radiation therapy involves a combination of external therapy and internal therapy. The external therapy is given to the whole pelvis to sterilize nodal disease. This is followed by one of the many internal techniques using radium or cesium. The internal sources deliver a large dose to the central tumor. Patients with Stage IIB, III, and IVA lesions are treated with radiation therapy as outlined above. Patients with distant metastatic disease are candidates for chemotherapy.

Once therapy is completed, the patient must be followed so that recurrence can be diagnosed quickly. Seventy-five percent of recurrences will occur in 2 years and 95 percent by 5 years posttreatment. Because of this, patients should be followed frequently during the first 2 years. Followup includes complete physical and pelvic examinations, Pap smears, chest x-rays, and periodic intravenous pyelograms. Signs and symptoms that suggest recurrence are pelvic and leg pain, leg swelling, a blocked or obstructed ureter, a positive Pap smear, and unexplained weight loss. Fifty percent of the recurrences occur with the disease still localized to the pelvis. Distant sites of recurrence of disease include the lung and the supraclavicular nodes. The diagnosis of recurrence needs to be confirmed by biopsy. Patients who are previously treated with radical surgery and who have disease localized in the pelvis, can be treated with radiation therapy for their recurrence. Patients who were previously treated with radiation therapy and now have pelvic recurrence are treated with ultraradical pelvic surgery. Because of 50 percent of patients have recurrent disease confined to the pelvis, these patients may be treated with pelvic exenteration which includes removal of the bladder, uterus, vagina, and rectum. This necessitates the formation of a urinary conduit and a colostomy. Survival after exenteration approaches 50 percent. Those with distant disease or disease outside of the surgical field are treated with chemotherapy. The most effective agent appears to be *cis*-platinum. Cervical adenocarcinomas are characterized by large, bulky lesions that can balloon out of the cervix and the lower uterine segment causing the so-called barrel shaped lesion. They spread like squamous-cell carcinomas of the cervix. They tend to have a somewhat higher recurrence rate in the pelvis. Because of this some authors have advocated combined radiation and surgical therapy for these lesions. Sarcomas of the cervix are very rare.

UTERUS

Uterine Leiomyomota (Fibroids)

Uterine fibroids are perhaps the most common disorder of the uterus occurring in 50 percent of women. Blacks have a five-fold greater incidence than whites. These benign tumors are made up of whorls of interlacing smooth muscle cells. They vary in size from a few millimeters to large tumors. There are no known etiologic factors but excessive estrogen stimulation has been implicated. They do tend to regress after menopause when estrogen levels are lower. They may be solitary but are more commonly multiple. They are named by their location—subserosal, intramural, or submucosal. Large subserosal fibroids may become pedunculated. They also can occur in the broad ligament and the round ligament.

Leiomyomas are most commonly discovered during routine pelvic examination and most of them are asymptomatic. Submucosal fibroids may cause bleeding as a result of venous edema and congestion. The tumor may also cause cervical dilatation and may be passed into the vagina (i.e., aborting fibroid). The pedunculated subserosal fibroid may undergo torsion and give pain and peritoneal irritation. Large lesions may outstrip their blood supply and undergo painful infarction. Pain with fibroids is more commonly due to large size and pressure on the rectum or bladder. Rarely fibroids are responsible for infertility or pregnancy wastage, particularly second trimester abortions. Rapid growth is worrisome and it may represent a leiomyosarcoma particularly in the postmenopausal patient.

Treatment of fibroids is surgical removal. Indications are symptomatic fibroids with pelvic pressure and pain. Bleeding is an indication but with the caution that a diagnostic curettage be undertaken prior to the surgery to rule out endometrial pathology. Rapid enlargement is another indication for surgery. In the postmenopausal years where it is important to be able to assess the ovaries for enlargement, fibroids may make it difficult. Therefore, inability to assess the ovaries is another indication for removal of fibroids. Removal is most easily accomplished by hysterectomy. Some women with fibroids presenting with infertility, and desirous to maintain their childbearing capacity, may be treated with multiple myomectomies.

Adenomyosis

Adenomyosis is the growth of ectopic endometrial tissue, glands, and stroma within the myomyetrium. This benign lesion occurs during the reproductive years. Adenomyosis is frequently an incidental finding in the uterus when hysterectomy is performed for other indications. These patients present with dysmenorrhea and heavy menstrual bleeding. On examination, the uterus is globular, enlarged, and tender. Asymptomatic enlargements suggest coexistent fibroids. The treatment of symptomatic cases is hysterectomy.

Endometrial Polyps

Endometrial polyps are localized, hyperplastic growths of the endometrium with a central fibrous stalk. The top can undergo inflammation and bleed presenting as postmenopausal or postmenstrual bleeding. These lesions can be found on D&C or visualized by hysteroscopy. Removal is curative and will also remove the rare polyp that harbors a malignancy.

Endometriosis

Endometriosis is a benign disease occurring in the reproductive years characterized by the findings of endometrial glands and stroma in areas outside the uterus. These ectopic implants are often hormonally responsive and the consequent menstrual bleeding explains the natural history and protean symptomatology. Sites of occurrence are varied. The uterosacral ligaments present as tender nodules. Ovarian involvement may lead to the formation of large cystic structures filled with old blood, the so-called chocolate cyst or endometrioma. Peritoneal implants on the cul-de-sac or pelvic peritoneum or bladder peritoneum appear as small 2 to 3 mm nodules that are brown to black in color (i.e., powder burns). Endometriosis is found n the cervix, in abdominal incisions, and episiotomy sites. Involvement of the gastrointestinal tract or urinary tract may present cyclical gastrointestinal bleeding or cyclical hematuria. Cyclical hemoptysis has been demonstrated secondary to lung endometriosis.

Many theories have been proposed to explain the histogenesis including tranportation via menstrual reflux, in situ formation, coelomic metaplasia, and a combination of these. Sampson proposed the reflux theory. During menses, viable endometrial glands and stroma can be transported via the fallopian tubes to the peritoneal cavity. Menstrual fragments have been found in the fallopian tubes and the peritoneal cavity. Experimental evidence with monkeys also supports this concept. The clinical finding of an increased incidence of endometriosis with cervical stenosis is also supportive. The menstrual fragments once passed into the peritoneal cavity can implant and grow. They are hormonally responsive and will proliferate with estrogen stimulation. They will also undergo bleeding with progesterone withdrawal. Coelomic metaplasia states that the peritoneum is a totipotential organ and can, under the appropriate stimulus, differentiate into functioning endometrial tissue. Supportive evidence for this comes from embryologic studies and by the frequent clinical observation of decidual changes in the peritoneal cavity during pregnancy. Combination theories state that menstrual reflux is the stimulus that causes the coelomic epithelium to differentiate toward endometrial tissue.

Classical teaching states that patients with endometriosis present with acquired dysmenorrhea of gradually increasing severity. The exact cause of the dysmenorrhea is unknown but may be related to cyclic bleeding into endometrial implants or the release of prostaglandins by the ectopic endometrial tissue. Large cysts may rupture causing acute pain. Abnormal uterine bleeding is also frequently associated with endometriosis but there is no specific bleeding pattern associated. Many patients are indeed asymptomatic. Large lesions may be without symptoms whereas tiny implants may cause severe pain. Other patients are discovered to have endometriosis when a workup for infertility results in laparoscopy and endometriosis is found.

Endometriosis can only be diagnosed by direct visualization of the intraperitoneal lesions. This necessitates laparoscopy or laparotomy. Laparoscopy is the technique most often utilized to confirm a clinical impression of endometriosis. Histologically the lesions show endometrial glands, endometrial stroma, and hemosiderin ladened macrophages in the wall of the lesions. However, the findings at not absolute. Frequently, the operative findings of typical endometriosis are not confirmed histologically.

Treatment of endometriosis can be surgical, hormonal, or conservative. Patients with mild endometriosis may be observed and treated with mild analgesia, particularly antiprostaglandin agents. Many feel that pregnancy will ameliorate the disease. Surgery is usually in the form of total abdominal hysterectomy, bilateral salpingo-oophorectomy which is very effective for older patients who no longer desire pregnancy. This removes the source of menstrual reflux and the ovarian estrogen source ablating the hormonal support of any remaining endometriosis lesions. Hysterectomy alone may help many patients even though the ovaries remain. Conservative surgery is indicated for patients who desire further child bearing. Conservative surgery involves removal of endometrial implants. Small powder burn lesions may be cauterized. Pregnancy rates of 50 percent are reported after conservative surgical procedures for endometriosis. Presacral neurectomy has been used for symptomatic relief of pain. Because the tissue of endometriosis is hormonally responsive, hormonal therapy has been used. This has included estrogens, androgens, and progestins. The most frequently utilized regime is combination estrogen and progesterone therapy in the form of oral contraceptive pills. This therapy suppresses ovulation and induces so called pseudopregnancy. Endogenous estrogen and progesterone levels are depressed. This prevents the stimulation of the endometrial implants and may help ameliorate the disease. Birth control pills are also frequently used in a continuous fashion for 6 to 9 months. Following a pseudopregnancy regime, the patient attempts pregnancy. Most patients have symptomatic relief and pregnancy rates of nearly 50 percent are reported. Progesterone alone has also been used. Some physicians feel that progesterone given for a few months prior to an anticipated surgical procedure for endometriosis makes the surgery easier. Recently a new agent, Danazol, has been used for endometriosis. This agent has little inherent steroid activity but is a potent inhibitor of gonadotropins. This induces a so-called pseudomenopause where the gonadotropin levels are very low. This prevents the ovarian secretion of estrogen and progesterone and may prevent stimulation of endometrial tissues. Seventy to 100 percent of patients receive symptomatic relief with Danazol and a pregnancy rate of 50 percent is seen. The major side-effects of Danazol therapy in addition to being expensive include hot flashes, nausea, vomiting, and vaginal dryness.

Endometrial Hyperplasia

Estrogen stimulation, endogenous or exogenous, causes proliferation of the endometrium. If sustained and unopposed as in exogenous use or secondary to anovulation, endometrial hyperplasia, focal or diffuse, can result. The endometrial hyperplasias are a spectrum of disorders which vary from entities with little potential for malignancy (cystic or Swiss cheese hyperplasia) to entities with a much greater malignant potential (adenomatous hyperplasia with atypia. Cystic hyperplasia is characterized by increased glands and stroma, with large epithelial lined cystic spaces. It carries a risk of subsequent endometrial carcinoma of less than 5 percent. Adenomatous hyperplasia is an increase in a number of glands per unit of stroma, crowding of glands, epithelial proliferation and carries a risk of endometrial carcinoma of approximately 25 percent. The risk of endometrial carcinoma doubles to nearly 50 percent when atypia of the glandular epithelium is present. Patients with endometrial hyperplasia present with abnormal uterine bleeding, either as post-menopausal bleeding or as increased bleeding in the premenopausal patients. The diagnosis is made by histologically studying the endometrium obtained via endometrial biopsy or by dilation and curettage.

Treatment of endometrial hyperplasia depends upon the type of hyperplasia and the patient's age. In healthy perimenopausal and postmenopausal patients total abdominal hysterectomy and bilateral salpingo-oophorectomy is the treatment of choice. Those who are not good surgical candidates can be treated with progestins. Young postmenarchal patients usually have hyperplasia secondary to anovulation. These patients are treated with cyclic progestins or ovulation induction.

Endometrial Carcinoma

Endometrial carcinoma has become the most common invasive gynecologic malignancy in the United States with 37,000 new cases annually and 3,000 deaths. It is predominantly a disorder of the postmenopausal years. Epidemiologic factors have been associated with an increased risk of endometrial cancer including obesity, nulliparity, diabetes, hypertension, and exogenous estrogen use. The central mechanism here seems to be persistent, unopposed estrogen stimulation of the endometrium. Obese patients convert a greater percentage of circulating adrenal androgens to estrogens, mainly, estrone in peripheral adipose tissue. Nulliparous patients tend to be anovulatory. Exogenous estrogen use for replacement and for the relief of postmenopausal symptoms has been shown to increase the incidence of endometrial cancer four to eight times. Clinical evidence that supports the estrogen hypotheses is the observation that estrogen-secreting ovarian tumors are associated with endometrial carcinoma in 5 to 25 percent of cases.

Patients present with abnormal vaginal bleeding, most commonly postmenopausal bleeding. Premenopausal patients who make up 25 percent of patients with endometrial carcinoma complain of menorrhagia or metrorrhagia. There are no pathognomic physical findings and diagnosis rests on sampling the endometrium for pathologic review. The classical method is the fractional dilatation and curettage. This consists of endocervical curettage followed by an endometrial curetting. The two specimens so obtained are submitted and reviewed separately. This is coupled with an examination under anesthesia to assess vaginal, parametrial, and adnexal involvement.

Once the diagnosis is obtained the patient undergoes a staging workup. This includes an intravenous pyelogram, barium enema, cystoscopy, and proctosigmoidoscopy. The gastrointestinal studies are particularly important due to the known association of endometrial and colon cancers. The staging criteria for endometrial cancers are listed below.

Stage I — lesions confined to the corpus
Stage IA — uterine cavity length less than or equal to 8 cm
Stage IB — uterine cavity length greater than 8 cm

Stage I lesions are sub-grouped based upon the histologic grade.

Grade I — well or highly differentiated
Grade 2 — moderately differentiated
Grade 3 — poorly differentiated
Stage II — cervical involvement
Stage III — spread outside the uterus but not outside the true pelvis
Stage IV — spread outside the true pelvis and/or bladder or rectal involvement and/or distant metastases

Endometrial cancer spreads by local invasion and by lymphatic dissemination. Hematogenous dissemination is less frequent but may account for most distant metastatic disease. Eighty percent of endometrial cancers are pure adenocarcinomas and adenoacanthomas in which there are also benign squamous elements. The remaining 20 percent are adenosquamous lesions in which there are malignant squamous elements. The histologic grade of the lesion is of great prognostic importance. As the lesion becomes more anaplastic (i.e., less well differentiated), the incidence of extensive disease, lymph node metastases, and recurrence increases.

Classically, endometrial cancer has been treated with a combination of radiotherapy and surgery, total abdominal hysterectomy and bilateral salpingo-oophorectomy. Radiation therapy is given to sterilize microscopic disease and to decrease vaginal vault recurrence. Hysterectomy is done to remove the central bulk of tumor. Patients with small well-differentiated lesions can be treated with hysterectomy alone. Large uteri or poorly differentiated lesions will benefit from radiation therapy. The tendency today is to treat stage I lesions with primary surgery, total abdominal hysterectomy, bilateral salpingo-oophrectomy and lymph node biopsies. It is on the basis of pathologic review of the operative specimen that the decision to use radiotherapy is made. The criteria to institute irradiation would be cervical involvement, adnexal involvement, deep myometrial invasion by the tumor, and all anaplastic tumors. Stage II lesions are treated with preoperative radiation therapy followed by surgery. Therapy for stage III and IV diseases needs to be individualized and may include surgery, radiation, and chemotherapy. The overall survival rate at 5 years is 68 percent. In patients with low-stage and low-grade lesions, the survival rate is much higher.

Most recurrent disease will occur within 2 years of treatment. The later the recurrence occurs, the better the patient's prognosis. Sites of recurrence are the vagina, parametrium, lung, and liver. For the past 20 years, hormonal therapy with progestins has been the main therapeutic modality employed for recurrent endometrial carcinoma. The exact mechanism of action is unclear but progestins have documented efficacy. Response rates of 30 to 35 percent are well known. Late recurrences respond better than earlier ones. Previously well differentiated lesions respond better than poorly differentiated lesions. Patients whose tumors respond, do live longer. Recently a great deal of interest has been generated in measuring estrogen and progesterone receptors in endometrial cancer to attempt the prediction of hormonal responsiveness. This concenpt has proven useful for breast cancer but remains a research tool for endometrial cancer. Patients who fail to respond to hormonal therapy can be treated with cytotoxic chemotherapy. Doxorubicin has a response rate of approximately 40 percent.

Uterine Sarcomas

There are many names and classifications for the uterine sarcomas. Essentially there are three main types: leimyosarcoma, endometrial stromal sarcoma, and mixed mesodermal sarcomas. Leimyosarcomas arise from the myometrium. These occur mainly in postmenopausal women and present with abnormal uterine bleeding or as a pelvic mass. The mitotic count of the lesion is correlated with aggressiveness. Lesions with greater than 10 mitotic figures per 10 high power microscopic fields have a worse prognosis. Leimyosarcoma is treated by TAH BSO. Adjuvant radiation therapy does not increase survival but may increase local control. Many advocate adjuvant chemotherapy. The overall survival is about 40 percent.

Endometrial stromal sarcomas occur predominantly in postmenopausal women. The stromal nodule is a well-circumscribed collection of endometrial stroma and is benign. Endolymphatic stromal myosis is a low-grade sarcoma that tends to occur in premenopausal women who present with abnormal uterine bleeding or pain. Treatment is TAH BSO. Recurrences are late. Endometrial stromal sarcoma presents with postmenopausal bleeding and pain. Diagnosis is made by curettage. Treatment is TAH BSO. Again, radiation therapy will increase local control. Widespread disease is treated with chemotherapy.

Mixed mesodermal sarcomas are tumors in which the endometrial glands and stroma are both malignant. If the malignant tissue contains elements that are usually found in the uterus, it is termed homologous type. It is called heterologous if it contains elements not normally associated with the uterus, like cartilage, fat, or muscles. These patients usually present with abnormal uterine bleeding and frequently a mass is seen to protrude from the uterus. Treatment is total abdominal hysterectomy, bilateral salpingo-oophrectomy. Radiation therapy will increase local control but may not increase survival. Many advocate chemotherapy for all mixed mesodermal sarcomas. Doxorubicin is presently the drug of choice.

FALLOPIAN TUBE

Salpingitis

The fallopian tubes are subject to a variety of infectious processes. Salpingitis is one aspect of the clinical problem of pelvic inflammatory disease. Acute salpingitis can be gonococcal or nongonococcal, about equally divided. Organisms other than *Neisserea* include anaerobic bacteria, particularly Bacteroides species, *E coli,* aerobic and anerobic streptococci, and the increasingly recognized *Chlamydia trachomitus.* Patients present with pelvic pain, fever, vaginal discharge, and less commonly, nausea, vomiting, and urinary symptoms. On examination there will be lower abdominal tenderness, adnexal tenderness and exquisite tenderness on cervical motion. The clinical diagnosis of salpingitis is confirmed in only 65 percent of cases. The diagnosis can be supported by culturing *Neisseria* from the endocervix. Endocervical cultures for other organisms are less reliable. Culdocentesis and culturing peritoneal fluid will in-

crease the diagnostic accuracy. In questionable cases, laparoscopy with visualization of the pelvic organs and cultures will confirm the diagnosis. The tubes appear reddened, edematous, swollen, and purulent material can be seen dripping from the tubes. Treatment is as outlined previously for pelvic inflammatory disease. Salpingitis compromises future fertility by increasing tubal scarring. The fertility rate decreases with increasing episodes of pelvic infection.

Salpingitis Isthmica Nodosum

Salpingitis isthmica nodosum (SIN) was felt to be the aftermath of previous pelvic infection but this is not universally accepted. SIN may be an incidental finding at surgery. The patients may be infertile. Hysterosalpingography reveals stippled diverticula in the isthmic portion of the tubes. Direct palpation will reveal nodules in the tubal isthmus.

Tuberculosis Pelvic Infection

Genital tuberculosis is almost always secondary to systemic infection of pulmonary or gastrointestinal origin. It is very uncommon in the United States. Tuberculosis pelvic infection can involve the tubes and endometrium and manifest itself as pelvic infection and infertility. The diagnosis is made by acid-fast staining and culturing curettage or surgical specimens. Antibiotic therapy with antituberculous drugs will spare life but the prognosis for normal fertility is very poor.

Actinomycoces

Actinomycoces infection of the tubes is caused by a bacterial organism *Actinomycoces israeli.* This agent has been found to be responsible for pelvic infection particularly in intrauterine device users. The diagnosis is frequently made by a Pap smear. Treatment is penicillin.

Ectopic Pregnancy

Ectopic pregnancy is any pregancy that occurs in a location other than the endometrial cavity. Sites include the abdomen, cervix, tube, and ovary. It is discussed with tubal disease because 95 percent of the cases occur in the tubes. Any condition that alters tubal motility may predispose to tubal pregnancy (i.e., previous tubal infection and scarring, pelvic adhesions, previous tubal surgery, congenital defects, and distorting tumors such as myomas or endometriosis). Any of these conditions can retard the passage of the fertilized ovum to the endometrial cavity. The zygote, so impeded, then implants in the tube, and trophoblastic tissue invades the tubal wall.

Maternal blood vessels are tapped. As the pregnancy grows, the tube distends. The tube is less distensible than the endometrial cavity and therefore cannot support an advanced pregnancy. The fate of a tubal pregnancy are two. The pregnancy can abort out the tubal fimbria. This situation probably occurs more commonly than it is clinically recognized. Tubal abortions are usually nonviable but an occasional one may reimplant as an abdominal pregnancy. The other fate is tubal rupture. This can occur between the leaves of the broad ligament leading to the so-called chronic ectopic. The most common situation is tubal rupture of the products of conception into the free peritoneal cavity. This can lead to profuse intraperitoneal bleeding.

The classical presentation of tubal pregnancy is a patient with a 6-week history of amenorrhea who then develops vaginal bleeding. Quickly the patient develops severe abdominal and pelvic pain and perhaps syncope. Examination reveals a tender unilateral adnexal mass or a bulge in the cul-de-sac secondary to intraperitoneal blood. These symptoms and signs are sufficiently variable such that is must be stated that ectopic pregnancy must be considered in any woman of reproductive age who has pelvic pain. In one-half of the cases, there is no history of delayed menses. Pain may be steady or crampy, dull or sharp, and there may or may not be any associated pregnancy symptoms. Pregnancy tests are positive in no greater than 50 percent of cases though the newer more sensitive tests will be positive more frequently. Pulse and blood pressure may be normal if the ectopic is not yet ruptured. A pelvic mass is palpable in only 50 percent of cases. The differential diagnosis includes salpingitis, ovarian torsion, appendicitis, and corpus luteum cyst. There are several diagnostic aids. Sonography if it reveals an intrauterine pregnancy makes an ectopic pregnancy extremely unlikely. Culdocenteses, the introduction of a needle into the cul-de-sac, is effective in demonstrating intraperitoneal blood. If nonclotting blood is obtained, immediate laparotomy is indicated. A negative culdocenteses does not rule out an ectopic. Laparoscopy is the introduction of a fiberoptic device into the peritoneal cavity via a small incision in the anterior abdominal wall. A tubal pregnancy will appear as an enlarged bluish area in the tube. In patients with intraperitoneal bleeding or abdominal catastrophe, laparotomy is the diagnostic technique of choice.

The treatment of ectopic pregnancy is surgical. The most frequently utilized technique is salpingectomy. This is in addition to blood and fluid replacement. The ipsilateral ovary need not be sacrificed. If the opposite tube is absent or damaged, a salpingostomy may be done, the pregnancy removed and the defect repaired. The chance of a repeat tubal pregnancy is high. The overall recurrence rate is between 10 to 25 percent.

Ovarian pregnancy comprises 1 percent of all ectopic pregnancies. Treatment is salpingo-oophrectomy. Cervical pregnancy is a rare situation. Treatment usually necessitates hysterectomy. Overall ectopic pregnancy occurs in 1 in 200 pregnancies in the United States. There are subgroups with higher incidences. Ectopic pregnancy unfortunately is responsible for 10 percent of maternal deaths. It is estimated that three-quarters of these deaths could be avoided by early diagnosis and prompt treatment.

Abdominal Pregnancy

Most ectopic pregnancies seldom survive beyond 2 to 3 months of gestation. Abdominal pregnancies can go to term. It may be discovered by abnormal fetal lie and by the failure of the cervix to dilate during labor. Treatment is laparotomy and removal of the fetus. Management of the placenta is controversial but most advocate leaving it in situ where it will be resorbed.

Tubal Neoplasia

Tubal neoplasia is more commonly malignant than benign. Tubal carcinomas are adenocarcinomas for the most part. The classic symptom of hydrops tubae profluens (colicky pain followed by watery vaginal discharge) is less common than vaginal bleeding as a presenting symptom. The diagnosis is usually made when surgery is undertaken for other reasons. The disease is staged as outlined below for ovarian cancer. Treatment is surgical excision, debulking, and chemotherapy.

OVARY

The ovary is subject to a wide variety of cystic and solid tumors, both benign and malignant. In general, there is an increased risk of malignancy of the ovary with advancing age.

Non-neoplastic Cysts

Follicular cysts of the ovary result from unruptured and enlarged follicles. The enlargements can rupture causing peritoneal irritation or undergo torsion leading to acute pain. More commonly they regress spontaneously. They are seldom greater than 10 cm in size and most are asymptomatic. Treatment is expectant. Most will regress within one to two menstrual cycles. Oral contraceptives may hasten resolution. If there is no resolution, laparotomy is indicated.

Corpus luteum cysts are less common and more often symptomatic. The menstrual period may be delayed.

Rupture will cause intraperitoneal bleeding. This picture is similar to that seen with tubal pregnancy. Management in unruptured cases is the same as that for a follicle cyst. Ruptured corpus luteum cysts need immediate laparotomy. Other nonneoplastic enlargements include endometriomas and polycystic ovaries.

Ovarian Neoplasms

The true ovarian neoplasms are outlined below. This classification is based on tissues normally found in the ovary.

    Neoplasms of the germinal epithelium
        Serous—cystadenoma, borderline, cystadenocarcinoma
        Mucinous—cystadenoma, borderline, cystadenocarcinoma
        Endometriod—cystadenoma, borderline, cystadenocarcinoma
        Clear cell—cystadenoma, borderline, cystadenocarcinoma
        Brenner tumor
    Neoplasms of the germ cells
        Teratoma—dermoid
        Immature teratoma
        Dysgermenoma
        Endodermal sinus tumor
        Embryonal carcinoma
        Choriocarcinoma
        Gonadoblastoma
    Neoplasms of the gonadol stroma
        Granulosa thecal tumors
        Sertoli-Leydig cell tumors
    Neoplasms of nonspecific mesenchyme
    Metastatic tumors to the ovary

Epithelial Neoplasms

The epithelial neoplasms are the most common group of ovarian tumors. They occur predominantly in the older age group. In each histologic group, there is a benign lesion (i.e., serous cystadenoma), a borderline lesion, and a frankly malignant cancer (i.e., mucinous cystadenocarcinoma). The benign lesions present as masses in the pelvis that do not regress over time. The serous cystadenomas are the most common and account for 25 percent of all benign ovarian neoplasms. They occur in the reproductive age group and are bilateral in 15 percent of cases. Mucinous cystadenomas make up 15 percent of all ovarian neoplasms and are as a rule, unilateral. They are the largest tumors of the ovary. Benign endometroid and clear cell tumors are rare. Treatment is surgical excision. The Brenner tumor is composed of a transitional-like epithelium in a fibrous stroma. It is frequently discovered as an incidental finding at laparotomy. It is rarely malignant.

For many years it has been known that there is a subgroup of ovarian epithelial lesions that clinically have a natural history which is less malignant than frankly invasive lesions. These borderline or low malignant potential lesions histologically have epithelial proliferation but no invasion of the stroma. They are slow growing and can recur late. Treatment is surgical excision for low-stage tumors. Higher stage lesions may benefit from adjuvant chemotherapy.

Ovarian cancers are staged by the operative findings as outlined below:

    Stage I   —tumors confined to the ovary
    Stage IA —limited to one ovary
    Stage IB —limited to both ovaries
    Stage IC —IA or IB lesions associated with ascites or positive peritoneal washings
    Stage II   —tumors with pelvic extension
    Stage IIA—extension to the uterus or tubes
    Stage IIB—extension to other pelvic tissues
    Stage IIC—IIA or IIB with ascites or positive peritoneal washings
    Stage III —peritoneal metastases above the pelvis or positive retroperitoneal lymph nodes
    Stage IV —distant metastatic disease or parenchymal liver metastases.

Malignant Epithelial Neoplasms

These tumors are the true ovarian epithelial cancers and make up 85 percent of all malignant ovarian neoplasms. They occur, in general, in the post-menopausal age group. Nearly three-quarters of patients will have stage III disease at diagnosis. Symptoms occur late and are nonspecific. Patients will have a history of nonspecific gastrointestinal complaints, weight loss, urinary complaints, and pelvic heaviness. Unfortunately, in many the diagnosis is not suspected until gross ascites occurs. Ascites in any postmenopausal woman must raise the suspicion of ovarian carcinoma. Examination will reveal a fluid wave and shifting dullness. Pelvic examination reveals pelvic masses that are typically multinodular. Nodularity may be felt on the uterosacral ligaments. The workup of patients with suspected ovarian carcinoma includes chest x-ray, intravenous pyelogram, and barium enema. The barium enema is particularly important to rule out colon cancer, which is a frequent lesion to metastasize to the ovaries, and to assess the invasion or lack of invasion of the colon by ovarian cancer.

The first step in the treatment of epithelial ovarian

malignancies is laparotomy. The goal of this sugery is to remove all tumor if at all possible. This usually involves TAH BSO and excision of metastatic implants. In younger women with Stage IA, Grade I mucinous lesions, unilateral salpingo-ophorectomy may be done. Prior to this decision, the patient must have had a complete staging workup. Areas known to have a high-risk of involvement must be histologically reviewed. These are the omentum, peritoneal surfaces, and undersurface of the diaphragm. The yield on biopsy of these areas even when there is no clinically apparent tumor, approaches 15 percent. It is becoming increasingly apparent that ovarian cancer can spread to the retroperitoneal lymph nodes, so these also should be biopsied and histologically reviewed. In actual fact, the ideal of total tumor removal is seldom possible. Most patients have Stage III diagnosis at presentation. The concept of surgical debulking is now well-established. This states that in patients with stage III or IV disease, in whom all tumors cannot be removed, it is of value to make any residual disease as small as possible. These patients respond better to subsequent therapy.

The majority of patients with epithelial ovarian cancer deserve further therapy. Radiation therapy to the whole pelvis was widely used in the past but much less frequently now. The major modality is cytotoxic chemotherapy. A variety of agents have been used. Classically alkylating agents were used. For Stage I and II lesions, alkylating agents are still used with proven efficacy. Patients with Stage III or IV disease or patients with residual disease are treated with multiple agent chemotherapy. Several combinations have been used and most include an alkylating agent. A very effective combination is doxorubicin, cyclophosphamide, and *cis*-platinum. Patients who achieve a complete response clinically are taken to second look laparotomy. At this surgery, the completeness of the response is assessed. If patients have no disease at second look laparotomy, chemotherapy can be stopped with the knowledge that 80 percent of patients will be alive in 5 years. Those patients with disease can be treated with second-line agents but the response is poor. The above therapeutic outline has been shown to increase the patient's quality of life and to increase the time to recurrence, but a 5-year survival advantage remains to be documented.

Germ Cell Tumors of the Ovary

Germ cell tumors constitute 15 to 20 percent of all ovarian neoplasms. They are a group with diverse clinical and biologic behavior. The ovarian teratoma or dermoid is a benign lesion with all three germ cell layers represented. The tumor can contain a variety of tissues, hair and teeth are very common. Ectodermally derived tissues are the most common germ layer to be repre-

sented. This occurs in less than 1 percent of dermoids. Dermoids are usually discovered as asymptomatic masses. Calcifications within the dermoid can be seen on x-ray of the abdomen. Most are unilateral. Only 5 percent are bilateral. Malignant transformation recurs in 1 percent of the cases. The malignancy most commonly found is epidermoid cancer. Treatment is surgical removal.

Immature teratoma is an ovarian malignancy of young women and children. These lesions are very aggressive. Most are Stage I at diagnosis and present with pelvic pain. Treatment is surgical removal usually by salpingo-oophorectomy. This is followed by chemotherapy. Using the treatment outlined, childbearing capacity has been preserved.

Dysgerminoma is also seen in young women. It is frequently found in intersex individuals associated with gonadoblastoma. This tumor is analogous to the seminoma in the male. It has a predilection for lymph node metastases. Treatment is surgical excision. Recurrences can be treated with radiotherapy to which the tumor is very sensitive.

Endodermal sinus tumor is also found in young women who present with pelvic pain of relatively brief duration. Most are stage I at diagnosis. This tumor secretes alpha-fetoprotein (AFP), which is a reliable indicator of disease. Treatment is surgical removal followed by chemotherapy.

Embryonal carcinoma occurs in very young women with an average age at diagnosis of 14 years. Patients present with pelvic mass or pain. Most are stage I. The tumor can secrete both AFP and HCG. Treatment is surgical removal followed by chemotherapy.

Ovarian choriocarcinoma is a very rare lesion which occurs in young women. Patients present with pain and a pelvic mass. The tumor secretes HCG. Treatment is surgical removal followed by chemotherapy.

Gonadoblastoma occurs in intersex individuals. These patients present with primary amenorrhea, virilization, and developmental abnormalities of the genitalia. They are themselves benign but are frequently associated with other malignant germ cell tumors. Hence the recommendation that the gonads be removed in intersex individuals.

The germ cell tumors frequently are mixed with dysgerminoma being the most common element. These tumors take on the biologic behavior of the most aggressive element.

Stromal Tumors of the Ovary

Between 5 and 10 percent of ovarian tumors rise from the gonadal stroma. They have a propensity to secrete steroids, thus, the designation functioning tumors.

Granulosa cell tumors should be considered low-grade malignancies. They usually secrete estrogens but occasionally secrete androgens. They usually present with estrogenic manifestations such as abnormal uterine bleeding or precocious puberty. Pain is secondary to rupture and they may present as an asymptomatic mass. In 15 prcent of cases, there is a coexisting endometrial cancer. Treatment is surgical removal. Recurrences can occur very late, greater than 20 years from treatment and they are treated with radiation or chemotherapy.

Thecomas are benign lesions that are typically unilateral and asymptomatic. Treatment is surgical excision.

Ovarian neoplasms that tend toward testicular differentiation are termed Sertoli-Leydig cell tumors or the older term arrhenoblastomas. These tumors secrete androgens and therefore masculinize or virilize female patients. They occur in women of reproductive age. Treatment is surgical removal. Many of the masculine features will resolve after removal but hirsutism and clitoromegaly may not.

Tumors of Ovarian Nonspecific Mesenchyme

The most common tumors of non-specific mesenchyme are fibromas and lymphomas. Ovarian fibromas are benign. An interesting clinical entity is Meig's syndrome in which an ovarian fibroma is associated with ascites and pleural effusions. These resolve with removal of the fibroma.

The most common metastatic tumors to the ovary are breast, colon, and endometrial cancers. Virtually any malignancy in the female has been found metastatic to the ovary. The Krukenberg tumor is a signet ring-cell lesion that is metastatic from a stomach primary. These bilateral lesions are also seen with colon cancers.

GESTATIONAL TROPHOBLASTIC DISEASE

Gestational trophoblastic disease is a triad of diseases including hydatidiform mole or molar pregnancy, chorioadenoma destruens, or invasive mole and choriocarcinoma. These entities are unique in that they universally secrete HCG, are extremely sensitive to chemotherapy, and that the karyotype though XX is of paternal origin.

Hydatiform mole is characterized by trophoblastic tissue that is grossly vesicular and by the absence of an embryo. The incidence varies throughout the world with the incidence in the United States of 1 per 2000 pregnancies. The etiology is unknown. Patients present with the passage of grape-like clusters of tissue or with bleeding during the first half of pregnancy. There may be nausea, vomiting, or preeclampsia in early pregnancy. Classi-

cally the molar pregnancy was stated to be large for expected dates but this occurs in only 50 percent of cases. There are no fetal heart tones audible. There may be enlarged ovaries bilterally, theca-lutein cyst. The diagnosis may be supported by a higher than expected level of HCG. Ultrasonography is the most reliable diagnostic tool. Treatment of molar pregnancy can be accomplished by a variety of techniques including dilatation and curettage, hysterectomy, hysterotomy, and suction evacuation. Suction evacuation of the uterine contents is the treatment of choice. If the patient desires no further childbearing, hysterectomy can be done. Following evacuation, the patient needs to be followed closely so that gestational trophoblastic disease can promptly be discovered and treated. This is aided by the measurement of Beta-HCG in the serum. The presence of Beta-HCG in the serum is a reliable marker for the presence of viable trophoblastic tissue. The Beta-HCG titer is measured weekly until the titers become undetectable and monthly thereafter for 1 year. Pregnancy during this period is proscribed. Pelvic examination is also done frequently to follow the resolution of theca-lutein cysts if they are present.

If the HCG titer rises or plateaus during the followup, it is indicative of persistent trophoblastic disease. These patients are evaluated for the presence of metastatic disease and are started on chemotherapy. If there is metastatic disease, it is termed metastatic gestational trophoblastic neoplasia (choriocarcinoma) and it is termed non-metastatic disease (invasive mole or chorioadenoma destruens) if there is no evidence of metastases. These entities make up the spectrum of malignant trophoblastic disease.

Nonmetastatic trophoblastic disease is the most common. These patients have disease limited to the uterus. They can be treated with single agent chemotherapy with either methotrexate or actinomycin-D. Patients are treated every two weeks until the HCG titer reverts to normal and one further course of chemotherapy is then given. If the titer rises or plateaus during this time, the patient should receive triple agent chemotherapy. This therapy for nonmetastatic thophoblastic disease is nearly 100 percent successful and fertility can be preserved.

Metastatic trophoblastic disease is divided into good prognosis (low-risk) and poor prognosis (high-risk) disease. The criteria are described in Table 10-5.

Patients with metastatic disease can be discovered during postmolar pregnancy surveillance by a rising titer, when vaginal bleeding persists after pregnancy or discovered in a variety of othr clinical situations. Metastatic trophoblastic disease or choriocarcinoma occurs after followup of molar pregnancy in 50 percent of cases, after a normal pregnancy in 25 percent of cases, or after a

Table 10-5. Criteria for Prognosis of Metastatic Trophoblastic Disease

Factors	Low-Risk	High-Risk
Duration	< 4 months from prior pregnancy	> 4 months from prior pregnancy
Pre-treatment titer of HCG	Urine: < 100,000 IU/24 hours Serum: < 40,000 IU/ml	Urine: > 100,000 IU/24 hours Serum: > 40,000 IU/ml
Site of metastases	Lungs—no brain or liver metastases	Brain or liver metastases
Prior chemotherapy	None	Significant

prior abortion or ectopic pregnancy in 25 percent of cases. Once disease is discovered, liver, and brain x-ray studies are undertaken. If lesions are found in these areas, they should immediately be irradiated. This is done for its hemostatic effect. Patients with low-risk disease can be treated with single agent chemotherapy as outlined above. Patients are treated with one course of chemotherapy after a negative titer is obtained. The overall success rate in good prognosis metastatic disease, approaches 100 percent. Patients with high-risk disease are begun on triple agent chemotherapy with methotrexate, actinomycin-D, and cyclophosphomide. These patients are followed with titers and are also treated with one course of chemotherapy after a negative titer is obtained. The success rate is approximately 66 percent.

FERTILITY CONTROL

There are three general methods of fertility control or family planning: contraception, abortion, and sterilization. Contraceptive methods include hormonal and nonhormonal methods.

Oral Contraceptives

The main hormonal method of birth control is the oral contraceptive pill. Birth control pills have theoretical effectiveness of 100 percent and actual use approaches this ideal. Birth control pills came about following the synthesis of orally active estrogens and progestins. Most birth control pills used today, contain a combination of an estrogen and a progestin taken for 21 days followed by 1 week of no medication. During this week, withdrawal uterine bleeding normally occurs. The birth control pills work by a variety of mechanisms including inhibition of ovulation, creating of hostile cervical mucus, creation of an unfavorable endometrial lining and alteration of tubal transport. The pill is begun on the fifth day of the menstrual period. Over the years, the dosage of estrogen in birth control pills has gradually decreased. This has

decreased the incidence of side-effects, as most side-effects are dose-related. Lower estrogen dosage may increase the incidence of bleeding or spotting while taking the pill because of low estrogen doses may not be sufficient to support the endometrium. The dosage must be adjusted for each individual patient.

Oral contraceptive pills have side-effects. Metabolic changes include changes in lipid profiles with an increase in total cholesterol and triglycerides. Plasma binding globulins are increased including thyroxin binding globulin and transcortin. Diabetics may have an alteration in their insulin dose and diabetes is considered a relative contraindication by many. Users have a somewhat increased incidence of gall bladder disease. Cardiovascular effects have received a great deal of attention. Users have an apparently sixfold greater risk of thrombosis and pulmonary embolism. This is due to alterations in blood coagulation factors. Arterial accidents including strokes and myocardial infarctions are estimated to be four times greater for users over nonusers. These effects are seen mostly in older women who are smokers. In women under age 35 who are not smokers, these risks are not significantly different for users versus nonusers. As women become older, after age 35 the incidence of these cardiovascular side-effects increases even more markedly for women who smoke.

Hypertension is associated with the use of birth control pill. The increased blood pressure occurs rarely and is in mild degrees in most patients. It is reversible with discontinuation of the medication. A variety of other effects including increased *Candida* infections, hyperpigmentation, acne, and weight gain may occur. Not frequently discussed are the health benefits of the birth control use, in addition to those obtained by preventing pregnancy complications. Users of birth control pills have been shown to have a lower incidence of pelvic inflammatory disease, rheumatoid arthritis, and malignancies of the endometrium and ovary.

Progestins have been used alone. Oral agents given continuously, the so-called mini pill, prevent pregnancy by causing an unfavorable endometrium and a hostile cervical mucus. Injectable progesterone agents (i.e., medroxyprogesterone acetate) have the advantage of three monthly injections. This agent is not marketed in the United States due to concerns over possible carcinogenicity. Postcoital contraception or the "morning-after pill" works by preventing implantation. High-dose oral estrogens are given after unprotected intercourse. The only agent licensed in the United States is Diethylstilbestrol.

Intrauterine Devices

Intrauterine devices IUDs have the advantage of being inserted and then needing no further action by the patient. She does not need to remember pills or barriers. There are two types: inert and drug-release devices. The mechanism of the inert devices is not well established but probably prevents implantation. Copper devices continuously release copper into the uterine cavity and by an unknown mechanism prevent implantation. They need to be replaced every 3 years. Progesterone-releasing devices appear to have less cramping and bleeding associated with their use and need to be replaced yearly. The theoretical effectiveness of IUDs in general is better than 95 percent.

IUDs do have side effects. The uterus can be perforated during insertion. When perforation is unrecognized, later peritonitis and bowel obstructions have been reported. Most women report increased cramping and menstrual bleeding. Pelvic infections have been described. Unilateral tubo-ovarian abscesses have been described with IUD use. It has been said that IUDs increase tubal pregnancies. This is probably not true but rather that the pregnancies that do occur with an IUD in situ are more apt to be ectopic. If pregnancy does occur with an IUD, it should be removed if the string is visible. This decreases subsequent late abortion and sepsis. If the string is not visible, it should be left in situ.

Local Methods

Local methods include diaphragms, condoms, vaginal spermicides in the form of foams or suppositories, and the recently marketed vaginal sponge. The effectiveness of condoms and diaphragms is increased by the concurrent use of a spermicidal agent. Barrier methods have success rates of greater than 80 percent if used correctly and with every act of intercourse. Spermicidal agents alone are less successful.

The ovum is suspectible to fertilization for only approximately 24 hours. The rhythm methods attempt to exploit this for contraception by avoiding intercourse during the so-called fertile period. Ovulation occurs 12 to 16 days prior to the subsequent menstrual period. The couple avoids intercourse around this time as judged by the previous cycle lengths. The addition of basal body temperature charts and observing changes in cervical mucus increases the effectiveness of rhythm methods. Overall success rates in motivated couples approach 80 percent.

Abortion

Abortion as a method of fertility control has increased in usage in the past decades. Indeed barrier birth control methods with first trimester abortion as backup is the safest method of birth control in terms of total mortality. First trimester elective abortions are best accomplished by suction curettage. This can occur with either general or local anesthesia. The major complications are uterine perforation and incomplete removal of the products of conception with possible late bleeding and sepsis. Suction evacuation techniques are now being used for pregnancies that are further along than the first trimester. Second trimester abortions can be accomplished by the intraamniotic injection of hypertonic saline or prostaglandins. The addition of intravenous Pitocin decreases the time to evacuation. Complications of hypertonic saline include sepsis, injury to each of the pelvic viscera, intravascular injection of saline, and disseminated intravascular coagulation. Live births have been reported after the use of prostaglandins.

Sterilization

Sterilization can be accomplished by tubal interruption or hysterectomy in the female and by vasectomy in the male. These methods are to be considered irreversible. Tubal interruption can be accomplished by a variety of techniques. All involve removing or destroying a portion of both fallopian tubes to prevent ovum transport. This can be accomplished after a delivery or as an interval procedure. Interval procedures can be done by laparotomy or via laparoscopy. Complications are mainly those of anesthesia and surgery. It has been stated that menstrual irregularities occur after tubal ligation. When factors such as previous menstrual history, previous birth control use and aging of the patient are considered, there does not apear to be any significant change. Success rates for tubal interruption are greater than 99 percent. Hysterectomy is a viable option for sterilization when other pelvic abnormalities are present.

Male sterilization or vasectomy has become increasingly popular. Vasectomy is a relatively simple and safe procedure. The major disadvantage is that sterility is not immediate. Complete expulsion of sperm from the distal reproductive structures may take weeks.

REFERENCES

Burrow GN and Ferris TN (eds): Medical Complications During Pregnancy, 2nd Ed. WB Saunders: Philadelphia, 1982
The second edition of this text is considered one of the most comprehensive and well written surveys of medical disorders complicating pregnancy. Although not limited to a discussion of medical diseases alone (there are sections on fetal surveillance, genetic disorders, and congenital infections), the discussion of cardiac, hematologic, and thyroid disorders complicating pregnancy are first-rate.

DiSaia PJ, Creasman WT: Clinical Gynecologic Oncology. CV Mosby, St. Louis, 1980
A readable text that begins each chapter with an outline of the entities to be discussed. The clinical manifestation of each disease are well outlined. Management of each disease is discussed in detail. Controversial areas are presented as such with literature reviews.

Pritchard JA and McDonald PC: Williams Obstetrics. 16th Ed. Appleton-Century-Crofts, New York, 1980
Williams Obstetrics has become the virtual cornerstone of obstetric written education since the turn of the century. It is well organized and illustrated to highlight strengths in discussing placental hormones and precursors, morphologic development of the placenta and fetus, initiation of parturition and techniques in providing obstetric care. It is an especially good text in dealing with prenatal, intrapartum and postpartum obstetric complications of mothers and fetus/infant.

Speroff, Glass, Kase: Clinical Gynecologic Endocrinology and Infertility. 2nd Ed. Williams & Wilkins, Baltimore, 1978
A very readable text that first reviews the underlying physiology and pathophysiology of gynecologic endocrinology. Specific problems are each given a chapter. Each problem has algorhythms presented that take one through an organized diagnostic and therapeutic program.

Romney SI, Gray MJ, Little AB, et al: Gynecology and Obstetrics—The Health Care of Women. 2nd Ed. McGraw-Hill, New York, 1981
This compendium of up-to-date information is the shared work of many active clinicians. It is attuned to studying women as individuals whose psycho-socio-sexual makeup is important in both health and disease. The text covers several areas of health and disease prevention quite well and has clearly written sections on maternal nutrition and reproductive genetics.

Romney SI, Gray MJ, Little AB et al: Gynecology and Obstetrics. The Health Care of Women. McGraw-Hill, New York, 1975
A multi-authored text that is organized in five major sections. The first is an overview of the specialty of obstetrics and gynecology. The second reviews the etiology of disease. The third approaches patient care in terms of different age groups. The fourth reviews signs and symptoms of disease. And the final section reviews specific problems in an organ related fashion.

MULTIPLE CHOICE QUESTIONS

Each question below contains four suggested answers of which one or more is correct. Choose the answer

A	if 1, 2, and 3 are correct
B	if 1 and 3 are correct
C	if 2 and 4 are correct
D	if 4 is correct
E	if 1, 2, 3, and 4 are correct

1. Tests of amniotic fluid that are clinically useful in evaluating the fetus include determination of
   1. Chromosomal abnormalities
   2. Fetal sex
   3. Metabolic disorders
   4. Amniotic fluid pH

2. A 24-year-old nulligravid woman who was exposed to diethylstilbestrol (DES) in utero wants to have children. She should be told that she is at increased risk for
   1. Preterm delivery
   2. Twins
   3. First trimester loss
   4. Abruptio placentae

3. A pregnant woman has macrocytic anemia and a low serum folate level. Which of the following should be expected?
   1. Hypersegmented neutrophils on maternal peripheral blood smear
   2. Fetal macrocytic anemia
   3. Megaloblastic maternal bone marrow
   4. Low fetal serum folate level

4. Preeclampsia is defined as severe if the preeclamptic woman develops
   1. Thrombocytopenia
   2. Pulmonary edema
   3. Epigastric pain
   4. Sustained blood pressure of 160/110 mm Hg or greater

5. Causes of vaginal discharge can be
   1. Monilia
   2. Trichomonas
   3. Gardenerella
   4. Syphilis

6. Sexually transmitted diseases include
   1. Herpes
   2. Gonorrhea
   3. Syphilis
   4. Condyloma accuminata

Choose the best answer

7. A pregnant patient with a congenital heart defect has no symptoms of dyspnea, angina, or palpitations at rest, but ordinary activity causes these symptoms. According to the New York Heart Association's functional classification, she is
   A. Class I

B. Class II
C. Class III
D. Class IV
E. Class intermediate

8. In the nursing mother, mastitis
   A. Usually occurs in the second or third week of the puerperium
   B. Is frequently caused by *Escherichia coli*
   C. Is best treated by weaning the infant
   D. Is usually bilateral
   E. Usually requires surgical drainage

9. Which of the following accounts for the largest amount of weight gain during a normal pregnancy?
   A. Uterus
   B. Placenta
   C. Amniotic fluid
   D. Blood
   E. Breasts

10. A pregnant woman at 15 weeks' gestation is found to have an elevated serum alpha-fetoprotein concentration. The next step in evaluating this patient should be
    A. Repeat serum alpha-fetoprotein determination
    B. Amniography
    C. Amniocentesis
    D. Abortion
    E. Ultrasonography

11. Thromboembolic episodes most commonly occur in association with which of the following?
    A. Oral contraceptive use
    B. Intrauterine device use
    C. Diaphragm use
    D. Puerperium
    E. Estrogen use for relief of vasomotor symptoms

12. The standard dose (300 µg) of Rh immune globulin (RhoGAM) is sufficient to neurtralize how many milliliters of Rh-positive erythrocytes?
    A. 5
    B. 15
    C. 30
    D. 45
    E. 60

13. All of the following are true about cervical intraepithelial neoplasia (CIn) except
    A. Multiple sexual patterns decrease the incidence
    B. The Pap smear is an appropriate screening test
    C. Younger age at first coitus is associated with an increased incidence
    D. Definitive diagnoses requires histology

14. The most common invasive genital malignancy in the United States is
    A. Cervical
    B. Vulvar
    C. Ovarian
    D. Endometrial

15. The most effective reversible form of birth control is
    A. Intra-uterine device (IUD)
    B. Oral contraceptive pill
    C. Barrier methods
    D. Sterilization

16. All of the following are true about the urogenital diaphragm except
    A. It lies superficial to the pelvic diaphragm
    B. It is bounded by the pubic symphysis and ischial tuberosities
    C. It is penetrated by the urethra
    D. Its major contributor is the levator ani

17. FSH, LH, β-HCG share a similar
    A. Alpha chain
    B. Beta chain
    C. Both
    D. Neither

18. The hormone responsible for a rise in basal body temperature is
    A. Estradiol
    B. Estrone
    C. Progesterone
    D. Cortisone

19. The first step in the work-up of amenorrhea in a 20-year-old patient is
    A. Progesterone challenge test
    B. Rule out pregnancy
    C. Endometrial biopsy
    D. Prolactin level

20. Galactorrhea can be caused by
    A. Pyridoxine
    B. Antibiotics
    C. Both
    D. Neither

Answers to Multiple-choice Questions

1 A	2 B	3 B	4 E	5 A
6 E	7 C	8 A	9 D	10 A
11 D	12 B	13 A	14 D	15 B
16 D	17 A	18 C	19 B	20 D

Pediatrics

John H. Straus and Mychelle Farmer

Pediatrics has changed drastically in the United States over the past 50 years. In 1930, infectious diseases accounted for over 60 percent of deaths, while today, this percentage has dropped to only 7 (Table 11-1). Accidents, mostly from motor vehicles, homicide, and suicide have become the new causes of death for children.

Although infant mortality has also dropped precipitously from 64.6 deaths per 100 live births in 1930 to 12.6 in 1980, the United States remains seventeenth on the list of countries with the lowest rates of infant mortality. Better prenatal care, the rise of neonatal intensive care units, and the emergence of the subspecialty of neonatology explain part of this decrease in infant mortality. However, more of the decrease in both infant and childhood mortality is related to improvements in the standard of living than changes in medical care. This chapter must deal in medical facts, but the student should remember that improvements in medical care will never equal the improvements in health achievable by better living conditions and healthier life-styles.

As serious infectious diseases have decreased, families have brought new concerns to the practitioner. Haggerty has termed these "the new morbidity" and they include behavior and family problems, learning problems, and problems of adolescence. Increasingly, training programs are stressing these areas.

PEDIATRIC HISTORY AND PHYSICAL EXAMINATION

In pediatric practices, the child, parent, or caretaker may provide the medical history. Each person brings their own perspective to a problem. Children begin talking at about age two to three and we often forget that the child may be an important source of information. The child may not answer direct history questions but will describe the problem in his own way. In addition, involvement of the child usually improves cooperation.

Pediatric Data Base

The proportion of time spent on each element of the pediatric data base will be tailored by the age of the child (Table 11-2). For many behavioral and chronic symptoms, having the parent describe a typical day is helpful to put the symptom into prospective.

For adults, the physical examination can proceed orderly from head to toe. With children, the examination should proceed from least to most invasive. Much information such as the general clinical state, degree of toxicity, appearance, and neurodevelopmental level are discernable from observation alone. Cardiac and abdominal exams are done early, while looking at the ears and mouth are left to last. For the younger child who exhibits stranger anxiety, the examination is best performed on the parent's lap. Relating appropriately to the patient and achieving cooperation remain major challenges in pediatrics.

GROWTH AND NUTRITION

Although nutrition is important to every physician, it is of special concern for those caring for children. They have the task of determining the nutritional needs of young, growing bodies. In addition, they must advise parents about meeting these nutritional needs. This is probably our most difficult job since the growth and

Table 11-1. Leading Causes of Death, United States 1975 (Ages 0 – 24)

Cause of Death	Percentage
Accidents	30
Neonatal Conditions	22
Congenital Anomalies	9
Infectious Diseases	7
Homicide	5
Neoplasms	5
Suicide	4
Cardiovascular Diseases	3
Other	15

Data from National Center for Health Statistics.

physical well-being of the child will depend heavily on food intake.

In infancy, the primary source of nourishment is either formula or breast milk. Breast milk has many advantages over formula, although it should be stressed that a formula fed baby is not compromised nutrition-

Table 11-2. Pediatric Data Base

Demographic data:
   Name (Nickname)   Date of birth
   Address   Telephone number
   Father   Age   Occupation
   Mother   Age   Occupation
   Insurance status

Chief complaint:

Present illness:

Past history:
   Prenatal (medications, illnesses, bleeding, toxemia)
   Birth (type of delivery, birth weight, complications)
   Postpartum (jaundice, feeding problems, other complications)
   Development
   Hospitalizations
   Operations
   Allergies
   Immunizations
   Usual childhood diseases

Routine areas of concern:
   Feeding
   Sleeping
   Stooling
   Behavior (temperament)

Family history:

Social history:
   Alternative caretakers
   Members of household (pets)
   Day care/school performance

Review of systems:

ally by this choice. Breast milk is preferred because it is readily available, sanitary, and generally less costly for the family. Human milk contains antibodies and other infection fighting substances which gives breast-fed infants a higher resistance to organisms entering the body through the gastrointestinal tract. Colostrum, the milk produced in the first week of life, is particularly high in anti-infective properties such as IgA. Breast-fed babies tend to have frequent, loose, yellow stools and are rarely constipated. Some physicians also believe that breast-fed children have fewer problems with allergies or obesity.

Both breast- and bottle-fed newborns are usually begun on a "demand" schedule feeding every 3 to 4 hours. Infants on formula initially take six 3 to 4 oz feedings per day. By 5 to 6 months of age, four 7 to 8 ounce feedings are usually adequate. The American Academy of Pediatrics recommends formula or breast milk through the first year of life. The addition of other food substances should not begin prior to 6 months of age. Whole milk is not introduced until the first birthday.

Formula as well as human milk contains 20 calories (cals) per ounce. A rule of thumb for calculating caloric requirements is as follows: 100 cals/kg for the first 10 kg, 50 cals/kg for the next 10 kg, and then 20 cals/kg for each additional kilogram. A 40 kg child would then require 1000 cals + 500 cals + 400 cals or 1,900 cals. Aside from calories, the diet must have the proper amount of vitamins and minerals as problems can arise from a vitamin or mineral deficiency or excess (Table 11-3). Vitamins

Table 11-3. Vitamin and Mineral Disorders

Nutrient	Disorder
Vitamin A	Deficiency causes loss of visual acuity, night blindness, and keratomalacia (softening and clouding of the cornea). Excess causes desquamation of skin, long bone pain, and pseudotumor cerebri.
Vitamin D	Deficiency causes bowing of lower extremities, frontal bossing, craniotabes, epiphyseal and costochondral widening (rachitic rosary), low serum phosphorus, elevated alkaline phosphatase. Excess causes nephorcalcinosis, nausea, anorexia, and elevated serum calcium.
Vitamin E	Deficiency state causes hemolytic anemia in the newborn.
Vitamin K	Deficiency usually occurs in newborns who do not receive a vitamin K injection, causing hemorrhagic disease of the newborn. Excess results in hemolytic anemia.
Iron	Deficiency produces a microcytic anemia.
Fluoride	Deficiency leads to less teeth with less caries. Excess causes fluorosis or mottling of the teeth.

A, D, E, and K described in Table 11-3 are fat soluble in contrast to the B complex and C vitamins which are water soluble. Iron fortified formula supplies the infant with a complete diet. Infants fed breast milk should be supplemented with vitamin D and fluoride. For humans the diet must also supply the essential amino acids and the essential fatty acid, linoleic acid.

With good nutrition, the child should grow normally. Appropriate growth is checked using standard height/weight charts. Continual assessment of height and weight, therefore, becomes an essential component of health maintenance visits. As long as the child follows a normal percentile, nutrition and growth are good. If the weight for height increases, obesity is recognized. If the weight drops off, then reasons for failure to thrive are assessed. A fall off in height raises the concerns of short stature (*see* p. 642). If growth curves are not handy, birth weights average 7 to 8 lbs. The infant can lose 10 percent of birth weight over the first several days, but the birth weight should be regained by 10 days of life. Babies then gain about one ounce per day. The birth weight is doubled by 5 months and tripled by 12 months. After 12 months, about 5 pounds are gained per year. Length at birth averages 50 cm, doubling by age 4 and tripling by age 13. The head circumference is also an important indicator of growth, especially brain growth. The head has reached 75 percent of its adult size by birth. Although six fontanels are present in the newborn period, only the anterior fontanel is open by 2 months of age and it closes before 18 months.

Puberty

The period of growth between 8 and 18 is known as puberty. During this time the child should achieve full adult sexual development accompanied by a growth spurt resulting in adult stature. Tanner has divided the changes of puberty into five stages from prepubertal, stage 1 to adult, stage 5 (Table 11-4). For males, Tanner staging includes evaluation of penile size, testicular size, and pubic hair type and distribution. For females, breast and pubic hair development are examined. Menarche occurs about 2 years after the start of breast development (thelarche). Girls generally are about 1 year ahead of boys in pubertal changes. Puberty should begin by age 14 in boys and age 13 in girls with menarche by age 16.

Failure to Thrive

Children who fail to gain weight need evaluation. Infants gain about 1 oz per day. Most failure to thrive is based on inadequate caloric intake either because of poverty, inadequate parental knowledge, parental neglect, or psychosocial deprivation. These children may need

Table 11-4. Stages of Sexual Development

Part of the Body	Development	Tanner Stage	Average Age of Onset (years)
Female			
Breasts	Breast buds develop	II	9–11
	Areolar development with breast enlargement	III–IV	12–13
	Adult breast without areolar projection	V	16–18
Genitals	Sparse and soft pubic hair	II–III	10–12
	Abundant coarse pubic hair	IV–V	11–15
	Vaginal secretions present		11–14
Axilla	Hair appears		12–14
Male			
Genitals	Enlargement of testes and scrotum	II	11–12
	Penile enlargement	III–IV	12–15
	Pubic hair sparse and long to slight curl	II–III	12–14
	Pubic hair abundant, coarse, curly	IV–V	13–16
Axilla	Hair appears		13–16
Facial and body hair	Hair appears		15–17

hospitalization to prove that growth is possible with normal nutrition. Various chronic diseases that may cause failure to thrive include hypothyroidism, cystic fibrosis and other diseases of malabsorption, metabolic diseases, renal, cardiac, and, liver disease, inflammatory bowel disease, mental retardation, and diencephalic syndrome.

PSYCHOSOCIAL DEVELOPMENT AND DISORDERS

In the last section, physical growth and development was discussed. In this section, we will focus on psychosocial development. Normal psychosocial development depends on the interaction between the child and his environment. This interaction should result in the child obtaining age-appropriate developmental skills and behaviors. The clinician first assesses the developmental level of the child and then determines whether the child is behaving appropriately for that developmental level.

Developmental Assessment

In the first approximately 4 years of life, intelligence testing is not possible and development is measured by assessing the child's progress in four areas: (1) gross motor; (2) fine motor; (3) language; and (4) personal-social. The more common developmental milestones used in each of the four areas and the average age that the particular milestone is usually achieved is given (Table 11-5). Table 11-5 also lists when 90 percent of children will accomplish the milestone. A delay past this age raises concern. Delays across all four areas usually suggest retardation (*see* p. 636) while a pure motor delay may occur with cerebral palsy (*see* cerebral palsy section) and a language delay may signify deafness. The Denver Developmental Screening Test is the most commonly used instrument to screen for abnormal development and the ages given in Table 11-5 are derived from this test.

Standard intelligence tests such as the Stanford-Binet and the Wechsler Intelligence Scale for Children (WISC) are available for use in children as young as age three.

Table 11-5. Developmental Milestones

Milestone	Age at Which 50% of Children Pass	Age at Which 90% of Children Pass
Gross motor		
Sit without support	6 months	8 months
Walks	12 months	14 months
Jumps	23 months	3 years
Hops on one foot	3.5–5 years	5 years
Fine Motor		
Reaches for object	4 months	5 months
Passes cube hand to hand	6 months	7 months
Pincer grasp	11 months	15 months
Copies circle	2.5 years	3.5 years
Copies cross	3.5 years	4.5 years
Copies square	4 years	6 years
Draw 3 part man	4 years	5 years
Language		
Laughs	2 months	4 months
Says dadda or mamma	10 months	12 months
Says three words, not dadda or mamma	13 months	20 months
Two word sentences	20 months	27 months
Gives complete name	27 months	3.5 years
Recognizes colors	3 years	4 years
Personal-social		
Initially shy with strangers	7 months	10 months
Drinks from cup	12 months	16 months
Uses spoon	15 months	25 months
Buttons	3 years	4 years

Children who are not achieving up to their grade level in school may be given one of these tests to determine the mental age level at which they are capable of learning.

Learning Disability

A learning problem exists when scholastic achievement testing falls behind mental age by greater than 1 to 2 years. For example, a 9-year-old fourth grader is achieving at the second grade level. On the WISC, a test of mental age, he scores at the 9 year level. This student would be classified as having a learning disability. If this same child had a mental age of seven, then he would be classified as retarded and functioning on an expected level. A learning problem may arise from an emotional disturbance or an inability to concentrate (attention deficit disorder).

Educational testing is used to identify the specific learning problem. For example, an inability to learn to read may be caused by a visual processing defect (dyslexia), an auditory processing defect, or the inability to associate visual and auditory information. For such a child, the practitioner can advocate to the school for a classroom setting that promotes the child's strengths and deals with his weak areas at the appropriate educational level. The physician also needs to be certain that the learning problem is not made worse by any auditory or visual loss.

Behavioral Problems

As serious infectious diseases have decreased, providers of health care to children are increasingly dealing with behavioral problems. The parent may not spontaneously complain about their child's behavior, but on questioning, the parent often has considerable concern. This section will discuss the more common behavioral problems.

COLIC

Colic is episodes of crying occurring in the first several months of life in an otherwise healthy baby. The parent often complains that the infant has increased amounts of gas or seems in pain, drawing up its legs. Colicky or "fussy" babies are now thought to be those with "difficult" temperaments. These babies are easily disturbed by external stimuli, have irregular sleep and feeding patterns, have increased activity levels, and are hard to calm. Mix a difficult temperament with a tense, hectic environment or a parent frantically trying to soothe their fussy infant and what is perceived as colic may result. Treatment is directed toward counselling the family that their infant's difficult temperament is not the result of poor parenting. Parents are also advised that crying behavior begins to diminish after 8 weeks of age and that a pacifier or infant swing may be calming. Occasionally brief usage of a sedative is necessary.

SELF-STIMULATING BEHAVIORS

Common self-stimulating behaviors include head banging, rocking, thumb sucking, hair pulling, nail biting, and masturbation. These habits are only abnormal during the preschool years if they occur in a setting of inadequate stimulation or in a child with retardation, deafness, or blindness. Parents are reassured that this behavior is normal and are advised to avoid negative reinforcement through restrictions, constant admonishments, or anger. If no underlying cause of tension is present, a program of positive reinforcement through the use of rewards or hypnosis is usually successful in decreasing the unwanted behavior.

NEGATIVE BEHAVIOR

Negative behavior may be the result of a normal psychological stage as the child attempts to define his ability to be independent. Between 6 and 12 months of age, the infant may become upset and negative when someone other than the parent gives him attention. The infant often cries when the mother leaves. This process is known as stranger anxiety. Between one and two, the infant varies from refusing to let the parent do the feeding as a sign of the need for independence to resisting bedtime as a sign of the need for dependence. Through well child visits, parents are counselled about such behaviors. For the 1-year-old refusing to be fed, the parent provides finger foods, a high chair, and a place to make a mess. For the 2-year-old resisting to go to bed, the parent is encouraged to develop a bedtime ritual to ease nighttime separation.

Other negative behaviors include temper tantrums beginning around 1 year of age which are handled by ignoring the child; oppositional behavior between age two and three ("the terrible twos"), and "passive-aggressive" behaviors such as not doing schoolwork and underachieving during school age.

When a negative behavior is not a response for a typical age and stage of parent-child relationships, the child is simply misbehaving. Children will misbehave as a means to get attention (acting out) or as a way to explore something about which they are interested. General suggestions for decreasing misbehavior include setting consistent rules, rewarding and giving attention to positive behavior, minimizing negative reinforcement or punishment, and using isolation or time out when the unwanted behavior does occur.

ENURESIS

Enuresis is the involuntary release of urine. Enuresis is subdivided into diurnal and nocturnal depending on when the wetting occurs. Primary enuresis exists when a child has never achieved dryness while secondary enuresis occurs when a child has been dry for 3 to 6 months and then relapses. Not being able to stay dry at night, primary nocturnal enuresis, is most common and should not be considered abnormal until age five. Even at age five, 15 percent of children will not be able to stay dry at night. By age 12, the percentage is down to three.

Secondary or diurnal enuresis usually happens as a result of an environmental change such as a move, birth of a new sibling, or a behavioral problem. Organic causes which include diabetes mellitus and insipidus, urinary tract infection, genital anomalies, and neurologic dysfunction are ruled out by examination, urinalysis, and urine culture. Although primary enuresis may be due to any of the above causes, it is usually due to a developmental delay in bladder control and will eventually resolve. Various behavioral modification schemes or the use of imipramine may speed up the spontaneous cure rate.

HYPERACTIVITY

Hyperactivity (also known as hyperkinesis, attention deficit disorder, or minimal brain dysfunction syndrome) is the most frequent behavioral complaint during the early school years. Typically, the teacher complains that the child has a short attention span and is easily distracted and frustrated to the point that learning progresses poorly. The child's impulsiveness and inability to pay attention can disrupt the entire class. Parents can become accustomed to the hyperactivity so that this behavior may not be a problem at home. Parents often find these children quick to get into trouble and hard to discipline. Psychometric testing often reveals a specific learning disability usually with average to above average intelligence. Children with this complex of behaviors frequently respond dramatically to treatment with stimulant drugs. These drugs have a paradoxical effect in prepubertal children, having a calming rather than stimulant effect.

CHILD ABUSE AND NEGLECT

The past two decades have seen a dramatic rise in the reporting of cases of child abuse and neglect. Few parents come into the office or emergency room stating that they have just injured their child. The physician must have a high index of suspicion with any injury or failure to thrive.

The suspicion often begins with an implausible history. The parent does not know how the injury occurred. There is a discrepancy between the histories offered by two supposed observors. The child is alleged to have done something that his developmental age would not allow. "The nine month old got into the tub and turned on the hot water." There may be a delay in seeking medical attention. The child supposedly consumes enough calories but is not growing. The parent often has a history of being abused or the family is in the middle of some crisis. The child may be considered "vulnerable" (i.e., was premature, has a chronic illness, or a difficult temperament).

On exam, the skin may show signs of a beating particularly lash marks, cigarette burns, or emersion burns of the buttocks with sparing of the hands or feet. Severe injury can occur with intra-abdominal hemorrhage and head injuries with skull fractures and subdural hematoma formation. A radiologic skeletal survey may reveal new or old fractures, particularly metaphyseal fractures of a long bone from a wrenching type injury. Be extra suspicious if multiple injuries at varying stages of healing are found. Failure to thrive usually requires hospitalization to document appropriate weight gain with adequate caretaking. Sexual abuse, often on an incestuous basis, also is increasingly being recognized.

Once the physician has a suspicion of abuse or neglect, the child must be removed from the abusive environment, often necessitating hospitalization. The physician can be most helpful to the parents by presenting the problem in a nonaccusatory manner so that the parents will be most open to getting counselling. The local protective service agency must be notified. A successful outcome for the child depends on the parents, social agencies, and medical and psychological professionals working together.

PSYCHOSOMATIC ILLNESS

Chronic headaches, abdominal pain, chest pain, and exacerbations of diabetes or asthma are common symptoms that often during childhood have a psychogenic origin. Ten to fifteen percent of school age children will complain of recurrent abdominal pain. Usually anxiety over some emotional stress leads to one of these symptoms. Rarely, a child will have a conversion reaction or be a malingerer, fabricating the symptom as a "ticket of admission" to get help for some other problem. Since the organic causes for these types of symptoms are numerous, the psychologic evaluation should progress parallel to the medical evaluation. Look for the symptom to (1) produce a psychological gain for the child, (2) have a "model" in the family, (3) occur at the time of some family crisis, especially a separation or divorce, and (4)

occur in the setting of overprotective, anxious parents who become preoccupied with the child's symptom instead of dealing with some problem of their own.

CHILD HEALTH MAINTENANCE

Pediatricians spend as much as 60 percent of their time doing health maintenance visits. The goals of these visits include (1) prevention of disease by immunizations and anticipatory guidance; (2) early detection of disease by screening tests, interval history, physical examination, and developmental assessment; and (3) development of a trusting, caring relationship between doctor, parent, and child. In the immunization schedule currently recommended by the American Academy of Pediatrics, note that tetanus boosters are needed only every 10 years and that smallpox vaccinations are no longer recommended (Table 11-6). Over the past several years, school systems have started to require full immunization upon school entry. This has led to high levels of immunization and near disappearance of all the immunizable diseases. Pneumococcal vaccine does not appear in Table 11-6, but it is recommended for children at risk for pneumococcal bacteremia such as following spleenectomy or in children with sickle cell disease.

Age appropriate screening tests and anticipatory guidance are administered at each well child visit (Table 11-7).

ACCIDENTS AND POISONINGS

As discussed in the introduction, accidents are now the leading cause of death for people less than 24 years old. In the United States, accidents cause 35,000 deaths and over 6 million injuries. Physicians to children are making accident prevention a major area of concern. While every effort should be made to treat injuries early, primary prevention is the ultimate goal.

Passive rather than active strategies are more successful in preventing accidents. Passive interventions do not require an individual to make a behavior change. Making safer designs for automobiles and other products is a passive strategy. The individual does not need to act differently to benefit from safer designs. Over the last 20 years, medications and toxic household products have been placed in child-proof containers. The parent no longer needs to remember to keep dangerous products out of the reach of the child. This has nearly eliminated deaths from ingestions in children under five.

On the other hand, educational programs about the advantages of wearing seat belts or pediatric counselling on the need to watch children so that they do not get into

Table 11-6. Recommended Schedule for Active Immunization of Normal Infants and Children*

Recommended Age	Vaccine(s)	Comments
2 mo	DTP,[a] OPV[b]	Can be initiated earlier in areas of high endemicity
4 mo	DTP, OPV	2-mo interval desired for OPV to avoid interference
6 mo	DTP (OPV)	OPV optional for areas where polio might be imported (e.g., some areas of Southwest United States)
12 mo	Tuberculin Test[c]	May be given simultaneously with MMR at 15 mo (see text)
15 mo	Measles, Mumps, Rubella (MMR)[d]	MMR preferred
18 mo	DTP, OPV	Consider as part of primary series—
4–6 yr[e]	DTP, OPV	
14–16 yr	Td[f]	Repeat every 10 years for lifetime

[a] DTP—Diphtheria and tetanus toxoids with pertussis vaccine.

[b] OPV—Oral, attenuated poliovirus vaccine contains poliovirus types 1, 2, and 3.

[c] Tuberculin test—Mantoux (intradermal PPD) preferred. Frequency of tests depends on local epidemiology. The Committee recommends annual or biennial testing unless local circumstances dictate less frequent or no testing (see Tuberculosis for complete discussion).

[d] MMR—Live measles, mumps, and rubella viruses in a combined vaccine (see text for discussion of single vaccines versus combination).

[e] Up to the seventh birthday.

[f] Td—Adult tetanus toxoid (full dose) and diphtheria toxoid (reduced dose) in combination.

* Committee on Infectious Diseases, American Academy of Pediatrics: 1982 Red Book. 19th Ed. American Academy of Pediatrics, Evanston, 1982.

dangerous situations are the types of active interventions that generally fail. An exception to the active-passive concept are changes which can be enforced by law or only require one-time actions. Purchase and use of infant car seats, turning down the temperature of hot water heaters, and putting gates on stairs are some examples. The physician should reinforce these actions in the office.

Despite increasing attempts at prevention, poisonings are still common accidents, particularly between the ages of one and five and as a means of adolescent suicide attempts. For the preschooler ingestions occur most commonly during busy times, when the family is dis-

tracted, stressed, or moving to a new home. Parents should know how to contact the local poison control center. Syrup of ipecac which can induce emesis should be kept in the home of all toddlers. Contraindications to inducing emesis include coma, corrosives, petroleum distillates, and strychnine. Common poisonings and the recommended treatment are listed (Table 11-8).

Lead Poisoning

Lead poisoning during childhood is usually a problem of chronic ingestion of lead-based paint and lead contaminated dust found in the old, poorly maintained housing of families of low socioeconomic status. The child may have obvious pica (the chronic ingestion of nonfood materials) for paint chips. High levels of ingestion can produce encephalopathy with seizures, coma, cerebral palsy, and significant retardation. Over the past 20 years, with the removal of lead from paint and with better screening for elevated lead levels, encephalopathy is rarely seen. Low levels of ingestion may produce nonspecific symptoms such as anorexia, vomiting, abdominal pain, and constipation. Of worry is the increasing evidence that low levels of lead to subtle neurologic changes with hyperactivity, mild behavioral change, and a small but significant lowering of intelligence. Treat-

Table 11-7. Health Maintenance Screening Tests and Anticipatory Guidance

Screening Tests	Age of Testing
Newborn screening (phenylketonuria, hypothyroidism)	Nursery, 1 month
Hematocrit	1 and 2 years
Tuberculin test	12 months
Lead poisoning testing	1 and 2 years
Hearing screen with pure tone audiometry	Annually beginning age 4
Visual acuity	Annually beginning age 3–4

Samples of Anticipatory Guidance

Safety:	Car seats, gates across stairs, prevention of poisoning, use of ipecac to induce vomiting, protection from falls from windows
Parenting:	Difficult temperaments, colic, stranger anxiety, parental support structure, approach to temper tantrums and discipline, toileting, enuresis
Cognitive stimulation	Provide age appropriate toys, language stimulation, fantasy play, school
Feeding:	Delay of solids until 6 months, breast or formula until 12 months, weaning, decreased appetite at 1 year, stopping of bottle at 18 months, food refusals

Table 11-8. Common Poisonings

Substance	Signs and Symptoms	Treatment
Acetaminophen	Nausea, vomiting Late complications include hepatic necrosis, death	Emesis, lavage Mucomyst (acetylcysteine)
Aspirin	Hyperventilation, respiratory alkalosis, hyperglycemia, metabolic acidosis, altered mental status, fever, shock	Emesis, lavage Fluids to correct metabolic imbalances Hemodialysis
Caustics (lyes, alkali)	Burns of skin and mucous membranes Ingestions cause gastrointestinal perforations and strictures	Administer milk, water Hospitalize for esophagoscopy
Hydrocarbons (gasoline, furniture polish)	Respiratory distress, central nervous system depression	Watch for respiratory distress Serial chest roentgenogram for aspiration pneumonia
Bleach (Chlorox)	Irritation of skin, mucous membranes but Chlorox is of low toxicity	Administer water
Iron	Nausea, vomiting, abdominal pain, gastrointestinal bleeding, convulsions, coma, shock Late complications include gastrointestinal strictures	Emesis, lavage Chelation therapy with desferoxamine

ment varies with the level of intoxication but should always include either repair of the home or removal of the child from the home.

DISEASES OF THE NEWBORN

The newborn infant presents a variety of special concerns to the pediatrician. The newborn period is traditionally defined as the first month of life, but evaluation of the newborn begins even before delivery. Many prenatal factors have an impact on the immediate neonatal course and the newborn evaluation requires careful attention to these factors. The expectant mother should receive comprehensive prenatal care to maximize the delivery of a healthy infant. High risk pregnancies may constitute 25 percent of an obstetric practice so that the pediatrician needs to know how prenatal complications may affect the newborn.

Teratogens including chemicals, radiation, and infectious agents may cross the placenta to cause malformations. Teratogens are considered most dangerous during the first trimester of pregnancy. The congenital infectious agents are remembered by the TORCH acronym standing for toxoplasmosis, other (syphilis, hepatitis B), rubella, cytomegalovirus, and herpes simplex. Congential rubella syndrome (deafness, growth retardation, cataracts, heart disease, microcephaly, and mental retardation) has nearly disappeared because of the rubella vaccination program. Well recognized chemical terato-

gens include alcohol, smoking, heavy metals, tetracycline, anticonvulsants, oral contraceptives, androgens, and thalidomide.

Maternal illnesses such as toxemia, diabetes, malnutrition, renal disease, hypertension, and sickle cell disease may lead to placental insufficiency and intrauterine growth retardation of the fetus. Maternal narcotic addiction, usually heroin or methadone, leads to withdrawal symptoms in the newborn characterized by irritability, jitteriness, high-pitched cry, tachypnea, diarrhea, poor feeding, and rarely convulsions.

Abnormal amounts of amniotic fluid should alert the physician to a potential problem. Increased amniotic fluid, polyhydramnios, is caused by gastrointestinal obstructions such as duodenal atresia or tracheoesophageal fistula. Decreased amniotic fluid, oligohydramnios, may be seen with renal anomalies or obstructive uropathies.

Many complications arise at the time of delivery. Fetal monitoring of the relationship between uterine contractions and fetal heart rate allows the obstetrician to intervene, for example, with a caesarean section before irreversible anoxic brain damage has occurred.

Upon delivery, an infant is evaluated by assigning an Apgar score at 1 minute and 5 minutes of life. The Apgar score assesses heart rate, muscle tone, respirations, color, and reflex irritability. Under normal circumstances the Apgar score is 8 to 10 indicating a vigorous infant. Apgar scores of 5 to 7 suggest some distress and Apgars less than 5 are indicative of a severely depressed infant. Although both scores at 1 and 5 minutes are important, the 5 minute score is the best predictor of neonatal outcome.

Most infants require some minor assistance to clear secretions from the oropharynx while a few will require resuscitation with stimulation, oxygen, suctioning, and possibly respiratory support.

Meconium is a tarry, thick material formed in utero in the intestine. An infant stressed before birth may pass this material into the amniotic fluid. If the amniotic fluid is meconium stained, the vocal cords are visualized and any meconium suctioned out before the first breath. This prevents meconium aspiration which can lead to a chemical pneumonia and respiratory distress. Depressed Apgar scores occur in the infant who has suffered intrauterine asphyxia or when the mother was given an analgesic late in labor. The asphyxiated infant may develop hypoglycemia, hypocalcemia, and seizures during the neonatal period and is at risk for neurologic deficits in the future.

All infants should have a complete physical examination during the first 24 hours of life. Gestational age is estimated by using various physical features or by using a Dubowitz score. The weight, length, and head circumference is measured. By combining gestational age and growth parameters, infants are classified as small (SGA), appropriate (AGA), or large (LGA) for gestational age. LGA indicates the risk of maternal diabetes and transient infant hypoglycemia. SGA infants are at risk for neonatal asphyxia, hypoglycemia, hypocalcemia, polycythemia (hyperviscosity), and persistent fetal circulation.

The skin is covered with a greasy white material called vernix. The skin should be assessed for pallor (indicating antenatal blood loss), plethora (indicating neonatal polycythemia), cyanosis (suggesting congenital heart disease, or temperature instability), or jaundice. Normal skin lesions seen on the first examination include mongolian spots, milia, erythema toxicum, forceps marks, and hemangiomas.

Molding of the head often occurs during the birth process as the head descends and exits from the birth canal. Molding resolves early in the newborn period without intervention. Caput succedaneum is an edematous area over the occiput, usually in the center of the head and crossing suture lines. Cephalohematomas represent subperiosteal bleeding over the skull and do not cross suture lines. The anterior fontanel is soft and measures 1 to 4 cm at birth while the posterior fontanel is open to about a fingertip. Epstein's pearls, white retention cysts on the gums or palate, are a normal newborn finding. A cleft lip or palate are midline defects which should be easily recognized. The eye is examined for gross anomalies. The fundus is observed for the red reflex as a means to rule out retinoblastoma.

Close attention should be paid to the respiratory pattern of newborns during the first examination. The respiratory rate during the newborn period is 40 to 60 breaths per minute. The breathing pattern may be irregular and vary from a rapid rate to periodic breathing. Rales and rhonchi can be present in the first day of life. Signs of respiratory distress include grunting, nasal flaring, increased respiratory rate, difficulty feeding and cyanosis. The possible etiologies of respiratory distress are listed (Table 11-9). Supernumerary nipples can be present on the thorax extending to the abdomen. A fractured clavicle due to birth trauma should be detected by tenderness and crepitus over the affected bone.

The newborn heart rate ranges from 120 to 160. A heart murmur is heard at some point in the first several days in many infants. The murmur is usually insignificant, often arising from a patent ductus arteriosus and will disappear spontaneously as the ductus closes. Coarctation of the aorta is detected by palpating for decreased femoral pulses.

Abdominal examination may reveal an umbilical hernia which generally resolves later in childhood. The spleen and liver may be palpated 1 to 2 cm below the costal margins. Kidneys can usually be felt in the newborn and if enlarged suggests a urinary tract anomaly. Genitourinary exam should include assessment in males for inguinal hernia, descent of testes and penile anomalies such as hypospadias. Females, likewise, may have inguinal hernias. A small amount of white or blood streaked vaginal discharge is common.

Several anomalies of the lower extremity are important to recognize. Infants with congenital dislocation of the hip appear normal but on abduction of the hip a "click" is felt as the femoral head passes back into the acetabulum. This is known as Ortolani's sign. Dislocations found in the newborn period and treated with abduction splinting (often by double diapering) can prevent permanent hip disease. Clubfoot (talipes equinovarus) is readily apparent on exam and requires early orthopedic evaluation.

Table 11-9. Causes of Neonatal Respiratory Distress

Transient tachypnea
Idiopathic respiratory distress syndrome
Meconium aspiration
Pneumonia
Pneumothorax/pneumomediastinum
Hypoplastic lung (Potter syndrome with absent kidneys)
Choanal Atresia
Diaphragmatic hernia
Aspiration secondary to tracheosophageal fistula
Congenital heart disease
Persistent fetal circulation
Hydrops
Hyperviscosity syndrome from polycythemia

Prematurity

Respiratory distress syndrome is the most common cause of morbidity and mortality in the preterm infant. The premature infant may present with mild grunting and tachypnea or prolonged apnea, cyanosis, and respiratory arrest. The disease reaches its peak at 36 to 72 hours of age. The condition is caused by inadequate pulmonary surfactant to keep the alveoli open. Chest roentgenogram shows air bronchograms and a ground glass appearance of the pulmonary parenchyma. Administration of oxygen and ventilation with continuous positive airway pressure (CPAP) is usually necessary. Complications of this disease are multiple and include pneumothorax, pneumomediastinum, bronchopulmonary dysplasia from oxygen toxicity, and retinopathy of the newborn (retrolental fibroplasia) also from excess oxygen administration.

Premature infants are at higher risk for jaundice, neonatal sepsis, hypocalcemia, and necrotizing enterocolitis (NEC). NEC is necrosis of the bowel wall from hypoxic injury. The injury can progress to perforation, sepsis, and death. NEC is more common after a birth with low Apgars and asphyxia. The baby develops abdominal distention and bloody stools. Abdominal x-rays reveal gas in the intestinal wall (pneumatosis intestinalis). Feedings are stopped and antibiotics started with the goal of preventing a perforation.

JAUNDICE

Jaundice is a frequent problem in the newborn period. It can have a multitude of causes (Table 11-10). In most cases neonatal jaundice is physiologic which is a transient rise in bilirubin over the first week of life due to the inability of the liver to metabolize bilirubin during this period. Certain infants are at increased risk for jaundice and they include newborns with sepsis, infants of diabetic mothers, severely bruised infants, premature infants, and the polycythemic newborn. Evaluation of jaundice is necessary if the bilirubin is above 5 mg/dl on the first day of life, 10 mg/dl on the second day, and 12 mg/dl on the third day. This evaluation should include a physical examination, direct and total bilirubin, mother and infant blood type and Rh, Coomb's test, hematocrit, and peripheral blood smear.

Blood type incompatibility between mother and baby is one of the more common reasons for neonatal jaundice. If the baby is Rh positive while the mother is Rh negative or the baby has type A or B blood while the mother has type O, the mother may make anti-Rh, anti-A, or anti-B antibodies. These antibodies cross the placenta resulting in hemolysis which if significant can lead to hyperbiliruninemia and anemia. Rh incompatibility is generally more severe with hemolysis often beginning in utero leading to profound anemia, congestive heart failure, and generalized edema (hydrops fetalis). The first pregnancy to a Rh negative mother with a Rh positive baby causes sensitization. The Rh incompatibility occurs in the second pregnancy. Giving anti-Rh immune globulin (Rhogam) after the first such pregnancy has nearly eliminated this disease over the past 20 years. The Coombs' test is positive with any blood type incompatibility. Significant hyperbilirubinemia is treated with phototherapy or exchange transfusion.

Table 11-10. Common Causes of Neonatal Jaundice

Physiologic jaundice
Hemolytic disease of the newborn (Rh, ABO, and other blood incompatibilities)
Congential Spherocytosis
Glucose-6-phosphate dehydrogenase (G6PD) deficiency
Sepsis
Congenital infection
Galactosemia

With prolonged neonatal jaundice
  Biliary atresia
  Neonatal hepatitis
  Hypothyroidism
  Breast milk jaundice
  Crigler-Najjar syndrome (congenital absence of glucuronyl transferase enzyme)

NEONATAL SEPSIS

Although rare, the physician needs to be particularly alert for neonatal sepsis because of its potential for a fatal outcome if not recognized. Because of the newborn's immature immune system, neonatal sepsis can occur up to 6 to 8 weeks of age. In the nursery, risk factors for sepsis include prematurity, prolonged rupture of membranes, maternal fever, and foul smelling amniotic fluid. During the first several days of life fever is rarely a presenting sign, but should fever occur in the newborn period or up to 6 weeks of age, it requires careful evaluation to rule out sepsis. Neonatal sepsis usually presents with nonspecific findings such as poor feeding, lethargy, vomiting, hypothermia, apnea. A bulging fontanel or respiratory distress may give a clue as to the source of the infection.

Bacteria picked up by the infant in its passage through the birth canal are the causative organisms. These include group B beta-hemalytic streptococci, *Escherichia coli, Klebsiella,* and *Listeria* organisms. Laboratory evaluation includes white blood cell count and differential, blood culture, urine culture, lumbar puncture, and chest roentgenogram.

DISEASES OF THE RESPIRATORY TRACT

In children, diseases of the respiratory tract are the most frequent cause of illness and visits to the physician. During the first 5 years of life, children average five to seven upper respiratory infections per year. Approach this group of diseases by first localizing the level at which the respiratory tract is involved and then consider which etiologies are possible for that location.

No reason is usually found for the occurrence of a lower respiratory illness. However, be aware that frequent or severe lower resiratory infections may signal an underlying disease of decreased immunity. For example, frequent pneumonias can be caused by cystic fibrosis or congenital heart disease with increased pulmonary blood flow.

Common Cold

Most common of all illnesses, the common cold has defied specific diagnosis and treatment. It is caused by a variety of viruses including the rhinovirus. Lasting 3 to 7 days, the initial watery rhinorrhea thickens after several days. Cough, chills, and fever, may accompany the rhinorrhea. Decongestants may bring symptomatic relief and antibiotics are not indicated. Frequent episodes of nasal congestion may be allergic rhinitis (hay fever).

Pharyngitis

Pharyngitis is most common in the midchildhood years from age two to eight. Etiology is usually nonbacterial (Table 11-11). Group A β-hemolytic *Streptococcus* (GABHS) causes only 10 to 30 percent of cases of pharyngitis with the higher incidence during the early spring. Diagnosis of GABHS is important because antibiotic treatment prevents (1) acute rheumatic fever, (2) supportive complications such as peritonsillar abscess and bacterial adenitis, and (3) spread of GABHS strains which cause poststreptococcal glomerulonephritis (*see* p 635). The presentation of pharyngitis is most often nonspecific, including sore erythematous pharynx, fever, enlarged tonsils, exudate, and anterior cervical adenopathy. Table 11-11 lists findings which may lead to a particular diagnosis. Because one of these specific findings is often absent, a throat culture needs to be taken to look for GABHS. Antibiotics are given only if the culture is positive.

Otitis Media

After upper respiratory tract infections (URI), otitis media is the second most common cause of illness visits to the doctor during childhood. Otitis media develops because of eustachian tube dysfunction which allows secretions and bacteria to accumulate in the middle ear. Otitis media and eustachian tube dysfunction are most prevalent in early childhood for reasons including the high frequency of URI's, hypertrophy of lymphoid tissue, and the angle of the eustachian tube.

Acute otitis media represents acute supportive infection of the middle ear. The offending organism is usually the pneumococcus or *Hemophilus influenza.* The symptoms are often nonspecific such as fever, irritability, rhinorrhea, vomiting, or diarrhea. Older children may complain of an earache and otorrhea is diagnostic. Treatment is a course of antibiotics.

Supportive complications (mastoiditis, brain abscess) are rare but fluid (serous otitis media) often persists after antibiotic treatment. Serous otitis media may even occur without a preceding acute infection. When this fluid lasts more than several months, the child may have enough hearing loss to delay language development or cause learning problems in school. Tympanostomy tubes or adenoidectomy may be employed to treat chronic serous otitis media but the timing of their use remains controversial. Some children are "otitis-prone" and require prophylactic antibiotics.

Problems of the Adenoids and Tonsils

Although removal of the adenoids and/or tonsils remains the most common operation done on children, its frequency has markedly diminished over the past 20 years. Enlargement of the tonsils and adenoids in the middle childhood years is normal. Infrequently, the enlargement causes upper airway obstruction, hypoxia, and cor pulmonale. The indications for tonsillectomy include airway obstruction or peritonsillar abscess, while adenoidectomy is done also for obstruction and perhaps for chronic otitis media.

Table 11-11. Pharyngitis

Cause	Specific Findings
Viral (usually an adenovirus)	Rhinorrhea, laryngitis
Group A β-hemolytic streptococci	Scarletinaform rash
Adenovirus type 3	Conjunctivitis
Herpangina (Coxsackie group A)	Pharyngeal vesicles or ulcers
Infectious mononucleosis	Splenomegaly, atypical lymphocytosis
Gonococcus	Sexually active adolescent

Croup and Epiglottitis

Croup and epiglottitis are the usual causes of upper airway obstruction in childhood (Table 11-12). Epiglottitis must be distinguished from croup because treatment needs to be initiated as soon as possible to prevent total airway obstruction and possible death. When epiglottitis is suspected, examination of the upper airway with a tongue depressor is contraindicated as this may trigger total obstruction. A lateral neck roentgenogram is used to make the diagnosis.

In the first several months of life, stridor may be caused by laryngomalacia, a condition in which the cartilage of the upper airway is not formed enough to prevent airway collapse. Recovery occurs over the first year. After early infancy consider the presence of a foreign body as the cause of upper airway distress.

Bronchiolitis

Bronchiolitis is a disorder unique to infants generally less than 1 year of age. It is a viral infection primarily at the level of the bronchioles, producing expiratory obstruction. The infants are tachypneic with variable degrees of respiratory distress including subcostal and intercostal retractions. The chest is hyperexpanded and on auscultation, wheezes, a prolonged expiratory phase, and occasional rales are heard. Fever is usually low grade. Bronchiolitis may last from 1 to 14 days.

Distinguishing bronchiolitis from asthma may be difficult. Age less than 1 year favors bronchiolitis while recurrent episodes of wheezing or a significant response to a trial of a bronchodilator favors asthma.

Pneumonia

Pneumonia, a disease which spans all ages, is an infection of the lung parenchyma which can be caused by almost any microorganism. The most common etiologies of pneumonia during childhood are listed (Table 11-13). The classic picture of high fever, shaking chills, pleuritic pain, productive cough, dullness on percussion, and rales on auscultation is less often seen in children. Young infants may only have tachypnea and fever. A chest roentgenogram reveals the diagnosis.

In the history, listen carefully for evidence of an aspiration which may cause either a chemical pneumonitis or a bacterial pneumonia secondary to obstruction by a foreign body. Peanuts are particularly notorious for this. Tuberculosis should be ruled out as a cause of pneumonia by doing a tuberculin test.

Asthma

Asthma is a condition in which bronchial hyperreactivity causes bronchospasm (wheezing) leading to reversible airway obstruction and respiratory distress. In the United States, with approximately 4 percent of children having asthma, it is the leading reason for the hospitalization of children and for school absences.

An asthma attack may be precipitated by infection, allergy, emotional factors, exercise, or meteorological change. Asthma, eczema, and hay fever are known as atopic diseases and tend to occur together in the same child. A family history of atopic disease is common.

Asthma may vary from an occasional attack to chronic wheezing, from no respiratory distress to respiratory failure, from requiring intermittent treatment to requiring chronic medication. Ninety percent of children "outgrow" asthma by the end of adolescence. Treatment consists of bronchodilators, good pulmonary toilet, hydration, and appropriate respiratory support. Rare causes of bronchospasm include congestive heart failure, foreign body aspiration, cystic fibrosis, and compression of a bronchus by tumor, node, or anomalous blood vessel.

Table 11-12. Upper Airway Obstruction in Childhood

	Croup	Epiglottitis
Cause	Viral (parainfluenza)	Bacterial (*Hemophilus influenza*)
Peak age	3 months to 3 years	3 to 7 years
Prodrome	Upper respiratory infection	None
Course	Variable, worse at night, 2 to 3 days	Rapidly progressive over several hours
Appearance	Nontoxic with severity from mild hoarseness to inspiratory stridor and retractions	Toxic, dysphagic, drooling, sitting with jaw forward
Fever	Low	High
Cough	Barky, spasmotic	None
Lateral neck roentgenogram	"Steeple" sign from subglottic narrowing of trachea	"Thumb" sign from swollen epiglottitis
Treatment	Respiratory support as needed, moist air	Endotracheal intubation, antibiotics

Table 11-13. Pneumonia in Childhood

Organism	Age
Streptococcus pneumoniae	All ages
Viruses	All ages
Mycobacterium tuberculosis	All ages
Group B β-hemolytic strep-tococcus	Neonate
Chlamydia trachomatis	0 to 4 months
Hemophilus influenza	2 months to 5 years
Mycoplasma pneumoniae	Late childhood, adolescence

DISEASES OF THE CARDIOVASCULAR SYSTEM

Congenital Heart Disease

The incidence of congenital heart disease is 8 to 10 cases per 1,000 births. The child may present with cyanosis, heart failure, poor growth, or a heart murmur on routine examination. Preliminary diagnosis is made by physical examination, electrocardiogram, and chest roentgenogram. These three tools demonstrate most common cardiac anomalies (Table 11-14). Echocardiography often provides a definitive diagnosis without the need for catheterization.

Ventricular septal defect (VSD) is the most prevalent cardiac malformation. High pulmonary vascular resistance at birth prevents left to right shunting across a VSD. Pulmonary vascular resistance falls over the first month and a clinically significant VSD presents around 1 month of age with congestive heart failure. A VSD causes a coarse, holosystolic murmur loudest at the left lower sternal border.

Tetralogy of Fallot consists of pulmonary stenosis, VSD, overriding aorta, and right ventricular hypertrophy. The infant may present in the first month with persistent cyanosis or at about 3 months with episodes of cyanosis known as "spells." These spells are caused by spasm of the right ventricular infundibulum and the child often learns to squat as a way to reduce right to left shunting.

About half of all children at some age will have a heart murmur heard. The majority of these murmurs have no hemodynamic significance. Such "innocent" murmurs are generally either midsystolic, short, vibratory murmurs located over the midprecordium or a venous hum which is a continuous, humming murmur near the clavicle.

Hypertension

In adults, hypertension is defined as a blood pressure over 140/90. In the past, using this definition, few children had hypertension, and in those that did, the hypertension was often secondary to renal disease, renovascular disease, or coarctation of the aorta.

Blood pressure standards are now available for children by age. Hypertension should be defined as three measurements over the 95th percentile for age and sex. Hypertension by this definition usually is found on routine examination which should begin at age three, and is idiopathic or "essential" hypertension in about 95 percent of cases. Family history, cultural influences, and obesity are risk factors.

Extensive evaluation of the child with hypertension is necessary only in the very young and when the blood pressure is very high. Normal growth, urinalysis, creatinine, and electrolytes are adequate to rule out renal disease. Normal femoral pulses and equal four extremity blood pressures rule out coarctation. In adolescents, oral contraceptives may cause elevated blood pressure. Treatment of the child with essential hypertension is controversial.

Rheumatic Fever

Acute rheumatic fever is an episode of carditis, polyarthritis, or chorea following a group A β-hemolytic streptococcal pharyngitis. The arthritis or carditis occurs 3 to 8 weeks after the pharyngitis while the chorea occurs after 2 to 6 months. Rare in children under three, a positive family history or a previous attack increases the incidence.

Diagnosis is based on the Jones criteria which require

Table 11-14. Common Congenital Cardiac Anomalies

	Oxygenation			
	Acyanotic		Cyanotic	
Pulmonary Blood Flow	Increased	Decreased	Increased	Decreased
Left ventricular hypertrophy	Patent ductus Ventricular septal defect	Coarctation Aortic stenosis		
Right ventricular hypertrophy	Atrial septal defect	Pulmonary stenosis	Transposition	Tetralogy of Fallot

evidence of a recent streptococcal infection (elevated antistreptococcal antibody titers) along with two major criteria or one major and two minor criteria. The major criteria include carditis, polyarthritis (usually migratory), chorea, erythema marginatum, and subcutaneous nodules. The minor criteria are fever, arthraliga without arthritis, prolonged P-R interval without carditis, previous rheumatic fever, and an elevated sedimentation rate or C-reactive protein.

Rheumatic fever is self-limiting so that its significance lies in its tendency for permanent valvular damage known as rheumatic heart disease. The mitral and less commonly aortic valves are effected.

Although antibiotic treatment of streptococcal infections prevents rheumatic fever, the near total disappearance of this disease today is probably more related to improved social conditions than medical treatment. Once an attack has occurred permanent streptococcal prophylaxis is instituted.

DISEASES OF THE GASTROINTESTINAL SYSTEM

Gastroenteritis

The most common gastrointestinal complaint is gastroenteritis. The child presents with vomiting and/or diarrhea. Accompanying symptoms may include fever, abdominal pain, and dehydration. Gastroenteritis is usually viral but a bacterial etiology such as salmonella or shigella should be considered if bloody stools or marked systemic symptoms are present. While other gastrointestinal causes of vomiting and diarrhea will be discussed, consider nongastrointestinal causes such as otitis, urinary tract infection, sepsis, and central nervous system disease. Treatment is aimed at resting the bowel either with clear liquids by mouth or parenteral hydration.

Constipation

Constipation is the formation of hard stools. In the infant, diet is the usual reason for constipation and the addition of water, sucrose syrup, or fruit juice relieves the problem.

For the toddler and older child, constipation results from a behavior pattern of stool retention. Emotional problems, traumatic toilet training, or a time of painful defecation from anal fissures, diarrhea, or other anorectal problems leads to stool retention. A child with severe stool retention may develop encopresis which is bowel movements occurring outside of the toilet. Treatment consists of an intitial cleanout, if necessary, mineral oil, high roughage diet, and behavioral therapy.

Hirschsprung's disease (congenital aganglionic magacolon) is a rare cause of constipation. The child is born with a segment of colon that has no parasympathetic innervation or ganglia. Infrequent stools from birth, little stool in the lower rectum, and little trouble around toileting, distinguish the constipation of this disease.

Pyloric Stenosis

Pyloric stenosis occurs in the first 2 months of life predominantly in males. The muscle of the pylorus hypertrophies resulting in obstruction with vomiting that classically becomes projectile. Since the vomitus is mostly gastric juice, the infant becomes dehydrated with hypochloremic hypokalemic alkalosis. On exam, the enlarged pylorus or "olive" is usually palpated in the right upper quadrant of the abdomen. Surgery is required to relieve the obstruction.

Acute Abdomen

The differential diagnosis of the acute abdomen varies depending on the age of the child. As in adults, outcome is improved with early diagnosis to prevent the progression from abdominal pain to obstruction and/or ileus to perforation. In the newborn period consider necrotizing entercocolitis, volvulus, malrotation, intestinal atresia, congenital bands, meconium ileus from cystic fibrosis, aganglionic megacolon from Hirschsprung's disease, and sepsis. Necrotizing enterocolitis was discussed in the newborn section.

From 1 month to 2 years, intussusception and incarcerated inguinal hernia are the likely causes. Intussusception is the invagination of one portion of the intestine into an adjacent portion. The infant develops colicky pain and may pass stool that has a "currant jelly" apperance. A barium enema not only is diagnostic but can be curative as it can reduce the intussusception.

After age 2, appendicitis is the leading reason for an acute abdomen. Appendicitis does not present differently during the pediatric years and will not be discussed further in this chapter. In girls, especially adolescents, pelvic inflammatory disease and ovarian problems and in boys, testicular torsion may present with acute abdominal symptoms.

Liver Disease

Although children get hepatitis from the same viruses as adults (hepatitis A and B viruses, Epstein-Barr virus), they become less ill, less jaundiced, and are less likely to develop chronic active hepatitis or fulminant hepatitis.

Remember that neonates may receive hepatitis B transplacentally.

Cirrhosis is rare in the pediatric age group. Most likely causes are biliary astresia, α_1-antitrypsin deficiency, and Wilson's disease, a disorder of copper metabolism.

DISEASES OF THE GENITOURINARY SYSTEM

Urinary Tract Infection

Recognizing urinary symptoms in infants is difficult so that a high degree of suspicion must be maintained when an infant presents with many nonurinary symptoms. Unexplained fever, irritability, lethargy, failure to thrive, jaundice, vomiting, and diarrhea, can signify a urinary tract infection. The older child may describe dysuria, urgency, frequency, low back pain. Females are more likely to get a urinary tract infection. Problems which predispose to recurrent urinary tract infections are listed (Table 11-15). After one infection in a male and two in a female, these disorders should be ruled out by an intravenous pyelogram and a voiding cystoureterogram.

Acute Poststreptococcal Glomerulonephritis

Acute poststreptococcal glomerulonephritis is an immune complex disease occurring 1 to 3 weeks after a skin or pharyngeal infection with a nephritogenic strain of group A β-hemolytic streptococcus. The child presents with mild edema usually of the face and eyelids and "rusty" colored urine. Renal failure is variable leading to oliguria and an increased vascular volume with hypertension and cardiovascular changes similar to congestive heart failure. Urinalysis shows hematuria with red cell casts. Serum changes include reduced C3 and C4 complement levels and elevated antistreptococcal antibody titers. Without these laboratory findings other types of

Table 11-15. Factors Predisposing to Urinary Tract Infections

Ureteral reflux from abnormal ureterovesicular junction
Uteropelvic junction obstruction
Uterovesicular junction obstruction
Urethral valves
Renal malformation
Chronic constipation
Neurogenic bladder
Diabetes
Poor hygiene in females
Urethral instrumentation

glomerulonephritis should be investigated. Supportive treatment usually results in a complete return to normal renal function.

Nephrotic Syndrome

The nephrotic syndrome consists of proteinuria, decreased serum protein (hypoalbuminemia), and increased serum lipids (cholesterol). The syndrome is caused by leaking of protein through the glomerulus. Although the disease is defined biochemically, clinical recognition comes from the insidious onset of edema, first periorbital and pedal, then scrotal and labial, and finally abdominal with ascites.

Over three-fourths of children with nephrotic syndrome have idiopathic or minimal change disease because of the appearance of the glomerulus by light microscopy. The onset of minimal change disease is usually between 2 and 6 years of age and has a good prognosis. The disease runs a relapsing course, responsive to corticosteroids, and ending by adolescence without renal damage. If significant hematuria or renal failure is present or if the child fails to respond to corticosteroids, a renal biopsy is obtained to look for other causes of the nephrotic syndrome.

In the nephrotic syndrome, the urinary loss of protein usually exceeds 1 g per day. A more common type of proteinuria is orthostatic proteinuria in which the loss of protein is less than 1 g per day and occurs when the patient is not recumbent. The first voiding in the morning should be free of protein. Orthostatic proteinuria is not a manifestation of any chronic renal disease.

Hemolytic-Uremic Syndrome

Hemolytic-uremic syndrome (HUS) is an acute illness consisting of thrombocytopenia, hemolytic anemia, and acute renal failure. Although relatively rare, HUS is a major cause of acute renal falure in infants and young children. HUS is usually preceded by a prodromal illness of bloody diarrhea in infants and an upper respiratory infection in older children. Etiology is unknown. Presenting manifestations may include fever, vomiting, anuria, purpura, pallor, petechiae, hypertension, edema, lethargy, seizures, and coma. Supportive therapy usually results in survival but 30 percent of cases go on to chronic renal failure.

Congenital Malformations

Hypospadias and undescended testes are congenital malformations visible at birth. Hypospadias occurs in males when the urethra opens proximal to the tip of the glans. Circumcision is contraindicated because the foreskin may be needed for corrective surgery. Undescended testis (cryptorchidism) is very common and usually unilateral. An extremely active cremasteric reflex may make a testis appear undescended. Surgical correction is performed by age five.

A hydrocele is an accumulation of fluid in the track (processus vaginalis) which the testes descend into the scrotum during development. An oval, fluid-filled swelling results which transilluminates and is easily palpated in the scrotum. Appearing in infancy, a hydrocele usually resolves spontaneously without surgery.

The first four entries in Table 11-15 encompass the most common of the obstructive malformations. These may present as recurrent urinary tract infections, an abdominal mass, or renal failure. Early surgical correction can prevent irreversible renal damage.

DISEASES OF THE NERVOUS SYSTEM

Mental Retardation

Normal development was described in the section on psychosocial development. Children with intellectual development two standard deviations below normal are defined as having mental retardation. Retardation has three levels of severity (i.e., mild, moderate, and profound). Mildly retarded children (IQ of 50 to 70) can learn elementary level reading and mathematics, should receive vocational training to hold simple jobs, and can live independently. Children with moderate retardation (IQ of 30 to 50) may learn simple routines of daily living such as cooking and shopping but they will need to live in a supervised environment (IQ below 30), for example, a group home. With profound retardation, self-help skills of toileting and dressing are learned but continuous supervision is necessary.

In only about one-third of the cases of retardation is a specific cause found (Table 11-16). Most retardation is mild with a high likelihood of a positive family history and low socioeconomic status. Children usually gain milestones in a progressive fashion. When a child loses

Table 11-16. Common Causes of Retardation

Prematurity
Birth asphyxia
Chromosomal and other syndromes (Down's syndrome)
Central nervous system malformations (hydrocephalus)
Metabolic diseases
Degenerative diseases
Trauma
Infection (meningitis, encephalitis, congenital infection)

skills (regresses), consider a degenerative disease such as Tay-Sachs or an acute problem such as trauma or meningitis.

Seizures Disorders

Seizure disorders are one of the most common chronic problems that pediatricians manage. While approximately 0.5 percent of children will have repeated afebrile seizures (epilepsy), another 5 percent will have seizures only with fever (febrile convulsion) or a seizure secondary to an acute illness. Seizures are classified by their clinical form and electroencephalographic pattern (EEG).

Grand mal or major motor seizures begin with loss of consciousness which is followed by tonic-clonic generalized movements. Tongue biting, salivation, and incontinence are common. The seizure is often followed by postictal drowsiness and transient focal neurologic findings (Todd's paralysis). The EEG may or may not show spike or spike and wave activity. Grand mal seizures account for more than half of all childhood seizures. Most seizures of this type have no specific cause and are labelled "idiopathic." Grand mal seizures may be caused by any form of cerebral injury such as that caused by infection, anoxia, dysgenesis, or metabolic and degenerative disease.

A febrile convulsion is a type of grand mal seizure that occurs during a febrile illness. The seizure lasts less than 20 minutes, the child is between the ages of 6 months and 5 years. The illness is not caused by a problem in the central nervous system and the child has no prior or residual neurologic abnormalities. Although 25 percent of children with febrile convulsions have additional febrile convulsions, these children have an excellent prognosis with fewer than 10 percent going on to having epilepsy.

A petit mal seizure or "absence" attack is characterized by a brief loss of awareness accompanied by eye blinking and a diagnostic EEG with 3/s spike and wave discharges. No postictal phase occurs and activities are usually not interrupted. Most children "outgrow" this type of seizure by puberty. Petit mal seizures are not caused by any underlying disease.

Psychomotor or temporal lobe seizures cause an episode of unusual behavior or automatic movements. An aura often precedes the seizure. The child is amnesic for the event but continues regular activity. There may be some postictal confusion or sleepiness. The EEG shows a temporal lobe focus.

Infantile spasms are sudden episodes of flexion or extension of the head and extremities similar to a Moro reflex. They start in the first year of life and are associated with profound regression of development in 90 percent of cases. The EEG pattern shows hypsarrhythmia. Infantile spasms may result from perinatal brain injury or an underlying disorder such as tuberous sclerosis or a congenital CNS malformation.

At the time of a first seizure, the evaluation focuses on ruling out any underlying disorder. These disorders would include meningitis, encephalitis, metabolic disturbances (hyponatremia, hypoglycemia, hypocalcemia), Reye's syndrome, intoxications (lead), and chronic neurologic diseases. The evaluation includes past medical history, developmental history, family history, full physical examination, glucose and calcium levels, electrolytes, and an EEG. A lumbar puncture and computerized axial tomography are necessary if any signs of infection or mass lesion are present. Seizure as a presenting sign of brain tumor is extremely unusual in children. Treatment is usually successful in controlling childhood epilepsy and often can be stopped after several years. The emotional impact of a seizure on the child and family needs careful attention.

Cerebral Palsy

Cerebral palsy (CP) is the name given to a group of motor deficits that arise from a nonprogressive lesion of the CNS occurring during the period of brain development. The child presents with a delay in motor milestones. On exam, cerebral palsy may take a spastic or athetoid form depending on the degree of pyramidal versus extrapyramidal involvement. There may be a hemiplegia, diplegia, or quadraplegia but the lower extremities are commonly more affected. Retardation and a seizure disorder are frequent concomitant findings. Any of the causes of retardation listed in Table 11-16 may also cause cerebral palsy. Prenatal insults are now the most common cause. Treatment involves close cooperation with physical therapy and orthopedics as well as evaluation for appropriate educational placement.

Congenital Malformations

Spina bifida arises from incomplete closure of the neural tube. The most serious form of spina bifida is the meningomyelocele in which the spinal cord and meninges protrude through the spinal defect and into a cystic sac on the back. The opening is most commonly in the lumbosacral area but the higher the level of opening, the greater the level of paresis. Associated problems include hydrocephalus with retardation, renal problems, and bowel and bladder incontinence. The spinal sac easily ruptures and early closure is necessary to prevent menin-

gitis. Whether to institute therapy in severe cases remains controversial.

Hydrocephalus may be recognized at birth or as an abnormally rapid growing head circumference over the first year of life. Hydrocephalus may occur alone (aqueductal stenosis, Dandy-Walker syndrome, Arnold-Chiari malformation) or in association with other anomalies such as spina bifida. A CT scan is diagnostic and treatment consists of placing a ventriculoperitoneal shunt.

Central Nervous System Infections

Meningitis continues as one of the most serious childhood infections with significant amounts of morbidity and mortality. The key to good outcome is early diagnosis. In the first 2 years of life a "stiff neck" may not be present with meningitis. In the infant, irritability, lethargy, poor feeding, or crying not relieved by cuddling may be the only symptoms. Fever and vomiting are often present but are nonspecific. Older children complain of headache. A seizure may be the presenting symptom at any age while an infant often has a bulging fontanel. A lumbar puncture not only confirms the diagnosis but may also distinguish a bacterial or viral etiology.

Most cases of bacterial meningitis occur before age 5 with 6 to 12 months being the peak age. *Hemophilus influenxae*, type B, causes most bacterial meningitis, followed by the pneumococcus and meningococcus. Petechial and purpuric skin lesions typically occur with meningococcal infection. Viral or aseptic meningitis occurs mostly in the summer when enterovirus, echovirus, and coxsackie virus infections are prevalent. These viruses can cause an encephalitis along with the meningitis. The agents which cause encephalitis are similar in children and adults.

GENETIC AND METABOLIC DISEASES

The human cell has 46 chromosomes which are subdivided into 22 pairs of autosomes and two sex chromosomes. Currently, the types of chromosomal abnormalities which are found most frequently are numerical abnormalities, nondisjunction and morphologic abnormalities, or translocations.

Down's syndrome, or trisomy 21, occurs in approximately 1 in 900 newborns. Diagnosis is suspected in a newborn with a small, brachycephalic head, flat nasal bridge, Brushfield's spots in the eyes, and a short fleshy neck. One may also note simian creases in the hands, a large tongue, and low set ears. Down's syndrome in-

Table 11-17. Patterns of Inheritance

Disease	Inheritance	Description of Disease
Neurofibromatosis	Autosomal dominant	Neurofibromas, café-au-lait's spots
Osteogenesis imperfecta	Autosomal dominant	Fragile bones, blue sclerae
Hemophilia A	Sex-linked recessive	Absent factor VIII
Duchenne muscular dystrophy	Sex-linked recessive	Progressive muscle weakness
Metabolic diseases of Table 11-18	Autosomal recessive	See Table 11-18 for description.
Sickle cell anemia	Autosomal recessive	See page 639 for description
Cystic fibrosis	Autosomal recessive	See page 644 for description

cludes mental retardation with IQs of 28 to 80. Approximately one-third of children with Down's syndrome have congenital heart disease such as endocardial cushion defect or ventricular septal defect. These children frequently have hypotonia, prolonged neonatal jaundice, or polycythemia. Leukemia is more common in patients with Down's syndrome and they are most likely to develop acute lymphocytic leukemia.

Trisomy 18 is characterized by mental retardation, failure to thrive, hypertonicity, low set ears, and "rocker bottom feet." Trisomy 13 consists of palatal abnormalities, mental retardation, congenital heart disease, genitourinary abnormalities, and digit anomalies. Children with trisomy 13 die by the second year of life, usually secondary to congenital heart disease.

About 0.35 percent of infants will have sex chromosomal anormalities. Indications for sex chromosomal examination include the presence of abnormal genitalia, infertility, females with primary amenorrhea, females with characteristics suggestive of Turner's syndrome (i.e., webbed neck, edema of the dorsum of the hands, increased carrying angle of the arms, delayed puberty, short stature), and females with inguinal (bilateral) hernia(s).

Diseases due to a single gene defect are expressed in an autosomal or X-linked (sex-linked) pattern depending on whether the same defect is on the X chromosone (Table 11-17). Autosomal dominant inheritance is present if the disease occurs when the defect presents in

the heterozygous or the homozygous state, while autosomal recessive inheritance occurs when the disease only appears when the defective gene is in the homozygous state. Characteristics of autosomal dominance include (1) the disease must be present in one parent; (2) each offspring has a 50 percent chance of being affected, and (3) individuals will be affected in each generation. Characteristics of autosomal recessive inheritance include (1) affected people are usually in the same generation; (2) the offspring have a 25 percent chance of contracting the disease and a 50 percent chance of being a carrier, and (3) the diseases tend to be rare. Sex-linked recessive diseases will follow a dominant pattern among males with 50 percent being affected.

Metabolic diseases result from a single gene defect which alters either the activity or quantity of an enzyme in a metabolic pathway. Phenylketonuria (PKU) is probably the best understood error of amino acid metabolism and is due to decreased activity of phenylalanine hydroxylase. This defect causes levels of phenylalanine to rise to toxic levels by 1 week of age. Untreated, PKU causes severe retardation. All infants in the United States receive within the first several weeks of life a blood test looking for elevated phenylalanine. If found, a low phenylalanine diet is started and the retardation prevented. This disorder follows an autosomal recessive inheritance pattern and occurs in 1 in 10,000 births. Metabolic diseases most commonly have autosomal recessive inheritance (Table 11-18).

Table 11-18. Metabolic Disorders

Disease	Defect in Metabolism	Clinical Manifestations
Maple sugar urine disease	Branch-chain amino acids	"Sweet" smelling urine, neonatal feeding problems, seizures, retardation
Galactosemia	Galactose	Neontal lethargy, vomiting, jaundice, hypoglycemia, retardation, galactosuria
Lesch-Nyhan syndrome	Purines	Retardation, choreoathetosis, self-mutilation, gout
Tay-Sachs disease	Lipid	Infant onset of CNS degeneration, cherry red spot of macula
Hurler's syndrome	Mucopolysaccharide	Coarse facies, kyphosis, dwarfism, spadelike hands, retardation, corneal opacity

DISEASES OF THE BLOOD

Normal blood cell values vary at different ages in childhood. Newborns have hemoglobin values (14 to 23 g/dl) and white cell counts (12,000 to 28,000/mm³ that are higher than an adult. Hemoglobin then drops at about 2 months of age to less than adult levels, the so-called physiologic anemia of 10 to 11 g/dl. It does not return to adult levels until between 6 and 12 years of age. All other types of hematologic results also need to be evaluated with careful attention to the patient's age.

The anemias of childhood may be divided into three categories: (1) those with decreased red blood cell (RBC) production (iron deficiency, aplastic anemia); (2) those with increased RBC destruction (hemolytic anemias such as sickle cell disease and thalassemia); and (3) those due to blood loss (hemorrhagic disease, gastrointestinal disease, or trauma).

Iron Deficiency Anemia

Iron deficiency anemia is the most common cause of anemia in children 6 months to 2 years of age. It generally occurs because the child outgrows his iron stores while simultaneously ingesting inadequate amounts of dietary iron. Because cow's milk has negligible amounts of iron, early introduction of cow's milk into the diet or excessive intake of cow's milk causes iron deficiency anemia. Signs and symptoms may include pallor, easy fatigability and increased irritability. The blood smear of children with iron deficiency anemia shows hypochromia and microcytosis. The mean corpuscular volume (MCV) is low, serum iron is low, total iron binding capacity (TIBC) is increased, and ferritin and transferrin are decreased. Free erythrocytic protoporphyrin (FEP) is also increased due to the lack of iron available to bind to protoporphyrin to make heme. Dietary modification and supplemental iron are the cornerstones of treatment. Hypochromic anemia may also be secondary to lead poisoning.

Aplastic Anemia

Aplastic anemia is a normocytic anemia with an associated white blood cell count less than 2,000/mm³ and platelet count less than 50,000/mm³. Approximately half of all cases are idiopathic, but toxins such as insecticides, heavy metals, benzene, and drugs such as chloramphenicol have been identified as the etiology in many cases. Pancytopenia coupled with congenital absence of the radii and thumbs is Fanconi's syndrome. Patients often present with unusual bleeding such as purpura, petechiae, or menometrorrhagia. Weakness, pallor, and unusual infections are also seen in newly diagnosed patients. The bone marrow shows a decrease in all cell lines with an increase in fat deposition. Therapeutic options include bone marrow transplant, androgens, corticosteroids, and supportive therapy with transfusions. In general, the prognosis is poor with most patients succumbing to overwhelming sepsis or hemmorhage.

Hemolytic Anemia

In the hemolytic anemias, the increased rate of destruction of red cells leads to the anemia. The hemolysis may be due to (1) an immune process from antibodies against the RBC membrane, (2) an unstable RBC membrane, (3) an RBC enzyme defect, or (4) an abnormal hemoglobin. An elevated reticulocyte count and often splenomegaly are the hallmarks of these disorders.

The most important immune hemolytic anemia is erythroblastosis fetalis which was described in the newborn section. Hereditary spherocytosis is a membrane defect causing increased sodium influx into the RBC with resultant hemolysis and splenic sequestration. This disease presents in young patients with a positive family history, splenomegaly, and neonatal jaundice. The osmotic fragility test will confirm the diagnosis.

G-6-PD deficiency is an example of a RBC enzyme defect causing hemolysis. This is a X-linked recessive defect so that males are usually affected. Hemolysis occurs at birth or upon exposure to an oxidant such as aspirin, sulfonamides, antimalarials, and fava beans. The hemolysis resolves spontaneously upon removal of the offending agent. G-6-PD has a high frequency in Mediterranean, African, and Oriental populations. American blacks have a less severe form.

Sickle Cell Anemia

Sickle cell anemia is the most common of the diseases caused by an abnormal hemoglobin occurring in 1 out of 600 black newborns. Sickle hemoglobin is characterized by a valine substitution for glutamate on the beta chain. Diagnosis is by hemoglobin electrophoresis. Sickle hemoglobin causes the RBC to sickle and produce episodes called "crises." Sickling crises include (1) vaso-occlusive crises which are manifested by abdominal, bone, or joint pain and fever; (2) hyperhemolytic crises, characterized by jaundice, increased anemia, and increased reticulocyte count; (3) sequestration crises with marked splenomegaly and increased anemia; and (4) aplastic crises, triggered by infection with decreased erythropoisis and life threatening anemia. Crises usually begin at about 6 to 12 months of age as fetal hemoglobin disappears.

Children under age 5 may develop overwhelming

sepsis or severe life threatening infections with pneumococci or *Hemophilus influenza.* Complications in older children include cerebrovascular accidents, pulmonary infarcts, leg ulcers, osteomyelitis with salmonella, cholelithiasis, and avascular necrosis of the femoral head.

Thalassemia

Thalassemia is due to a genetic defect causing a decrease in the synthesis of one of the hemoglobin chains. Children with thalassemia minor or trait are asymptomatic and have a mild microcytic anemia with increased reticulocyte count and elevated hemoglobin A_2. Children homozygous for this genetic defect have thalassemia major or Cooley's anemia. This disease results in a severe anemia starting in the second year of life. Repeated transfusions are necessary leading to hemochromatosis which prevents these patients from surviving past age 30.

Bleeding Disorders

Hemophilia A, or classic hemophilia, is caused by a decrease in factor VIII (antihemophilic factor). Hemophilia B, or Christmas disease, is characterized by factor IX deficiency. Both disorders have X-linked recessive inheritance and are found in males. Hemophilia A is treated with cryoprecipitate and hemophilia B is treated with factor IX concentrate. Long-term problems include hemarthroses, complications of frequent transfusions of blood products, and the development of antibodies to factor VIII or IX.

Idiopathic Thrombocytopenic Purpura

Idiopathic thrombocytopenic purpura (ITP) presents with bruises, petechiae, and purpura often following a viral illness. Platelet counts are less than $100,000/mm^3$. Gastrointestinal, genitourinary, or mucous membrane bleeding is common, and in 1 to 3 percent of children with ITP intracranial hemorrhage occurs. Corticosteroids are used with very low platelet counts. A few children will go on to have chronic ITP requiring splenectomy.

CHILDHOOD MALIGNANCY

Leukemia is the most common form of cancer in childhood. Children usually have acute leukemia and 90 percent of children have acute lymphocytic leukemia (ALL). Leukemia is a great masquerader of many diseases and may present with fever, pallor, hemorrhage, bone or joint pains, lymphadenopathy, or hepatosplenomegaly. Onset can be at any age but peak onset is 3 to 5 years of age. Down's syndrome children, children postradiation therapy, and identical twins of children with leukemia are at higher risk to develop leukemia. Although blasts may appear in the peripheral smear, diagnosis is confirmed by an increased percentage of blasts in the bone marrow. Modern therapy has increased survival to over 50 percent at 5 years so that achieving a "cure" is now very possible. Because of immune suppression from the treatment, death usually comes from overwhelming infection due to unusual organisms such as pseudomonas, candida, or pneumocystis carinii.

Central nervous system tumors comprise the second most common group of childhood malignancies with peak incidence between 5 and 10 years. In childhood most CNS tumors are infratentorial (medulloblastoma, astrocytoma, and brain stem glioma). Common supratentorial tumors are gliomas and craniopharyngiomas. Symptoms of CNS tumors include signs of increased intracranial pressure, papilledema, and for cerebellar tumors, ataxia.

Neuroblastoma is the next most common neoplasm in childhood. Approximately half of all cases are diagnosed before age 3. Neuroblastoma often presents as an abdominal mass, as 37 percent arise from the adrenal gland and another 20 percent arise from other intra-abdominal sites. Since 70 percent have metastasized at the time of diagnosis, look for signs and symptoms of metastatic involvement. Bone pain, fever, weight loss, "raccoon eyes" (black eyes from periorbital metastases), elevated blood pressure, and lymphadenopathy are among the presenting complaints. Neuroblastoma causes an elevation of catecholamines and vanillylmandelic acid (VMA) in the urine.

Lymphoma (Hodgkin's and nonHodgkin's) arise in older children usually in the second decade. They may present with painless cervical adenopathy, intermittent fever, malaise, and weight loss. Depending on the stage of disease, curability rates are generally high.

Wilms' tumor is a malignant solid tumor of the kidney and 90 percent are diagnosed before the seventh birthday. There are a host of associated anomalies seen in patients with Wilms' tumor including other genitourinary anomalies, congenital aniridia, congenital hemihypertrophy, and Beckwith's syndrome. Wilms' tumor is usually found during the evaluation of an abdominal mass which may or may not be painful.

DISEASES OF THE IMMUNE SYSTEM

Allergic Disorders

An allergic reaction involves an antigen-antibody reaction which may lead to a systemic or a focal response. Urticaria (hives) is a hypersensitivity reaction due to release of histamine. This reaction is localized to the dermis and is usually of short duration. Potential causes include medications or vaccines, infectious agents of any kind, insect bites, certain foods (shellfish, egg albumin), inhalants, and physical factors (cold, heat, sunlight, trauma).

Atopic dermatitis (eczema) is a chronic recurring inflammation of the skin which can be seen at any stage of childhood. The dermatologic changes consist of erythema, oozing of transudate, scaling, and pruritis. Late changes include lichenifiction. Eczematoid skin changes occur on the face in early infancy, extensor surfaces in later infancy, and flexor surfaces during the rest of childhood.

Allergic rhinitis is another common atopic disorder whose primary symptoms include recurrent nasal congestion and discharge. The symptoms are brought on by inhaled allergens. Diagnosis is confirmed by the presence of recurrent nasal discharge, usually with seasonal variation in severity, conjunctival erythema, and tearing. Eosinophilia is found in the nasal secretions.

Immunology

Immune functions are carried out by the lymphoid family of blood cells. The plasma (B-cells) synthesize antibody (IgG, IgM, IgA, IgE, and Igd) while the lymphocyte (T-cell) lines are responsible for cellular immunity. Within the lymphocyte line, different functions are performed by the following types of cells: (1) long life memory cells; (2) effector cells (delayed hypersensitivity); (3) proliferating cells (release lymphokines); (4) helper cells; and (5) suppressor cells.

At birth the normal infant has IgG which was acquired transplacentally. This donated IgG will protect the fetus against bacteria (pneumococci, streptococci), viruses (measles, rubella, mumps), and toxins (diphtheria, tetanus). Breast-fed infants will have intestinal IgA which is secreted in the breast milk. Over the first year IgM, then IgG, and finally IgA and IgE rise to adult levels. IgM will rise in utero in response to a congenital infection.

Should an immunologic deficiency be suspected, B-cell competency is measured by immunoglobulin levels determined by immunoelectrophoresis and elevated antibody levels to dipththeria and tetanus in response to immunization. Cellular or T-cell immunity is demonstrated by skin tests to detect delayed hypersensitivity. Tuberculin, candida, trycophytin, and mumps skin tests are commonly used.

Infantile X-linked (Bruton) agammaglobulinemia occurs primarily in males and is associated with an increase in pyogenic infections such as those caused by staphylococci, pneumococci, and streptococci. Diagnosis is made by finding a marked decrease in immunoglobulins, a paucity of lymphoid tissue, and an absence of adenoid tissue on lateral nasopharyngeal x-rays. Patients are treated with monthly gammaglobulin injections. Children with DiGeorge's syndrome have a congenital absence of the thymus and parathyroid glands. They have a deficiency of cellular immunity but normal antibody levels. Delayed hypersensitivity reactions are absent. Severe combined immunodeficiency syndrome includes both absent immunoglobulins and absent cellular immunity. Infants with this disorder have recurrent severe bacterial, fungal, and viral infections.

DISEASES OF THE ENDOCRINE SYSTEM

Diabetes Mellitus

Diabetes mellitus has traditionally been divided into two types, juvenile onset (JDM, type I) and adult onset (type II). JDM is characterized by complete lack of insulin production while in adult onset disease resistance is found with normal or increased amounts of insulin. The cause of JDM is not known. A positive family history plays a role but the pattern of inheritance is unclear. Epidemiologic studies have implicated a viral cause. A viral agent may start an autoimmune process against the pancreatic β-cell in a genetically predisposed child.

Unlike adult onset disease, JDM has a short prodromal phase with the child often presenting with coma and ketoacidosis and a brief history of polyuria, polyphagia, polydipsia, and weight loss. The finding of hyperglycemia and glucosuria is diagnostic provided aspirin poisoning or Reye's syndrome is not present. Insulin therapy is always required in JDM although many children go through a brief "honeymoon" period after diagnosis in which they may need minimal insulin.

As in adult onset diabetes, after 15 to 20 years, JDM becomes complicated by a microangiopathy mostly affecting the retina and kidneys, a peripheral neuropathy, and premature atherosclerotic disease. Better control is increasingly being thought to prevent these complications. Tighter control is achievable through glucose monitoring with hemoglobin A_{1c} and home blood glucose measurements, and more physiologic insulin administration with two or three injections per day or an insulin pump. How these changes will affect the outcome of JDM in the future is unknown.

Thyroid Diseases

Hypothyroidism can be due to congenital or acquired diseases (Table 11-19). Congenital hypothyroidism (cretinism) leads to severe retardation, coarse facial features, large tongue, large fontanelles, lethargy, and prolonged neonatal jaundice. Older children with acquired hypothyroidism present with growth failure, constipation,

Table 11-19. Causes of Hypothyroidism in Childhood

Congenital hypoplasia
Hereditary hypothyroidism (inborn error of metabolism)
Iodide deficiency
Autoimmune disorder (Hashimoto's thyroiditis)
Irradiation
Hypopituitarism
   Decreased thyroid releasing factor (TRF)
   Decreased thryoid-stimulating hormone (TSH)
End-organ defect
Idiopathic

sluggish behavior, dry skin, and delayed puberty. T-4 is decreased and the bone age is delayed. Newborn screening detects congenital hypothyroidism early enough so that treatment with exogenous thyroid will prevent retardation.

Hyperthyroidism is characterized by nervousness, increased sweating, heat intolerance, increased appetite, proptosis, and tachycardia with increased pulse pressure. It is more common in females and beings to appear in the second decade of life. Thyrotoxicosis (Graves' disease) and Hashimoto's thyroiditis are the usual causes. Treatment for children is similar to the adult.

Adrenogenital Syndrome

Adrenogenital syndrome is a group of autosomal recessive disorders caused by an enzymatic defect in cortisone metabolism. Female infants present with virilization while males may have precocious puberty. In some forms of adrenogenital syndrome, aldosterone is not produced resulting in severe salt wasting in the neonatal period. Other defects lead to increased desoxycorticosterone and hypertension along with the virilization. All forms of adrenogenital syndrome have increased urinary 17-keto steroids.

Short Stature

In most cases, short stature is a variation of the normal growth patterns which have been influenced by familial stature, sex, race, psychosocial interaction, or nutrition (Table 11-20). Growth hormone deficiency is an un-

Table 11-20. Common Causes of Short Stature

Familial or genetic short stature
Constitutional delay
Genetic syndrome (Turner's syndrome, dwarfism)
Intrauterine growth retardation (fetal alcohol syndrome)
Psychosocial deprivation
Chronic disease (especially renal, gastrointestinal, and cardiac)
Hypothyroidism (*see* Table 11-19)
Hypopituitarism (growth hormone deficiency)

common reason for short stature. A good rule of thumb is that as long as growth is greater than 5 cm per year, a progressive disorder such as an endocrinopathy or psychosocial deprivation is unlikely. In the absence of a progressive loss of height growth or another primary disease, the first two causes in Table 11-20 become the most likely explanations for short stature. The bone age is normal with genetic short stature while it is delayed with constitutional delay. Children with constitutional delay will eventually achieve catch up growth.

INFECTIOUS DISEASES

We have already discussed many infectious diseases under the specific organ system affected. This section will cover those infectious agents not fully described in other sections of this chapter.

Group A β-hemolytic Streptococcus

Group A β-hemolytic *Streptococcus* (GABHS), the most common type of streptococcus leading to pediatric disease, may cause pharyngitis skin infections (impetigo), and scarlet fever. Impetigo presents with pruritic, weeping, honey-colored crusted lesions often beginning around the nose. Two-thirds of cases are mixed infections with both GABHS and staphylococci.

Scarlet fever usually occurs in middle childhood and results from a GABHS infection with a strain that produces an erythrogenic toxin. Scarlet fever presents with fever and a fine, erythematous, papular rash. Other associated findings include a strawberry tongue, palatine petechiae, Pastia's lines, and desquamation of the hands and feet (a late finding). GABHS may also cause cellulitis and adenitis. Rheumatic fever and glomerulonephritis are the two nonsuppurative diseases occurring after a GABHS infection.

Other types of streptococci may produce infections in children. Group B stretptococcal infections appear in the newborn period as the primary cause of sepsis, pneumonia, and meningitis. *Streptococcus viridans* is the most frequent cause of bacterial endocarditis.

Staphyloccal Infections

Staphyloccal infections may occur in a variety of locations. Cutaneous infections include impetigo, cellulitis, and staphylococcal scalded-skin syndrome (also known as toxic epidermal necrolysis or Ritter's disease). The *Staphylococcus* organism, when it is the sole invader, causes a bullous type of impetigo. Exfoliatin-producing strains of staphylococcus produce the scalded skin syndrome. The child begins with erythematous areas that are susceptible to necrolysis, a peeling off of the skin upon lateral pressure. These areas then progress to exfoliation and desquamation. The staphylococcus is the most common cause of osteomyelitis in children. Infants may get a rapidly progressing pneumonia characterized by pneumatocele formation. Staphylococcal food poisoning arises from an enterotoxin produced by the organism in contaminated food.

Pertussis

Pertussis, or whooping cough, can be a serious respiratory disease for children less than 2 years of age. It is caused by the bacterium, *Bordetella pertussis,* and is transmitted via the air with an incubation period of 7 to 14 days. Illness begins with a catarrhal stage of 1 to 3 weeks with cough, coryza, and vomiting. This is followed by the paroxysmal cough phase which may last 2 to 4 weeks. The white cell count is typically high with 70 to 80 percent lymphocytes. In infants complications include severe pneumonia and pneumothorax, asphyxia, and cerebral edema from the paroxysmal attacks. This is one of the diseases preventable by immunization.

Tuberculosis

Tuberculosis in children is usually asymptomatic and when clinically apparent most commonly presents as pulmonary disease. Children less than 3-years-old and females within 2 years of menarche are the most susceptible. Follow up of contacts of active cases and routine screening with the tine test or the Mantoux test with PPD are the main tools of prevention.

Viral Diseases

The most common viral diseases in childhood cause upper respiratory illnesses and gastroenteritis, have already been discussed, and do not have a unique enough clinical presentation to allow a specific species of virus to be identified. On the other hand, some viruses produce a specific syndrome. Some viruses including measles, rubella, and chickenpox are identifiable by the rash they produce (Table 11-21). Several Coxsackie viruses also produce a distinctive rash.

Mumps

Mumps is another common infectious disease of childhood that has been nearly eliminated by a vaccination program. The child presents with unilateral or bilateral swelling and tenderness of the parotid glands. The parotitis is preceded by fever, headache, and malaise for about 1 day. The incubation period is 16 to 18 days. Meningoencephalitis, pancreatitis, and orchitis may also occur. The serum amylase is often elevated.

Herpes Simplex Infections

Herpes simplex type 1 infections are extremely common in childhood presenting with several days of high fever and gingivastomatitis with ulcerations in the lips and buccal mucosa. Type 2 infections usually occur during the neonatal period to a baby born vaginally to a mother with active genital lesions. A vesicular rash appears at 1 week of age with hepatosplenomegaly, jaundice, and severe encephalitis that often leaves the infant profoundly retarded. This illness is preventable by deliv-

Table 11-21. Common Childhood Viral Diseases with Rashes

Disease	Incubation Period	Signs, Symptoms
Rubeola (measles)	2 weeks	3 day prodrome of cough, coryza, conjunctivitis, fever Maculopapular, generalized rash, spreads head to toe Koplik's spots (small white papule on buccal muscosa) may appear several days before rash
Rubella	2–3 weeks	Rapidly spreading pink, maculopapular rash Lymphadenopathy (postauricular, cervical) Low grade fever, resolves 3–5 days
Roseola	2 weeks	Prodrome of 3 days of high fever Rapidly appearing pink macular rash
Chicken Pox (varicella)	2–3 weeks	Papulovesicular pruritic rash with crusting May involve mucous membranes, mild fever
Fifth disease	1–2 weeks	"Slapped cheeks," confluent red rash on face Mild systemic symptoms
Pityriasis rosea	?	Begins with large annular lesion (herald patch) After 5–10 days, generalized, pruritic, papular, oval lesions in "Christmas tree" distribution lasting as long as 6 weeks

ering the baby by a caesarean section rather than vaginally.

Fungal Infections

Fungal infections may be cutaneous or systemic. While systemic infections are rare during the pediatric years, cutaneous fungal infections are very common. "Ringworm" or tinea corporis appears as a circular raised lesion with central clearing. Tinea versicolor is caused by fungi which produce a flat, scaling, patchy rash that is either hypo- or hyperpigmented. A scaling, erythematous rash on the upper thighs during adolescence is tinea cruris. Fungal infection with red, peeling, fissuring lesions between the toes is tinea pedis or "athlete's foot." On the scalp, tinea capitis appears as areas of alopecia with the broken ends of hair at the level of the scalp. Tinea capitis may involve the deeper tissues forming a tender, boggy lesion known as a kerion. The other common fungal infections are caused by *Candida albicans*. White curdlike plaques on the oral mucosal surfaces during infancy (thrush) is a candidal infection. Candida thrives on moist, warm intertriginous areas such as the diaper region where it produces a red, moist rash with satellite pustules. Chemical irritation and seborrhea may also cause diaper rashes.

MISCELLANEOUS DISEASES

Cystic Fibrosis

Cystic fibrosis (CF) is a disease of the exocrine glands that results in abnormal mucus production. CF has an autosomal recessive mode of inheritance and is found primarily in Caucasians with an incidence of between 1 : 1000 and 1 : 2000. It is the most common lethal genetic disease of Caucasian children with death usually occurring before age 30. About 5 percent of the Caucasian population are carriers (heterozygotes). No reproductive advantage is known to explain the continuation of such a high carrier rate. Heterozygote or prenatal detection are presently not possible.

Chronic pulmonary disease and pancreatic insufficiency are the most common manifestations of CF. Pulmonary disease presents with recurrent infection (usually pneumonia, often from various Pseudomonas strains) and small airway obstruction (wheezing) due to the abnormal bronchial mucus. The airway obstruction progresses to bronchiectasis and hypoxia with clubbing and cor pulmonale. Severe hypoxia and right heart failure are the causes of the early death in patients with CF.

Eighty percent of children with CF have pancreatic insufficiency which presents with fat and protein malabsorption with foul-smelling bulky, greasy stools and failure to thrive. Meconium ileus, rectal prolapse, cirrhosis, nasal polyps, pansinusitis, diabetes, and aspermia are other problems that CF may cause.

Diagnosis is made by measuring the elevated salt content of the sweat by performing a "sweat test." Early diagnosis along with pancreatic enzyme replacement and vigorous pulmonary treatment have raised mean survival to late adolescence.

Juvenile Rheumatoid Arthritis

Juvenile rheumatoid arthritis (JRA) has five major types (Table 11-22). Unlike adult rheumatoid arthritis, JRA most often involves the large joints, rarely leads to joint damage, and carries a good prognosis. No laboratory test is pathognomonic. Aspirin is the mainstay of treatment with close ophthalmalogic examination being critical in several of the forms of JRA with iridocyclitis.

Henoch-Schönlein Purpura

Honoch-Schönlein purpura (HSP) is a type of vaculitis affecting the arterioles that is unique to childhood. No specific etiology is known but the disease often follows an upper respiratory tract or streptococcal infection. The first sign is usually an urticarial or papular rash which becomes flat and then purpuric. The distribution is predominantly below the waist. Angioneurotic adema of the scalp, eyelids, and legs may occur in younger children and arthritis of the large joints is common.

Table 11-22. Juvenile Rheumatoid Arthritis Syndromes

Type	Characteristics
Systemic (Still's disease)	Diurnal fever Erythematous, maculopapular rash with fever Lymphadenopathy and hepatosplenomegaly Arthritis may occur after systemic symptoms
Pauciarticular	Female > male Chronic iridocyclitis, often leading to decreased vision ANA positive
Polyarticular	Chronic continuing polyarthritis HLA-B27 antigen present
Ankylosing spondylitis	Male > female Pauciarticular Acute self-limiting iridocyclitis HLA-B27 antigen present
Adult type	Rheumatoid nodules present Boney erosions Positive rheumatoid factor

Colicky abdominal pain is frequent and may be severe enough to mimic an acute abdomen. Rectal bleeding results from hemorrhage into the bowel wall and rarely intussusception or perforation occurs. The kidneys are involved in up to half of the cases with hematuria and proteinuria which can occasionally lead to a chronic nephritis. HSP generally resolves over 7 to 14 days and steroid treatment is reserved for severe gastrointestinal involvement.

Reye's Syndrome

Reye's syndrome is a disease of children discovered over the past 20 years that consists of encephalopathy and fatty degeneration of the viscera. Although mitochondrial dysfunction appears as the common pathway of this multiorgan failure, the cause remains obscure. Three to seven days after a mild respiratory illness (influenza B) or the chickenpox, the child presents with vomiting followed shortly by increasing signs of encephalopathy progressing from agitation to delirium to decerebrate coma. Liver function is markedly abnormal with elevated serum SGOT, SGPT, and ammonia levels while the bilirubin remains normal. A normal cerebrospinal fluid rules out encephalitis.

The course of Reye's syndrome may vary from minimal illness to death. Supportive treatment of hepatic failure and cerebral edema improves the outcome.

Sudden Infant Death Syndrome

Sudden infant death syndrome (SIDS), also known as crib or cot death, is the leading cause of postneonatal mortality, from 1 month to 1 year. Most cases occur between 1 and 6 months of age during sleep. The parent usually goes to awaken or check their child only to find the child dead. In about half the cases, an upper respiratory infection was present. On autopsy, no specific cause of the death is determined. SIDS is more frequent during the winter, in premature infants, and in lower socioeconomic groups. Theories abound but no etiology for SIDS is known. The physician can play a critical role in supporting the family and counselling to relieve the guilt felt by families who usually believe themselves to be responsible.

REFERENCES

Behrman RE, Vaughan VC III (eds): Nelson Textbook of Pediatrics. 12th Ed. WB Saunders Co., Philadelphia, 1983

Hoekelman RA (ed): Principles of Pediatrics. McGraw-Hill, Inc., New York, 1978

Roberts KB (ed): Manual of Clinical Problems in Pediatrics. Little, Brown, and Company, Boston, 1979

Rudolph AM: Pediatrics. 16th Ed. Appleton-Century-Crofts, East Norwalk, 1977

MULTIPLE CHOICE QUESTIONS

For each question choose the best answer.

1. Over the last decade, the leading cause of death in childhood is
   A. Accidents
   B. Congenital malformations
   C. Cancer
   D. Infections

2. An infant is born weighing 6 lbs. At 4 months this infant should weigh
   A. 9 lbs
   B. 12 lbs
   C. 15 lbs
   D. 18 lbs

For each nutrient, select the correct nutrient deficiency.

3. Vitamin D   A. Hemolytic anemia

4. Vitamin E   B. Microcytic anemia

5. Vitamin K   C. Bowed legs

6. Iron   D. 2-day-old born at home with hemorrhaging

7. Global development delays are indicative of
   A. Cerebral palsy
   B. Mental retardation
   C. Learning disability
   D. Hyperactivity

8. A learning disability
   A. Is indicative of an emotional disturbance
   B. Is best determined by the WISC test
   C. Is another term for hyperactivity
   D. Is present when scholastic achievement falls behind mental age by 2 years

9. Which of the following is abnormal behavior for a 3 year old?
   A. Thumb-sucking
   B. Masturbation

C. Head-banging
D. None of the above

10. The most frequent behavior problem during grades 1 to 3 is
    A. Truant behavior
    B. Hyperactivity
    C. Encopresis
    D. Thumb-sucking

11. The suspicion of child abuse necessitates all of the following *except*
    A. Reporting one's suspicion to the police
    B. Skeletal survey
    C. Discussion of your concerns with the parents
    D. Reporting one's suspicion to the local protective services
    E. Documentation of any failure to thrive

12. Which of the following is most effective in preventing poisoning in young children?
    A. Ipecac
    B. Poison control centers
    C. The usage of child proof containers
    D. The use of aggressive media campaigns

13. Which of the following is not a component of lead poisoning?
    A. Encephalopathy
    B. History of pica
    C. Macrocytic anemia
    D. Seizures
    E. Intellectual deficits

14. All of the following are variants of a normal newborn *except*
    A. Mongolian spot
    B. Respiratory rate of 48
    C. Erythema toxicum
    D. Hip click
    E. Cephalohematoma

15. A premature infant has respiratory distress syndrome. Sequelae may include all of the following *except*
    A. Necrotizing enterocolitis
    B. Pneumothorax
    C. Retrolental fibroplasia
    D. Bronchopulmonary dysplasia

16. Neonatal sepsis is not likely to be recognized by
    A. Poor feeding
    B. Apnea

C. Fever
D. Hypothermia

17. Which of the following is not true about epiglottitis?
    A. It is usually caused by *H influenza* type B
    B. Roentgenogram shows "steeple" sign
    C. Child responds to antibiotic
    D. Disease has rapid onset with fever, drooling, and dysphagia

18. Asthma attacks may be associated with
    A. Emotional stress
    B. Exercise
    C. Atopy
    D. Meteorological changes
    E. All of the above

19. The most common congenital cardiac malformation is
    A. Tetralogy of Fallot
    B. Atrial septal defect
    C. Pulmonary stenosis
    D. Ventricular septal defect

20. Which of the following is *not* a major Jones criteria for rheumatic fever?
    A. Arthralgia
    B. Subcutaneous nodules
    C. Chorea
    D. Carditis

21. Pyloric stenosis is frequently associated with
    A. Cystic fibrosis
    B. Gastrointestinal obstruction is early infancy
    C. Hyponatremic dehydration
    D. Palpable "olive" in the abdominal right lower quandrant

Match the clinical findings in the first column with the offending agent in the second column.

22. Conjunctivitis   A. Adenovirus

23. Rhinorrhea, laryngitis   B. Clamydia

24. Splenomegaly, atypical lymphocytes   C. Coxsackie A

25. Scarletinaform rash   D. Gonococcus

26. Pharyngeal vesicles and ulcers   E. Infectious mononucleosis

27. Sexually active teenager

F. Group A β-hemolytic *Streptococcus*

28. Acute otitis media

G. Hemophilus influenza

29. All of the following may cause cirrhosis *except*
    A. Cystic fibrosis
    B. Gallstones
    C. Wilson's disease
    D. α_1-Antitrypsin deficiency

30. The most common cause of nephrotic syndrome is
    A. Proteinuria
    B. Streptococcal infection
    C. A virus
    D. Idiopathic

31. All of the following are true about cryptorchidism *except*
    A. Requires repair by age 12 years
    B. Can be caused by an active cremasteric reflex
    C. Is usually unilateral
    D. Is a contraindication for circumcision

32. Severe mental retardation is defined by an IQ below
    A. 30
    B. 40
    C. 50
    D. 55

33. Which is *not* a feature of a simple febrile seizure?
    A. Generalized seizure
    B. Lasting 10 minutes
    C. Occurred in a 3 month old child
    D. Most common presentation of viral meningitis in a preschool child

34. Cerebral palsy
    A. Is defined as a nonprogressive lesion of the brain causing a motor deficit
    B. Is usually associated with a seizure disorder
    C. May resolve with intensive physical therapy
    D. Is caused by a focal lesion within the extrapyramidal tracts

35. An 18 month old child would be unlikely to have anemia because of
    A. Sickle cell disease
    B. Thalassemia
    C. Blood loss
    D. Inadequate dietary iron

36. All of the following are at increased risk of leukemia *except*
    A. Child with sickle cell disease
    B. Child with Down's syndrome
    C. Child with history of radiation treatment
    D. Identical twin of child with leukemia

37. Causes of short stature include all *except*
    A. Hypothyroidism
    B. Adrenogenital syndrome
    C. Turner's syndrome
    D. Chronic renal disease

38. Which of the following is not prevented by routine immunizations?
    A. Chicken pox
    B. Measles
    C. Rubella
    D. Pertussis

39. After a viral illness, a child presents with vomiting and disorientation. Which of the following is unlikely?
    A. Elevated serum ammonia level
    B. Recent history of aspirin use
    C. Elevated serum ketones
    D. A normal cerebral spinal fluid exam

Answers to Multiple Choice Questions

1 A	2 B	3 C	4 A	5 D
6 B	7 B	8 D	9 D	10 B
11 A	12 C	13 C	14 D	15 A
16 C	17 B	18 E	19 D	20 A
21 B	22 B	23 A	24 E	25 F
26 C	27 D	28 G	29 B	30 D
31 D	32 A	33 C	34 A	35 C
36 A	37 B	38 A	39 C	

12

Preventive Medicine and Public Health

Donald A. Kennedy

In modern society, there are two major branches of scientific inquiry and professional practice associated with the preservation and restoration of health and the relief of suffering. They are the fields of medicine and public health. The practice of clinical medicine is primarily concerned with responding to individual requests for professional consultation and treatment. The field of public health is primarily concerned with preventing the occurrence of disease, injury, and disability. Public health deals with the sciences and professional skills needed to maintain and improve the health status of population groups.

The fields of public health and preventive medicine and important because there are a number of disease and injuries that can be more effectively controlled by prevention rather than by curative therapies or rehabilitative procedures. This has been demonstrated in the case of diphtheria, cholera, malaria, hepatitis, typhoid fever, smallpox, and poliomyelitis. There is growing evidence to support a preventive strategy for diseases such as cancer, heart disease, and stroke, and for injuries due to accidents.

PUBLIC HEALTH

Public health activities in the United States trace their origin back to the sanitary reform movement which began in England in the nineteenth century. Public health activities emerged in close association with patterns of industrialization and urbanization. These societal changes had a negative impact upon health status and produced premature death for significant numbers of people. The most visible danger was in the form of epidemics of communicable disease. Significant advances in controlling these epidemics were achieved through environmental sanitation—control of the purity of water supplies and changes in the handling of sewage and waste materials.

In the United States, there were public health developments beginning in the 1830s—a time of increase in immigration and urban growth. These activities produced situations that required urgent attention. There were shortages of adequate housing, poor water quality, and poor handling of waste water. This resulted in recurrent epidemics of smallpox, typhoid, typhus, cholera, and yellow fever in the mid to late 1800s.

New York established the Metropolitan Board of Health in 1866, an important event in the development of public health in the United States. Other states and communities soon established health departments—Massachusetts (1869), California (1870), District of Columbia (1871), Minnesota (1872), Virginia (1872), Michigan (1873), Maryland (1874), Alabama (1875), Wisconsin (1876), and Illinois (1877). At the national level, Congress created the National Board of Health in 1879, but it was not viable and disappeared after 1883. In 1953, the Federal government established a cabinet-level Department of Health, Education, and Welfare. This included the Public Health Service, the Children's Bureau, and the Food and Drug Administration. In 1946, the World Health Organization (WHO) was established.

Perhaps the most dramatic recent accomplishment of WHO has been the worldwide eradication of smallpox. This event occurred on October 26, 1977, nearly 200 years after Jenner developed smallpox vaccine.

Since the turn of the century, there has been a significant shift in the profile of disease and causes of preventable death in the United States. Infectious and communicable diseases, such as tuberculosis and influenza have been replaced by chronic diseases such as heart disease, cancer, stroke, and accidents as the major causes of death.

Throughout history, public health actions have been closely linked to both public education and political action. During the past decade, there has been growing recognition in Canada and in the United States about the importance of preventive strategies to complement the development of highly sophisticated diagnostic and therapeutic services. A report was issued in the United States in 1979 on this subject titled, "Healthy People, the Surgeon General's Report on Health Promotion and Disease Prevention." Fifteen categories of health problems were identified along with specific plans for action and control. The fifteen areas were family planning services, prenatal and infant care, immunizations, sexually-transmitted disease services, control of high blood pressure, toxic agent control, occupational safety and health, control of accidental injury, fluoridation of community water supplies, infectious agent control, cessation of smoking, reducing misuse of alcohol and drugs, improving nutrition, exercise and fitness, and stress control. These areas of program priority were selected because of the significance of the health problems and the potential for application of effective control measures.

EPIDEMIOLOGY

The scientific research methodology utilized most frequently in the field of public health is called epidemiology. It can be defined as the study of changing patterns of disease in a population. The emphasis is upon the study of populations, not individual patients.

Epidemiologic methods are used to search for the etiology of a variety of disease states, to identify factors which influence susceptibility, to locate environmental factors that facilitate the transmission of disease, and to identify modes of transmission, especially for infectious disease. The epidemiologic method was developed to study the natural history of the disease process in populations, including the preclinical phase before the disease state is identified by the host or by practicing physicians. The method is used to monitor the health status of populations through time and to determine which major dis-

eases need attention in terms of the allocation of resources. The method is also used in clinical field trials when new drugs or therapies are being tested. The method complements the research focus on individual patients in clinical medicine.

Both time and space are significant dimensions of the epidemiologic method. Time considerations include short intervals of time when there is a sudden outbreak of disease, the clustering of onset of disease in relation to an hypothesized cause, secular disease patterns that run over long periods of time, and seasonal patterns related to the annual cycle. In terms of geographic space, the epidemiologic method makes comparisons between populations located in different geographic areas. The overall mortality rate from cancer is about equal in Japan and the United States, but the mortality rate from stomach cancer in Japan is five times greater than that in the United States. The reverse is true for cancer of the colon. Cancer of the breast and prostate, which are major causes of death in the United States, have very low mortality rates in Japan. The use of maps to identify residential location of persons suffering from specific illnesses often has assisted in the identification of the cause. Snow used such a method to identify cases of acute cholera in London in 1854. The discovery that these cases were clustered around the water pump on Broad Street led to the discovery of contaminated water as the source of transmission of the bacteria.

In making comparisons, it is necessary to develop quantitative measures — the concept of rate is a key part of epidemiological studies. The rate is expressed in the form of a formula as follows:

$$\text{rate} = \frac{\text{number of events in a specified period}}{\text{population at risk of experiencing the event}} \times 10^n$$

The multiplier 10^n (1,000; 100,000; etc.) produces a rate that is a manageable number. There are several important factors used in calculations of vital statistics. The birth rate equals the number of live births divided by the midyear population. The crude death rate is the number of deaths divided by the midyear population. The infant mortality rate is the number of live-born infants who die before age 1 year divided by the live births in the year.

There are two basic kinds of rates — incidence and prevalence. An incidence rate is the number of new events in a specified time period divided by the population at risk of experiencing the event during that time. A prevalence rate is the total number of all individuals who have an attribute or disease at a particular time (or during a specified period) divided by the population at risk of having the attribute or disease.

The distinction between incidence and prevalence is important. The incidence rate indicates the probability that a new case of disease will occur during a time interval, whereas prevalence rate measures the probability that an individual will have the disease at a single point in time, as on a given day during the year. Incidence rates are useful for studying the disease causation and the evaluation of preventive measures. Prevalence rates estimate the magnitude of the health problem and are especially useful for administrative and planning purposes. The duration of an episode of illness or disease is the key to this distinction. If we assume that the population is stable and the incidence and duration are not changing, then the relationship can be expressed as prevalence equals incidence times mean duration. For example, if the incidence of a particular disease is at a constant level of 60/100,000 per year and the mean duration is 6 years, the prevalence is 360/100,000.

For some purposes, it is valuable to use an annual prevalence figure, meaning the total cases existing at any time during a year divided by the population. This measure includes cases arising before, but extending into or through the year, as well as those that have their inception during the year. In studies of acute infectious disease, it is often useful to estimate the lethality of an acute disease by estimating the case-fatality rate. This is simply the ratio of deaths to cases. An additional measure is the secondary attack rate. This was devised to measure the dissemination of contagious disease within families. It is calculated by observing families from the time of the onset of the first case of the disease for a period over which related cases might occur. The secondary attack rate is calculated by dividing the number of secondary cases by the number of susceptibles at risk.

There are a number of personal characteristics strongly associated with patterns of health and disease. They include age, gender, ethnic group, occupation, economic status, marital status, and family history.

Certain diseases have been linked to groups working in specific occupations. This is true for people working with asbestos, coal dust, lead, and certain chemicals, such as organic solvents or pesticides.

Patterns of disease and death are strongly associated with marital status. In general, married people are less disease-prone than unmarried persons. Recent studies have shown a sharp rise in death for those who have just entered widowhood. Some disease conditions run in families, due to a common residential environment and common genetic background.

This list of characteristics is not a complete list. Other characteristics, such as size of family, birth order in family, mother's age at birth of child, body build, and blood group have been shown to be associated with patterns of disease and injury.

RESEARCH DESIGN

The basic methods and frame of reference of epidemiology can be used in a variety of scientific studies. There are two major types: observational and experimental studies. In terms of actual practice, most studies are observational because of the ethical problems associated with conducting experimental studies in human populations. There are exceptions to this general rule and they are usually found in controlled clinical trials of new therapeutic procedures or drugs. A comparison is made between a standard therapy and a newly developed therapy to see which is more effective. Such trials were conducted during the 1950s in testing the efficacy of the newly developed polio vaccines. They are currently in use with a variety of drug therapies and surgical procedures.

Observational studies can be divided into descriptive and analytic categories. Descriptive studies are useful for identifying disease outbreaks, assessing the impact of diseases on a community, and finding control measures that are effective with certain subgroups in the population.

Analytic studies are organized to explore one or more hypotheses about a disease process. There are three kinds of analytic epidemiologic studies: cross-sectional, prospective, and case-control.

The simplest form of study is the cross-sectional study, in which a set of individuals is chosen from a general population or from a particular subgroup, such as military personnel or workers in a particular industry. These individuals are selected without regard for what may be known of their health status and are investigated concerning the attributes of interest. The research question may have to do with variations in blood pressure, patterns of behavior that are health-related, vital capacity of the lungs, presence of infections, and the like. For example, it is possible to study the presence of chronic bronchitis by such a study. A cross-sectional survey can be designed to produce simple descriptions: occasionally it can be used to test a specific hypothesis.

The prospective study deals with the identification of a defined population in which there are individuals or groups with differing levels of exposure to risk. The population group is then followed through time to some suitable end point. The aim is usually to test hypotheses about suspected risk factors or presumed causes of a chronic disease. The longitudinal heart disease study in Framingham, Massachusetts, is an excellent example of a prospective study that is focused on the measurement of biologic variations in relation to the onset of heart disease. Often it is necessary to follow a population for 5 or 10 years or longer in order to accumulate sufficient numbers of events to demonstrate statistically significant differences between the groups exposed to different levels of risk.

Case-control studies often develop out of clinical observations by physicians caring for patients. An example of this is the work of Percivall Pott when he described cancer of the scrotum in 1775 and attributed it to exposure to soot, an occupational hazard of chimney sweeps. These were the only people he had seen with this condition.

A case-control study is a carefully designed extension of clinical history taking in a defined subgroup. The subgroup consists of cases of persons who have the disease and of cases of persons who do not have the disease and can therefore serve as controls. The other names used for this kind of study are retrospective study or case history study. A case control study may demonstrate a significant difference in patterns of disease between two groups of individuals that are matched on all characteristics except presence of the disease or exposure to a particular risk factor. Studies of this kind can often produce results quickly and at little expense. It is also possible to study more than one risk factor at the same time.

The objective of case-control studies is to demonstrate whether a significant statistical association exists between the condition and a presumed risk factor. Unlike a prospective study, which can produce incidence rates with reference to exposed and unexposed groups, a case-control study does not provide data from which one can calculate incidence rates. The case-control study does produce the odds ratio. This is the exposure ratio in the cases divided by the exposure ratio in the controls. If the condition is uncommon, the odds ratio is a close approximation to the relative risk. Relative risk is the ratio of incidence rate in the exposed group compared to the incidence rate in the unexposed group.

Both prospective and retrospective studies can be used to test a variety of hypotheses about suspected etiological factors. Although none of these methods can provide absolute proof, they are capable of providing sufficient evidence so that decisions can be made and public actions taken. This was certainly the case with the early studies of the statistical association between cigarette smoking and lung cancer.

Factors that should be considered in making a judgment about the empirical findings include the following: the strength of the association, similar findings by different investigators, finding a quantitative relationship between the amount of the risk factor and the frequency of the disease, noticing a significant chronological relationship between exposure and onset of disease, isolation and specificity of the factor in producing changes in the incidence of the disease, and having evidence fit the facts that are thought to be related.

In experimental studies, a population group is selected for a deliberate trial of a preventive or therapeutic treatment. The effects are measured by comparing the outcome of the two treatment techniques. Members of the experimental and control groups are selected so that they are as close to identical as possible. Members of the total population group are chosen randomly to receive, or not receive, the experimental treatment. Those who do not receive the treatment are given some type of substitute or placebo therapy or a previously tested method of therapy. In ideal terms, neither the people who participate in the experiment nor the attending physician should know who is receiving the experimental or control treatments. If these conditions are met, the experiment is known as a double blind trial. The double blind method serves to reduce, as far as possible, the effect of bias and the power of suggestion in determining the outcome. When it is possible to meet the ethical requirements, controlled clinical trials provide valuable new scientific knowledge. Examples of this form of study are the major clinical field trials in 1954 of the polio virus vaccine and the study of fluoridation of the water supply in the towns of Newburgh and Kingston, New York, during the 1940s.

BIOSTATISTICS

The field of biostatistics is a specialized branch of the general field of statistics. It deals with the application of statistical methods to biological and medical phenomena. Concepts and techniques from the closely related field of social statistics are often used in health care studies dealing with patterns of human behavior.

The field of biostatistics can be divided into descriptive statistics and analytic or inferential statistics. Descriptive statistics involves the presentation of data in graphs and tables and the calculation of numerical summaries, such as frequencies, averages, medians, percentages, and ranges. Inferential or analytic statistics provide a methodology for arriving at conclusions or making decisions about a population by reasoning from the evidence of observed numerical data in a sample of that population.

Biomedical data may be classified according to four measurement scales. Measurement at the simplest level involves giving a category assignment to specified events of a given variable. For example, measurement of the variable known as "blood type" consists of the classifications "type O," "type A," "type B," and "type AB." When names, numbers, or symbols are used to specify the groups to which various subjects belong, the measurement scale is called a nominal or classificatory scale. Other variables that can be measured on nominal scales are gender, race, and marital status. It is essential that the categories be exhaustive and mutually exclusive, meaning that each individual event must fall into one and only one category.

The second type of measurement scale is called the ordinal scale. It differs from the nominal scale because there is a relationship and graded order between the categories. Episodes of illness can be classified according to the variable of "getting worse," "stable," "getting better." The variable of patient satisfaction with hospital care can be classified according to an ordinal scale. The ordinal scale requires that categories be arranged from low to high or high to low so that the subjects or events are ranked according to their scores along a dimension.

The third measurement scale is the interval scale. It may be used when it is possible to identify units of equal size along the scale dimension. With this scale, it is necessary to specify how much more one variable is when measured against another. The Fahrenheit temperature scale uses degrees that are a variable measured on an interval scale. An important weakness of the interval scale is the absence of a true zero point.

When measurement begins at a true zero point, and the scale has equal intervals, then the ratio scale of measurement has been achieved. Variables such as length, time, volume, mass, and temperature in degrees Kelvin are variables that can be measured on a ratio scale. Temperature measured on the Kelvin scale starts with absolute zero temperature.

The type of measurement scale used in a study determines the kinds of descriptive statistical measures that can be used in a meaningful way. Data that are measured on nominal or ordinal scales usually require nonparametric statistical methods. Most of the traditional parametric statistical techniques require at least an interval scale of measurement.

Data that have been collected in a scientific study may be arranged to produce frequency tables or frequency diagrams. The basic categories for classifying the data are arranged in a column, and a parallel column is generated showing the number of times that each of these events is represented in the sample. An important feature of the shape of a frequency diagram is its symmetry or lack of symmetry. Distributions that are considered symmetric are nearly equal at points on either side of a central value. Skewed distributions do not show a relationship to a central value in the same manner.

It is possible to classify data into intervals to simplify the preparation of a frequency table. Measurements of a variety of biological substances can be accurately measured to one or two decimal points. It is possible to group these data according to established intervals without distorting the frequency pattern that is generated. The frequency diagram for grouped data using intervals is called a "histogram."

Once the data have been recorded and displayed in a frequency table or histogram, it is necessary to describe the distribution in terms of central tendency or location and dispersion or spread.

The mean of a sample is the arithmetic average of the sample values and it represents the center of the data according to the size of the values. The mean is sometimes called the "expected value" or the "center of gravity." The median divides the sample so that half the observations are below it and half of them are above it. This means that the median locates the center of the data by count and disregards size.

The mode is related to the pattern of peak or peaks in the frequency distribution. If there is only one peak, the distribution is said to be unimodal and the sample value corresponding to this peak is called the "mode." The mode is the most frequent sample value.

Once the characteristics of location and central tendency have been accurately identified, it is necessary to describe the variation. Variation can arise from intrinsic differences among the subjects being measured. Examples of this are the biological variation from patient to patient. There are also extrinsic factors, such as the failure of the measuring techniques to yield the same result when measuring the same subject on repeated occasions. These two sources of variation combine to determine the spread among the observed values in a particular table.

There are two common measures of variation. One is the range of sample values and the other is the standard deviation of the sample. Tables are usually easy to interpret and compare. The number of observations falling into each interval is presented as a fraction or percentage of the total number of observations. The absolute frequency divided by the total number of observations is the relative frequency. The relative frequency is expressed as a percentage.

The cumulative frequency is the fraction, or percentage of observations, below the upper boundary of each successive interval. It is obtained by adding the relative frequencies.

The standard deviation of the sample, is an indication of how spread out the sample is. It is calculated from deviations of individual sample values from the sample mean. Because the sum of the deviations from the sample mean will be zero, it is necessary to square each of the deviations, calculate their average, then take the square root. The resulting figure gives the standard deviation of the sample.

The level of measurement achieved in recording the data is the key to the selection of appropriate, descriptive statistical measures. For nominal data, there are very few descriptive statistics. Even if numerical codes are used to define categories, it is not appropriate to perform numerical operations on nominal scale variables. The only summary that is appropriate is the frequency of observations in the various categories, the percentages, and the mode. The descriptive statistics most appropriate for describing ordinal data are frequency counts, the median, and the mode.

Both the interval and ratio scales allow the use of ordinary operations of arithmetic. All of the basic methods of descriptive statistics can be employed.

It is essential for anyone dealing with statistical analysis to recognize the importance of the relationship between samples and populations. When selecting the sample, care must be taken to be sure that each observation or unit in the population has an equal chance of being included in any sample. The usual way to accomplish this is to collect the sample data by using a simple random sample method. This method protects against conscious or unconscious bias on the part of the investigator. The best method for random sampling is to use some kind of mechanical means or a table of random numbers. Another sampling technique that is used is the nonrandom predefined system. This sample is developed by obtaining events from predetermined subpopulation groups. A representation of all significant subsections of the population will be included in the sample.

The frequency distribution that is calculated from data in a sample is called an empirical distribution. It is used to make estimates on the true distribution in the total population. The frequency distribution of all the values in the total population is called the theoretical distribution. The most frequently used continuous theoretical distribution is the normal distribution. The normal distribution, or bell curve, is particularly useful in making studies of a large number of naturally occurring phenomena. The distribution of height, weight, and blood pressure in a population fall on a normal distribution curve.

The concepts and mathematical methods of inferential statistics are based upon the basic concepts of descriptive statistics, plus an understanding of probability and the relationships between samples and populations.

HEALTH DATA

Data about health events in the United States come from two basic sources; from routine administrative reports of a variety of health service organizations and agencies and from special population studies.

The United States Bureau of the Census conducts an extensive survey of the total population of the United States every 10 years. This procedure has been in operation since 1790 and it produces a sizable body of data about the total population. This information is essential to provide information for the denominator of epidemiologic formulas. Data collected in the census include a

count of all individuals and enumeration of age and gender, marital status, household membership, ethnicity, family income, immigration status, service in the armed forces, and related information. These data on population characteristics are categorized according to geographical areas using political units such as states, counties, municipalities, townships, and units known as census districts.

Data are developed at the local level and this information is forwarded through channels to a state governmental agency and then to the national government. Data are collected, compiled and published by the National Center for Health Statistics (NCHS). The Center provides tabulations that are published annually. Data on marriage, divorce, and birth are useful in planning a variety of health care services. In recent years, special surveys have been conducted to supplement the data obtained through the registration process.

Survey data collected in recent years include the information on family socioeconomic characteristics, pre- and postmedical care, dental care, infant immunization, health care financing, and other factors related to maternal and infant health.

For many years, the data produced by the Death Registration System have been used for studying changes in the health characteristics of the population. The present registration system has provided data on virtually 100 percent of all deaths since 1933.

The United States uses the international classification of diseases, injuries, and causes of death for categorizing cause of death in its vital statistics. The WHO has taken the initiative in obtaining cooperation from a large number of nations to collect data on cause of death in a consistent fashion. The NCHS publishes life tables for each individual state and for the whole country. Changes in expectation of life at various ages constitute an important indication of the progress of medical and public health programs.

Patterns of illness and injury in the population are more difficult to collect on a regular and systematic basis. In the United States, cases of reportable diseases are given by physicians to local or state health authorities and the data are compiled on a weekly basis. Weekly reporting of reportable diseases is a data collection system authorized by Congress in 1893 and used by all of the states since 1925. The information is transmitted to the United States Centers for Disease Control (CDC). The Public Health Service and the CDC publish state and national data in a weekly morbidity and mortality report. Lists of diseases include specified communicable diseases, foodborne diseases, and diseases transmitted by mammals, birds, and insects. This disease reporting system is used to initiate local case investigation in order to detect and investigate potential epidemic situations.

Since 1965, the NCHS has maintained a system for collecting patient data from hospitals. The Center also maintains inventories on nursing homes, personal care homes, chronic illness institutions, and other long-term care facilities. Since the establishment of funding for medical care under Medicare in 1966, the Health Care Financing Administration has been collecting data on hospitalization, outpatient care, and extended care. Since 1946, data on mental health and mental illness have been assembled by the National Institute of Mental Health. Over the years, most of the record-keeping systems have dealt with patient services in hospitals or long-term facilities rather than in physicians' offices. To correct this imbalance, the National Center for Health Service Statistics initiated an ambulatory medical care survey in 1973.

The most comprehensive single source of data about health status in the United States is the health interview survey conducted by the NCHS. This survey program was initiated in 1957. It is based upon a scientifically designed national sample of 130,000 persons each year. The sample for data collection each week is representative of the population of the United States. Findings from the weekly samples are accumulated and compiled as quarterly and annual findings. The questionnaire requests information on demographic variables such as education, employment, veteran's status, family income, and family organization. Health variables include acute illness, injuries, specified chronic conditions, days of disability, work loss, and long-term limitations of activity. There are items that request information on use of health services such as frequency and place of visits to physicians and dentists, as well as frequency and duration of hospitalization.

Recently, the health interview survey has been supplemented by the health examination survey. This program was started in 1960 to provide greater precision of information on diagnostic classification, examination procedures, and biological abnormalities. This series of surveys is also based on national population samples. The surveys are organized to collect information on various age groups. The content of the examinations differs with each survey cycle. Emphasis has been placed upon chronic disease among adults and studies of children and adolescents. Primary emphasis has been placed on physical growth and development and performance on a variety of psychological tests for the younger age groups.

All data-collecting cycles have provided information concerning the following areas: prevalence of chronic conditions that can be determined by a single examination; distribution of a range of physiologic characteristics such as blood count, cholesterol, blood glucose, blood pressure, bone age, levels of hearing, and vision acuity; and anthropometric distributions of height, weight, skinfold, and other anatomical characteristics. These data are analyzed and then published in a series of monographs by the NCHS. Data are also available to medical reserachers who may wish to use the information for different kinds of analysis.

COMMUNICABLE DISEASES

The history of public health and preventive medicine is associated with the study of infectious disease and its control. A large number of disease conditions can be categorized as infectious or communicable. There is no satisfactory way to classify all communicable diseases, but it is useful to classify them by process of transmission — person-to-person, animal-to-man, insect-to-man, or transmission through water, air, or food; by infectious agent — virus, bacteria, fungus, parasites, etc.; or by name of the disease — rabies, tetanus, etc.

Methods of control are related to the conceptual scheme that identifies the relationship between host, vector, and environment. Strategies of prevention and control fall into the following categories: (1) increasing host resistance by the use of vaccines and other forms of immunobiologics, by breaking the chain of transmission of infection, or by deactivating the infectious agent; or (2) interrupting the transmission of infection by quarantine of persons suffering from the disease, control of animals or insects that serve as vectors of the disease, use of septic techniques in care of patients, improving general sanitation, avoiding certain environments, and by wearing protective clothing.

Physical or chemical means are used to deactivate infectious agents. Heat is used to provide pasteurization or sterilization. Refrigeration is used to maintain food at a temperature that will not support growth of bacteria or parasites. Chlorine is used to purify water supplies, and other chemicals are used as disinfectants.

There are a large number of communicable diseases. The ones selected for presentation here are relatively well known and are considered relevant to public health practice in the United States. In addition, there are certain diseases presented because of their significance in the history of communicable disease control.

Smallpox

Smallpox has been eradicated by a concentrated public health program, organized and managed by the WHO between the years 1967 and 1977. This represents the ultimate in terms of disease control.

Smallpox was caused by the variola virus. The virus was transmitted by infectious persons to susceptibles and indirectly through contaminated clothing or bed linen.

During recent years, when the disease was restricted to the Asian subcontinent, the death rate varied from 15 percent to 40 percent of those afflicted. Site of entry for the virus was the respiratory tract. Smallpox was a disease of man because no animal host was known.

A proposal for eradication of smallpox was made in 1949 and a program was begun in 1950 by the Pan American Health Organization with the idea of eliminating smallpox from North and South America. In 1958, the Soviet Union proposed to the World Health Assembly that a global program be undertaken to eradicate smallpox. The proposal was approved the following year. These events led to the intensified program by the WHO that was launched on January 1, 1967. The program used a potent, stable vaccine and an inexpensive method of vaccination to contain and control the disease. It required the development of a very effective surveillance and communication network. The last known indigenous case of smallpox occurred on October 26, 1977, in the town of Merka, Somalia. This achievement is a landmark in the history of public health. The experience gained from this program has been used to launch a worldwide immunization program to prevent six childhood diseases—diphtheria, pertussis, tetanus, poliomyelitis, measles, and tuberculosis.

Influenza

Influenza has the distinction of being largely uncontrolled due to its mutable virus. Influenza infection can range from inapparent to severe epidemics that occur regularly in all parts of the world. From a historical perspective, epidemiologists compare current epidemics with the serious pandemic that occurred internationally in 1918 to 1919. It was estimated that 500 million people were affected during that epidemic and that the disease killed 20 million.

One of the most carefully studied epidemics of influenza began in February 1957 in China. The distinctive strain of type A influenza virus rapidly spread through the South Pacific, Southeast Asia, and Middle East by June. Cases began to appear in Europe and North America in early summer, but peak incidence did not occur until midautumn. By the end of 1957, the disease was identified in all parts of the world. In the United States, the epidemic waves experienced in fall and winter were thought to have contributed to nearly 70,000 deaths.

Influenza viruses are divided into three antigen types (A, B, and C). It is believe that antigen shifts are due to mutations from animal, avian, and human reservoirs. The WHO has established a system to collect laboratory specimens and epidemiologic information on influenza. Because of the time it takes to develop a new vaccine and the speed of transmission of the disease, it often proves impossible to develop and distribute vaccine to innoculate subpopulations in time to control epidemic patterns.

Influenza is not a reportable disease in most parts of the United States. It is estimated that between 10 and 25 percent of the people in the United States can have clinical influenza during a mild to moderately severe epidemic. School-age children are particularly susceptible, and the first evidence of influenza in a community often is found by a sudden increase in absenteeism from school.

There are four major characteristics of epidemiologic patterns for influenza. They are very widespread epidemic potential, high morbidity and low mortality rates, excess mortality for predictably high-risk groups, and periodic recurrences of the epidemics. Elderly and infirm persons are particularly susceptible to severe or fatal influenza. Vaccines and antiviral drugs are available. Optimal preventive impact is related to administration of biologics prior to onset of illness. The best current strategy for prevention control requires careful surveillance and forecasting, annual immunization of high-risk groups, and study of vaccine efficacy with reference to future research.

Measles

Measles has been identified as a distinctive disease for over 1,000 years. Measles is caused by an RNA virus of the paramyxovirus group. Man is the only natural reservoir. In many parts of the world, measles is feared because of its high mortality rate among children. In most geographic regions, nearly everyone experiences measles at some point during his lifetime.

Since 1963, two types of measles vaccine have been available in the United States. At first, there were difficulties in terms of side-effects. Beginning in 1965, vaccines were developed from further-attenuated strains of measles virus. These vaccines produced fewer side-effects and have been widely used in the United States.

Before the widespread use of vaccine, measles infections were essentially universal in the United States. Nearly 95 percent of all persons living in urban areas had antibodies to measles by the age of 15. The disease appeared in cycles with major peaks every 2 to 3 years. Measles epidemics were most likely to occur in April or May, and the highest specific incidence was to be found in children aged 5 to 9 years.

Beginning in 1963, widespread use of virus vaccine has brought a dramatic reduction in reported cases of measles. Within 5 years, the level of reported cases dropped more than 90 percent. During the period 1960 to 1964, the number of cases fluctuated between 400,000 and 450,000. In 1968, there were only 27,000 cases reported in this country. In the United States, the measles

PREVENTIVE MEDICINE AND PUBLIC HEALTH

case rate per 100,000 decreased from 245.42 in 1960, to 23.23 in 1970, and to 5.96 in 1980. The effectiveness of this immunization program led to plans for eliminating measles from this country. Total eradication of measles, however, will not be possible in any country until an effort is made to bring it under control throughout the world.

Typhoid Fever

Typhoid fever is an acute bacterial disease caused by *Salmonella typhi,* the typhoid bacillus. This disease was initially confused with typhus.

Studies show that the incubation period usually varies from 7 to 21 days; the average is 14 days. Antibiotic therapy terminates the clinical illness. Most clinical symptoms subside within 2 days and the fever within 4 to 5 days.

Since man is the only carrier, outbreaks must originate from human carriers. Most typhoid epidemics can be traced to injestion of food or water contaminated with human waste.

Typhoid fever has a worldwide distribution. There has been a steady decline in incidence in western Europe and the United States due to the development of protected water supplies, pasteurization of milk, and improved sewage systems. In the United States, there are now fewer than 150 clinical cases reported each year, and 33 percent of these cases are associated with foreign travel. Immunization against typhoid fever has been available for more than 70 years.

Cholera

Cholera is a disease caused by the bacteria *Vibrio cholerae.* Cholera has been known and feared for many centuries because of its epidemic potential and high mortality rate. Worldwide spread of cholera began in the early 1880s and was associated with trade and travel between major continents. Robert Koch first isolated the bacteria in 1883. Fortunately, the North American continents has been spared from cholera since 1911, although a single case was detected in Texas during 1975 and eleven cases were identified in Louisiana in 1978.

There have been important improvements in therapy over the past 20 years. With prompt treatment, there should be few deaths. Effective treatment is based upon prompt and complete replacement of water and electrolytes.

Water is considered an important vehicle of transmission. Some outbreaks are related to eating contaminated foods, such as shellfish, raw vegetables, or fish. The provision of safe water supplies and adequate sewage disposal reduces the rate of cholera and other diarrheal diseases. Any effective control program requires a surveillance system and epidemiologic investigation of cases. Cholera vaccination is no longer recommended by the WHO as a requirement for foreign travel, although some individual nations require evidence of immunization. Quarantine and mass immunization programs are not recommended.

Rocky Mountain Spotted Fever

The spotted fevers are caused by a tick-borne typhus disease. Despite a variety of names, there is a clearly identified clinical pattern and a single etiological agent, *Rickettsia rickettsii.* In the United States, the spotted fever that is most widely known is called Rocky Mountain Spotted Fever. It has been known since the late 1800s. The illness has an abrupt onset 3 to 12 days after exposure to a tick. The patient is often unaware of contact with ticks.

The overall fatality rate is about 7 percent. The fatality rate is higher for children, the elderly, and for those persons who receive inadequate treatment. Death is uncommon when there is prompt recognition and treatment. Prompt removal of the complete tick without crushing is imperative since the case fatality rate is 20 percent or higher in untreated cases. Prompt treatment with tetracyclines or chloramphenicol is usually effective. It is important to provide careful clinical management to avoid complications.

There has been a marked increase in spotted fever cases in the United States during the past 25 years. In 1960, there were 204 cases reported and in 1977, a total of 1,115 cases. The largest number of cases are reported in Virginia, Maryland, North Carolina, South Carolina, and Georgia. Ticks transmit the infectious agent between animals, such as ground squirrels, chipmunks, mice, and rabbits by bloodfeeding. No disease process is apparent in these transmissions. Dogs are important in bringing the infected ticks into contact with humans. Dogs can be adversely affected by the disease process.

Plague

Plague is a reportable disease according to international regulations sponsored by the WHO. Until recent times, human plague was a very serious epidemic disease; the disease has gradually begun to disappear. The causative agent is a bacillus known as *Yersinia pestis.* Fleas are the only arthropods known to transmit the bacillus in nature. Rodents serve as the primary hosts. Other mammals such as rabbits, carnivores, and man are incidental hosts. The most feasible control procedures are to kill rodents and avoid flea bites. There are vaccines available and these should be used by persons working regularly around the disease agent.

Malaria

Malaria is caused by four different species of the Plasmodium parasite (*Plasmodium falciparum, P malariae, P vivax,* and *P ovale*). Each of these species generates its own pattern of disease. Malaria parasites are carried by the female anopheles mosquito. When an infected mosquito bites a human, the parasite eggs are carried by the human circulatory system to the liver where they develop.

The most virulent of the human malarias is *P falciparum.* It is distributed throughout the world, is the dominant species in tropical Africa, and is responsible for a high mortality rate. Response to drug therapy is differential based upon the parasite species. Resistant strains of *P falciparum* are found in South America, in Southeast Asia, and in certain western Pacific countries, including Indonesia and the Philippines.

In recent years, there has been limited success in developing a vaccine. The standard prevention is a weekly administration of chloroquine. This treatment should be started approximately 2 weeks prior to scheduled exposure and should be continued for at least 6 weeks after exposure.

Near the end of World War II, a new antimalarial drug, chloroquine, became the drug of choice throughout the world. If taken once a week, it gives complete protection with very few side effects.

Malaria is a rare event in the United States. Indigenous malaria ceased to be a health problem in the United States with the last reported case in 1957. There have been 11 documented outbreaks of introduced malaria (malaria acquired abroad) since World War II. Between 1959 and 1977, a total of 3,346 cases of imported malaria were reported to the CDC. There were 466 cases reported in 1977 and approximately 650 in 1978. In terms of disease control, the most effective methods are chemoprophylaxia and control of contact with mosquitoes. With the development of synthetic insecticides, an effort was made in the 1950s to eradicate the disease in many parts of the world. This program was only partially successful.

The current global incidence of malaria is estimated by the WHO to be 150 million cases. It is estimated that there are 1 million deaths annually in Africa, where there are no effective control programs. During the past decade, there has been an increase in malaria cases.

Rabies

Rabies is a disease transmitted primarily from animal to man. In man, the disease produces an acute and serious dysfunction of the central nervous system, nearly always causing death. The causative agent is a virus.

The incidence of rabies in man in western Europe, Canada, and the United States has been reduced to a small number of cases per year, but the incidence rate is higher in other parts of the world. For example, in India, several hundred thousand persons are treated each year because of possible exposure to rabies. The WHO estimates that thousands die each year and nearly 1 million are given the extensive treatment regimen each year. The treatment causes great discomfort and often serious side effects. It is estimated that approximately 30,000 persons are treated for potential rabies exposure each year in the United States. The total number of reported rabies cases in the United States was 10,883 in 1946, 3,276 in 1970 and 3,182 cases in 1977. In 1978, there were four human deaths, and in 1979, there were five.

In nature, rabies is found in two basic epidemiologic forms—the urban type in domesticated dogs and the wildlife type associated with wolves, foxes, mongooses, weasles, skunks, and bats. Fox rabies is a serious problem throughout North America. In the United States, the disease is found principally among skunks and bats. The decrease in dog and cat cases of rabies is related to the widespread use of immunization programs for domestic pets and the application of other rabies control measures.

The virus, once innoculated in a wound, travels along a nerve from the peripheral site of innoculation to the central nervous system. The incubation period in man is highly variable due to the location of the bite and the distance the virus must travel to the brain. The most frequent incubation period is approximately 6 weeks. The disease in man usually runs its course within 1 week.

The diagnosis of rabies is based on a number of factors. When a dog or cat is involved, it should be held under veterinary supervision for at least 10 days. If the animal shows symptoms of rabies, then it should be destroyed and its brain examined. Testing should be conducted as quickly as possible.

Prompt treatment of all skin wounds is important. Recent studies have shown that a five-dose regimen of the human diploid cell vaccine provided protection against rabies in over 70 persons bitten by proven rabid animals. Both rabies immune globulin of human origin or antirabies serum of equine origin are recommended for administration to all persons bitten by animals in whom rabies cannot be excluded. It should be given as soon as possible after exposure. The major control developed in recent years has been the vaccination of animals. Vaccines are available that provide an immunity lasting three years. Immunization of dogs and cats is considered an important public health preventive measure.

Anthrax

From an historical perspective, anthrax has been recognized as an infectious disease in animals and man for many centuries. There were epidemics of significant proportion in nineteenth century Europe. The presence of this disease stimulated the work of Pasteur and others to identify the etiologic agent and to provide control measures. The etiologic agent is *Bacillus anthracis*. It is a large gram-positive bacterial rod that grows in a variety of culture media. The bacillus lives in the soil and is not communicable directly between animals. The disease is found in animals in the lower Mississippi River Valley of the United States. Outbreaks can occur nearly anywhere. A warm temperature is often associated with outbreaks among grazing animals.

Prevention of human anthrax is dependent on control of animal anthrax. Annual immunization of livestock is recommended. Livestock should be vaccinated 2 to 4 weeks before the season when outbreaks may be expected. Fewer than 10 cases of human anthrax have occurred annually in the United States during the past decade. Human anthrax vaccine is available in the United States and is usually used for persons having ongoing risk of infection.

Nosocomial Infections

Nosocomial infections are defined as those infections acquired during hospitalization and unrelated to the patient's primary complaint. The presence of nosocomial infections does not indicate that hospital personnel made any errors. Many nosocomial infections cannot be prevented with techniques that are currently available. In hospitals during the 1970s, the nosocomial infection attack rate was estimated to be between 5 and 6 percent. This represented approximately 2 million infections annually. Collectively they account for more than 6 million excess days of hospital stay each year. Studies conducted by the CDC indicate that at least 1 percent of infected patients die as a direct result of infection and that nosocomial infections are a major contributing factor in the deaths of an additional 2 to 3 percent of patients. The risk of infection is related to the patient's inherent susceptibility to infection. Various medical treatments can alter a patient's susceptibility, and environmental exposure to potentially dangerous microorganisms can occur during hospitalization. Infection rates differ among hospitals. Differences appear to be related to the different characteristics of patients being treated and the types of procedures being performed.

Urinary tract infections account for 40 percent of nosocomial infections. Infections are generally mild and are easily resolved. In some cases, serious infection may occur because of kidney involvement or spread into the blood stream. Surgical wound infection is the next most common infection. It represents about 21 percent of all nosocomial infections.

The third most frequent nosocomial infection is lower respiratory infections. These infections represent 16 percent of the nosocomial infections. Many of these infections (pneumonia, lung abscess, emphysema, and bronchitis) are acquired by aspiration of oropharyngeal secretions and are difficult to prevent. The risk of aspiration can be reduced by identifying patients who are particularly prone to aspiration and by using simple patient care measures.

Other types of nosocomial infection include nonsurgical cutaneous (6.1 percent), primary bacteremia (4.7 percent), gynecologic (2.2 percent), and upper respiratory (1.6 percent).

Gram-negative bacteria, especially *Escherichia coli,* represent 51 percent of the infections, gram-positive bacteria, 20 percent, and of the remainder, 29 percent are caused by a variety of agents.

Food Poisoning

There are seven types of agents that can cause foodborne disease: bacterial infection, bacterial poison, viral infection, parasitic infection, chemical poisons, poisons of plant and fungal origin, and poisons of animal origin.

The traditional means of surveillance and control of foodborne diseases emphasizes the location and removal of contaminated products from the market, the identification and correction of improper food handling practices, and the identification and treatment of cases and carriers of foodborne disease.

In 1976, there were 438 reported outbreaks involving 12,463 cases of food poisoning in the United States. The etiology for these 438 outbreaks was identified in only 30 percent of the outbreaks. When the etiology was known, the distribution of causes were as follows: bacterial (70 percent), chemical (21 percent), parasitic (7 percent), and viral (3 percent). Most of the cases due to bacterial cause involved *Salmonella* (33 percent), *Staphylococcus* (26 percent), and *Clostridium perfringens* (14 percent).

Staphylococcal food poisoning produces symptoms within 2 to 4 hours after ingestion. The onset of the disease is generally abrupt. The symptoms include salivation, nausea, vomiting, abdominal cramps, prostration, diarrhea, and occasionally hypotension. There is generally no fever. Diarrhea occurs less frequently than vomiting. Gastrointestinal symptoms commonly last several hours and generally less than a day. The mortality rate is extremely low for otherwise healthy persons.

Clostridium perfringens is a frequent cause of food-borne disease in developed countries. The organism is a common, anaerobic spore-forming rod that is found widely in nature and can be found in most raw meat and meat products. The implicated food is usually a meat dish prepared in bulk for a large group. The spores that survive the initial cooking temperature can germinate once the meat cools to a specific temperature. A critical dose of organisms can be produced under optimal conditions in 8 to 9 minutes. After an incubation period of approximately 12 hours, abdominal cramps and diarrhea develop. Nausea is sometimes present. Vomiting and fever are infrequent. The illness usually lasts only a day. Good preventive control can be provided by immediate consumption of food while it is still hot, prompt refrigeration and then high temperature reheating.

Sexually Transmitted Diseases

Sexually transmitted diseases are defined as infectious diseases whose primary mode of transmission is through sexual contact. Although there are approximately 24 diseases known to be transmitted sexually, only two of these will be presented here. They are the diseases of syphilis and gonorrhea.

Syphilis is a chronic infection caused by the spirochete *Treponema pallidum*. The course of the disease is classified into primary, secondary, and tertiary stages of syphilis. It is possible for pregnant women with latent syphilis to transmit the disease to the fetus in utero. Infection of the fetus can produce intrauterine death or premature stillbirth, an infant born with active secondary lesions, a child who will develop secondary lesions during infancy, or an infected child with late manifestations of infection in puberty.

The data available on the incidence of syphilis are incomplete because men seek medical attention more frequently than women, physicians do not report all of the cases they diagnose, and the effectiveness of control programs is highly variable. From the data available, it is clear that primary and secondary syphilis are conditions characteristic of young persons living in major metropolitan or urban areas. In 1978, the disease rate per 100,000 in communities over 200,000 in size was 23.6; 10.7 in communities between 50,000 and 200,000 population; and 3.4 in smaller towns and rural areas. The average rate was 10.0. In terms of age distribution, persons between the ages of 20 and 24 have the highest rate for primary and secondary syphilis. This rate is followed very closely by persons in the age group 25 to 29. The number of syphilis cases reported for men is twice that reported for women.

It is also known that homosexual males in large cities have become an important source of early syphilis. In 1978, approximately 50 percent of men in the country who had early infectious syphilis were bisexual or homosexual males. Over the past 30 years, important changes have been noted in the incidence of syphilis. There have been steady declines in congenital and late syphilis cases. These two categories are at their lowest levels ever recorded in the United States. After a 20 percent drop in primary and secondary syphilis between 1975 and 1977, there was a slight rise of 5.6 percent reported in 1978.

Fluctuations in the incidence of syphilis are known to be closely associated with the level of intensity of venereal disease control programs conducted by state health agencies.

Gonorrhea is caused by the bacterium *Neisseria gonorrhoeae*. Gonorrhea starts in the adult males as a purulent infection of the mucous membranes of the genitourinary tract. Early symptoms are painful urination and mucopurulent discharge. The disease is, however, capable of involving certain other body structures. The incubation period is usually 2 to 8 days. It is more difficult to find recognizable symptoms in females during the early stage of the disease. A large fraction of women with gonorrhea are completely without symptoms. Symptoms, when they occur, include abdominal discomfort, vaginal discharge, and dysuria. Men are at risk of gonococcal invasion of the prostate, seminal vessels, and epididymis. Women are at risk from gonococcal pelvic inflammatory disease (PID). Approximately 15 percent of women with endocervical infection develop this complication. Penicillin and tetracycline are used for treatment.

The incidence of gonococcal infection is highest among young persons residing in major metropolitan areas. There were over 40 times more cases of gonorrhea than of primary and secondary syphilis reported in 1977. Gonococcal infection is also found in persons of younger age than those who have syphilis. The highest age-specific rates were found in the 20- to 24-year-olds and the 15- to 19-year-olds.

There has been a significant rise in the reported incidence of gonococcal infection in the United States since the late 1950s. Factors thought to be associated with this increase are population mobility and mixing, the development of oral contraceptives and the development of positive attitudes about premarital sexual behavior and sexual activity with a variety of partners. Strains of gonorrhoeae resistant to penicillin were first detected in England and the United States in 1976. Surveys have shown that the prevalence of this strain of the bacterium have been generally low—between 0 and 2 percent of gonococcal isolates. The current preventive emphasis is upon identification of asymptomatic infected women and men.

CHRONIC DISEASES

Since the turn of the century, there have been significant improvements in the control of infectious diseases. Both the mortality and the morbidity patterns for the United States have shifted accordingly. Since 1900, the life expectancy of newborn infants has increased on an average from 47 years to 74.4 years. In contrast, persons who are 40 years today do not have a life expectancy that is significantly different from those persons who were 40 years old in 1900.

Coronary Heart Disease

Coronary heart disease (CHD) is a serious disorder of epidemic proportion in the United States, especially for elderly and middle-aged persons. Heart attack, or myocardial infarction, is the most frequent and the most important clinical expression of CHD. Nearly a million heart attacks occur annually in the United States, and there are approximately 550,000 CHD deaths each year. The age-adjusted death rate for all causes in 1980 was 594.1 per 100,000 population. Diseases of the heart ranked first among causes of death and accounted for 34.6 percent of all deaths in that year. This represented an age-adjusted death rate for diseases of the heart in 1980 of 205.3. A National Institute of Health Task Force estimated the direct costs of the heart disease epidemic for 1967 at $2.1 billion and the indirect costs at $13.5 billion. Premature CHD rates in the United States are among the highest in the world. A male in the United States has a one in five chance of having a major myocardial infarction or coronary death before the age of 65. In terms of trends, the age-adjusted death rate from heart disease has been declining slowly since 1950 (307.6 in 1950 to 205.3 in 1980). Within that set of diseases, the trend for CHD increased from 1950 to 1965, and then in 1966 began a downward inflection that has continued to the present time. In 1978, an estimated 114,000 fewer deaths occurred among people aged 35 to 74 than expected based upon 1968 mortality rates. The downward trend has been consistent for males, females, blacks, and whites.

A number of risk factors that have been identified as associated with cardiovascular disease. Among the established risk factors are hypertension, hypercholesterolemia, advanced age, male gender, cigarette smoking, diabetes, and obesity. Suspected risk factors include physical inactivity, a high concentration of glucose without overt evidence of diabetes mellitus, and certain personality traits.

Findings from a series of studies have shown a strong and consistent association between cigarette smoking and cardiovascular disease, especially sudden cardiac death. The rate of sudden cardiac death in young people is four times greater for smokers compared to nonsmokers. In older age groups, smoking is associated with a two-fold greater incidence of sudden cardiac death. Smoking is also associated with an increased rate of ischemic heart disease and its complications. A smoker who consumes a pack a day has twice the risk of a heart attack as a nonsmoker. A smoker who consumes two packs a day has three times the risk. When people stop smoking, there is an immediate decline in their risk for cardiovascular disease. High blood pressure is also strongly implicated as a risk factor for cardiovascular disease. It is clear from epidemiologic research that chronic conditions of high blood pressure increase the risk of ischemic heart disease. Figures from the Framingham studies showed that young men followed for 24 years had twice the risk of developing CHD if they were hypertensives. High blood pressure is also related to the development of myocardial infarction and angina pectoris.

There is a considerable body of evidence that supports an association between an elevated concentration of cholesterol in the blood and the progressive advancement of atherosclerosis. The relative risk of a major coronary event for men with serum cholesterol levels of 250 to 274 mg per 100 ml after 10 years was 2.5 times as high as that for men with initial levels less than 175 mg per 100 ml. As the level of serum cholesterol rises, there is a steady curvilinear increment in premature atherosclerotic disease, at least from levels of 220 mg per 100 ml on up. There is a marked increase in risk for those with levels greater than 240 mg per 100 ml. The relationship is apparently continuous with no evidence of a critical threshold. Clinical practice defines levels of less than 220 mg per 100 ml as normal 220 to 239 as borderline, and 240 or greater as seriously abnormal for adults over 30 years of age. Recent research suggests that the risk of cardiovascular disease is directly related to total cholesterol and cholesterol in the form of low-density lipoprotein. High-density lipoprotein may provide positive protection.

It is important to recognize that dietary habits have been shifting in the United States. During the period 1950 to 1980, patterns of food consumption changed in the direction of lower intake of saturated fat and cholesterol. The mean levels of serum cholesterol in the population has also shown a decrease.

Another risk factor is obesity. There is a cluster of

relationships involving weight gain, increase in serum cholesterol, increase in blood pressure and the onset of diabetes. Data from the Framingham studies show that weight gain since youth was strongly related to the 7-year incidence of new hypertension.

Several carefully designed studies indicate that physical activity decreases the risk of developing CHD. The Framingham study showed that the rate of coronary disease for men with sedentary life-styles was about three times higher than that for active men. There is, of course, a significant coupling between physical activity and consumption of food in relation to weight control. Further research is needed to determine how physical exercise interacts with other risk factors in relation to the etiology of cardiovascular disease.

There is a relationship between diabetes, CHD, and atherosclerotic manifestations. This has been documented clinically, pathologically, and epidemiologically. But the relationships between insulin and glucose regulation, lipid and uric acid metabolism, obesity and hypertension, and atherosclerosis are not well understood at this time. The evidence suggests that behavioral changes involving weight loss through exercise and modified diet could have beneficial effects.

At the community level, preventive programs usually emphasize health education. Two important community education programs have demonstrated effective behavior changes in terms of disease prevention and health promotion. The studies are the Stanford Heart Disease Prevention Program in California and the North Karelia Project in Finland. Both of these projects used mass communication, improved organization of community resources, enhancement of preventive services, and some regulatory modification of the environment.

The Stanford program was designed to determine whether risk factors for coronary heart disease would be reduced through a combination of media and face-to-face instruction. Factors included were cholesterol intake, smoking, blood pressure, and plasma cholesterol. The directors of the study concluded that risk factors can be substantially reduced in an asymptomatic population and that results can be achieved rapidly with persons who know they are at risk. At the end of 2 years, the results achieved through the use of media alone were almost as good as those achieved through use of face-to-face instruction.

The North Karelia program was organized to focus on high cholesterol intake in the local diet, smoking, and high blood pressure. The program was intensive and used a variety of educational methods, involving the media, health professionals, voluntary community groups, women's groups, agricultural associations, and industrial organizations. After 5 years, the incidence of myocardial infarction had decreased by 14 percent, and

strokes in persons aged 30 to 64 had decreased by 40 percent.

Hypertension

The medical condition of hypertension has been extensively studied over the past 25 years. Epidemiologic studies in many population groups have consistently found continuous, unimodal distributions of both systolic and diastolic blood pressure. The shape of the statistical distribution generally varies with the mean level of blood pressure in the population under investigation. Despite many studies, there is no evidence for a threshold value that clearly identifies hypertension as a disease process. The evidence does lead to the conclusion that higher levels of blood pressure are associated with risk in terms of both morbidity and mortality.

The choice of specific blood pressure levels is arbitrary in terms of designating a person as hypertensive, but it is customary practice to designate adults with sustained blood pressure readings greater than 160/95 mm Hg as definite hypertensives. Persons are defined as borderline when the pressure readings vary between 140 to 159/90 to 94 mm Hg. A diastolic pressure that averages 95 to 104 mm Hg is defined as evidence of mild hypertension. Diastolic pressures of 105 to 114 mm Hg are defined as moderate and pressures equal to or greater than 115 mm Hg are considered as indicating severe hypertension. These criteria are used for adults aged 30 and over. Lower criteria are appropriate for adolescents and young adults.

Hypertension can produce pathologic changes in the kidneys, brain, heart, and other organs. Recent epidemiologic studies consistently demonstrate an association of level of blood pressure with risk of CHD, stroke, congestive heart failure, and peripheral arterial disease.

Two major screening programs were conducted in the 1970s: the Hypertension Detection and Follow-up Program (158,000 adults) and the Community Hypertension Evaluation Clinic Program (1 million adults). In both studies, an estimated 18 percent of the population aged 18 to 74 had definite hypertension and an additional 18 percent had borderline hypertension. Prevalence increased steadily with advancing age. More than 50 percent of all adults with definite hypertension had never been told by their physicians that they were hypertensive. Beyond the age of 30, blacks had higher prevalence rates than whites. Both studies showed a significant increase in the proportion of hypertensive persons who knew they had the condition and had brought it under control (12 percent in 1960 increased to 38 percent in 1974 and 45 percent in 1975).

With primary hypertension, there is a large body of scientific evidence from clinical trials on the effectiveness of drug treatment for severe and moderate forms of the disease. It has been demonstrated that treatment of hypertension reduces morbidity and mortality from stroke, congestive heart failure, retinopathy, and renal failure. Hypertensives can achieve control with a relatively simple pharmacologic regimen.

A variety of animal, epidemiologic and clinical studies have shown a statistical association between high salt intake and increased prevalence of hypertension. These findings are based upon populations in various parts of the world. Some studies suggest that it is necessary to study the intake of both sodium and potassium in relation to hypertension. The evidence is incomplete, but it seems prudent to recommend a general reduction of salt intake for all persons and to initiate moderate to extreme restriction for persons who have hypertension.

Modification of behavior has also been studied. Biofeedback techniques have been reported to induce small decreases in blood pressure. Studies have also been done with a variety of relaxation techniques. The results show that some reduction of blood pressure is possible with relaxation therapies. More studies need to be done on both dietary and relaxation therapies. Preventive control of hypertensive disease requires close integration of public health practice with primary medical care services. The morbidity and mortality risks associated with hypertension are well known and documented. The effectiveness of chemotherapy is clearly demonstrated. Now it is necessary to establish collaborative programs that produce more effective intervention.

In 1979, a report was published giving the results of a 5-year demonstration project dealing with methods to reduce mortality associated with hypertension. This was a randomized clinical trial that involved 10,940 men and women 30 to 69 years of age. The program achieved a 17 percent reduction in 5-year "all causes" mortality rate among persons who received the intensive care program. The project showed that it was possible to improve the mortality rate for mild hypertensives using drugs and a comprehensive program of intensive medical care.

Cancer

In terms of both mortality rate and incidence rate, cancer is a significant disease in the United States. In 1980, cancer ranked second as a cause of death in the United States, with an age-adjusted death rate of 134.2 per 100,000. This rate has increased gradually since 1950 when it was 125.4. The age-adjusted death rate for diseases of the heart was 205.3 in 1980 and 307.6 in 1950.

In terms of morbidity, it is estimated that there were approximately 700,000 new cases of cancer identified in 1978. For males, lung cancer is responsible for 20 percent of the incident cases and approximately 30 percent

of cancer deaths. Studies indicate that nearly 85 percent of lung cancer events can be attributed to cigarette smoking, alone or in conjunction with other causes. Prostate and colon cancer are in second and third place as causes of cancer mortality among males. These two forms of cancer account for 9.8 percent and 9.0 percent of cancer deaths, respectively. Prostate cancer has an incidence rate of 48 per 100,000 population, or 16.3 percent of cancer cases. The incidence rate for colon cancer is 27.7 per 100,000 and 9.3 percent of cancer cases.

For women, breast cancer is the most important site. Breast cancer represents almost 30 percent of the incident cases and 20 percent of the deaths. Among women, colon cancer represents the second most likely cancer site with a death rate of 19 per 100,000 in 1973. The incidence for cancer of the colon was 30.7 per 100,000 in the same year.

In terms of trends over the past 50 years, the age-adjusted death rates for cancer of the stomach, uterus, and liver have been declining steadily. Breast cancer has remained at approximately 22 per 100,000 from 1930 to 1976. Under the age of 45 years, the age-adjusted death rate for malignant neoplasms has decreased slightly while the rate has increased for most age groups over 45 years. For example, the rate for persons 35 to 44 years has decreased from 62.7 in 1950 to 48.8 in 1980, while the rate for persons 45 to 54 years has increased from 175.1 to 178.9 in the same time period. The rate for persons 65 to 74 years increased from 692.5 to 814.8, and the rate for persons 85 years and older decreased from 1,451.0 to 1,413.1.

Lung cancer is the exception to the basic trends. The age-adjusted death rate for males with lung cancer shows a rise in the rate from 21.6 in 1950 to 57.8 in 1979. Lung cancer in women increased from an age-adjusted death rate of 4.6 in 1950 to 17.3 in 1979 per 100,000 resident population. Epidemiologic studies in various geographic locations throughout the world show that there is considerable variation among cancer incidence and prevalence.

The exact etiology of various forms of cancer is still unknown, but a number of risk factors have been identified as being associated with the presence of cancer at various sites in the human body. A number of chemical agents have been identified as having carcinogenic propteries. They include arsenic, vinyl chloride, combustion products of coal, asbestos, nickel, radium, and uranium. Exposure to these agents on a continuing basis is frequently related to specific occupations. For example, tanners, smelters, and pesticide workers are frequently in contact with arsenic.

In all of the studies that have been conducted to date, no specific chemical structure has been determined as being associated with carcinogenesis. Very small changes in the structure of a chemical compound may transform it into a carcinogen. With the exception of arsenic, no chemical has been identified as being carcinogenic in human beings without being carcinogenic in animals as well. Some chemicals may produce cancers at different sites within the body. Exposure to two or more chemicals may have an additive or synergistic effect in generating cancer. It is also recognized that ionizing radiation can induce cancer. Persons receiving high doses of radiation have a substantially increased risk of acquiring acute leukemia or the chronic myeloid form. Chronic lymphatic leukemia is not related to radiation exposure.

The use of hormones in medical therapy has been demonstrated to be associated with specific forms of cancer. Estrogens given for the treatment of menopausal symptoms in women can increase the risk of endometrial cancer between four and eight times. There is some evidence that conjugated estrogens may also increase the risk of breast cancer.

During recent years, research studies have indicated a possible relationship between dietary factors and various forms of cancer. Alcohol consumption has been linked by epidemiologic studies to cancers of the mouth, larynx, tongue, and esophagus. It may also play a role in liver cancer.

Lung cancer is the most serious form of cancer in terms of the number of deaths and the morbidity and disability associated with it. A large number of studies have shown that smokers have a greatly increased risk of dying of lung cancer as compared to nonsmokers. Risk is much greater for cigarette smokers than for smokers who use a pipe or cigars. The risk of dying of lung cancer is between 8 and 15 times higher in the cigarette smoker than the nonsmoker. It is currently estimated that cigarette smokers have a reduced life expectancy of 5 to 6 years. Life expectancy decreases with the number of cigarettes smoked per day.

Lung cancer mortality rates for women have been much lower than the rates for men. This difference seems to be due to lower cigarette consumption by women. Since 1955, there has been a strong increase in the age-specific and age-standardized rates for lung cancer in women. Cancers of the respiratory, gastrointestinal, and urinary tracts all show significantly higher incidence rates among smokers, especially cigarette smokers. Although there was considerable skepticism expressed at first about linking cigarette smoking with lung cancer, the body of research accumulated over the past 30 years has demonstrated the etiologic link.

Secondary prevention of cancer consists of the early detection of individuals with the disease. Methods have been developed to screen fairly large population groups. This has proven to be successful for early detection of breast cancer. Data collected in a screening study showed that 31,000 screened women, aged 40 to 64 years of age, had a mortality from breast cancer that was about 40 percent lower than those in the unscreened control group. The current guidelines for breast cancer screening recommend that mammography and physical examination be carried out on an annual basis for women 50 years of age and older. The use of routine mammography for women 40 to 49 years of age should be restricted to those with a personal history of breast cancer, or those with a mother or sister with a history of breast cancer. The use of mammography in women below 40 years of age should be limited to those persons who have a personal history of breast cancer.

Another successful screening technique has been the use of cytologic examination of exfoliated cancer cells. Specimens containing such cells can be obtained from a variety of tissues. The Papanicolaou or Pap test, used for early detection of cervical cancer, is an example of this technique.

Diabetes

Approximately 5 million Americans are known to have diabetes, and it is quite possible that an additional 5 million people may have undiagnosed or latent diabetes. The annual prevalence rate is 5 percent for persons age 45 to 64 years. The rate is 1 in every 12 persons for those over 65 years. Diabetes accounted for 35,000 deaths in 1976 and was a contributing factor in another 90,000 deaths. Blindness is 25 times more common in the diabetic than in the nondiabetic population. Approximately 500,000 women of childbearing age have diabetes. These women, during pregnancy, face a probability of fetal death that is five times greater than for nondiabetic women. The risk of bearing an infant with congenital abnormalities is three times greater than for the general population. Nearly 25 percent of diabetics have heart disease and diabetes.

Annual direct and indirect costs of diabetes were estimated at $6.8 billion in 1977. Approximately 5 to 10 percent of the Americans with diagnosed diabetes require one or more daily injections of insulin. Juvenile-onset diabetes usually develops before the age of 20 years. It is the most common endocrine disease in children. Eighty percent of the diabetic population has maturity-onset diabetes mellitus. This disease typically develops in individuals over age 40 who are overnourished or obese. Symptoms can often be controlled by oral hypoglycemics, exercise, and restricted diet. More than 1 million patients with maturity-onset diabetes take insulin for better control of their symptoms and blood glucose levels.

Though all body systems can be affected by complications of diabetes, the most serious problems are blindness, atherosclerosis, and gangrene. Diabetics experience a 100-fold increase in the prevalence of peripheral vascular problems as compared with persons without diabetes. The major blood vessels of diabetics show premature aging. The average life span for juvenile diabetics is about 35 years from the time of diagnosis.

There is an important connection between diabetes and obesity. Obesity is a risk factor for both diabetes and cardiovascular disease. Approximately 90 percent of the people who become diabetic are overweight. For these people, a crucial problem is how to control excessive caloric intake. As body weight increases, more insulin is needed to keep blood sugar at a normal level. With weight loss, glucose tolerance returns to normal or near-normal.

ACCIDENTS AND INJURIES

All accidents involve harm resulting from one of five types of physical energy: kinetic, chemical, thermal, electrical, or radiation. These same energy forms are also etiologic agents for a variety of chronic occupational and environmentally related diseases. The difference is the speed with which the energy is transmitted to the human body.

In 1980, unintentional injury was the third leading cause of death in the United States, resulting in a death rate of 43.4 per 100,000 resident population. The rate for deaths due to motor vehicle accidents was 23.7 — a rate close to that of 21.3 in 1975. There are important differences in death rate associated with gender and race. The 1979 age-adjusted death rate per 100,000 resident population was 64.5 for white males, 22.0 for white females, 82.3 for black males, and 24.6 for black females.

Between the ages of 1 and 40, injuries are the leading cause of death. Among the young, accidents are responsible for more deaths than all other causes combined. In the United States, approximately 75 million people are injured each year. There were 110,000 injury deaths in 1978. Approximately 30 percent of the population has an injury sufficient to cause loss of 1 day or more of usual activity or to require medical attention. Estimates of financial cost of injury and property damage in the United States in 1977 was estimated at $62 billion, of which $47 billion was the cost of personal injuries alone. The potential time of work lost due to accidents and injuries is greater than the loss due to cancer or to heart disease. The following categories of accidents and injuries are frequently used: highway crashes, other transportation accidents, home injuries, falls, poisonings, recreation, and occupational injuries.

By far, the most significant category of accident in-

volves motor vehicles and highway crashes. In 1980, highway crashes in the United States produced an age-adjusted death rate of 23.7 per 100,000 population. This rate has fluctuated between a low of 21.3 in 1975 to a high of 27.4 in 1970. In 1977, traffic crashes produced 49,500 deaths and 1.9 million disabling injuries. A total of 150,000 persons suffered permanent impairments. Males have much higher fatality rates from highway crashes than do females. In 1979, the age-adjusted death rate per 100,000 population was 36.2 for white males, 12.6 for white females, 34.2 for black males, and 8.9 for black females. In 1979, people between 15 and 24 years of age experienced the highest fatality rate — 46.8 per 100,000 — compared to 29.8 per 100,000 for persons 25 to 34 and 10.0 for persons 5 to 14 years. White males between 15 and 24 years of age have a very high death rate of 77.3 per 100,000 population. The rate drops to 47.4 for the age group 25 to 34 and to 30.8 for the interval 35 to 44 years. The use of alcohol has been identified as a significant behavioral factor associated with a large percentage of fatal crashes.

The need to protect infants and children from injuries and death in highway crashes also is widely recognized. The preventive control measure most widely advocated is the use of special carriers and safety belt restraints.

In recent years, it has been estimated that the number of injuries taking place in the home has averaged 36 million per year. There were 24,000 deaths in the home environment in 1978. Approximately 7,000 of these deaths were from falls, 5,000 from burns and fire, 4,700 from unintentional poisonings, 2,700 from suffocation, 1,200 from firearm mishaps, and 3,400 caused by miscellaneous events. Impairment related to alcohol consumption has been identified as being associated with approximately 50 percent of the injuries for persons 15 years or older in the home. The age-standardized death rate was 9.7 per 100,000 persons in 1977.

There were 14,000 deaths due to falls in the United States during the year 1974, and 54 percent of these occurred in or around the home. Falls cause approximately 13.6 million injuries per year. The injury rate is highest for children. The fatality rate is highest for elderly persons. Deaths from falls in 1977 showed a strong association with age. The rate per 100,000 persons, for all ages, was 6.5, but the rate for children 0 to 4 years was 1.1; for persons 65 to 74 was 13.7 and for elderly 75 years or more was 88.7.

Thermal injuries result from contact with fire, hot surfaces, hot substances, or electricity. Approximately 5 million fires in residential homes occur each year. There were 6,600 deaths related to fires in 1977. This represented a rate of 3.1 per 100,000 population — an improvement over the rate of 3.6 in 1969.

Occupational Injuries

During the past 40 years, there has been a substantial decrease in the number of deaths associated with occupational injuries. In 1937, there were 19,000 deaths for an annual rate of 43 per 100,000 employees in a work force of 44 million people. In 1977, there were 13,000 deaths for a rate of 14 per 100,000 employees in a work force of 91 million workers. On an annual basis, it is estimated that there are 2.3 million work injuries that are disabling beyond the day of the event. Disabling work injuries resulted in an estimated loss of 45 million worker days during 1977. Nondisabling injuries produced a loss of 200 million worker days.

Prevention of occupational injuries uses both an educational approach with workers and a modification of environment and equipment to reduce the possibility of injuries. Major improvements have been made by reducing the number of high-risk tasks to be performed by workers by the use of protective equipment and clothing and by imposing physical barriers between workers and dangerous equipment. Experience in the railroad industry showed that the use of air brakes with automatic couplers significantly reduced the number of worker deaths associated with coupling and uncoupling railroad cars. Installation of roll-over bars and safety straps on tractors could provide improved safety for farmers. There is considerable evidence to support the belief that an increased application of knowledge to high priority areas of potential risk could significantly reduce the injury rate in various occupational fields.

ENVIRONMENTAL HEALTH

Many of the difficulties in understanding and controlling environmental health hazards are associated with the long time period of clinical latency. After initial exposure to certain chemicals, it takes 15 to 20 years for the first manifestation of serious clinical disease to appear. It is often difficult to scientifically measure exposure of persons to suspected toxic agents, chemicals, or radiation in the environment. The exposure may be continuous at very low levels for long periods of time or it may be intermittent and the degree of exposure may fluctuate. When certain chemicals enter the body, they may become incorporated in a variety of metabolic processes which, in turn, may generate health risks. Interactions among combinations of risk factors may produce a negative impact on health status. Both a person's age and gender may be associated with significantly different health effects. For example, it is known that older persons will manifest lung problems faster after breathing asbestos dust than will younger workers. Despite the ap-

parent difficulties concerning scientific research in the field of environmental health, considerable progress has been made in recent years.

The way to preventive action in the field of environmental health is usually through the control of exposure. Once there is scientific evidence that links a specific chemical to a disease, then it is possible for regulatory agencies to make decisions to ban or restrict chemicals. This knowledge also provides important information for practicing physicians and for the public at large. The same control procedures are applicable in the physical environment dealing with such energy sources as noise and ionizing radiation.

It is possible to classify physical and chemical environmental factors by the mode of exposure (e.g., air, water, food); the organ system that is exposed (e.g., respiratory tract, skin, eyes, ears); the organ system primarily affected (e.g., lungs, liver, kidneys, brain); or by the adverse effect (e.g., irritation, behavioral change, carcinogenesis).

There are a number of physical factors in the environment that can affect the health status of individuals. These factors include temperature, barometric pressure, vibration, noise, and electromagnetic radiation. These physical factors operate in both the natural and manmade environments. People do not usually experience negative health effects until these factors operate at extreme energy levels. People living in modern industrial societies are more likely to experience these physical factors operating at high energy levels than are persons living in developing countries.

It is estimated that ambient urban noise levels have increased about one decibel per year for the past 30 years. Adverse effects include interference with personal activities and such psychological effects as headache, irritability, nervousness, and insomnia.

Because of the increasing amounts of radiation generated by man-made activity, this field promises to remain a significant one over the next several decades. The field of radiation can be categorized into two major areas— nonionizing radiation and ionizing radiation. In order of increasing wavelength, nonionizing radiation includes ultraviolet radiation, visible light, infrared radiation, microwave radiation, and radiofrequency radiation.

Electromagnetic radiation produces biologic effects that are photochemical and thermal. The biologic effects of radiation exposure depend on the type and duration of exposure and on the amount of absorption by the organism. Visible light and ultraviolet light are not harmful at normal intensities, but shorter wavelength ultraviolet radiation is generally harmful to organisms. The organs that are affected are primarily the skin and the eyes. Over 90 percent of skin cancers occur on parts of the body exposed to sunlight. Rates for skin cancer vary from fewer than 2 cases per 100,000 in dark-skinned populations to more than 100 per 100,000 in white populations. There is a greater frequency of skin cancer in persons who work in outdoor occupations. Persons working in the following occupations are at risk in terms of exposure to ultraviolet radiation: construction workers, electricians, farmers, fisherman, ranchers, and welders. Protection is available by the appropriate use of shields and barriers, including goggles and clothing.

Microwave radiation is of importance to the field of public health because the rapid growth in this field and the increased exposure of the population. Microwave radiation presents a thermal hazard to hypersensitive tissues, such as the avascular ocular lens of the eye and the male gonad. Heating of the lens of the eye has been associated with cataract formation. Microwave radiation can interfere with the electronic operation of pacemakers. In the United States, there is an occupational standard set for microwave radiation, but there is no standard for exposure for the general public.

Ionizing forms of radiation pose a serious threat to human health. These forms of energy are capable of splitting atoms into positively and negatively charged particles as they pass through biological tissue or air. The radiations of greatest medical interest are very high frequency electromagnetic waves such as x-rays and gamma rays and particles moving at extremely high velocities. There are several biological effects resulting from ionizing radiation. Radiation disrupts the macromolecules of the cell. Their disruption can lead to the death of the cell, or to delay in mitosis and alteration of chromosomes. Some damaged cells may later undergo transformation into a malignant form. This means that radiation injury has two effects—a somatic effect on individual cells and a genetic effect on subsequent generations of cells.

The sources of ionizing radiation are usually divided into four groups—natural radiation and radioactivity, applications in medicine and dentistry, the production and use of nuclear power, and a variety of consumer and industrial products. In terms of natural sources, cosmic radiation enters the earth's atmosphere and can provide adverse effects in terms of human exposure. This is particularly true for people living at high altitudes or traveling in aircraft at high altitudes. Terrestrial radiation comes from radioactive materials present in varying amounts in soils and rocks in the atmosphere and the water. This is transferred to human beings from food chains and inhaled as gases. Dosage rates are relatively constant. External dosage rate varies on the nature of the soil and composition of building materials used for shelters.

It is important to recognize that natural sources of radiation are still the largest sources to which most people are exposed. The annual dose of ionizing radiation received from natural background sources at sea level averages 80 to 100 mrem, of which 20 to 40 mrem come from the earth's crust, 30 to 40 mrem from cosmic rays, and 20 to 25 mrem from radionuclides within the human body. Recent increases in the mining of coal, phosphates, and other materials are adding small amounts of radioactivity to the environment.

The greatest man-made source of exposure is related to medical practice. The use of radiation in diagnostic procedures has been increasing steadily. Between 1964 and 1970, the estimated mean dosage rose from 16 to 20 millirads per year. This increase occurred despite many improvements in techniques designed to minimize stray radiation and reduce radiation levels. Man-made equipment is estimated to contribute an average per capita dose of 75 mrem per year to the population. Most of this comes from medical diagnostic x-rays. To limit potential risk, there is an established standard for maximum permissible dose to the whole body. The limit is 5 mrem per year for radiation workers and 170 mrem per year for the general population. The 170 mrem limit does not include diagnostic x-rays that are considered necessary for medical purposes.

There is additional production of radiation through the use of nuclear power for generating electricity. With increased use of radioactive materials, there is increased dissemination of radioactive leakage into the environment. This is associated with the entire industrial process starting with mining and milling uranium, fabricating fuel units, installing and operating reactors, and then reprocessing and disposing of spent fuel. The perpetual storage of radioactive waste materials adds a further element of hazard.

There are a number of consumer products that use radioactive materials or generate ionizing radiation. Included in this list are color television tubes. Considerable progress has been made in controlling exposure for these products within recent years.

Environmental radiation, especially of the ionizing form, is sure to continue to be a major public health issue during the next few decades. Shortly after Roentgen discovered the x-ray in 1895, it was known that radiation could cause cancer and other biologic effects. It is now well known that there is no threshold dose of radiation below which carcinogenic effects are absent. This means that unnecessary exposure to ionizing radiation should be reduced to an absolute minimum.

Persons at occupational risk should always use dosimeters to monitor exposure and comply with regulations about exposure limits. Man-made sources should be shielded and operated according to recommended safety procedures.

Episodes of intense air pollution have been associated

with adverse health effects for over 50 years. Persons with chronic respiratory and cardiac disease and the elderly are particularly vulnerable when exposed to smog conditions. Many studies have shown adverse effects of air pollution on the respiratory tract. There is, however, still some uncertainty about specific health hazards associated with exposures to specific pollutants, at various levels of concentration, for varying amounts of time.

Increased amounts of smog in urban areas are linked to increased use of internal combustion engines and the use of fossil fuels to produce electricity and to heat buildings. Current estimates show that approximately 50 percent of the pollutants are produced by the transportation sector. It has been estimated that the daily output of 1,000 automobiles operating in an urban community burdens the air with 3.2 tons of carbon monoxide, 400 to 800 pounds of organic vapors, 100 to 300 pounds of nitrous oxides, and smaller amounts of sulfur and other chemicals.

A major concern at the present time is the presence of sulfur compounds in the atmosphere. At the time of the intense pollution episodes in Donora and London, sulfuric acid droplets or acid sulfate aerosols were considered harmful agents. In animal studies conducted since that time, it has been found that certain acid aerosols of very small particle size are much more toxic than sulfur dioxide. Unfortunately, no method has been developed to analyze sulfuric acid droplets in the air over cities. More recent studies show that sulfur dioxide gas goes through a chemical change in the atmosphere. Most of the SO_2 ends up as neutral or acid sulfate aerosols. This conversion process may take 1 or more days. This means that it is necessary to monitor all atmospheric sulfate compounds and to study their potential adverse health effects upon vegetation, and human health.

On the basis of increases in air pollution levels and growing evidence of adverse health effects, governmental action took the form of setting up regulatory agencies to monitor concentrations of pollutants, to establish standards of air quality, and to develop methods for reducing the discharge of pollutants into the atmosphere. Congress has passed air pollution control laws since 1955, but the most important law was the Clean Air Act amendment of 1970. This statute assigned responsibility for air pollution control to the Environmental Protection Agency (EPA), established in 1970.

EXPOSURE TO CHEMICALS

From a public health perspective, the most significant chemical substances are those known as organic solvents, pesticides, and halogenated polyaromatic hydrocarbons. The organic solvents include a large group of

compounds — alcohols, ketones, ethers, esters, glycols, aldehydes, carbon disulphide, and other chemicals with similar structures. These chemicals are used as solvents in a large number of industrial processes. They can dissolve and disperse oils, waxes, paints, pigments, varnishes, rubber, fats, and other materials. Some solvents are well known for their specific toxic effects on the liver, kidney, and bone marrow. A few organic solvents are particularly toxic to the nervous system. Once a danger to health status has been discovered, it is often possible to find engineering solutions so that exposure is significantly reduced or eliminated. Control is possible largely because most of these materials are used in a limited number of industrial work settings.

Pesticides are some of the most toxic materials that are deliberately added to our environment. One billion pounds of pesticides were used in the United States in 1975. Pesticide compounds are now very widely dispersed contaminants in our environment. Pesticides made from organophosphorous compounds have been responsible for more deaths than any other group of chemical compounds. One of these, called Parathion is responsible for most of the pesticide fatalities. Organophosphates are readily metabolized by the body. If there is early and proper treatment, most individuals poisoned in occupational settings will recover. Permanent nerve damage, due to exposure to these compounds is well documented.

There is no well organized system for reporting pesticide morbidity and mortality events. It was estimated in 1971 that there had been 2,600 hospital admissions, or a rate of 8.2 per 100,000 hospital admissions for pesticide poisoning. The following year the rate was estimated at 8.8 and in 1973, the figure was 8.5. Deaths from pesticides in the United States were 152 in 1956; 111 in 1961; 87 in 1969 and 52 in 1974. The WHO estimates that there are approximately 500,000 pesticide poisonings annually throughout the world and that the mortality rate is 1 percent.

Some of the chemical compounds known as halogenated polyaromatic hydrocarbons are of particular concern in public health. Of particular interest, are the polychlorinated biphenyls (PCBs), polybrominated biphenyls (PBBs), and chlorinated dibenzo-*p*-dioxins (CDDs). All of these compounds have strong environmental penetrance and persistence, and show bioaccumulation throughout the food chain. Once a toxic dose is attained in humans, manifestations of disease are similar and include persistent halogen acne, eye irritation often associated with metaplasia of the meibomian glands, reproductive dyscrasias in females, neurologic effects, including decreased velocity of conduction in peripheral nerves, and liver toxicity. Production of PCBs was halted in the mid-1970s, but exposure will continue because of the 200,000 tons of PCB compounds to be found in products currently in use.

Preventive actions include careful monitoring, control of exposure, safe disposal of these compounds, and education of the public.

A major category of environmental diseases can be identified as respiratory diseases associated with occupational activities. The major occupational respiratory diseases are associated with the inhalation of asbestos, coal dust, silica, silicates, and organic dust. A discussion of health problems associated with the use of asbestos materials is presented to illustrate the problems associated with occupational respiratory disease.

Although health hazards associated with the use of asbestos have been known since 1907, most of the definitive research has been conducted during the past 20 years.

Asbestosis was the first disease associated with exposure to this material and it is the most common disease condition. The clinical characteristics of asbestosis are interstitial fibrosis, pleural scarring, and pulmonary insufficiency. Abnormal physical signs also include finger clubbing, fine rales, and mild cyanosis. In early days, exposure was so intense, it often caused death by lung scarring and pulmonary insufficiency. People did not live long enough for the cancerous forms to develop. It should be noted that most patients who die of asbestosis do not necessarily succumb to the progression of the fibrosis, but rather to pulmonary infection.

The most common asbestos-induced neoplasm is lung cancer. The latency for this form of lung cancer starts at 10 years from onset of exposure and hits a peak between 30 and 34 years. Treatment is usually ineffective with fewer than 1 person in 20 surviving 5 or more years. Asbestos workers who smoke cigarettes add considerable risk. A 9-year prospective study of 12,051 asbestos workers showed the following age-standardized death rates per 100,000 man-years: men who neither worked with asbestos nor smoked cigarettes had a death rate of 11.3; asbestos workers who did not smoke, 58.4. Smokers who were not asbestos workers showed a rate of 122.6 and men with exposure to both cigarettes and asbestos had a rate of 601.6.

The disease of mesothelioma is, in addition to lung cancer, seen as a specific result of exposure to asbestos. The mechanism by which asbestos fibers induce mesothelioma in the pleura or the peritoneum is not known at this time, but it has been definitely established that the asbestos fibers do reach these tissues and remain there. The neoplasms that are generated have an unusual and striking appearance. They are usually diffuse, spreading rapidly and widely over the large surfaces of the thoracic and abdominal cavities. They invade the underlying organs only superficially. There is no satisfactory treat-

ment for mesothelioma, and most people afflicted with the disease die within 1 year after diagnosis.

It has taken a long time to develop regulations for control of asbestos exposure. In 1968, an expert committee of the British Occupational Hygiene Society recommended a standard of 2 to 12 fibers per ml of air. Experience since then has shown that it is necessary to reduce that level. In 1976, the National Institute for Occupational Safety and Health recommended a level of 0.1 fiber per ml for industrial exposure.

HYGIENE AND SANITATION

There are four areas of environmental health that need to be mentioned because of their potential contribution to serious outbreaks of disease. They are the monitoring activities and preventive controls associated with the acquisition and use of water, food, and milk, plus the disposal of liquid and solid wastes. Because of the long-standing experience with environmental sanitation and the high level of regulatory performance in this field, most people are unaware of this nearly invisible health-related infrastructure.

Causes of food poisoning or infection can be grouped into eight categories: preformed bacterial toxins; preformed mycotoxins (aflatoxins); microorganisms such as *Salmonella, Clostridium perfringens,* and *Shigella;* animal parasites such as *Trichinella spiralis* and tapeworms; chemical poisons such as arsenic, nitrites, mercury, and a wide variety of organic compounds; inherently poisonous foods such as certain mushrooms and shellfish; contamination with radioactive materials, and toxic elements in the soil where food is grown.

By far the largest number of outbreaks involving foodborne diseases are related to bacterial contamination. Food poisoning in this country is underreported. In 1976, the CDC estimated there were 4,000 outbreaks of which only 430 were reported. Based on studies, the estimate is that 70 percent of foodborne disease is due to bacterial agents. Chemical poisoning accounts for 21 percent. Parasites and viral agents are involved in 9 percent.

The organization of food controls in the United States is very complicated. It involves all levels of government and considerable voluntary participation and self-inspection by major organizations responsible for the production or processing of foodstuffs. Federal agencies involved in food control include the Food and Drug Administration, Department of Agriculture, the EPA, and the Bureau of Commercial Fisheries in the Department of the Interior.

Food control procedures are required at every stage from growing foods on land or in the water, all the way through harvesting, transportation, processing, preserving, to food preparation prior to consumption. The food system of this society is large and complicated due to the tremendous variety of foodstuffs grown, distributed, and consumed. The health-related problems vary considerably, depending upon the foodstuff and the way in which it is managed. Examples are control of pesticide contamination of vegetable and meat products and the contamination of shellfish by mercury or microorganisms in the seawater. In more recent years, there has been a growing threat from radionuclides in the contamination of food. Nuclear weapons testing in the atmosphere prior to the test-ban treaty of 1963 generated environmental fallout of Strontium 90 and Cesium 137. These radioactive compounds entered the foodchain and were concentrated at high levels in milk.

Another area of potential health hazard is the control of sanitary conditions in public eating places. Public food service establishments such as restaurants, cafés, cafeterias, fast food outlets, soda fountains, and taverns produce an estimated 117 million consumer transactions per day. Schools, hospitals, industrial plants, and institutions provide an additional 33 million meals each day. The basic essentials of cleanliness in food preparation in public eating places are as follows: avoid hand contact with food as far as is practical; keep perishable food below 40 degrees or above 140 degrees Fahrenheit; keep food protected from personal contact and contaminating insects, dusts and animals; discard all food and food products that are not of high quality; clean and disinfect equipment that comes into direct contact with food, and keep the environment in sanitary condition at all times.

The sanitary control of milk is very important because milk is a highly perishable food and is an excellent medium for the multiplication of pathogenic bacteria. Milk is a major item of food for infants and children and is available in all parts of the country throughout the year. The milk production and distribution system is long and complicated.

Sanitation control of milk is based upon collaboration between the U.S. Public Health Service (USPHS) and the health departments of each state. The USPHS interest goes back to 1896. Studies established the role of milk in the spread of gastrointestinal disease and set the standards for heat levels to be used in pasteurization. The current guide is called the Pasteurized Grade A Milk Ordinance and Code developed by the USPHS in 1965. Surveillance of the health of dairy cattle and compulsory pasteurization are included among other health safety provisions of this law. These guidelines are used within this country and by other countries of the world. The effectiveness of these guidelines is evident in the steady decrease in the number of foodborne outbreaks due to milk. There were 43 outbreaks in 1940, 10 in 1950, 4 in 1970, and 3 in 1975. In contrast, outbreaks due to other foods increased in the same time period — 218 in 1940 to 497 in 1975.

The major diseases that can be transmitted in the milk of infected cows are tuberculosis, brucellosis, streptococcal infection, and Q fever. Monitoring the health of dairy cows and preventing the introduction of bacteria at the time of milking are necessary first steps in the disease prevention process.

Prompt cooling immediately after production is essential if the bacterial count is to remain low. This stage is followed by some type of heat treatment. The efficiency of heat used as a bactericide is a function of the intensity or the temperature and the length of exposure time. Thermal disinfection by a milk heat treatment is known as pasteurization. The pasteurizing process consists of three steps — heating to 145°F for 30 minutes, holding, and then cooling rapidly to 50°F or lower. There are alternate heat treatments that use higher temperatures for short durations. Dairy products such as ice cream mixes and chocolate milk need slightly higher temperature treatment.

Effective sanitary control of milk and milk products requires careful testing on a routine basis. Properly pasteurized milk has a bacterial count of less than 50,000/ml and most regulations limit the standard plate count to 30,000/ml. It is also necessary to monitor milk for contaminants such as antibiotics, insecticides, and radionuclides.

Solid Waste Disposal

Our society produces solid wastes at the rate of 260 million tons per year, 7 pounds per person per day, or 1 ton per person per year. These wastes, handled by street collection, are only part of the total disposal problem. In addition, there are wastes generated by various sectors of the economy — mining, ore refining, manufacturing, and agriculture. The disposition of toxic and radioactive wastes pose special health and safety problems as well. Because the production of solid wastes has shown an exponential growth over the past 60 years, we can anticipate continuing economic and health problems in this area.

The traditional method of waste disposal was surface dumps in remote or hidden locations. Now it is necessary to change from that method to a combination of three other methods: burning, land burial, and transformation for reuse. The best preventive measures require the development of safe disposal methods and the control of insect and rodent vectors. Disposal methods currently in use are incineration, open dumps, dumping at sea, grinding and adding to sewage sanitary landfill, composting, and salvage. With the exception of open dumps and dumping at sea, these disposal methods can provide effective control of most serious health hazards.

Water Quality

The amount of water used in American communities is quite large. The average per capita consumption averages 600 L per day. Residential use represents 40 percent of the total consumption. Within the home, the allocations in percentages are as follows: toilet flushing, 40; bathing, 30; laundry, 15; drinking and cooking, 5; dishwasing, 5; and miscellaneous, 5.

Approximately 80 percent of the United States population is served by water supply and sewerage systems in 40,000 communities. Only a small fraction of the water supply is actually consumed by people, but most water supply systems are designed to deliver potable water for all purposes.

Water quality is measured by a combination of physical, chemical, and biologic standards. Potable water is free of any harmful substance or pathogen and is acceptable in terms of taste, odor, and appearance. Contaminated water is water polluted with human wastes and capable of serving as a vehicle to spread infection. Polluted water contains one or more foreign substances — organic, inorganic, radiologic or biologic — that tend to degrade water quality so as to produce a hazard or impair the usefulness of the water.

The initial public health concern with water quality was related to the prevention of waterborne diseases such as cholera and typhoid fever. In more recent years, it has been necessary to expand the scope of concern to include contaminants such as inorganic chemicals, organic chemicals, and radioactive materials. It was also discovered that chlorination, the standard method for controlling bacterial contamination, could produce potential toxicants such as chloroform. Chloroform and other trihalomethanes are capable of causing cancer in laboratory animals.

Water pollution reached a critical phase in the 1950s. Nearly all major river systems were seriously polluted. Industries were discharging toxic chemicals and other contaminants directly into rivers and municipal sewage systems. Many sewage treatment plants had become obsolete. Beginning in the mid-1950s, Congress made grants available to the states for modernization of waste-treatment facilities. In 1972, the Federal Water Pollution Control Act was passed. Its purpose was to eliminate the discharge of all pollutants into navigable waters by 1985. By the end of the 1970s, the control of water pollution had become the biggest public works program. The regulations established three broad categories of pollutants, set priorities, and produced scheduled dates for com-

pliance. Control of 65 classes of toxic pollutants, such as arsenic, mercury, lead, and zinc, were given the highest priority. Conventional pollutants, such as human waste and organic matter, were assigned second priority. Nonconventional pollutants, such as pesticides and some organic solvents, were given the third and lowest priority.

PUBLIC HEALTH SERVICES

Public health services are designed to prevent disease, promote health, and measure and evaluate the health status of populations. Many preventive health services are provided to communities without the residents being aware of them. Services such as the provision of pure water supply, sanitary sewage disposal, air pollution control, and surveillance of food services are examples of this kind of public health service. In addition, there are preventive services that are directed to individual persons. Programs of health education concerning risk factors in cigarette smoking, consumption of alcoholic beverages and the adverse health effects of being overweight fall in this category. Another example is baby clinics operated by public health nurses.

From a historical perspective, public health services have traditionally been concerned primarily with preventive services that would affect the community as a whole. In recent years, there has been a widening of scope of public health activities to include more participation in the area of preventive aspects of personal health care.

In the United States, most public health services are provided by government agencies at the federal, state, and local levels. There is no provision in the Constitution regarding the federal government's responsibilities and power in relation to matters of health. The Constitutional basis of authority for the federal government's participation in health activities is based upon the authority to tax and spend in order to provide for the general welfare and to regulate interstate and foreign commerce.

The largest government agency dealing with health is the Department of Health and Human Services (HHS). It is also the largest federal governmental department in terms of budget and number of employees. This department was established in 1979 and grew out of the Department of Health, Education, and Welfare (HEW) established in 1953. Reorganization in 1979 created a separate department of education. HHS retained most of the health service responsibilities of HEW, including nearly all programs for health manpower education.

Within HHS, there are two principal health agencies — the Health Care Finance Administration (HCFA) and the USPHS. The primary responsibility of the HCFA is to run two major financing programs, Medicare and Medicaid.

The USPHS is responsible for six major areas. In 1981, the major bureaus within USPHS were the CDC —disease prevention; Food and Drug Administration (FDA)—consumer protection; National Institute of Health (NIH)—biomedical research; Health Resources Administration (HRA)—facilities, manpower training, and planning; Health Services Administration (HSA)—direct care or access to care; Alcohol, Drug Abuse and Mental Health Administration (ADAMHA)—care and prevention of mental illness, alcoholism, and substance abuse.

The unit within the USPHS that has disease prevention as its primary mission is the CDC, which came into existence as a malaria control program during World War II. It was designated the Communicable Disease Center in 1946. At that time, its scope of responsibility was extended from vector-borne infections to a broad range of communicable diseases. The center became involved in international as well as domestic infectious disease control programs during the 1960s and was renamed the Center for Disease Control in 1970. Again its scope of responsibility was expanded to include prevention and control of certain noninfectious diseases. In 1980, additional responsibilties were added and the agency was renamed Centers for Disease Control. The Centers are the Center for Infectious Diseases, Center for Preventive Services, Center for Environmental Health, Center for Health Promotion and Education, Center for Professional Development and Training, and National Institute for Occupational Safety and Health.

In 1970, the FDA became a part of the USPHS. This was also the year for the establishment of the National Health Service Corps. The Corps is responsible for provision of medical services to medically underserved areas of the country.

In 1979, an Office of Health Research, Statistics, and Technology was established. This office was organized to include the National Center for Health Services Research (NCHSR), the NCHS, and the newly-created National Center for Health Care Technology (NCHCT).

There are other federal agencies with important responsibilities in the field of public health. The Department of Defense has chief medical officers at each of its installations. These medical officers are responsible for provision of both personal health services and public health services. The Department of Agriculture has important responsibilities for human and animal health. The Department of Labor contains the agency known as Occupational Safety and Health Administration (OSHA). This agency attempts to set a minimum level of protection for workers against specified hazards and to

achieve this through education, persuasion, and legal enforcement.

There is one additional federal agency concerned with environmental health in a major way. It is the Environmental Protection Agency that was established in 1970. This agency is independent and not part of one of the major departments.

The EPA is the largest federal regulatory body concerned with health and safety. Its mission is to mobilize a coordinated attack on the environmental problems of air and water pollution, solid waste management, pesticides, radiation, and noise. The agency conducts research and establishes and enforces environmental standards. One of the agency's most important programs is the control of toxic substances, including pesticides.

Other federal agencies concerned with the general area of health and safety include the Consumer Product Safety Commission which was created in 1973; the Federal Aviation Administration (FAA) which has broad powers to ensure safe conduct of air travelers; the National Highway Safety Traffic Administration, established in 1966, whose responsibility is to reduce the number of deaths and injuries on highways; and the Nuclear Regulatory Commission, established in 1974, whose responsibility is to ensure that public health and safety is protected when nuclear energy is used for commercial purposes.

The Department of Labor administers the Federal Mine Safety and Health Act. The Department of Transportation administers the Federal Railroad Safety Act and the Federal Trade Commission insures that information provided by manufacturers to consumers is not false or misleading.

The trend in recent years has been to add programs to this basic list. Examples of new functions are radiation control, noise pollution control, accident prevention, occupational health and safety, hazardous waste management, and health resource planning.

With few exceptions, nearly all areas of the United States are served by local health units. These units are part of activity at the county and municipal levels of government. Many of the larger local health departments have also sponsored community health centers and home health agencies to facilitate the provision of personal health services to underserved residential populations. Some counties and large cities operate general purpose hospitals.

Most states have departments of mental health. The director, or commissioner, is usually a psychiatrist who is appointed by the governor. The traditional responsibility of these departments has been the operation of large hospitals for the mentally ill and institutions for the mentally retarded. In recent years, there has been a trend toward development of community mental health centers, halfway houses, and treatment programs for alcohol and drug abuse.

It is important to realize that there is a lack of detailed information about the services provided by state and local health units. Surveys initiated in 1977 are beginning to correct this deficiency. Some public health services are provided by private commercial firms. This is especially true in solid waste disposal and the provision of pure water supplies.

The evolution of public health services in the United States is tied closely to voluntary actions taken by groups of citizens. It is estimated that there are 100,000 voluntary health agencies now operating on the national, state and local levels.

PERSONAL HEALTH CARE

The large number of different health care services can be categorized according to the type of health problems and the setting in which the care is provided.

Emergency Health Care

In 1970, it was estimated that nationwide, there were 44,000 ambulances, of which 19,000 were operated by morticians, 11,000 by volunteer groups, 4,700 by commercial firms, 4,500 by police and fire departments, and 1,300 by hospitals. Fewer than one-third of these ambulances carried the equipment recommended by the American College of Surgeons. During the 1970s, efforts were made to improve emergency medical services throughout the country.

In 1971, the United States Department of Transportation sponsored a training program to professionalize ambulance personnel by providing training at various levels for emergency medical technicians. In 1973, Congress enacted the Emergency Medical Services Systems Act to set standards and to work to facilitate the development of improved emergency medical service systems within all of the states. As a result of these activities, there was better organization and coordination of emergency medical services and a legal basis for the supervision of ambulance squads.

Closely linked to the ambulance services are the hospital emergency departments in hospitals. The practice of using full-time salaried emergency room (ER) physicians is growing rapidly. There has been strong growth of interest in the field of emergency medicine. The field was recognized as the newest medical specialty in 1979 and there is an American College of Emergency Physicians. The American Medical Association (AMA) has proposed classifying hospital emergency service units into four levels according to the immediate availability of physicians, nurses, and allied personnel with various grades of technical skill in the field of emergency medicine. The transition from primary to secondary and even to tertiary levels of care can occur in a relatively short span of time.

Ambulatory Care

The term "ambulatory care" refers to personal health care services provided in physicians' offices, clinics, health centers, and hospital outpatient departments.

Physicians' offices represent the setting for the largest volume of ambulatory care visits. According to survey data for 1975, patient visits to office-based physicians totaled 567,600,000. This represented an estimated 45.2 percent of all patient-physician encounters. Since there were 215,000 physician's offices, that means an average of 2,640 office visits per physician per year. In 1975, the distribution of ambulatory visits to place of visit was estimated to be as follows: individual doctor's office, 55.5 percent; group practice clinics, 25.0 percent; hospital outpatient departments, 12.9 percent; industrial health units, 0.9 percent; patient's home, 0.8 percent; and other places or unknown, 5.0 percent.

The hospital outpatient department (OPD) is probably the most important type of organized clinic in the nation. In 1977, there were scheduled clinics in 30 percent of all hospitals, a total of 1,955 facilities. A great majority of these clinics were located in community hospitals. Many hospitals which do not operate scheduled clinics do provide emergency care to outpatients at various hours. This was true for 90 percent of 4,860 community hospitals in 1977. The number of outpatient visits to hospitals has grown steadily in recent years—from 126 million visits in 1965 to 264 million visits in 1977. It is customary to classify OPD services into three types: general—nonemergency services given to an ambulatory patient who has not been referred by a private physician; referred—services given to a patient who was referred by a private physician and expected to return to that physician for subsequent care; and emergency—health services given for a condition which the patient considers in need of immediate care. Ambulatory health care services are also provided by schools, colleges, industrial plants, government agencies, voluntary health agencies, and health maintenance organizations (HMOs).

During the past 20 years, there has been a considerable growth in new patterns of ambulatory care. Examples include neighborhood health centers, rural health centers, women's clinics, abortion clinics, birthing centers, short-stay surgical centers, renal dialysis centers, drug rehabilitation centers, community mental health centers, walk-in emergency centers, and free clinics. This trend can be expected to continue.

Hospitals

In 1980, there were approximately 7,000 hospitals of all kinds in the United States. Most of these hospitals were short-stay hospitals (6,229). The ownership of the short-stay hospitals was distributed as follows: federal, 325; nonfederal, 5,904; nonfederal nonprofit, 3,339; state-local government, 1,835; and proprietary, 730. The trends show a slow growth in the number of short-stay hospitals from 5,768 in 1960 to 6,307 in 1977 and a gradual decline since that time.

The total number of beds in short-stay hospitals has grown since 1980. The percentage of beds occupied in these hospitals fluctuated between 73.7 and 75.6 during 1975 to 1980. The number of admissions to short-stay hospitals increased from 30.7 million in 1970 to 38.1 million in 1980. The average length of stay decreased from 8.7 to 7.8 days in the same decade.

Hospitals can be classified in different ways, including title of ownership, type of problem treated, average length of stay, type of medical orientation (allopathic, osteopathic), role of education, and size. Hospitals, especially voluntary hospitals, are complicated in their function and management. The group with legal responsibility for the hospital is the Board of Trustees.

The medical or professional staff consists primarily of physicians, but may also include dentists, psychologists, and other professionals with doctoral degrees. An "open" staff is one where any licensed physician may admit his private patient to the hospital and care for the patient there. The practice used to be widespread, but it is now relatively rare. A "closed" staff is one where only those physicians whose applications for staff membership have been reviewed and approved by the Board of Trustees may admit and care for patients.

Many hospitals have categories of medical staff, including the following:

Active staff — regular membership
Associate staff — physicians newly appointed or physicians who work in the outpatient department
Consulting staff — those who can consult, but not admit patients
Courtesy staff — Physicians who only occasionally use the hospital
House staff — Resident physicians still in training

Usually staff appointments are renewed on a yearly basis. Medical staff by-laws are the rules that govern

physicians on the medical staff. The staff usually has an elected president or chief of staff. Larger hospitals have physicians in major specialties responsible for their area of practice.

Hospitals are organized both as functional departments and as patient care units. Patients are usually grouped by age and the nature of the major medical problem for which they were hospitalized. One of the functional departments is nursing services. This is the single largest component of the hospital. There are also medical specialty departments where physicians and technical personnel provide diagnostic and therapeutic procedures, but do not have primary, ongoing responsibility for patients. Nearly all hospitals have departments of anesthesiology, pathology, and radiology. Some have departments of physical and rehabilitative medicine.

There are a number of important professional services that supplement medical care of patients. The pharmacy provides drugs and medications. The social service department provides services to reduce the environmental, social, and emotional obstacles to the recovery of the patient by working with the patient's family. In some hospitals, there is a special discharge planning unit.

The dietary service department includes the kitchen, inpatient food service, cafeteria, food storage and purchasing, catering for special events, and a special diet kitchen.

There are also departments for general administration and overall support services. They usually include administration, financial affairs, public relations, admissions, medical records, medical library, personnel department, purchasing and stores, communications, central supply, housekeeping, maintenance, security, and volunteers.

There has been a growing volume of medical technology to be found in hospitals. This includes x-ray, surgical and laboratory equipment, as well as electronic patient monitoring devices. Some of the more complex and expensive pieces of equipment are the computerized axial tomography x-ray (CT scanners) and special radiation therapy equipment.

The activity and performance of hospitals is monitored by using a certain set of parameters. The following statistics are used to report performance characteristics of hospitals. Patient "bed" days refers to the total number of inpatient days of care given in a specified time period. Hospital beds refer to the average number of beds, cribs, and pediatric bassinets regularly maintained for inpatients during the period of time. Admissions refers to the number of patients accepted for inpatient service in a period of time, excluding births. Discharges and deaths refer to the number of inpatients leaving the hospital in a period of time. This usually excludes newborn babies. Average daily census refers to the number of inpatients receiving care on an average day (excluding newborns). This is usually calculated by counting the number of patients in the hospital every midnight. Occupancy refers to the ratio of census to beds, and usually is the percentage of available beds in use. Average length of stay is measured in days of inpatients over a given time period and can be calculated by dividing the number of patient days by either the number of admissions or the number of discharges and deaths. Available bed days is the average number of beds available for use times the number of days in a given time period. For example, a 100-bed hospital would have 36,500 available bed days per year.

The staffing ratio is the total number of hospital employees measured in full-time equivalents divided by the average daily census. The per diem cost per patient day is calculated as the cost of running the hospital divided by the number of patient days in that time period. The waiting list is an ordered list of patients who are awaiting admission to the hospital. The hospital service charge, or per diem charge, is the basic price per day for inpatient care. This usually includes food, basic nursing care, administrative overhead, the use of services by all patients. Ancillary charges are for special diagnostic and treatment services such as lab tests, x-rays, and operating rooms. Case mix refers to the distribution of types of cases or patients cared for in the hospital.

A special category of hospitals provide physician residency training programs. In 1980, 1,372 hospitals offered residency programs for a total of 64,600 resident physicians. Teaching hospitals have physician faculty and most of them have affiliation agreements with medical schools.

Nursing Homes

Patients with certain levels of disability associated with chronic illness and advancing age need the services of nursing homes. Approximately 5 percent of people aged 65 years or over are in nursing homes. In 1980, there were 14,316 certified nursing homes in the United States, with a total bed complement of 1,416,757. This provided a bed rate of 57.5. The bed rate is the number of nursing home beds per 1,000 population 65 years of age and over. The number of nursing home beds has increased significantly in the past 20 years — from .57 million in 1963 to 1.3 in 1976 to 1.4 in 1980. There were 1.3 million nursing home residents in 1977. Their age distribution was under 65 years, 177,100; 65 to 74 years, 211,400; 75 to 84 years, 464,700; and 85 years or more, 449,900.

There are different types of nursing homes. The terminology and the criteria vary. The basic principle behind the classification scheme is an attempt to indicate the levels of technical health care services required by nursing home residents. A skilled nursing facility is usually a nursing home or may be a special section of an acute hospital or an infirmary in a home for the aged. To qualify for Medicare reimbursement, the facility must provide skilled nursing or other skilled rehabilitation services on a daily basis. An intermediate care facility is for long-term care, usually at a level of nursing care where the services offered are of lesser intensity than those available in a skilled nursing facility. The domiciliary care facilities comprise a category that includes homes for the aged, personal care homes, boarding homes, and similar institutions. Residents are ambulatory and require only minimal visiting, nursing, or medical attention.

Intermediate care facilities must have a supervising registered nurse or licensed practical nurse full-time on each day shift. Rehabilitation services by qualified therapists or assistants must be available. These facilities provide services for persons who do not require hospital or skilled nursing care, but whose mental or physical condition requires services above the level of room and board. Intermediate care services are included, to some degree, in all state Medicaid programs, but Medicare does not provide coverage for intermediate facility care.

A single nursing home facility may have both skilled and intermediate care services within the same building. In terms of certification, in 1977, there were 3,600 skilled nursing facilities (19.2 percent); 6,000 intermediate care facilities (31.6 percent); and 4,600 skilled nursing facilities and intermediate care facilities (24.2 percent).

The great majority of nursing homes are smaller than community hospitals — only 900 out of 14,000 facilities had 200 beds or more in 1977.

Unlike the ownership pattern for hospitals, proprietary facilities dominate the field of nursing care homes. Proprietary facilities make up approximately 77 percent of the total; voluntary/nonprofit, 18 percent; and government, 6 percent.

According to a nursing home survey conducted in 1974, most nursing homes were small-scale operations, with an average size of 75 beds. Nursing homes were not heavily staffed; the average staffing ratio was 0.67 full-time equivalent staff per bed. Two-thirds of the staff were nursing personnel. Most nursing homes were full and 70 percent had waiting lists.

According to a survey conducted in 1977, the residents of nursing homes had the following characteristics: 70 percent of the population was female; 15 percent were less than 65 years of age and 71 percent of residents were over 75 years of age. Widowed persons represented 58 percent of the population and never-marrieds, 21 percent.

The principal reason for admission to a nursing home

is illness and the need for treatment and nursing care. This category accounts for over 80 percent of total admissions and for an even larger proportion of admissions for residents over age 75. Lack of family support capability accounted for 6 percent and lack of financial resources for only 1 percent of admissions. Disruptive behavior or mental deterioration accounted for 12 percent for those under age 65.

Approximately 40 percent of patients enter the nursing home directly from their residences and 35 percent are transferred from general hospitals. The remainder come from other institutions, such as mental hospitals, and long-term care specialty hospitals (8 percent); other nursing homes (14 percent); or boarding homes (2 percent).

Patients in a nursing home frequently suffer from more than one chronic illness problem. The prevalence of chronic impairments is indicated by the following functional limitations: 32 percent of the residents could not hear a telephone conversation, 46 percent could not read ordinary newsprint, 28 percent had lost bowel and bladder control, 51 percent had problems with mobility, and 31 percent were either chair-bound or bed-ridden.

According to a 1973 to 1974 survey on chronic conditions and impairments of nursing home residents, the most frequent conditions in terms of prevalence per 1,000 residents were senility, 583.0; arthritis or rheumatism, 342.5; heart trouble, 335.1; and mental illness, 186.3.

Most nursing homes do not offer a wide range of health care services to their residents. There is, however, a growing trend for greater involvement of physicians, especially those who are specialists in the field of geriatrics. The recent development of the specialty of geriatric nursing and the training of nurse-practitioners and physician-assistants offer new professional resources to provide improved care for nursing home residents.

Home Care

Patients with chronic illness, especially the disabled elderly, are frequently discharged from hospitals to receive care in their home. Several varieties of home care service exist, ranging from single services to organized comprehensive programs. There are a variety of home care programs, but the term "Home Health Agency" is defined in federal legislation as an agency authorized to receive payment under the federal Medicare program for services provided in the home of patients.

Under Medicare regulation, all home health agencies must provide, under medical supervision, nursing care plus at least one other health service. Many programs provide physical therapy, social services, speech therapy, occupational therapy, podiatry, nutritional guidance,

and homemakers' services. Either the patient's own physician or a hospital-based home care physician may attend the patient. In the hospital-based programs, nursing services are generally obtained through a contract with the local visiting nurse association. The physician in a federally reimbursed program must supply a plan of treatment and periodically reassess the patient and update the plan. The plan must also specify the types of skilled services required for treatment of the patient. Admission to a home care program is indicated when a person requires short-term convalescence from acute illness or long-term care for chronic illness. Patients who live alone or who live with family members are eligible for home care services. It is important to have physicians and nurses participate in the hospital discharge planning process if an organized home care program is to successfully provide services.

HEALTH CARE COSTS

Health care costs in the United States have risen sharply in the past 30 years. National health expenditures in billions were $12.7 in 1950, $26.9 in 1960, $74.7 in 1970, $249.0 in 1980, and $322.4 in 1982. National health expenditures also account for a growing share of the gross national product (GNP). This percentage has risen from 4.4 in 1950 to 5.3 in 1960, 7.5 in 1970, 9.5 in 1980, and 10.5 in 1982. The proportion of the GNP devoted to health care in the United States makes this country one of the largest spenders on health care in the world.

The proportion of all health care expenditures paid by public funds has increased from 27.2 percent in 1950 to 42.4 percent in 1982. The proportion of federal health funds in relation to national health expenditures has increased from 12.8 percent in 1950 to 28.9 percent in 1982.

In 1982, private expenditures were $185.6 billion and public expenditures were $136.8 billion. Federal sources spent $93.2 billion and state/local government sources spent $43.7 in the same year.

The great majority of health expenditures are for personal health care. Total expenditures for government public health activities in 1982 were $8.6 billion. The federal total for that activity was $1.4 billion and the state/local government expenditures were $7.3 billion. In contrast, total expenditures for personal health care in 1982 were $286.9 billion. Public funds for personal health care totaled $115.7 and the federal government was responsible for $83.7 billion of that amount.

In terms of national health expenditures of all kinds, per capita expenditures have risen from $82 in 1950 to $359 in 1970, $1,075 in 1980, and $1,365 in 1982. The annual percentage change in national health expenditures was 11.5 percent for 1970 to 1971, 12.8 percent for 1975 to 1976, and 12.5 percent for 1981 to 1982.

Within the category of personal health care, the major expenditures are for hospital care and physicians' services. Table 12-1 shows the amounts and the percentages spent on major categories of expenditure in the field of personal health care. Trends recorded over the past 30 years show expenditures for hospital and nursing home services have increased 10 and 7 percent, respectively. Percentages of expenditures for drugs and physician services have decreased by approximately 6 and 2 percent, respectively.

There have been significant increases in expenditures for the Medicare programs since it began in 1966. Expenditures in billions of dollars have been as follows: $1.1 in 1966; $7.5 in 1970; $16.3 in 1975; $36.8 in 1980, and $52.2 in 1982. The recent rate of increase requires major decisions by Congress on new plans for financing this program. The Medicaid program has also experienced increases in expenditures as shown in Table 12-2.

Another perspective on health care costs is provided by the use of per capita amounts spent on various kinds of services. Table 12-3 shows trends in per capita amounts for selected categories of expenditures. The per capita amounts for nursing home care were $10.48 in 1965; $22.54 in 1970; $46.47 in 1975, and $79.13 in 1979.

Age distribution within the population has a bearing on the amount and distribution of health care expenditures. Data collected in 1976 showed that there were great differences when three age groups were used. Per capita expenditures for personal health care for all ages in 1976 was $551.50. Table 12-4 shows the age-related data (financial data in dollars per capita).

The Consumer Price Index (CPI) compiled by the Bureau of Labor Statistics is the major source of information about price changes in the American economy. Historically, medical care price increases have exceeded the increase registered by the total of all items in the CPI.

Table 12-1. The Amounts and Percentages Spent on Major Categories of Personal Health Care in the Year 1982

Category	Amount (in billions of dollars)	Percentage
Hospital Care	135.5	47.2
Physicians' Services	61.8	21.5
Nursing Home Care	27.3	9.5
Drugs and Medical Sundries	22.4	7.8
Dentists' Services	19.5	6.9
Other Health Services	7.6	2.6
Other Professional Services	7.1	2.5
Eyeglasses and Appliances	5.7	2.0
Totals	286.9	100.0

Table 12-2. Rate of Increase in Expenditures for the Medicaid Program on Federal and State and Local Levels (in billions of dollars)

	1966	1970	1975	1980	1982
Federal	0.7	3.0	7.9	14.6	18.0
State and Local	0.8	2.5	6.2	12.2	16.0
Total	1.5	5.5	14.1	26.8	34.0

From the period 1950 to 1977, the overall CPI increased at an average rate of 3.5 percent per year. During the same time interval, the price of medical care increased at an annual rate of 5 percent per year. Charges for hospital rooms increased at an annual rate of 8.9 percent. Doctors' fees increased at an annual rate of 5 percent and drug prices rose an average 1.6 percent per year. The Bureau of Labor Statistics has recently completed a comprehensive revision of the CPI. This revised index was introduced in January 1978. The list of items priced for the medical care index has undergone considerable expansion.

These increases in personal health care expenditures can be explained in terms of three factors: price, population, and intensity of services. For the time period 1965 to 1981, price increases accounted for 59 percent; population growth for 9 percent, and intensity of services accounted for 32 percent of the change. It is clear that price inflation has been the major factor in the recorded increases in health care spending.

During the past 20 years, there has been strong support for medical and health-related research. Table 12-5 shows the annual expenditures for selected years since 1960. This represents an average annual percentage change of 11.6 for the period 1960 to 1980.

FINANCING METHODS

One of the distinctive features of health care in the United States is the complexity of its financing methods. Some care is paid for directly by patients, some is provided free, and an increasing proportion is paid for indirectly by a variety of insurance or prepayment plans.

Table 12-3. Per Capita Expenditures for Selected Categories of Health Services (in Dollars)

Category	Year			
	1960	1970	1980	1982
Hospital Care	49	133	433	574
Physicians' Services	31	69	202	262
All Other Personal Care	48	111	311	379
Personal Health Care Totals	128	313	946	1,215

Table 12-4. Per Capita Age-related Expenditures for Personal
Health Care (in Dollars Per Capita)

Category	All Ages	<19 Years	19–64 Years	65+ Years
Hospitals	254	90	268	689
Physicians	121	77	121	256
Drugs	51	30	51	121
Nursing Homes	49	2	20	351

The four basic methods are described below.

1. Direct Pay—The patient pays directly for the health care service received. Direct pay is the method used frequently for dental services, drugs, eyeglasses, and appliances. This category also includes deductible and coinsurance payments associated with insurance plans.

2. Services Without Charge—Some groups of people in the population are eligible to receive health care services without charge. Programs administered by the Veterans Administration, the Indian Health Service, and the Armed Forces of the United States provide a comprehensive range of health services for specified population groups. Many states provide services without charge in their state mental hospitals. Some counties and municipalities provide services without charge through their county and municipal hospitals. Tax revenues are used to support annual budgets for these programs, and there may be some income from insurance, Medicaid, and/or direct payment.

3. Free Care—Some free care is still provided by many nongovernmental hospitals and physicians. This care is provided either without charge or sometimes in the form of write-off of uncollectible debts. Hospitals that have received federal funds for the Hill-Burton Construction Program are required to give a certain percentage of free care.

4. Indirect Payment—This category includes various types of insurance and prepayment programs. There are governmental insurance programs, such as Medicare and Medicaid, nonprofit Blue Cross and Blue Shield prepayment programs, commercial insurance (for profit) plans, and health maintenance organizations that use prepayment methods of financing. Some large companies provide their own insurance for their employees.

Table 12-5. Annual Expenditures for Health Research and Development for Selected Years Since 1960 (in Millions of Dollars)

Sources	1960	1970	1980	1981
Private nonprofit	139	215	313	329
Industry	253	795	2433	2864
State/Local Govt.	44	169	473	507
Federal Government	448	1667	4723	4898
Totals	884	2846	7942	8598

There is some ambiguity with the use of the terms "prepayment" and "insurance." The primary purpose of the traditional insurance approach is to provide financial protection for people against the risk of large and unusual costs or losses. The prepayment concept is more recent in origin and refers to a payment method associated with actual rendering of a comprehensive set of health care services. The concept of prepayment is often linked to capitation payment—the payment to providers of a fixed monthly fee on behalf of insured persons, whether or not services are rendered.

Insurance can be defined as protection by written contract against the costs of various kinds of health care services and lost income due to illness or injury. Individuals make a contractual agreement either as single persons or in groups with an insurer who promises to pay for a set range of services under specified conditions. The insurance carrier can then pay the money directly to the person insured or to the provider of services. In 1934, the American Hospital Association gave official support to this insurance program, issued a set of standards and established the Blue Cross name and symbol. The guidelines for Blue Cross programs are as follows. The Blue Cross-Blue Shield organizations are independent, private, nonprofit tax-exempt corporations. They provide insurance protection against the cost of hospital care (Blue Cross), and surgery and other types of physician care (Blue Shield).

They were to be nonprofit organizations; their boards of directors were to represent hospitals, physicians, and the public; they were to be supervised by state insurance departments; they were to hold low cash reserves; and they were to emphasize hospital benefits in the form of service rather than cash indemnities. The plans were not to be in competition with each other and, therefore, would not operate in overlapping geographic areas. Employees were to be on salary; salesmen were not paid a commission.

By 1937, the State Medical Societies of California, Michigan, and Pennsylvania were sponsoring physician service plans. In 1946, the AMA financed the development of associated medical care plans, which became the National Association of Blue Shield Plans. Although Blue Cross and Blue Shield programs have worked in close cooperation for many years, they were legally independent until 1978. In recent years, they have merged at the national level and in many states.

There are approximately 1,100 private insurance companies in the United States writing many different kinds of health insurance policies.

The key principle in commercial health insurance is indemnification of the policy holder for a stated dollar amount in relation to a specified schedule of hospital and ambulatory medical services. Since there is no contractual relationship between the health care provider and the insurance carrier, the charges for services may be greater than the amounts available through the policy. The patient is responsible for providing the difference as direct payment. Most commercial insurance policies are designed to constrain medical service utilization by using deductibles and coinsurance or percentage payments. There is strong competition among all health insurance carriers, including the Blue Cross-Blue Shield plans.

Many business firms, industrial corporations, government agencies, and other nonprofit organizations provide financial contributions to health insurance premiums as a fringe benefit for their employees. The amount of the contribution varies, but the trend has been to increase the employer's contribution. Between 1953 and 1970, the percentage of employers paying the total premium increased from 10 to 39; those paying part increased from 49 to 53; and those paying none decreased from 41 to 8. In 1976, the estimated total amount of employers' contributions was about $21 billion.

In 1977, between 80 and 90 percent of the population under the age of 65 had some form of nongovernment health insurance and 97 percent of persons 65 years and older were insured under Medicare. In that year, nearly 60 percent of the people over 65 had policies supplementing Medicare. The kinds and amounts of insurance coverage varied widely among the plans and policies.

Since 1930, there has been a trend away from direct payment toward payment through third parties. Table 12-6 shows the trends in terms of percentage distributions. Similar trends are evident in the changing balance between private and public sources of third party payments. In 1981, the balance between private and public third parties was 26.2 percent and 40.4 percent. Within the public sector, the balance was 29.3 percent federal

and 11.1 percent state and local. The percentage contributed by the state and local public sector has not changed more than 2 percentage points in 40 years.

The federal category increased suddenly from 10.1 percent in 1965 to 21.4 percent in 1967. The changes since 1967 have been gradual—29.3 percent in 1981. The dollar amounts have been very large.

Health Maintenance Organizations

The name "Health Maintenance Organization" (HMO) was introduced by Paul Ellwood in 1971. It refers to a particular type of health care organization that uses an independent, comprehensive health insurance plan, coupled to medical group practices and one or more hospitals. HMOs can be broadly defined as organizations that are responsible for the provision of comprehensive health care services for an enrolled population in return for a set monthly fee or premium. The HMO actually provides ambulatory and hospital services directly or through contract with specific providers.

In recent years, there has been a rapid growth in the establishment of HMOs. In 1980, it is estimated that there were 235 HMOs enrolling 9.1 million persons. Approximately half of these were established following federal guidelines.

Although there is a great variation in the pattern of programs and relationships in the general field of HMOs, the United States government defines them in the following terms. They are to provide basic health services to enrollees and supplemental benefits for additional payment. Enrollment fees are fixed uniformly without regard for the patient's medical history. Basic health services include physician services, in-patient, out-patient and emergency care, crisis mental health care, care for drug abuse and alcohol addiction, x-ray and laboratory tests, home health care, and preventive services. Supplemental care may include long-term care, vision care, dental services, other mental health services, long-term physical medicine, and prescription drugs. Services are provided by HMO staff professionals under contract. Essential services are available 24 hours a day, 7 days a week. Reimbursement is provided for emergency care obtained outside the HMO service area. The physicians must have a prearranged method for distributing HMO income. There must be a quality assurance program. Education services must be provided. One-third of the board of directors must be enrollees. There must be open, annual enrollment. Any HMO that can fulfill these conditions is eligible to be defined as federally qualified and obtain certain benefits under Public Law 93-222.

Starting with the Health Maintenance Organization

Table 12-6. Trends of Payment Methods Used in the Health Care Industry in Terms of Percentage Distributions

Payment Method	Year			
	1940	1960	1970	1981
Direct	81.3	54.9	39.9	32.1
All Third Parties	18.7	45.1	60.1	67.9

Act of 1973, the federal government has pursued a policy that encourages and facilitates the growth of HMOs.

Workmen's Compensation

Workmen's Compensation is a form of government social insurance dealing with industrial injuries, both in terms of costs of medical care and in terms of lost earnings. The first plan was developed by New York State in 1910. By 1950, all states had workmen's compensation plans. In 1980, nearly 9 out of 10 wage and salary workers were covered by workmen's compensation programs. This is a no-fault arrangement. Employers are required to pay compensation to their employees for job-related injuries and illnesses without regard to who caused the injury. Most of the insurance is carried by private insurance companies to which employers pay premiums. The premiums average about 1 percent of payrolls, but the amounts vary according to levels of hazards in different industries. About 7.8 million workmen's compensation claims were paid in 1978. Six million were paid for disability or death. Approximately 30,000 of the disability and death claims paid for occupational diseases. The number of claims submitted for occupational diseases is increasing. Many of these claims are contested and the average payments are much smaller than for comparable accident/injury cases.

Charitable Contributions

Prior to the widespread use of health insurance and the advent of the Medicare and Medicaid programs in 1965, philanthropic gifts were an important source of funds for health care, especially for the poor. Hospital trustees were expected to contribute both time and money to their hospitals. Physicians were expected to contribute professional services to the care of the poor. Many religious organizations provided financial support for medical care services.

Despite these trends, philanthropic support for personal health services increased from $261 million in 1960 to $756 million in 1976. As a proportion of total health expenditures, philanthropy declined from 1.1 to 0.6 percent. Charitable support for short-term hospitals increased in amount from $135 million in 1950 to $424 million in 1970, but the percent of the total decreased from 6.1 to 2.2 percent during the same time period.

Charitable funds are also contributed to support medical research. These contributions were estimated to be $121 million in 1960 and $258 million in 1976. The share of expenditures for research declined from 13 percent in 1960 to 5 percent in 1976. In 1974, charitable funds totaled $375 million for the construction of hospitals making up 9.8 percent of the total construction funds.

HEALTH CARE PERSONNEL

A large number of people are employed in the health care industry. In 1981, there were 7.5 million people employed in this field. During the past 30 years, the increase in the number of people employed has been extraordinary. In 1950, there were 1.5 million; in 1960, 2.3 million; in 1970, 4.3 million; in 1975, 5.9 million. Between 1950 and 1975, the number of people employed in the health care field increased by 215 percent, while the total number of persons in the workforce of the United States increased from 63 million to 91 million — a gain of 44 percent. Of the total of 7.5 million employed in 1981, the great majority are employed in hospitals (4.1 million). Convalescent institutions employed 1.2 million and the offices of physicians and dentists employed 1.2 million. These totals do not include pharmacists employed in drugstores, school nurses, and nurses working in private households.

At the present time, there are over 200 occupations in the health field. A significant trend in the field of health care personnel is toward increased specialization in occupational groups and the requirement of longer periods of training. In 1977, there were 35 health professions licensed in one or more states. Educational programs leading to licensed professions are usually approved and accredited by state agencies or boards of registration.

There are two major classes of occupational groups that deal with a wide range of health care problems. They are physicians and nurses. In 1980, there were 449,992 active M.D. physicians in the United States. This represented 197 active physicians per 100,000 population. The ratio was 125 per 100,000 in 1930 and it grew slowly to 133 in 1940. The ratio began to increase rapidly after 1960: 136 to 156 in 1970, 174 in 1975, and 197 in 1980. This increase was due in large measure to an increase in the number of medical school graduates and the immigration of physicians trained in foreign countries. The number of medical school graduates increased from 5,553 in 1950 to 7,081 in 1960, and to 15,346 in 1980. The number of medical schools increased from 79 in 1950 to 126 in 1982. In the decade 1965 to 1974, 75,000 foreign-trained physicians entered the United States.

Physicians are engaged in a variety of specialties and practice locations. In 1980, there were 16,585 physicians employed by the federal government, and 393,407 non-federal physicians. Table 12-7 shows the distribution of the nonfederal physicians by major specialty and/or practice location. The process of specialization in medicine has continued to develop.

Table 12-7. The Distribution (in Thousands) of the Nonfederal Physicians by Major Specialty and/or Practice Location

Specialty or Location	1970	1980
Office-based practice	187.6	269.0
General and Family Practice	50.4	47.3
Internal Medicine	22.8	40.3
Pediatrics	10.2	17.2
General Surgery	18.0	22.3
Obstetrics/Gynecology	13.7	19.3
Other Specialties	72.5	122.7
Hospital-based practice	65.1	89.5
Resident Physicians	45.5	59.1
Full-time hospital staff	19.6	30.3
Other professional activity	26.1	34.9

There are now 23 American specialty boards recognized and approved by the American Board of Medical Specialists in conjunction with the AMA Council on Medical Education. The 23 specialty boards are the following: (1) Ophthalmology—1917; (2) Otolaryngology—1924; (3) Obstetrics and gynecology—1930; (4) Dermatology—1932; (5) Pediatrics—1933; (6) Radiology—1934; (7) Psychiatry and neurology—1934; (8) Orthopedic surgery—1934; (9) Colon and rectal surgery—1934; (10) Urology—1935; (11) Pathology—1936; (12) Internal medicine—1936; (13) Anesthesiology—1937; (14) Plastic surgery—1937; (15) Surgery—1937; (16) Neurological surgery—1940; (17) Physical medicine and rehabilitation—1947; (18) Thoracic surgery—1948; (19) Preventive medicine—1948; (20) Family practice—1969; (21) Nuclear medicine—1971; (22) Allergy and immunology—1971; and (23) Emergency medicine —1979. There are additional areas of subspecialty within a number of the board certified specialties. For example, special certifications are available within internal medicine for the subspecialties of cardiovascular disease, endocrinology, gastroenterology, hematology, infectious disease, oncology, nephrology, pulmonary disease, and rheumatology.

After World War II, there was a decline in the number of general practitioners and an increase in the number of medical specialists. This continuing trend triggered strong interest in comprehensive medicine and primary care.

Recent projections by an expert committee indicate that there should be an appropriate number of family practitioners and other primary care physicians by 1990.

Allopathic physicians (MDs) and osteopathic physicians (DOs) are often listed together because their education and styles of practice are very similar. Osteopathy started as a reform movement in American medicine and was originally established in 1874. It was a school of medical practice that held that muscular skeletal dysfunctions, especially of the spine, disrupt the body's resistance to disease. It also considered medication to be overemphasized by allopathic physicians. The field has now evolved so that osteopathic physicians use basically the same diagnostic and therapeutic measures as their colleagues in the field of allopathic medicine. There are currently 15 colleges of osteopathy accredited by the American Osteopathic Association. In 1980 there were approximately 17,000 professionally active osteopathic physicians.

Physicians trained in foreign countries have been entering the United States in growing numbers. The total number of new foreign medical graduates entering practice in the United States was 6,628 in 1966 and 7,316 in 1975. The number of United States trained physicians entering practice in 1966 was 7,574 and in 1975 was 12,714.

By 1978, approximately 80,000 physicians in this country were graduates of foreign medical schools. Most of these physicians were originally educated in countries that could scarcely afford to lose their valuable services through migration to the United States. With the growth in the number of graduates from United States medical schools, Congress took action to reduce occupational preference for physicians entering the country. Implementation of this action started in 1978 and is now beginning to be put into effect.

Nurses

Nursing began as a helping profession in the United States with training programs associated with general hospitals. Students entered these 3-year training programs directly after high school graduation. They were awarded a diploma upon successful completion of the course; then after passing the state licensing examination, they were referred to as "registered nurses" or RNs. Approximately 75 percent of the RNs practicing today are graduates of hospital-based diploma schools of nursing.

The second type of training is in baccalaureate programs. These programs are 4 to 5 years in length and based in colleges or universities. Clinical experience is obtained in university or affiliated teaching hospitals. Graduates of these programs take state licensing examinations and receive the designation, "Registered Nurse." These programs were responsible for graduating 32.5 percent of new nurses in academic year 1978 to 1979.

The third form of training for graduates or registered nurses is called the associate degree program. Associate degree programs are 2-year programs usually based in junior or community colleges. These programs lead to an associate in arts degree and practical experience is obtained in affiliated hospitals. These programs were first established in 1952 and have increased rapidly since that time. In 1978 to 1979 these programs graduated 47.2 percent of the new nurses. Graduates of these programs are also eligible to take the state exams and to be designated registered nurses.

All states and the District of Columbia have licensure statutes for nurses. The first statute was passed in 1903 and all of the states had licensure laws by 1923. These statutes are called nursing practice acts and are administered by state nursing boards.

There are three kinds of nurse-specialists that deserve brief descriptions. They are nurse-midwives, nurse anesthetists, and nurse practitioners. Nurse anesthetists are RNs who have received special training in the administration of anesthesia. They have been employed in hospital/surgical departments since 1900. The first formal training program was established in 1910. The programs now generally require 18 months of training and lead to certification. Nurse-midwives are RNs with special training in prenatal and postpartum care, as well as in the management of normal labor and delivery. They practice in collaboration with obstetricians. The first United States training school in this field was established in New York City in 1932. Programs leading to certification are from 8 to 24 months in duration. The longer programs lead to a master's degree in midwifery. Nurse-midwives are separately licensed in many states. Their legal right to manage normal deliveries, with obstetricians available as needed, has been established by all states.

Nurse practitioners are RNs who have received additional training in clinical skills. Programs range in duration from 6 to 24 months. There are both certificate and master's degree programs. Physician supervision and accountability in some form is required when nurse practitioners perform tasks traditionally performed by physicians.

Practical nurses are recognized in all states as licensed practical nurses (LPNs). In California and Texas, they are known as licensed vocational nurses (LVNs). The first educational programs in practical nursing were established in 1917. The training programs are based in vocational and technical schools, hospitals, and community colleges. The program usually lasts for 8 to 15 months. Most practical nurses work in hospitals (65 percent) and nursing homes (20 percent). They are usually supervised by RNs. In 1974, there were 492,000 practical nurses employed in the country. The increase in numbers of practical nurses has been rapid — from 137,500 in 1950 and 206,000 in 1960 to 492,000 in 1974.

Nurses aides are important personnel in most hospitals and nursing homes because they perform many tasks related to the personal care of patients. There are a variety of training programs, many of them located in high schools and hospitals. Nurses aides are supervised by registered nurses and practical nurses.

Nursing is largely a hospital-based profession. In 1972, 74 percent of the RNs worked in hospitals and nursing homes, 7 percent in public health and in schools, 3.6 percent in nursing education, 2.6 percent in occupational health, and 12.7 percent in private duty, doctors' offices, and other settings.

The number of registered nurses employed in the United States has grown from 504,000 in 1960 and 750,000 in 1970 to 1.2 million in 1980. The number of RNs per 100,000 population has grown from 282 in 1960 and 369 in 1970 to 520 in 1980.

The fraction of registered nurses working part-time was 40 percent in 1970 to 1974.

PATTERNS OF MEDICAL PRACTICE

Physicians may organize their practices in several different ways in terms of legal and economic arrangements. There is solo practice where the physician is a sole proprietor of an unincorporated business. There is a professional partnership. This is based upon a legal agreement between two or more physicians to share income and assets in an unincorporated business. Each partner becomes the agent of the other. A physician joining a partnership may receive a salary for a time prior to being invited to become a junior or senior partner.

There is also a professional corporation. This is a legal entity that is distinct from its professional members. There is limited liability for corporate debts, but physician members are liable for their own negligent acts in patient care.

The most widely accepted definition of group practice is the one provided by the American Medical Association: "Group medical practice is the application of medical services by three or more physicians formally organized to provide medical care, consultation, diagnosis, or treatment through the joint use of equipment and personnel and with the income from medical practice distributed in accordance with methods previously determined by members of the group." There are three categories of group practice: single specialty groups, general or family practice groups, and multispecialty groups (providing services in two or more specialties).

The growth of medical group practices was slow at first, but it has accelerated in recent years. The trend is described in Table 12-8. If one calculates the ratio of group practice physicians not in relation to all active physicians but in relation to active, nonfederal physicians in office-based medical practice, the proportions

Table 12-8. The Growth of Medical Practices for Selected Years Since 1932

Year	Number of Groups	Physicians in Group Practice	Percent of all Active MDs
1932	239	1,466	0.9
1946	368	3,084	2.6
1959	1,546	12,009	5.2
1969	6,162	38,834	12.8
1975	7,733	59,809	17.1
1980	—	88,290	—

were 21 percent in 1969 to 1970, 31 percent in 1975, and 33 percent in 1980.

The distribution of single specialty and multispecialty groups is interesting. Originally, the composition of medical groups emphasized multispecialty combinations. Then in the 1950s, the number of single specialty groups began to increase. This pattern grew so rapidly that by 1975, single specialty clinics represented 54.2 percent of the group clinics and 35.3 percent of the group practice physicians. Table 12-9 shows the distribution for 66,842 physicians and 8,483 group clinics in 1975.

Since family practice groups are capable of providing a more comprehensive range of services than single specialty clinics, they are, in a sense, more like multispecialty groups. A combination of these two groups produces a total of 45.8 percent of the clinics and 64.7 percent of the physicians engaged in the provision of comprehensive medical services. Single specialty groups are typically smaller in size (75.5 percent having 3 to 5 physicians) as compared to multispecialty groups (41.8 percent having 3 to 5 physicians).

Historically, group practices are associated with the development of health maintenance organizations. These health care organizations have been described in a previous section of this chapter. Their rapid development and expansion represents one of the major, new organizational patterns in American medicine.

During the past 20 years, there has been a significant growth in numbers and kinds of organized clinics in the United States. In the mid-1970s, approximately one-half of all medical services provided to ambulatory persons were given in an organized setting of some type, as distinguished from the pattern of private solo medical prac-

tice. The estimates for patient visits to organized clinics in 1975 are listed in Table 12-10. The total number of patient visits to physicians in 1975 was estimated to be 1.2 billion.

A new form of organized ambulatory care emerged in the mid-1960s. It was the Community Health Center, often known as the neighborhood health center in an urban area. These health centers were organized to provide programs of comprehensive health services to defined residential populations.

Rural health centers have developed in parallel with the urban health centers. Many of them have been developed with federal financing, some with state funds, and others with funds raised by local community groups. Many of these rural health centers are located in small towns that have insufficient population to support a physician, which means that many of these health centers are staffed by nurse practitioners or physician assistants. These midlevel health practitioners are supervised by physicians who make weekly visits to the health centers and are available for telephone consultation.

For patients of all ages, Table 12-11 describes the most frequent medical problems in office visits to physicians on an average annual basis for 1975 to 1976.

The patterning of medical problems in ambulatory care shifts significantly in relation to the age of the patient. Persons under 15 years visit for medical exams and acute URI; persons 15 to 24 years visit for prenatal care, medical exams and URIs; persons 25 to 44 years visit for prenatal care, neuroses, and medical exams; persons 45 to 64 years visit for hypertension, arthritis and ischemic heart disease; and persons 65 years and over visit for ischemic heart disease, hypertension, and arthritis. This means that with the exception of treating URIs, the most frequent medical problems require diagnosis, treatment, and monitoring of chronic diseases.

Traditionally, personal health services have been organized as a complaint-response system. In years past, the bulk of illness presented to the physician consisted of acute, self-limited conditions that progressed rapidly to

Table 12-9. The Distribution for 66,842 Physicians and 8,483 Group Clinics in 1975

Type	Percentages of: Group Clinics	Physicians
Multispecialty	35.1	58.8
Family Practice	10.7	5.9
Single Specialty	54.2	35.3
	100.0	100.0

Table 12-10. The Estimates for Patient Visits to Organized Clinics in 1975

Clinic Sponsorship	Number of Visits (in millions)	Percent
Private group practices	282.3	47.4
Hospital outpatient departments	236.0	39.7
Federal beneficiary clinics	23.0	3.9
Health Department clinics	20.0	3.4
School and college health services	14.0	2.4
Industrial health units	10.0	1.7
County health centers	4.7	0.8
All other clinics	5.0	0.8
All clinics (Total)	595.1	100.0

Table 12-11. The Most Frequent Medical Problems Requiring Office Visits to Physicians on an Average Annual Basis for the Years 1975 to 1976

Common Principal Diagnosis	Office Visits per 1,000 population (all ages)
Medical or special exams	205.2
Acute upper respiratory infection (URI), excluding influenza	175.6
Medical and surgical aftercare	135.1
Hypertension	110.9
Heart disease	103.5
Prenatal care	101.3
Neuroses	100.1
Arthritis and rheumatism	86.7
Infections of skin	85.1
Diseases of ear and mastoid	84.2
Bronchitis, emphysema, asthma	76.6
Sprains and strains	68.6

death or to recovery. Now a large part of professional practice requires dealing with abnormalities that affect various subsystems of the body for long periods of time. This pattern of health maintenance requires routine use of clinical procedures associated with a strategy of secondary prevention. Health maintenance may become the primary emphasis in personal health care. This requires monitoring immunologic susceptibility to various infectious diseases; anatomic abnormalities, such as obesity and lumps in the breast; chemical changes, such as elevated blood glucose or cholesterol; physiologic changes, such as elevated blood pressure or EKG abnormalities; and behavior patterns that increase risks to health status, such as smoking, excessive use of alcohol, or overeating. While the complaint-response pattern continues, emphasis is shifting toward health maintenance in response to the dominant profiles of disease and disability in the society.

There have been important developments in the attempt to improve effectiveness and quality of medical care. It is generally agreed that there are three main measures used in the review of the quality of personal health care programs. These measures deal with structure, process, and outcome. The key elements of structure are personnel, facilities, equipment, organization, information systems and records, and financing methods. The basic assumption is that better care is likely to be provided when the staff, facilities, and organizational arrangements meet established standards. The information required for structural assessment is relatively easy to collect, classify, and evaluate.

Process refers to the activities of physicians and other health care personnel in patient care management. Here the key elements for the physician are problem recognition, diagnostic procedures, diagnoses, therapy,

management, and reassessment. The key elements for patients or clients are utilization, acceptance, understanding of service offered, and compliance with professional recommendations. Standards used to evaluate process can be based on scientific clinical trials, patterns of care observed in practice, or norms recommended by recognized leaders in the profession.

Outcome refers to discernible changes in health status. The key parameters are longevity, activity, comfort, satisfaction, disease, achievement, and resilience—or the outcome measures can be expressed as avoidance or reduction of death, disease, disability, discomfort, and dissatisfaction. Health status can be defined as a person's position with reference to all of these parameters considered simultaneously. It is assumed that structure and process are linked in a predictable way to outcomes.

The operational review of medical care programs have utilized a variety of methods, including tissue committees, direct observation of physicians engaged in clinical practice, and audits using medical records.

In 1972, Congress mandated the formation of Professional Standards Review Organizations (PSROs) to provide a continuing assessment of the quality of medical care. Quality was defined as the extent to which scientifically established procedures in the diagnosis and management of serious common and treatable disorders are properly applied to patients who can benefit from their application. Given a list of procedures considered appropriate for the diagnosis and treatment of a given disease or disorder, it is possible to check this list against the record of actual procedures carried out with a particular patient.

A medical audit system called criteria mapping has been developed. In this system, criteria are developed to reflect sequential clinical decision-making based on specific findings for the individual patient at a particular time. This method is believed to be superior to the use of protocols that mandate the sequencing in the clinical process. This technique more accurately reflects the intentions of the physicians and more closely relates process to outcome. Development and application of methods for quality assurance in medicine is likely to receive continued emphasis in the years ahead.

HEALTH LAW

The legal structure of the United States has four major components: Constitutional law, statutory law, administrative law, and common law or case law. The Constitution is the supreme law of the land. All other laws, including state constitutions, must be consistent with it. Although the Constitution does not contain the words "medicine" or "health," the federal government has developed important activities concerning health by using institutional powers to regulate interstate and foreign commerce and to promote the general welfare. Laws passed by legislative bodies are called statutes. Congress and state legislatures pass a number of laws dealing with the field of general health and safety of the public. Administrative law refers to the rules and regulations when statutes are implemented by administrative agencies. Common law is the set of legal principles that have evolved from court cases based on precedent and custom. Most legal actions taken by one person or group against another are called civil actions and are carried out under common law. Conflicts concerning professional negligence or medical malpractice are handled in this legal area.

Professional practice of physicians is sanctioned by society through state licensure laws. Once a license has been granted to a physician, it cannot be revoked without the physician having an opportunity to answer charges brought against him. Valid reasons for revocation or suspension of license are conviction of serious crimes, unprofessional conduct in the practice of medicine, and physical or mental incapacity to practice safely as a physician.

Once a physician establishes a professional relationship with a particular patient, he is obligated to care for that patient until the patient's illness is adequately treated or the patient is referred to and accepted by another physician for care. When a physician wishes to withdraw from the care of a patient, he must give reasonable notice and an opportunity for the patient to find an alternative source of professional care. Violation of this duty to provide care for a patient during a present illness is called "abandonment" and is grounds for medical malpractice action.

The physician is required, by both legal and ethical standards, to keep confidential any information received from a patient. This includes findings from medical tests and diagnostic information provided by the physician. Control over the confidentiality of the information belongs to the patient who can instruct the physician to disclose the information to a particular person. When this occurs, the physician must comply with the patient's request. If a physician communicates confidential information improperly, he runs the risk of revocation of license to practice. There are two exceptions to the confidentiality requirement. One is when testimony is required in a court of law, and the other is when reporting of certain diseases is required by public health regulations. The intent of these regulations is to protect the health of the public by control of communicable diseases.

Professional negligence of medical malpractice occurs when the physician fails to provide medical care of an acceptable level of quality. The individual physician's performance is evaluated in terms of what other physicians in a similar practice would do under similar circumstances. It is usually difficult for patients to prove and to win a malpractice action against a physician. The patient must be able to show a clear relationship between a physician's breech of duty and the patient's condition after treatment. The patient also must prove that there was injury or damage, increased pain and suffering, and financial loss.

During the past 20 years, there has been increased concern about medical malpractice actions. Unfortunately, there were no empirical studies made on malpractice litigation until a national commission was established in 1971 and gave its final report in 1973. The report concluded that there were far fewer malpractice cases than most people assumed. Of those cases that were processed through the courts, there were few awards made to patients. A survey of all claims filed in 1970 showed that 60 percent of all payments to patients in out-of-court settlements or court awards were less than $3,000 each. Over 88 percent of the awards were less than $20,000. Only 3 percent of the awards were for amounts over $100,000. A total of 16,000 claims were closed in 1970. No money was awarded in 55 percent of these claims. In most cases, no law suit actually took place.

State laws and public health regulations require physicians to report certain events and medical conditions to government agencies. A physician who attends the birth of an infant is required to fill out a birth certificate. A similar procedure is required for completing a death certificate.

Determinations of time and cause of death are important for legal, insurance, and public health reasons. Certain deaths raise legal questions and are, therefore, considered to fall within the jurisdiction of coroners or medical examiners. The medical examiner has the power to remove the body and to order an autopsy without consent of spouse or next of kin in the following situations: suspected homicide, suspected suicide, deaths where the cause is uncertain or unknown, deaths that occur in a hospital within 24 hours after admission, and deaths where there may be a possibility of contagious disease.

Each state has a list of notifiable diseases, and physicians are responsible for reporting cases of the listed diseases on a weekly basis. Most of the notifiable diseases are contagious or related to occupational health hazards. The most demanding laws concern venereal diseases. These laws may require identification of contacts and treatment status.

Physicians are required to promptly report cases of gunshot or knife wounds. All states have laws to protect children from neglect or cruelty inflicted by parents or guardians. Many states require physicians and hospitals to report suspected cases of child abuse to the police or to social agencies.

A person has no control in deciding the disposition of his or her body after death. The surviving spouse or next of kin has the authority to make burial arrangements and to give permission for autopsy. There are statutes in all states that authorize persons before death to make gifts of their bodies for dissection or for organ transplantation. These laws also authorize next of kin to make organ donations if the person did not express his objection to donation before death. Persons who participate in the anatomical gift procedure usually carry a donation card. The physician attending at time of death is authorized to effect the donation if he finds such a card.

In traditional view, death is a natural process associated with cessation of respiration and heartbeat. It is customary practice to have a physician examine the person and to declare that the person has died. This is done to fix the time of death and cause of death for the death certificate. With the development of mechanical respirators and heart-lung machines, the determination of death in some situations becomes more difficult. In 1968, an expert committee at Harvard Medical School developed new criteria to be used in dealing with patients with irreversible coma. The committee's definition of brain death was widely adopted. The criteria are unreceptivity and unresponsivity to externally applied stimuli, no movement or breathing over a period of at least 1 hour, no reflexes, a flat electroencephalogram (EEG) for a minimum of 10 minutes, and no changes in the patient's condition when all of the preceding tests are repeated at least 24 hours later. The brain death definition is particularly useful in situations of organ transplantation.

Physicians caring for patients suffering from serious mental illness may find it necessary to arrange the procedure of legal commitment to a psychiatric hospital. This legal control is justified when the patient may be a danger to either the community or to himself. There are four categories of hospitalization: voluntary admission, commitment for temporary observation, emergency commitment for a short time, and compulsory commitment for an indefinite period of time. Statutes require that patients be given notice and opportunity to be heard prior to hospitalization using compulsory commitment procedures.

After World War II, there was a significant increase in medical research in the United States. During most of this time period, there were no legal controls on the research activity involving either human or animal subjects. The Drug Amendments Law of 1962 made it a requirement to obtain written, informed consent from all human subjects who participated in clinical investigation of new drugs. In the next few years, the National Institutes of Health and other agencies involved in funding medical research established strict controls for all clinical investigation involving human subjects. The guidelines require the establishment of human rights review committees in institutions conducting research with human subjects. These "Institutional Review Boards" (IRBs) review research grant proposals and monitor procedures used to protect the welfare and safety of all human subjects.

The basic elements of informed consent procedures in medical research are (1) an explanation of the procedures to be followed, including identification of those that are experimental; (2) a description of discomforts and risks; (3) a description of benefits to be expected; (4) disclosure of alternative procedures that would be advantageous to the subject; (5) an offer to answer any inquiries concerning the procedures; and (6) the instruction that the research subject is free to withdraw his consent and to discontinue participation in the project at any time.

MEDICAL ETHICS

With the continuing production of scientific discoveries in biology and medicine, there are new ethical and legal questions to be dealt with. There is also a need for improved skills in ethical reasoning on the part of physicians, scientists, administrators, legislators, patients, and members of the public at large. Each physician must learn to identify key ethical issues within his daily clinical practice. He then needs to develop and practice a certain form of ethical reasoning so that the patient and those who are associated with the care of the patient can have a clear understanding of the value conflicts that emerge.

When a physician engages in ethical reasoning, he should keep in mind the physician-patient relationship, the issue of informed consent, the value of life and personhood, and the question of who has the right to participate in the decision-making process. The physician must also learn to detect and correct errors in ethical reasoning and argument. Some of the errors that are frequently encountered are (1) appealing to empirical data to settle an ethical question; (2) arguing backward from successful results to the original ethical question; (3) assuming that a person will have good motives because of his social or professional role; (4) assuming that good motives will lead to good actions; (5) arguing the ethics of a position by definition without reference to actual real-life consequences; (6) basing one's ethical claims on a right without stating where the right originates, on what authority it is based, or who has the responsibility to fulfill the right; (7) arguing that an ethical statement or action is wrong because it may lead to bad consequences, without showing that those consequences are probable; (8) arguing on the basis of a slogan that is either inherently devoid of meaning or so vague as to be inapplicable in real-life circumstances; and (9) placing great weight on a possible consequence of very low probability to the exclusion of more probable consequences.

There are a large number of ethical issues to be found in current medical research and medical practice. Five important areas have been selected for presentation here.

A number of important ethical issues are associated with conception and birth of a human being. Historically, procedures of contraception, sterilization, and abortion have been linked in strong ways to conflicting values and to decisions that physicians and their patients face on a continuing basis. The development of new diagnostic and therapeutic procedures, such as amniocentesis and in vitro fertilization add both new hopes and new ethical problems.

The central ethical issues in this field relate to establishing the precise time at which the developing embryo or fetus is defined as a human being. Once this defined stage occurs, then the organism is granted a series of rights. The mother, the father, and the attending physician have protective responsibilities once the event of conception occurs and an embryo begins to develop. At the present time, there are different positions taken as to when the developing embryo or fetus achieves human status.

In 1973, the Supreme Court of the United States decided that abortions were legal up to the end of the second trimester, or about 28 weeks. The decision was based on the woman's right to a private decision about her pregnancy. During the last 3 months of pregnancy, the state can intervene to protect the life of the fetus. This decision is based upon the stage of development at which the fetus is likely to survive outside the woman's body. In a subsequent court decision in 1976, the Supreme Court ruled that a father could not overrule a decision made by the mother with her attending physician. A woman has the right to reach a decision without interference.

New developments, such as genetic screening and prenatal diagnostic techniques, raise additional issues for both ethical and legal consideration and decision-making. If we know that a developing fetus has a congenital disorder or is the recessive carrier of a serious inheritable disease, we have new knowlege and this, in turn, raises the consideration of proper ethical behavior in conducting an abortion as a form of neonatal euthanasia.

The second major area of ethical issues is associated with death and dying. Both the process of dying and the death event itself have been topics of attention and interest in all societies for a long period of time. Now modern technical developments, such as the mechanical respirator and the heart-lung machine make it possible to extend life and to modify the dying process. New capabilities in the field of organ transplantation force consideration of ethical, moral, and legal issues similar to those associated with the beginning of human life. The earlier definition of death was associated with the cessation of essential cardiopulmonary functions. Now there is a new definition that includes "brain death." This was discussed in a previous section of the chapter.

Many of the significant ethical issues concern euthanasia, a word which derives from the Greek expression for "good death." The central need has been to avoid prolonged suffering on the part of a dying person. According to current definition, euthanasia means putting to death or failing to prevent death in cases of terminal illness or injury. The motive is to relieve the person from physical suffering, anxiety, or a serious sense of burdensomeness to self and others. In euthanasia, at least one other person causes or helps to cause the death of one who desires death, or in the case of an incompetent person, makes a substitute decision either to cause death directly or to withdraw something that sustains life.

Euthanansia decisions can be analyzed in terms of two dimensions: voluntary-nonvoluntary and active-passive. Voluntary decisions about death are those in which a competent and mature person requests or gives formal consent to take a particular course of treatment or nontreatment. The decision reflects a person's conscious intent. Nonvoluntary euthanasia decisions involve situations in which a person is incompetent to make choices for himself because of age, mental impairment, or unconsciousness. The person who makes the decision about life and death is not the patient himself. The second dimension involves a degree of action on the part of the person who will die and some other person. It is often difficult to make clear distinctions, but a lethal injection is an active form of euthanasia. Leaving a newborn infant with severe congenital defects alone in its crib to die is considered a passive form of euthanasia. It has been argued that the intention is to hasten the death of a person in comparison to what would happen naturally. The only debate is the means by which this intention is to be accomplished.

One of the productive results in recent years has been the development in 1968 of the "living will." This document is prepared for people who want to leave written instruction to members of their family, their physician, and their lawyer, expressing their desire that extraordinary medical technologies not be used in the face of imminent death. In contrast, the official position of the American Medical Association was that intentional termination of life of one human being by another is contrary to that for which the medical profession stands and is contrary to the policy of the American Medical Association. This statement also says that the decision to cease extraordinary treatment is the decision of the patient and the members of the patient's family. This leaves the physician in the undefined role of advisor to the patient.

Several groups are working on guidelines for hospitals to follow with reference to resuscitation procedures. Until recently, there has been relatively little open discussion about the process by which the decision is made not to resuscitate a patient. One guideline in current use states that it should be a general policy of hospitals to act affirmatively to preserve the life of all patients, but to respect the patient's expressed wish to reject specific kinds of treatment, incuding cardiopulmonary resuscitation. The statement shows the balance between two equally valid concerns; mainly, the preservation of life and the patient's right of self-determination.

The present public debate concerning these technical principles and proposals for statutory law is part of the process by which an open democratic society makes important choices. Not only physicians, their patients, and their patients' families, but the public at large has an important stake in the way in which these problems come to be understood and be resolved in terms of specific guidelines for decision-making and action.

The third area of important ethical concern deals with informed consent in the physician-patient relationship. There is a basic dilemma to be faced in the choice between two valued duties—telling the truth and caring for the patient when care includes not telling the complete truth. The concept of therapeutic privilege justifies a physician in withholding information, or even lying when, in his medical professional judgment, serious harm could be caused to a patient by a disclosure of certain information.

There are a number of new developments that have required professionals concerned with the practice of medicine to study the informed consent dimension of the relationship between physicians and their clients. (1) There is the fact that medical information is increasingly sophisticated and a special effort is required to translate and to convey essential information about technical matters to patients who have no medical training. (2) Diagnostic procedures can provide information to physicians long before there are symptoms and before the patient has an awareness of any future medical difficulties. (3) Specialization among physicians often results in a patient dealing with a group of specialists. (4) We live in a time when difficulties of communication and misunderstanding are frequently brought to a court of law for settlement. (5) There is a social movement to provide consumers with more complete information so that they can make more informed decisions. This social movement is now being experienced in the field of health care. (6) The traditional sense of authority, technical knowledge, and paternalism that characterized the doctor-patient relationship in earlier years is now being challenged more frequently by patients and family members. (7) There has been clarification about self-determination and individual rights in actions taken by courts and legislatures over the past decade. (8) There has been considerable publicity about abuses in the use of informed consent procedures in the field of medical research. (9) There is a difference between the medical and legal professions in terms of their concept of therapeutic privilege and discretionary use of information. Lawyers treat therapeutic privilege in a very narrow and strict sense, and physicians consider therapeutic privilege a highly valued generic feature of the professional practice of medicine.

The President's Commission for the Study of Ethical Problems in Medicine and Biomedical and Behavioral Research issued a report in 1982 dealing with ethical and legal implications of informed consent in the patient-practitioner relationship. The report stated that the ethical foundation of informed consent can be traced to the promotion of two values: personal well-being and self-determination. These values are to be respected and enhanced in the practice of clinical medicine. The Commission then went on to state that the informed consent doctrine has substantial foundations in law, but it is essentially an ethical imperative. Ethically valid consent is a process of shared decision-making based upon mutual respect and participation.

The fourth major area involving physicians and other health care professionals is the value placed on the "right to health." This ethical and moral issue differs in several ways from those considered up to this point. This is a decision that involves the use of scarce resources at the societal level of decision-making. Here, the basic conflict is between high levels of costs associated with the achievement of improvements in health status for a majority of the members of the society and national principles devoted to the promotion of the general welfare. Mixed in with this is our long-standing support for individual rights and self-determination.

The country now devotes ten percent of is gross national product to health care. How does the nation decide what level of expenditure is enough for the field of health in competition with other needs such as education, transportation, and national defense? In the public arena of expenditures for medical research and for medical services, what is the appropriate balance between these two priorities? Is the allocation of resources to personal health services and public health services in proper balance in terms of current national expenditure? Funds are finite; no government-sponsored program, such as Medicare, can be expanded indefinitely without reaching a limit. The percentage of the elderly in the population continues to grow larger. In 1930, 5 percent of the population was over 65 years of age. In 1960, it was 9 percent; in 1990, it is projected to be 13 percent; and in the year 2040, it will be 23 percent. This is important because elderly persons utilize large amounts of medical services. In 1976, the 10 percent of people who were 65 years or older required 36 percent of our national health expenditure. It is possible that at some point in the future, we may face policy decisions about witholding certain life-saving health care resources from citizens who are older than a given age.

Man-made diseases have become of significant concern in recent years. The control of environmental health hazards is costing billions of dollars. New research knowledge about the etiology of important diseases, such as cancer and heart disease where there is a link to man-made environmental pollutants, is going to mobilize strong resistance in major sectors of the business and industrial economy. As economic transactions with other countries increase, there will be greater need for maintaining low production costs so American companies can effectively compete with goods from foreign countries.

The recent attempts to make stringent federal laws concerning environmental pollutants are likely to continue to represent an area of public responsibility for the medical profession and for scientists engaged in health research.

Differences between special interest groups and competing values in society will be managed through the political process. The resultant statutes and administrative regulations will significantly influence the way Americans view their health status in relation to other requirements for fulfillment of a rich and rewarding life.

The final topic in the area of ethics deals with the field of applied genetics. With the discovery in the 1950s of the structure of the deoxyribonucleic acid (DNA) molecule, there has been a rapid acceleration of new knowledge in the field of human biology. Once the structure of

DNA had been discovered and its language deciphered, the next step was to manipulate genetic material itself. The engineering phase, known as DNA recombination, began in the early 1970s. The public name for this stage of applied research is genetic engineering or "gene splicing." These procedures involve actually cutting and rearranging genetic material. The result is that the subsequent development of the organism can be altered in a significant way. This technique was first used to develop rare biological chemicals, such as insulin, hormones, and interferon.

By testing adults and newborns, it is possible to detect individuals who have inherited some specific genetic diseases, even though no symptoms have appeared. By the use of the amniocentesis procedure and other prenatal genetic testing techniques, it is possible to identify fetuses that will experience genetic disorders or will be carriers of disorders. Through selective abortion, such fetuses could be destroyed. Through an intensive, routine genetic prenatal screening program and selective abortion process, we could eliminate certain genetic disorders from the population. Such possibilities raise important moral dilemmas.

New knowledge in this area reactivates the discussion of balance of influence from genetic inheritance and the process of environmental learning and influence. The pursuit of scientific knowledge has produced a number of benefits for mankind, and it also has produced a number of important moral and political dilemmas. Nuclear energy can be used for peaceful purposes, and it also can be used to support a set of military weapons that are capable of destroying all life on the planet. We may be facing similar potentialities for benefit and risk in the development of genetic engineering. Our society is now entering an age of intervention which requires open public discussion and debate. Through future applied genetic techniques, the evolution of the human species and its environment will be influenced, either intentionally or accidentally. To be effective and intentional, efforts to control evolution will, by necessity, have to be international in scope. The social interaction of individuals operating within the framework of a variety of social institutions have brought us to this point in human history. We can expect these institutions to serve as facilitators for discussions and decisions that must be made by physicians, scientists, and the public concerning the field of applied genetics.

REFERENCES

Benenson AS ed: Control of Communicable Diseases in Man. 13th Ed. The American Public Health Association, Washington, D.C., 1981
  This book provides an official source of information on communicable diseases. The diseases are listed alphabetically. Data are

included on identification, infectious agents, occurrence, reservoir, mode of transmission, incubation period, period of communicability, susceptibility and resistance, and methods of control for each of the disease categories.

Brody H: Ethical Decisions in Medicine. 2nd Ed. Little Brown and Co., 1981
> This book is organized around 66 problem cases and is presented in a self-instructional format.

Clark DW, MacMahon B: Preventive and Community Medicine. 2nd Ed. Little Brown and Co., Boston, 1981
> This is one of the basic textbooks in preventive medicine and public health. It covers methods in preventive medicine, disease etiology and prevention in clinical practice and a section on health services and health legislation.

Curran WJ, Shapiro ED: Law, Medicine, and Forensic Science. 3rd Ed. Little, Brown, and Co., Boston, Massachusetts, 1982
> An excellent source book covering a wide range of content in health law.

Duncan RC, Knapp RG, Clinton MM: Introductory Biostatistics for the Health Sciences. 2nd Ed. John Wiley and Sons, New York, 1983
> This book is designed to enable health science professionals to apply basic descriptive and inferential statistical techniques to problems in the medical field.

Gibson RM, Waldo DR: "National Health Expenditures, 1981," pp. 1–35 in Health Care Financing Review, Vol. 4, Number 1 September 1982
> Comprehensive statistics on health care costs in the United States are presented annually in this journal, published quarterly by the U.S. Health Care Financing Administration.

Gold R, Yankaskas BC eds: Epidemiology and Public Health: Pretest Self-Assessment and Review. 2nd Ed. McGraw-Hill, New York, 1980
> This is a good practice volume. There are 500 questions in the formats used by the National Board of Medical Examiners and explanations are given for the correct answers.

Hamburg DA, Elliott GR, Parron DL eds: Health and Behavior, National Academy Press, Washington, D.C., 1982
> This report presents the finding that much of the world's burden of illness is behavior-related. About half the mortality from the 10 leading causes of death in the United States is strongly linked to long-term patterns of behavior or life style. Evidence is presented on major diseases.

Harron F, Burnside J, Beauchamp T: Health and Human Values: A Guide to Making Your Own Decisions. Yale University Press, New Haven 1983
> This monograph provides a succinct description of the legal, ethical, and moral issues associated with abortion, prenatal procedures, euthanasia, death, informed consent, the right to health, and applied genetics.

Hill AB ed: Controlled Clinical Trials. Charles C Thomas, Springfield, 1960
> This is a collection of professional papers that provides a clear understanding of the methods used in controlled clinical trials.

Hill AB: Principles of Medical Statistics. 9th Ed. Oxford University Press, New York, 1971
> A very well written introduction to statistical reasoning in the field of biomedical research.

Jonas S: Health Care Delivery in the United States. Springer Publishing Co., New York, 1977
> One of the widely used texts in the field. It has good chapters on data for health care, nursing, hospitals, mental health services, the federal legislative process, and control of health care quality.

Last JM, ed: Maxcy-Rosenau Public Health and Preventive Medicine. 11th Ed. Appleton-Century-Crofts, New York, 1980
> This compendium of 1,926 pages covers nearly all of the major fields of public health and preventive medicine. It is the best single source published in recent years.

National Center for Health Statistics: Health, United States, 1982, DHHS, Publication Number (PHS) 83.1232, Public Health Service, U.S. Government Printing Office, Washington, D.C., December, 1982
> Starting in 1975, the U.S. Public Health Service has produced an annual report on the health of the nation. This report provides up-to-date statistical information and current information on a comprehensive range of topics in the health field.

President's Commission for the Study of Ethical Problems in Medicine and Biomedical and Behavioral Research. Making Healthcare Decisions, Vol. I, U.S. Government Printing Office, Washington, D.C., October, 1982
> This is the first of a series of reports dealing with significant ethical problems in the field of medicine and related research areas. The first volume deals with ethical and legal implications of informed consent in the patient-practitioner relationship.

Roemer MI: Ambulatory Health Services in America. Aspen Systems, Rockville, 1981
> This book provides a comprehensive set of information about patterns of ambulatory care in the United States.

Shouldice RG, Shouldice KH: Medical Group Practice and Health Maintenance Organizations. Information Resources Press, Washington, D.C., 1978.
> This book provides a comprehensive description of the development of medical group practices in the United States and the development of health maintenance organizations.

U.S. Public Health Service: Promoting Health and Preventing Disease: Objectives for the Nation, Department of Health and Human Services, Washington, D.C., 1980
> This publication identifies 15 health problems that have a high priority for preventive attention. It also provides recommendations for specific prevention and control programs.

Veatch RM: Case Studies and Medical Ethics. Harvard University Press, Cambridge, 1977
> This book deals with major issues in the field of medical ethics by presentation and analysis of 112 problem cases.

Wilson FA, Neuhauser D: Health Services in the United States. 2nd Ed. Ballinger Publishing Company, Cambridge, 1982
> This book provides a comprehensive description of health care services in the U.S. It covers a broad range of areas, including hospitals, nursing homes, ambulatory care, health manpower, paying for care, the federal government and health, the role of state and local governments, voluntary agencies and organizations, pharmaceutical firms, clinical laboratories, blood banks, review and control of quality and costs, health law, and medical ethics.

MULTIPLE CHOICE QUESTIONS

Choose the best answer.

1. What percentage of drivers killed in automobile accidents have blood alcohol levels over 0.1 percent?
   A. 80 percent
   B. 50 percent
   C. 30 percent

D. 20 percent
E. 10 percent

2. According to the Centers for Disease Control, how many legal abortions were performed in the United States in 1979?
   A. 1.3 million
   B. 0.9 million
   C. 0.7 million
   D. 0.5 million
   E. 0.3 million

3. All of the following statements about Medicare and Medicaid are true except that . . .
   A. In 1982, Medicare and Medicaid financed 29 cents of every dollar spent for personal health care in the United States.
   B. The combined Medicare and Medicaid programs paid 35 percent of all hospital expenditures, 23 percent of all physician expenditures, and 50 percent of all nursing home expenditures in 1982.
   C. Nearly 55 million people, 90 percent of whom were 65 years of age or over, were enrolled in Medicare in 1982.
   D. Medicare has two parts, each one with its own trust fund.
   E. The federal government contributed 53 percent of the funds used in the Medicaid program in 1982.

4. All of the following are correct statements except that . . .
   A. Medical licensure is on a state-by-state basis.
   B. All states now have mandatory controls called medical licensure laws.
   C. In most states, a court finding of medical malpractice is grounds for revocation or suspension of a license to practice.
   D. Surveys show very little disciplinary activity by state medical licensure board for the period 1963 to 1972.
   E. Recent revisions in medical licensure statutes often specify an investigative system to monitor professional activities relating to misconduct and lack of quality in medical practice.

5. The following are correct statements about trends in long-term hospitals (1970 to 1980) except that . . .
   A. The number of general care beds decreased from 43,000 to 8,250.
   B. The number of psychiatric beds declined from 552,000 to 218,000.
   C. The number of psychiatric beds in hospitals

owned by state and local governments declined from 498,000 to 185,000.
   D. The number of tuberculosis and other respiratory disease hospitals declined from 103 to 10.
   E. The number of proprietary psychiatric hospitals decreased and the number of nonprofit psychiatric hospitals increased.

6. All of the following statements about the new prospective reimbursement system are correct except that . . .
   A. The key concept of the DRG system is to replace per diem reimbursement with payment of set fees for 467 identified major medical problems.
   B. Psychiatric hospitals are exempt from the new regulations, but long-term care facilities and rehabilitation centers are included.
   C. The acronym DRG stands for "diagnosis-related groups."
   D. On October 1, 1983, the federal government implemented a new prospective reimbursement method for hospitals receiving Medicare and/or Medicaid funds.
   E. New Jersey, New York, Massachusetts, and Maryland are exempt from the federal DRG system because they have their own cost-containment programs.

Each question below contains four suggested answers of which one or more is correct. Choose the answer:

    A   if 1, 2, and 3 are correct
    B   if 1 and 3 are correct
    C   if 2 and 4 are correct
    D   if 4 is correct
    E   if 1, 2, 3, and 4 are correct

7. Which of the following statements about births are correct?
   1. The number of live births for the U.S. population in 1950, 1970, and 1979 were nearly equal.
   2. The crude birth rate decreased from 24.1 in 1950 to 15.9 in 1979.
   3. The number of live births per 1,000 women for the age groups 20 to 24 years and 25 to 29 years have been nearly equal since 1977.
   4. The number of live births per 1,000 women for women aged 35 to 39 showed a decline from 1950 to 1975 and has been stable since that time.

8. Which of the following statements about physician visits in 1980 are correct?
   1. The number of physician visits per person was 4.7.

2. In 1980, the physician visit rate for persons in families with income less than $7,000 was higher than for persons in families earning $25,000 or more.
3. In 1980, the rate of physician visits per person for blacks was nearly equal to the rate for whites—4.6 and 4.8, respectively.
4. The physician visit rate for males is slightly higher than for females.

9. Which of the following statements about acute rheumatic fever in the United States are correct?
   1. The number of first cases are estimated to be 5,000 to 8,000 on an annual basis.
   2. Prevalence rates are much higher in socioeconomically depressed populations.
   3. Beta hemolytic streptococcus infection is the cause of initial and recurrent attacks.
   4. Mortality statistics show a continuing upward trend since 1900.

10. Which of the following statements about inpatient days of care in mental health facilities are correct?
    1. There was an annual decrease of 7.3 percent of inpatient days for all facilities.
    2. Private hospitals showed an increase of 2.3 percent in inpatient days.
    3. State and community hospitals experienced a 10.3 percent decline in number of inpatient days.
    4. There was a 5 percent average increase per year in the number of inpatient days in Veterans Administration psychiatric services.

11. Which of the following statements about suicide are correct?
    1. In 1980, death rate for white males was nearly three times the rate for white females.

2. The death rate for white males 15 to 24 years of age increased from 6.6 in 1950 to 21.0 in 1979.
3. The death rates for white males 45 years and older have declined since 1950.
4. The age-adjusted death rate for white males has remained stable for the past 30 years.

The group of questions below consist of lettered choices followed by several numbered items. For each numbered item select the one lettered choice with which it is most closely associated. Each lettered choice may be used once, more than once, or not at all.

Between 1950 and 1980, there have been significant changes in the rates of certain notifiable diseases among the United States population. For each disease, select the trend in number of cases per 100,000 population.

A. Measles (rubeola)
B. Pertussis
C. Tuberculosis
D. Syphilis
E. Gonorrhea
12.   192.5 – 443.3
13.   80.5 – 12.3
14.   79.8 –   0.8
15.   146.0 – 30.4
16.   211.0 –   6.0

Answers to Multiple Choice Questions

1 B	**2** A	**3** C	**4** C	**5** E
6 B	**7** E	**8** A	**9** B	**10** A
11 E	**12** E	**13** C	**14** B	**15** D
16 A				

Psychiatry

Igor Grant

INFORMATION GATHERING: HISTORY AND MENTAL STATUS EXAMINATION

Despite considerable research on possible biochemical correlates of behavioral disorders, there are still no generally agreed upon biochemical or physiologic markers which are specific for particular psychopathologic entities. Therefore, we must rely almost exclusively on careful gathering of indirect (history) and direct (mental status observations) data to arrive at a proper diagnosis, and thereby, a treatment plan. The validity (i.e., whether our data correspond to something demonstrably real) and reliability (i.e., whether other suitably trained observers will arrive at the same conclusions) of our information will be influenced by our notions of normality, our biases, and our techniques of gathering information.

Normality

Offer and Sabshin (1966) describe four ideas of normality. Normality as health means that we call phenomena normal so long as they are not manifestly pathologic. Thus, a person who does not have an obvious illness would be called normal, even though he might have minor problems such as dental caries or acne. Normality as ideal suggests that we do not call somebody normal unless they are essentially perfect. In psychiatry, this would mean that virtually no one is normal, since we all have the potential to improve. Normality as average takes a statistical viewpoint. A person whose behavior falls within a certain confidence interval from the mean would be considered normal. Normality as process introduces a time frame into the definition. For example, being tearful and sad might be "normal" in the context of a grief reaction following death of a loved one; it would not be normal if there were no reasonable explanation for that behavior.

Bias

Bias refers to the influence of preconceptions on the manner in which we send, receive, and interpret information. Since our diagnosis and treatment depend heavily on data gathered at an interview, we must always be aware of the potential distorting effect of bias. Examples of bias include appearance bias (i.e., how we are influenced by the appearance of another person, including their dress and grooming), contextual bias (means we might be misled by the behavior of a person in a clinic or office setting, which might be very different than behavior at home), and psychiatric interview bias (people who know that they are coming to a psychiatric interview might selectively present "psychiatric complaints" to the exclusion of other, potentially important medical problems). Identification bias means that we are more likely to identify with patients similar in age and social position to ourselves. While such identification can help in establishing rapport, it also presents the risk that the interviewer might not question certain behaviors based on values he shares with the patient.

Techniques of Gathering Information

THE PSYCHIATRIC INTERVIEW

In a properly conducted interview two or more people exchange meaningful information in an atmosphere of relative trust and comfort.

Role of the Interviewer. The interviewer is a participant observer interacting actively with the patient while at the same time observing and thinking about the patient's behavior, his own behavior, and the interaction between himself and the patient.

Phases of the Interview. The interview has three phases. The task of the initial phase is to achieve rapport which means establishing an emotional resonance, or getting on the same "wavelength." The initial phase also gives the patient an opportunity to state his concerns in his own words, and gives the interviewer a chance to introduce some operational ground rules. The body of the interview is that phase in which most of the data are gathered. To be successful, the therapist must be empathetic (i.e., show that he or she has an insightful understanding of the thoughts and feelings of the patient). Generally, the first part of the interview tends to be more open-ended, which means the patient is allowed to tell his story in his own words. As the interview progresses, the interviewer imposes more structure so that a complete history can be gathered. The termination phase serves the dual purpose of summarizing and planning for the future, and bringing the patient back "down to earth" after a potentially difficult emotional experience.

HISTORY

History is the data gathered from the patient supplemented by other sources of information, as necessary. When there are questions about the reliability of a patient, then relatives and other informants need to be consulted. The history consists of identifying information (name, age, sex, ethnic background, etc.), the problem statement (the patient's major concerns in his own words, if possible), the history of present illness (recent evolution of the problem or problems), past psychiatric history (more remote information on the present difficulty as well as other potentially unrelated psychiatric episodes), medical history (with specific emphasis on changes in health or medication regimens which might be contributing to the patient's disorder), personal history (family history, personal developmental history, occupation, social history, sexual and marital history, financial status, present life situation, and plans for the future), and alcohol/drug use history.

MENTAL STATUS EXAMINATION

The mental status examination (MSE) consists of direct observations made during the interview, and recorded in written form. The mental status write-up is generally organized as follows.

Attitude and General Behavior. This includes the patient's dress, posture, facial expression, attitude, and motor activity. Some of the specific phenomena include: psychomotor retardation, indicating a paucity of body movement and general physical slowing; catatonic phenomena, which consist of posturing, waxy flexibility (modest resistance to attempts at passive limb motion), and mutism. Very occasionally there may be catatonic excitement (i.e., wild hyperkinetic state). Extrapyramidal phenomena can also be noted here. These neuroleptic induced symptoms include dystonia (prolonged spasm of muscle groups, especially neck muscles), parkinsonism (slowed body movements, rigidity to passive movement of limbs, masklike face, tremor of hands and feet most prominent at rest, shuffling gait, excessive salivation), and akathisia, a form of motor restlessness.

Stream of Mental Activity. Here we observe organization and rate of speech. Organizational difficulties can be seen as circumstantiality (inclusion of excessive detail and peripheral information before eventually reaching the point), tangentiality (gradually moving off the point into irrelevant ideas, and never coming back), loose association (loss of connections between ideas), word salad (illogical sequencing of words), and verbigeration (groups of sounds with no logical meaning).

Regarding rate of speech, speeding up of thoughts is generally called push of speech, suggesting the patient has so many ideas that he has difficulty expressing them all quickly enough. Flight of ideas is an extreme form of acceleration such that ideas might be expressed only partially before moving on to the next. Flight of ideas and loose associations are distinguished by definite acceleration in flight of ideas, and relative preservation of logical connections between ideas in flight of ideas. Interruption of thought is termed blocking; it is as though an idea is inexplicably lost and the patient is left momentarily speechless. Thought progression can also be slowed in severe depressions, to the extent that total lack of speech (mutism) can occur.

Emotional Reaction. By affect we mean the minute to minute change in emotional reactivity; by mood we refer to long-term emotional tone. The major qualitative dimensions of mood and affect are sadness/depression *v* happiness/elation; anger/hostility *v* affection/love; and fear/anxiety versus tranquillity/courage.

Lability refers to rapid shifts in affect; flatness connotes an inappropriate unchangingness with poverty of emotional response.

We can also assess a person's emotional response to the environment. For example, nonreactive refers to affect (usually profoundly depressed) which does not respond to cues from the surroundings. Inappropriate affect describes idiosyncratic emotional response which is out of keeping with the social context (e.g., giggling and making jokes at the sight of a fatal accident).

Mental Content and Special Preoccupations

Perceptual disorders can be grouped as distortions, illusions, and hallucinations. Distortions are imprecise perceptions. For example, objects may appear to be smaller (micropsia) or larger (macropsia) than they really are. Illusions represent premature or improper labeling of aspects of the perceptual field. For example, a pattern on wallpaper might be misinterpreted as crawling insects; or a curtain as a robed figure. Hallucinations are perceptions occurring in the absence of adequate sensory stimulation. They can occur in any sensory modality, but schizophrenics generally report voices, whereas patients with delirium generally see visions. Hallucinations can also involve experiencing foul tastes, bad odors, and strange sensations in the skin or other parts of the body.

A common ideational disturbance among psychotic patients is the delusion, or false belief. Often such delusions have a paranoid (i.e., pathologically suspicious) flavor, with beliefs that persons, social agencies, or extraterrestrial forces have a malevolent intention toward the person. There can also be delusions of alienation (i.e., of nonownership of thoughts, feelings, or behavior), of control (i.e., one's thoughts, feelings, or behavior being under the direct control of someone or something outside the self), of thought broadcasting (i.e., thoughts audibly "leaking" out of one's mind), of grandeur (beliefs that one has unusual or supernatural powers) and of nihilism (belief that one is utterly without hope). Two other terms that are sometimes used to describe delusions are ideas of reference (i.e., the belief that events which most people would consider to be neutral actually have some special meaning or significance to the patient, for example, special messages from television programs) and ideas of influence (i.e., either a belief that one has special power over another person or event, or that other people or agencies have special power over the patient, this latter usage being comparable to delusions of control).

Nonpsychotic ideas and preoccupations also belong under mental content. These include suicidal ideas, homicidal ideas, hypochondriasis (paying inappropriate attention to normal bodily sensations and attributing disease to these), obsessions (intrusive, unwanted ideas which a person has difficulty dismissing), compulsions (irresistible impulses to do unwanted things), and phobias (irrational fears and avoidance responses associated with various objects and situations).

Dissociations and conversions are also included under mental content. Dissociation refers to the unconsciously operating mental mechanism which splits an aspect of mental information away from its normal associations. Examples of dissociations include selective inattention ("not noticing" an event which one might find disturbing if one were aware of it), hypnotic anesthesia (lack of awareness of an incoming sensation, usually pain), trance states (selective changes in consciousness as in a hypnotic trance), amnesia ("forgetting" of emotionally charged events), fugue (finding oneself in a new location or activity without awareness of how this occurred), pathologic intoxication (outbursts of uncharacteristic violence precipitated by small amounts of alcohol or drugs), somnambulistic trances (waking up, entering a trance state, and acting out emotionally charged material); to be distinguished from sleepwalking, which is a physiologic event occurring during EEG confirmed sleep and consisting of uncoordinated wandering and barely comprehensible mumbling. Other complex dissociations include estrangements (feelings of unreality), derealization (a feeling that an inexplicable change has occurred in one's environment), and depersonalization (a feeling that an inexplicable change has occurred in oneself, for example, feeling that one has stepped outside one's body, seeing a part of one's body detached or somehow transformed). Dissociations of entire sectors of personality have been termed multiple personality.

Sensorium. Here are considered mental functions which are thought to reflect the physical health of the brain.

State of consciousness refers to a general level of alertness and awareness of the surroundings. Terms that describe progressive disturbance of consciousness include confusion (person is generally alert and responsive, but has difficulty thinking clearly, following instructions, or recalling information), obtundation (definite reduction in alertness, confused, disoriented, but able to follow simple commands), stupor (responsive only to painful or vigorous stimulation), and coma (unresponsive to any stimulation). Attention is the process of focusing on meaningful aspects of the phenomenal field. Difficulty in sustaining attention, and excessively broad attentional field with consequent distractability occur in several mental disorders, including schizophrenia, depression, mania, and various organic brain syndromes. Orientation describes accurate awareness of self in environment. Disorientation can be in relation to time, place, person (identity of others), or personal identity. Whereas the first three forms of disorientation tend to occur with organic brain disease, disturbance of personal identity is more often a sign of nonorganic psychopathology, such as the dissociation involved in fugue or multiple personality.

Intelligence is a multifaceted concept which refers to a person's ability to manage information. Crystallized intelligence refers to "overlearned" information such as vocabulary, general fund of knowledge, and simple computational skills. Fluid intelligence connotes ability to manage novel information, to see unusual relationships, and to problem solve. On standard intelligence tests, such as the Wechsler Adult Intelligence Scale (WAIS), crystallized intelligence generally corresponds to the verbal intelligence quotient (VIQ) whereas fluid intelligence tends to be reflected by the performance intelligence quotient (PIQ). With brain diseases, there tends to be a dissociation between crystallized and fluid intelligence, with relative preservation of the former. One aspect of fluid intelligence has been termed abstracting ability, or the ability to group symbols into concepts and to manipulate such concepts in meaningful ways. Failure of abstracting ability is termed concreteness. Perseveration describes an inability to shift flexibly from one idea to another, with a resultant repetition of one or a small group of ideas or symbols.

In accessing language ability, aphasia refers to impairment in spoken and written language. There are many kinds of aphasia, the two most frequently recognized are Wernicke's aphasia in which semantic difficulties dominate (i.e., the patient has difficulty understanding the meaning of words and produces words which are imprecise, incorrect, or frankly nonsensible), and Broca's aphasia, which is primarily a syntactical disorder (i.e., meaning is preserved, but structure and flow of language are altered, grammar suffers, and there is a paucity of language which loses its normal rhythm).

Sound memory requires efficient input of information (learning) and retrieval of previously stored data. Brain disease generally affects both learning and retrieval, although there are now recognized a number of amnestic syndromes which have various patterns of deficit. Memory is often divided into immediate (i.e., repetition of letters or numbers), short-term (i.e., recollection of new material after a few minutes to a few hours), and long-term (i.e., remembering things from a year or more ago). Generally speaking, brain diseases affect short-term memory the most, long-term memory next, and immediate recall the least. Anterograde amnesia refers to a period of defective memory which follows a brain insult. Retrograde amnesia describes memory deficit for a period preceding the insult. Generally speaking, in cases of reversible brain injury, the durations of anterograde and retrograde amnesia are comparable, with the most severe memory deficit occurring in the period immediately surrounding the injury.

Judgement refers to soundness of decision making based on accurate appraisal of self, environment, and their interrelationships. Clinically, this is assessed by understanding how a patient handles work, interpersonal situations, recreation, finances, and plans for the future.

Insight. The sixth and last area of the MSE is termed insight, and refers to the degree of understanding a patient has about his or her difficulties, their cause, and their possible solutions.

DIAGNOSIS

In psychiatry, diagnoses serve several purposes. The most obvious is that they provide the clinician an opportunity to form a conceptual understanding of the patient's symptoms in the context of history and present situation. If a diagnostic scheme is valid and reliable, then such a use of diagnosis should lead to understanding of prognosis and suggest a treatment. Diagnoses are also used as shorthand to facilitate communication among physicians and researchers, and can be helpful in matters of health policy and health economics.

Because the specific causes of most mental disorders are not known, psychiatric diagnosis has attempted to provide diagnostic categories which have clinical utility in terms of predicting outcome or suggesting treatment. The scheme in current use is embodied in the *Diagnostic and Statistical Manual of Mental Disorders,* third edition, of the American Psychiatric Association (1980). The shorthand for this is DSM-III.

DSM-III is a multiaxial system. Axis 1 consists of the major clinical syndromes such as the organic mental disorders, schizophrenia, and the affective disorders. Axis 2 contains the long-standing personality disorders such as antisocial personality and compulsive personality, plus certain specific developmental disorders of childhood and adolescence. Axes 1 and 2, as a group, comprise all of the recognized mental disorders. Axis 3 allows for taking note of associated physical medical disorders; Axis 4 permits the clinician to estimate the role of psychosocial stress in the present symptomotology, while Axis 5 identifies the highest level of adaptive functioning in the past year. For practical purposes, students need to be concerned with Axes 1 and 2 diagnoses (Table 13-1). (Note: this is *not* an exhaustive list — rather is a *complete* listing of *major* categories plus certain subcategories which are of importance.) In the sections which follow, the diagnostic features, prevalence, natural history, and treatment of the major mental disorders will be considered.

AFFECTIVE DISORDERS

The affective disorders are characterized by episodic or relatively long lasting disturbances of mood. The commonest mood disturbance is depression, and the other is mania. Persons who have periodic depressions are termed unipolar; those with both depressive and manic episodes are called bipolar.

Table 13-1. Major Diagnostic Categories from Axes 1 and 2 of DSM-III, with selected illustrative examples from these categories

Disorders usually first evident in infancy, childhood, or adolescence (note: children and adolescents can also be diagnosed from the remaining "Adult" categories, as appropriate: e.g., Schizophrenic or Affective Disorders can apply to children)

Mental retardation
Attention deficit disorder
Conduct disorder
Anxiety disorders of childhood or adolescence
  Separation anxiety disorder
  Overanxious disorder
Other disorders of childhood or adolescence
Eating disorders
  Anorexia nervosa
  Bulimia
Stereotyped movement disorders
  Transient tic disorder
  Tourette's disorder
Other disorders with physical manifestations
  Functional enuresis
Pervasive developmental disorders
  Infantile autism
Specific developmental disorders (Axis 2)
  Developmental reading disorder

Organic mental disorders
  Dementias arising in the senium or presenium
    Primary degenerative dementia
    Multi-infarct dementia
  Substance induced organic mental disorders
  Organic brain syndromes of other cause

Substance use disorders
  Abuse (classified by specific substance)
  Dependence (classified by specific substance)

Schizophrenic disorders
  Disorganized
  Catatonic
  Paranoid
  Undifferentiated
  Residual

Paranoid disorders

Affective disorders
  Major affective disorders
    Bipolar disorder
    Major depression
  Other specific disorders
    Cyclothymic disorder
    Dysthymic disorder
  Atypical affective disorders
    Atypical bipolar disorder
    Atypical depression

Anxiety disorders
  Phobic disorders
  Anxiety states
  Posttraumatic stress disorder

Somatoform disorders
  Somatization disorder
  Conversion disorder
  Psychogenic pain disorder

Hypochondriasis

Dissociative disorders
  Psychogenic amnesia
  Psychogenic fugue
  Multiple personality
  Depersonalization disorder

Psychosexual disorders
  Gender identity disorders
  Paraphilias
  Psychosexual dysfunctions
  Other psychosexual disorders

Factitious disorders

Disorders of impulse control not elsewhere classified

Adjustment disorder

Psychological factors affecting physical condition

Personality disorders (Axis 2)
  Paranoid
  Schizoid
  Schizotypal
  Histrionic
  Narcissistic
  Antisocial
  Borderline
  Avoidant
  Dependent
  Compulsive
  Passive aggressive
  Atypical or mixed

Clinical Aspects of Depression

EMOTIONS

Depressed people feel some combination of sad, blue, gloomy, dejected, worthless, or guilty. Occasionally, anger and irritability are prominent, the so-called hostile depressions. In other cases, anxiety is prominent, "anxious depression." The affect can be nonreactive (i.e., does not change in response to the environment), or restricted at the lower range (i.e., flat).

COGNITIVE DISTURBANCES

Beyond these readily identifiable mood changes, depression can be accompanied by various *cognitive disturbances.* These can include the following:

Attention: The patient may be distractible, preoccupied, have difficulty focusing, and complain of difficulty in concentrating.

Thinking: The organization of thought can be disrupted by intrusion of unwanted pessimistic, guilty, self-deprecatory, or self-destructive thoughts. The flow of thought can be slowed, labored, and can lapse into mutism. The content of thought can be dominated by the "cognitive triad" of depression; a negative view of self, others, and the future. Furthermore, there can be delusions, self-deprecatory, somatic (e.g., parts of the body decaying), and sometimes paranoid. Concept formation can occasionally suffer, especially among elderly depressed persons. Such disturbance in abstracting can be part of "pseudodementia" which describes a dementialike state, usually among elderly depressed persons, which, however, improves with treatment of depression.

Perception: Depressed people can experience illusions involving the dead, and hallucinations of voices expressing deprecatory or nihlistic ideas. Visual, olfactory, gustatory, and other somatic hallucinations are also possible, usually involving themes of worthlessness and decay.

Memory: Depressed people frequently complain of difficulty in remembering. Significant loss of memory, as identified in neuropsychological tests, is uncommon except in the "pseudodementia" syndrome of the elderly. Such defects in learning and memory which are attributable to profound depression recover with alleviation of depression.

MOTIVATION

There is a motivational shift in depression from activity to passivity, independence to dependence, interest and curiosity to apathy, and a wish to live to a wish to die.

SOCIAL FUNCTIONING

Work, family, and recreational life can all suffer. Employed persons become indecisive, unreliable, and ineffective. The family can experience the patient as withdrawn, uninterested, guilt-provoking, or angry. Hobbies and recreation suffer from loss of interest and absorption in inner life.

BIOLOGICAL SYMPTOMS

These include psychomotor retardation, loss of appetite and weight, early morning awakening, loss of energy and sex drive, and, occasionally, restricted consciousness (in profound depressions there is an uncommunicative stuporous state, resembling catatonia).

PHYSIOLOGIC FINDINGS

Sleep. Sleep EEG studies have confirmed that depressed people take longer to fall asleep, spend less time asleep, and have disruptions during sleep. Interestingly,

once a depressed person falls asleep, the latency between sleep onset and first episode of rapid eye movement (REM) sleep is shortened. There is also some evidence that durations of REM periods decrease as the night goes on, a pattern opposite that seen in normals.

Endocrine Changes. About 50 percent of severely depressed persons show increased excretion of cortisol in the urine. This observation led to studies with the dexamethasone suppression test (DST) in affective disorders. Normal people, when given a small amount of dexamethasone, will show a lowered level of plasma cortisol in the following 24 hour period because of down-regulation of the pituitary. Many depressed persons do not show this expected suppression and are called "nonsuppressors." Recent data suggest that about 45 percent of unipolar patients and 85 percent of bipolar (depressed) patients show DST nonsuppression. A related observation is that some patients with affective disorder may have an enhanced ACTH response to CRF (corticotropin releasing factor).

Other, less firmly established endocrinologic abnormalities in depression include reduced growth hormone response to insulin induced hypoglycemia and blunted thyroid stimulating hormone (TSH) response to infusion of thyrotropin releasing hormone (TRH). A metabolite of norephinephrine, 3-methoxy-4-hydroxy phenylethylene glycol (MHPG) has been reported to be excreted in reduced amounts in the urine of depressed patients with bipolar histories.

Clinical Aspects of Mania

The manic state is characterized by increased energy. The accompanying mood can be either optimistic, happy, elated, and jovial; or, the predominant mood can be irritable, angry, and impatient. Mania can be accompanied by cognitive shifts in the direction of suspiciousness and frank paranoia. Under such circumstances hallucinations and delusions can be present. These tend to differ from the delusions and hallucinations of schizophrenic patients by being mood congruent (i.e., the false beliefs, voices, and visions are generally compatible with the patient's grandiose self-assessment). Bizarre delusions such as delusions of control by alien forces are uncommon in mania and are more suggestive of schizophrenia.

The behavior of manics is characterized by hyperactivity, intrusiveness, rapid-fire speech (push of speech), and flight of ideas. Excessive spending and hopeless social overcommitment, including increased sexual behavior, are common. In severe mania, patients often do not have time to eat or sleep, and a state of physical exhaustion can supervene.

Diagnostic Criteria for Affective Disorders

DSM-III provides three major groupings for the affective disorders, but stipulates that a diagnosis of affective disorder should not be made if the mood disturbance is secondary to organic pathology (alcoholism, drugs, delirium, dementias, metabolic-endocrine disorders, neoplasia, infectious diseases, collagen-vascular diseases, and the like). The three principal groups of affective disorders are major affective disorders, other specific affective disorders, and atypical affective disorders.

MAJOR AFFECTIVE DISORDERS

To qualify for a diagnosis of major affective disorder, a patient must experience either a major depressive episode, a manic episode, or both.

Diagnosis of Major Depressive Episode. The following five conditions must be satisfied. (1) A prominent, persistent dysphoric mood (or loss of interest or pleasure). (2) At least four of the following critical symptoms present nearly every day for a period of at least two weeks:

Significant appetite or weight disturbance (decreased or increased)
Insomnia or hypersomnia
Psychomotor agitation or retardation
Loss of interest or pleasure in usual activities
Loss of energy or fatigue
Feelings of worthlessness, self-reproach, or excessive or inappropriate guilt
Difficulty concentrating, slowed thinking, or indecisiveness
Recurrent thoughts of death, suicidal ideation, or suicide attempt

(3) The clinical picture is not dominated by preoccupation with mood-incongruent delusions or hallucinations or by bizarre behavior (mood-incongruent psychotic features are those which are not readily understood as natural extensions of profound depression or mania). (4) The disorder is not superimposed on schizophrenia, schizophreniform disorder, or paranoid disorder. (5) The depressive episode is not due to any organic mental disorder or uncomplicated bereavement.

A major depressive episode with melancholia describes an episode characterized by loss of pleasure in almost all activities, lack of reactivity, and features such as profound or inappropriate guilt, significant anorexia or weight loss, marked retardation or agitation, marked early morning wakening, diurnal variation in mood (worse in the morning), and a definite difference in the quality of the mood which distinguishes it from grief.

Diagnosis of Manic Episode. Here DSM-III also specifies five criteria, which are largely parallel in structure to those of a major depressive episode: (1) Prominent and relatively persistent elevated, expansive, or irritable mood. (2) At least three (or four if mood in #1 is principally irritable) critical symptoms lasting a minimum of a week:

Increase in activity/physical restlessness
Increased talkativeness
Flight of ideas (or subjective experience that thoughts are racing)
Inflated self esteem
Decreased need for sleep
Distractability
Excessive involvement in self-defeating activities such as spending sprees, foolish business investments, sexual indiscretions, reckless driving, and the like

(3) If there is not a clear-cut affective syndrome then there cannot be preoccupation with mood incongruent psychotic features or bizarre behavior. (4) The syndrome is not superimposed on schizophrenia, schizophreniform disorder, or paranoid disorder. (5) The syndrome is not due to any organic mental disorder (e.g., stimulant abuse).

A patient who has either a major depressive episode or a manic episode is classified by DSM-III as having a major affective disorder. If a patient has experienced only a major depressive episode (with no previous history of mania) then the diagnosis is major depression. Major depression can be single (one time only) or recurrent.

Patients who meet the criteria for a manic episode either during the current illness or at some previous time are classified as having a bipolar disorder. If the current episode is major depression, then the diagnosis is bipolar disorder depressed; if the current episode is manic, then bipolar disorder manic; and if the current episode has had both manic and depressive episodes then the diagnosis is bipolar disorder mixed.

OTHER SPECIFIC AFFECTIVE DISORDERS

These disorders are characterized by long-standing disturbances of mood (at least two years duration). If the mood disturbance is intermittent, characterized by highs and lows (which, however, are not of sufficient intensity to qualify for major depressive episode or manic episode), then a diagnosis of cyclothymic disorder is made. If the prominent mood disturbance is one of chronic depression or loss of interest (the depression is also not of sufficient severity to qualify as a major depressive episode) then the diagnosis of dysthymic disorder is met. This condition is synonymous with the older term "depressive neurosis."

ATYPICAL AFFECTIVE DISORDERS

Some patients experience one or more episodes of major depression interspersed with episodes of manic-like symptoms which, however, are not of sufficient intensity to qualify as a manic episode. Such patients are given the diagnosis of atypical bipolar disorder, which is synonymous with the term bipolar II disorder.

Atypical depression is a catchall category for depressions which cannot conveniently be classified in any of the other categories. Examples include a depressive episode in a schizophrenic who has recovered from psychosis (i.e., the depression is not part of a psychotic picture), a person with dysthymic disorder who has some sustained periods of normal mood, and a person who experiences a brief episode of depression which is not of sufficient severity to qualify as a major depressive episode nor is part of either of the specific affective disorders.

Prevalence of Affective Disorders

According to DSM-III, 18–23 percent of adult females and 8–11 percent of adult males have had a depressive episode at some time in their lives. The prevalence of bipolar disorder is considerably lower, approximately 0.6 percent.

Causes of the Affective Disorders

Setting aside secondary affective disorders (i.e., those due to drugs, intoxications, physical illnesses, and other psychiatric illnesses such as schizophrenia or alcoholism), the primary affective disorders are generally thought to be caused by a combination of hereditary predisposition, developmental events, and current life stresses.

GENETICS

Data on inheritability of the affective disorders come from consanguinity studies (examining relatives of affected persons), twin studies (comparing rates in monozygotic and dizygotic twins), and adoptive studies (i.e., offspring of affective disorder parents adopted away

shortly after birth). There is a general convergence of evidence to suggest that a hereditary factor is strongly operative in the major affective disorders. For example, whereas the morbidity risk for bipolar disorder in the general population is about 0.6 percent, it rises to 11.5 percent in a first degree relative of a bipolar proband. The risk for unipolar disorder among first degree relatives of unipolar patients is about 14 percent, and only 2 percent in the general population.

Pairwise rates from pooled data from nine twin studies show that whereas the concordance rate for dizygotic twins is approximately 20 percent, concordance for monozygotic twins is approximately 75 percent. Finally, adoptive studies also show increased rates of unipolar and bipolar affective disorder in adopted away offspring of patients with affective disorder (Schlesser and Altschuler, 1983).

BIOCHEMICAL HYPOTHESES

The manner in which this hereditary predisposition expresses itself is unknown. The catacholamine hypothesis states that there is excess noradrenergic activity in mania and reduced noradrenergic activity in depression. Similarly, it has been speculated that mania and depression are accompanied by increases and decreases in activity of serotonin. Since some of the effective antidepressant drugs principally inhibit reuptake of norepinephrine, and others principally inhibit reuptake of serotonin, some investigators have postulated that there may be two kinds of affective disorders based on specific disturbances in each of these amines. There is also a theory which combines serotonin and norepinephrine effects. In this case it is speculated that the predisposition to affective disorder is characterized by reduced availability of brain serotonin; the development of the specific syndrome (mania or depression) depends either on elevation or reduction of norepinephrine in the context of such a serotonin deficiency.

There is also a cholinergic theory of the affective disorders. Here, it is posited that excess activity of acetylcholine at muscarinic brain receptors is accompanied by depression, whereas reduced activity is related to mania.

In summary, there are many interesting biochemical speculations on neurotransmitter abnormalities in the affective disorders; at this time, however, none has sufficient evidence to be firmly established.

PSYCHOLOGICAL THEORIES

From a classical psychodynamic standpoint severe melancholic depressions were thought to be related to pathologic mourning. It was speculated that the self-deprecatory thoughts and self-revilings of such melancholics were in reality expressions of "retroflexed rage" (i.e., anger directed at the image of the lost person or object carried within the person's own mind). More recent psychodynamic theories have focused on collapse of self-esteem in depression.

The cognitive-behavioral view holds that disturbed learning, thinking, and behavior are important in the genesis and maintenance of the affective disorders. For example, Beck has postulated that depressed people have a negative "cognitive triad" (i.e., pessimistic view of self, others, and future) brought into play by aberrant thinking processes involving inappropriate magnification of reverses, minimization of assets, arbitrary jumping to conclusions, and the like. Other behaviorists have argued that depression results from faulty learning (i.e., such faulty learning can produce either a state of "learned helplessness" or an inability to extract "goodies" out of the environment). People who do not know how to get their needs met in positive ways might resort to depressed behavior in order to regain love, gain sympathy, and the like. Still other behaviorists believe that depressed behavior can be reinforced by those around the patient (e.g., by being excessively solicitous and sympathetic, or responding only when a person is sad, such significant others might maintain depressed behavior).

The role of early loss in depression is not well established, although the literature generally suggests that early losses of parents and other adverse early experiences do predispose to later affective disorder.

With respect to timing of onset of affective disorder, life circumstances sometimes predispose. Although major affective disorders apparently can come on without any environmental precipitants (thereby earning the name "endogenous"), in many cases there are environmental precipitants. These are generally losses or other threatening or undesirable life events.

Treatment of the Affective Disorders

There are biological and psychosocial treatments for the affective disorders. Most of the milder forms (e.g., the specific affective disorders, or the atypical affective disorders) tend to be managed with counselling or psychotherapy. The same can be said for affective reactions which are part of adjustment reactions (i.e., responses to major life stresses). Although many forms of psychotherapy have been proposed, the general tendency now is to employ some combination of cognitive-behavioral strategies which focus on pessimistic thinking, teach more satisfactory appraisals of self and circumstances, and encourage adaptive behaviors.

PSYCHOPHARMACOLOGIC TREATMENT

The more severe affective disorders generally require psychopharmacologic treatment, sometimes coupled with hospitalization and/or electroconvulsive therapy (ECT).

Three major groups of drugs have antidepressant properties. These are the tricyclic/tetracyclic compounds; the monoamine oxidase inhibitors (MAOI), and lithium. The latter seems to be primarily effective in depression which is part of a bipolar disorder, and may be most useful in preventing recurrences of depression rather than as an acute treatment. Examples of tricyclic drugs include imipramine (Tofranil), amitriptyline (Elavil), desipramine (Norpramin, Pertofrane), and doxepin (Sinequan). Norpramin is primarily an inhibitor of norepinephrine reuptake; amitriptyline of serotonin; while imipramine and doxepin have both properties. Although some have speculated that specific kinds of depressions might be particularly responsive to one or the other reuptake inhibitor, there is not conclusive research on this. Furthermore, since the reuptake inhibition is not a prominent feature of chronic therapy, it is believed that some other pharmacologic mechanism must be responsible for efficacy. For example, long-term antidepressant treatment usually decreases β-adrenergic and serotonin type II receptor binding in animal studies. The tricyclics, certain of the newer nontricyclic antidepressants (e.g., iprindole, trazadone, bupropion), the MAOIs, and ECT all appear to share this property.

Dose, Duration of Treatment, and Side Effects. For cases of moderate to severe depression in healthy adults, the usual starting dose of a tricyclic is 75 mg per day escalating over a period of a week or more to a maximum of 150–300 mg daily. A typical daily dose for an adult is 200 mg. The tricyclics require 2 to 4 weeks to exert their action, and maximum benefit is generally achieved at 4 to 6 weeks. There are no hard and fast rules about discontinuing treatment. Most therapists will continue treatment for 3 to 9 months, with gradual decrease of the drug after that time, assuming a stable response.

The principal side effects of the tricyclic antidepressants are anticholinergic. In this regard, amitriptyline has the most prominent anticholinergic properties, and desipramine the least. The anticholinergic side effects include dilated pupils, blurred vision, dry mouth, tachycardia, constipation, urinary retention, and, in severe cases, a delirium termed the "central anticholinergic syndrome." The latter, an atropinelike psychosis, is characterized by confusion, dry mouth, racing heart rate, mild blood pressure elevation, dry skin, amnesia, and occasionally hallucinations and delusions accompanied by agitation. The specific treatment is the cholino-mimetic drug, physostigmine.

The tricyclics are also membrane stabilizers. This accounts for their quinidinelike effect on the heart. They can precipitate complete heart block under certain circumstances.

Monoamine Oxidase Inhibitors. Although these were the first of the effective antidepressants to be discovered, they are generally not used as front-line drugs in the treatment of major affective disorders. However, patients who have failed tricyclics sometimes do respond to MAOI. They can be useful in treatment of atypical depressions and dysthymic disorder. The MAOI can also be useful in panic attacks. The MAOI can produce many of the same side effects as the tricyclics. Additionally, patients must be warned not to eat foods which are rich in the naturally occurring amine tyramine, since a severe hypertensive crisis can be produced by this amine in the context of reduced MAO activity.

Lithium Carbonate. The principal use for lithium is as an antimanic agent. As was mentioned, there is some evidence for its efficacy in treating some forms of depression in a bipolar disorder, and, more specifically, in reducing the likelihood of future episodes of depression.

In treating mania, patients are generally begun on a dose of approximately 900 mg per day, with increases up to approximately 1,500 mg per day. The therapeutic plasma level of lithium is in the range of 0.8 to 1.2 mEq/L although some patients respond at levels as low as 0.5 mEq/L and others require levels as much as 1.8 mEq/L. Levels of 2 mEq/L are generally accompanied by toxic signs and symptoms, and fatalities occur at 2.5 mEq/L. Response of manic symptoms should become apparent after 5 to 10 days. Often, to control severe mania in the short-term, neuroleptic drugs (such as chlorpromazine) are used adjunctively.

Early signs of lithium toxicity include tremor, polyuria, polydipsia, gastrointestinal upset, and sometimes sedation. More severe signs of toxicity include ataxia, somnolence, and obtundation. High doses can lead to cardiovascular collapse. Patients treated with lithium occasionally develop skin rash and acne. A nontoxic goiter occurs in a minority of patients; in most instances this is not accompanied by clinical hypothyroidism. Cases of interstitial fibrosis of the kidney have been reported, but this is not firmly established.

How long to treat with lithium is not clearly established. Some investigators have advocated very long-term treatment since relapses are clearly less frequent in treated patients. Others have feared that there could be long-term deleterious effects on the thyroid, kidneys, and other organ systems; such authorities would recommend discontinuation of therapy after the patient has remained asymptomatic for a year or so.

Prognosis of the Affective Disorders

With modern treatment, patients with bipolar disorder can be expected to have productive lives, although some relapses are likely. Lithium therapy has reduced the number and severity of relapses, but is unlikely to eliminate these completely. The same can be said for treatment of major depression (i.e., combinations of psychopharmacology and specific psychotherapy show promise of returning depressed people relatively quickly to productive living). It is not clear how successful such treatments are in eliminating or markedly reducing the chance of relapse. The prognosis of the specific affective disorders (cyclothymia and dysthymia) and the atypical disorders is unclear.

Suicide occurs more frequently in people with affective disorders. It is estimated that approximately 15 percent of persons with bipolar disorder will commit suicide.

SCHIZOPHRENIA

Schizophrenia is a syndrome associated with multiple symptoms in the biological, psychological, and social spheres, leading to a deterioration in a person's level of functioning. The key features usually include a typical cognitive disorder and marked disturbance in interpersonal relationships.

Related Concepts

PSYCHOSIS

Schizophrenics are often termed psychotic. Psychosis means a break with reality. Schizophrenia has been called a "functional psychosis" on the basis that no clear-cut organic brain pathology has yet been reliably identified. Schizophrenics are *not* always psychotic, although DSM-III states that psychotic features must be present at some point in the course of the disorder, in order to make the diagnosis.

SCHIZOID PERSONALITY

Schizoid personality refers to a long-standing personality disorder characterized by an incapacity to form meaningful social relationships, an insensitivity to the feelings of others, and a distant or aloof response to warm feelings from others. Put another way, the schizoid person shares with the schizophrenic some of the interpersonal incapacities without having a typical cognitive disturbance.

SCHIZOTYPAL PERSONALITY

On the other hand, schizotypical personality describes a person with cognitive disturbance, but adequate interpersonal capacities. The cognitive disturbance can include strange beliefs, imprecise and fuzzy thinking, and ideas of reference, but these are generally not of the severity found in schizophrenia. Thus, schizotypals can be seen as having a mild form of some of the cognitive difficulties of schizophrenics without their interpersonal incapacities or deteriorating course.

BORDERLINE PRSONALITY

Borderline personality describes a long-standing instability in interpersonal relationships and in the control of mood, motivations, and identity. Borderlines experience impulsive and potentially damaging behavior, and marked shifts in mood that cause their relationships to fluctuate from intense attachment to intense anger and rejection.

PARANOID PERSONALITY

Paranoid personality, another life-long pattern, is characterized by chronic suspiciousness or jealousy. Such people tend to be very sensitive to what they consider to be slights or criticism, and they tend to blame others for their difficulties. There are no delusions or hallucinations.

It will be seen that the above four personality disturbances have some features in common with schizophrenia. The difference is that these are relatively stable, enduring life-long patterns of adaptation, they do not deteriorate into schizophrenia in most instances, and the symptoms are milder than typically seen in schizophrenia.

Two psychotic disorders are also related. Paranoid disorders are characterized by persistent persecutory or jealous delusions without other cognitive disorders (e.g., loose associations). Schizoaffective disorder has features of both schizophrenia and the affective disorders (i.e., delusions, hallucinations, or loose associations coupled with depression or mania of sufficient intensity to qualify as depressive or manic episodes). Whether schizoaffective disorder is a separate condition from both bipolar disorder and schizophrenia is not clear. Family history studies have shown that some schizoaffectives have relatives with affective disorders, others have relatives with schizophrenia, and still others do not have either. Thus, schizoaffective disorder may be a variant of schizophrenia in some instances and a variant of bipolar disorder in others.

Diagnosis of Schizophrenia

DSM-III specifies six criteria for diagnosis of schizophrenia. (1) There must be at least one critical symptom chosen from a list of six possibilities. These critical symptoms include several types of delusions, auditory hallucinations, and thought disorder (incoherence, loose associations, illogicality, poverty of thought); (2) deterioration from a previous level of functioning; (3) duration of symptoms must be at least 6 months; (4) no preexisting depressive or manic syndrome; (5) onset of illness before age 45; and (6) not due to organic mental disorder or mental retardation.

Additionally, DSM-III specifies five subtypes of schizophrenia. These include the disorganized type (frequent incoherence, no systematized delusions, blunted, inappropriate, or silly affect); catatonic type (catatonic phenomena are prominent); paranoid type (delusions of persecution, jealousy, grandiosity); undifferentiated type (does not fit neatly into the first three types, but has prominent delusions, hallucinations, incoherence, or grossly disorganized behavior); and residual type (reserved for persons who have had a history of a schizophrenic episode with prominent psychotic symptoms, but who now are not floridly psychotic, but show some evidence of continued illness such as blunted or inappropriate affect, social withdrawal, or thinking disturbance). It should be noted that these subtypes of schizophrenia are principally diagnostic shorthands; patients diagnosed as one type at one point in their illness might have symptoms of another type at a subsequent relapse.

General Symptoms of Schizophrenia

Schizophrenics experience many symptoms not all of which are covered in the DSM-III criteria. In the cognitive sphere, associational disturbances can incude tangentiality, loose associations, word salad, and verbigeration. Flow of thought can be punctuated by blocking. Abnormal content can include bizarre or persecutory delusions, often with ideas of alienation (i.e., nonowner-ship of mental processes) or control (mental processes under control of an outside agency). Abstracting ability can be impaired (e.g., concrete or peculiar interpretation of proverbs).

Affective disturbances include flat affect or, in some cases, labile or inappropriate affect. Depression is common during the recovery phase from a psychotic episode. Anger and hostility frequently accompany paranoid schizophrenia. Anhedonia (pleasurelessness) has also been described.

An important motivational disturbance is ambivalence. Some schizophrenics have such strong "equal but opposite" feelings about people or situations that they seem paralyzed into inaction.

In the social sphere schizophrenics often behave awkwardly; misreading interpersonal cues. Often they read "too much into" a social situation, or miss the nuances entirely. The onset of schizophrenia is generally accompanied by deterioration in school, work, leisure time activities, and interpersonal relationships. Social withdrawal is common.

Biological Markers of Schizophrenia

Although schizophrenia has been thought of as a "functional" psychosis, many investigators believe that it is fundamentally a biologic disease or set of diseases. Hence, there has been a search for biological markers. Several have shown some promise recently. Disturbances in cerebral structure and function are suggested by (1) the presence of dilated ventricles and cortical atrophy in the brain CT scans of at least some schizophrenics; (2) neuropsychologic deficit suggestive of mild, generalized brain disorder in about half of schizophrenics; (3) EEG and evoked potential abnormalities suggesting left hemispheric abnormalities in some schizophrenics; (4) positron emission tomography evidence for frontal "hypometabolism" in some cases; (5) defects in smooth pursuit eye movements in some cases; and (6) diminished pupillary response to light in some cases. Other biological findings from some studies of schzophrenics include (1) reduced platelet MAO activity in some chronic schizophrenics; (2) elevated serum creatine phsophokinase (CPK) in many acute schizophrenics; (3) presence of antibrain antibodies (IgA) in the cerebrospinal fluid (CSF) of some schizophrenics; and (4) differences in HLA antigens in some schizophrenics. So far none of these laboratory or biological tests has been found to be specific for any particular form of schizophrenia.

Theories of Etiology

GENETICS

Consanguinity studies have shown an increased risk for schizophrenia in first degree relatives of schizophrenic patients. Pooled results from many twin studies suggest that the concordance rate for schizophrenia among monozygotic twins is in the order of 50 percent, while for dizygotic twins it is in the order of 20 percent. Studies of adopted away offspring of schizophrenics indicate a higher incidence of schizophrenia among offspring of affected than nonaffected parents. Thus, there is a moderately strong case for a hereditary component to schizophrenia, though this seems like a less powerful influence than in the case of the major affective disorders.

BIOCHEMICAL THEORIES

The manner in which this hypothesized biological vulnerability expresses itself in the individual patient is not known. The most important hypothesis is the dopamine hypothesis. This states, in effect, that overactivity in mesolimbic dopamine pathways is associated with schizophrenic phenomena. This theory is consistent with the observation that effective antipsychotic (neuroleptic) drugs tend to be potent dopamine antagonists, while dopamine agonists, such as amphetamine, can produce a paranoid schizophrenialike psychosis. One variant of the dopamine theory which attempts to take into account some of the CT scan findings that have been mentioned, suggests that schizophrenics with noraml CT scans are the ones who have the dopamine abnormality (perhaps an increased number of receptors), that they tend to have "positive" symptoms (i.e., hallucinations, delusions), and it is they who are responsive to the dopamine blocking neuroleptic drugs. According to this hypothesis, schizophrenics with CT scan abnormalities probably have brain damage, and not necessarily a dopamine circuit abnormality. This would explain some observations that such patients are less likely to benefit from neuroleptics.

There have been a number of other biological theories for the causation of schizophrenia. For example, it has been suggested that phenethylamine (PEA), a compound structurally related to amphetamine and produced in the metabolism of phenylalanine, might accumulate in schizophrenics because of their lowered levels of MAO. Another theory has suggested endorphin abnormalities. Yet other theories have sought explanations in viral and related immunolgic theories. The transmethylation hypothesis has suggested that there might be abnormal metabolism of serotonin or norepinephrine, resulting in accumulation of compounds with hallucinogenic properties (e.g., serotinin to N,N-dimethyltryptamine).

PSYCHOSOCIAL THEORIES

Psychosocial theories of etiology have focused on disturbances in communication within the families of schizophrenics. For example, it has been suggested that vague and imprecise thinking and idiosyncratic logic are more prevalent among parents of schizophrenics. The existence of "double bind" communication (verbal and nonverbal communications disqualify each other) has been suggested. Among children of schizophrenics, the risk of the children themselves becoming ill seems to increase if the psychotic parent actively involves the child in his belief system.

Although older notions that socioeconomic disadvantage and inner city life were causally related to schizophrenia are now generally rejected, there is evidence that poor prenatal care and adverse obstetrical and perinatal events increase the risk of schizophrenia in genetically predisposed persons.

Prevalence

In the United States and Canada the prevalence of schizophrenia is about 0.5 percent. Low prevalence groups include the Mennonites of North America (0.1 percent) while high risk has been found in parts of Ireland and northern Scandinavia (1 percent). Generally speaking, however, schizophrenia seems to have a roughly similar prevalence in most countries and cultures in which careful epidemiolgic studies have been done.

Natural History

Schizophrenia is typically diagnosed first in young adults (i.e., from late teens to early thirties). Men tend to be diagnosed somewhat earlier than women, although there is no sex related difference in prevalence. There is no typical premorbid personality, although many schizophrenics have been described in their childhood as eccentric, withdrawn, friendless, and lonely. Others have been described as quarrelsome, with severe school adjustment difficulties. The typical case of schizophrenia results in a deterioration from previous level of social functioning with only relative recovery. There tend to be relapses and remissions. A minority of cases proceed to complete recovery (10–25 percent). Another minority deteriorates steadily (10 percent).

Treatment

Most schizophrenics are hospitalized at some point in their lives. Most also receive neuroleptic drug treatment. There is also generally a psychosocial treatment regimen consisting of individual or group supportive counselling and/or more structured arrangements such as day hospital programs. Some patients require semistructured life situations (e.g., "board and care" facilities). Chronic hospitalization is now rare, although repeated hospitalization is frequent.

NEUROLEPTIC (ANTIPSYCHOTIC) AGENTS

The seven chemical categories of drugs with antipsychotic properties, along with the generic name of a typical compound from that class, are provided (Table 13-2). In practice, the most commonly used drugs come from the phenothiazine and butyrophenone categories. The actual choice of drug depends on the familiarity of the

Table 13-2. Classes of Neuroleptic Drugs

	Approximate Equivalent Dose (mg)
Phenothiazines	
Aliphatic	
Chlorpromazine	100
Piperidine	
Thioridazine	100
Piperazine	
Fluphenazine	2
Butryrophenones	
Haloperidol	2
Thioxanthines	
Aliphatic	
Chlorprothixene	65
Piperazine	
Thiothixene	5
Dibenzazepines	
Loxapine	15
Indolones	
Molindone	10
Diphenylbutylpiperidines[a]	
Pimozide	0.5
Rauwolfia alkaloids[b]	
Reserpine	2

[a] Still experimental
[b] Less efficacious than other classes; no longer recommended as an antipsychotic

clinician with particular drugs, the patient's previous favorable experience with a particular drug, the ancillary effects desired, and the side effects experienced. All the neuroleptics have antipsychotic efficacy when given in proper dose. Some neuroleptics are more potent (i.e., fewer milligrams produce the desired effect), but none (except perhaps the rauwolfia compounds, which are less efficacious) is known to have better efficacy. Generally speaking, the low potency compounds such as chlorpromazine and thioridazine have more anticholinergic and antiadrenergic side effects; thereby, producing greater autonomic dysfunction.

Neuroleptics are not equally effective in treating all of the symptoms of schizophrenia. Hallucinations, agitation, and some of the more florid delusions respond best; these are the so-called positive symptoms. "Negative symptoms" (i.e., apathy, withdrawal, poverty of ideation) respond least well. Suspiciousness, chronic paranoid ideas, and social inappropriateness respond at an intermediate level. The general principles of treatment are to give sufficient quantity of drug in the first instance to bring about rapid control of the positive target symptoms. This means that more drug is prescribed at the beginning of therapy than during the maintenance phase later. A particular drug may have to be prescribed for as long as 6 weeks before it is clear that it is ineffective. Much unnecessary drug switching occurs from failure to give a particular compound an adequate trial.

The principle of long-term treatment should be to give the least number of neuroleptic molecules that is necessary to maintain a remission. For some patients this may mean that after a period of months or perhaps years a neuroleptic can be discontinued entirely while the patient is carefully monitored on a regular basis. Drug discontinuation has its risks; 40–50 percent of patients typically will relapse 6 months after abrupt cessation of a neuroleptic on which they had been stabilized.

The neuroleptics have many side effects. These can be grouped as idosyncratic, dose related, and long-term. Idiosyncratic effects are not dose related and are specific allergiclike reactions of a particular patient which disappear if the drug is discontinued. Examples are skin rash, jaundice, and agranulocytosis. Dose related side effects include sedation, dry mouth, low blood pressure, blurred vision (accommodation difficulties), constipation, urinary retention, weight gain, and extrapyramidal symptoms (EPS). All of these symptoms, with the exception of EPS, are more common with the lower potency aliphatic and piperidine neuroleptics. EPS increase in frequency with the potency of the neuroleptic drug. EPS include dystonia, akathisia (purposeless motor restlessness), and parkinsonism (masklike face, reduced blinking, salivation, "pill rolling" tremor, shuffling gait). Since the EPS appear to represent an imbalance in the cholinergic-do-

paminergic tone as a result of dopamine blockade by the neuroleptics, these symptoms can be treated with anticholinergic drugs (e.g., benztropine or procyclidine), or with the dopamine agonist, amantadine. Generally speaking, however, it is preferred to reduce the amount of neuroleptic drug, or switch to one which is less likely to produce EPS than to embark on a chronic course of antiparkinsonian drug treatment. Specifically, "prophylactic" treatment with antiparkinson drugs is no longer favored. Acute dystonic reactions can be treated with parenteral benztropine or diphenhydramine.

Irreversible neuroleptic effects include tardive dyskinesia, pigmentary retinopathy, lenticular deposits, and purplish discoloration of the skin. Of these the first two are the most serious. Tardive dyskinesia includes grimacing and lip smacking as well as an athethoid movement of the limbs. It is a permanent effect for which there is no treatment at present. The best prevention is to use the fewest number of neuroleptic molecules possible during a person's life to control the schizophrenia. Because tardive dyskinesia is thought to represent a dopamine supersensitivity state, neuroleptic drugs can, paradoxically, temporarily relieve the syndrome, whereas antiparkinsonian agents tend to make it worse.

Pigmentary retinopathy has been reported with thioridazine prescribed chronically in doses exceeding 800 mg per day. To prevent this side effect, thioridazine should not be prescribed in doses exceeding 800 mg daily. Lenticular deposits, while visualizable on slit lamp examination, do not impair vision; purple skin discoloration, while unsightly, does not produce any other harmful effects.

Neuroleptic drugs have a wide margin of safety (i.e., very large doses can be consumed over a short period without lethal effect). A rare exception is the neuroleptic malignant syndrome in which high doses of neuroleptics have resulted in hyperthermia, limb rigidity, stupor, coma, dysphagia, tachycardia, labile blood pressure, sweatiness, dyspnea, and incontinence.

Efficacy of Treatment of Schizophrenia

Placebo controlled outcome studies have shown that after 2 years approximately 50 percent of neuroleptic treated patients will relapse. The rate of relapse for placebo treated patients is about 80 percent. There is some evidence that combination of sociotherapy plus neuroleptics produces better results than neuroleptics alone. To be effective, such sociotherapy must be focused on helping patients acquire basic social skills that will allow them to cope more effectively with day-to-day demands of living.

ORGANIC MENTAL CONDITIONS

The organic mental conditions are disturbances of thinking, feeling, and behavior produced by metabolic or physical changes in the brain. DSM-III distinguishes between organic mental syndromes and organic mental disorders. Syndromes are symptom complexes which do not connote any specific disease etiology. In other words, they are used primarily as descriptive entities. Examples of syndromes are delirium, dementia, intoxication, withdrawal, amnestic syndrome, and affective and personality organic syndromes.

The term disorders, on the other hand, connotes a known (or presumed) etiology. Thus, alcohol withdrawal delirium is a specific disorder under the general syndromatic category of delirium. Similarly, dementia is a syndromatic designation while multi-infarct dementia is a specific organic mental disorder.

Among the most prevalent of the organic conditions are the syndromes of delirium, dementia, intoxication, and withdrawal. The former two will be covered in this section; the latter will be described in the section on alcohol and drug abuse. Delirium and dementia have in common global cognitive impairment as a central feature. In some of the other syndromes, cognitive impairment is selective (e.g., principally memory in the amnestic syndromes). In still other syndromes cognitive functioning might be relatively intact, but affective disturbance or personality change may predominate, hence the designations organic affective syndrome or organic personality sydrome.

Delirium

Delirium is synonymous with the older term "acute brain syndrome." The key features are rapid onset of global cognitive impairment characterized by features such as marked perceptual disturbance (vivid visual hallucinations are common), disorientation, impairment of memory, and disorganization of thinking. Clouding of consciousness is a cardinal feature. This decrease in alertness can be accompanied by drowsiness, somnolence, sometimes ranging to stupor, or by bursts of paradoxical agitation, and insomnia. Fluctuations between drowsiness and agitation are common. Reversibility of the syndrome is implied, if the cause is corrected promptly.

ETIOLOGY OF DELIRIUM

Virtually any influence which can broadly affect the physicochemical integrity of the brain can result in delirium. The most common cause is drugs; these include prescribed and "recreational" drugs which have psychotropic properties. Among the prescribed drugs, the worst offenders are those which have central anticholinergic effects. These include the tricyclic antidepressants, aliphatic and piperidine phenothiazines, antihistamines, antiparkinsonian drugs, and other agents with atropinic properties (e.g., certain over-the-counter sleeping pills which contain scopolamine).

Drugs which are capable of altering central monoamines can also produce delirium. The antihypertensive agents are the best example. Drugs with sedative-hypnotic properties can produce delirium both by their intoxicating effects and by inducing withdrawal phenomena. These include hypnotics, minor tranquilizers (e.g., diazepam), and many of the antiepileptic drugs (e.g., phenytoin). All of the "recreational" drugs are capable of producing deliria, the specific characteristics of which are touched on in a later section. The most common offenders ar alcohol, cannabis, cocaine, the sedative-hypnotics, and phencyclidine.

Aside from drugs, common causes of delirium include: (1) systemic metabolic derangements (e.g., hypoxemia, hypoglycemia, electrolyte imbalance, uremia, hepatic encephalopathy, hypo- and hyperthyroidism, and other endocrinopathies). High fever and complex metabolic derangements accompanying major surgery are also common culprits. (2) Trauma; head injuries can produce brain contusions, subarchnoid hemorrhage, and subdural hematoma. (3) Infections, particularly viremias leading to meningoencephalitis. (4) Circulatory-vascular disorders including cerebral arteriosclerosis, arrhythmias, severe hypertension, and collagenvascular disease, and (5) intrinsic brain disease including epilepsy, demyelination, and intrinsic tumors.

INFLUENCES PREDISPOSING TO DELIRIUM

Beyond the strength (dose) of the noxious influence, there may be predisposing factors that make the evolution of delirium more likely. These include age (young children and old adults are more vulnerable), underlying brain damage, sensory deprivation (loss of sight, hearing, or disconnection from natural light-dark cycle), sensory overload (intensive care unit, extreme pain), sleep deprivation, malnutrition, and general poor state of health.

NATURAL HISTORY

Deliria typically have rapid onset (hours to days), and the recovery (assuming successful institution of specific treatment) takes several days to a week. There is generally amnesia surrounding the events of a severe delirium. This memory impairment can encompass hours or days preceding the delirium (retrograde amnesia) as well as some time period following onset of delirium (anterograde amnesia).

TREATMENT

The key is to identify the specific cause and institute specific therapy. In most instances this involves removing of the noxious influence (e.g., treating the infection, correcting the metabolic disturbance). In some instances specific medications are helpful (e.g., physostigmine to reverse central anticholinergic syndrome, or diazepam in the management of alcoholic delirium). If delirium is accompanied by severe psychosis and agitation, neuroleptic drugs can be helpful. Finally, it is important to correct any environmental predisposing influences that can be aggravating the delirium (e.g., pain, sensory deprivation).

Dementia

In contrast to delirium, the global cognitive impairment of dementia tends to evolve gradually. Confusion, clouding of consciousness, and vivid hallucinations are uncommon except in very late stages. Whereas most deliria reverse with specific treatment, most dementias are not curable.

DIAGNOSTIC CRITERIA

DSM-III specifies five diagnostic criteria: (1) a loss of intellectual abilities of sufficient severity to interfere with social or occupational functioning; (2) memory impairment; (3) at least one critical symptom chosen from impairment in abstracting ability, impairment in judgment, other cognitive disturbances such as aphasia, apraxia, or agnosia, and personality change; (4) clear state of consciousness; and (5) either identification of a specific etiologic factor or global cognitive change with no other reasonable explanation.

Dementias are sometimes grouped as "senile" (affecting those 65 and over) and "presenile." Although Alzheimer's disease used to be classified as a presenile dementia, it is now generally accepted that "senile dementia" and Alzheimer's disease are one in the same, and that in some people it presents earlier and in others later. Hence the term, dementia of the Alzheimer type (DAT) is now used for this most common form of dementia.

CLASSIFICATION OF DEMENTIA

Dementia is most commonly diagnosed in people 65 years and older. Among such dementias of old age, 70 percent will be of the Alzheimer type, 20 percent of the multi-infarct type, and the remaining 10 percent will contain innumerable possible causes including late Parkinson's disease, Wernicke-Korsakoff syndrome, chronic subdural hematoma, neurosyphilis, and neolasia. Dementia is extremely rare in people under 50. Huntington's disease, transmissible virus dementias (e.g., Creutzfeld-Jakob disease), chronic sequelae of head injury or infection, and Pick's disease are some possible causes.

It is now generally recognized that there are some slowly reversible dementias. These are disorders which may mimic primary degenerative dementia (a DSM-III term equivalent to dementia of the Alzheimer type), but which can be improved with specific treatment. Examples include chronic infections such as miliary tuberculosis or neurosyphilis, trauma (subdural hematoma), certain metabolic endocrine disorders (especially hypothyroidism and vitamin B_{12} deficiency), normal pressure hydrocephalus, and pseudodementia.

Pseudodementia describes a dementialike picture occurring in an older person who is deeply depressed. The signs and symptoms of depression may be atypical, for example, sadness, suicidal ideas, and psychomotor retardation might not be prominent features. Nevertheless, these are people whose "dementia" improves with antidepressant therapy. Although some authors have suggested that profound affective disturbance alone can produce a dementialike picture in an elderly person, there is increasing evidence that severe depression can markedly worsen a mild underlying organic brain syndrome, and that many cases of pseudodementia represent combinations of affective and organic causation.

DEMENTIA OF THE ALZHEIMER TYPE (DAT)

DAT encompasses what used to be called senile dementia and Alzheimer's disease. About 6 percent of persons over 65 have it. The disorder is slowly progressive with death occurring within a period of 2 to 10 years. The etiology is unknown. First degree relatives of cases have slightly increased morbidity risk. Some cases are compatible with autosomal dominant transmission.

Pathology. The Alzheimer brain is small with thinning of the cortex (especially in the frontoparietal areas) enlargement of sulci, and dilation of ventricles. Microscopically, one observes neuritic (senile) plaques consisting of degenerating neural processes, reactive cells, and amyloid; neurofibrillary degeneration (tangles) within neurons; and granulovacuolar degeneration of the neurons. Congophilic angiopathy (amyloid deposits around smaller cerebral blood vessels) has also been observed in many cases.

NEURORADIOLOGICAL FINDINGS

On brain CT scan one observes dilated ventricles, and widened sulci. Glucose metabolism is noted to be markedly decreased in all brain areas, especially in the frontal cortex on positron emission tomography (PET). Similarly, regional cerebral blood flow (rCBF) is decreased, especially in the frontoparietal areas.

BIOCHEMICAL FINDINGS

Activity of the enzyme cholineacetyltransferase is lowered in many parts of the brain, with reduction in the hippocampus especially prominent. This enzyme is involved in the synthesis of acetylcholine. Since postsynaptic muscarinic cholinergic receptor activity has generally been found to be unchanged, it is assumed that one of the principal biochemical lesions in DAT is a presynaptic cholinergic defect. Other neurotransmitters have also been found variably to be decreased.

TREATMENT

There is no specific treatment, although the findings of a presynaptic cholinergic defect led to trials of acetylcholine precursors (lecithin and choline) and to trials of the anticholinesterase drug, physostigmine. So far the data have been inconclusive, although there is some suggestion of mildly improved memory when lecithin and physostigmine are combined.

Most treatment, therefore, is palliative and supportive. The principles are to relieve aggravating conditions (e.g., superimposed medical problems or drug intoxication; depression), substitute for lost cognitive functions (e.g., reduced reliance on memory or compromised language skills), and to provide support for the family.

ANXIETY DISORDERS

Anxiety Defined

Anxiety is an unpleasant psychological experience colored by fearfulness, foreboding, and a sense of impending doom. Coupled with this intensely unpleasant psychological experience are a variety of physiologic changes reflecting autonomic arousal. These include sweatiness, dry mouth, hyperventilation, tachycardia, tension or trembling, epigastric discomfort, diarrhea, dizziness, and faintness.

Classification of Anxiety Disorders

SECONDARY ANXIETY

As with depression, it is convenient to think of anxiety as being primary or secondary. Secondary anxiety can be a concomitant of another major psychiatric disorder such as affective disorder or schizophrenia, can be induced by certain drugs (e.g., caffeine, amphetamine, cocaine, cannabis), may be part of an abstinence syndrome from physical dependence on alcohol, other central nervous system depressants, or opiates, or may be part of a physical disease (e.g., hyperthyroidism, mitral valve prolapse).

PRIMARY ANXIETY

There are three major groupings of primary anxiety disorders. In the first group, consisting of panic disorder and generalized anxiety disorder the anxiety is experienced directly as the major symptom. In panic disorder the anxiety comes on intermittently, often without warning. The most common symptoms are breathlessness, dizziness, a choking sensation, chest pain, sweatiness, and fears of dying or going crazy. Between attacks a person functions normally unless frequent panic attacks cause him to develop elaborate avoidance patterns (see phobia section). In generalized anxiety disorder the actual symptoms are less dramatic, but persist for months or years. The characteristic features are apprehensive expectation (i.e., a tense, worried state, constantly expecting something bad to happen); motor tension (i.e., muscle aches, inability to relax, shyness, and jitteryness); and autonomic hyperactivity (i.e., sweating, heart pounding, dry mouth, tingling in hands and feet, and upset stomach).

By way of contrast, the phobic disorders, though often predated by panic attacks, consist primarily of fears of various situations, and elaborate mechanisms of avoidance. Agoraphobia is fear of open spaces; social phobia refers to fear of being scrutinized, embarrassed, or humiliated by others; whereas simple phobia describes more circumscribed fear/avoidance reactions such as fear of flying, fear of snakes, fear of heights, etc.

In obsessive compulsive disorder anxiety is linked to frequent experience of undesired, uncontrollable thoughts (obsessions) which are sometimes associated with irresistible urges to engage in certain kinds of behaviors (compulsions). Common obsessions are thoughts of harming someone else, thoughts of becoming contaminated by germs and dirt, and repeated doubts. Common compulsions include hand washing, repeated checking that gas jets are turned off or that doors are locked, counting, and touching parts of the body.

Etiology

The cause of primary anxiety disorders is not understood. Genetic and family studies have been inconclusive. Anxiety can be triggered by life stresses, in which case, if it is relatively short-lived, the term "adjustment disorder with anxiety" is used. The term "posttraumatic stress disorder" has been used to describe reaction to very severe life stresses such as combat, natural disasters, internment in a concentration camp, and the like. Here the severe life stress is followed by a period of withdrawal and apparent emotional numbness to the world around. Later, the individual may experience anxiety, depression, and various autonomic and cognitive symptoms. The latter can include nightmares, intrusive thoughts, "flashbacks," and feelings of guilt.

Prevalence and Natural History

DSM-III states that 2–4 percent of the population has at sometime experienced an anxiety disorder. Panic attacks and generalized anxiety are often self-limiting, with about half of persons experiencing them expected to improve after a period of 5 years. Many phobic disorders improve as well; some, however, become persistent, and can undergo generalization (evolution of simple phobia to the more pervasive agoraphobia). Obsessive compulsive disorders wax and wane in intensity, but tend to be of long duration. The prognosis of severe obsessive compulsive disorder is poor. Posttraumatic stress disorders generally remit spontaneously, although follow-ups of Vietnam era veterans have shown long-term persistence in some patients.

Treatment

Panic disorders respond well to tricyclic antidepressants and MAO inhibitors. Beta blockers (propranolol) and benzodiazepines (e.g., diazepam) have also been used, but these are less effective and have undesirable side effects. In particular, the benzodiazepines can produce tolerance and dependence. Generalized anxiety is best treated with behavior therapy with an emphasis on teaching systematic relaxation. Agoraphobia responds well to systematic desensitization. This technique teaches patients first to achieve a state of calmness through muscle relaxation exercises and then gradually introduces the feared stimulus to him in a graded fashion. Tricyclics and MAOI are helpful in controlling the panic attacks that can accompany agoraphobia, but are probably not useful for the phobic disorder itself. Forced

immersion techniques have also been successful with agoraphobia. This technique attempts to force a maximal confrontation with the feared situation either in imagination (implosion therapy) or through actual confrontation with the feared object (flooding therapy). Social phobia is probably best managed through a combination of teaching relaxation techniques, role modeling, and other more traditional cognitive-behavioral psychotherapeutic strategies. Obsessive compulsive disorder can be very difficult to manage, although there is some evidence that the tricyclic chlorimipramine is relatively effective in controlling obsessions. Thought stopping (the patient or the therapist shout "stop," or make a loud noise by clapping hands, or otherwise produce a distraction whenever the patient reports an obsessive thought) also has been promising.

SUBSTANCE ABUSE DISORDERS

Definition

A substance abuse disorder exists when a person's preoccupation with psychoactive drugs impairs health or psychosocial functioning. Examples of psychosocial impairment are school failure, difficulties at work, marital, family, or other interpersonal difficulty, and trouble with the law. Health difficulties can occur from impairment of perception, judgment, or psychomotor skills during acute intoxication (e.g., automobile accidents, head injury from a fall or from getting into a fight), or can represent an accumulation of chronic toxic effects of long-term use of the drug (e.g., brain damage or cirrhosis from chronic alcohol abuse).

Intoxicaton

Intoxication describes the acute behavioral and physiolgic effects of the substance (Table 13-3).

Overdose

This refers to acute toxicity resulting from accumulation in the body of substantially more drug than is necessary to produce "desired" effects. Examples are convulsions from LSD, severe psychosis from PCP, and respiratory depression or coma from opiate or sedative-hypnotic overdose (*see* Table 13-3).

Dependence

Psychological dependence exists when a person "needs" his drug in order to function at a level he considers to be desirable. Psychological dependence is an

Table 13-3. Substances of Abuse

Drug Class	Intoxication	Overdose	Withdrawal Symptoms	Treatment of Withdrawal	Long Term Adverse Biological Effects
Alcohol	Conviviality, light-heartedness, silliness, emotional lability, sadness, anger, recklessness, cognitive impairment, psychomotor slowing, ataxia, sedation	Somnolence, obtundation stupor, coma, death	Mild include tremor, insomnia. Severe: delirium tremens: convulsions, tremulousness autonomic instability (e.g., fever, sweats, cardiovascular collapse), hallucinations, especially visual and tactile; can be fatal if untreated	Administer a sedative-hypnotic (e.g., diazepam) in sufficient dose to block symptoms, then gradually withdraw. Thiamine for Wernicke's encephalopathy	Dementia, Wernicke-Korsakoff syndrome, chronic hallucinosis, paranoia, cirrhosis, myopathy, various cancers, pancreatitis, ulcer disease, proneness to infection, early death
Sedative-hypnotics Barbiturates (e.g., secobarbital) nonbarbiturate hypnotics (e.g., methqualone glutethimide) Benzodiazepines shorter acting (flunitrazepam, temazepam, aprazolam, triazolam) longer acting (chlordiazepoxide, diazepam, flurazepam)	As for alcohol above, sedation, cognitive inefficiency (e.g., memory difficulty), psychomotor retardation, nystagmus	As for alcohol, respiratory depression a common cause of death	As for alcohol, can be fatal if untreated. Time to develop physiolgic dependence is weeks to months, rather than months to years, as in alcohol. Anxiety, depression, sleep disturbance, irritability, emerging subtly and persisting for weeks	For barbiturates, nonbarbiturate sedative hypnotics, and shorter acting benzodiazepines: Use pentobarbital, phenobarbital, or short acting benzodiazepines in doses sufficient to reverse symptoms then reduce 10 percent per day. For longer acting benzodiazepines: Recommence benzodiazopine and withdraw gradually over weeks	Accidents, fractures, head injuries, neuropsychologic deficit (?), increased likelihood of infections
Opiates Heroin Morphine Propoxyphene	Sedation, euphoria, analgesia, nausea, vomiting, pinpoint pupils, constipation, impotence	Obtundation, stupor, coma, respiratory depression. *Rx* naloxone or other "antagonist"	Craving, piloerection, rhinorrhea, sweating, diarrhea, irritability, aches and pains, sleep disturbance. Despite severe discomfort, withdrawal is not life-threatening	None, if not severe; if severe, administer longer acting opiate (e.g., methadone) to reverse symptoms then withdraw over 7 to 10 days.	Earlier death, neuropsychologic deficit (?), susceptibility to blood borne infection [e.g., hepatitis, acquired immunodeficiency syndrome (AIDS), bacterial endocardatis, syphilis, malaria, septic emboli]
Hallucinogens Indoleamine type LSD Psilocybin	Marked perceptual distortion, hallucinations, detachment, dissociation, passivity, tachycardia, increased temperature, nausea	Psychosis, fever, vomiting, chills, convulsions	None	None	Flashbacks (recurrences of drug experiences) and possibly triggering of schizophrenia in susceptible individual
Phenthylamine type Mescaline STP (or DOM) MDA Nutmeg (TMA) PMA	Mescaline: like LSD Other phenethylamines: perceptual distortions, arousal, hallucinations, sleeplessness, dry mouth, blurred vision	Mescaline: like LSD Other phenethylamines: hyperpyrexia, labored respiration, delirium; central anticholinergic syndrome, convulsions, coma, death	Mescaline: none Others: (?)	None	As for LSD

(cont.)

Table 13-3. Substances of Abuse

Drug Class	Intoxication	Overdose	Withdrawal Symptoms	Treatment of Withdrawal	Long Term Adverse Biological Effects
Central Stimulants	Euphoria, reduced need for sleep or food, increased energy, increased sexuality, improved concentration (in low doses), distractibility (higher doses)	Suspiciousness, paranoia, delusions, hallucinations, especially visual and tactile, irritability, violence, stereotyped behavior, fever, convulsions, cardiovascular collapse, death	Hunger, lethargy, depression, excess sleep	Nonspecific supportive	Microvascular damage (?), increased susceptibility to stroke (?), dyskinesias, ulceration of nasal membranes. For intravenous users, *see* consequences of intravenous opiate use
Cannabis Marihuana Hashish	Highly dependent on mental set and setting, calmness, silliness, time distortion, psychomotor slowing, mild cognitive impairment, dissociation (rare: panic, paranoia, hallucinations), dilation of conjunctival blood vessels, lowered ocular pressure	Nausea and vomiting, arrhythmia in persons with heart disease, headache	Uncertain in humans, possibly insomnia, irritability, fever, and chills, restlessness (after abrupt discontinuation or chronic high dose)	None	Bronchitis, susceptibility to COPD and lung cancer, impaired T-cell immunity, lowered testosterone (?)
Phencyclidine (PCP)	Disorientation, analgesia, dissociation, perceptual distortion, hallucinations, hostility, bizarre posture, outbursts of violence, loose associations, drowsiness, blank stare, sweating, increased heart rate and blood pressure	Psychosis, delirium, uncontrollable violence alternating with catatonia, paranoid delusions, respiratory depression, fever, convulsions, coma, death	None	None	Memory impairment, other neuropsychologic deficits, prolonged anxiety or depression
Volatile substances Toluene containing glue and paint Aldehydes and ketones in glue and solvents	Euphoria, disorientation, cognitive impairment, light headedness, sedation, ataxia, incoordination	Obtundation stupor, convulsions, amnesia	Not known	None	Cerebral atrophy (toluene) Peripheral neuropathy (aldehydes and ketones)

imprecise concept, and, by definition, people diagnosed as having substance abuse disorders must be psychologically dependent on their drug.

Physiologic (physical) dependence exists when a drug has been consumed in sufficient amount and duration to produce adaptive biochemical/physiologic changes in the organism. Abrupt drug withdrawal disequilibrates this physiologic adaptation causing "rebound" symptoms which are generally in the direction opposite to the effects of acute intoxication with the substance in question. The two principal classes of drugs which produce serious withdrawal (abstinence) phenomena are the CNS depressants (alcohol and the sedative-hypnotic drugs) and opiates (heroin, morphine, etc.).

Abstinence (Withdrawal) Syndrome

This describes symptoms consequent on abrupt withdrawal of a drug capable of producing physiologic dependency from an organism that is physiologically dependent. Tremors, convulsions, and hallucinosis are examples (*see* Table 13-3).

Tolerance

Tolerance exists when increasing amounts of a substance are required to produce the same neurobehavioral effects. Tolerance is a necessary precondition to the development of physiolgic dependence, but the opposite is not true: there can be tolerance without physiologic dependence. For example, the hallucinogens produce tolerance rapidly, but there is no physiologic dependence nor abstinence syndrome. Tolerance develops rapidly with constant use of hallucinogens and central stimulants (days) and opiates (days to weeks), more slowly for the sedative-hypnotic drugs (weeks to months), and even more slowly to alcohol (months to years). It is not known whether and to what extent tolerance develops to volatile substances (toluene, aldehydes, and ketones contained in glue and paint), cannabis, or PCP.

Epidemiology and Natural History

There are said to be approximately 10 million alcoholics and half a million other substance abusers in the United States. The majority of abusers are male. The age at first use for most substances is during the teenage years, although abuse of alcohol, cannabis, and volatile substances is occasionally reported in late elementary school. After the middle 20s, persons who have not taken substances recreationally are unlikely to become abusers in later life (abuse of sedative-hypnotics by older adults who have problems with anixety, insomnia, or pain, is an exception to this general rule).

There are many ways to classify the progression of drug use. After a few "experimental" uses, some people go on to more regular "recreational" use, usually dictated by a particular social context (e.g., weekend parties, rock concerts, and the like). Some proportion of such recreational users will then become more regular "needful" users, thereby entering the arena of dependent drug use. Dependent drug use tends to have a waxing and waning course, that is, periods of regular or heavy use will alternate with periods which are relatively or completely drug-free. Even with no specific treatment, some proportion of dependent drug users will spontaneously achieve stable abstinence. This is particularly likely after people reach their 40s.

Etiology

The cause of drug abuse is not known. Although some genetic studies favor a genetic mechanism for alcoholism (see section on alcoholism), similar studies have not been accomplished for other substance abuse. We are still left with the homily that substance abuse requires an addicting drug, a susceptible person, and some mechanism to bring the two together. The nature of "susceptibility" is particularly preplexing. Drug abusers have often been described as immature, unstable, passive-aggressive, and antisocial. Some have been thought to have

attention deficit disorders. Still others are known to have affective disorders. Nevertheless, the fact remains that many persons with personality disorders and other major mental illnesses do not become drug abusers, thus, the specific nature of the causal link remains obscure.

Treatment of Substance Abuse

The specific interventions for overdose and withdrawal are shown in Table 13-3. The management of established substance abuse generally requires specialized facilities and know-how. The first step is detoxicaton. Detoxification means withdrawal of the drug in question. For most drug classes removal of the drug can be done abruptly. For sedative-hypnotics and opiates, gradual detoxification is necessary since severe abstinence phenomena can ensue from abrupt withdrawal.

Substitution maintenance is used in some instances for the treatment of opiate addiction. Here, a long-acting opiate such as methadone or L-alpha acetyl methadol (LAAM) is administered daily or several times a week to maintain a sufficient degree of opiate receptor blockade that use of heroin will not produce a markedly pleasurable effect. Methadone and LAAM are opiate agonists (i.e., they have some morphinelike actions). Another biological approach is to give an opiate which blockades receptors but has few or no agonist (morphine-like) properties. Naltrexone and cyclazocine are examples of such drugs. They have been used with some success with opiate addicts who have first been completely detoxified. Naloxone, a "pure antagonist," is too short-acting for long-term treatment but useful in reversing opiate overdose.

Psychosocial treatments consist of various types of inpatient, residential, and outpatient programs. Inpatient units are generally reserved for assessment and detoxification. Residential treatment units generally stress drug-free existence while acquiring new behavioral skills. A "therapeutic community" model is used stressing openness, confrontation, mutual responsibility, and prohibition against drug use or violence. Although many people do well while they actually live in such therapeutic communities, the long-term outcome is unclear. There are also many types of outpatient and day treatment programs which stress acquisition of new skills, drug-free existence, and, sometimes, vocational retraining.

Occasionally, drug abuse is complicated by some other major mental disorder. In this case, treatment of that disorder must go on concurrently with management of the drug abuse. This may mean prescription of lithium, antidepressants, or antipsychotics, as appropriate.

Alcohol Abuse and Alcoholism

DSM-III distinguishes between alcohol abuse and alcohol dependence. Alcohol abuse is defined as (1) a pattern of pathologic alcohol use (e.g., need for daily use of alcohol, inability to cut down, binges, etc.); (2) impairment in social or occupational functioning due to alcohol use (i.e., troubles with work, the law, or family); and (3) duration of disturbance of at least 1 month. Alcohol dependence requires a pattern of pathologic alcohol use, impairment in social or occupational functioning, *and* signs of either tolerance or withdrawal.

Epidemiology

In the United States approximately 4 percent of the population (about 10 million people) are thought to be alcoholic. Men are so diagnosed more frequently than women. Subgroups at risk include the American Indian and urban ghetto males under age 25. Most alcoholics continue to function with some modicum of social success; only 3–5 percent of alcoholics are the classic "skid row" type. Although the majority of alcoholics abuse only alcohol, a substantial subgroup also abuses other substances, particularly the sedative-hypnotic drugs and marihuana.

Natural History

The first drink is generally in teenage years. "Normal drinkers" tend to consume their maximum amount of alcohol in their early or middle 20s and gradually taper off thereafter. Those destined to become alcoholics apparently do not reach this natural peak in their 20s, but rather continue to escalate into their 30s, peaking in the late 30s or early 40s. As with other drug abuse, alcohol abuse presents with a relapsing and remitting pattern. Many alcoholics become abstinent spontaneously for varying periods of time. Approximately one-third will achieve stable abstinence without treatment.

In terms of negative effects, modest social problems consequent on alcoholism begin in late teen years or in the 20s (e.g., violence, drunk driving, rows with family or friends). More severe social sequelae appear in the 30s (job loss, divorce, loss of driver's license, etc.), while physical health problems begin to appear in the 40s and 50s (gastritis, liver disease, heart disease, neurologic and neuropsychiatric sequelae).

Etiology

The cause of alcoholism is not known, although investigators now commonly divide alcoholism into primary and secondary groups. Secondary refers to alcoholism which follows on some other disorder (e.g., affective disorder, antisocial personality, schizophrenia). Primary alcoholism appears *de novo* without major psychiatric antecedents.

There is increasing evidence for a genetic contribution to primary alcoholism. There is more than a five-fold increase in the risk of alcoholism among the relatives of alcoholics. Twin studies have suggested an increased concordance for extensive alcohol consumption (though not alcoholism per se) among monozygotic *v* dizygotic twins. Adoptive studies indicate that adopted away male offspring of alcoholic parents are at higher risk to become alcoholic than the general population, although the same has not been established for adopted away girls. There is some evidence that sons of alcoholics (who are not themselves alcoholic) may have different neuropsychologic and neurophysiologic response to alcohol than do young men without a family history of alcoholism.

Various psychological and social theories have also been propounded over the years. These will not be reviewed here, since none has received powerful emprical support.

Organic Mental Disorders Associated with Alcohol Abuse and Dependence

DSM-III defines two disorders related to acute ingestion of alcohol. The most common is alcohol intoxication which consists of physiologic, psychological, and behavioral concomitants of ingesting an amount of alcohol sufficient to cause most people to become intoxicated (*see* Table 13-3). On the other hand, alcohol idiosyncratic intoxication is characterized by marked behavioral change (usually to aggressiveness) in response to amounts of alcohol which would not intoxicate the average person. Also termed "pathologic intoxication" this disorder might reflect either an unusual sensitivity to alcohol (e.g., a consequence of brain damage) or might reflect a tendency on the part of some people to dissociate under the influence of alcohol.

There are three principal disorders associated with alcohol withdrawal. Simple alcohol withdrawal consists of tremor, irritability (or anxiety, or depression), autonomic hyperactivity, and gastrointestinal upset, coming on several hours after cessation of a period of drinking and lasting several days or longer. There can also be headache, dry mouth, disturbed sleep, vivid bad dreams, and misperceptions. Consciousness in not clouded.

Alcohol withdrawal delirium is the more severe abstinence syndrome characterized by clouding of consciousness, tremulousness, agitation, autonomic instability, sleeplessness, beginning within a day to as long as a week after cessation or reduction of heavy alcohol consumption. Several convulsions can occur; these generally being early in the course of the delirium. Vivid visual hallucinations can begin on the second or third day of withdrawal. These visions are often frightening, sometimes ridiculous, and may be accompanied by voices and tactile sensations (e.g., of bugs crawling or burrowing in the skin – "formication"). Untreated, this syndrome has a 10–15 percent fatality rate.

Alcohol hallucinosis, the third major withdrawal disorder, consists of vivid auditory hallucinations following abrupt cessation or reduction of prolonged drinking. Usually the voices carry a disturbing or unpleasant content. Although the disorder is typically short-lived (hours to days), it can last weeks to months in a minority of people and become a chronic disability in a few. In the latter case it may be indistinguishable from a schizophrenic disorder.

A number of long-term neuropsychiatric consequences of alcoholism have been identified. The most common is an intermediate duration organic mental disorder characterized by some impairment in memory, abstracting ability, and perceptual-motor skills which reverses slowly over a period of months to years if stable abstinence is maintained. The next most common is alcoholic dementia, varying in severity from subtle but permanent neuropsychologic disturbance to severe dementia mimicking Alzheimer's disease. A less common, but dramatic form of organic mental disorder, is the Wernicke-Korsakoff syndrome (termed alcohol amnestic disorder in DSM-III). The key feature is severe memory loss usually accompanied by an effort to fill in the gaps with fictitious facts (confabulation). Associated features are other neuropsychologic disturbances such as impairment in abstracting ability and disturbed perceptual-motor skills, plus ataxia and peripheral neuropathy.

Other Medical Complications of Alcoholism

Other medical complications include cirrhosis of the liver (in about 50 percent of persons who have been alcoholic for 20 years or longer), cardiomyopathy, peptic ulcer disease, chronic pancreatitis, susceptibility to a variety of infections, including tuberculosis, susceptibility to cancer, and the consequences of various types of accidents. Death from a wide variety of medical causes occurs 10 to 15 years earlier in alcoholics than in the nonalcoholic population. The risks of suicide and accidental death are also increased.

Social Consequences of Alcoholism

Alcoholism also has negative effects on family, offspring, and society. Alcoholism is major factor in divorce, spousal abuse, and child abuse. Alcoholic mothers can give birth to undersized babies some of whom may have the features of fetal alcohol syndrome (i.e., dysmorphism, growth deficiency, and neurologic dysfunction).

The other social costs of alcoholism are increased violence, accidents, and loss of productivity from work. A 1975 study estimated the economic cost at 10 billion dollars annually.

Treatment of Alcoholism

BIOLOGICAL THERAPIES

Biological therapies are effective in management of alcohol withdrawal. Beyond the usual supportive care of assuring adequate hydration, nutrition, and control of infection, the specific therapy of withdrawal rests on adminstering sedative-hypnotic agents which are crossreactive with the depressant effects of alcohol, and then withdrawing these gradually. Diazepam (Valium) is commonly used, although other benzodiazepines are also effective. Benzodiazepines can also be used for brief periods, particularly on inpatient units, to manage anxiety and dysphoria related to the withdrawal state. Longterm prescription is not advised because of the possibility of substituting a benzodiazepine dependence for an alcohol dependence. Lithium and the tricyclic antidepressants are useful in some subgroups of alcoholics who may have an underlying affective disorder. Similarly, neuroleptics are indicated when schizophrenia is present.

Disulfiram (Antabuse) can be administered as a deterrent to drinking. The drug impedes degradation of acetaldehyde, a by-product of the metabolism of alcohol, causing that substance to accumulate in the bloodstream. Acetaldehyde produces nausea, vomiting, hypotension, vasomotor changes, and other unpleasant symptoms. Thus, alcoholics tend not to drink while taking Antabuse in order to avoid such a reaction. Unfortunately, most are clever enough to stop their Antabuse for a few days if they wish to resume drinking.

PSYCHOSOCIAL THERAPIES

Psychosocial therapies include inpatient hospitalization (for diagnosis and initial management), group, individual, and family psychotherapies, and various selfhelp groups. Of the latter, Alcoholics Anonymous has been the most effective, but generally requires an alcoholic to "commit" himself to a new quasireligious thinking pattern. Alcoholics Anonymous also have self-help groups for families (Alanon) and for teenage alcoholics.

Various forms of aversion therapies have been attempted. For example, alcohol intake has been coupled with apomorphine, which produces nausea and vomiting. Alternatively, alcohol intake has been juxtaposed to painful electric shocks. The theory is that through a process of classical conditioning a mental association is formed between drinking and the unpleasant consequence. Aversion therapies have had only limited success.

OTHER AXIS 1 DIAGNOSES OF ADULTHOOD

Dissociative Disorders

These are disorders which involve "disconnection" of aspects of cognition, affect, or behavior. Psychogenic amnesia involves sudden inability to recall important memories, which cannot be explained by ordinary forgetfulness or some organic mental disorder. Psychogenic fugue involves sudden unexpected travel away from one's home or customary place of work with inability to recall one's past. A new identity is assumed. The disturbance is not part of an organic mental disorder. Depersonalization disorder involves a major disturbance in perception of self, to the extent that social or occupational functioning is impaired. Examples include a sense that parts of one's body have somehow undergone a change in shape or size, or that a person somehow feels "mechanical" or "outside of himself." Derealization (a sense that the environment has undergone some inexplicable change) sometimes accompanies.

Multiple personality involves dissociation of entire sectors of thinking-feeling-behavior. Different "personalities" might operate under differing social circumstances. The "personalities" may be wholly or partially unaware of each other's existence.

Psychosexual Disorders

These are divided into disorders of gender identity and paraphilias. Gender identity disorder is also known as transsexualism, which involves a deep discomfort with one's anatomic sex, and a sense that one has somehow been "misassigned" sexually. Transsexuals will generally cross-dress and seek out same sex sexual partners not because of a homosexual preference, but because the transsexual himself has a strong wish to function in the opposite gender. Some transsexuals have been treated successfully with hormonal therapy consistent with their preferred orientation. Surgical treatments have also been undertaken, ranging from cosmetic surgery (e.g., breast augmentations for men or excisions for women) to more major surgery involving attempts to convert the genitalia to the desired morphology. Such "gender reorientation" surgery has proved to be problematic in many cases,

both from a technical and psychological standpoint, hence is now recommended much less frequently than in the 1960s.

The paraphilias are a group of disorders characterized by preoccupation with fantasies, wishes, behaviors, or sexual object choices which are distinctly atypical. Transvestism involves dressing in clothes of the opposite sex to achieve sexual arousal. A minority of transvestites progress to living primarily as "charicature women;" in this instance they may be difficult to distinguish from transsexuals. Generally speaking, however, transvestites do not repudiate their own genitalia the way transsexuals do. Fetishism involves use of inanimate objects to aid in sexual arousal. The object choice extends beyond clothing from the opposite sex (otherwise the term transvestism is more properly used). Exhibitionism involves compulsive display of one's genitalia to unsuspecting strangers. Voyeurism involves achieving sexual excitement by observing other people disrobing, or in sexual activity. In sadomasochism physical or psychological suffering become necessary prerequisites for sexual excitement. A sadist derives gratification from inflicting physical injury or humiliation; a masochist derives pleasure from being so victimized. In extreme cases masochists can suffer severe physical harm and even death. Pedophilia defines persons whose exclusive or preferred sexual activity is with prepubertal children, while zoophilia defines preferences for animals.

DSM-III also defines several psychosexual dysfunctions, which are more properly seen as disturbances of "normal" sexual functioning, rather than profound aberrations. Desire phase disturbances suggest an absence (or inhibition) of ordinary interest in a particular sexual partner, or sexual activity generally. Excitement phase disturbances occur in people who have normal desire, but difficulties in arousal. In men this is manifested by impotence and in women by vaginal nonlubrication, which can lead to pain and vaginismus (muscular contractions constricting the vaginal orifice leading to coital pain). Orgasmic dysfunctions include inability to achieve orgasm in women (primary or secondary anorgasmia, frigidity), and premature or delayed ejaculation in men.

Homosexual behavior is not classified as a disorder in DSM-III, so long as it is "ego syntonic" (i.e., does not cause inner conflict). Ego dystonic homosexuality is reserved for persons who are distraught by their sexual orientation and wish to change it.

Somatoform Disorders

These disorders are characterized by prominent physical complaints whose origin is partly or predominantly psychogenic. Somatization disorder is characterized by multiple physical complaints involving many organ systems and leading to multiple consultations or hospitalizations. The disorder usually begins before age 30, has a chronic course and rarely remits. Somatization disorder is more common in women than in men, although some authors believe that antisocial personality in males expresses the same predisposition that manifests itself as somatization disorder (also known as Briquet's syndrome) in women.

Conversion disorder involves more circumscribed symptoms, usually of a neurologic nature, but lacking an adequate pathophysiologic explanation. Psychological theories of conversion include "primary gain" (anxiety is expressed in physical terms rather than consciously experienced), "secondary gain" (the symptom allows the patient to "escape" a conflict laden situation), and "communication" (the symptom allows the patient to make a statement without having to risk consequences). Conversion disorder tends to have a good prognosis, especially when treated early. Often conversions accompany major physical or mental disorders (e.g., early signs of a neurologic disturbance, or part of an affective disorder).

Psychogenic pain disorder is characterized by persisting complaints of pain for which there is not an adequate pathophysiologic explanation. Sometimes there is, indeed, a physical disorder, but it is the severity of pain and the psychosocial disability which it wreaks which allow classification as a psychiatric disorder. Dependence on sedative-hypnotic drugs and analgesics is a common complication.

Hypochondriasis is a chronic disorder in which patients pay undue attention to normal physiologic events, and ascribe morbid meaning to them. Hypochondriacs generally do not respond to reassurance and explanation and may become severely disabled in social and occupational functioning.

Factitious Disorders and Malingering

Factitious disorders are uncommon conditions characterized by a "mimicking" of psychiatric or physical disorder. Also known as Munchausen's syndrome, patients present with dramatic physical complaints (sometimes complicated by self-induced bleeding, fever, vomiting, etc.) or symptoms resembling a psychotic disorder. Although factitious disorders appear to be under volitional control, the "gain" is unclear, other than the goal of being a patient. In contrast, malingerers, who also exhibit physical or mental symptoms that are volitionally produced, generally have a clearly discernible "gain" in terms of insurance compensation, being excused from work or military service, and the like.

Psychosomatic Disorders

These disorders, which DSM-III entitles "Psychological Factors Affecting Physical Condition," are characterized by the fact that psychological determinants play a role in the causation, pathogenesis, or nonresponse to treatment of a particular physical disease. Diseases which are commonly thought to have psychosomatic components include migraine headache, neurodermatitis, peptic ulcer disease, ulcerative colitis, rheumatoid arthritis, hypertension, hyperthyroidism, and bronchial asthma. Beyond these "classic psychosomatic disorders," virtually any other physical disease can be complicated by psychological factors which may aggravate the physical problem or retard recovery (e.g., depression delaying recovery from myocardial infarction).

Eating Disorders

Although in previous nomenclatures they were considered as part of psychosomatic (psychophysiologic) disorders, two eating disorders are singled out by DSM-III as separate conditions. One is anorexia nervosa, characterized by a morbid fear of fatness, misperception of self as overweight despite being thin, and major weight loss (exceeding 25 percent of original body weight). Anorexia is uncommon among men, and usually has its onset in teen years. Many cases require repeated hospitalization for severe inanition, and a substantial proportion of cases ultimately die of the disorder. Treatment involving combinations of behavior therapy, family therapy, and neuroleptic or antidepressant drugs have had only modest success.

Bulimia consists of episodes of binge eating terminated by intense uncomfortable fullness, sleep, or vomiting, and alternating with efforts to lose weight by restrictive diets, use of cathartics, or vomiting. Bulimics are aware that their eating pattern is abnormal, and tend to feel badly about it. The disorder is more common among women than men, has its onset in teen years, and usually has a chronic remitting and relapsing course. Various forms of psychotherapy have been attempted, but the long-term efficacy is unknown.

Personality Disorders (DSM-III Axis 2)

All of us have a personality which is a shorthand for underscoring that we tend to think, feel, and behave in somewhat predictable ways under various circumstances.

In contrast to these personality traits, which everyone possesses, are the personality disorders which consist of relatively inflexible and maladaptive behavioral repertoires. Personality disorders are sometimes described as "ego syntonic," meaning that they do not cause internal distress in their own right (as might, for example, depression), but rather get people in trouble with the world around them. Such social friction can of course lead to personal suffering as a result of rejection, conflicts with others, and the like.

DSM-III suggests that personality disorders can be grouped into three clusters. One cluster is characterized by eccentricity. The disorders include *schizoid, schizotypal,* and *paranoid* personality disorders. These have been discussed earlier under schizophrenia and related concepts.

The second personality cluster is characterized with preoccupation with self, and erratic, impulsive, or dramatic behavior. Persons with *histrionic* personality present in a dramatic attention seeking manner, overreacting to events, and craving activity or excitement. Their interpersonal relationships, although superficially warm and charming, tend to lack depth, and are colored by vanity, manipulativeness, excessive dependency, and irrational emotional outbursts, which sometimes include suicide attempts.

Persons with *narcissistic* personality tend to hold excessively high opinions of themselves, are preoccupied with their self-worth, seek attention and admiration, tend to be indifferent to the feelings of others (or react excessively to "narcissistic injuries"), and may exploit others for their own benefit.

With *antisocial* personality disorder there is a pattern of repeated violation of the rights of others, ususaly leading to troubles with the law. Onset is early in life (DSM-III requires that certain traits be present prior to age 15, for example, misconduct at school, delinquency, persistent lying, substance abuse, theft, vandalism) and there is familial disposition. Antisocial men tend to have antisocial or alcoholic fathers. Antisocial people tend not to have long-term interpersonal relationships, but drift from one sexual partner to another, and usually lack any caring relationship for their offspring. Secondary alcoholism and other substance abuse are common.

The final personality disorder in the second cluster is termed *"borderline."* This disorder was described in the section on schizophrenia and related concepts.

The theme of anxiety runs through the third cluster of personality disorders. The *avoidant* person is excessively sensitive to potential rejection, will not enter into close ties with others unless sure of acceptance, and has a tendency to be withdrawn socially while feeling a need for affection and acceptance. People with *dependent* personality tend to rely on others for major life decisions, and subordinate their needs to those of people on whom they depend. In *passive-aggressive* personality, social and occupational functioning is compromised by tendency to procrastinate, dawdale, "forget," and be inefficient, or stubborn. When faced with demands to perform tasks which they are unable (or unwilling) to do, such people, rather than refusing directly, will employ "passive resistance" (e.g., forgetting, misunderstanding, misfiling, etc.). *Compulsive* personality is characterized by limitation in a person's ability to respond warmly and spontaneously to others, and by a tendency to be rigid, perfectionistic, excessively work oriented, and, sometimes, indecisive.

Having described these personality disorders, I should emphasize that most do not exist in "pure culture," rather, certain personality features might predominate, but these usually are mixed with features of other personality disorders as well. For this reason, the term *"mixed personality disorder"* is commonly used to describe people with severe personality disturbances.

PSYCHOPATHOLOGY OF CHILDHOOD AND EARLY ADOLESCENCE

In contrast to adults, children do not commonly manifest their psychopathology by subjective complaints (i.e., they will not generally complain of feeling depressed, anxious, tense, or conflicted). Rather, their psychopathology will manifest itself in disturbance of adaptive behavior (e.g., difficulties in school, family life, relationships with peers, and troubles with the law).

Childhood psychopathology has many causes, and can express itself as many syndromes. A partial listing of these, based on DSM-III, is provided in Table 13-1. For the purposes of this review it will be useful to consider childhood psychopathology under two general headings (i.e., maladaptations in which a cognitive disorder is primary, or at least significant; and maladaptations which are disturbances of affect, conduct, personality, identity formation, or biological functioning but which do not have a substantial cognitive deficit).

Disorders With Substantial Cognitive Components

SPECIFIC DEVELOPMENTAL DISORDERS

The specific developmental disorders are among the most common dysfunctions of childhood. Ten to twenty percent of elementary school children are estimated to have one or another of these specific disorders, which are sometimes also called "learning disabilities."

Developmental reading disorder is the most common. It is characterized by reading ability which lags significantly below the expected level for the child's age, schooling, and mental age based on achievement tests.

Reading disorders are sometimes caused by sensory deficits (deafness, visual disturbance), but more often involve disturbances in central ability to discriminate heard vowels and consonants, or seen language symbols.

Developmental language disorder means that acquisition of language lags behind. It may involve difficulties in comprehending, expressing, and/or articulating language.

Developmental arithmetic disorder, which often is associated with developmental reading disorder, means that a child's mathematical abilities lag substantially behind what would be expected for the level of schooling and age.

Finally, some children have developmental articulation disorder which involves difficulty pronouncing certain consonant sounds. This, and the other specific developmental disorders are more common in boys than girls.

MENTAL RETARDATION

In mental retardation the cognitive impairment is generalized, such that overall intellectual functioning is significantly substandard. Although to diagnose mental retardation specific subnormalities in IQ are required, the diagnosis should not be made unless there are also accompanying deficits in adaptive behavior (i.e., difficulties in school, work, or general social functioning).

Mental retardation can be subgrouped according to IQ achievement. Mild retardation (IQ 50–70) is the most common, affecting as many as 3 percent of schoolchildren. Generally, no specific etiology is found, and most mildly retarded people are said to have "primary retardation." Mild retardation comprises 80 percent of all retardation. Most people in the mild category are able to achieve independent functioning, although they exhibit scholastic difficulties and may manifest behavioral disorders when stressed by being put into settings with which they cannot cope intellectually.

Moderate retardation (IQ 35–49) is less common, about 12 percent of the retarded group, and consists of individuals who do require supervision in dealing with complexities of society, although they can perform ordinary activities of daily living such as feeding, grooming, and simple tasks which can be broken down into component sequences. Severe retardation (IQ 20–34) affects about 7 percent of the retarded. These individuals can achieve some independence in very basic domestic functions, but require a protected setting. Profound retardation (IQ below 20) occurs in less than 1 percent of retarded people, who usually have very substantial communication difficulties, and require supervision by others.

The category of borderline intellectual functioning comprises persons with IQ between 71 and 84. These are people who may have scholastic difficulties, but generally do not have major behavioral abnormalities except when stressed beyond their intellectual limits.

Causes of Mental Retardation. For the largest group (i.e., mild retardation), the cause is unknown; there being no specific physical or physiologic pathology. More severe forms of mental retardation are produced by natal and prenatal infections (e.g., cytomegalic inclusion body disease, rubella, toxoplasmosis), metabolic disturbances (e.g., fetal alcohol syndrome, hyperbilirubinemia), hypoxia, trauma, inborn errors of metabolism (e.g., Tay-Sachs disease), chromosomal abnormalites (e.g., Down's syndrome), and various disorders in the development of the neuraxis (e.g., microcephaly, congenital hydrocephalus).

As mentioned before, many cases of mental retardation do not have a defined organic etiology. Some of these are classified as having cultural-familial mental retardation. In these instances mental retardation is often found in other blood relatives and may be due either to accumulated environmental factors or hereditary influences. Sensory deprivation and highly disturbed family environment can also produce retardation.

ATTENTION DEFICIT DISORDER

About 3 percent of school children have difficulties in school and social relationships on the basis of disturbances in attending and impulse control. The attentional difficulties can manifest by difficulties in concentrating, inability to finish things, having trouble listening, etc. The impulsiveness manifests itself as difficulty in organizing activity, severe impatience, inability to wait one's turn, or inability to stick to one activity for any length of time. Some children with attention deficit disorder also display hyperactivity (i.e., running and climbing excessively, fidgeting and squirming, excessive restlessness, etc.). Some children with attention deficit disorder (ADD) can also have "soft neurologic signs" and the specific learning disabilities that were described previously.

The etiology is unknown, although some of the specific factors listed for mental retardation can sometimes underlie. Psychophysiologic studies demonstrate that some children with ADD are physiologically "underaroused," whereas others are physiologically "overaroused." Because many have a positive response to central stimulants (e.g., methylphenidate), disturbances in monoamine neurotransmitters have been postulated.

Treatment of ADD consists of specific behavioral interventions, often coupled with special education classes, family therapy, and sometimes, use of psychopharmacologic agents. Of the latter, methylphenidate (Ritalin) appears to have been the most effective.

Prognosis remains uncertain, and depends in part on the severity of the attention and impulse disorders, and presence of specific learning disabilities. Many children with ADD appear to "mature out" by late teenage years. Others may continue to have ADD into adulthood, and there is speculation that some psychopathologies of adulthood (e.g., polysubstance abuse, antisocial behavior) might, in fact, be on the basis of underlying ADD.

INFANTILE AUTISM

Autistic children have profound disturbances in forming relationships, in reality testing, and often have a number of cognitive deficits. The diagnosis requires a generalized unresponsiveness to people, severe disturbance in language development, and bizarre responses to surroundings. Many children have stereotyped and repetitive behavior such as rocking, exhibit inappropriate laughing or giggling, show lack of eye contact, and may engage in self-mutilative acts. Typical age of onset is before 30 months, and the prognosis is poor. The etiology is unknown, although abnormality of serotonin and uric acid metabolism have been suggested for some subgroups.

Behavioral Disorders Without Major Cognitive Components

CONDUCT DISORDERS

As with antisocial personality of adulthood, conduct disorders of children are characterized by chronic violation of the rights of others and disregard of societal norms and rules. These disorders are considered along two major dimensions (i.e., the degree of ability to form meaningful social relationships, and the degree of aggressiveness). The four resultant conduct disorders are summarized (Table 13-4).

The etiology is unknown. Criminal behavior and alcohol or drug abuse in parents is frequent. Beyond the likely role of adverse environment, there is recent evidence of genetic transmission of antisocial behavior. Conduct disorder can also be superimposed on another major disturbance, for example attention deficit disorder.

The prognosis of conduct disorders is not well delineated. It is clear that such children are at risk to develop adult psychopathology, including antisocial personality, affective disorders, and schizophrenia. At the same time, others seem to remit spontaneously and have uneventful adulthoods.

ANXIETY DISORDERS OF CHILDREN AND ADOLESCENTS

Separation anxiety disorder has features in common with the agoraphobia of adults, except that the central fear concerns being separated from a parent or that harm will befall the parent. Most common in elementary school children, the disorder manifests itself by anxiety, often to the point of panic, at the prospect of being separated from a parent (e.g., to go to school, to sleep at someone else's house, when parents go out for the evening or on a trip, etc.). School phobia is a special case of separation anxiety disorder.

The disorder tends to be self-limiting, with symptoms subsiding by adolescence. Specific treatment generally involves explanation and reassurance to the child, play therapy to assist with mastery, and family therapy (or mother-child therapy) in selected cases. Rarely, antidepressants may be indicated.

Overanxious disorder is similar to the generalized anxiety disorder of adults. Rather than being concerned with separation per se, such children have pervasive worry about their adequacy and performance, can be markedly self-conscious, and experience somatic signs of tension and anxiety.

The natural history of overanxious disorder is unclear, although many children seem to "mature" out of it. Some go on to develop adult anxiety disorders. The treatment can involve combinations of individual and family therapy, as described for separation anxiety disorder. Minor tranquilizers or beta blockers are occasionally indicated.

Table 13-4. Conduct Disorders of Children and Adolescents

	Socialized	Undersocialized
Aggressive	Has meaningful peer relationships, sense of loyalty. Attacks on persons and property involve violence or confrontation.	Is a loner, unconcerned with welfare of peers. Attacks on persons and property involve violence or confrontation.
Nonaggressive	Has meaningful peer relationships, sense of loyalty. Covert violation of rules, norms, and rights of others (e.g., drug abuse, running away from home, truancy, lying, cheating, stealing).	Is a loner, unconcerned with welfare of peers. Covert violation of rules, norms, and rights of others (e.g., drug abuse, running away from home, truancy, lying, cheating, stealing).

AFFECTIVE DISORDERS

Affective disorders, particularly depression, are increasingly recognized among children and young adolescents. Sometimes the symptoms are similar to those of adults, but many younger children do not complain specifically of dysphoric mood. Rather, they experience loss of appetite and weight, sleep disturbance, disturbance in mobility, or loss of interest in their usual activities. Withdrawal, irritability, and school difficulties can also be signs of depression. Some children exhibit alternations in levels of energy and activity which are suggestive of a bipolar picture.

Although the etiology is not known, many children with affective disorders have parents with psychopathology, often affective disorder. Sometimes, when a depressed parent is treated to the point that effective parenting is restored, the depressed child also improves. Individual psychotherapy centering on building self-esteem can be helpful. Antidepressants and lithium are occasionally indicated. Suicidal children and adolescents will probably need hospitalization, although this decision needs to be based on the degree of support and understanding available in the family.

SCHIZOPHRENIA

Childhood schizophrenia is probably an early expression of adult schizophrenia. Many of the symptoms are similar (i.e., hallucinations, delusions, bizarre behavior, withdrawal, and catatonic phenomena). The disorder generally does not manifest itself before kindergarten years. Therapy involves use of neuroleptic drugs and combinations of individual and family therapy. Depending on the severity of the presenting symptoms, such children may need to be hospitalized in units specializing in behavior modification of severely disturbed youngsters.

OTHER DISORDERS OF CHILDREN

Eating disorders, including anorexia nervosa and bulimia, can have their onset in late latency or early adolescence. These have been discussed previously.

Children can have a variety of movement disorders. Tics are intermittent involuntary purposeless movements which can involve muscle groups of the face, extremities, or vocal cords. Simple tics are generally transient and require no treatment. Gilles de la Tourette's syndrome is a chronic disorder characterized by multiple tics and vocal utterances. The latter can be simple grunts or obscenities. The disorder has its onset in early adolescence, usually affects boys. Many cases respond to haloperidol.

Children sometimes have disturbance of control of bowel and bladder. Enuresis is bedwetting, and occurs more often in boys than in girls, sometimes is a manifestation of developmental delay, and other times represents "regression" in response to life stress (e.g., birth of a younger sibling). Effective treatments have included explanation, teaching children to retain urine for longer periods of time while awake, nighttime wakenings to empty the bladder, electrical sensors to awake the child whenever the bedwetting occurs, and imipramime in low doses.

Encopresis means passing of normal (or essentially normal) feces into inappropriate places (usually underclothing). Cases with onset after age four generally are psychogenic in nature. In some instances there is no major psychopathology; children simply get into cycles of avoiding passing large painful stools, thereby creating retention and leakage. At other times the encopresis is part of a severely maladaptive family pattern involving coercion, punitiveness, and passive aggression.

Children can experience several sleep disorders, including night terrors, sleepwalking, and nightmares. Night terrors are generally seen in children between 4 and 12 years of age, and are characterized by abrupt awakening with a scream, evidence of severe anxiety, inability to be comforted, disorientation, and perseverative movements. There is autonomic arousal, including pupillary dilation, sweating, piloerection, and rapid heart rate and breathing.

Sleepwalking involves getting up and walking about, often stumbling. Both sleepwalking and night terrors occur during the first half of sleep, during stages 3 and 4 (as measured by the sleep EEG). In the morning, children generally do not recall episodes of either. In contrast, nightmares tend to occur in the last half of the night, and their content can be recollected, at least partially. They occur during stage REM.

TREATMENTS IN PSYCHIATRY

Treatments can be divided into biological, psychological, and social.

Biological Treatments

These include psychopharmacologic agents, electroconvulsive therapy, biofeedback, and psychosurgery. The latter is rarely used, and will not be discussed here. Various psychopharmacologic treatments have been discussed in the appropriate sections earlier.

Electroconvulsive therapy (ECT) can be useful in the management of severe depressions. Generally speaking, 6 to 12 treatments are given. Patients are first provided with a skeletal muscle relaxant followed by a short acting barbiturate so that the experience is not painful nor frightening. A period of confusion follows awakening from ECT. Anterograde and retrograde amnesia surround the treatment. The periods of amnesia become longer with increasing number of treatments, but tend to disappear in the year following cessation of treatment. Some patients continue to complain of memory loss, but objective neuropsychologic tests have yet to uncover unequivocal evidence of such a deficit, particularly when unilateral ECT is used (i.e., application of electrodes to the nondominant hemisphere).

Psychotherapies

Psychotherapies can be classified by theoretical orientation (psychoanalytic, cognitive, behavioral, client centered, etc.), by unit of service (individual, conjoint, family, group), by intent of the therapist (e.g., support or reassurance *v* exploration or attitude change), and by degree of control exerted by the therapist (directive *v* nondirective). Generally speaking, the more disturbed and disorganized a patient is, the more the therapy will focus on support, reassurance, reality testing, and constancy of the relationship; whereas patients who are better integrated will receive treatment that is less directive, requiring more self-exploration and marshalling of personal resources.

Among the theoretical positions, psychodynamic therapy follows the teachings of Freud and his followers. The central notions involve a belief that behavior is motivated, that there is an unconscious, and that patients can be helped to gain insight through a combination of establishing a close relationship with the therapist and free association. The latter means, roughly speaking, letting one's mind wander, out loud, in an uncensored fashion. The special relationship with the therapist involves transference which means that the patient unconsciously assigns to the therapist feelings and attitudes he has had toward important persons in the past. By exploring the vagaries of transference neurosis with the therapist, the patient gradually learns about himself, and undergoes a corrective emotional experience. For heuristic purposes, the mind is often thought of as a tripartite structure, consisting of the id (containing drives and impulses), the superego (containing conscience and ego ideal), and ego (the executive portion of the personality, which is responsible for elaboration of adaptive coping mechanisms, among other things). Psychodynamic therapy and psychoanalysis have been used in many settings, but appear to be most appropriate in the management of neurotic disorders.

Behavior therapies are rooted in one of the three principles of learning, which include operant conditioning, respondent (classical) conditioning, and modeling. Operant principles have been applied with considerable success to the treatment of eating disorders, substance abuse, chronic schizophrenia, and severely disturbed children. Classical conditioning underlies some of the successful treatment of phobias, including systematic relaxation with imagery, implosion, and flooding. Aversion therapy of alcoholism also utilizes respondent conditioning. Modeling is an element of many psychotherapeutic strategies where therapists use role playing, observation of the consequences of a behavior on others, or discussions to exemplify behavioral alternatives.

Cognitive therapy is concerned principally with beliefs and ideas. For example, the cognitive therapy of depression focuses on pessimistic ideas about self, others, and future. The treatment also tries to unearth distortions in cognitive processes (e.g., the tendency to overgeneralize, minimize, make arbitrary inferences, etc.). Several studies indicate that in the treatment of moderate depression cognitive therapy is about as effective as the tricyclic antidepressants.

Conjoint therapies are applicable to married couples in distress. Sexual therapies are a subset of these. Family therapies are indicated for many disorders of children, although individual attention to the child is usually necessary as well. Group therapies are useful for persons who have difficulties in interpersonal relationships. They are also a cost beneficial treatment for persons who share problems in common (e.g., phobia, eating disorder, sexual disorder, or substance abuse). Group treatment can be oriented toward providing support (as in support groups for alcoholism, chronic disease, or parents or spouses of ill persons), or may focus more on behavior modification or insight. Any of the theoretical schools previously discussed can be applied in a group setting.

Social Treatments

Although the less severe psychopathologies are generally managed through some combination of psychotherapy and psychopharmacology, the more severe disorders require hospitalization, day treatment, or some other protected setting. Hospitalization is indicated for psychotic patients who present a danger to themselves or others, or who become so gravely disabled that they can no longer look after themselves. Actively suicidal patients should likewise be hospitalized. Hospitalization is usually indicated for severe disorders such as anorexia nervosa, schizophrenia, profound depression, mania, and dependence on drugs likely to cause an abstinence syndrome. The general purposes of hospitalization are to isolate the patient from environmental stressors, to permit a careful evaluation, and to begin treatment under close observation. Beyond beginning treatments which can be extended to the outpatient setting, well-run hospital units also exert therapeutic benefit by organizing themselves into therapeutic milieus (i.e., patients and staff coordinate their activities in a systematic fashion in the service of getting maximum learning and understanding accomplished by using each other as resources and observers).

Community Psychiatry

The 1960s brought with them a national movement to organize the United States into comprehensive mental healthcare networks, called catchment areas (Community Mental Health Centers Act of 1963). The lynchpin of each catchment area was to be the community mental health center, which was intended to provide inpatient, outpatient, emergency services, community consultation, day care, and research and education. Although community mental health centers do exist in many areas, funding has not been sufficient to actualize the ideals of the 1960s. Consequently, many community mental health centers are delivering rudimentary inpatient and outpatient services, with inadequate staffing and facilities.

PSYCHIATRY AND THE LAW

Psychopathology can alter a person's ability to manage his life in his usual way; furthermore, some psychiatric interventions involve denial of liberty and other rights to patients. For these reasons it is not surprising that a complex relationship has evolved between psychiatry and the law. Some of the key issues have been (1) the circumstances under which patients can be detained, (2) the rights of detained patients, (3) how one judges mental competency, (4) the relationship of insanity to criminal justice, and (5) the requirements and limts of the physician patient relationship.

Involuntary Admission of Patients

Most patients enter psychiatric hospitals voluntarily. Since many inpatient units do not have locked doors, no special procedures are required other than those which would be followed in any ordinary hospital. Units with locked doors generally require a more formal voluntary admission mechanism. This involves signing a document formally requesting admission, and may require notification by the patient in writing before discharge can be effected.

Temporary emergency involuntary admissions can be effected in most jurisdictions by medical personnel upon certifying a person is in imminent danger to himself and others or is "gravely disabled." Usually, such emergency detention is for no more than a few days. Longer involuntary detentions require court proceedings. Again, such longer involuntary hospitalizations (sometimes called commitments) are generally for a period of several weeks to several months with review thereafter.

In the area of involuntary commitment, an important guiding principle was set by the United States Supreme Court in 1975 in the case of O'Connor v Donaldson. The Court found that involuntarily committed persons could not be kept detained indefinitely, simply because they were mentally ill, if they were not dangerous to themselves or others, and capable of surviving safely in the community by themselves.

Right to Receive or Refuse Treatment

Several court cases have now dealt with "right to treatment" and "right to refuse treatment." The former means that patients have a reasonable expectation, while hospitalized, to receive those forms of therapy which are thought to be effective. Right to refuse, on the other hand, means that a patient, even if hospitalized involuntarily, need not be forced to take treatment (this usually means drugs or ECT) unless it can be shown that the patient is "incompetent" to decide on his care. It should be noted that most jurisdictions recognize two types of competence (i.e., competence to care for self; and competence to care for one's estate). Only the person who is judged incompetent to look after his own health can generally be "forced" to accept treatment.

Competency

A court can judge a person to be incompetent either to look after himself or his estate. Although some persons are incompetent on both counts, there can be a dissociation. For example, a person might be very self-destructive (therefore unable to take care of himself), and yet be fully competent to manage his estate. On the other hand, a person might, by virtue of brain damage, be unable to manage his financial affairs, yet be capable of cooking for himself, clothing himself, and generally looking after his house. Generally speaking, to be judged incompetent to look after one's own estate requires a determination that a person is likely to squander his estate unwisely, or be a prey to designing others. When a person is judged incompetent a guardian (called a conservator in some jurisdictions) is appointed to manage those activities which the patient is incompetent to do.

Competency to stand trial is a special determination which requires that a patient be able to understand the nature of the proceedings against him, what his legal situation is, and assist in his own defense.

Criminal Responsibility

There are several legal "tests" which could lead to diminished legal responsibility for a crime.

The oldest of these, the M'Naghten rule states that a person can be found not guilty by reason of insanity if he did not know (1) the nature of his act; (2) the quality (harmfulness) of his act; and (3) that the act was generally considered wrong; provided that this lack of knowledge was the result of a mental disorder.

A broader test has been called the Durham decision. Here a person is not held criminally responsible if his unlawful act was the product of mental disease or mental defect.

Another test, the American Law Institute Standard, states that a person is not responsible for criminal conduct if at the time of such conduct, as a result of mental disease or defect, he lacked substantial capacity either to appreciate the criminality of his act, or to conform his conduct to the requirements of the law.

Different jurisdictions have used different tests of criminal responsibility. Nevertheless, the general theme is that all jurisdictions recognize that under certain circumstances the mentally ill should be treated differently than other persons who commit unlawful acts.

Doctor Patient Relationship

As in other fields of medicine the relationship between psychiatrist and patient constitutes an implied contract. This means that the psychiatrist must possess an acceptable level of competence, deliver at least the standard level of care, and take steps to prevent his patient from being subjected to unreasonable risks based on substandard care. Failure in these areas can provide grounds for malpractice suits. Further, and in common with the rest of medical practice, the psychiatrist is obliged to secure informed consent based on informing his patient of what will be done and what risks will be involved, including side effects or drugs.

The issue of confidentiality is of special concern in psychiatry. Virtually all jurisdictions recognize that the psychiatrist-patient communication should be kept confidential, and that a psychiatrist who divulges such information without the patient's consent is liable to suit. Some jurisdictions regard privileged communication between psychiatrist and patient as a statutory right, which means, in effect, that the patient owns the information, and that it cannot be released without the patient's permission. In jurisdictions where statutory right does not

exist courts can compel psychiatrists to divulge confidential information.

Psychiatrists have certain "social duties" which go beyond the limits of confidentiality. For example some jurisdictions require psychiatrists to warn intended victims of a patient's threats. In virtually all jurisdictions psychiatrists and other physicians are also required to report child abuse.

REFERENCES

American Psychiatric Association: Diagnostic and Statistical Manual of Mental Disorders. APA Press, Washington DC, 1980
    The current classification "Bible" in psychiatry.
Barsky AJ, Klerman GL: Overview: Hypochondriasis, bodily complaints and somatic styles. Am J Psychiatry 140:273, 1983
Cavenar, JO, Brodie HKH: Signs and Symptoms in Psychiatry. JB Lippincott, Philadelphia, 1983
    Multi-author book with excellent scholarly reviews of a number of key topics in psychiatry, including normality, anxiety, obesity, and hypochondriasis.
Goodwin DW, Guze SB: Psychiatric Diagnosis. Oxford University Press, New York, 1984
    Short, practical, heavily nosological and biological in emphasis. Excellent brief review of psychopathology.
Grant I: Behavioral Disorders. Spectrum, New York, 1979
    Single author text for medical students. Good sections on mental status schizophrenia, affective disorders, and drug abuse. Note: published before DSM III, therefore not useful for classification.
Gregory I, Smeltzer DJ: Psychiatry. Little Brown & Co., Boston, 1983
    Joint authored text for medical students. Excellent sections on childhood psychopathology, community psychiatry and forensic psychiatry.
Insanity Defense Work Group. American psychiatric association statement on the insanity defense. Am J Psychiatry 140:681, 1983
Kendler KS: Demography of paranoid psychosis (delusional disorder). Archives Gen Psychiatry 39:890, 1982
Kendler KS: A current perspective on twin studies of schizophrenia. Am J Psychiatry 140:1413, 1983
Kessler KA, Waletzky JP: Clinical use of the antipsychotics. Am J Psychiatry 138: 202, 1981
Lader M: Dependence on benzodiazepines. J Clin Psychiatry 44:121, 1983
Leigh H: Psychiatry in the Practice of Medicine. Addison-Wesley, Menlo Park, 1983
    Multicontributor volume from Yale group. Readable, considerable emphasis on intervention. Parts may be more useful for nurses and medical practitioners.
Lipowski ZJ: Transient cognitive disorders (delirium, acute confusional states) in the elderly. Am J Psychiatry 140:1426, 1983
McAllister TW: Overview: Pseudodementia. Am J Psychiatry 140:528, 1983
Nelson JC, Charney DS: The symptoms of major depressive illness. Am J Psychiatry 138:1, 1981

Schneck MK, Reisberg B, Ferris S: An overview of current concepts of Alzheimer's disease. Am J Psyschiatry 139:165, 1982

Strayhorn JM: Foundations of Clinical Psychiatry. Year Book Medical Publishers, Chicago, 1982

Single author text. Aimed at senior medical students. Excellent coverage of biological psychiatry, pharmacotherapy, and systems of psychotherapy.

Waldinger RJ: Psychiatry for Medical Students. APA Press, Washington DC, 1984

Single author text. Very readable, DSM III — oriented handbook for students on clinical psychiatry rotations. Less depth than Strayhorn.

MULTIPLE CHOICE QUESTIONS

For the following questions select the best answer. Although several answers might be partially correct, you will receive credit only for the best *answer.*

1. Mimicing of a physical or psychiatric disorder without apparent gain, other than the wish to be a patient is:
   A. Conversion disorder
   B. Hypochondriacal disorder
   C. Malingering
   D. Factitious disorder
   E. Somatization disorder

2. DSM-III diagnostic criteria for schizophrenia include all of the following *except:*
   A. A typical cognitive disorder
   B. Deterioration from a previous level of functioning
   C. Duration of symptoms at least 12 months
   D. No preexisting depressive or manic syndrome
   E. Onset before age 45

3. Belief that one does not own one's own thoughts is:
   A. Idea of alienation
   B. Idea of control
   C. Idea of reference
   D. Paranoid idea
   E. Nihilistic idea

4. The polka dot pattern on a curtain beginning to undulate, taking on the appearance of bugs crawling represents:
   A. Hallucination
   B. Dissociation
   C. Illusion
   D. Derealization
   E. Delirium

5. Inclusion of excessive detail into the report of an incident is:
   A. Tangentiality
   B. Loose associations
   C. Flight of ideas
   D. Circumstantiality
   E. Perseveration

6. A psychiatrist concludes, on the basis of a favorable impression gained from an office visit, that a young man is not a drug abuser, despite complaints to the contrast by the boy's parents. The psychiatrist is showing:
   A. Appearance bias
   B. Contextual bias
   C. Psychiatric interview bias
   D. Identification bias
   E. Conceptual bias

7. A young woman has mood swings, but they do not impair her performance. A psychiatrist says that her mental state is "essentially normal:"
   A. Normality as health
   B. Normality as utopia
   C. Normality as average
   D. Normality as ideal
   E. Normality as process

8. Of the following, the most common condition among school-age children is:
   A. Mild mental retardation
   B. Specific developmental disorder
   C. Conduct disorder
   D. Attention deficit disorder
   E. Infantile autism

From the lettered answers select the one which forms the best completion to the statements below. An answer may be used once, more than once, or not at all.

DSM-III

A.	Axis 1
B.	Axis 2
C.	Axis 3
D.	Axis 4
E.	Axis 5

9. Histrionic personality
10. Severe anxiety worsens a patient's congestive heart failure

11. Infantile autism

   Personality disorders:
   A.   Passive aggressive
   B.   Avoidant
   C.   Dependent
   D.   Narcissistic
   E.   Histrionic

12. Excessive sensitivity to possibility of rejection, but feel a need for affection
13. Excessive reliance on others for major life decisions
14. When unwilling to do something will resist by dawdling, procrastination, and inefficiency

   A.   Transsexualism
   B.   Transvestism
   C.   Exhibitionism
   D.   Premature ejaculation
   E.   Homosexuality

15. Not a mental disorder according to DSM-III
16. Cross-dressing to achieve sexual arousal
17. A disturbance of core gender identity

   A.   Panic disorder
   B.   Generalized anxiety disorder
   C.   Social phobia
   D.   Agoraphobia
   E.   Obsessive compulsive disorder

18. Fear of being contaminated by germs, frequent hand washing
19. Thought stopping has shown promise of efficacy
20. Chronic tension, worry, and apprehension

   A.   Schizophrenia, paranoid type
   B.   Schizoaffective disorder
   C.   Schizotypal personality
   D.   Paranoid disorder
   E.   Schizoid personality

21. Onset at age 50 of persistent persecutory or jealous delusions without loose associations, bizarre behavior, or other cognitive disorder
22. Lifelong pattern of eccentricity, aloofness, insensitivity to feelings of others, lack of meaningful interpersonal relationships
23. Flight of ideas, loose associations, delusions of grandeur, thought broadcasting, previous history of depression

For the questions that follow select "A" if "A" only is correct; completions "B" if "B" only is correct; completion "C" if both "A" and "B" are correct; and completion "D" if neither "A" nor "B" is correct

   A.   Anterograde amnesia
   B.   Retrograde amnesia
   C.   Both
   D.   Neither

24. Seen after electroconvulsive therapy
25. Forgetting events that occurred in the two days which followed a head injury

   A.   Validity
   B.   Reliability
   C.   Both
   D.   Neither

26. A 6-year old is diagnosed schizophrenic. At age 18 he is severely disabled by thought disorder and inability to relate to others
27. Neuropsychologic tests indicate an elderly woman is brain damaged. A brain CT scan shows dilated ventricles and widened sulci
28. After viewing a videotape of an interview, two psychiatrists agree that the patient is alcoholic

Each question below contains four suggested answers of which one or more is correct. Choose the answer:

   A   if 1, 2, and 3 are correct
   B   if 1 and 3 are correct
   C   if 2 and 4 are correct
   D   if 4 is correct
   E   if 1, 2, 3, and 4 are correct

29. DSM-III criteria for alcohol dependence include:
   1. Pattern of pathological alcohol use
   2. Impairment in social or occupational functioning
   3. Signs of either tolerance or withdrawal
   4. Duration of disturbance for at least 6 months

30. Opiates which have few or no agonist properties, and which have been used in treatment of heroin addicts:
   1. Methadone
   2. Cyclazocine
   3. LAAM
   4. Naltrexone

31. Concerning substance abuse disorders it is correct to say:
    1. All persons properly diagnosed as having substance abuse disorders are psychologically dependent on their chosen drug
    2. Tolerance precedes physiologic dependence
    3. Withdrawal symptoms can be psychological and physiological
    4. Drugs with the greatest capacity to produce rapid tolerance cause the most severe abstinence syndromes

32. DSM-III diagnostic criteria for dementia include:
    1. Presence of senile plaques and neurofibrillary tangles
    2. Slow progression
    3. Confusion
    4. Memory impairment

33. In elderly people anticholinergic syndrome is commonly associated with use of:
    1. Tricyclics (e.g., imipramine)
    2. Benzodiazepines (e.g., diazepam)
    3. Antiparkinsonian drugs (e.g., benztropine)
    4. Butyrophenones (e.g., haloperidol)

34. Points which help to differentiate delirium from dementia:
    1. Whether behavior worsens at night
    2. Whether consciousness is clouded
    3. Whether memory is impaired
    4. Whether onset was sudden

35. Idiosyncratic (allergiclike) reactions to neuroleptics:
    1. Dystonia
    2. Agranulocytosis
    3. Leuticular deposits
    4. Jaundice

36. Factor(s) dictating choice of neuroleptics for a particular patient diagnosed as schizophrenic are:
    1. Clinician's familiarity with the properties of the drug
    2. Patient's previous therapeutic response to the drug
    3. Whether or not sedation is desired
    4. The side effects a patient has experienced with the drug

37. Recent studies of brain function in schizophrenia have found that many (but not all) cases present with:
    1. Dilated ventricles on brain CT scan
    2. Increased metabolic activity in the frontal lobes (using positron emission scanning)
    3. Defects in smooth pursuit eye movements
    4. EEG and evoked potential abnormalities localized to the right hemisphere

38. A definite genetic predisposition has been demonstrated for:
    1. Affective disorders
    2. Schizophrenia
    3. Primary alcoholism
    4. Dissociative disorder

39. In a person with major depression, which of the following is (are) criteria to make the additional diagnosis of melancholia:
    1. Suicidal ideas
    2. Marked retardation
    3. Difficulty remembering
    4. Inappropriate guilt

40. Endocrine finding(s) in affective disorder are:
    1. Reduced urinary methoxy hydroxy phenylethylene glycol (MHPG)
    2. Nonsuppression of cortisol after dexamethasone administration
    3. Enhanced ACTH response to CRF
    4. Enhanced TSH response to TRH

41. Dissociation:
    1. Fugue
    2. Trance
    3. Psychogenic amnesia
    4. Sleepwalking

42. Parkinsonism involves:
    1. Masklike face
    2. Akathisia
    3. Tremor, more prominent at rest
    4. Dystonia

43. Patients who are detained involuntarily in a psychiatric hospital following a court hearing:
    1. Have the legal right to sign out of the hospital by giving 3 days written notice to the hospital superintendent
    2. Have a legal right to refuse neuroleptic treatment

3. Are legally incompetent to manage their estate while under involuntary detention
4. Must receive regular court review if their detention is to be prolonged

44. A child is irritable, moody, and has academic difficulties in school. This can be a reflection of:
    1. Childhood depression
    2. Attention deficit disorder
    3. Conduct disorder
    4. Specific developmental disorder

Answers to Multiple Choice Questions

1 D	**2** C	**3** A	**4** C	**5** D
6 B	**7** A	**8** B	**9** B	**10** A
11 A	**12** B	**13** C	**14** A	**15** E
16 B	**17** A	**18** E	**19** E	**20** B
21 D	**22** E	**23** B	**24** C	**25** A
26 A	**27** A	**28** B	**29** A	**30** C
31 A	**32** D	**33** B	**34** C	**35** C
36 E	**37** B	**38** A	**39** C	**40** A
41 A	**42** B	**43** C	**44** E	

14

Surgery

William E. DeMuth

WOUND HEALING

Wound healing is the fundamental mechanism which makes surgical therapy possible. Surgical procedures inflict local trauma to which the body responds with a process which depends upon systemic and local factors known as healing. The three types of wound healing are by (1) first intention when separated tissues are approximated and repair occurs without complication, (2) second intention when open wounds are permitted to heal spontaneously, and (3) third intention when the wound is allowed to remain open for days and is then reapproximated secondarily.

Immediately after injury a brief period of local vasoconstriction is followed by vasodilatation and increased permeability of vessels, allowing plasma to enter the area of injury. White cells migrate through the vessel wall, and the wound fills with red cells, white cells, fibrin, and plasma proteins collectively, called an inflammatory exudate. The polymorphonuclear leukocytes engulf debris and cell fragments, and within a few days monocytes invade to perform this function. The presence of foreign material or necrotic tissue prolongs this process, which may be shortened by surgical débridement. The basal cells of the epidermis start to migrate across the defect by rapid mitotic division, with the new cells moving across a scaffolding of fibrin strands. In time, the surface cells keratinize and the skin covering becomes visible. On the second or third day fibroblasts appear in the wound depths, and by 10 days the wound is highly cellular with fibroblasts dominating. About 5 days after injury collagen fibers appear, proliferate, and are asso-

ciated with invasion by capillaries. By 6 or 8 weeks the fibroblasts are markedly reduced in number, collagen fiber bundles predominate, capillaries are marked reduced, and the scar is the result.

Highly specialized tissues such as the brain and kidney do not regenerate but develop simple scar tissue at the site of injury. Bone and tendon do have regenerative capacity so that as the wound heals the normal functional state is restored.

Systemic factors which affect wound healing are diabetes, blood dyscrasias, or deficiency states such as ascorbic acid, protein, or lysine deficits which are essential for collagen synthesis. Hypoproteinemia fosters poor healing as well. More important are local factors such as crushed tissue, foreign materials, inadequate hemostasis, and bacterial contamination, all of which delay healing and predispose to wound complications. Corticosteroids and heparin retard healing only if given before and during the initial injury, but not postoperatively.

At about the third day after injury, cells in the wound start synthesizing glycosaminoglycans. Hyaluronic acid is the initial mucopolysaccharide to be synthesized but chondroitin-4-sulfate and dermatan sulfate gradually become the principal glycosaminoglycans in dermal wounds. Collagen fibers seem to vary in size and orientation depending upon the types and concentrations of different glycosaminoglycans. Collagen is the major structural protein produced. It is insoluble, aggregates as long fibers, and becomes progressively stronger in the maturation process. New collagen deposition reaches a maximum between 2 and 4 weeks after injury but remains elevated for months. Collagenases, which also destroy collagen, are present and this turnover may explain changes in scar shapes over time.

The development of wound strength varies greatly depending upon the tissue involved. Strength progresses for a year or more. Muscle and tendon wounds gain strength more slowly than skin. Strength increase seems to occur as a result of an architectural rearrangement of collagen fibers and an increase in the density of intermolecular covalent bonding.

Complications of wounds depend upon several factors, some which are avoidable. In the surgical wound hematoma formation will retard healing. Careful hemostasis will help avoid this. Bacterial contamination, common to all wounds, may lead to infection. Preoperative and intraoperative antibiotic administration may help prevent infection and are indicated in circumstances where infection may compromise a surgical result. Heart valve and joint replacement or vascular procedures involving prosthetic devices are illustrative of such situations. Most infections in surgical wounds become manifest within a week of operation, and fever, local tenderness, redness, and swelling are suggestive signs. Early invasive infections respond to antibiotics and the presence of pus requires drainage. Wound separation (dehiscence) is usually caused by abdominal distention, wound sepsis, or nutritional deficiencies. Premature suture removal in all wounds will predispose to separation. Abdominal wound dehiscence is usually suggested by the drainage of serosanguinous fluid. Resuture using large full-thickness sutures of the abdominal wall is indicated.

From a clinical point of view, the most effective way to promote healing is by good surgical technique. Local blood supply must be adequate and a reasonable level of nutrition is vital. Intravenous hyperalimentation has added greatly to improved nutrition.

METABOLIC RESPONSE TO INJURY

ACTH and cortisol secretion are increased following injury. This neuroendocrine response is ablated if the injured part is denervated. Loss of circulating blood volume leads to sequestration of fluids in the injured region ("third space"). Sympathetic neural activity increases secretion of epinephrine and norepinephrine from the adrenal, renin from the kidney, and glucagon from the pancreas.

The juxtaglomerular apparatus of the renal afferent arterioles secrete more renin after most injuries as a result of sympathetic stimulation, decreased renal artery perfusion pressure, and decreased delivery of NaCl to the distal tubule. Vasopressin, angiotensin II, and potas-

sium, all increase after injury and tend to suppress renin formation, but usually their influence is overshadowed by the stimulatory ones.

The adrenal cortex responds to injury by an increase in aldosterone secretion which acts in the distal nephron to increase reabsorption of sodium, partly for exchange for potassium and hydrogen. This response makes possible the critical excretion of potassium and acid, which increase greatly following severe trauma.

Antidiuretic hormone (ADH) secretion is increased after most major injuries due to stimulation of the hypothalamus. Hypovolemia produces the same effect. Head injuries sometimes cause excessive increases in ADH called "inappropriate ADH secretion," meaning more than is required for homeostasis. This causes a marked dilutional hyponatremia along with low urine volume with high osmolarity. The opposite effect, diabetes insipidus, may be seen with basilar skull fractures. Diabetes insipidus produces severe dehydration and hypernatremia.

Glucagon, a diabetogenic hormone produced by the pancreas, stimulates glucose production. Insulin secretion is not usually increased in response to trauma. The net effect is a diabetic glucose tolerance curve after injury.

These endocrine changes tend to produce a maintenance of blood pressure, gluconeogenesis, general mobilization of carbohydrate, water and salt conservation, and lipolysis to provide ready energy for the heart and brain.

Protein Metabolism After Trauma

Severe injury or complicated operative procedures result in a marked protein breakdown with a resulting three-fold or more increase in excretion of nitrogen (urea). The cause is not well understood since synthesis and breakdown are known to occur simultaneously. The greatest change in body composition is in muscle, which seems to be sacrificed to maintain the integrity of vital organs. Protein supplies 15 percent or less of caloric requirement. It rarely exceeds 20 percent even with major injury and marked increases of nitrogen excretion. Alanine, the chief amino acid released from muscle, may contribute to the hyperosmolality of trauma.

Fat Metabolism

Fat is the main source of energy in trauma and starvation. The activity of lipolytic enzymes is enhanced to increase hydrolysis of triglycerides to fatty acids and glycerol in the presence of cortisol. Fatty acids are burned in the liver to supply energy for organ use and gluconeogenesis. Glycerol forms a substrate for gluconeogenesis. Liver ketone levels are increased due to the increased fatty acids and glucagon and, in themselves, may be important in supplying energy to the brain.

NUTRITION IN SURGICAL PATIENTS

Surgical diseases and the operations employed to correct them impose nutritional deficits which, in many patients, have led to protracted convalescence or death. The better understanding of nutrition in general and the development of efficient methods of providing nutrition in the patient incapable of sustaining himself by ingestion of food is one of the most significant advances in medicine in this century.

Nutrition depends upon a balance between energy expenditure and protein requirement for maintaining body cell mass (protein), and available protein, fat, and carbohydrate. That portion of the protein intake required for building body cells must be discounted as an energy source. The basal metabolic rate (BMR) may be measured by oxygen consumption at rest. In states such as hyperthyroidism, the BMR may be increased by more than 50 percent. Added to this, minimal metabolic requirement is the energy needed to cover temperature adjustment to a cold environment and that needed to implement the digestive process. The latter is known as the specific dynamic action. Amounts involved in performance of mechanical work (may be very high in the restless, agitated patient) and, to a lesser degree, mental activity must be added to determination of nutritional requirement. Patients with major burns are unable to prevent evaporation of water from the skin and must metabolize rapidly enough to replace heat absorbed by evaporation. Perspiration likewise accounts for heat (energy) losses by evaporation.

If the body does not receive a sufficient number of calories to meet expenditure requirements, the body cells will be broken down to meet the deficit. A small quantity of carbohydrate (glycogen), a large store of fat, and an intermediate quantity of protein (plasma and body tissue, especially muscle) are available. Protein breakdown may be measured by nitrogen loss. Consumption of body protein and fat leads to weight loss.

The quality of ingested nutrients is as important as the quantity. Man is unable to digest cellulose, and therefore a large proportion of the carbohydrate available in nature is unassimilable. He is capable of digesting starch and sugars by virtue of gastrointestinal enzymes which hydrolyze appropriate carbohydrates to glucose, galactose and levulose. Ten amino acids are essential for protein synthesis, and these must be available simulta-

neously. They are generally abundant in meat, fish, milk, and eggs, but some foods such as cereals may be incomplete in this regard. Fat is a major source of calories (9 calorie/g as opposed to 4 calorie/g from proteins and carbohydrates) and is present mostly as triglycerides comprised of three fatty acid molecules combined with one molecule of glycerol. Body protein is "spared" (not broken down) in the presence of adequate carbohydrate and/or fat ingestion, and often because of injury or operation this protein breakdown is a major contributor to the metabolic decline of the patient.

Vitamins must be provided for, especially in substances used for parenteral nutrition. Vitamin K is of special interest to surgeons since maintenance of the prothrombin level depends upon it. It is synthesized by intestinal bacteria, and therefore ingestion is not required. Like vitamins A and D, which also are fat soluble, bile is required for its absorption. When obstructive jaundice is present, the absence of bile in the gastrointestinal tract precludes absorption and vitamin K must be given parenterally. Patients with external gastrointestinal fistulas are also vulnerable.

Water and electrolytes are required to sustain nutrition and are considered in the section on fluids and electrolytes.

Protein depletion is of great concern to surgeons, especially in the treatment of patients with gastrointestinal disease. The reduction in colloid osmotic pressure associated with hypoproteinemia leads to edema, especially when the serum albumin is low. Anastomoses in the gastrointestinal tract fail to function owing to the edema. Wounds tend not to heal and dehiscence may result. Calcification of fractures may be delayed. Hypoproteinemia interferes with the immune response, and infections of wounds, lung, and urinary tract are prone to develop.

The realization of the importance of nitrogen balance stems from the early observation that injured patients lose nitrogen at a markedly increased rate. Most of the nitrogen lost by the body is represented in the nitrogen found in the urine. Since about 16 percent of the protein molecule is nitrogen by weight, multiplying excreted nitrogen in grams by 6.25 will indicate the number of grams of protein participating in metabolism. It was formerly believed that a negative nitrogen balance was inevitable in certain diseases and after injury, but newer methods of supplying nutrients to the patient unable to eat has proven this to be incorrect. For many reasons, the best method for supplying calories and protein is by the enteral route. It is physiologic and cheap. When food ingestion or enteral feeding by a tube placed in the gastrointestinal tract is not possible, intravenous alimentation becomes very beneficial and, indeed, all nutritional requirements may be met at considerable monetary cost.

Parenteral Nutrition

The basic ingredients for intravenous feeding are glucose, essential amino acids, and certain fat emulsions. The usefulness of these substances evolved from work extending back to the turn of the century, but work done in the 1960s by Rhoads and Dudrick showed that a positive nitrogen balance could be maintained in animals and man when infusions into the central nervous system were used. Hyperosmolar solutions could be injected into the circulation without the constant development of thrombophlebitis when peripheral veins were used.

Several basic types of solutions are available. Protein hydrolysates derived from casein or fibrin used in conjunction with 20–25 percent glucose solutions are commonly used. The limiting factors are the volume required to deliver the required caloric content and the hypertoxicity of the solution. One liter of a typical solution contains about 23 g of protein equivalent from casein hydrolysate, 230 g of dextrose (or 23 percent), and appropriate quantities of potassium, magnesium, and vitamins. One liter yields 900 calories and 2.5 g of utilizable nitrogen. Sodium acetate or sodium chloride may be added by the pharmacy if required. The average total intravenous diet usually ranges from 2,500 to 4,000 ml containing about 60–90 g of protein equivalent and 575–900 g of dextrose.

The placement of a central venous line, usually by the subclavian vein route, is required and infusion begun at about a 1.5–2 L/day rate, depending upon the cardiovascular reserve. The usual limiting factor is the quantity of glucose tolerated. The maximum amount of utilizable glucose ranges from 0.5 to 0.85 g/kg/hr. Most patients require less than 5 L per day.

Fat emulsions in 10 percent solutions are available and may be administered through peripheral veins. One liter provides 1,100 calories, and essential fatty acids, absent in standard parenteral solutions, are present.

Indications for parenteral alimentation may be considered primary or supportive. In the primary category, the most frequently utilized is in treatment of enterocutaneous fistulae. More than half such fistulae will close with parenteral therapy alone. Complete rest of the gastrointestinal tract may be desirable in the presence of such disorders as Crohn's disease, and in some healing may be accomplished without resort to operation. It may be lifesaving in the case of multiple organ failure after trauma or operation.

If a patient has only a short segment of small intestine remaining, intermittent hyperalimentation may help to sustain life. A supportive role is found in some patients requiring radiation or chemotherapy and in such conditions as carcinoma of the esophagus where the chance of survival is enhanced by preoperative parenteral alimentation.

COMPLICATIONS OF PARENTERAL NUTRITION

Several potentially serious complications exist. Technical problems usually relate to difficulties with central venous catheter placement. At the time of insertion, brachial plexus or arterial injury, air embolism, pneumothorax, hydrothorax, and thoracic duct injury, are possibilities. Careful attention to detail avoids most of these complications. After catheter insertion, a chest roentgenogram should always be made before fluid is infused. The catheter tip should lie in the superior vena cava and should not be permitted to remain in the heart or out of the thorax.

Metabolic complications include glucose intolerance, the hyperosmolar state, fluid overload, and electrolyte acid-base imbalances. Glucose intolerance is the most frequently encountered. In previously normal patients, glycosuria most adequately assesses tolerance for glucose. If significant glycosuria appears, insulin must be added or the rate of infusion must be slowed. Patients with diabetes, pancreatic or liver disease, and those on corticosteroid therapy are most likely to develop glycosuria. Hypoglycemia occurs in about 10 percent of patients due to hyperinsulinemia which develops in response to a high glucose load. Infusion should be at a relatively constant rate to achieve maximum utilization, and slowing of the infusion may result in severe hypoglycemia with marked symptoms or even death. This dreaded complication is best avoided by close monitoring and a constant infusion pump. Rapid acceleration of the infusion rate results in glycosuria and an osmotic diuresis. Fluid overload is avoided by careful intake-output records. Most patients begin to gain weight within a few days but gains over one-half pound per day usually represent fluid retention. Slowing the infusion and the judicious use of diuretics overcome the problem. Uncontrolled hyperglycemia may lead to the hyperosmolar state, which leads to dehydration of brain cells. The infusion rate must be curtailed, isotonic solutions must be administered, and the hyperglycemia treated with insulin. Electrolyte balance should be managed in the same way as those not on parenteral regimens.

Septic Complications. Most septic complications are those due to contaminated solutions or delivery equipment or delayed catheter sepsis. Careful aseptic technique in preparing solutions and daily changes of infusing equipment best avoid infection except for delayed catheter sepsis, which is minimized by careful care of catheters. The elements of successful parenteral alimentation are the following:

1. Maintenance of sterile conditions during catheter insertion with the placement of an airocclusive dressing.

2. Povidone-iodine ointment used at skin-catheter junction.
3. In-line Millipore filter (no stopcocks).
4. No blood or drugs administered via catheter.
5. Intravenous tubing changed daily, sterile dressings every other day.

Management for a patient with fever without other cause consists of removal of the catheter and culturing of blood. If no growth occurs on blood culture and fever abates, antibiotics are not required; otherwise, they are indicated.

FLUIDS AND ELECTROLYTES IN SURGICAL PATIENTS

Nature attempts to maintain body fluid chemistry by maintaining concentration while varying volume. The amount of solute is the product of the volume multiplied by concentration.

Total body water comprises about 60 percent of body weight in young normal males and 50 percent in females because of a smaller muscle mass. This is comprised of 20 percent in the extracellular space and 30–40 percent in the intracellular compartment. Further divided, the extracellular compartment contains about 5 percent of the fluid as plasma and 15 percent in the interstitial space. Thus, the functional compartments of body fluid in a 70 kg man would be 3,500 cc plasma, 10,500 cc interstitial fluid, and 28,000 cc in the intracellular space.

Cell membranes are completely permeable to water, and therefore the osmotic pressures of the intracellular and extracellular compartments are considered to be equal. There are about 290–310 mosm in each compartment. The cell membrane is semipermeable to various electrolytes and other substances. The interstitial fluid contains about 144 mEq/L of sodium, while the intracellular fluid contains only 10 mEq/L. Conversely, the potassium cation in the intracellular fluid is maintained at 150 mEq/L, while it normally is about 4 mEq/L in the interstitial fluid and plasma.

Disease and trauma (including operations) may result in the sequestration of fluid in the extracellular space as edema and fluid in the gastrointestinal tract, peritoneal, or pleural cavities, the so-called third space. These fluids contribute nothing to homeostasis but must be considered because during recovery they are reinfused into the circulation and may tend to overload the circulation as they become mobilized. Antidiuretic hormone secretion is increased in surgical patients and the injured, leading to fluid retention in the extracellular space with decreased urine production. The kidneys very effectively conserve sodium but do not restrain potassium excretion. Nasogastric suction increases potassium losses.

Fluid requirements are determined by urine output, and losses due to water in expired air and perspiration (insensible loss), gastrointestinal losses in fecal material, vomitus, and gastrointestinal suction material. Each degree of rise in body temperature increases fluid requirements by about 7 percent. About 2,500 ml of fluid is required to provide for a 1,200 ml urine output and insensible losses. Electrolyte replacement must be met by the addition of potassium and sodium, the latter to be given sparingly if renal, hepatic, or heart disease is present. Abnormal losses should be replaced quantitatively, and determination of electrolytes in urine or lost gastrointestinal fluid will help in determining required replacement. When urine output is satisfactory, 20 mEq of potassium/L of solution covers usual losses.

Prolonged gastric suction or vomiting results in protein losses which may be significant and may require albumin administration.

Electrolyte deficits usually occur from gastrointestinal losses due to obstruction or inflammation. Diarrhea, gastric suction or vomiting, or fistula drainage are common causes. Increase in hematocrit and plasma protein and decrease in plasma volume follow. If the loss is gastric juice, metabolic alkalosis is manifested by a decrease in plasma chloride and a rise in bicarbonate concentrations. Normal saline administration corrects the alkalosis. Potassium will be required but should be withheld until urine output is adequate. Losses from the lower intestinal tract produce a reduction in plasma CO_2. One-sixth M $NaHCO_3$ given as one-third of the replacement volume should be administered. Chronic losses from the gastrointestinal tract result in azotemia and low serum sodium with a low urine output. Electrolyte replacement is the first consideration and when acidosis is present, 200–300 cc of hypertonic (2–3 percent) saline and 5 percent $NaHCO_3$ tend to rapidly correct electrolyte disturbances. Replacement of losses should follow and when urine output is established, potassium should be given. Alkalosis usually responds to like volumes of hypertonic saline.

Excess fluid administration and secretion of excessive antidiuretic hormone may result in serious water overload. Patients with renal and cardiac disease are especially prone, and edema, pulmonary edema, and hyponatremia supervene. Treatment is by water restriction. Diuretics are valuable and digitalis, when indicated, may be lifesaving. If pulmonary edema is not present, hypertonic saline infusion will correct the sodium deficit. The measurement of central venous pressure will give an estimate of heart function before sodium is administered.

If insufficient water is administered in intravenous solutions, the plasma becomes hypertonic and plasma sodium increases. Urine volume may be normal or high in an effort to excrete the excess electrolyte load. Adding water to the intravenous solution reduces the solute load and corrects the disorder.

Homeostasis is largely determined by the ability of the organism to ward off acidosis and dehydration. When body functions are unable to maintain acid-base balance, we must correct disorders by therapeutic means.

Respiratory acidosis results from a buildup of CO_2 secondary to decreased alveolar ventilation from any cause. Lung disease, muscle weakness, or depression of the respiratory center are the possible causes. Blood gas determinations reveal an elevated PCO_2 (over 45 mm Hg) and a normal plasma CO_2. The kidneys compensate by conserving bicarbonate and excreting hydrogen in an acid urine. Increasing ventilation provides the only lasting relief. Bicarbonate administration may temporarily reduce the acidosis.

Respiratory alkalosis results when hyperventilation eliminates CO_2 to a degree sufficient to reduce PCO_2 to 30 mm Hg or less. Plasma CO_2 falls and the kidneys respond by excreting bicarbonate and conserving hydrogen ions. Pain, hysteria, and fever are usual causes and reduction in ventilation may be accomplished by narcotics, but the danger of hypoxemia must be guarded against. Ammonium chloride may be given carefully to provide chloride ion to compensate for bicarbonate replacement.

Metabolic acidosis is caused by lactic acidosis (reduced perfusion during shock), renal failure, diabetes, starvation (ketosis), or loss of bicarbonate from intestinal or pancreatic secretions. The PCO_2 is normal but plasma CO_2 content falls below 24. Serum potassium is usually elevated. Hyperventilation occurs in an attempt to lower PCO_2 and the kidneys excrete hydrogen and conserve bicarbonate to produce an acid urine. Treatment consists of overcoming the cause by treatment of shock, diabetes, or the lesion producing gastrointestinal losses. Sodium bicarbonate best corrects the disturbance temporarily with a goal to keeping the plasma bicarbonate above 15 mEq/L.

Metabolic alkalosis is usually caused by loss of gastric juice. Alkalis given to reduce gastric acidity and diuretic administration may be at fault. Plasma chloride and potassium are low. Isotonic saline should be administered and after urine output is adequate, potassium as required should be administered.

PHYSIOLOGIC MONITORING OF THE SURGICAL PATIENT

Sophisticated physiologic monitoring of surgical patients began in the 1950s with the advent of open heart operations. Monitoring devices permit the rapid evaluation of cardiopulmonary function upon which important therapeutic decisions can be made. Monitoring has been shown conclusively to save lives in coronary care units; in other areas of care, the benefits are less obvious. Nonetheless, monitoring is here to stay in surgical practice.

Central venous pressure and cardiac output determinations started to be useful at about the same time as electrodes were developed for the rapid determination of partial pressure of oxygen and carbon dioxide in blood. Indicator dilution techniques were made possible by the invention of the densitometer, thereby permitting continuous recording.

The ideal monitoring system would be noninvasive, would not be psychologically upsetting to the patient, and would not interfere with careful observation of the patient. The recording of data in no way should take the place of careful clinical evaluation. Physiologic processes often generate dynamic potentials, tensions, pressures, and electromagnetic emissions which may be measured. Electrocardiography (ECG), electroencephalography (EEG), and thermography are examples.

RESPIRATORY MONITORING

Recordings of respiratory rate and depth are useful tools and may be all that is required in uncomplicated situations. However, blood gas measurements must be available to safely operate mechanical ventilators so that the levels of ventilation and gas exchange are appropriate for the specific patient. The Clark and Severinghaus electrodes permitted measurement of oxygen and carbon dioxide, respectively. Small quantities of blood can be drawn, heparinized, kept in ice, and stored as long as an hour with accurate results. Gas exchange may be measured by determining the alveolar-arterial oxygen tension gradient $[P(A_aDO_2)]$. Normal man breathing room air will show a $P(A_aDO_2)$ of 10–15 mm Hg owing to ventilation-perfusion imbalance and shunting of blood into the left atrium, and when breathing pure oxygen the gradient ranges between 25 and 65 mm Hg. An increased gradient on breathing 100 percent oxygen is useful in predicting pulmonary edema, atelectasis, pneumonia, etc., and the change is noted before radiologic evidence of lung consolidation appears.

About 2 percent of oxygen consumption is used to power the act of breathing in man. This may be 50 percent in postoperative patients, and since much of this may be saved by mechanical ventilation it would be useful to know how much work is being done just to breathe. Patients with chronic obstructive lung disease (COPD) spend most of their work of breathing on expiration and ventilators are not helpful. Bronchodilators, antibiotics, and physiotherapy are more effective and should be applied before operation where possible.

Table 14-1. Typical Values in Pulmonary Function Tests

Ventilation	
Tidal volume, ml	500
Respiratory/Min	12
Minute Volume, ml/mm	6,000
Respiratory dead space, ml	150
Alveolar Ventilation, ml	4,200
Lung Volumes	
Vital capacity (VC), ml	4,800
Functional residual capacity (FRC), ml	2,400
Residual volume (RV), ml	1,200
Total lung capacity (TLC), ml	6,000
Expiratory rescue volume, ml	1,200
Inspiratory capacity,ml	3,600
RV/TLC × 100, percent	20
Mechanics of Breathing	
FEV_1, percent	85
Maximum breathing capacity (L/min)	125 – 170
Compliance of lungs and thorax, L/cm H_2O	0.1
Airway resistance, cm H_2O/L/se	16
Arterial Blood	
Oxygen tension, torr	100
CO_2 tension, torr	40
O_2 tension (100 percent inhaled O_2), torr	640
Alveolar-arterial PO_2 difference (100 percent inhaled O_2), torr	33
O_2 Saturation hemoglobin, percent	97.1
pH	7.4

Compliance is the change in pressure associated with each cubic centimeter of lung volume and it decreases with lung stiffness or consolidation of the lung. Volume is measured by a transducer which corrects pressure differences across a screen to an electrical signal related to flow. Work per breath is the power expended during the respiratory cycle where power is the flow times the transpulmonary pressure. Sophisticated bedside monitors are available which measure transpulmonary pressure, inspired oxygen concentration, air flow, expired oxygen, and carbon dioxide content. Thereby tidal volume, rate, resistance, oxygen consumption, work, compliance, alveolar-arterial oxygen gradient, carbon dioxide output, and dead space can be calculated. The battery of results provides more accurate information regarding the necessity for mechanical ventilatory assistance than do single tests. In practice, much simpler tests such as tidal volume, vital capacity (VC), and functional residual capacity (FRC), used in conjunction with blood gas determinations, are usually employed. The level of carbon dioxide in arterial blood is a sensitive, simple test of the adequacy of ventilation. Inadequate ventilation is rapidly reflected by a high level, and hyperventilation by a diminished level, owing to the efficiency of diffusion of this gas in the lung. The dynamic measurement of a patient's ability to move volumes of air during units of time is important in determining the need for mechani-

cal assistance and, indeed, the prospect for recovery. The forced expiratory volume in one second (FEV_1) is a useful measurement and 80 percent or more is considered normal.

Some useful values of pulmonary function tests are depicted (Table 14-1).

ANESTHESIA

The aim of satisfactory anesthetic administration is to provide the least anesthesia consistent with performance of the proposed operation with the greatest margin of safety. This must be a highly individualized procedure based upon the physical status of the patient and an estimate of the extent and length of time of the anticipated operation. A careful history will often suggest limitations of cardiopulmonary function and the physical examination may discover problems with dentition, airway, or availability of peripheral veins, in addition to obvious signs of heart failure. The chest roentgenogram, ECG, blood count, urine analysis, glucose and blood urea nitrogen, electrolyte determination, and other tests suggested by circumstances are very helpful in determining risk of anesthesia administration. Blood gas and spirometric determinations may quantify deficits otherwise not fully appreciated.

Premedication

A wise choice of premedication can only be made if the anesthetist evaluates the patient before operation. The level of apprehension, body habitus, and physiologic age are invaluable guides. Two or more drugs are usually employed. Narcotics, barbiturates, and/or tranquilizers are used to subdue anxiety; they tend to reduce anesthesia requirements. One of the disadvantages of narcotics is that they cause respiratory depression which may extend into the postoperative period. Phenothiazines are potent antiemetics, but they may cause hypotension. Anticholinergics reduce vagal activity and tend to reduce secretions.

Local Anesthesia

Local anesthetics work by making the neural membrane impermeable to ion exchange. Epinephrine added to the solution prolongs anesthesia by vasoconstriction. Systemic reactions are rarely allergic, and many so-called reactions are due to the added epinephrine. Most reactions are due to overdosage. Overdosage results in central nervous system or vascular symptoms. Anxiety, somnolence, scotomata, and even grand mal seizures may result. Treatment must be directed to preventing hypoxemia. Seizures may be controlled with short-acting barbiturates.

Maximum dosages are the following:

Cocaine	160 mg
Procaine	1 g
Tetracaine	100 mg
Lidocaine	500 mg
Bupivacaine	225 mg
Mepivacaine	500 mg

If these doses are not exceeded, few reactions will occur. No local anesthetics should be administered unless means of providing artificial ventilation and administration of a rapid-acting drug (barbiturates or diazepam) are available.

Solutions containing epinephrine should not be injected into digits, ears, or penis because of the danger of gangrene.

Spinal and Epidural Anesthesia

Spinal anesthetics act by injecting a local anesthetic into the subarachnoid space to block spinal nerve roots and ganglia. An L3–4 to L4–5 interspace puncture avoids the spinal cord. By weighting the anesthetic solution with a 10 percent glucose solution, the specific gravity of the fluid exceeds that of spinal fluid. Gravity and positioning are used to adjust the level of anesthesia. Sympathetic blockade, in addition to sensory and motor blockade, occurs; significant hypotension may ensue. Added epinephrine prolongs duration of anesthesia. High spinal anesthesia blocks thoracic sympathetic fibers, and bradycardia may ensue because of parasympathetic (cranial outflow) predominance. An intravenous line should always be placed prior to anesthetic administration so that fluids and drugs may be rapidly administered should hypotension occur. Headache is the most frequent complication and will be reduced in incidence by the use of small (22–25 gauge) needles.

Epidural anesthesia is produced by injecting an anesthetic drug into the space between the dura and periosteum of the spinal canal and extending from the fifth sacral vertebra to the foramen magnum. If injected at S5, it is called caudal anesthesia; if at L3–5, it is called epidural anesthesia. Its advantages over spinal anesthesia are absence of headache and the possibility of introducing a catheter to produce continuing anesthesia for long procedures. It is technically more difficult than spinal anesthesia to induce.

Intravenous Anesthesia

Barbiturates are the most commonly used intravenous anesthetics. Very short-acting drugs are used to induce anesthesia or in conjunction with other agents to allay apprehension. They do not abolish reflexes, consequently are not satisfactory for major procedures. They are myocardial and cerebral depressants. Intra-arterial injections often lead to gangrene; if it occurs, the needle should be left in place and intravenous lidocaine or tolazoline injected.

Innovar produces neuroleptic analgesia (tranquilization and intense analgesia). It is a combination of fentanyl (narcotic) and droperidol (tranquilizer). Fentanyl is a profound respiratory depressant. Innovar is a useful adjunct to nitrous oxide anesthesia. Postoperative hypertension may require treatment.

Ketamine produces profound analgesia while maintaining reflex activity. It does not relieve visceral pain so it is not suitable for abdominal or thoracic operations. Ketamine causes marked secretion formation; consequently, an anticholinergic drug should be administered before induction. It is useful in burn treatment.

Inhalation Anesthesia

Nitrous oxide is a weak anesthetic and must be used in high concentrations. It is contraindicated in hypoxemic patients. It is often used to potentiate other inhalation anesthetics.

Ethrane is a potent halogenated nonflammable ether. Muscle relaxation is profound, and muscle relaxant dosages may therefore be reduced.

Penthrane is another nonflammable ether which provides good muscle relaxation and analgesia. Nephrotoxicity is an undesirable side effect which is related to duration and depth of anesthesia.

Halothane was the first nonflammable, nontoxic anesthetic agent to be introduced. Because of its potency, special vaporizors are required. Its parasympathomimetic effect may cause nodal rhythm with marked reduction in cardiac output, which may add to the depressing effect on the vasomotor center. It is well adapted to asthmatics because bronchial smooth muscle is relaxed and is an excellent choice for pediatric anesthesia. Splanchnic blood flow is increased; therefore, its use in patients in shock is widely accepted. Because of uncertainty about its relationship to liver necrosis, halothane should not be given if prior administration has been followed by jaundice.

Cyclopropane and diethyl ether are little used because of their flammability. They are relatively nontoxic.

Muscle Relaxants

Muscle relaxants provide the relaxation required to perform abdominal operations or to make tracheal intubation easier. They block impulses passing from motor nerves to skeletal muscle by competing with acetylcholine. Depolarizing drugs such as succinylcholine produce muscle fasciculation followed by a depressed response to stimulation. Nondepolarizing relaxants cause no fasciculation but cause the face to twitch. These relaxants also cause tetanic stimulation. Nondepolarizing agents may be reversed by prostigmine.

Succinylcholine is very short-acting and is widely used to facilitate intubation. Prolonged respiratory depression may require ventilatory support.

D-Tubocurarine produces quick relaxation which lasts about 1 hour. It is the agent of choice if renal failure is present.

Pancuronium enjoys the advantages of absence of histamine release and ganglionic blockade. It is reversed by anticholinesterases and is very useful in shock states because it lacks cardiovascular depression.

POSTOPERATIVE CARE

Good postoperative care provides psychological and physical support to assure a smooth recovery from operation. Reassurance diminishes stress and enhances the patient's cooperation in his care. The usual postoperative patient is routed through the recovery room, from which he may return to an intensive care unit (ICU) or his own room, depending upon requirements for monitoring and complexity of care. Intensive care units should be equipped with devices required for measuring and recording cardiovascular and respiratory functions as a minimum. Respirators, hypothermia equipment, defibrillators, and pacemakers are used in the ICUs as support devices in the critical time following operation. This highly sophisticated setting is extremely valuable in providing physical support of physiologic functions, but in the conscious patient the constant stimulation can lead to severe psychological stresses. Therefore, the patient should be moved to a less anxious environment as soon as possible. Furthermore, the cost of an ICU bed is several times that of an ordinary hospital bed and costs of thousands of dollars per day are commonplace.

The recording of information vital to the patient's care by many members of the hospital staff is of great importance. A brief operative note should be placed upon the patient's chart when the operation is completed. Special hazards should be noted along with precautions to be taken. The postoperative orders should be written in the operating room. These orders automatically cancel preexisting orders.

Postoperative orders should include the following:

1. Sedatives and routes by which they are to be administered.
2. Intravenous fluids including route of administration.
3. Medications with stop orders.
4. Instructions for care of catheters, drains, tubes, etc.
5. Instructions for taking vital signs.
6. Orders for required laboratory procedures (electrolytes, blood counts, etc.).
7. Other appropriate items.

Medication for the continuing treatment of preoperative conditions (cardiac, endocrine, metabolic, etc.) must be continued postoperatively. Pain relief by the least amount of appropriate drugs is desirable, thereby avoiding depression of respiration and gastrointestinal function. Body size, age, and frequency and rate of administration are considered in choice of drug and dose. It is better to use smaller doses at frequent intervals than larger doses less frequently. Morphine, meperidine, and other potent narcotics are replaced by codeine or less potent analgesics as soon as the level of pain diminishes. Long-term antibiotic administration, and regimes of bowel preparation in anticipation of intestinal resection may eliminate the bacteria which synthesize vitamin K in the gut lumen. Depressed liver function or biliary fistulas also promote deficiency of this vitamin. Vitamin K, administered 10 mg/day intramuscularly (IM) or orally, will prevent this potential cause of prothombin deficiency.

Monitoring

The extent of monitoring is determined by the preoperative physical state and age of the patient and the operative procedures. Blood pressure, pulse, and respiration should be recorded; in severe situations these can be continuously recorded by ECG and intra-arterial catheter, the latter sufficing to obtain blood for gas and pH determination. Blood volume and cardiac output determinations are possible as well. Central venous pressure lines and Swan-Ganz catheters are important devices to estimate cardiac function and blood volume requirements.

Urine output is an excellent indication of the state of the circulation, and an output of about 50 ml/hour in adults is a minimum target value. Adequate fluid administration to assure coverage of insensible losses and a 1,200 ml urine output is provided by 500 ml of normal saline (NS) and 2,000 ml of 5 percent glucose in water (G/W). When urine output is satisfactory, 40 mEq potassium (as KCl) are added to these fluids, the potassium being diluted to 20 mEq per L of solution. Each degree of temperature increase requires about a 7 percent increase in fluid administration. Sodium and potassium administration is based upon serum electrolyte determinations, which should be done daily while abnormal fluid losses (e.g., nasogastric suction, fistulas) are occurring. Further details are found in the section on fluid and electrolytes.

Nutrition

Convalescence is improved if nutritional deficits are corrected preoperatively. This is not always possible if the disease precludes the establishment of optimal nutrition. Extracellular fluid volume is brought to normal, vitamin deficiencies are corrected, a normal urine output is obtained, and electrolyte deficiencies are corrected. After operation a negative nitrogen balance ensues and body tissues are utilized to provide calories required for muscle function and temperature regulation. Fever, sepsis, and continued starvation all interact to deplete the patient. For every gram of nitrogen found in the urine, 6.5 g of protein have been broken down, mostly at the expense of skeletal muscle. Intravenous glucose, even in small amounts, affords a significant effect in sparing nitrogen loss and preventing starvation ketosis. Achieving nitrogen balance requires 35 calories/kg/day. Fortunately, most wounds heal even in the presence of a negative nitrogen balance.

When starvation is prolonged, as in major gastrointestinal tract operations, recourse to intravenous hyperalimentation is desirable. Basically, hypertonic glucose solutions and 5 percent solutions of protein hydrolysate or amino acids can provide as much as 5,000 calories/day, with restoration of nitrogen balance.

Another option useful in some situations is the use of elemental diets which are completely free of bulk. These materials contain amino acids, sugars, essential fats, vitamins, and minerals. They are entirely absorbed in the upper intestine with very little stimulation of digestive secretion.

If convalescence is prolonged, it is wise to furnish intravenous vitamins in excess of needs. Standard solutions contain 500 mg of ascorbic acid (vitamin C), 50 mg of thiamine hydrochloride (B_1), 10 mg of riboflavin (B_2), and assorted others.

SHOCK

Shock due to any cause is one of the most serious disorders confronting the surgeon. It is characterized by hypotension and may be classified according to cause. Blood pressure is maintained by the pumping action of the heart, an adequate circulating blood volume, and the peripheral vascular resistance. The ultimate function of the circulatory system is to furnish oxygen and nutrients to body cells and to remove the waste products of metabolism. Inadequate blood flow leads to hypoxia which, in turn, leads to metabolic acidosis, then eventually leads to death if uncorrected.

Shock may be conveniently classified according to major causes (i.e., cardiogenic, hypovolemic, and septic

shock). It should be emphasized that these shock types may be present singly or in combination.

The basic cause of cardiogenic shock is a failure of the pump action of the heart which may be precipitated by a myocardial infarction or congestive heart failure. In the perioperative period it is a grave threat to life. Its treatment is that of the underlying disorder.

Hypovolemic shock results from an inadequate circulating blood volume and is the type most frequently encountered by surgeons. The volume deficit may be due to blood loss (trauma, operation), loss of fluid to the environment (diarrhea, vomiting, diuresis, sweating, etc.), or sequestration of fluid in the extravascular spaces (intestinal obstruction, edema, effusions, or ascites).

Septic shock, unlike cardiogenic and hypovolemic shock, is usually difficult to diagnose. Septic shock may be very subtle in its onset and it is less well understood. Infection may produce an increase in capillary permeability which probably results from an interaction between bacterial products, probably an endotoxin, and polymorphonuclear leukocytes. The temperature control mechanism of the midbrain is affected and the systemic hemodynamic change results from vasodilatation. The resulting fall in peripheral vascular resistance with pooling of blood in peripheral vessels sets the stage for decrease in venous return to the heart with a reduction in cardiac output when compensatory mechanisms fail. The hypermetabolic state that follows sepsis probably results from increased production of catecholamines and the increase in protein catabolism. Chills and fever are frequently encountered and are often signs of impending shock. Shivering and increased muscular activity greatly increase heat production. Increase in oxygen demand only partially explains the marked increase in cardiac output. If the underlying sepsis is not controlled, the elevated cardiac output leads to cardiac fatigue. Eventually the output can no longer overcome the effects of the falling peripheral resistance and hypotension ensues. Most patients in septic shock have been sick for a time and often have been the victims of blood loss and malnutrition, which complicated treatment. In many, an underlying disease such as leukemia is present. Septic shock is uncommon in children and is most commonly encountered in urinary tract infections in elderly males.

Clinically, septic shock is usually encountered in situations where gram-negative septicemia may be suspected (e.g., peritonitis, urinary tract infections, etc.). Initially the skin may be warm and flushed, and the patient may be quite responsive despite the presence of hypotension. Urine output may be satisfactory initially. Sudden drop in blood pressure and oliguria follows. A marked tachycardia is present. Measured blood volume is usually in normal range, and central venous pressure is slightly reduced or normal. The hematocrit is usually within normal range and the white blood count may be normal. Hyperventilation may produce hypocardia, and pulmonary venous admixture may lead to hypoxemia. Total peripheral resistance is usually less than 500 dyne s/cm and cardiac indices often exceed 3.75 L/min/m². Myocardial failure often develops and attempts at volume expansion may only increase central venous pressure without augmenting cardiac output. If the initial cardiac index is less than 2.5 L/min/m², mortality exceeds 75 percent, probably the result of inadequate perfusion in the face of peripheral vasodilatation.

Treatment of shock depends upon the basis for its presence. Cardiogenic shock requires attention to factors such as preload and afterload, and myocardial contractility and pulse rate. It is discussed in detail elsewhere in this volume. The basis of treatment of hypovolemic shock is volume replacement to increase circulating blood volume. In general, fluid therapy should approximate that of the fluid lost. In the case of blood loss, Ringer's lactate solution may be used initially until blood is typed and crossmatched. When fluid loss is due to vomiting or sequestration of fluid in obstructed intestine, saline or Ringer's solution suffices. If blood loss is a liter or less, Ringer's solution may be all that is required. Since Ringer's solution fills the extracellular fluid space as well as the vasculature, more solution must be given than is lost, and about 2.5 times the volume of shed blood is required to maintain a normal blood volume. Substantial evidence exists to show that the use of such crystalloid solutions results in improved function of kidneys and lungs over that experienced when colloid solutions are employed. The limit in the volume of electrolyte solution to be used for blood loss depends upon the extent of anemia which the patient will tolerate. When the hematocrit decreases below 30, there is a progressive decline in the oxygen carrying capacity of the blood. Most blood loss beyond 1,000 ml will require blood transfusion. If time is unavailable for crossmatching, the administration of uncrossmatched type specific blood or low titer type-O-negative blood is acceptable practice. It goes without saying that ongoing blood loss must be controlled concomitantly. Other volume expanders including concentrated serum albumin and hydroxyethyl starch; dextran and plasma may be useful at times. During operation, autotransfusion may be used to return shed blood to the patient but it is not widely used.

In the presence of shock, volume replacement must at least keep up with the rate of ongoing loss, and the more rapidly circulating volume is restored the more quickly will the metabolic abnormalities be corrected.

Appropriate monitoring of the patient being treated for shock includes the recording of arterial blood pressure and electrocardiographic monitoring. Urine output is a very useful indicator of circulatory sufficiency and the central venous pressure is useful in determining the adequacy of blood volume. More sensitive indicators of the adequacy of volume restoration are the pulmonary wedge pressure as measured by the Swan-Ganz catheter and the cardiac output determinations (thermal or dye dilution techniques).

Additional treatment measures might include sodium bicarbonate infusion if indicated by the arterial pH, but in no circumstances must this be considered to replace adequate volume replacement to restore perfusion to correct acidosis. Vasoconstrictors are contraindicated except in dire circumstances where a blood pressure of 40 or 50 mm Hg may be life-threatening. They should be discontinued as soon as the blood volume is sufficiently increased to improve the blood pressure to more reasonable levels. The administration of oxygen, the use of pneumatic trousers where appropriate, and the elevation of the lower extremities are useful adjuncts.

Clinical responsiveness to treatment is the best gauge of success, and in most instances unresponsiveness is the result of ongoing blood loss or inadequate replacement of losses.

MULTIPLE ORGAN FAILURE

The support systems now available to treat seriously sick patients are so effective that death due to failure of a single organ in a patient hospitalized for a time is unusual. Hemodialysis for renal failure, mechanical ventilatory assistance for lung failure, and parenteral nutrition for gastrointestinal failure are taken for granted as systems sequentially fail. Failure of one organ or system predisposes to failure in others, and the advent of new failures may be almost imperceptible.

Elderly patients with preexisting disease are most prone to develop multiple organ failure (MOF), and the absence of these adverse factors explains the increased survival rate of young over old patients with similar injuries. Coronary artery disease, chronic lung disease, diabetes, and kidney disease, all common in the aged, set the stage for MOF. Depressed immunity, also common in the elderly, is another major feature not usually shared by youthful patients.

Events which predispose to MOF are the development of shock, technical errors related to operation or treatment, and the use of potent therapeutic agents such as multiple transfusions, vasoactive drugs, antibiotics, mechanical ventilation, and other potent treatment modalities which may damage kidneys, lungs, liver, or central nervous system. High oxygen concentrations in inspired air may damage the lungs, and antibiotics may cause renal failure to compound the damage induced by shock in the first instance.

The sequence of organ involvement cannot be predicted, as opposed to specific organ susceptibility in some lower animals, but the kidney and lung seem most vulnerable in man. Sepsis in the pleural and abdominal cavities seems to be the most common cause of MOF, and its prevention is paramount in prevention. Technical errors which result in intestinal anastomotic leaks or vascular compromise are major causes as are accidents associated with insertion of vascular lines, catheters, etc.

Treatment should be directed to the underlying cause (i.e., undrained abscesses, anastomotic leaks, etc.) rather than merely supporting the failing individual organs. Operation should not be delayed in the belief that they will "get in shape" by further supportive treatment. These patients usually require repeated transfusions and fluid-electrolyte balanced must be maintained. Digitalis, diuretics, and mechanical support of lungs and kidneys are frequently necessary.

PREOPERATIVE CARE

Assuming that an adequate diagnostic work-up has been completed, further evaluation to assess risk of operation and to determine required treatment to bring the patient to the best possible state to withstand surgery is necessary. Preexisting diseases of the cardiovascular, respiratory, and genitourinary systems are those most likely to adversely affect smooth convalescence. In elderly patients, the physiologic rather than the chronologic age is the important determinant in survival. Because of the frequency of degenerative and malignant diseases in the elderly, evaluation must be more detailed than in youth.

Cardiovascular System

History and physical examination will suggest heart failure, detect hypertension, and assess reserve based on exercise tolerance. The ECG should be obtained in all elderly patients to rule out myocardial damage and conduction defect. Appropriate medication (i.e., digitalis, diuretics, α and β blockers, etc.) should be administered if disorders are found.

Respiratory System

Dyspnea, exercise intolerance, a smoking history, productive cough, and asthmatic attacks are of great concern in postoperative management. Pulmonary function tests should be obtained if doubt exists since the risks of operation may be estimated based upon experience with these tests. Operations upon the thorax and abdomen

cause the greatest reductions in lung function and pulmonary complications are most frequent with these procedures. Briefly, some values of pulmonary function testing known to be associated with high risk are (1) vital capacity (VC) < 1 L, (2) a maximum voluntary ventilation (MVV) < 50 L/min, (3) forced expiratory ventilation of 1 s (FEV_1) < 0.5 liters, (4) maximal expiratory flow rate (MEFR) < 100 L/min, (5) PaO_2 < 55 mm Hg, and (6) $PaCO_2$ > 45 mm Hg.

Significant reduction in risk due to pulmonary disease may be accomplished by cessation of smoking, sputum culturing with antibiotic administration, inhalation therapy, bronchodilators, and chest physical therapy. Shock and sepsis enhance the risk of developing the respiratory distress syndrome, and vigorous treatment to establish an adequate blood volume and overcome infection preoperatively is mandatory.

Renal Function

A complete urine analysis, serum blood urea nitrogen (BUN) and creatinine, albumin, and BUN combined with physical examination will detect most renal disease likely to affect convalescence. Hematuria, proteinuria, and elevations of BUN or creatinine are suggestive of significant disease but they rarely require the delay of elective surgical procedures. In patients with chronic renal failure who do not require maintenance dialysis, preoperative hydration and transfusion to get the hematocrit to a level of 32 percent are desirable. During and after operation, strict attention to fluid balance is necessary since dehydration often precipitates acute renal failure. If on maintenance dialysis (glomerular filtration rate below 5 ml/min), transfusion to achieve a 32 percent hematocrit should be given. Diabetics with renal failure are especially prone to infection. Jaundiced patients appear to suffer renal failure more often than nonicteric patients.

Some drug dosages must be modified in the presence of renal failure. They are the antibiotics, analgesics and anesthetics, hypoglycemic agents, anti-inflammatory agents, and antineoplastic drugs. Gentamycin, amphotericin B, methicillin, and tetracyclines are the worst offending antibiotics in this regard. Digitalis toxicity is more prone to occur in renal failure because excretion is by the renal route.

Liver

Adequate liver function is essential to many phases of recovery from the stress of operation. Although operative mortality following a major operation in cirrhotic patients may be small, both acute and chronic forms of liver failure may threaten life in patients subjected to anesthesia and operation. Prognosis depends upon the degree of hepatic damage, the rate of change in hepatic function, and the magnitude of the procedure. The fundamental issue is the degree of cellular function impairment. Chronic low grade jaundice and mild ascites may be an almost stable condition in cirrhotics. Recent onset of jaundice and ascites suggests a recent advancement of disease which is more serious. Ascites resistant to control, a serum protein under 3.0 g percent, and a serum bilirubin over 3.0 mg percent are recognized bad prognostic signs, especially when neurologic signs coexist. Malnutrition, likewise, favors a poor prognosis. These findings are especially pertinent in the selection of patients considered for portacaval shunting for portal hypertension.

Hematologic System

Most derangements of the hematologic system which might prejudice outcome can be corrected preoperatively if they are recognized. Coagulation is especially important, but estimates of blood volume and red cell abnormalities should be known. Most patients do well with a hematocrit over 30 percent. It was formerly believed that patients with chronic anemia had contracted blood volumes. In truth, many have expanded plasma volumes and transfusion of whole blood sufficient to raise the hematocrit to normal levels may overload the circulation. Packed cells should be administered up to a hematocrit of about 30 percent.

Coagulopathies are best discovered by the history and physical examination. Routine bleeding and clotting times are so inaccurate that they are almost worthless as screening devices. Most postoperative bleeding is due to inadequate hemostasis. Once bleeding occurs, the problem is more complicated. The best screening tests are the one-stage prothrombin time (PT) and the partial thromboplastin time, in addition to bleeding and clotting times. Platelet counts and clot retraction are measures of platelet function, and fibrinolysis is estimated by the level of fibrin split products. Specific deficits are corrected preoperatively by appropriate components.

MISCELLANEOUS INFECTIONS OF SURGICAL INTEREST

Infections complicating surgical procedures or traumatic injury are the major cause of morbidity and mortality. Peritonitis and intraabdominal abscess formation are discussed in another section, and the importance of anaerobes in these processes is discussed. A few specific, infrequently encountered infections will be discussed since they are largely in the domain of surgical care.

Tetanus

Tetanus is caused by infection with the anaerobic, gram-positive *Clostridium* tetani. The toxin diffuses and stimulates neuromuscular end-organs causing tonic contraction, and it systemically acts on cells in the central nervous system to produce trismus, rigidity, and convulsions. External stimuli such as noise and movement often precipitate these seizures. The spore-bearing bacillus is found largely in the gastrointestinal tract of animals and soil. Puncture wounds and those having considerable contamination are most prone to develop the infection but about one-third of patients with tetanus have no demonstrable wound.

Treatment consists of complete local excision when possible and 250 units of human antitetanus globulin (TIG) to neutralize circulating toxin. In addition, the patient should be activity immunized. Antibiotics do not control the effects of the toxin but they should be given in high doses intravenously in an attempt to eradicate the bacteria. Ventilatory support and sedation are important adjuncts in treatment.

The efficacy of serotherapy in established infections is uncertain but TIG, 5,000–10,000 units given intravenously, would seem to be reasonable. Sodium pentothal is indicated to control seizures and is continuously administered to produce light sleep. Diazepam (Valium) 10–20 mg/kg of body weight per 24 hours may be sufficient to control seizures. Succinylcholine or methocarbamol may be used with mechanical ventiatory support. Tracheal intubation is very useful in severe cases and tracheostomy may be helpful if the course is prolonged. The care of these patients is constant and complex. Assurance of ventilation, avoidance of external stimuli, nutritional support, and maintenance of fluid and electrolyte balance are crucial.

Immunization, properly executed using tetanus toxoid, virtually eliminates the chance of subsequently getting tetanus.

Treatment of wounds in previously immunized patients is the following:

1. When the patient has been actively immunized within the past 10 years and has a severe, neglected, or old (>24 hours) tetanus-prone wound, give 0.5 ml of adsorbed toxoid unless it is certain that a booster injection was received within the previous 5 years.
2. When immunized more than 10 years previously and has received no booster in that time, give 0.5 ml adsorbed tetanus toxoid to all. In tetanus-prone wounds

give 250 U of TIG (human), using different needles in different injection sites.

3. Those with severe or neglected wounds should be given 500 U of TIG in addition to a toxoid booster. Consider antibiotic prophylaxis in any patient with tetanus-prone wounds.

Clostridial Myositis (Gas Gangrene)

Clostridial myositis is a virulent infection caused by one of several clostridia with a predilection for wounds with a compromised blood supply and devitalized muscle. High velocity missile wounds and compound fractures which have been contaminated by foreign material are especially prone, especially if treatment has been delayed.

In clinical gas gangrene, wounds will often yield multiple species of clostridia, the commonest being *C perfringens* (welchii). Both vegetative and spore forms are widespread in soil, the gastrointestinal tract, and clothing. They are strict anaerobes and the bacteria possess little invasive ability. However, in the presence of dead or injured tissue, ischemia, and pyogenic bacteria, the oxidation-reduction potential of the wound is reduced favoring transition from the spore to vegetative forms, which produce the powerful toxins (lecithinases and others) which account for the clinical picture. These toxins destroy cell membranes and increase capillary permeability, tissue digestion, muscle necrosis, and bacterial invasion.

Prevention is best accomplished by early and adequate operation with thorough debridement of all dead or potentially devitalized tissue and removal of dirt and foreign bodies. These wounds should be left open for several days to be closed only after no evidence of local sepsis is present. Antibiotics including penicillin, cephalothin, and clindamycin are effective against most clostridia, but they should not be considered as the sole treatment but only adjuncts to thorough debridement. There is no evidence that prophylactic antitoxin is of any use.

Treatment of established gas gangrene will be facilitated if the wound is carefully inspected at frequent intervals. Casts, splints, and dressings must be removed promptly if fever, local pain, and toxicity suggest a problem. The average incubation period of *C perfringens,* the most common organism, is 48 hours but it may be far shorter. Fever may not be present; when toxicity supervenes its absence may be a bad prognostic sign. Stupor and delirium are late signs. Early, the skin may look normal. A dirty-brown discharge with a peculiar odor usually drains and the skin becomes dusky or bronze. Crepitation is a late sign.

Laboratory studies and roentgenogram may be useful. The hematocrit usually falls; leukocytosis usually does not exceed 15,000 mm³. Gram stain will show large gram-positive rods and few pus cells. Gas in muscle planes seen on roentgenograms helps confirm the diagnosis.

TREATMENT

Early, adequate debridement is the basis of treatment. Amputation may be avoided by wide incision and drainage and excision of devitalized tissue. If amputation is required, the wound should be left open. Penicillin G, cephalothin, and clindamycin are the drugs of choice (given in large doses intravenously). The efficacy of hyperbaric oxygen therapy and antitoxin are unknown but their use in this desperate condition will undoubtedly continue.

Clostridial Cellulitis

Clostridial cellulitis is caused by the same organisms, but its virulence is somewhat less, its onset more gradual, and it usually has fewer systemic effects than are seen in clostridial myositis. The same care of wounds as for clostridial myositis is indicated and debridement and wide drainage of wounds along fascial planes is indicated. Antibiotic therapy is indicated.

Anaerobic Cellulitis

Anaerobic cellulitis is a mixed gas-forming infection occasionally seen following wounds of the perineum, buttocks, hip, and abdominal wall as well as in other locations, especially if the areas are contaminated by material from the genitourinary, gastrointestinal, or respiratory tract. Coliform organisms, anaerobic streptococci, and bacteroides species predominate. Spread along fascial planes leads to thrombosis of skin vessels with resulting gangrene of the skin. The purulent material is thin and foul-smelling. Wide excision of devitalized tissue and drainage of fascial planes is indicated. Penicillin and broad spectrum antibiotics should be used.

Infections Resulting From Human Bites

Human bite infections are produced by mouth organisms that cause invasive infections. Aerobic nonhemolytic streptococci, staphylococci, spirochetes, and anaerobic streptococci are usually responsible. When infection occurs, debridement and wide decompression of tissue spaces are vital in treatment. Local heat, immobilization, and elevation of the extremity tend to localize the infection. Penicillin G or other suitable antibiotics should be administered.

Actinomyces

Actinomyces bovis is a fungus which produces a granulomatous process which is prone to suppurate and discharge pus through sinus tracts. The discharge contains characteristic "sulfur granules," which are masses of mycelia which are visible to the unaided eye. The commonly affected sites are the thorax and cervicofacial areas and the abdomen, and the infection usually develops at a site of previous injury. Excision and drainage and prolonged penicillin therapy are accepted elements of treatment.

Rabies

Occasionally the surgeon becomes involved in the care of animal-bite victims in whom the possibility of developing rabies must be considered. Skunks, foxes, raccoons, bats, and dogs are most likely to harbor the virus in their saliva. Since clinically evident rabies is uniformly fatal, prophylaxis is the only useful intervention. The wounds should be immediately copiously washed with soap and water followed by 70 percent alcohol. The current method of immunization involves the use of rabies immune globulin (RIG) and human diploid cell rabies vaccine (HDCV).

If the animal is a household pet (dog or cat), it should be held for 10 days, and no immunization is required if clinical rabies does not develop in the animal. At the first sign of rabies in the animal, the patient should be treated with RIG and HDCV. The symptomatic animal should be killed and tested under the supervision of a veterinarian. Public health officials should be notified. If the animal is unknown or escaped, or if the bite was inflicted by a skunk, bat, fox, coyote, bobcat, etc., RIG and HDCV should be administered. Bites from livestock, rats, squirrels, rabbits, and hares should lead to inquiry to local and state public health officials to determine the advisability of active immunization.

MISCELLANEOUS POSTOPERATIVE COMPLICATIONS

The recognition and management of postoperative complications ranks in importance with the technical skill with which the operation is performed. Indeed, in many circumstances the outcome will depend more upon this aspect of surgical care than the operative procedure itself. Some of the important complications will be considered.

Posttraumatic Pulmonary Insufficiency

Postoperative and posttraumatic pulmonary insufficiency are terms which embrace a wide spectrum of disorders due to many causes. All progress to hypoxia to a greater or lesser degree and threaten life. These changes may affect normal lungs in young patients, but when superimposed upon chronic lung disease it is even more serious. The syndrome follows severe trauma, even extrathoracic, with early spontaneous hyperventilation and alkalosis which leads to a free interval of apparently good pulmonary and circulatory function. Consolidation of the lung follows with venoarterial shunting, which ultimately may lead to a marked decrease in arterial oxygen content despite inhalation of high concentrations of oxygen. Interstitial edema and hyaline membrane formation ensue to interfere with diffusion of oxygen from alveolus to capillary. Infection in other sites appears to hasten the process, and when it proceeds to a fatal outcome, pneumonia is always present.

Treatment consists of mechanical ventilation, the control of sepsis, and the restoration of other visceral function. Formerly, renal failure killed many of these patients before the pulmonary problems mounted to threaten life. Hemodialysis now makes renal failure less threatening. Ventilation itself poses problems since it may "wash out" carbon dioxide so effectively that cerebral vasoconstriction and myocardial irritability may result. If the arterial carbon dioxide tension (PCO_2) falls below 32 mm Hg, dead space should be added to the system to overcome the low PCO_2.

Wound Sepsis and Dehiscence

Wound infections are among the most serious complications and operation. All wounds, even those healing primarily, are contaminated by bacteria, so the mere presence of bacteria does not mean that infection will occur. The development of infection depends upon the types and numbers of organisms, the presence of significant amounts of devitalized tissue in the wounds, the presence of foreign substances, and the general and local immunity of the patient. The advent of immunosuppressive therapy for use in transplantation and the treatment of malignant disease has led to a better appreciation of the importance of the immune system in combating infection.

Although local factors are of greater importance in the

development of wound complications, the general status of the patient is of great importance. Malnutrition, dehydration, shock, uncontrolled diabetes, and anemia are some factors favoring infection.

Most wound infections begin as cellulitis without suppuration and are characterized by hyperemia, pain, and edema. When local liquefaction of tissue ensues, an abscess forms. Most infections spread by way of the veins and lymphatics in the subcutaneous tissue, muscle, and tendon sheaths. Certain streptococci, *Staphylococcus aureus,* and *Bacteroides* tend to favor the development of septic thrombophlebitis and septicemia. Staphylococcal infections tend to localize.

DEHISCENCE

Dehiscence is the disruption of a wound, usually of the abdomen. It always leads to further morbidity. It represents a failure of wound healing and may involve any or all layers of the wound. When incomplete dehiscence occurs, an incisional hernia develops; when dehiscence is complete, the abdominal (or thoracic) viscera protrude and a mortality in excess of 10 percent may be expected. Dehiscence is best avoided by wise choice of incisions, avoidance of hematoma formation, and proper technique of closure with appropriate suture material. The avoidance of abdominal distention and vomiting, and attention to nutrition reduce the likelihood of this serious complication.

The drainage of serosanguinous fluid from a postoperative wound strongly suggests impending disruption. Loops of bowel may protrude through the fascial defects and still be contained beneath the skin. When intestine protrudes through the wound, great care should be taken to cover the viscera with sterile dressings while preparation for operation is made.

Treatment is best accomplished by wound closure with through-and-through heavy wire sutures.

Thrombophlebitis and Pulmonary Embolism

Homeostasis in surgical patients demands a delicate balance between coagulability and maintenance of the fluid state of the blood. Coagulation of blood in small vessels is necessary for healing to occur, but increased clotting tendency, tissue injury, and blood stasis are associated with operation and the danger for clotting of blood in large vessels, most commonly the veins. Clotting in large veins is often a silent process and massive pulmonary embolism may be the first sign of its presence.

Blood stagnation is probably the most important factor in the development of thrombus in veins. Congestive heart failure, shock, immobilization, and aging are important factors in stasis. The inactivation of muscle pumping action during anesthesia and at bed rest stagnates venous flow. Contrast material clears leg veins four times faster during walking than while at bed rest.

Collagen exposed to blood by intimal damage releases platelet ADP which causes platelet aggregation, which in turn become foci of coagulation. Thrombin formation further aggregates platelets by the release of ADP, which promotes fibrin formation to form stable clots. An activator substance in endothelium converts plasminogen into plasmin, which degrades fibrin. If fibrinolysis is sufficient to prevent fibrin deposition platelet aggregates disperse and thrombosis is prevented. If an intraluminal thrombus forms, it may break off to be swept to the lungs as a pulmonary embolus. If it becomes adherent to the vein wall, it may gradually dissolve or become fibrotic and adherent to the vein wall. Chronic obstruction may go unnoticed or give rise to the postphlebitic syndrome.

PULMONARY EMBOLISM

Pulmonary embolism is associated with a high mortality, yet it is diagnosed in less than half of fatal cases coming to autopsy. Clinical manifestations are often vague and, even when typical, other common disorders may be suspected. Most emboli originate in the deep veins of the leg, so swelling, pain, or tenderness may give a clue, but these findings are present in less than half of the victims.

The abrupt onset of dyspnea is the most common presentation. Faintness may occur if the embolus is massive. Chest pain occurs in about one-third and hemoptysis in less than 10 percent. Wheezes and pulmonary friction rub may be present on auscultation of the chest and cyanosis, if present, is usually mild.

Serum lactodehydrogenase (LDH), glutamic oxaloacetic transaminase activity (SGOT), and serum bilirubin may be useful in diagnosis. Most commonly, the LDH is elevated and SGOT and bilirubin are normal. LDH may require three or four days to be elevated and therefore the test is of limited utility. Chest roentgenograms may be normal but radiolucency due to ischemic lung may be evident early. A triangular density based on the pleura is possibly the most typical.

Pulmonary scanning is a rapid, simple method of assessing regional pulmonary blood flow even in very ill patients. Intravenous radioactive isotopes are injected and nonperfused areas of the lung are demonstrated. Pulmonary arteriography will demonstrate more than 80 percent of emboli, but it is not without risk.

Anticoagulation is the primary method of treatment, with a goal of maintaining a two- to three-fold increase in normal clotting time. Intravenous heparin is used in a carefully controlled hospital setting using the partial thromboplastin time (PTT) as a guide to therapy with a goal of at least twice normal values. In patients unsuitable for anticoagulation therapy, surgical procedures designed to filter clots in the inferior vena cava may be required. Pulmonary embolectomy may be lifesaving, but the procedure carries a high mortality. Partial bypass procedures in which the femoral artery and vein are cannulated are useful in procedures designed to remove pulmonary artery emboli.

Postoperative Hepatic Failure and Jaundice

Jaundice in the early postoperative period is most frequently related to operations on the biliary tract, stomach, pancreas, or duodenum. Stones in the common bile duct are the most frequent cause but common duct injury and cholangitis must be considered. Operative cholangiography done on a routine basis at the time of cholecystectomy best avoids overlooking stones at the initial operation. Frequently, stones are removed from the common duct and a T-tube is inserted. Postoperative tube cholangiogram then may show one or more retained stones which may produce jaundice if left in place. While the T-tube is draining, external decompression of bile avoids the development of icterus. By leaving the T-tube in place for several weeks, the radiologist may be able to remove retained stones by manipulation through the established tract after T-tube removal. If unsuccessful, reoperation is advisable to avoid the serious consequences of cholangitis.

Another possibility is the oversight of an ampullary or pancreatic cancer causing common duct obstruction. This most frequently occurs in instances where stones are removed which were thought to be the cause of jaundice. Common duct injury may be suspected if early postoperative jaundice is associated with bile drainage from the wound. Hepatic necrosis may follow ligation of the hepatic artery or its branches, especially if portal blood flow is compromised by hypotension or cirrhosis.

Acute suppurative cholangitis and acute postoperative pancreatitis are serious causes of jaundice early after operation. Cholangitis usually means infection and at least partial obstruction of the bile ducts, while a variety of manipulations of the biliary system may produce pancreatitis. The mortality of both of these complications is over 35 percent.

Other causes of jaundice occasionally may include the use of halogenated hydrocarbon anesthetics (halothane, methoxyflurane, fluroxene, enflurane, etc.). Hepatic necrosis may be slight or massive. Jaundice usually develops between 4 and 7 days after operation and is usually accompanied by fever, eosinophilia, and pro-

gressive elevation of SGOT. Other drugs including antibiotics, tranquilizers, and steroids may be hepatotoxic. Cholestasis, fatty infiltration, and frank necrosis are the most common findings.

Jaundice is frequently associated with sepsis in any location. Some infections, such as those due to *Costridium welchii,* cause hyperbilirubinemia due to massive hemolysis. The cause of jaundice associated with infections due to *E coli, Bacteroides,* and *Staphylococcus aureus* is not clear. Acute cholecystitis may cause jaundice with no common duct obstruction being present. The localized liver infection associated with it may produce elevations in SGOT and alkaline phosphatase, which may briefly continue to rise after cholecystectomy.

Hemolysis must be ruled out by performance of tests including serum bilirubin, Coombs' test, serum haptoglobin, and urinary urinobilinogen. Elevations of serum and urine hemoglobin are indicative of hemolysis. Heart operations sometimes produce hemolysis whether or not prosthetic valves are used.

Liver biopsy in the jaundiced patient may be risky owing to the possibility of bleeding due to prothrombin deficiency. If jaundice persists and duct obstruction is suspected, endoscopic retrograde cholangiopancreatography will demonstrate the biliary tract in more than 75 percent of patients. Percutaneous transhepatic cholangiography using an ultrathin needle is useful but carries with it the risk of hemorrhage.

Jaundice due to hepatitis B virus may be detected by a positive HBAg (Australia antigen). Stool examination is very useful. If hepatocellular dysfunction or hemolysis is responsible for jaundice, the stool usually contains bile. With deepening jaundice due to mechanical obstruction, stools will be light-colored or even gray.

Postoperative Bleeding Problems

Acute, unexpected bleeding during or shortly after operation in the absence of an accountable surgical source may require early action without the benefit of time-consuming tests. In the absence of preexisting defects, the possibilities are (1) inadequate hemostasis, (2) fibrinolysis, (3) defibrination, (4) thrombocytopenia due to massive transfusion, (5) anticoagulants and their antagonists, and (6) mixed clotting problems. The first consideration is to be sure that blood loss is not due to inadequate hemostasis incident to operation. When continuous bleeding requires constant transfusion to avoid shock, the problem is usually surgical.

A few rapid tests are useful and include the following:

1. Partial thromboplastin time (PTT). This will diagnose previously undetected hemophilia, coagulation de-

ficiencies, and anticoagulants. It should take the place of the old clotting time.

2. Platelet count. Counts under 100,000 may be the cause of bleeding.

3. Bleeding time. If the bleeding time exceeds 4 min, platelet abnormalities or von Willebrand's disease is a probable cause.

4. Prothrombin time. Prolongation may indicate fibrinolysis, intravascular coagulation, or liver disease.

5. Thrombin time. This will uncover overheparinization, fibrinolysis, or defibrination. If the thrombin time is prolonged, a plasma fibrinogram is useful since low levels of fibrinogen preclude clotting.

If the patient is receiving a blood transfusion during operation, the earliest sign of a transfusion reaction may be diffuse bleeding due to defibrination. Hemoglobinuria is an additional useful sign in the anesthetized patient. The transfusion should be stopped immediately, an osmotic diuretic (mannitol) should be given to wash out hemoglobin deposits in nephrons, and blood volume should be maintained by infusion of crossmatched blood or other fluids.

If fibrinolysis is the cause, epsilon-aminocaproic acid (EACA) will inhibit the action of plasmin. If intravascular clotting (disseminated intravascular coagulation–DIC) is present, heparin must be administered as well to avoid further DIC. Hypofibrinogenemia will respond to fresh plasma. Anticoagulant antagonists such as protamine may produce paradoxical bleeding. Further heparin (25,000 units) should be given.

If an explanation of the cause of bleeding cannot be given, fresh frozen plasma, EACA with heparin or fibrinogen with heparin may be the best approch to therapy. Although the absolute efficacy of calcium administration following massive blood transfusion is unproved, many clinicians advise its administration after a five-unit transfusion.

CARDIAC COMPLICATIONS

Myocardial Infarction

Myocardial infarction (MI) occurs in about 5 percent of elderly patients undergoing operation. Diagnosis is difficult because chest pain, dyspnea, or other symptoms are attributed to the operation. All elderly patients should be carefully monitored throughout the operation and postoperative ECG should be done if unexplained hypotension, cyanosis, or changes in cardiac rhythm occur. Angina, hypertension, previous MI, aortic disease, or diabetes are at high risk for MI.

Arrhythmias

Changes in heart rate or rhythm are common after operation. Some arrhythmias are life-threatening if untreated. Sinus tachycardia is often related to fever, pain, or hypoxia but may be caused by pulmonary embolus, infection, or anemia. Treatment of these causes is indicated. Most atrial arrhythmias are not serious, but ventricular arrhythmias may require immediate treatment. Premature ventricular contractions (PVC) exceeding 5/min require treatment of 50–100 mg of lidocaine intravenously as a single bolus followed by an IV drip at a rate of 1–4 mg/min. Ventricular tachycardia usually presents as hypotension and a rapid rate. Lidocaine, phenytoin (Dilantin), procainamide hydrochloride (Pronestyl), or propranolol are used to treat the arrhythmia. If digitalis toxicity is present, IV potassium chloride given at a rate of 20 mEq/hour is given in 500 mg of 5 percent glucose in water.

Cardiac Arrest

Ventricular fibrillation and ventricular standstill are indistinguishable clinically. Sudden loss of consciousness, absence of pulse, absence of or gasping respirations, and dilatation of the pupils are easily recognized signs. Immediate cardiac massage and ventilation of the lungs are imperative. Th ECG must be used to check ventricular activity. Ventricular fibrillation is much more common than standstill. Defibrillation is best performed by a direct current defibrillation using 100–400 J. If unsuccessful at first, further massage should be given, and defibrillation should then be repeated at higher energy levels. Ventricular standstill is usually treated with intracardiac adrenalin. Sodium bicarbonate (two ampules, 88 mEq) should be given intravenously and another ampule every 10 minutes until there is an effective beat.

URINARY TRACT COMPLICATIONS

Acute renal tubular necrosis (ATN) is one of the most serious renal complications following operation and trauma. Basically, it results fron renal ischemia in the course of shock. Dehydration is a common cause (prerenal) of oliguria and azotemia, and must be distinguished from it. Tissue damage and prerenal azotemia favor the development of tubular damage, but if urine flow is maintained, kidney damage is averted. The best way to treat the disorder is to prevent it by assuring kidney blood flow and maintaining a diuresis. Vasoconstrictors such as levarterenol are contraindicated in the treatment of shock because they cause a decrease in renal perfusion. ATN is usually marked by a urine specific gravity below 1.018, osmolality under 300 mosm/L, and urine sodium level of less than 20 mEq/L. Treatment of ATN consists of restricting fluid intake to replacement of urine and gastrointestinal losses plus 500–1,000 ml of water for insensible losses. Replacement losses should contain glucose but no potassium. High serum potassium may require hemodialysis. High output renal failure is a less severe form of ATN and azotemia with high serum potassium is found.

Urinary Retention

Urinary retention is the most common postoperative complication of the urinary tract. It is most frequently encountered in aged males due to prostatic hypertrophy. It may be the cause of diminished urine output. Bladder distention may be detected by palpation if the abdominal wound permits. Catheterization using sterile technique is indicated.

Urinary Tract Infection

One of the most common causes of postoperative fever is urinary tract infection (UTI). Many such patients have had prior catheterization. A very serious cause of "gram-negative shock" is urinary tract instrumentation. Chills, fever, and hypotension suggest its presence. Urine and blood cultures will identify the organism but treatment with high doses of antibiotics should be started immediately.

PSYCHIATRIC COMPLICATIONS

Severe psychotic disturbances may seriously jeopardize recovery and may lead to fatality. Their subtle prodromes may go unnoticed by surgeons. Metabolic disturbances, medications, especially barbiturates and narcotics, and electrolyte disturbances are common causs. Delirium tremens, a complication of severe alcoholism, carries a mortality ranging from 5 percent – 15 percent. Sleeplessness, confusion, agitation, and overactivity mark its presence. Hallucinations are common before the development of the full-blown syndrome. Treatment consists of sedation, paraldehyde or chlordiazepoxide HCl (Librium), restraint, careful fluid balance, and nutritional support.

The seriousness of these disorders makes psychiatric evaluation desirable if abnormal behavior is suspected.

INFECTION OF VASCULAR PROSTHETIC GRAFTS

Infection of arterial prosthetic grafts is fortunately low in incidence, but if it occurs the mortality rate is very high. Primary infection may be due to contamination at the time of implantation from skin contamination, most often in the groin, and usually the coagulasepositive *Staphylococcus aureus.* Inadvertant opening of the bowel is another source of contamination and operation such as appendectomy, gastrectomy, or cholecystectomy incidental to the procedure is not advisable. Prophylactic antibiotic administration is established as efficacious in reducing the incidence of postoperative infection.

Secondary infection of an actual prosthesis is caused by erosion into the bowel, usually the duodenum, with aortic replacement prosthesis. These infections track to the suture lines, where suture line breakdown occurs, often with catastrophic hemorrhage. Graft thrombosis, spontaneous wound abscess drainage, septic emboli, and low grade fever suggest its presence.

Treatment is complete removal of the prosthesis with restoration of blood flow by an alternate route. Sometimes these methods result in leg amputation(s), which is preferable to death from exsanguination.

EARLY CARE OF THE SERIOUSLY INJURED

This section is mainly devoted to the early phases of care, with emphasis on the patient with multiple injuries. One physician, preferably a general surgeon, should function as the "captain of the ship." The mnemonic A,B,C calls attention to the priorities in the order in which attention must be focused. Assurance of the airway (A) takes priority and it is easily attainable in over 90 percent of cases by bringing the mandible forward, care being taken to avoid aggravation of a cervical spine injury with consequent spinal cord damage. The insertion of an endotracheal tube provides the best airway and frees the physician for other duties. The control of external bleeding (B) is next in order and is almost always possible by pressure applied with fingers or pressure dressings, the latter more effective with large wounds. If unable to control extremity bleeding by the above, a pneumatic tourniquet placed above the wound and inflated well above systolic pressure is indicated. It is rarely necessary. Restoration of an adequate circulation (C) is carried out simultaneously to correct hypovolemic shock. Most patients with multiple injuries have severe deficits of red blood cell volume (RBCV), plasma vol-

Table 14-2. Amounts of BES Administered at Different Levels of Blood Loss

	Blood Volume Loss	Signs	Fluid Required
Mild blood loss	10–15% (750 ml)	Tachycardia	BES 2,000 ml
Moderate blood loss	20–25% (1,000–1,250 ml)	Tachycardia Decresed BP	BES 3,000–4,000 ml
Severe blood loss	30–35% (1,500–1,750 ml)	Tachycardia Tachypnea Narrow pulse pressure Hypotension Oliguria	BES 4,000–6,000 ml (Start blood as soon as crossmatch)
Catastrophic blood loss	>40%	Most will sustain cardiac arrest	BES and type specific whole blood

ume (PV), and interstitial fluid (IF). Normally, the RBCV averages 2 L, PV about 3 L, and IF about 11 L. The total extracellular fluid space (ECF), the sum of PV and IFS, measures about 14 L.

In severe hypovolemic shock, the RBCV has been reduced by about half. Refilling of the PV from the IF compartment occurs rapidly, resulting in a reduced hemoglobin and hematocrit over time. During the bleeding episode, the IF is a buffer to loss of blood volume and the quickest way to correct the deficit is by administering a balanced electrolyte solution (BES) to which $NaHCO_3$ (44 mEq) has been added (Table 14-2). BES requires no crossmatching, it is readily available, and it is inexpensive. Two large bore intravenous lines should be placed in peripheral, subclavian, or internal jugular veins as required. One line can be used to measure venous pressure, a valuable index of volume sufficiency. Two liters of BES are given over 15 to 30 minutes.

Blood is withdrawn for crossmatching, and baseline complete blood cell count (CBC) and chemistry determinations.

Patients in severe shock have poor peripheral perfusion and should be given sodium bicarbonate to overcome the severe metabolic acidosis. When many units of blood are required, fresh frozen plasma should be adminstered (1 U/5 transfusions) to supplement coagulation factors.

Some patients will arrive in the emergency room with pneumatic trousers (MAST) in place. This device should not be removed until blood pressure is restored; if the blood pressure falls, the suit should be reinflated. The MAST garment provides for autotransfusion from peripheral veins into the central vascular system and, very importantly, tends to slow blood loss due to pelvic fractures and visceral injuries.

SPECIFIC ORGAN INJURIES

Cervical Spine Injury

One must assume that the cervical spine has been injured, especially in deceleration injuries. Avoidance of manipulation and the application of a rigid collar (Philadelphia collar) or other support are indicated until a cross-table lateral roentgenogram of the neck has ruled out fracture. All seven cervical vertebrae must be visualized.

Hemothorax and Pneumothorax

Pleural space air or fluid interfere with ventilation. Auscultation reveals diminished breath sounds and, if the accumulation is large, tracheal shift to the unaffected side will be apparent. Open (sucking) thoracic wounds produce lung collapse by atmospheric pressure, and occlusion of the wound and the insertion of a chest tube temporarily control the physiologic disorder. Chest tubes properly applied serve as final treatment in the majority of these injuries.

Internal Bleeding

The source of internal bleeding depends to a significant degree upon the mechanism of injury. Automobile accidents produce fractures and solid viscera (liver and spleen) damage which may account for massive blood loss. In penetrating injuries, losses into the chest may be massive due to major vessel or cardiac injuries. Intercostal and internal mammary artery injuries are common with stab wounds.

Fractures are associated with major losses of blood. Closed pelvic and extremity fractures may account for several liters of blood loss, which usually largely abates within several hours. These sites tend to be overlooked as sources of hypovolemia.

The peritoneal cavity may contain a large quantity of blood before it is detected on clinical grounds. This is especially so in the obtunded patient. The presence of shock in the presence of a head injury usually means blood loss unless the patient is moribund due to the head injury. Peristaltic activity and abdominal distention are unreliable signs, and when in doubt, peritoneal lavage affords an accurate method of assessment. A catheter inserted, under local anesthesia, into the peritoneal cavity is much more reliable. If gross blood or intestinal contents are not recovered, a liter of saline (300–500 ml in children) instilled into the catheter by means of an intravenous tubing and allowed to drain by gravity will give the required information. If the drainage fluid contains more than 100,000 RBCs/ml, if the hematocrit is greater than 1 percent, of if bacteria are present, operation is indicated. If newsprint cannot be read through the plastic drainage tube, the test may be considered positive. With penetrating injuries, even lower levels of blood recovery may be associated with significant injuries. If leukocytes in the peritoneal drainage exceed 500 WBCs/ml, laparotomy may be indicated. Peritoneal lavage is contraindicated if a decision has already been made to do a laparotomy or if extensive adhesions from prior operations are suspected.

INDICATIONS FOR OPERATION

In addition, the decision to perform a laparotomy may be based on clinical information. Most surgeons now advocate laparotomy for gunshot wounds of the abdomen. Stab wounds may be treated conservatively if clinical signs of visceral injury do not supervene. Some perform laparotomy if the peritoneum has been perforated. Time-honored indications for operation are tenderness, rigidity, or distention of the abdomen, free air on roentgenogram, enlarging abdominal masses, or evidence of a developing peritonitis.

OPERATIVE TREATMENT

When urgency is not great, hours may be taken to correct acid-base or metabolic disturbances. The induction of anesthesia is often hazardous because of the dangers of hypotension caused by vasodilatation and aspiration of vomitus due to retained gastric contents.

A midline incision is perferred because of the access it provides. It may be extended into either hemithorax or directly through the sternum if further exposure of liver or intrathoracic parietes becomes desirable. When hemorrhage has produced abdominal tamponade, laparotomy with rapid decompression may permit further bleeding. Consequently, one must be prepared to immediately occlude the aorta at the diaphragm. The liver, spleen, aorta, and inferior vena cava are the likely sites of massive bleeding, and direct pressure applied to sponges overlying the injured structure may afford sufficient time for resuscitation and orderly repair of the injuries. Single holes in viscera must be viewed with suspicion since embolization, in the case of missiles, or hidden perforations which may be missed may account for the single apparent defect. Retroperitoneal hematomas must be investigated unless easily explained by intravenous pyelography suggesting minor injury or if a pelvic fracture is present. If hematomas overlying pelvic fractures are opened, uncontrollable bleeding may ensue. Major pelvic vessels may account for the hematoma, and they require repair after proximal and distal control.

Spleen

The spleen is the intra-abdominal organ most frequently injured by blunt trauma. It is often accompanied by rib fractures of the left side. The WBC is often markedly elevated. Radiographic signs include increased density in the left upper quadrant, obliteration of the left psoas shadow, displacement of the stomach bubble, and elevation of the left hemidiaphragm. Angiography and isotopic scanning may be very useful in poor risk patients in whom laparotomy may carry great risk.

Splenectomy is now known to increase susceptibility to serious sepsis, especially in children under the age of four, and because of this an effort should be made to control bleeding other than by splenectomy. In children, splenic injuries are often the only significant injury, and it is justified to carefully monitor patients suspected of having a splenic injury if ongoing bleeding is not evident. Ultrasonography, angiography, and isotopic imaging are very useful in following such injuries.

In adults, about half of the injured spleens can be preserved. In patients in deep shock and with multiple injuries, it is usually better to remove the spleen than to prolong the operation greatly. Pneumovax should be given to all patients undergoing splenectomy, with a booster dose being given every 3 years. The patient should be alerted to the need for early treatment should symptoms of sepsis occur.

Liver

About 90 percent of liver injuries are associated with injuries to other organs. Hemostasis is the main problem, and the inability to control bleeding accounts for most of the deaths. Sometimes the bleeding has stopped by the time laparotomy is performed and often local suturing techniques suffice. On occasion, liver resections are necessary to gain control of bleeding. Hepatic artery ligation may be necessary to save life if other methods fail. Large doses of broad spectrum antibiotics should be administered.

Pancreas

Injuries of the pancreas may not be apparent for days or weeks after the injury occurs, and a normal serum amylase may be present with major injuries. About one-third of pancreatic injuries are due to blunt trauma, the remainder due to penetrating injuries. Most are associated with other injuries. Operative treatment depends upon the magnitude of injury and, in a few, pancreato-duodenectomy may be required.

Stomach

In most stomach injuries blood will be recovered from the nasogastric tube, which in itself is an indication for laparotomy. Closure of the wound is indicated.

Duodenum and Small Intestine

Duodenal wounds are usually due to blunt trauma or gunshot or stab wounds. Very frequently, the pancreas, bile ducts, or inferior vena cava are injured as well. Delay in treatment beyond 12 hours results in high morbidity and mortality. Roentgenograms may show retroperitoneal air and contrast studies may show a leak. Hematomas of the duodenum may cause obstruction, which will usually resolve with time. Simple closure may result but much more extensive procedures may be required if the pancreas is injured.

Small intestinal injuries usually result from penetrating injuries but blunt injuries, including seat belt trauma, may be slow in manifesting themselves.

Large Intestine

Wounds of the colon are very serious injuries owing to the possiblity of serious sepsis. Prophylactic antibiotics should be given before operation. Treatment depends upon the presence of shock, the time since injury, age of the patient, the extent of injury, and the degree of fecal contamination. If any of the above circumstances exist, externalization of the colon is the wisest choice. Small perforations treated early with minimal contamination may be closed.

Rectum

Even very small rectal injuries may be lethal. Wounds of the extraperitoneal rectum should be repaired and drainage through the perineum established. A proximal diverting colostomy should be done. The distal colonic segment should be irrigated with antibiotic solutions to wash out fecal material.

LUNG, CHEST WALL, PLEURA, AND MEDIASTINUM

Congenital Disorders

Pulmonary agenesis results from failure of development. The remaining lung fills the entire thorax. Congenital tracheoesophageal fistulas are usually associated with esophageal atresia. Pulmonary arteriovenous aneurysms are fistulas between the pulmonary arteries and veins. The resulting right-to-left shunt can cause cyanosis, clubbing, congestive heart failure, and polycythemia. Infantile lobar emphysema involves mild to marked overdistention of the upper or middle lobes with compression of the remaining ipsilateral and the contralateral lung. Some require lobectomy if respiratory distress is marked. Occasionally congenital blebs and bullae occur and may become infected.

SPONTANEOUS PNEUMOTHORAX

Subpleural blebs at the apices may rupture to cause spontaneous pneumothorax. They usually occur in young adults. Reexpansion of the lung may occur spontaneously or reexpansion may be accomplished by inserting a chest tube and attaching it to a valve or water-seal drainage. Bleb resection and pleural abrasion or pleurectomy are acceptable methods for control of recurrent episodes.

Pulmonary Infections

Lung abscess usually follows aspiration of stomach contents. Parenchymal necrosis leads to bronchial communication and the abscess may be "coughed up," resulting in purulent sputum. *Staphylococcus aureus, Klebsiella,* and tuberculosis are common aerobes involved, while the anaerobic *Bacteroides* group is commonly cultured. Foreign bodies in bronchi, septic emboli, infected hematomas, or bronchial obstruction due to malignant tumors are less frequent causes.

BRONCHIECTASIS

Bronchiectasis is a dilatation of bronchi associated with bronchial and parenchymal infection. Except for the lingula, upper lobe involvement is unusual. Its highest incidence is in late childhood to middle age. Productive sputum, recurrent pneumonias, hemoptysis, and clubbing are common alone or in combination. The basic cause is unknown. Bronchography is the only accurate method of confirming the diagnosis. Most are treated medically, but operation may be offered if the disease is sufficiently localized. Resection of the involved lobe or segments is the procedure of choice.

TUBERCULOSIS

In the 1960s there was a sharp decline in the indications for operation in pulmonary tuberculosis. More effective antibiotics and chemotherapeutic agents made this change possible. Less than 10 percent of patients will require operation and, when done, should always be preceded by a course of intensive antimicrobial therapy. Principal indications are (1) persistently active disease with resistant organisms, (2) bronchopleural fistula, (3) pulmonary hemorrhage, (4) suspected associated carcinoma, and (5) bronchostenosis. Some patients with "open-negative" cavities are best operated upon if continued medical surveillance is a problem.

FUNGUS INFECTIONS

Fungal lesions may occasionally require pulmonary resection for diagnostic purposes since they may be difficult to differentiate from malignant neoplasms. Sometimes they mimic tuberculosis. Histoplasmosis is common in the Mississippi Valley, and chest roentgenogram often shows granulomas and hilar node calcification. Amphotericin B is effective in controlling progressive disease, although treatment is not often required. North American blastomycosis can resemble tuberculosis or carcinoma. Coccidioidomycosis, endemic in California, may resemble tuberculosis. Aspergillus fumigatus tends to invade other lesions, especially those possessing cavities. Such cavities tend to bleed and hemoptysis may be a reason for resection.

LUNG CANCER

Lung cancer is the leading cause of death due to cancer in the United States. There is a strong relationship to prolonged cigarette smoking. The majority of carcinomas are of the squamous cell, small cell, and adeno-

carcinomas, but many other cell types occur. Less than 10 percent survive 5 years after diagnosis.

Although mainly a male disease, women are increasingly afflicted due to smoking prevalence. Cough, hemoptysis, or chest pain may be the only symptoms. Hoarseness, weight loss, and signs of superior vena caval obstruction are ominous signs. Chest roentgenogram and bronchoscopy are the basic diagnostic tools but peripheral lesions may require open biopsy.

Pulmonary resection offers the chance of cure in a minority of patients with localized lesions. Radiotherapy and chemotherapy may offer good palliation.

Tumors metastatic to the lung may be amenable to cure by resection in a significant percentage of patients, provided the primary tumor has been eradicated. Sarcomas of extremities, renal carcinomas, and colon carcinomas seem to offer the best outlook.

Mediastinal Tumors. The nature of mediastinal neoplasms can be estimated according to their location. Neurogenic tumors and enteric cysts tend to occupy the posterior mediastinum. Substernal goiter and thymic tumors and cysts lie anteriorly, and lymphomas and other lesions involving lymph nodes appear at the hila. Most lesions found except those known to be benign (sarcoid, etc.) are best treated by excision, usually to rule out a malignant process.

THORAX

Traumatic Injury

Most serious thoracic injuries result in a reduction of ventilating capacity. A few serious thoracic injuries result in severe blood loss which threatens life. Statistically, the large majority can be treated without performing a major operation.

VENTILATORY COMPROMISE

Except for pulmonary contusion, most injuries resulting in decreased ventilation are the result of bellows failure (chest wall or diaphragm) or lung collapse due to intrapleural air or blood, frequently both. Simple rib fractures may cause enough pain to inhibit chest wall excursion and multiple rib fractures may cause flail chest, resulting in paradoxical motion of the chest wall. Similarly, ventilation is impaired by pneumothorax and hemothorax. The obstructed airway, especially in the unconscious or obtunded patient, has first priority in the management of all injured patients. Blood, mucus, teeth, dentures, or vomitus may obstruct the larynx or trachea and the tongue may prolapse into the hypopharynx to block the airway.

When lung injury permits air to escape into the pleural space, pneumothorax occurs. When air is forced into the space by vigorous inspiration due to a ball-valve mechanism, tension pneumothorax results. This is a highly lethal injury which must be relieved quickly or death ensues. Absent breath sounds, shift of the trachea away from the involved hemithorax, and a distended hyperresonant hemithorax are diagnostic. Insertion of a needle or chest tube or merely incising a short wound in the interspace gives quick relief.

Open chest wall wounds become "sucking" wounds due to the sound produced by the passage of air into the pleural space. The atmospheric pressure collapses the passive lung and ventilation is impaired. Wound closure by dressing or the gloved hand relieves the problem. When chest wound closure is accomplished and a chest tube inserted, the lung reexpands.

Hemothorax caused by bleeding chest wall vessels or lacerated lung causes parenchymal compression and may be relieved by chest tubes placed on water seal drainage. Massive bleeding due to major vessel disruption will be the indication for operation in about 10 percent of major injuries. Another small group will have tracheal or bronchial disruptions requiring operation.

About 10 percent of patients with aortic rupture survive long enough to reach the hospital alive. A wide mediastinum and deviation of the trachea or esophagus to the opposite side, seen on roentgenogram, is suggestive and requires angiography to rule out. If present, immediate operation is advisable.

SURGERY OF THE HEART AND GREAT VESSELS

The modern era of cardiac surgery began in the 1950s with the invention of the heart-lung machine. Many congenital and acquired lesions, formerly untreatable, became amenable to treatment. Some traumatic injuries, constricting pericarditis, arotic coarctations, and patent ductus arteriosis still are usually treated without extracorporeal circulation.

Congenital heart and vessel defects which are amenable to operation are enumerated (Table 14-3). It is convenient to classify according to prominent features of the anatomical and clinical alterations. Obstructive, cyanotic, and acyanotic congenital anomalies are recognized.

When abnormal communications between the two sides of the heart are present, blood is shunted from the high pressure to the low pressure system. Initially this will be from the left to right, but in time pulmonary

vascular changes lead to pulmonary hypertension which raises right-sided pressure. Added to this is the increased work required of the right heart. Dyspnea and exercise intolerance ensue. Cyanosis is not present unless right heart pressures rise far enough to produce a shunt to the systemic circulation (right to left). Four such abnormal communications that occur are patent ductus arteriosus, aortopulmonary window (communication between pulmonary artery and aorta at root of aorta), atrial septal defect, and ventricular septal defect. The extent of shunting can be determined by cardiac catheterization and significant shunts require operation.

Other abnormalities may produce cyanosis because of abnormal position of the great vessels. In total pulmonary venous return, the pulmonary veins empty into the right atrium only to recirculate into the lungs instead of the systemic circulation. Usually blood is shunted to the left heart via a septal defect. In transposition of the great vessels, the vessels are switched so that the aorta originates from the right heart and the pulmonary artery from the left. Unoxygenated venous blood returns to the right heart and is pumped to the aorta. Infants cannot survive unless a shunt exists to afford communication between the two sides of the heart. If the shunt is small a palliative septoplasty, using a balloon technique may enlarge it to sustain life until total surgical correction is feasible.

Congenital valvular defects can produce obstruction or insufficiency. Congenital stenosis impedes blood flow, resulting in work hypertrophy of the ventricular myocardium and, in turn, heart failure. With insufficiency, the unidirectional flow pattern is upset and more pumping is required to produce flow to the lungs or systemic circulation. The aortic and pulmonary valves are usually those affected, but rarely the tricuspid is displaced and malformed (Ebstein's anomaly). Obstructions above and below the valve may be responsible for outflow tract obstructions. The ECG, chest roentgenogram, and cardiac catheterization are helpful in demonstrating the effects upon the heart, and pressure readings indicate gradients.

Coarctation of the aorta is a congenital narrowing of the aorta which usually is found just distal to the left subclavian artery. Pressure proximal to the narrowing is high; distally it is low. Hypertension noted by high arm pressures and absent or diminished femoral pulses suggest its presence. The major complications are related left heart failure and the effects of hypertension upon the brain. Roentgenograms show left ventricular hypertrophy and notching of the lower borders of the ribs produced by pulsations of the enlarged tortuous intercostal arteries which act as major collateral pathways. Because of markedly diminished life expectancy, operative correction is indicated. Unless uncontrollable heart

Table 14-3. Common Forms of Congenital Heart Disease

Congenital Lesion	Defect	Physiologic Deficit Signs, Symptoms	Correction	Method of Diagnosis– Laboratory	Clinical Diagnosis
Obstruction					
Pulmonic valvular stenosis	Stenosis valve and/or infundibulum	Right ventricular hypertension	Operation if gradient > 50 mm Hg, valvostomy, infundibular resection	Roentgenogram– Right ventricular hypertrophy ECG–Right ventricular hypertrophy	Systolic murmur, weak pulmonic second sound, dyspnea, fatigue
Congenital aortic stenosis	Fusion of commissures	Cardiac failure	Commissurotomy	ECG–Left ventricular hypertrophy Cardiac catheterization	Systolic murmur, narrow pulse pressure, fatigue, dyspnea
Coarctation of aorta	Stenosis of aorta with prominent collaterals	Left ventricular failure, hypertension	Resection and repair	Chest roentgenogram ECG–Left ventricular hypertrophy Cardiac catheterization and aortography	Hypertension, upper left heart failure
Left-to-right shunt (acyanotic)					
Atrial septal defect	Septal defect with/without pulmonary veins, valve defect	Shunt from systemic circulation	Closure and correction associated defect	ECG–Left axis deviation Cardiac catheterization	Fatigue, palpitations, dyspnea, often none in first years of life
Ventricular septal defect	Left-to-right shunt, increase pulmonary blood flow	Cardiac failure, pulmonary hypertension	Closure	Cardiac catheterization	May close spontaneously first few years of life, loud systolic murmur
Patent ductus arteriosus	Aortic, pulmonary artery shunt	Aorta to pulmonary artery shunt (may be 50–70% of left ventricular output)	Closure after 2 to 3 years	Aortography, cardiac catheterization	Continuous murmur
Right-to-left shunt (cyanotic)					
Tetralogy of Fallot	Obstruction outflow tract right ventricle, ventricular septal defect, dextroposition of aorta, hypertrophy right ventricle	Large left-to-right shunt, right ventricular pressure = left ventricular pressure, chronic anoxia	Shunt in infancy, correction with open procedure after infancy	ECG–Right ventricular hypertrophy Chest roentgenogram– heart normal size, decreased vascularity of lungs, sabot-shaped heart Cardiac catheterization and angiography	Cyanosis, severe exertional dyspnea, squatting, heart normal size, and systolic murmur
Transposition of the great vessels	Aorta originates frim right ventricle, pulmonary artery from left ventricle	Severe anoxia and progressive cardiac failure, systemic arteries carry unoxygenated blood	Increase right-to-left shunt-balloon septostomy, create septal defect (palliation), pulmonary artery banding, total correction after 2 to 3 years	Chest roentgenogram– enlarged heart, "egg-shaped" heart Cardiac catheterization and angiography	Cyanosis, cardiac enlargement, congestive failure

failure supervenes, operation is best delayed until 10 or 12 years of age when the aorta approximates adult size.

Pulmonary stenosis of high resistance, overriding aorta, ventricular septal defect, and right ventricular hypertrophy are combined to form the tetralogy of Fallot. The high pulmonary outflow resistance shunts a portion of the blood into the left heart and systemic circulation, resulting in cyanosis or hypoxemia. Dyspnea, cyanosis, and convulsions may occur and squatting is common. Fingertip clubbing and stunting of growth often appear. The chest roentgenogram shows diminished vascularity of the lungs and the right ventricular hypertrophy produces a boot-shaped heart. Palliation may be afforded by anastomosing a systemic artery to the pulmonary system (e.g., subclavian artery or aorta to pulmonary artery). Total correction requires an open heart procedure in which the right ventricular outflow tract obstruction is relieved and the septal defect is repaired.

ACQUIRED HEART DISEASE

Heart Injuries

Most injuries of the heart are due to penetrating objects (e.g., knives, bullets, etc.) but blunt injuries may produce severe injuries as well. The chamber most involved by a penetrating object is the right ventricle. If the pericardial defect produced is large, exsanguination usually occurs if the myocardial injury is large. Pericardial tamponade will occur if this structure contains the blood, giving rise to an inhibition of cardiac output because of interference with right heart filling. A high venous pressure, hypotension, and a quiet heart to auscultation in the presence of a suggestive wound makes the diagnosis, and pericardiocentesis may be lifesaving. Surgical repair is indicated. Blunt injuries may produce a myocardial contusion with a clinical picture reminiscent of myocardial infarction, but it may be asymptomatic. The ECG may show S–T segment deviation or heart block, and an ECG should be done in the presence of all blunt thoracic injuries. Most recover spontaneously.

Intracardiac foreign bodies may embolize to lymph or peripheral vessels.

Neoplasms

Most primary neoplasms are benign (e.g., myxomas, rhabdomyomas, fibromas). About 20 percent are malignant, almost all sarcomas. Most myxomas occur in the left atrium. They may be silent or produce valvular obstruction or embolization. Most clinical signs depend upon the location of the tumor rather than its cell types. Metastatic disease of the heart is found in about one-quarter of cancer victims coming to autopsy. Breast, lung, kidney, and esophageal cancers as well as melanomas are frequently the primary tumors involved.

Coronary Artery Disease

Operation for coronary arteriosclerosis has become the cardiac operation most frequently done. Genetic factors, cigarette smoking, diabetes, and hypertension seem to be involved in most patients. Angina pectoris is the most common symptom leading to diagnosis. Myocardial infarction is the end stage of the process. Left main coronary stenosis and unstable angina are firm indications that infarction is imminent and revascularization by balloon dilatation or coronary bypass should be considered. Although angina is relieved in many of those operated upon, the prolongation of life has been more difficult to prove. When infarction has led to myocardial aneurysm formation, cardiac output may be seriously jeopardized and resection may be feasible.

Acquired Valvular Disease

The most common cause of acquired valvular disease is rheumatic fever (RF), followed by degenerative calcification, bacterial infection, syphilis, and other rare causes. RF usually involves the aortic and mitral valves and an interval of years or decades usually intervenes between the acute episode and the apperance of hemodynamic changes. Calcification of the aortic valve leads to stenosis but RF and acquired stenosis of a tricuspid valve also occur. Leaflet fusion is the result. Aortic regurgitation usually is due to RF. A wide pulse pressure, loud diastolic murmur, and a large left ventricle are present. Mitral stenosis (MS) is almost always due to RF, which causes leaflet fusion and shortening of the chordae tendiniae. Fatigue, dyspnea, hemoptysis, and atrial fibrillation are frequently present and embolization of atrial thrombi may occur. Mitral regurgitation (MG) usually results from RF, and tricuspid valvular disease rarely is found.

In all of the above, prosthetic or heterologous valvular devices may be used to replace diseased valves, the procedure being done using an extracorporeal circulation device to substitute for heart and lung function.

Heart transplantation and the use of the artificial heart are currently being employed for uncontrollable myocardial failure.

Pericardium

Inflammation of the pericardium, pericarditis, may be due to viruses, bacterial infection including tuberculosis, uremia, radiation, rheumatoid arthritis, and other disorders. Pericardial effusion may go on to tamponade, which might be fatal if untreated. Treatment is usually by medical means, or surgical drainage if this is ineffective. Chronic constrictive pericarditis is usually caused by tuberculosis or other bacteria or *Histoplasma* capsulatum. Lupus or chest trauma may be the precursor. When venous return becomes sufficiently impaired, pericardiectomy is indicated. Recurring effusion may be treated by creating a pericardial "window" by excising a small area of pericardium behind the xiphoid.

PERIPHERAL ARTERIAL DISEASE

Acute Arterial Occlusion

The usual causes of acute arterial occlusion are embolism, trauma, or thrombosis. Prominent features are pain, pallor, paresthesias, paralysis, and absence of pulses (five Ps). Paralysis and paresthesias signify severe occlusion with nerve anoxia. Emboli frequently originate in the diseased heart, atrial fibrillation, or myocardial infarcts favoring the clotting in the left heart chambers. Acute occlusions associated with fractures call for early arteriography and repair if indicated. Most acute arterial occlusions require prompt investigation (i.e., arteriography and treatment with embolectomy, thrombectomy, or vessel repair). Streptokinase infusion by intraluminal catheter placement after angiography is being widely used to reestablish patency of thrombosed arteries. Sources of emboli should be sought after the occluded vessel has been treated.

Chronic Arterial Occlusion

Chronic arterial obstructions usually occur in the abdominal aorta and its branches. Arteriosclerosis is the most common cause and diabetics frequently have more distal disease in tibial and feet vessels. Intermittent claudication is the most common symptom associated with chronic peripheral arterial occlusions. The pain of claudication characteristically comes on with exercise and gradually subsides with rest. Collaterals frequently develop sufficiently rapidly to lead to stabilization or even disappearance of pain. In the absence of diabetes, patients with claudication usually do not go on to amputation. Pain at rest and skin gangrene usually presage severe disease requiring angiography and bypass of obstructions or endarterectomy. Most such patients have smoked and continued use of tobacco is strongly contraindicated. Patients with peripheral occlusive disease have a high incidence of other cardiovascular catastrophes which often lead to death.

Impotence, claudication, and absence of femoral pulses or gangrene are characteristic of the Leriche's syndrome, which results from gradual occlusion of the abdominal aorta distal to the renal arteries. Vessel bifurcations are favored sites for atheromatous occlusion.

Another distinctive clinical picture centers about the propensity for occlusive disease at the carotid artery bifurcation. When the internal carotid artery narrows sufficiently, blood flow to the brain falls and stroke may ensue. More commonly, the atheromatous plaque may ulcerate to form a crater, which may form the nidus for a clot to form, break off, and embolize to the cerebral circulation. These tiny emboli give rise to the transient ischemic attack (TIA) which may give brief lapses of consciousness, memory, confusion, or temporary blindness (amaurosis fugax). Cervical bruits may be associated. Oculoplethysmography or arteriography (direct and venous) define the presence of the lesion.

The ulcerated plaques in the presence of symptoms usually indicate surgical correction. Endarterectomy usually suffices.

Several noninvasive testing devices are helpful in diagnosing varying degrees of arterial obstruction. Various Doppler devices and pressure recording devices identify levels and degrees of occlusion. The angiogram is the most reliable method of confirming the diagnosis and is required if operation is anticipated.

SURGICALLY CORRECTABLE HYPERTENSION

In the United States about 30 million people have hypertension. Less than 10 percent have lesions which can be corrected by surgical means. Recognized causes are the following:

1. Primary aldosteronism
2. Cushing's syndrome
3. Pheochromocytoma
4. Coarctation of the aorta
5. Renovascular hypertension
6. Unilateral renal parenchymal disease

Logistically, it would be almost impossible to study every hypertensive patient to exclude causative surgical lesions, to say nothing of the economic considerations. Many amenable to surgical correction may be suspected by careful history and physical examination and the use of simple laboratory and roentgenographic tests. Many hypertensives are given a trial of therapy, and successful control usually is taken as evidence of essential hypertension.

A history of urinary tract infections or peripheral vascular disease suggests renal parenchymal disease or renal artery stenosis. Flushing, sweating, and intermittency of hypertension leads one to suspect pheochromocytoma. Decreased femoral pulses suggest coarctation of the aorta, and an epigastric bruit may be due to renal artery stenosis.

The chest roentgenogram is often diagnostic for coarctation of the aorta (i.e., rib notching). Routine urine analysis may show proteinuria or urinary tract infection in advanced kidney disease. Hyperaldosteronism may be suspected by ECG or serum determination which show effects of hypokalemia.

Primary Aldosteronism

Primary hyperaldosteronism may be caused by hypersecretion of an adrenal adenoma or hyperplastic cells. Rarely adrenal carcinoma may be its cause. Aldosterone regulates extracellular fluid volume by controlling the excretion of sodium and water by the kidney. Females predominate three to one. Hypokalemia, low plasma renin activity, and increased serum sodium and CO_2 are usual laboratory findings. Treatment consists of resection of an adenoma or, in the case of hyperplasia, the adrenal shown to have the highest secretion on testing.

Pheochromocytoma

Pheochromocytoma is a rare but dramatic cause of hypertension. These tumors elaborate epinephrine and norepinephrine. The 24 hour urinary excretion of catecholamines (normally less than 10 $\mu g/24$ hrs) and the catecholamine metabolite VMA (usually over 7 $\mu g/24$ hrs) are frequent findings in patients with pheochromocytoma.

Aortography is very helpful in diagnosis, but not without danger in precipitating a hypertensive crisis. Therefore, catecholamine determinations should be made before this study is done. Treatment is surgical, but the preoperative preparation is exceedingly critical. Alpha and beta adrenergic blockade and assurance of adequate blood volume are critical.

Cushing's Syndrome

Cushing's syndrome is due to a chronic excess of cortisol. Central obesity ("buffalo hump" and "moon face"), amenorrhea, osteoporosis, abdominal striae, and hypertension characterize the clinical picture. Bilateral adrenal cortical hyperplasia is the most common cause (60–70 percent), but an adenoma may be at fault. Hyperplasia results from chronic ACTH stimulation from the pituitary. Occasionally a nonendocrine ACTH-secreting tumor of lung or other viscera is the cause. Secretion of 17-hydroxycorticosteroids, in normals, ranges from 3–12 mg in 24 hours. Patients with Cushing's syndrome usually secrete more than 12 mg/day. Aortography is a very useful adjunct in diagnosis.

Treatment depends upon the causative lesion. Adrenal tumors require complete resection. Bilateral lesions are present in about 10 percent of cases so bilateral adrenal exploration is desirable. Control of the parent ectopic ACTH tumor source (lung or pancreas) may result in improvement. When adrenal hyperplasia is responsible for a severe manifestation of the syndrome, bilateral adrenalectomy is required. Pituitary irradiation may control symptoms in less severe cases.

Coarctation of the Aorta

Coarctation of the aorta is suspect in any instance of hypertension in the young. Almost all occur in the first portion of the descending aorta. The cause of hypertension is debatable. Diminished or absent pulses in the lower extremities associated with normal pulses in the arms strongly favor the diagnosis. Untreated, coarctation leads to death in two-thirds of the patients before 40 years of age. Relief of the obstruction by resection results in remission of hypertension in 95 percent of cases.

Renovascular Hypertension

Renovascular hypertension results from activation of the renal-pressor mechanism (renin-angiotensin system). In about 70 percent, arteriosclerosis is the responsible lesion; most of the others are due to fibromuscular dysplasia of the renal artery, mostly in young women.

Except for an upper abdominal bruit, no distinctive physical findings are usually found. Ordinary laboratory tests are not helpful in diagnosis. Rapid-sequence urography, isotope renography, renal arteriography, and split renal function tests are very helpful. Split renal venous renin assay yields a 1.5 renin ratio of the involved to the uninvolved kidney. When split renal function tests and/or renin determination lateralize to one side, the rate of hypertension remission following renal artery reconstruction is about 90 percent.

Unilateral Renal Disease

Renal disease associated with hypertension and amenable to operation is limited to unilateral disease such as that produced by pyelonephritis, radiation fibrosis, congenital hypoplasia, or traumatic fibrosis. The cause of hypertension is thought to be activation of the renal pressor mechanism. Renal vein renin determination best identifies candidates for nephrectomy.

THE ACUTE ABDOMEN

Most diseases of the abdominal viscera which come to the attention of surgeons have the potential for causing pain sometime in their course. Indeed, the diagnosis of the "acute abdomen" usually requires the identification of the cause of abdominal pain and it must be emphasized that making an early diagnosis without adequate history is virtually impossible.

Pain impulses from the abdominal cavity reach the CNS by three routes. Visceral afferents travel *with* the sympathetic and parasympathetic nerves, and from the parietal peritoneum, body wall, and root of the mesentery and diaphragm via somatic afferents that travel in the segmented spinal nerves or phrenic nerves. The autonomic nervous system (ANS) includes the sympathetic and parasympathetic nerves which are efferent nerves. Afferent nerves do accompany the ANS but are not part of the system. The usual route of nervous impulses is from the axons of nerve endings in the wall of the viscus, which course with the visceral artery, thence to the aorta and through the collateral sympathetic ganglion without synapsing, and into the splanchnic nerves. The fiber proceeds (without synapsing) to the paravertebral sympathetic ganglion to then join the spinal nerve by way of white ramus communicans. The cell body of this primary visceral afferent neuron is located in the spinal ganglion, from which processes are sent to the posterior horns of the spinal cord via the posterior root. The central processes of the primary neurons synapse with at least three spinal tracts as sensory neurons which cross in the anterior commissure to the spinothalamic (antherolateral) tract and two others, the function of which is not entirely clear. Sensory tracts synapse in the thalamus which project to the cerebral cortex. The area(s) of the cortex which perceives pain is not well defined and, indeed, the hypothalamus, the limbic system, and the reticular formation of the brains stem are involved in pain perception.

There are three recognized types of pain involved with abdominal disorders (i.e., visceral, somatic, and referred).

Visceral Pain

Visceral or splanchnic pain arises in abdominal organs which are covered with visceral peritoneum. Viscera are normally insensitive to stimuli (e.g., cutting, burning, etc.) which cause pain when applied to the skin. Stimuli causing visceral pain are distention (tension) and ischemia. Visceral pain tends to be diffuse and is poorly localized. Autonomic reflexes such as nausea and vomiting, sweating, bradycardia or tachycardia, hypotension, and involuntary contractions of abdominal wall muscles are common.

Somatic Pain

Pain arising in the root of the mesentery, the diaphragm, and parietal peritoneum is carried by somatic afferents in segmental spinal nerves and therefore is more sharply localized and more intense than visceral pain. The pain of appendicitis is an excellent example of generalized visceral discomfort (distention) followed by somatic pain (peritoneal irritation) which is localized in the right lower quadrant.

Referred Pain

Diseases of viscera may cause pain localized in more superficial areas of the body. This probably results from convergence of skin and visceral afferents upon the same neuron in the pain pathway, which is interpreted by the brain as originating in the skin.

The causes of abdominal pain amenable to surgery can be broadly grouped as inflammatory, mechanical obstruction, and vascular causes.

Inflammation usually results from peritonitis, localized or generalized, owing to an underlying visceral disorder. On occasion, primary peritonitis (e.g., pneumococcal, tuberculous, or streptococcal) occurs without evident visceral disease. Chemical nonbacterial peritonitis may produce great pain. Ruptured ulcer, perforated ovarian cyst, or ruptured gallbladder are examples. Both hollow and solid viscera are frequent sources of pain and none is exempt. Operations for cholecystitis, appendicitis, endometriosis, and diverticulitis are among the most commonly performed.

Mechanical obstruction causing distention of hollow viscera such as the gallbladder, colon, small intestine, and ureter are among the most common of surgical emergencies. Acute enlargement of the liver and spleen produces pain by capsular distention.

Vascular disorders leading to arterial or venous obstruction or intraperitoneal bleeding cause pain, and the bleeding associated with traumatic injury of the spleen or liver is manifest by the peritoneal irritation they cause. Infarction of the bowel due to mesenteric thrombosis is among the most serious of surgical disorders. Early recognition is of special importance in situations where surgical intervention can eliminate the serious consequence of infarction of major portions of the intestinal tract. Arterial embolism and torsion due to adhesions or volvulus, when treated before bowel infarction occurs, is associated with marked reduction in morbidity and mortality.

Extraperitoneal Causes of Abdominal Pain

The surgeon must be acutely aware of a variety of disorders which cause abdominal pain but which do not require operation. Indeed, unnecessary operation may lead to death owing to the added stress. Intrathoracic disease such as myocardial infarction, pulmonary embolism and pneumonia are the most serious with which a surgical disease may be misidentified. Chest roentgenograms, ECG, and taking a careful history lessen the risk of misdiagnosis. Genitourinary disease such as pyelonephritis, prostatitis, and epididymitis, and neurogenic sources such as osteomyelitis of the spine, cord tumors, herpes zoster, and tabes dorsalis are often mistaken for abdominal problems. Hematologic and metabolic diseases including sickle cell anemia, leukemia, uremia, diabetic acidosis, and porphyria may mimic peritonitis. Toxins, venoms, and lead poisoning add to the list.

Evaluation of Abdominal Pain

The appreciation of pain requires consciousness and an intact sensory nervous system. Sensitivity to pain tends to diminish with old age. Hyperthyroidism seems to increase sensitivity to pain, and there appears to be ethnic differences in sensitivity to pain (i.e., Latins and Jews appear to be more sensitive). Severe pain may cause bradycardia and hypotension, and superficial pain often leads to epinephrine outpouring with tachycardia.

The history is of great importance, and most abdominal pain lasting more than 5 or 6 hours is surgical in implication. The character, severity, location, and exacerbating factors should be noted. Colic, high intensity, intermittent pain usually means intestinal, ureteral, or biliary obstruction. Pain due to a penetrating ulcer may be "burning" in character, while pain produced by inflammation tends to be less intense, and pain due to peritonitis is usually commensurate with the amount of rigidity present and tends to be continuous.

The location of pain (initial and present) is helpful in suggesting its origin. Small intestinal pain usually is midabdominal, and colon disorders usually cause pain in the lower abdomen. The patient's age suggests the likely presence of cancer or other disorders prone to occur in the age group. Appendicitis usually occurs in the young, cholecystitis in middle age, and diverticulitis and cancer usually in older age groups. The menstrual history may lead to a diagnosis of ectopic pregnancy. Previous operation makes adhesions a likely cause of intestinal obstruction. Bowel history is of great importance in intestinal obstruction.

Examination of the patient by inspection usually suggests illness owing to restriction of movement. Patients with peritonitis move cautiously. Auscultation may reveal borborygmi due to mechanical intestinal obstruction or absence of peristalsis due to peritonitis. Palpation should begin away from the area of maximal discomfort and must include a search for hernia. Gentle percussion best determines the site of maximum tenderness, and masses may be obscured by abdominal wall rigidity. Pelvic and rectal examinations are mandatory parts of the examination.

Laboratory Procedures

Elaborate laboratory tests are rarely required in the presence of an acute abdomen. Blood studies to include the hematocrit and white blood cell count with differential are useful in determining the presence of anemia of inflammation. The urine analysis helps to detect diabetes, urinary tract infection, or porphyria, and red cells may suggest calculi. A high serum amylase is usually related to acute pancreatitis, but perforated viscera, cholecystitis, and other inflammatory processes often cause elevations. In blacks, a sickle cell preparation may indicate sickle cell disease.

Appropriate roentgenographic studies include a chest roentgenogram to rule out intrathoracic disease, and supine and upright or decubitus films to demonstrate free air and intestinal distention. In patients over 40, an ECG is advisable to rule out myocardial ischemia, which may be very useful in instances of suspected pancreatitis or cholecystitis. Peritoneal lavage and culdoscopy are very useful in discovering intrperitoneal blood. Laparotomy may be required if the clinical situation suggests an acute abdomen in the presence of negative studies.

STOMACH

Duodenal Ulcer

Duodenal ulcer forms as a result of excess acid-peptic gastric secretions. Pepsin must act with excess acid to form the chronic duodenal ulcer. Acid hypersecretion appears to depend upon vagal activity. There appears to be a predilection among siblings of peptic ulcer patients, in subjects with blood group O, and in those patients with pulmonary emphysema, cirrhosis, and chronic pancreatitis. The relationship between the hypergastrinemia of the Zollinger-Ellison syndrome and gastroduodenal ulceration is well known and is the most virulent form of gastrointestinal ulcer disease.

Pain is the most frequent symptom, and when conservative treatment fails the intractable ulcer is the prime indication for operation. Bleeding, obstruction, and perforation are the most common other indications for operation.

Operations currently used most widely as definitive therapy for duodenal ulcer are based upon reduction in acid-secreting capacity of the stomach. Removal of a major portion of the parietal cell mass by gastrectomy and the removal of the stimulation of gastric secretion by vagotomy are currently in greatest use. Vagotomy combined with a procedure designed to promote gastric emptying is now most used.

Gastric Ulcer

Pyloric canal ulcers behave much like duodenal ulcers and clinically they are similar. High-lying stomach ulcers seem to occur in a different setting (Table 14-4).

About 25 percent of chronic gastric ulcers are associated with duodenal ulcer. Stasis caused by the duodenal ulcer may account for gastric ulceration.

Symptoms of gastric ulcer often are very similar to those of duodenal ulcer. They are often asymptomatic until a complication (i.e., bleeding or perforation) occurs. The recurrence rate after healing is higher with gastric ulcer than with duodenal ulcer.

Duodenal ulcers are very rarely malignant, while gastric ulcers not infrequently are.

The indications for operation are the following:

1. Pyloric channel ulcers
2. Gastric ulcers associated with duodenal ulcers
3. Gastric ulcers with deep penetration (bleeding and perforation common)
4. Prior bleeding
5. Healing less than 50 percent over 3 week trial of treatment
6. Giant ulcers
7. Recurrence after initial healing
8. Multiple gastric ulcers
9. When any doubt about malignancy exists

Partial gastrectomy or vagotomy plus pyloroplasty are the usual operations performed for gastric ulcer. If a duodenal ulcer is present as well vagotomy should be part of the procedure done.

Diagnosis of both duodenal ulcer and gastric ulcer is by roentgenogram and endoscopic examination. Cytologic examination and endoscopic biopsy are important adjuncts in ruling out malignancy in gastric ulcer.

Stress Ulceration

Trauma, pulmonary insufficiency, and sepsis are important causes of acute mucosal ulcerations of the stomach and duodenum. These ulcerations are multiple, tend to occur in the fundus, and are superficial. The serious complication is severe bleeding and some may perforate.

Early endoscopy aids in diagnosis. Transfusion, gastric cooling, and buffering by antacids are important adjuncts of treatment. Occasionally operation will be required and "ulcer" operations are usually employed.

Mallory-Weiss Syndrome

Longitudinal mucosal tears along the gastroesophageal junction characterize this syndrome. Most cases seem to be related to acute alcohol intoxication with violent retching. Bleeding from such tears can be massive. Occasionally full thickness tears can result in perforation.

Gastric Cancer

For unknown reasons, the incidence of stomach cancer has been declining in the past two or three decades in the United States, England, Norway, and Holland. Although the cause is essentially unknown, some risk factors are the ingestion of smoked fish, blood type A, and atrophic gastritis and achlorhydria. Malignant transformation of gastric ulcer probably does not occur.

Symptoms are vague and nonspecific. Antral lesions may obstruct and cause vomiting. Dull pain, weight loss, anorexia, and anemia are frequently associated and usually signify that the lesion is beyond surgical cure. More than half will have metastasized to regional nodes, and direct extension of the gastric tumor to liver and pancreas is common. Gastric resection offers the only prospect for cure but less than 20 percent survive 5 years.

Other malignant tumors are uncommon and are mostly of lymphomas and leiomyosarcomas. Surgical treatment is indicated. Benign tumors are not so un-

Table 14-4. Differences of Duodenal and Gastric Ulcers

	Duodenal Ulcer	Gastric Ulcer
	Young and Middle Age	Old
Stress relationship	High	Low
Blood type association	Type O	Type A
Gastric acid secretion	High	Low

common. Some benign polyps may undergo malignant degeneration. Leiomyoms, neurogenic tumors, fibromas, and lipomas occur and are often found on gastrointestinal roentgenograms done for other suspected lesions.

PANCREAS, LIVER, AND BILIARY SYSTEM

Pancreas

Congenital lesions of the pancreas are rare, the most frequent being annular pancreas, which tends to encircle the second portion of the duodenum. When they cause obstruction, bypassing by duodenojejunostomy is the preferred treatment.

Pancreatitis, an inflammatory process, may be acute or chronic. Acute episodes in the course of chronic pancreatitis may be called relapsing pancreatitis. The cause may be obscure, but some situations predispose. Gallstones are frequently present, but less than one-fifth have common duct stones. The relationship is uncertain. Alcoholism is a frequent precursor, but the exact mechanism is unknown. Postoperative pancreatitis may be related to direct trauma during operations upon the biliary tract or stomach; often the cause is obscure, but mortality approaches 50 percent. Metabolic causes such as hyperparathyroidism and hereditary conditions that cause aminoaciduria or hyperlipidemia may be associated.

Diagnosis is usually made following the onset of acute epigastric pain which may radiate to the back. Vomiting is common. Frequently, pain is triggered by the ingestion of a heavy meal. Epigastric tenderness and guarding are found, and fever and tachycardia are common. Elevations of serum amylase are confirmatory, but by no means all patients have marked elevations. The urine amylase determination is a more sensitive test. Renal clearance of amylase is enhanced with pancreatitis. Low serum calcium levels often indicate a poor prognosis since it is associated with extensive disease with fat necrosis. Abdominal roentgenograms may reveal a "sentinel loop," a segment of localized small bowel ileus, but it is not specific. The chance for error in diagnosis is present and sometimes laparotomy may be the only certain method.

Treatment consists of meticulous support by fluid and electrolyte correction and necessary transfusions, calcium, and insulin replacement provided for. The stomach must be kept empty by nasogastric suction. Occasionally, debridement of the necrotic pancreas is indicated.

Complications consist of pseudocyst formation and secondary hemorrhage. Diabetes, calcification, and steatorrhea occur almost exclusively in alcoholic pancreatitis.

Chronic pancreatitis is most common in alcoholics and often narcotic addiction is present as well. Chronic pain due to segmental ductal obstruction may be relieved by pancreatojejunostomy.

Pancreatic trauma may be caused by penetrating or blunt injuries. Most blunt injury disruptions occur at the neck because of the prevertebral fixed retroperitoneal position. Most have associated visceral injury. Partial or complete resections and drainage procedures may be employed. The indications for operation may be on clinical evaluation or peritoneal lavage, where blood or elevated amylase may be detected in lavage fluid.

Most tumors involving the pancreas are adenocarcinomas arising in the gland or in the periampullary region. Ductal carcinomas predominate, often are small, and often become clinically manifest because of their location in the head of the pancreas, which lies in proximity to the common bile duct. Perineural and lymph node spread is very common. Weight loss and dull pain often precede jaundice. Examination may reveal a distended gallbladder, but it is by no means constant. Laboratory tests to detect obstructive jaundice are the most reliable. Serum bilirubin rarely exceeds 35 mg/100 ml (may be much higher with hepatic disease), the alkaline phosphatase is usually elevated, and a decrease in fecal urobilinogen is highly suggestive. Most will show radiographic signs with contrast studies such as a "reverse 3" sign and widening of the duodenal loop. Computerized tomography (CT) scan may clearly show the lesion and its presence in relation to the bile ducts and vessels, and is especially useful in lesions of the body or tail of the pancreas when jaundice is not present.

Operative resection affords the only opportunity for cure and biliary bypass may provide substantial palliation in relieving jaundice. Obtaining an accurate diagnosis at the time of operation is a major problem and the decision for pancreatoduodenectomy must often be made on the basis of gross findings. Five year survivorship does not exceed 20 percent at very best and many patients can be offered only jaundice-relieving palliation.

ISLET CELL TUMORS

Hyperinsulinism results from the presence of tumors of pancreatic beta cells. Profound hypoglycemia results with most manifestations seen in the CNS, which depends mostly on glucose for its metabolism. Confusion, convulsions, mental deterioration, and even death may ensue. Glucose administration rapidly reverses the hypoglycemia and the symptoms disappear.

Most of the tumors are benign adenomas but the severity of the hypoglycemia bears little relationship to the severity of symptoms.

The diagnosis is suggested by the presence of Whipple's triad: (1) attacks precipitated by fasting or exertion, (2) fasting blood sugar below 50 mg/100 ml, and (3) relief of symptoms by administration of oral or intravenous glucose. Hepatogenic hypoglycemia and functional hyperinsulinism may account for hypoglycemia as well and must be ruled out. Serum insulin level determinations, angiography, and CT scanning are valuable adjuncts in diagnosis.

Early resection of islet cell tumors is indicated to avoid permanent CNS changes. If a tumor is not found, subtotal resection of the body and tail may remove an undiscovered adenoma or hyperfunctioning islets.

Ulcerogenic Islet Cell Tumors. Nonbeta islet cell tumors may provide virulent gastrointestinal ulceration due to gastric hypersecretion (Zollinger-Ellison syndrome). Markedly elevated gastrin levels tend to confirm the suspicion that the Zollinger-Ellison syndrome is present.

If cimetidine therapy is ineffective, most will require operation. The multiplicity of tumors often makes resection of the target organ, the stomach, advisable. Total gastrectomy is usually required unless the tumor is located in the duodenal wall.

Liver

Surgical procedures involving the liver largely are concerned with trauma, tumors, cysts, and infections. Portal hypertension, a complication of hepatic cirrhosis, is importantly related but does not involve direct surgical procedures upon the liver.

Trauma of the liver is especially dangerous because of its vascularity. Blunt injuries are especially hazardous. Blood loss and associated injuries account for the morbidity and mortality. Diagnosis is made by the peritoneal tenderness and guarding, hypotension, and, in many instances, by peritoneal lavage. The important consideration is whether operation is required since valuable time may be lost if specific organ injury diagnosis is sought.

Treatment consists primarily of control of bleeding by suture ligation. Resection of liver tissue may be required and bile leaks must be controlled.

Tumors of the liver in North America are mostly metastatic from other structures. Primary liver tumors are unusual in Western countries. Most are malignant but benign adenomas and hemagiomas do occur, and adenoma formation appears to be related to ingestion of oral contraceptives in young women. Cirrhosis predisposes to malignant liver tumors, and a racial factor in Oriental and African cultures is apparent. Resection is indicated when the process is sufficiently confined to permit extirpation. Intra-arterial and systemic chemotherapy have a place in unresectable malignant lesions.

Abscess usually is metastatic from an infective process or as a result of trauma. Drainage and antibiotic therapy are indicated. Amebic abscess should first be treated with iodoquinol (Diodoquin), chloroquine, and emetine; in ineffective, open drainage within 2 or 3 days is indicated. The CT scan is a valuable diagnostic adjunct.

Cysts are best treated by resection. Hydatid cysts may be enucleated after injection of a formalin solution, which tends to reduce contamination by dissemination of the scoleces and capsules.

Portal hypertension is caused by obstructed portal outflow. Collateral circulation frequently develops at the gastroesophageal junction, at the umbilicus and anus. Esophageal varices are prone to massive hemorrhage. Congestive splenomegaly may lead to hypersplenism. Ascites is common and serum proteins tend to be low. Aldosterone secretion is increased and sodium retention abets the process. Disturbed nitrogen metabolism results in ammonia accumulation in the blood, resulting in hepatic encephalopathy. Bleeding is temporarily controlled by a balloon-tube, and sclerotherapy by injection. Portosystemic shunts provide amelioration of the bleeding tendency. Sclerotherapy is being used more frequently as definitive treatment.

Biliary System

The gallbladder is among the most common of organs treated by surgeons. Over 10 percent of the population have gallstones, women predominating. Most stones are composed of cholesterol or bilirubin and may be mixed. Hemolytic anemias produce bilirubin stones. In most cases, stones form from an imbalance of concentrations of cholesterol, bile salts, and lecithin. Stones may be silent, cause ductal obstruction or lead to infection. Cystic duct obstruction promotes the development of the acute gallbladder, and stones passing into the common duct may obstruct to give rise to jaundice or infection (cholangitis). Chronic calculous cholecystitis as seen by the clinician typically results in repeated attacks of right upper quadrant pain which may radiate to the right scapular area. Attacks tend to occur after food, especially fat, ingestion. Peptic ulcer, coronary heart disease, and hiatal hernia may cause similar episodes and must be carefully eliminated prior to recommending operation. Acute cholecystitis occurs when stones obstruct the cystic duct. The tender gallbladder may be palpable and tenderness is present. Perforation and gangrene are possible, but unusual, complications. Fever and leukocytosis suggest such impending complications and operation may be advisable.

Choledocholithiasis may lead to obstruction, producing jaundice with or without cholangitis. Bile darkens the urine and stools may lack pigment. Serum direct bilirubin is elevated and alkaline phosphatase is usually markedly elevated.

Calculous disease is best diagnosed by ultrasonography, which additionally shows ductal size.

Most patients with symptomatic gallstones should be treated by cholecystectomy. The acute gallbladder may be safely treated conservatively, if improvement is rapid, thereby avoiding the hazards of operation in an acutely inflamed field. Small common duct stones may be removed by endoscopic retrograde techniques carried out through the ampulla of Vater.

Cancer of the gallbladder is a virulent tumor which usually occurs in the presence of stones. Symptoms are not specific and usually are suggestive of gallstone disease. Occasionally, in situ tumors are resectable for cure. Bile duct tumors may occur anywhere in the system, and those found at the confluence of the hepatic ducts or below may be amenable to removal, usually by pancreatoduodenal resection.

SMALL INTESTINE

The small bowel differs from the large intestine in remarkable ways, one of the most notable being the differences in susceptibility to tumor formation, inflammatory conditions, and mechanisms of obstruction. They vary greatly in function. The upper gastrointestinal tract secretes a variety of digestive enzymes and is involved in the early stages of digestion. Approximately 5,000 ml of secretions enter the small bowel in a 24-hour period. Saliva (1,500 ml), gastric juice (1,000 ml), pancreatic juice (2,000 ml), and bile (500 ml) containing electrolytes of varying composition contribute to the fluid flux of the intestine. These substances contribute to the digestion of carbohydrates, proteins, and fats, which are absorbed as sugars, amino acids, and fatty acids, respectively. The colon, by contrast, functions mostly as a storage compartment for fecal material and as a principal site of water absorption.

Small intestinal obstructions comprise one of the most frequent disorders surgeons must treat. The causes of small bowel obstructions differ sharply between childhood and the mature years. Hernial incarcerations account for about 40 percent in both groups, while adhesions, mostly secondary to earlier operations, are common in adults and quite unusual in children. Volvulus and intussusception are shared by both, while py-

loric stenosis, congenital atresias, and annular pancreas are seen almost exclusively in children. Cancer causes about 10 percent of small intestinal obstructions in adults.

Profound physiologic changes result from small bowel obstructions. Pyloric obstruction results in vomiting with major losses of hydrogen and chloride ions, with resulting hypochloremic alkalosis. Obstruction below the ampulla of Vater results in loss of Na^+, K^+, and HCO_3^-, with generalized electrolyte and water depletion. Distention due to gas and fluid gives rise to painful peristaltic rushes of intermittent (colic) character. High-pitched peristalsis is heard. Pain is generally in the periumbilical area due to the vague nature of afferent visceral nerve stimulation as opposed to sharper localization associated with somatic nerve stimulation when parietal peritoneum becomes inflamed. When both ingress and egress are blocked, a "closed-loop" obstruction exists and will cause varying degrees of vascular obstruction, which, if it progresses, results in strangulation obstruction with gangrene, usually reflected in tenderness of the abdomen overlying the involved bowel. Although leukocytosis, fever, progression of pain, and metabolic acidosis are characteristic of vascular compromise, a significant number of patients lack one or more of these features and it is often better to do a laparotomy than to risk an oversight with extensive loss of small bowel or even death being the result.

Intestinal paralysis (ileus) is a common disorder which is frequently seen after abdominal operations or as part of other disease processes such as uremia and diabetic acidosis or following opiate administration. It is important to differentiate ileus from mechanical obstructions since the latter usually require operation while ileus rarely would require it. Peristalsis is diminished and abdominal roentgenograms usually suggest the diffuse intestinal atony in contradistinction to the ladder sign associated with mechanical obstructions in which fluid levels in the distal segment of a visible loop are higher than in the proximal segment.

Treatment of intestinal obstruction must be vigorous in restoring fluid and electrolyte balance. Intestinal decompression by intubation of stomach or small intestine should be provided but should not be considered a substitute for operation. The critical issue is the possibility that gangrene will supervene, which carries with it a 25 percent mortality rate. Therefore, operation is the mainstay of treatment early rather than too late. Antibiotic coverage to include agents effective against anaerobes should be given preoperatively. In those instances where conservative treatment, usually by long tube (Cantor, Miller-Abbott, etc.) insertion, seems indicated, a substantial number will respond (usually in patients with adhesions) without operation. Careful watching is required to be certain that vascular compromise is not occurring.

Small Intestinal Fistula

Fistulas of the small intestine are among the most formidable complications of abdominal operations. When the fluid output is high, serious fluid and electrolyte and nutritional deficits occur. Fistulas are classified as internal when the communication is between hollow viscera, or external when the communication is to a body surface. When the tract is to surrounding tissue it may be considered a sinus tract into an adjacent cavity. The leaking duodenal stump is an example of the latter.

Most fistulas result from operative trauma but injury, regional enteritis, foreign bodies, or neoplasms may also be causative.

The most serious fistulas are the external ones, and those with a fluid output greater than 500 ml/24 hours are considered high output fistulas. Most high output fistulas involve the upper small intestine. Persistent pain, tenderness, fever, and leukocytosis are suggestive early signs of fistula development, and when drainage of bile-stained fluid through the wound occurs the diagnosis is confirmed. Radiographic visualization following the ingestion of contrast material may confirm and even identify the site of leakage.

The outcome depends largely upon the age and nutrition of the patient and the associated disease duration (i.e., one present many weeks is less likely to close).

Treatment consists of monitoring fluid and electrolyte balance along with nutritional support. Intravenous hyperalimentation leads to healing in most patients. If it fails, operation may be required. Protection of the skin using appropriately applied bags and skin care are important nursing considerations. At operation, closure of the fistulous tract of defunctionalizing procedures best achieve a good result. Failure of both conservative and surgical methods of treatment is most often due to neoplasm, granulomatous disease, local infection, foreign body, or epithelialization of the tract, and relief of these problems by resection may be required before healing will occur. Intravenous hyperalimentation provides the nutrition and bowel defunctionalization which has revolutionized the treatment of fistulas.

Inflammatory Small Bowel Disease

Crohn's disease (regional enteritis) is the most common inflammatory disease affecting the small intestine. The terminal ileum is most often involved but all other areas of the intestinal tract may be involved. The Jewish population appears to have a significant increased incidence and it is rare in blacks, hispanics, and American Indians. The cause is unknown. Malnutrition due to protein loss and decreased food intake is common. Diarrhea and abdominal pain, the presence of palpable abdominal mass, and sometimes fistulization into the bladder or vagina may be presenting findings. A third or more demonstrate carbohydrate or fat malabsorption, which may be made worse by intestinal resection. Contrast roentgenograms studies demonstrate disturbances of peristaltic activity, irregularity of mucosa, and thickening of the valvulae conniventes. Fibrosis and obstruction are late findings. Angiography reveals mesenteric arterial vessels which are dilated and abruptly tapered.

Medical treatment includes drugs to control diarrhea, steroids, and immunosuppressive therapy. Intravenous hyperalimentation leads to remission in about 75 percent of patients.

Surgical treatment, advised for disabling symptoms, fistulae, and obstruction, is best provided by resection with restoration of continuity or, when this is not practical, by bypass procedure. Recurrence is frequent and reoperation is often necessary.

Small Bowel Tumors

Neoplasms of the small intestine are rare, in sharp contrast to the colon. When involved with tumor, the duodenum, upper jejunum, and terminal ileum are most susceptible. Malignant carcinoids and polyps are associated with the carcinoid syndrome and Peutz-Jeghers syndrome.

Most benign tumors are polyps, lipomas, leiomyomas, and hemangiomas which may cause obstruction, bleeding, and rarely perforation. More than half are detected at laparotomy. Contrast roentgenograms and angiography are the only worthwhile studies and these lesions are often missed.

The Peutz-Jeghers syndrome consists of intestinal polyposis and melanin spots on the lips or oral mucosa transmitted as a simple mendelian dominant with a high degree of penetration. The polyps are hamartomas and therefore not malignant. Intestinal bleeding or obstruction is the most common presentation.

Primary malignant tumors are rare, adenocarcinoma being the most common. The others are malignant carcinoids, lymphomas, and sarcomas. Obstruction and bleeding call attention to them.

The carcinoid syndrome is characterized by episodes of flushing of the skin, abdominal pain, diarrhea, and asthmalike spells suggesting massive liver involvement with tumor. Right-sided cardiac lesions often are present. Serotonin is deaminated in the liver, and when massive hepatic replacement occurs, 5-hydroxyindole acetic acid (5-HIAA) is excreted in the urine which, when detected, is the basis for diagnosis. The small bowel harbors the malignant carcinoid in about 30 percent of patients, with most of the remainder originating in the colon or appendix.

COLON, RECTUM, ANUS, APPENDIX

The colon differs substantially from the small intestine in several ways. It is much shorter, partly retroperitoneal, and much more subject to tumor and inflammatory diseases. Its blood supply comes from both superior and inferior mesenteric arteries which anastomose via the marginal artery of Drummond. Lymphatics follow the intermediate arteries to the preaortic nodes at the origins of the superior and inferior mesenteric arteries. The nerve supply is autonomic with sympathetic fibers from the thoracolumbar portion of the spinal cord synapsing in the preaortic sympathetic ganglia. Here the postganglionic fibers originate and follow the major arteries to terminate in the submucosal (Meissner's) and myenteric (Auerbach's) plexuses. The presacral nerve originates below the aortic bifurcation and joins the parasympathetic nerves (nervi erigentes) to form the pelvic plexuses which supply fibers to the pelvic viscera. If the pelvic autonomics are damaged during operation, impotence and poor bladder function may result. The levator ani, external sphincter, and coccygeus are supplied by fibers from the fourth sacral segment to control these voluntary muscles.

The function of the colon is to absorb water and electrolytes and to store and expel feces. Most of the absorption occurs on the right side, while storage and expulsion functions reside on the left. Bile acids are absorbed by passive diffusion.

Inflammatory Diseases

Granulomatous colitis (Crohn's disease) involves all layers of the colon. The cause is unknown and, characteristically, the distal ileum is involved. Clinically it shares many of the features of ulcerative colitis. Abdominal pain and diarrhea are prominent symptoms. Perianal fistulas and granulomas are often present as well as internal fistulas to the bladder, vagina, or other intestinal sites.

Ulcerative colitis primarily involves the mucosa but full-thickness involvement may occur with the development of dilatation (toxic megacolon), possibly perforation due to full-thickness destruction. Diarrhea, bleeding, and abdominal pain are frequently present. Iritis, uveitis, arthritis, pyoderma gangrenosum, and ery-

thema nodosum are systemic complications sometimes present.

There is a distinct tendency to develop cancer of the colon in ulcerative colitis if the process has been present for over 10 years. This along with massive hemorrhage and perforation comprise the absolute indications for operation. Obstruction, fistula formation, chronic blood loss, chronic pain, and disability are indications for operation with transmural colitis. Formerly it was believed that granulomatous colitis caused no increased risk of cancer; this is probably not true.

Elective operation for failing to respond to medical management is commonly done, and the decision is based upon duration and severity of symptoms. Proctocolectomy is curative if ulcerative colitis is present. Colon resection for Crohn's disease often leaves small intestinal disease behind, with an uncertain future.

Toxic megacolon is the most dreaded complication of ulcerative colitis. Gaseous distention of the colon on roentgenogram in a patient with rising fever, tachycardia, and abdominal pain and distention strongly suggests this diagnosis. Most agree that early operation (before 5 days) is indicated instead of prolonged medical therapy.

Other types of colitis include pseudomembranous colitis due to various antibiotics (e.g., clindamycin, lincomycin, and chloramphenicol) and amebiasis.

Diverticular Disease

Diverticulosis is a common disorder in which outpouchings occur through areas of weakness due to increased intraluminal pressure. The sigmoid and left colon are most prone to develop these false diverticula covered only by mucosa and serosa. True diverticula containing all layers are rare and mostly occur in the right colon. Inflammation, with or without abscess formation or perforation, bleeding, and obstruction are complications which may require operation. Free rupture with widespread peritonitis is a very serious complication requiring early operation. Simple inflammation may be treated conservatively. Fistulas to the bladder, vagina, or other viscera may require operation. Resection is the fundamental definitive operative procedure, but anastomosis may only be safely done if inflammatory changes are minimal. Free perforations are best treated by resection of the involved segment, end-colostomy and exteriorization, or closure of the distal colon segment. Subsequent anastomosis can be done weeks later when inflammatory changes have subsided. Massive bleeding is a rather rare complication which may sometimes be controlled by barium enema. About 5 percent of colon obstructions are due to diverticulitis. Relief of obstruction, often by proximal colostomy followed by resection and anastomosis, is appropriate.

Traumatic Injury of Colon and Rectum

Because of the potential for virulent infection, colon and rectum wounds are the most serious of the hollow viscera. Blunt injuries may result in delayed perforation days after injury. Any suspicion calls for the administration of broad spectrum systemic antibiotics. The decision for the specific type of operative procedure depends upon the time between injury and operation, degree of fecal spillage, and type and extent of colonic wound. Simple small perforations may be closed primarily after debridement if done within a few hours of injury. Major wounds are best treated by exteriorization (transverse or left colon), end-colostomy with closure of the distal segment (Hartmann's procedure), or resection with proximal diversion of ileum or colon. If the rectum is injured, drainage of the presacral space is indicated, with proximal colostomy and repair where possible. Associated genitourinary injury must be excluded and appropriately managed.

Volvulus of the Colon

Volvulus is a twisting of a mobile segment of the bowel about its mesentery. Partial or complete obstruction results, and circulatory compromise and gangrene may follow. About three-quarters involve the sigmoid and then the cecum. Volvulus is the most common cause of colon strangulation. Advanced age and neurologic disease appear to predispose. Initial treatment depends upon whether strangulation is suspected; if it is, operative intervention is indicated. Sigmoidoscopic reduction should otherwise be attempted and barium enema may reduce the volvulus as well. Cecal volvulus is managed by operation and resection or fixation.

Abdominal pain and distention associated with a characteristically dilated colon on roentgenograms are highly suggestive of this diagnosis.

Tumors of the Colon and Rectum

POLYPS

Polyps may be neoplastic, hamartomatous, or inflammatory. Adenomatous polyps are neoplasms and may be sessile (broad base) or pedunculated (on a stalk). It is the most common of all polyps. About 75 percent occur in the rectum or sigmoid. Bleeding is the usual symptom, many are silent, and malignant transformation occurs in 1–2 percent.

Villous adenomas usually occur after 50 years of age and their soft, diffuse character makes them very difficult to palpate. Invasive cancer occurs in 25–30 percent. Bloody mucus may be passed and rarely hypokalemia,

hypochloremia, or hyponatremia may result if the discharge is copious.

Juvenile polyps usually occur in children under 12 and are almost all pedunculated. They are not premalignant but, if within reach of the colonoscope, should be excised.

Multiple familial polyposis is an inherited autosomal dominant which appears in about half the children of the affected parent, and almost all those affected will develop colorectal cancer by 40 to 50 years of life if left untreated. These polyps usually develop about puberty. Removal of the involved colon is indicated. If only a few rectal polyps are present, the rectum may be spared if very close proctoscopic surveillance and polyp removal are practiced. Gardner's syndrome is a variant in which, in addition to colon polyps, the patient has osteomas of the skull or mandible, soft tissue sebaceous cysts, or desmoid tumors alone or in combination. In Peutz-Jegher's syndrome, colon polyps may be present but small intestinal polyps predominate. Melanin spots on the lips and buccal mucosa complete the clinical syndrome. Intussusception is a common complication. Other lesions such as carcinoids, hyperplasias, and pseudopolyps associated with ulcerative and granulomatous colitis all may assume a polypoid configuration.

Air contrast barium enemas and colonoscopy are very useful in diagnosis in all polypoid lesions.

Cancer of the Colon, Rectum, and Anus

Adenocarcinoma of the colon is the most common visceral cancer in the United States, accounting for 50,000 deaths/year. Right- and left-sided lesions differ in occurrence rate, gross appearance, signs, symptoms, and ease of diagnosis. The usual right-sided tumor is a fungating, ulcerating tumor which projects into the lumen, while on the left side it is characteristically annular and constricting with a greater tendency for obstruction. Anemia due to chronic bleeding is usual with right-sided lesions, while left-sided ones often produce obstipation, crampy pain, weight loss, and gross blood in the stool. Sigmoidoscopy or colonoscopy and barium enema must be done to rule out these lesions.

Metastasis occurs by lymphatic or venous routes and prognosis depends upon whether such has occurred.

If both gross and microscopic penetration of the tumor are superficial, the survival rate is excellent. When deep bowel wall penetration or lymph node spread is present, survival at 5 years falls sharply. When distant metastases are present, almost none survive. If the cancer is confined to the bowel wall, about 60 percent live 5 years. Lymph node metastases (Dukes' C) is associated with survival of about 25 percent. Cancer of the rectum tends to have spread further before diagnosis and the 5-year survivorship is about 45 percent despite the fact that it is more accessible for diagnosis. Spread of rectal cancer tends to be proximal, and in many instances rectum-saving operations are being done instead of abdominoperineal resection, formerly the standard procedure.

Rectal prolapse or procidentia occurs when part of all layers of the rectum extrude through the anal sphincter. Children and the elderly are most susceptible, and about half suffer neuropsychiatric disorders. Many operative procedures, ranging from minor sphincter-tightening techniques to resections and suspensions requiring major operations, are available options.

The anorectum and the adjacent area is subject to a number of disorders not shared by the colon. Infections of the anal glands may lead to abscess and fistula formation in the subcutaneous space or further out in the ischiorectal fossa. Abscess drainage is indicated and medical therapy has no place in management.

Fissure-in-ano is a tear in the anoderm, usually midline posteriorly, which usually heals spontaneously. Constipation predisposes and they often accompany Crohn's disease and ulcerative colitis. Excruciating pain during and after defecation is present in the acute phase. Division of the lower fibers of the internal anal sphincter is usually curative by relief of spasm. In children, most respond to gentle anal dilatation which can be done by the mother.

Hemorrhoids are enlargements of either or both the internal or external hemorrhoidal plexus of veins. Pain and bleeding are common complaints when hemorrhoids become symptomatic. Prolapse of hemorrhoids leads to exacerbation of symptoms. Hemorrhoidectomy is indicated if symptoms warrant. All patients subjected to hemorrhoidectomy should first have a sigmoidoscopic examination since one must be certain that a rectal cancer is not responsible for the symptoms

Anal carcinoma represents about 2 percent of large bowel cancers. The large majority are of the squamous or basal cell varieties and they tend to metastasize to inguinal nodes. Abdominoperineal resection is the preferred treatment, with radiotherapy being a useful adjunct.

Appendix

The narrow appendiceal lumen surrounded by voluminous lymphoid follicles sets the stage for one of the most common causes of an acute abdomen. It may lie in a variety of positions about the hub formed by its base, and more than half are retrocecal. Appendicitis, its most common affliction, affects about 6 percent of the population, with the maximum incidence in the teen years. It comes about by obstruction either by hypertrophy of

lymphoid follicles or fecalith impaction. Rarely, worms or tumors may obstruct. The classical history of diffuse abdominal discomfort becoming localized in the right lower quadrant reflects the stimulation of visceral afferent nerve fibers followed by pain due to peritoneal irritation when inflammation involves the serosa. Characteristically, tenderness is present over the appendix. Guarding and rigidity due to spasm of abdominal vessels ensue. Palpation of the opposite quadrant may cause pain over the appendix (Rovsing's sign). Pain and spasm may vary depending upon the location of the appendix-pelvis, retroperitoneum, etc. Rectal examination may reveal tenderness when a pelvic appendix is present, and this examination is vital in all instances. Should perforation occur, findings become more diffuse and the changes associated with peritonitis supervene. Abscess may ensue and an abdominal mass or one found on rectal examination may be the sole residual of an acute appendix days or weeks before. An elevated white blood cell count with a shift to the left is usually present. Abdominal roentgenograms show no pathognomic changes but a fecalith in the right lower quadrant is suggestive. The differential diagnosis depends upon the age and sex of the patient. Salpingitis, tubal pregnancy, endometriosis, and mittelschmerz in young women; ureteral calculi, Crohn's disease, epididymitis or testis torsion in young men; and gastroenteritis or mesenteric adenitis in infants and young children are likely alternatives. If acute appendicitis cannot be ruled out, it is better to operate than to risk the consequences of perforation and peritonitis.

Tumors and congenital anomalies are rare.

HERNIA

A hernia is a protrusion of viscera through an abnormal opening or through a normal opening which is enlarged. By no means do all have to be treated surgically.

Groin Hernia

Groin hernias include direct and indirect inguinal hernias in addition to femoral hernias. Groin hernias occur more frequently in males, but more women than men develop femoral hernias. Indirect inguinal hernias are congenital and descend through a patent processus vaginalis which accompanies the spermatic cord. Its exit through the internal inguinal ring is lateral to the inferior epigastric vessels, a useful landmark separating them from direct hernias. In females, the peritoneal vagination occurs along the round ligament. Although the processus is patent from birth, these hernias may only become manifest late in life. Direct inguinal hernias result from fascial disruption of the posterior inguinal wall, usually medial to the inferior epigastric vessels, and is therefore an acquired lesion. Femoral hernias, also acquired, protrude through the femoral canal medial to the femoral vessels. In most groin hernias, gradual enlargement is the rule and pain and disability are highly variable. The most serious complication is incarceration, especially in indirect inguinal and femoral hernias, due to the narrow hernial sac neck.

The diagnosis of groin hernias is often made by the patient, who notices the protrusion. Discomfort may be the earliest sign. In babies, the mother usually notices the bulge first. Physical examination is not conclusive in diagnosis among the three types of groin hernia, but since most come to operation, this is not a critical factor. Most direct hernias occur at an older age, tend to be round in configuration, and tend not to enter the scrotum. Femoral hernias are the most difficult to diagnose since one might have the impression that they lie above the inguinal ligament. The accuracy of diagnosis in incarceration is critical, however, since gangrene is a possibility. Not infrequently, patients having intestinal obstruction are operated upon without the hernia having been detected as its cause beforehand. The reduction of an incarcerated hernia may be hazardous owing to the possibility that nonviable bowel was returned to the peritoneal cavity, and it is wise to visualize the bowel at operation.

Treatment is usually surgical unless the patient's general condition precludes it. Many times the general status of the patient may be improved by medical therapy sufficient to permit safe operation. Local anesthesia permits operation in almost all.

Ventral Hernia

EPIGASTRIC HERNIA

Epigastric hernia is a defect through the linea alba between the xiphoid and umbilicus. There may be a true hernial sac or only protrusion of preperitoneal fat. They often produce striking symptoms considering their size; they rarely incarcerate. Detection by palpation may be difficult and having the patient lift his head may make it more apparent. Repair is rarely followed by recurrence.

UMBILICAL HERNIA

Most umbilical hernias detected during childhood close spontaneously. In adults, most occur in obese women who have had children. They are prone to incarceration, often with omentum being involved, and elective repair is indicated.

INCISIONAL HERNIA

Incisional hernias follow operations. Wound infection, obesity, and vertical incisions predispose. Ascites and chronic cough also favor their development. These hernias tend to enlarge but the risk of incarceration is inversely proportional to the size of the abdominal defect. These tend to be bothersome because of their size. Treatment must be individualized depending upon the defect size (small usually more dangerous), symptoms, and general condition of the patient. Repair is effective, especially if tension is avoided, often by the use of a prosthesis.

ESOPHAGEAL HIATUS HERNIA

There are two types of esophageal hiatus hernias, sliding and paraesophageal. The sliding is much more common than the paraesophageal lesion. The upper stomach is retroperitoneal and may enter the chest by sliding retroperitoneally as well as through the dilated hiatus. In children they are considered to be congenital, while in adults they are acquired. Sliding hernias in this position rarely incarcerate and the principal concern is the development of esophagitis due to reflux which may proceed to scarring and esophageal stricture. Barium swallow roentgenograms, endoscopy, and esophageal manometry are useful diagnostic aids. Many also have duodenal ulcers and a complete gastrointestinal roentgenograms series is indicated.

Medical treatment consists of elevation of the head of the bed to reduce esophageal reflux, antacids, weight loss, etc. Intractability and severe reflux with symptoms of aspiration or esophagitis are the primary indications for surgical repair. Operation should be directed to reducing reflux and, if gastric or duodenal ulcer is present, an acid-reducing operation should be combined with hernia repair.

In paraesophageal hiatus hernias, the stomach fundus protrudes through the hiatus beside the esophagus or through a separate diaphragmatic defect adjacent to the hiatus. The gastroesophageal junction is in its normal position. Incarceration is common and repair by closure of the defect is indicated. The diagnosis is usually made by roentgenogram.

SPLEEN

The normal adult spleen weighs approximately 75–100 g. The splenic artery arises from the celiac axis and the splenic vein joins the superior mesenteric to form the portal vein. Accessory spleens are present in about one-quarter of individuals and usually lie in supporting splenic ligaments, although they may be present in the female pelvis. Three pulp zones (i.e., white, marginal, and red) exist. The white pulp is analogous to a lymph node and consists of lymphocytes, plasma cells, and macrophages. The marginal zone contains sequestered foreign material and plasma elements. The red pulp contains cords and sinuses to form a vascular space. The spleen is the most vascular of all viscera. Under normal circumstances, red cells pass from terminal arterioles directly into splenic sinuses as well as from terminal arterioles into pulp cords and splenic sinuses.

The nature of splenic function has been slow in unfolding but newer techniques have led to better understanding. From the fifth to eighth months of embryonic life, the spleen contributes both white and red cells to the circulation. About 30 L of blood pass through the spleen hourly, and abnormal and aged red cells, normal and abnormal platelets, and cellular debris are cleared in a process in which the spleen is able to discriminate between normal and abnormal components. In pathologic states the reduction of cellular elements has been ascribed to excessive destruction of cellular elements, splenic inhibition of marrow, and splenic production of antibody which results in destruction of blood cells. Hypersplenism is the term applied to the accelerated removal of any or all of the formed blood elements by overactivity of the spleen. Leukopenia, thrombocytopenia, and anemia alone or in combination may result. The spleen removes nuclear remnants from circulating erythrocytes (Howell-Jolly bodies) and after splenectomy this function is lost with resulting presence of these elements in the circulating blood. Normally, red cells survive 105–120 days, after which they deteriorate and are phagocytosed by reticuloendothelial cells and splenic macrophages. Most neutrophils migrate into tissues or are destroyed within 24 hours. Splenomegaly may hasten the process leading to neutropenia. Platelets survive about 10 days and almost a third of the platelets reside in the spleen. With spleen enlargement, up to 80 percent of the platelets may be sequestered in the spleen which, along with accelerated destruction, may cause thrombocytopenia. Postsplenectomy, a marked increase in platelets often occurs but this is usually temporary.

Increased red cell destruction results in a rise of reticulocytes in the circulating blood. If blood loss is not responsible for reticulocytosis, it may be assumed that red cell destruction is present. If the spleen is involved in a hemolytic anemia, a spleen/liver ^{51}Cr-tagged erythrocyte ratio greater than 2:1 detected on uptake studies indicates that splenectomy may be of benefit.

The normal spleen is not palpable, but examination affords only a rough estimate of its size. Radiocolloid scans using 99 m Tc-sulfur, or other isotopes, affords a more accurate estimate of splenic size.

Indications for splenectomy evolve about traumatic injury, hematologic disorders, and, more recently, in patients in whom kidney tranplantation is anticipated. In recent years the dangers of serious sepsis in splenectomized patients, particularly children, has led to a more conservative approach in managing the injured spleen. When severely injured spleens threaten to jeopardize life, splenectomy is still indicated; however, hemostatic methods now available will afford the opportunity to save most of them. Spontaneous ruptures of the normal spleen are rare; usually such ruptures involve spleens enlarged by disease processes. If splenectomy is required, pneumococcal vaccine should be given and care exercised in providing antibiotic coverage for those at risk.

Some hematologic disorders in which splenectomy may be useful in therapy are well known.

Idiopathic thrombocytopenic purpura (ITP) may represent an autoimmune disorder. Subnormal platelet counts in the presence of normal or increased megakaryocytes without known causes of thrombocytopenia suggest the disorder. Splenomegaly is rare and its presence suggests other causes. Steroid administration is an alternative, usually less effective, form of treatment.

Thrombotic thrombocytopenic purpura (TTP), fortunately a rare disorder, causes a high mortality. Fever, purpura, hemolytic anemia, and renal and neurologic disorders accompany the syndrome. Splenectomy and steroids are indicated.

Primary hypersplenism is a syndrome in which formed blood elements, any or all, are reduced. Splenomegaly is usually present, females predominate, and clinical manifestations depend upon which elements are involved. Steroids are ineffective and splenectomy is indicated. Secondary hypersplenism, associated with portal hypertension due to liver disease, should not be treated by splenectomy alone, without consideration of a shunting procedure.

Myeloid metaplasia is associated with miniature forms of red cells with poikilocytosis in the peripheral blood. Platelets may exceed one million. Some patients benefit from splenectomy for control of anemia and thrombocytopenia or for symptoms associated with splenomegaly, but it is not the mainstay of therapy, which is medical. Postoperative infections are common.

Hemolytic anemias of several types may respond to splenectomy. Both congenital and acquired types show reduced erythrocyte survival as measured by disappearance of labeled ^{51}Cr erythrocytes and the spleen's contribution may be demonstrated by determining relative uptake by the spleen and liver. *Hereditary spherocytosis* is the most common of the symptomatic familial hemolytic anemias. The erythrocyte membrane is defective and the red cell becomes spherical. Fragility is increased. Anemia, reticulocytosis, splenomegaly, and jaundice characterize the syndrome. Gallstones occur in almost half. Splenectomy is effective and cholecystectomy can be done concomitantly if stones are present.

Other anemias due to hereditary elliptocytosis, thalassemia, sickle cell disease, idiopathic autoimmune hemolytic anemia, and hereditary nonspherocytic hemolytic anemia may be helped by splenectomy.

Splenectomy may be useful in a variety of disorders such as chronic leukemia, reticular cell sarcoma, and Hodgkin's disease for relieving hypersplenism or as an addition to therapy. It has been useful in staging Hodgkin's disease but newer imaging techniques (e.g., CT scan) may be replacing this function.

Patients with Felty's syndrome, sarcoidosis, porphyria erythropoietica, Fanconi's anemia, and Gaucher's disease may also benefit in a palliative sense by relieving blood element destruction or in relieving symptoms due to splenic enlargement.

Splenic artery aneurysms and a spectrum of cysts and tumors also are indications for splenectomy.

The hematologic indications for splenectomy will be discussed in more detail in chapter 9.

Most of the postoperative complications are rare. Infection has already been mentioned. Trauma to the tail of the pancreas is a consideration. Although platelet counts may be markedly elevated, thrombosis seems not to be increased.

PERITONITIS AND INTRA-ABDOMINAL ABSCESSES

Despite vast improvements in antibiotics, intraperitoneal infections still account for death in over 60 percent in some populations of patients, especially the aged. Peritonitis may be primary or secondary. Primary peritonitis may be caused by pneumococci, streptococci, gram-negative bacteria or *Mycobacterium* tuberculosis. Secondary peritonitis arises from injuries or lesions of the gastrointestinal or genitourinary system.

The site of origin of infection significantly influences mortality. If strangulation or perforation of the small intestine is the source, mortality is about 20–25 percent. Gastric or duodenal ulcer perforation leads to a mortality of 5–10 percent, while large intestinal sources (diverticula, etc.) may have a much higher mortality. The presence of associated renal failure adds greatly to mortality.

The peritoneal cavity is a potential space containing a few milliliters of fluid which may increase enormously in the presence of infection. Peritonitis is the equivalent of a cutaneous burn, and may result in the sequestration of fluid lost to the circulation which might be the equivalent of a 50 percent burn. The lymphatic drainage plays a great role in removing bacteria from the peritoneal cavity. Lymphatics underlie the peritoneal mesothelium on only the diaphragmatic surface and diaphragmatic motion acts as a pump to move bacteria into the central lymphatic circulation aided by the negative intrathoracic pressure associated with spontaneous inspiration. Fluid and bacteria tend to move upward and, when clearing is inadequate, abscesses tend to occur beneath the diaphragm, in the paracolic gutters, and in the subhepatic space. Although Fowler's position may favor gravitational migration of bacteria into the pelvis, the migration of bacteria through diaphragmatic lymphatics is to be preferred since exposure to systemic antibiotics tends to avoid bacterial sequestration and abscess formation.

Secondary peritonitis, that most frequently encountered, is sharply related to the gastrointestinal bacterial flora. The normal empty stomach discourages bacterial growth by virtue of gastric acidity; food or blood in the stomach favors bacterial growth. Lactobacilli and streptococci commonly inhabit the upper jejunum. In the distal ileum, bacterial population approaches that of the colon, where anaerobes and aerobes abound. Cultures of peritoneal fluid in the presence of peritonitis are almost always polymicrobial, and *B fragilis* and *E coli* are the most common pathogens, and about one-third result in positive blood cultures. Feces, barium, bile, and necrotic tissue all enhance bacterial growth. Competition among different bacterial species (as many as 400 exist in the gastrointestinal tract) leads to restricted growth of many organisms with survival of the most pathogenic species. *E coli* and *B fragilis* appear to act synergistically to act as copathogens. Coliforms lower redox potential, which favors the growth of anaerobes, and abscesses result because of failure of mechanisms which provide for destruction of bacteria. When bacterial contamination is severe or ongoing and uncontrolled by phagocytes and opsonins, abscesses form. Fibrinous loculations prevent passage of bacteria into the diaphragmatic lymphatics to further reduce bacterial eradication. When they degenerate, neutrophils release lysosomal enzymes which act to increase abscess size and to dissect through new tissue planes. Abscesses frequently rupture into pleura, pericardium, or peritoneum, where rapid absorption may cause septic shock, or they may rupture into a hollow viscera or through skin, whereby they decompress themselves. Foreign bodies such as sutures and drains enhance the possibility of abscess formation.

Treatment of peritonitis must provide for restoration of fluid and electrolyte balance and assurance of adequate oxygenation. A urine output of at least 30 ml/hour is desirable, and blood determinations of gases, and creatinine and electrolytes are vital. Caloric intake must be maintained to satisfy the increased metabolic demand, and more than 4,000 calories/day may be required. Catecholamines, glucocorticoids, and insulin are increased. High glucagon levels cause insulin resistance. Intravenous hyperalimentation using amino acids and other nutrients in mixtures with 1 calorie/ml are most suitable.

Initial antibiotic therapy must be presumptive, and the choice is based upon the suspected organisms. Upper gastrointestinal perforations are primarily associated with gram-positive organisms but delay in treatment enables gram-negative and gram-positive anaerobes to multiply. In lower perforations, aminoglycosides in combination with clindamycin and ampicillin provide the coverage for enterococci, coliforms, and anaerobes, especially *B fragilis.* The early use of effective antibiotics administered as soon after the insult as possible may prevent abscess formation. Polymicrobial infections are best treated as if each pathogen existed in pure culture.

Operation is always indicated early in secondary peritonitis unless the evidence suggests that the initial process is well walled off and ongoing contamination is controlled. The treatment of primary peritonitis is nonsurgical. Control of continued contamination is the goal. Drains become walled off by fibrin and probably add little except where ongoing leakage (e.g., pancreatic injuries) is expected. Peritoneal lavage has limited usefulness.

Intraperitoneal abscess may be suspected postoperatively if fever and leukocytosis continue through a course of antibiotics. Ultrasound and the CT scan may localize intraperitoneal abscesses and the latter may assist in positioning needles for drainage of abscesses. Gallium 67 scintillation imaging has limited usefulness. Neutrophils absorb gallium 67 complexes and may show up on this test. The liver-lung scan may show subphrenic collections.

Abscesses require drainage, usually best done by laparotomy. Needle drainage is increasing in usefulness and may substitute for laparotomy. Drains are helpful in avoiding recurrences of abscess but must be kept away from anastomoses where they may cause disruption.

UROLOGY

Hematuria

Gross or microscopic blood in the urine may be due to systemic disorders or urinary tract lesions. Bleeding may indicate a life-threatening disorder; consequently, the cause must be determined in all instances. One must be certain that there is, indeed, blood in the urine to be ascertained by microscopic examination and that the bleeding is not arising from the vagina or rectum.

Major systemic causes of hematuria include hemoglobinopathies such as sickle-cell anemia, hemophilia, and leukemia. Anticoagulation therapy is a prominent cause but may signal an already present lesion which is prone to bleed.

The urethra may be the source of bleeding due to stricture, urethritis, prostatis, or prostatic cancer or trauma. Ureteral sources include calculi, tumors, or strictures. Renal causes include infections, glomerulonephritis, hydronephrosis, and tumors. Bladder infections, tumors, foreign bodies, varices, and calculi may cause bleeding.

In children up to 5 years of age, Wilms' tumor and infections are likely causes of hematuria, and between 5 and 15 years glomerulonephritis, pyelonephritis, and calculi predominate.

A careful family history is very important in detecting blood dyscrasias, predisposition to stone formation, and polycystic disease. All patients with hematuria should have a urine analysis, hematologic studies, blood urea, and serum creatinine determinations and an intravenous pyelogram (IVP) as a minimum.

Malignant tumors of the urinary tract are serious causes of hematuria and deserve further consideration. Bladder cancer occurs mostly in males over 50 years of age. Most arise in transitional epithelium. Smoking and occupations in the aniline dye and textile industries are predisposing factors. These tumors are usually multifocal, and because of the predisposition of transitional epithelium, the upper urinary tract must be evaluated to rule out additional lesions. Diagnosis is best achieved by IVP and cystoscopy and Papanicolaou cytology testing. Treatment ranges from instillation of chemotherapeutic agents into the bladder to total cystectomy. Follow-up should include reexamination of the upper tract because of the possibility of recurrence in the kidney, pelvis, and ureters. Prognosis depends upon the depth of bladder wall invasion and the extent of surgical treatment.

Carcinoma of the kidney is almost always an adenocarcinoma. Elderly male smokers are most commonly afflicted. The classic presentation of hematuria, flank pain, and the presence of a mass, is evident in less than half the patients, and many first present with metastatic lesions of lung or bone.

Valuable diagnostic tools include IVP with tomograms, angiography, and ultrasound, the latter of which is valuable in ruling out renal cysts.

Radical nephrectomy offers the best chance of cure. Radiotherapy and chemotherapy are usually ineffective.

Hydronephrosis

Dilatation of the collecting system may result from obstructions of any type from ureters to urethra due to tumor, stones, vascular anomalies, infections, strictures, or congenital malformations. When bilateral, bladder outlet obstruction is the usual cause, backpressure results in decreased blood flow in the kidney, and glomerular filtration is reduced. Complete ureteral obstruction is tolerated for a week or two or less before irreversible renal damage occurs. Consequently, early recognition and treatment are required.

Prostatic hypertrophy is the major cause of bladder neck obstruction in adults. Hesitancy, reduced stream, nocturia, and frequency are common symptoms. On rectal examination, if nodularity of the prostrate is found, cancer is suspected. Prostatitis, urethral strictures, and bladder stone or tumor are less common causes of bladder outlet obstruction. The bladder musculature hypertrophies, but eventually bladder emptying is incomplete and residual urine becomes infected because of stasis, and hydronephrosis will ensue if the obstruction is not relieved. IVP and cystoscopy are basic diagnostic procedures and serum acid phosphatase determination should be done to rule out carcinoma. Transrectal or transperineal needle biopsy is required if prostatic carcinoma is suspected since that portion of the prostate accessible by transurethral resection is rarely the site of malignancy. Treatment of benign hypertrophy is by transurethral or open prostatectomy, the former preferred in most cases. Acute retention is best treated by urethral catheterization; if unable to do this, trocar drainage with catheter insertion into the bladder may be used. Prostatic cancer may be treated by several methods including radical operative resection, implantation of radioactive pellets, or palliative procedures depending upon the stage of disease. Since the tumors are androgen-dependent, orchiectomy, which tends to reduce progression of metastatic lesions, and estrogen administration, which blocks the formation of testicular androgen, are useful adjuncts in treating metastatic disease.

Urinary calculi may cause acute symptoms or may be silent, depending upon size and location. Metabolic disturbances are responsible for some stone formation and treatment may be directed toward the cause or composition of the calculi. Uric acid stones may be prevented and dissolved by the administration of allopurinol, which reduces excretion of uric acid, and by giving a diet low in purines. Magnesium ammonium phosphate calculi are usually associated with urinary tract infections which do not respond unless all calculi are removed. Patients with cystinuria are prone to cystine stone formation. D-Penicillamine combines with urinary cystine to form a more soluble compound to inhibit calculi formation, especially if the urine is kept alkaline.

Operative removal of resistant calculi which do not pass spontaneously depends upon location and the extent of interference with function. Both open operation and endoscopic removal are effective.

Masses of the Scrotum

Masses in the scrotum may be caused by congenital abnormalities, infections or tumors of the epididymis or testicle, or as part of a systemic disease. Hernias, varicoceles, and changes associated with vascular compromise, such as in testicular torsion, and spermatoceles are additional considerations.

Torsion and strangulated hernias require early operation to avoid loss of testicle or incarcerated hernia contents. Because of the frequency of bilateral inadequacy of testicular fixation in instances of torsion, bilateral exploration with orchiopexy is the preferred treatment. Sudden pain with scrotal mass in young people is the classic setting. The testis tends to lie high and scrotal ecchymosis and edema are usual signs. Epididymitis may be confused with it, but when present in children, torsion should be considered to be the cause.

Varicoceles are varicose veins of the pampiniform plexus, predominantly on the left side. Except in instances of infertility, operation is not required.

Testicular tumors usually occur in males under 40 except when secondarily involved, as with lymphoma. Increased size and firmness of the testicle usually are found but pain is uncommon. Undescended (cryptorchid) testes are 30–40 times more prone to develop tumors than are normals, presumably due to dysgenesis which predisposes to both nondescent and tumor. Lymph node and vascular spread are common. Two types, germinal and nongerminal, occur. Germinal tumors predominate and the most common germinal tumor is the seminoma. Characteristically, it spreads to retroperitoneal nodes and is very radiosensitive. Embryonal carcinoma is more malignant and contains immature elements. Teratomas and teratocarcinomas contain tissues of various origin, commonly cartilage, thyroid, lung, etc. Choriocarcinomas are composed of cytotrophoblastic cells and are the most virulent of all testes tumors.

Most nongerminal tumors are of Leydig cell type, which produce estrogen and may lead to gynecomastia.

Diagnosis and treatment are urgent. Any hard, painless, testicular mass should be operated on promptly. Hydroceles commonly accompany these tumors and epididymitis may be confused with them.

Patients suspected of having such tumors should have IVP, chest roentgenogram, and urinary chorionic gonadotrophin assay. If the latter turns negative after operation, the likelihood is that all tumor has been eradicated.

Operation through an inguinal approach with early clamping of the cord and orchiectomy with high cord transection is appropriate when a testicular tumor is found. Further therapy depends upon the cell type found on permanent sections.

BREAST

Infections

Breast abscesses are usually associated with lactation and nursing. Nipple fissures afford access of organisms, often *staphylococcus aureus,* and subsequent abscess. If antibiotics are not effective within a few days, surgical drainage is indicated.

Tuberculosis is an uncommon breast infection and may be confused with carcinoma. Painful masses may be due to inspissated material in ducts causing plasma cell mastitis, a nonpyogenic lesion. Biopsy may be required to differentiate it from carcinoma. Paget's carcinoma of the nipple and areola may be mistaken for dermatitis.

Breast Tumors

Most breast lumps in old women are due to carcinoma and most are found by the patient. Fibroadenomas and cysts are common in the young. Intraductal papillomas are the most common cause of nipple discharge. Biopsy of all suspicious lesions is indicated.

CYSTIC DISEASE

This is the most common tumor of the breast and is related to variations in response to the neuroendocrine sequence of the ovary and menstruation. Ductal dilatation may occur with cyst formation. Needle aspiration is useful in determining the nature of cysts (i.e., failure to disappear with aspiration is an indication for open biopsy). There seems to be an increased incidence of carcinoma in patients with cystic disease. Fibroadenomas are usually single, sharply defined, and mobile. Excision is the treatment of choice.

CARCINOMA

Cancer is the second most common tumor of the breast, and it is the most common malignant tumor in women. There is a strong family tendency. A dominant mass, firmness of one breast, skin dimpling, shrinkage of the breast, and skin redness are obvious signs of carcinoma. Axillary lymph nodes are found to contain metastatic deposits in more than two-thirds of patients subjected to radical mastectomy, and internal mammary nodes are usually involved as well. The majority are scirrhous adenocarcinomas with predilection for the upper outer quadrant. Systemic spread is very common, with lung, liver, and bone being favored sites for metastatic deposits. Median survival for untreated patients from time of first symptom is a little over 3 years.

Prognosis is related to tumor size and cell type, involvement of axillary nodes and other metastatic lesions, and estrogen and progesterone receptor status. Patients believed to have their disease confined to the local area, and patients with three or fewer positive axillary lymph nodes, have a better prognosis than those with more extensive involvement. Estrogen receptor (ER)-positive tumors appear to be better differentiated and slower growing, but this relationship is uncertain. Second primary breast cancers may be more prevalent in patients with ER-positive first tumors. The estrogen receptor

assay is highly useful in determining which patients with metastatic breast cancer may benefit from hormonal therapy.

Over the past two decades surgical treatment has undergone considerable change, with less extensive procedures gaining favor. The removal of axillary lymph nodes assists in defining prognosis and in determining the advisability of radiotherapy or chemotherapy.

Although a variety of operations, varying in magnitude alone or in combination with radiotherapy and/or chemotherapy, are being used currently, the modified radical mastectomy is the one most employed for tumors thought to be curable. If axillary nodes are involved, adjuvant roentgenogram therapy or chemotherapy is frequently employed. Some evidence suggests that postoperative chemotherapy may cause a delay in the appearance of recurrent tumor in those patients not cured by initial treatment.

Several biochemical manipulations have evolved for treatment for metastatic carcinoma of the breast. Antiestrogens may cause regression of lesions and tamoxifen has been used with therapeutic response in about one-third of patients. Adrenalectomy has been shown to cause temporary regression and aminoglutethimide, a drug known to suppress corticosteroid synthesis, may substitute for adrenalectomy. Patients who fail to respond are spared the necessity to take cortisol-replacement therapy for the rest of their lives.

The use of chemotherapy in metastatic breast cancer is undergoing constant change. Single drug therapy has resulted in about a 20 percent response rate. Recently, cyclophosphamide or doxorubicin (Adriamycin) were shown to produce a response in more than half. The drugs used most are cyclophosphamide, doxorubicin, methotrexate, and 5-fluorouracil, and they apparently demonstrate no cross-resistance. The evidence suggests that multiple drug therapy programs have resulted in higher rates of regression than when single agents are used.

ENDOCRINE SURGERY

Pituitary Gland

The pituitary gland provides control of internal secretion and is the "master" gland. The anterior lobe secretes thyroid stimulating hormone (TSH), adrenocorticotropic hormone (ACTH), and growth hormone (GH). The posterior lobe, or neurohypophysis, secretes oxytocin and antidiuretic hormone (ADH). Both have neurohumoral connections with the hypothalamus and psychic stimuli act through the hypothalamus to release corticotropin releasing factor (CRF), which releases ACTH by the anterior pituitary lobe. Metabolic balance is maintained through the pituitary, and pathologic state resulting in excess hormone production results in distinctive clinical syndromes. The anterior pituitary is necessary for normal growth and homeostasis, and the posterior lobe is required for water balance by its secretion of ADH. ACTH controls the secretion of cortisol and a sensitive feedback mechanism inhibits excess ACTH production depending upon the cortisol plasma level. ACTH also stimulates androgen and aldosterone release. Other anterior lobe hormones include thyroid stimulating hormone (TSH), gonadotrophins (follicle stimulating hormone FSH), and luteinizing hormone (LH). FSH causes graafian follicles to secrete estrogen, and LH induces the luteinizing of theca cells after follicle rupture. In males, LH stimulates Leydig cells (interstitial cells causing androgen secretion). FSH stimulates development of the spermatic tubules, so both FSH and LH are required for sptermatogenesis. Prolactin influences the breast to lactate.

ADH and oxytocin are produced by the hypothalamus and are passed into the bloodstream through the posterior lobe. Osmotic pressure of the blood controls the rate of ADH secretion, which stimulates the reabsorption of water by the kidney. Excessive ADH secretion causes water retention (water intoxication), and pituitary destruction by operation or trauma results in water loss with severe dehydration (diabetes insipidus).

Certain malignant tumors may produce compounds closely related to pituitary hormones, giving rise to syndromes mimicking those due to overreactive states of pituitary function.

Pituitary tumors comprise about 10 percent of brain tumors and may manifest themselves by changes due to size or function. Pituitary enlargement sufficient to press upon the optic chiasm produces visual field cuts. Formerly most surgery on the pituitary focused upon this problem, but now functional disturbances are appreciated and earlier treatment may restore secretory function and avoid the visual consequences of tumors. Most commonly, tumors cause hypofunction with alteration in menstruation or sterility, and in males and postmenopausal women thyroid hypofunction may become evident. Lack of growth and sexual maturity in the young may be the first indication. Excess hormone production may produce gigantism (GH excess) in prepubertal patients and acromegaly in older patients, with resulting hyperplasia of nose, joints, and extremities. Less commonly, ACTH excess may produce Cushing's syndrome with hypertension, hirsutism, abdominal striae, etc. Prolactin secreting tumors produce galactorrhea. Headache is the most common symptom of pituitary tumor. Skull roentgenograms may show sella enlargement (late sign) and the CT scan may be helpful.

Management of pituitary tumors includes roentgenogram therapy and surgical excision alone or combined.

The availability of adrenocortical hormones has allowed hypophysectomy, which has also permitted ablation for the management of hormone-dependent metastatic breast cancer.

Cushing's syndrome is caused by excess circulating cortisol due to excessive production of glucocorticoids by the adrenal cortex or by the administration of steroids given for arthritis, renal disease, or a variety of other disorders. A tumor of the adrenal cortex or excessive secretion of ACTH by the anterior pituitary may be the cause. Ectopic production of ACTH by malignant tumors, usually bronchial carcinoma, may produce similar changes and is responsible for about 1 percent of cases. There is a normal diurnal fluctuation of plasma cortisol levels which compares with a high, sustained level in patients with Cushing's syndrome.

Obesity is the most common finding which, when accompanied by thin extremities, is suggested. The cervicodorsal "buffalo hump" may be present. Rounding of the face ("moon face") is present in most. Hypertension, decreased glucose tolerance, menstrual and sexual dysfunction, weakness, striae of abdominal skin, and acne may be present in varying proportions. Occasionally an abdominal mass is palpable.

The dexamethasone suppression test (DST) is a valuable diagnostic adjunct, based upon the fact that this highly potent synthetic steroid suppresses ACTH in normals with a much lower dose than that witnessed in Cushing's syndrome. The need for ACTH release to preserve a given level of cortisol production is reduced and the urinary excretion of 17-hydroxycorticosteroids, the metabolites of cortisol and related compounds, falls sharply. A much higher dose of DST is required to effect such a fall in Cushing's syndrome.

Treatment depends upon the specific cause. Bilateral adrenalectomy for adrenocortical hyperplasia is the preferred method, and resection of adrenocortical tumors is appropriate. When complete excision is impossible, debulking is indicated in the hope that benefit will accrue. When excessive ACTH by the pituitary is at fault, irradiation by external source or implantation of radioactive yttrium into the pituitary fossa is indicated. About one-third of patients benefit, making adrenalectomy a more attractive option. Great care to supply sufficient exogenous cortisol is mandatory during the following operation.

Primary aldosteronism is a cause of hypertension in about 1 percent of hypertensive patients. Other features include hypokalemia, mild metabolic alkalosis, polyuria resistant to vasopressin, and weakness. Aldosterone is normally produced by zona glomerulosa cells of the adrenal cortex, which, when excessive, produces the syndrome by acting on the distal tubule of the kidney to promote sodium retention with consequent water retention, thus increasing total blood volume. Single benign cortical adenomas usually are found. There is a female predominance and there is no relationship between tumor size and degree of hypertension. Complete resection must be accomplished to produce a cure. Bilateral cortical hyperplasia may produce the syndrome, but adrenalectomy is less commonly curative than when a single adenoma is present.

Diagnosis is suggested by increased urinary aldosterone and potassium levels. If the patient is not on diuretics and on a regular diet, a urinary potassium loss of more than 40 mEq/day in the presence of hypokalemia is supportive of the diagnosis. Arteriography, pyelography, and CT scanning are indicated. Iodocholesterol labeled with radioactive iodine 131 concentrates on the side involved or bilaterally if hyperplasia is at fault. Adrenalectomy is the preferred treatment.

Virilism and feminism due to adrenal cortical influence may result in ambiguous genitalia in children and other clinical pictures in adults. Adrenal hyperplasia results in excess production of adrenal androgens. In female infants it causes incomplete differentiation of the external genitalia and, after birth, progressive virilization in both sexes. Virilizing and feminizing adrenal tumors are much less frequent than hyperplasia. The surgical correction includes corrective surgery upon the external genitalia in females and, if adrenal tumors are present, adrenalectomy is indicated.

In adults with hyperplasia, corticosteroid administration for suppression of ACTH is indicated. Tumors should be surgically removed.

Pheochromocytoma

Pheochromocytomas are adrenal medulla or sympathetic chain tumors which usually secrete epinephrine and norepinephrine. They characteristically cause episodic hypertension which may be associated with headache, dyspnea, ocular hemorrhages, stroke, etc., all related to hypertension. About 10 percent are malignant. These tumors arise in chromaffin tissue. Physical examination may be negative including blood pressure determination. The presence of von Recklinghausen's neurofibromatosis suggests its presence. Rarely is the tumor palpable, a maneuver which may initiate a paroxysm of hypertension.

Diagnosis by laboratory means includes measurement of epinephrine, norepinephrine, metanephrine, normetanephrine, and VMA, which are elevated in almost all instances. IVPs and CT scanning are useful and lateralizing by selective sampling of vena caval blood and on the two sides with assay is possible.

Treatment is surgical. Bilateral tumors are present in 10 percent. Phentolamine and phenoxybenzamine, both alpha-adrenergic blockers, control blood pressure pre-

and intraoperatively. Tachyarrhythmias are best controlled by propranolol. Because of chronic vasoconstriction, blood volume is reduced and blood transfusion may be required to avoid shock. Anesthetic management is critical, especially during tumor manipulation. Preoperative phenoxybenzamine administration usually avoids marked elevation of blood pressure. Phentolamine infusion at the appearance of elevated blood pressure provides control.

Because of bilaterality, both adrenals and sympathetic chains should be carefully explored. If metastases are present, debulking may be useful, but usually oral phentolamine or phenoxybenzamine are required since sufficient reduction of catecholamine to avoid symptoms is not usually possible.

Thyroid

Thyrotoxicosis is a state of hypermetabolism caused by thyroid hormone excess. Thyroxine (T_4) and triiodothyronine (T_3) are involved in endogenous thyrotoxicosis. Most such patients have a diffuse toxic goiter associated with exophthalmos (Graves' disease). Less commonly, multinodular toxic goiters are at fault.

The adult thyroid weighs about 20 g. The blood supply is so generous that ligation of the major vessels rarely results in necrosis. The recurrent laryngeal nerves and parathyroid glands are intimately associated and the most serious long-term complications of thyroidectomy are related to injury to these structures.

Thyroidal iodine metabolism is the central point to be considered. T_3 and T_4 production involves iodine transport into the gland followed by a reaction with tyrosine to yield monoiodotyrosine (MIT) and diiodotyrosine (DIT), which separately are inactive. When coupled, they form T_3 and T_4. TSH promotes all stages of hormone production and facilitates release. These hormones are stored in the thyroid colloid as thyroglobulin, which releases the hormones by proteolysis. Iodine inhibits this release and thereby checks the release of thyroxin, with abatement of symptoms. T_3 and T_4 inhibits TSH release by the pituitary, thereby reciprocally controlling hormone level. Diagnosis is aided my measurement of T_3 and T_4, which are characteristically elevated. The normal range for T_4 is between 4 and 13.5 μg/100 ml and for T_3 is 75 to 220 ng/100 ml.

Symptoms of Graves' disease result from the multisystem involvement in the hypermetabolic state. Weight loss, increased appetite, palpitation, nervousness, emotional lability, and increased sweating are usual. Fatigue and weakness are often present. All of these result from heightened sensitivity to adrenergic stimuli and adrenergic blockers are effective in controlling these symptoms. The gland may weigh up to 200 g or more and is diffusely enlarged. Microscopy shows hyperplastic follicular epithelium, marked vascularity, and diminution of follicle size. Lid lag and globe lag on downward and upward gaze are seen. True infiltrative ophthalmopathy with proptosis is present in about half and bears no relationship to the degree of toxicity. Sometimes proptosis is extreme and requires operative decompression of the orbit.

Treatment of thyrotoxicosis ranges from long-term antithyroid therapy, ^{131}I ablation, to major resection of the thyroid gland. Examples of antithyroid drugs for control are propylthiouracil and methimazole. Thyroidectomy controls toxicity in over 90 percent and is preferred in adolescents and adults up to 40 years of age. Bleeding, parathyroid and recurrent nerve injuries are important complications of operation.

Thyroid crisis is, fortunately, a rare complication which carries with it a high mortality. It results from a runaway of the hypermetabolic state leading to severe anxiety and agitation, disorientation, delirium, coma, and death. Hyperpyrexia is present and heart failure common. Antithyroid drugs, iodides, and reserpine or propranolol should be adminstered promptly.

Thyroiditis may be of the struma lymphomatosa (Hashimoto's) subacute (granulomatous) or Riedel's type. Struma lymphomatosa is the most common found and is probably an autoimmune disorder. The process tends to destroy the thyroid, resulting in myxedema. Lymphocytic infiltration or oxyphilic epithelium are characteristic. Both lobes are involved. Needle biopsy usually is diagnostic and desiccated thyroid administration is indicated.

Subacute thyroiditis may be viral in origin. Pain and tenderness of the thyroid are usually present and pain often radiates to the ears. Signs mimicking those of thyrotoxicosis may appear. The entire gland or only part of a lobe may be involved in the indicated process. The disease is self-limited and relief can usually be obtained promptly by prednisone administration. Operation is not required.

Riedel's struma is a fibrotic process which may involve all or part of the gland. Little vascularity is apparent. Sometimes an adenoma is associated and, when present, should be resected.

GOITER

Adenomatous goiter is the most common cause of thyroid enlargement. It occurs most commonly in women and probably results from abnormal TSH stimulation. Iodine deficiency (rare in North America) and errors of thyroid synthesis may be causative, and initial diffuse enlargement followed by localized hyperplasia results in a thyroid scan showing diffuse uptake with areas of hypofunction or nonfunction (cold nodule).

Hemorrhage, fibrosis, and calcification are common. When a solitary cold nodule is present, the chance of malignancy is enhanced and operation (lobectomy) is indicated to rule this out. Early in the course of nodular goiter, thyroid given to suppress TSH may result in regression. High substernal extension may give rise to anterior mediastinal tumors.

Adenomas are localized benign tumors which may be hyperfunctioning (hot nodule). Hormone production may be high enough to block TSH, to produce atrophy in the remaining thyroid. Resection is the treatment of choice. Cysts represent degenerated adenomas and have a low incidence of malignant change. Ultrasound and needle aspiration are helpful diagnostic tools.

THYROID CANCER

Four types (i.e., papillary, follicular, anaplastic, and medullary) occur. Mixtures also occur.

Papillary carcinoma is the most common and may be found in conjunction with follicular tumors. The pure and mixed types behave similarly. Papillary cancers occur at all ages, but in young adults they account for 90 percent of thyroid cancers. Most are asymptomatic but hoarseness, pain, and dyspnea may occur. A single mass is usual, and 20–30 percent have palpable metastatic nodes, formerly sometimes called "lateral aberrant thyroid." Most infiltrate adjacent thyroid tissue, and "warm" or "cold" nodules are found on scan. At operation about half are found to have metastases to nodes and the tumor is multicentric in up to 80 percent. Vascular invasion is present in only about 15 percent. Metastases tend to go to lung and bone.

Follicular adenocarcinoma is a more virulent malignancy, occurring at all ages. Hematogenous metastases predominate and may be the first indication of a malignant process. Nodes are infrequently involved. Some follicles may contain colloid, and capsular and vascular invasion are important prognosis features.

Anaplastic carcinoma usually occurs in old age and is highly malignant. Dysphagia, shortness of breath, and hoarseness are common due to local invasion. Lung and other viscera and node metastases are often present.

Medullary carcinoma is a C-cell calcitonin-producing tumor which may be familial as part of the multiple endocrine neoplasia (MEN) syndrome. They comprise about 10 percent of thyroid cancers and about one-quarter are familial (autosomal dominant). Multiple or single nodules may be present. Diarrhea is commonly present and serotonin, calcitonin, or prostaglandins may be responsible. A few have adrenal cortical hyperplasia and may be found associated with Cushing's syndrome. Diagnosis is best made by an elevated serum calcitonin concentration (radioimmunoassay) and is valuable to determine ablation of the tumor.

Treatment of thyroid cancer depends upon cell type. Papillary and follicular carcinomas are best treated by thyroid hormone administration followed by resection (total or subtotal) or both thyroid lobes with unilateral modified lymph node dissection on the involved side if nodes are involved.

In patients with a history of external irradiation of the neck, as much thyroid tissue as possible should be removed because of the danger of carcinoma developing in the remnant. After operation, thyroid substance to suppress TSH is indicated. Differentiated metastases may take up ^{131}I, which may be useful in controlling metastases. Anaplastic carcinomas are lethal and operation does not alter their course.

Parathyroids

The upper parathyroids arise embryologically from the fourth branchial pouch, the lower from the third. They usually lie on the posterolateral aspect of the thyroid lobes but may be in other locations including the mediastinum. A few are intrathyroidal. Most people have four; a few have more or less. The chief cell is the major cell type and is responsible for parathyroid hormone (PTH) synthesis and secretion. Oxyphil cells, the other cell type, may be a degenerative form of chief cell.

PTH is an 84-amino acid polypeptide, the secretion of which is primarily controlled by the concentration of calcium in the circulation. Its effect is inhibitory, a property shared by magnesium. PTH influences calcium reabsorption in the nephron but it enhances phosphate excretion as well. PTH also mobilizes calcium from bone and stimulates bone formation.

Hyperparathyroidism is a disorder of parathyroid glands leading to an inappropriately high rate of PTH secretion, the most important manifestation of which is hypercalcemia. In its extreme, marked demineralization of bone (osteitis fibrosa cystica) may result. More commonly now, recurrent kidney stones favored by hypercalciuria and hyperphosphatemia, are seen. Skeletal muscle weakness, psychologic changes and, in the extreme, coma and death are manifestations of hypercalcemia. Pancreatitis is a serious complication. Hypercalcemia is always accompanied by hypomagnesemia. Many cases are found in the course of routine blood chemistry determinations when an elevated serum calcium is found. Hyperparathyroidism may be secondary to chronic renal failure which causes elevation of PTH owing to phosphate retention, which lowers free calcium, thereby stimulating PTH formation and release.

An interesting syndrome involving multiple endocrine adenopathies (MEA) includes hyperparathyroidism in both so-called MEA I and MEA II types. MEA I consists of hyperparathyroidism, the Zollinger-Ellison syndrome, and chromophobe adenoma, while it accompanies medullary thyroid carcinoma, pheochromocytoma, and adrenal cortical tumors in the MEA syndrome. These seem to be transmitted as autosomally dominant characteristics with partial penetrance.

The differential diagnosis of hypercalcemia, as is illustrated by the following, is of greatest importance in directing appropriate investigation and treatment.

> Malignancy
> Hyperparathyroidism
> Sarcoidosis
> Hypervitaminosis D
> Paget's disease of bone
> Milk-alkali syndrome
> Renal acidosis
> Protein metabolism abnormalities
> Immobilization

Treatment of hyperparathyroidism is removal of the hyperactive parathyroid tissue. Preoperatively, very high serum calcium levels can be reduced by intravenous saline infusions to induce diuresis. Dehydration must be avoided to prevent precipitation of calcium in the renal tubules. Hypokalemia must be corrected.

Technically, identification of the parathyroid glands is the greater challenge. Preoperatively, the CT scan may be useful in locating adenomas. The location of an adenoma may be determined by venous sampling of PTH in neck veins. Less than 2 percent require a thoracic approach for excision. All of the parathyroids should be visualized and, if no adenoma exists, many advocate resection of three and one-half glands. If an obvious adenoma is present, it alone should be resected. All resected tissue should be examined by frozen section to avoid resection of thyroid of lymph nodes in the mistaken belief that parathyroid tissue is being excised.

Postoperatively, hypocalcemia must be watched for. The Chvostek's sign and perioral numbness may occur. Serum calcium determinations at intervals are indicated and calcium infusions given if values are low. Hypocalcemia may be temporary.

Hyperinsulinism Amenable to Surgical Management

Only about 60 percent of patients having hypoglycemia are amenable to surgical treatment. The beta cells of the pancreatic islets produce insulin and, when beta cell adenomas, hyperplasia, or carcinomas are responsible for hyperinsulinism, surgical resection is indicated. A variety of functional disorders also may cause hypoglycemia and must be carefully excluded before operation is considered.

Confusion, seizures, bizarre behavior, and stupor brought on by fasting associated with low blood glucose levels are tentatively diagnostic. Whipple's triad includes the above plus relief of symptoms by glucose administration but is not diagnostic of surgical hyperinsulinism. Some extrapancreatic tumors elaborate insulin or insulinlike substances, and these must be excluded before operation on the pancreas is decided upon. Resection of such tumors may ameliorate symptoms, but they must first be identified.

Diagnosis depends upon measurement of immunoreactive insulin with concomitant blood glucose determination. In patients with beta cell lesions, the normal feedback control of insulin with respect to glucose is lost and the autonomous release of insulin results in further depression of blood glucose levels. The usual overnight fast may not be sufficiently long to produce hypoglycemia and occasionally 72 hours are required.

Unless there is clear evidence that functioning metastases are responsible for hypoglycemia, removal of the source of autonomous insulin secretion is indicated, with care being taken to preserve as much normal pancreas as possible. Excision of adenomas, or an 80 percent resection of the distal pancreas if islet hyperplasia is the cause, is indicated. Adenomatosis is another form of the disorder and may require excision of a major portion of the pancreas. If surgical control is not possible, dietary adjustment and diazoxide (inhibits insulin release) administration are helpful.

THE LYMPHATIC SYSTEM

The lymphatic system consists of the lymphatic vessels and lymph nodes. Lymph vessels anatomose with veins to provide for the passage of lymph into the vascular system. The fine lymphatic capillaries are distributed throughout the body, where they collect interstitial fluid and its constituents in a selective way. The capillaries join larger vessels containing valves essential for the unidirectional movement of lymph. Before emptying into the venous system, these vessels pass through a number of lymph nodes which act as barriers to lymph flow. The nodes are highly vascular and are supplied by arteries and veins which traverse the hila of the nodes.

The main connections between the lymphatic and venous systems are in two principal locations. (1) The thoracic duct joins the left subclavian vein where the latter joins the jugular vein. Lymphatic vessels draining the left side of the head and neck also converge here. (2) The great lymphatic vein on the right side joins the right subclavian vein.

The transfer of fluid from the interstitial tissues into the lymphatics is determined by the quantity of interstitial fluid, the pressure within the interstitial space, and the concentration of molecules within the fluid. Large molecules are more readily retained in the lymph vessels than are smaller ones. The mechanical factors affecting lymph flow are active muscle contraction, changes in pressure around lymphatic vessels, and changes in venous pressure which, when high, impedes lymph flow. The laws of osmotic pressure affect the flow in the direction of high molecular concentration.

Pathologic conditions of the lymphatic system which are of surgical interest are congenital malformation, tumors, and injuries. Little has been accomplished in the direction of surgical attack on the lymphatic system itself, but many disorders involving the system are amenable to surgical therapy.

Congenital Abnormalities

Congenital abnormalities often involve specific sites and therefore may present characteristic clinical findings. Lymphedema of the upper or lower extremities is one of the more common abnormalities. Lymphangiectasis involving the intraperitoneal structures may become evident by the presence of chylous ascites or chyluria. Congenital lymphatic cysts of the mesentery may compress adjacent viscera with associated symptoms. The neck and mediastinum are favored sites for the development of cystic hygromas (see Pediatric Surgery section) from lymphatic anlage.

Injuries

Injuries of the lymphatic vessels occur due to direct or blunt trauma. Thoracic and abdominal operations may produce injuries of the major lymphatic vessels. Lymphadenectomy may be followed by local collections of lymph in a minority of patients. An explanation as to why it occurs in only a small percentage of patients is lacking. Penetrating wounds of the base of the neck may damage the thoracic duct. The must common sites of thoracic duct injury are in the neck and lower two-thirds of the thorax.

Tumors

Both benign and malignant tumors occur in many locations. Lymph node tumors are essentially malignant tumors of lymphoid origin, more commonly encountered in children and young adults. Hematopathologists now favor a classification consisting of Hodgkin's disease and nonHodgkin's lymphoma. By and large, therapy is nonsurgical, consisting of radiation therapy and chemotherapy, with surgery playing a minor role except in diagnosis and staging. Laparotomy for staging of Hodgkin's disease will probably be replaced by newer imaging techniques such as computerized tomography.

Miscellaneous Lymphatic Disorders

Chylothorax may follow many intrathoracic operations and be associated with intrathoracic inflammatory lesions and neoplasms of the lung or mediastinum. The diagnosis is usually made by thoracentesis which yields milky fluid. The fluid may be clear if the patient has been taking no food. Treatment consists of tube drainage of the pleura which, if unsuccessful, should be followed by thoracic duct ligation. Lymphography may be helpful in identifying the site of leakage. Intravenous hyperalimentation may provide nutritional support if the patient is critical and not suitable for immediate operation. Chylopericardium may accompany chylothorax.

Fistulous communications between lymphatic vessels and various organs and cavities may be caused by malignant tumors, congenital malformations, inflammatory conditions, or trauma. Ascites, chyluria, chylothorax, and lymphoenteric fistulas might appear. Chylous ascites occurs more in males, and pancreatic and gastric neoplasms are major causes. Chyluria may occur with filiariasis and lymphedema is usually present. Chylous diarrhea associated with a protein-losing enteropathy is usually due to congenital malformation.

Lymphedema

Lymphedema is the accumulation of protein-rich fluid in the soft tissues and is usually present in the extremities. It is due to obstruction to the flow of lymph. Primary lymphedema is considered to be idiopathic and of obscure origin and underdevelopment of the lymphatic vessels is thought to be the cause. The vessels are dilated and tortuous. When edema develops early, it is referred to as praecox, and if late, tarda. These changes are probably present at birth. Edematous tissue is prone to bacterial invasion and infection. The lower extemities predominate in frequency. The familial type is referred to as Milroy's disease.

Secondary lymphedema results from a specific cause, most commonly due to surgical interruption of major lymphatic pathways such as with radical mastectomy. Postmastectomy angiosarcoma may develop in the edematous arm.

Lymphangiography is the best means of diagnosing disorders of the system. Nodal architecture may thereby be shown and metastatic desposits and other abnormalities may be appreciated.

Treatment is usually provided by conservative means such as compression bandages or pneumatic devices as well as intermittent elevation. Operative means, less than completely satisfactory, include the excision of edematous subcutaneous tissue, omental implantation, and other procedures designed to remove edema accumulations.

VENOUS DISEASES OF SURGICAL INTEREST

Varicose Veins

The treatment of varicose veins is based upon Trendelenburg's demonstration of a relationship between distended veins and valvular insufficiency. In the erect position the leg veins are subjected to a hydrostatic pressure of about 125 cm of water, which approximates the distance from the right atrium. The supine pressure is about 5 – 10 cm of water. The main superficial channels are the long and short saphenous veins. The long saphenous begins anterior to the medial malleolus and extends upward in an anteromedial position to the fossa ovalis in the groin, where it joins the femoral vein. The short saphenous arises behind the lateral malleolus and ascends the posterio aspect of the leg to enter the popliteal vein in the popliteal fossa. These large vessels communicate freely by small tributaries. These veins contain valves which prevent downward flow.

The deep venous system begins as vena comitantes of the posterior tibial, peroneal, and anterior tibial arteries which converge to form the popliteal vein behind the knee. The popliteal vein continues upward in the thigh as the superficial femoral and is joined near the femoral triangle by the deep femoral vein to become the common femoral vein. The common femoral passes under Poupart's ligament to become the external iliac vein. The deep venous system contains valves as far cephalad as the external iliac vein. Flow directed centrally is facilitated by muscular contractions in the extremity which produce a powerful propulsive force. A network of communicating veins connects the superficial to the deep system, providing for emptying of the superficial veins.

The pathogenesis of varicose veins probably stems from proximal valvular incompetence due to defective valves in conjunction with vein wall weakness, which yield to hydrostatic pressure in the erect state. There is a strong hereditary component, with females being much more susceptible. Pregnancy and occupations requiring prolonged standing seem to predispose, and the long saphenous vein is the most prone to develop varicosities. As the process extends distally, it even involves the intracutaneous veins. If the perforating valves become involved, the muscle pump fails and the surrounding tissue is exposed to a constant high hydrostatic pressure with subsequent stasis dermatitis and, in some instances, ulceration. These ultimate changes are usually associated with postphlebitic changes, and ulcers are unusual with primary varicose veins.

Even huge varicose veins are not often symptomatic, and when pain is present there usually is another cause. Heaviness and nocturnal leg cramps may be present. If ulcers appear, they usually occur above the medial malleolus if the long saphenous is at fault. If the short saphenous is involved, ulcers may be present over the lateral lower third of the leg. Superficial varicosities may rupture, with significant hemorrhage.

A variety of tourniquet tests are available to test the competency of perforating veins which connect the superficial with the deep venous systems. They are useful in establishing the site of incompetent perforators, which should be ligated to avoid recurrence.

Treatment is usually by vein excision and high ligation of the involved vein. Stripping is now the treatment of choice. Small recurrent varicosities may be treated by injecting with sclerosing solutions.

Thrombophlebitis

Thrombophlebitis is an inflammatory reaction in veins, usually in afferent veins leading into the inferior vena cava. Thrombus formation is usually associated with the inflammatory process. Surgeons have great interest in this process because of the threat of thrombus detachment and consequent pulmonary embolism. Surgical operations predispose to the development of thrombus formation but there are many other causes such as direct trauma, the infusion of fluids into veins, infections, and a larger number in which the cause is not known. Stasis due to the absence of the pumping mechanism provided by leg muscles, recumbency, pregnancy, low cardiac output, and other causes combine to set the stage for its development. Drug addicts inject contaminated substances into their veins with resulting septic phlebitis.

In most instances, phlebitis involving superficial veins is easily treated by elevation and warm compresses. When the deep venous system of the lower extremities is involved, however, there is a potential for both pulmonary embolism and the postphlebitic syndrome to develop. If the initial thrombotic process is severe, massive edema may be present. Clot lysis usually occurs, but, when incomplete, it adds an element of obstruction to blood flow, intensifying the effect of valvular insufficiency.

Treatment of deep phlebitis is best carried out by prolonged intravenous heparin administration and elevation of the extremity. Not infrequently, the location of thrombosis is not clinically apparent and pulmonary embolism may call attention to its presence. Venography is the most reliable test but it requires an invasive technique. Other noninvasive tests using plethysmography and radioisotope uptake studies are useful if the clinical diagnosis is not apparent.

The basic treatment for pulmonary embolism is long-term heparin therapy. Occasionally, however, emboli continue to migrate to the lungs and mechanical means are required to control the process. Inferior vena caval occlusion by direct ligation or by filtering devices passed into the cava by way of the neck veins are appropriate if medical treatment fails.

Massive thrombosis of the venous system of a lower extremity with involvement of the iliac vein may produce massive edema and cyanosis, which may threaten the limb. On occasion, thrombectomy carried out through the common femoral vein may avoid amputation. There is a marked tendency for thrombus formation to recur, however, and the postphlebitic syndrome frequently follows irrespective of treatment.

MOUTH, JAWS, NECK, LARYNX, PHARYNX AND SINUSES, EAR, AND NOSE

Diseases of the mouth, jaws, and neck may be congenital, traumatic, inflammatory, neoplastic, or metastatic. Neoplasms are benign or malignant.

Lip

The majority of mouth lesions occur on the lip. The embryogenesis of the facial region predisposes to developmental anomalies, and clefts of the lips and palate are the most common major anomalies to occur. They are more frequent in males, are more common on the left side of the lip, and may be bilateral. There is hereditary tendency. Unless extreme difficulty requires special treatment, operative repair of the lip at 8 to 10 weeks is usually advised, with palate repair some months later.

Hemangiomas of the lips are common at birth. Capillary hemangiomas usually regress but may grow rapidly, and when they become infected, bleed, or develop arteriovenous fistulas, excision may be indicated. Cavernous hemangiomas generally do not regress and may require excision, intralesional cautery or injection of sclerosing agents. Mucoceles are best excised to exclude malignancies.

Squamous cell carcinomas of the lip account for about 25 percent of oral cancers. Males who smoke or who are exposed to severe actinic radiation are prone, and alcoholism and poor oral hygiene commonly accompany this tumor. It almost always involves the lower lip and is usually low grade with first route of metastases to the submental nodes. Treatment is surgical, radiation, or a combination of both.

Tongue

Anterior tongue lesions are easy to examine, while posteriorly they may be difficult to detect. Congenital lesions include lingual thyroid, hemangioma, and lymphangioma. Vitamin deficiencies and inflammatory lesions such as syphilis or tuberculosis are part of systemic processes. Benign ulcers are painful lesions of viral origin. Benign tumors include granular cell myoblastoma, and less common lesions such as glossitis rhomboidica and pregnancy tumor of the tongue.

Cancer of the tongue is the second most common of oral cancers. The anterior two-thirds of the tongue is mobile, differs embryologically from the posterior one-third, and malignant lesions under the anterior tongue tend to be of lower grade malignancy. Alcoholism, tobacco use, syphilis, and poor oral hygiene appear to predispose to tongue cancer. Irradiation, surgery, or combinations are accepted treatment modalities. Speech is usually quite good even after major glossal resections.

Floor of Mouth

Lesions here arise in the mucosa anterior to the tongue and posterior to the lower gingiva. Partial obstruction of a salivary duct by stone may produce a cyst (ranula). If symptomatic, excision or marsupialization is indicated.

Squamous cell carcinoma is the major lesion and surgical excision is indicated. They may metastasize early.

Tonsil

Inflammation is the most common affliction of this structure. Malignancies may be lymphomas or, more commonly, squamous cell carcinomas. Treatment is primarily by radiotherapy.

Jaws

Congenital epignathus is a teratoma of the jaws and trapped epithelial cell nests may produce cysts at time of fusion. Odontogenic cysts are epithelial appendages which grow with the teeth. The most common ectodermal neoplasm is the adamantinoma (ameloblastoma) which arises from the enamel organ. These may occasionally metastasize. Excision is the treatment of all these lesions.

Burkitt's tumor is a highly malignant neoplasm of undifferentiated lymphoreticular cells. They respond

well to cyclophosphamide. Sarcomas and chondrogenic tumors of the jaws are unusual and often highly malignant.

Salivary Glands

Mikulicz's syndrome is characterized by enlargement of the parotid and lacrimal glands due to invasion by lymphoma. Mikulicz's disease refers to a syndrome of rheumatoid arthritis, keratoconjunctivitis, and xerostomia with salivary and lacrimal gland swelling which is probably due to an autoimmune disorder.

Mumps parotitis is common and self-limited. Suppurative parotitis is seen in sick or postoperative patients and *Staphylococcus aureus* is the usual causative organism. Parotid duct stone may obstruct to cause gland infection.

Tumors of the parotid are usually benign, most being mixed tumors. Most occur in the superficial lobe. Parotidectomy is the preferred treatment. Warthin's tumor (papillary cystoadenolymphomatosum) comprises about 5 percent of parotid lesions and is most frequently seen in older men. Malignant lesions demonstrate a spectrum of virulence and resection is indicated in all. Seventh nerve involvement usually indicates malignancy. If resection of a portion of the facial nerve is required, a nerve graft may reduce facial paralysis.

Sialolithiasis may occur in any of the salivary ducts. Sialography may be useful if the stone is neither palpated nor visualized by roentgenogram. Stone removal may avoid infection.

Neck

Masses in the neck occur in all age groups and clinical diagnosis may be easy or very difficult. Midline tumors and cysts are usually benign. In adults, lateral lesions are often malignant. A thorough history and physical examination are extremely important in diagnosis before biopsy is performed. Mouth lesions should be carefully sought because of the possibility that the neck mass is metastatic. In children, ectopic thyroid, dermoid cysts, thyroglossal duct cysts, lipomas, and thyroid nodules are midline lesions to consider. Lateral lumps might be thyroid or mucogenic tumors, cystic hygromas, or sarcomas. Branchiogenic cysts lie in the anterior triangle of the neck and arise from the second branchial groove. If infected, drainage is indicated; if not, excision is curative.

The cervical lymph nodes are prone to enlargement in a wide variety of infections and malignant processes. When a single node is enlarged malignancy must be suspected. Inflammatory lesions range from acute nonspecific lymphadenitis to tuberculosis (scrofula). "Cat scratch disease" is a granulomatous lymphadenitis due to minor skin trauma, with or without cat contact.

RADICAL NECK DISSECTION

Radical cervical lymph node dissection is an established therapeutic modality which deserves brief mention. Many malignant lesions of the head and neck metastasize to cervical nodes in a predictable manner. They may be contained therein for some time and may therefore be amenable to resection with improved therapeutic results. Neck dissection may be offered under the following circumstances:

1. The primary lesions should have been controlled clinically, or if not controlled, should be amenable to resection at the time the neck dissection is performed.
2. There should be a reasonable chance for complete removal of cervical metastases.
3. There should be no evidence of distant metastases.
4. Neck dissection should offer a better chance of cure than alternate procedures (e.g., radiotherapy or chemotherapy).

The operation is designed to remove the lymph node bed en bloc, to remove all lymphatic tissue between the platysma and deep cervical fascia from mandible to clavicle and posteriorly to the border of the trapezius to the lateral border of the strap muscles. Prophylactic node dissections remain controversial with some primary tumors such as those of the tongue.

Larynx

Trauma to the larynx may cause death due to airway obstruction. The external wound, hemoptysis, loss of voice, and dyspnea suggest the injury. Repair should always be accompanied by tracheostomy. Hematomas due to contusion are lesser injuries and the signs are correspondingly milder. Intubation granulomas from inlying endotracheal tubes result when pressure on the vocal cords results in necrosis with granulation tissue formation. They usually respond to local excision by direct laryngoscopy. A more serious injury due to prolonged intubation is tracheal ulceration due to cuff pressure. When extensive, cicatricial stenotic tracheal lesions go on to obstruction. Resection of stenosis, difficult under the best circumstances, may be impossible with permanent tracheostomy being required. Large low pressure endotracheal tube cuffs tend to lessen the incidence of this dreaded complication.

Laryngeal paralysis may result from injury to the recurrent laryngeal nerve during operation or other trauma or by pressure due to tumors such as lung cancer. The vocal cord is immobilized near the median position since all intrinsic muscles except the cricothyroid are affected. Sometimes paralysis is idiopathic. When both recurrent nerves are involved (bilateral "abductor paralysis"), dyspnea may not occur at rest but inspiratory stridor ensues with exertion.

Benign laryngeal tumors include infantile laryngeal papillomatosis, adult papilloma, hemangiomas, fibromas, etc. Excision is usually recommended.

Laryngeal cancers are usually squamous cell tumors and predominate in male smokers who use alcohol. Persistent hoarseness is the symptom most likely to be present. Treatment depends upon the stage of the lesion and consists of surgery, radiotherapy, and chemotherapy. With an early lesion confined to the midportion of one cord, radiotherapy usually cures. Laryngofissure and chordectomy also cures but leaves the patient with dysphonia. Small supraglottic lesions are amenable to supraglottic hemilaryngectomy. Total laryngectomy is required when the cord becomes fixed. Radical neck dissection is added when cervical adenopathy is present. Laryngectomy obliterates vocal function, and training and mechanical devices are necessary to assist in communication.

Pharynx

The pharynx is one of the structures most commonly treated by operation. Tonsillectomy and adenoidectomy rank high in incidence among surgical procedures. Briefly, tonsillectomy may be indicated if marked hypertrophy leads to dyspnea or dysphagia, if repeated attacks of tonsillitis are disabling, or if peritonsillar abscess or chronic cervical adenitis, especially with abscess formation, occurs. The indications for operation have been more sharply defined and it is likely that tonsillectomy will be performed less often in the future. The adenoids are also part of Waldeyer's ring of lymphoid tissue surrounding the pharynx and, if hypertrophied, may produce nasal obstruction and recurrent otitis media, both of which are indications for adenoidectomy.

Of the malignant tumors of the pharynx, squamous cell carcinomas are the most frequent, but lymphoepitheliomas, transitional cell tumors, and adenocarcinomas occur as well. Radiation is the basic form of treatment.

Benign pharyngeal tumors include juvenile angiofibroma, chordoma (notochord remnant), and choanal polyps.

Tumors and abscesses also affect the hypopharynx and may be difficult to diagnose because of inaccessibility to direct examination.

Paranasal Sinuses

The frontal and ethmoid sinuses and the antra are paired structures which drain into the nose beneath the middle turbinate. The posterior ethmoids and sphenoids drain into the superior nasal meatus above the middle turbinate. Acute sinusitis usually starts as a virus infection followed by bacterial superinfection. Pain, headache, and local tenderness, along with inflammation of the nasal mucosa, suggest its presence. Sinus roentgenograms demonstrating dullness or fluid levels are confirmatory. Decongestants may promote drainage and antibiotics are indicated. Surgery should be delayed if possible during the acute episode. Complications include osteoma, mucocele, and frontal osteomyelitis, which are indications for operation.

Trauma to the cribriform plate with leak of cerebrospinal fluid may require operation and broad spectrum antibiotics should be given to avoid meningitis.

The Ear

The ear is comprised of the external ear (sound collector), the middle ear (ossicles which transmit sound), and inner ear (utricle and three semicircular canals, which is the balance mechanism). The outer ear is prone to infections, obstruction by cerumen, and foreign body impaction. Exostosis of the bony canal may obstruct the canal and require removal, and other benign and malignant tumors may appear in skin or ceruminal glands. Surgery and radiotherapy may be required.

Middle ear disorders include infections, common in children, drum rupture due to perforating or barotrauma, tumors, and otospongiosis (otosclerosis). When infection extends to the temporal bone, mastoidectomy may be required. Otosclerosis leads to conductive hearing loss. It is more common in women, progressive with each pregnancy, and begins in the third decade of life.

The inner ear is subject to a wide variety of disorders, many hereditary, resulting in sensorineural hearing loss. Disorders of balance, nystagmus, vertigo, and Meniere's disease are frequently due to disorders of the middle ear.

The Nose

The nose functions to humidify inspired air, to smell, and to provide vocal resonance. The external nose is frequently operated upon for deformity and tumors. Basal cell carcinomas are usually curable with excision or irradiation. Squamous cell tumors tend to metastasize early to preauricular, parotid, or submandibular nodes. Wide excision is the best treatment. Epistaxis is a common disorder which reflects local or systemic disorders (blood dyscrasias, hypertension, etc.) The area of Kiesselbach and branches of the internal maxillary artery posteriorly are sites of predilection. Pressure devices such as packing and pneumatic balloons may be required to control bleeding, but ligation techniques may be required if simpler methods fail.

The inner nose has surgical interest because of septal deviations which may obstruct breathing, hematomas, polyps, and malignant tumors.

CENTRAL NERVOUS SYSTEM

Head and spinal cord injuries account for most of the deaths due to deceleration injuries and account for a major proportion of disabled survivors. Because the brain will tolerate only a few minutes of anoxia before irreversible changes occur, the emergency management of head injuries is extremely important. Oxygenated blood must reach the cerebral cortex rapidly and the most critical correctable problem is the obstructed airway. This is easily restored by manipulation of the mandible, removal of obstructing objects (dentures, vomitus, blood, and mucus) and intubation, care being taken to avoid cervical cord injury in the presence of cervical spine fractures. A cross-table lateral roentgenogram of the neck early in the course of resuscitation is valuable in ruling out cervical spine injury (all seven cervical vertebrae must be seen). Correction of thoracic injuries to thereby provide adequate ventilation or the reinstitution of mechanical ventilation manages this problem.

Shock is almost never associated with the survivable head injury. Its presence mandates the necessity for identifying the cardiovascular deficit, usually hypovolemia, usually due to intra-abdominal bleeding. High cervical cord injury may cause hypotension due to sympathetic denervation, so-called spinal shock.

Evaluation of the head injured patient must be systematically done in order to guide treatment. The level of consciousness is the most important sign and changes in level of consciousness must be carefully recorded. The Glasgow coma scale is one of several schemes used to objectively evaluate these patients (Table 14-5). This scale requires only recording of best response to verbal and noxious stimuli. Severity of injury is the inverse of the score. The use of a flow sheet with time and findings recorded is very important in following these patients, especially when different individuals are examining them.

After assessment of the level of consciousness, focal signs should be sought. Pupillary response is highly significant in that this may indicate dangerous shift of the brain. A dilated pupil usually indicates compression of the oculomotor nerve by the ipsilateral temporal lobe. Stimulation of the cornea with a wisp of cotton resulting

Table 14-5. Glasgow Coma or Responsiveness Scale
(Score Sum 3 – 15)

Eye opening	Spontaneous	4
	To speech	3
	To pain	2
	None	1
Verbal response	Oriented	5
	Confused conversation	4
	Inappropriate words	3
	Incomprehensible sounds	2
	None	1
Best motor response	Obeys commands	6
	Localizes pain	5
	Flexion withdrawal	4
	Flexion abnormal	3
	Extends	2
	None	1

in lid closure indicates an intact corneal reflex, and conjugate deviation of the eyes in a direction opposite to that in which the head is being sharply rotated indicates an intact oculocephalic reflex (doll's eye movement). This latter test must not be done until cervical spine films demonstrate absence of a spine fracture. These tests of brain stem function elicit important prognostic signs.

The skull must be inspected and palpated for evidence of fracture. Blood in the auditory canals, nonclotting blood in the nares and mastoid, or upper eyelid ecchymosis suggests basal skull fracture.

Lacerations are debrided and carefully repaired. Open fractures require operating room facilities.

Brain swelling is a dreaded complication of head injuries, and steroids and diuretics are often used in an attempt to reduce edema. Mannitol, 500 ml of a 20 percent solution, given over 15 minutes causes a rapid decrease in intracranial pressure. Hyperventilation tends to quickly reduce intracranial pressure due to the effect of alkalosis upon the cerebral circulation. Catheters inserted into the ventricles are valuable in following intracranial pressure changes.

After the patient's condition is stabilized, investigation should be carried out to determine whether an operable lesion is present. The CT scan does this best and will show depressed fractures and collections of blood which may benefit by craniotomy. Lacking the CT scan, skull roentgenograms and cerebral arteriography are very useful. Indications for operation are as follows:

Open fractures: Remove foreign bodies (sometimes metallic foreign bodies removed from the site are not removed). Remove depressed fragments of the cranium. Hemostasis (close carefully, especially dura).

Epidural hematoma: Usually "clear interval" after injury followed by deepening level of consciousness.

Middle meningeal artery usually injured by fracture. Evacuate hematoma and control bleeding.

Subdural hematoma: Symptoms early or delayed. Deteriorating neurologic status. Evacuate hematoma by craniotomy.

Subarachnoid hemorrhage: Most common type of intracranial hemorrhage. Meningeal signs. Usually requires no operation.

Cerebrospinal fluid leak: Most close spontaneously. If rhinorrhea or otorrhea persist over 2 weeks, surgical repair. Antibiotic coverge to avoid meningitis.

Intracerebral hemorrhage: May require craniotomy if condition is deteriorating. Often found with subdural hematoma.

Spinal Cord Injuries

Spinal cord injuries are among the most serious of all injuries and may result in permanent total paralysis. Fatal injuries of the cervical cord paralyze intercostal respiratory effort, and injuries above C5 involve the diaphragm. Above C4, death is the usual outcome.

Therapy is aimed at reducing neurologic deficit and especially to prohibit manipulations from making the deficit worse, as during intubation during resuscitation. Traction and rigid cervical collars are very useful in protecting the cord. Arterial blood gas determinations are important in monitoring the adequacy of ventilation. Patients with brain and cord injuries are especially prone to infections, pulmonary embolism, and other pulmonary complications.

Intracranial Tumors

Intracranial tumors arise from the brain or its coverings and are mimicked by vascular accidents, hematomas, granulomas, parastic cysts, and pseudotumor cerebri. Brain tumors occur mostly in children under 10 and in adults over 40 years of age. In childhood, tumors arising in congenital defects and cell rest beneath the tentorium predominate; in adults, supratenorial tumors are common. Pituitary tumors and meningiomas usually affect adults and gliomas occur in both age groups.

Classical symptoms are headache and vomiting associated with papilledema. Papilledema reflects venous obstruction of retinal vessels. Convulsions, especially adult onset, are common. Focal signs may include contralateral weakness, paralysis of extraocular muscles, and speech defects. Memory loss, personality changes, and changes in smell are suggestive.

Gliomas, meningiomas, and pituitary tumors comprise about 75 percent of brain tumors. Metastatic tumors are common, and primary tumors must be excluded before embarking on therapy. Astrocytomas (75 percent of gliomas) spread to the opposite hemisphere and glioblastomas are highly malignant invasive tumors. Oligodendrogliomas may grow very slowly and long survival is possible. Meningiomas are benign but their location may make removal impossible. Neuromas may involve the acoustic nerve, giving rise to deafness, impaired corneal reflex, and vestibular dysfunction. Resection is tedious but results are good. Metastatic tumors may respond to radiotherapy or chemotherapy.

Cerebrovascular Disorders

Partial or complete obstruction of the carotid or vertebral arteries may produce symptoms. With complete obstruction, flow can rarely be restored. A small number of patients have had bypass procedures done by microsurgical procedures in which extracranial vessels are anastomosed to intracranial arteries directly or by graft.

Temporal arteritis, a curious disorder in which giant cell inflammation of the arterial wall is found, is associated with cerebral infarction or loss of vision due to retinal artery occlusion. Steroids control the disorder.

Hemorrhage due to vascular disease is usually due to abnormalities about the base of the brain such as aneurysm. Arteriovenous (AV) malformations, blood dyscrasias, and neoplasms are other causes. Control by surgical procedures and antihypertensive medication is indicated, depending upon the site of aneurysm. AV malformations are sometimes resectable and therapeutic embolization is coming into use.

Cranial and intracranial infections often are secondary to infection in other structures such as sinuses, heart, lung, etc. Veins of the face and orbit emptying into the cavernous sinus may lead to thrombosis with ophthalmoplegia, ptosis, and papilledema. Cranial bone infections may originate in ear infections, and extradural and subdural empyema may result from sinusitis. Drainage by craniotomy is indicated. Children are prone because of hemophilus and pneumococcal meningitis, which are not uncommon. Brain abscess is usually bloodborne (gram + cocci + anaerobes most common). Treatment is by systemic antibiotics and drainage or excision when indicated.

Surgery of the Spine

Pain due to herniated intervertebral disks is one of the most common complaints seen in patients referred to neurosurgeons. The lumbar and cervical spines are most vulnerable in the third to fifth decades. Symptoms and signs are produced by compression of the cord or nerve roots by protruding disks and the bony excrescences associated with them. In the lumbar area, pain radiating down the distribution of the sciatic nerve is common.

Back pain, stiffness, and spasm are commonly experienced. Less of the lordotic curve, motor weakness, and reflex loss involving the specific distribution are objective signs. When conservative therapy fails, operation to relieve nerve root and cord pressure is indicated. At times spondylolisthesis, the displacement of lumbar vertebra anteriorly or posteriorly, causes pain, and spine fusion may be indicated.

Correction of scoliosis and removal of cord AV malformations, tumors, etc., are less frequently employed surgical procedures.

The neurosurgical relief of pain is often required for incurable malignant processes. The aim is pain relief with a minimum of functional dysfunction, often hard to achieve. The sectioning of posterior nerve roots and spinothalamic tract section (cordotomy) is employed.

Trigeminal neuralgia (tic doloreaux) is a severe form of pain involving the distribution of the fifth cranial nerve. Intractable cases are best treated by injection, avulsion of nerve branches, or section between the gesserian ganglion or pons.

ONCOLOGY

About one in four persons now living will develop cancer and about one-third of those who develop cancer will survive 5 years after treatment. Certain cancers are declining in incidence, but overall the disease is increasing. Lung cancer is the leading cause of cancer death when both sexes are considered, and in men the incidence is about 18 times as great as it was 40 years ago. Pancreatic cancer has shown a steady increase in both sexes, but stomach cancer declined more than two-thirds since 1930. In decreasing order of frequency for males are lung, colon and rectum, prostate, pancreas, and stomach. In women the order is the breast, colon and rectum, uterus, lung, and ovary.

Etiology

The causes of many cancers in lower animals are known, and there are many reasons to believe that multiple factors act in humans to produce neoplasia. Some of these are known or are highly suspect.

HEREDITARY FACTORS

A number of cancers developing in special situations suggest strong hereditary influence. Familial polyposis of the colon is associated with a high incidence of colon cancer. Breast cancer shows high frequency in certain families and daughters developing breast cancer tend to develop it earlier than did their mothers. Gardner's syndrome (epidermal inclusion cysts, bony exostoses, colon polyposis, and benign connective tissue tumors) are prone to develop colon cancer in those afflicted. There is a high incidence of skin cancer in patients with xeroderma pigmentosa. Some families have a tendency to polyendocrine adenomas and there is a tendency to develop adenocarcinomas in the gastrointestinal and genital tracts in these patients. Lymphatic system tumors tend to occur in rather sharply defined age groups, melanoma postpubertal, acute lymphocytic leukemia in children, etc.

PHYSICAL CARCINOGENS

The best recognized physical carcinogen is ionizing radiation. Cancers of the skin and thyroid are known to be related to radiation. Schistosomiasis predisposes to liver and bladder cancer, and irritation may be at fault. Cancers developing in scars (Marjolin's ulcer), and development of skin cancer in those exposed to prolonged ultraviolet light are believed to be induced by such physical agents.

Chemical Carcinogens

Certain systems show a predilection for development of cancers in response to exposure to specific chemical agents. Asbestos is known to produce bronchial tumors and mesotheliomas. Aromatic amines affect the urinary tract, coal tar and creosote products affect the skin and bronchi, benzene affects the blood and lymphatic organs, etc. Most occur in industrial workers exposed over prolonged periods of time. Agents such as the tar in cigarette smoke are clearly cancer producing but additional factors such as heredity, hormonal states, etc., may be required before cancer occurs.

VIRUSES

The strong relationship between viruses and cancer in lower animals is not evident in man in most instances. However, the Epstein-Barr virus (the cause of infectious mononucleosis) is related to the occurrence of Burkitt's lymphoma in Africa and to cancer of the nasopharynx in China, and evidence is mounting that sexually transmitted malignant diseases may be viral in origin.

Biological Behavior of Tumors

Most malignant tumors arise from malignant transformation of a single cell to form a malignant clone. After transformation, the malignant cell differs from the normal in morphology, antigenic expression, and biochemistry. The tendency is to dedifferentiation to more primitive cell types, and orderly tissue patterns are replaced by an aggregation of malignant cells in no organized orientation. Mitoses increase, nucleus and nucleoli tend to hyperchronicity, and pleomorphism is evident. No single biochemical aberration characterizes malignant change, but changes in DNA and RNA seem linked to loss of inhibition to intercellular adhesiveness and proliferation. Hyperfunction of malignant cells may suggest evidence of hyperfunction of the parent cell (e.g., hyperparathyroidism). The biochemistry of normal cells may revert to that of embryonal cells with the advent of malignant change. For example, the carcinoembryonic antigen associated with gastrointestinal cancers and the α-fetoglobulin associated with hepatoma and embryonal cancers are useful markers used to detect malignancy in these structures.

Immunity is undoubtedly related to the development and sustaining of tumor growth although the evidence is still sketchy in man. Spontaneous regression of tumors, the presence of malignant cells in peripheral blood in patients who do not develop metastases, and the rapid recrudescence of growth many years after apparent arrest all suggest an immunologic mechanism.

If assumed that cancer arises from a single cell, it is apparent that most of the growth of human cancers occurs before they become clinically detectable. It requires about 30 exponential divisions to produce a 1 cm tumor (one billion cells). Growth rate is expressed as doubling time or the time required to double in volume. Most tumors double in volume between 20 and 100 days (some more than 600 days), and the speed of doubling bears a roughly inverse relationship to survival. Doubling time is useful in determining response to treatment. Most tumors appear to be present at least 1 year before detection, and it is in the prediscovery phase of growth where promise exists for screening methods for detection and treatment by surgery.

Of great importance are carcinomas in situ, the detection of which has been most effective in a large number of people. The Papanicolaou smear used to detect early cancer of the cervix is the outstanding example of a useful screening test. It often requires more than 10 years for in situ carcinomas of the cervix to become invasive, an interval affording virtual assurance of prevention by appropriate treatment. The stomach and bronchus are other sites amenable to detection by cytologic examination.

Malignancies have been graded based upon their degree of differentiation, number of mitoses, and the appearance of their cells and nuclei. They are usually graded progressively from 1 to 4, with 1 being the best differentiated and least malignant. Such grading is useful in a general way in predicting the clinical course, but actual growth (doubling time) and the presence or absence of metastases are most useful.

Neoplasms are best classified on the basis of cell of origin. Carcinomas arise in epithelial cells and sarcomas have a mesenchymal origin (connective tissue, bone, muscle, vascular or fatty tissue). Teratomas indicate an origin in immature somatic cells and they show different degrees of differentiation into somatic cells of endodermal, epidermal, and mesodermal types. The latter occur mostly in the testis, ovary, and mediastinum.

Without the potential for spread before clinical detection, most cancers would be easy to eradicate. The routes of spread are direct, vascular, lymphatic, and implantation. Many tumors show a distinct tendency to spread by one or more of the above routes and the search for metastases is based upon these patterns. Stomach and esophageal carcinomas and soft tissue sarcomas tend to spread great distances beyond the grossly apparent limits of the lesion. Tumor cells easily enter the lymphatics and embolize in regional nodes, and this mode of spread is common in cell epithelial neoplasms except basal cell carcinomas of the skin, which tend only to be locally invasive. Sarcomas tend not to metastasize to nodes. Vascular spread occurs by way of the thoracic duct or by direct venous invasion. Arteries are rarely invaded. Peritoneal and pleural "seeding" are examples of spread by implantation.

Clinical Manifestations of Cancer

Clinicians frequently classify cancer as early or late depending upon the possibility of effecting a cure, and there may be little relationship to length of time the tumor has been present. Clinical manifestations depend upon where the tumor is located, and the so-called seven warning signals enunciated by the American Cancer Society are based upon the prevalence of the most common tumors. Palpable lumps, change in bowel or bladder habits, chronic cough or hoarseness, indigestion or dysphagia, changes in skin lesions, unusual bleeding, and nonhealing sores are typical. In the gastrointestinal and genitourinary tracts and the respiratory system, obstruction is often the first symptom. Vomiting, jaundice, urinary retention, and pneumonia distal to an obstructing bronchial lesion are manifestations of obstruction. Brain tumors cause pain and paralysis owing to the expansion of the tumor in the unyielding cranial cavity. When tumors impinge upon or infiltrate nerves, pain results, and direct extension of breast cancer may fix the breast to the chest wall. Tumor necrosis may cause bleeding (e.g., cecum) and infection may result in fever, which may be the presenting symptom. Palpable nodes may be the first sign. Palpable nodes in the neck may indicate a primary lesion in the thyroid, oral cavity, larynx, or pharynx, and lymphomas often present in this way. The primary source of metastatic deposits in axillary nodes is usually the breast, but melanomas and lymphomas may be the cause. Tumors most likely to metastasize to the

central nervous system are breast, lung, kidney, and colon. Implantation of tumors on peritoneal and pleural surfaces most likely arise in the lung, breast, and ovary, and lymphomas often behave in this manner. Ascites or pleural effusions may be the first objective evidence. Breast, prostate, bronchial, and thyroid tumors are the most likely sources of tumors metastasizing to bone. The lung favors metastatic growth of a large number of tumors principally from the breast, colon, melanomas, thyroid, kidney, and stomach, and sarcomas of all types may spread to the lung by the hematogenous route. Colon, breast, stomach, pancreatic, and lung cancers tend to metastasize to the liver.

Some interesting systemic manifestations may result from the production of hormones by the tumor, some of which may mimic known hormones in their physiologic activity. Some include the following:

Cushing's disease (increased ACTH)	Lung, thymus, pancreas
Hyperparathyroidism (increased PTH or bone destruction)	Lung, breast, kidney sarcomas
Hyponatremia (increased ADH)	Lung, brain
Precocious puberty	Adrenal, lung, testicle, liver
Zollinger-Ellison syndrome (increased gastrin)	Pancreatic nonbeta cell adenomas
Hypoglycemia	Liver and mesenchymal tumors

A variety of cutaneous, hematologic, neurologic, and vascular diseases may suggest an underlying neoplasm. Myasthenia gravis suggests a thymic tumor and hyperuricemia hematopoietic neoplasms.

Cancer Staging

A variety of staging classifications for malignant tumors have developed over the years and some are organ specific. A basic classification long in use is the following:

Stage I   — Tumor confined to primary site
Stage II — Metastases to regional nodes
Stage III — Metastases to distant sites

The TNM classification now in favor is based upon tumor size, node metastases, and distant metastasis, respectively. T_1, T_2, T_3, and T_4 indicate lesions of increasing size. N_0 indicates absence of nodal metastases and

N_1, N_2, etc., indicate extent of nodal metastases. Distant metastatic status is M_0 (no evidence for metastases) or M_1 (if distant metastases evident). Therefore, a small lesion with no evidence of spread would be classified at $T_1N_0M_0$, and a far advanced tumor which has metastasized to nodes and other sites might be $T_3N_1M_1$.

Specific staging systems have been developed for Hodgkin's disease and other lymphomas. Treatment protocols rely strongly on the accuracy of clinical staging. In this instance, symptoms (i.e., fever, night sweats, weight loss) are taken into account in staging. Stage I relates to disease localized to one lymph node-bearing area, and stage II indicates extension into adjacent regional areas but confined to one side of the diaphragm and restricted to lymph node-bearing areas including Waldeyer's ring and spleen. Stage III denotes involvement of nodes on both sides of the diaphragm, and stage IV is assigned to situations where there is diffuse involvement of one or more extralymphatic sites including the liver. Stage III is divided into III_1 and III_2. III_1 indicates involvement of upper abdomen only, and III_2 is designated if para-aortic, iliac, or inguinal involvement is present whether or not the upper abdomen is involved. The suffix B indicates the presence of fever, night sweats, or weight loss, and A their absence.

Surgeons have become involved in operative procedures designed to obtain information regarding the extent of tumor and the histologic characteristics. Operation is rarely depended upon as a therapeutic measure. Staging laparotomy is done to sample lymph nodes from all locations, and to perform splenectomy and liver biopsy. Since the development of computerized tomography (CT), lymphangiography and laparatomy are being employed less frequently, but in situations where therapeutic decisions depend heavily upon precise information regarding extent of involvement, surgical staging has a place. Bone marrow biopsy is useful, especially in stage III and IV lesions, and generous iliac crest biopsies seem best.

Treatment

Surgery is the primary treatment of most malignant tumors. Specific indications are discussed under respective organ systems. Cancer treatment by an interdisciplinary team of surgeons, radiologists, and internists is well established.

CHEMOTHERAPY

The treatment of cancer by drugs dates from 1941 when Huggins discovered that estrogens were useful in treating prostatic cancer. A large number of agents have been developed. Most affect cell enzymes or enzyme substrates and, in most instances, relate to DNA synthesis. The antimetabolites inhibit nucleic acid synthesis. Alkylating agents work by substituting alkyl groups for hydrogen ions in DNA, which break the DNA molecule, and this action resembles that seen in ionizing radiation. Some antibiotics form complexes with DNA, inhibiting synthesis of DNA and RNA.

Hormonal manipulation is an additional form of chemotherapy applicable in patients with hormone-dependent tumors such as breast and prostate cancer. Castration benefits metastatic prostatic cancer patients, and ablation of adrenals, ovaries, or pituitary has been used in breast cancer. Newer drugs are being developed which simulate the effect of ablation and their usefulness will increase.

RADIATION THERAPY

Radiation treatment, like surgery, can cure ony localized cancer. Its overall use extends far beyond its usefulness in curing localized cancers, and more than one-third of cancer patients receive it as curative, adjunctive, or palliative treatment. Some neoplasms are best treated by radiation, others by operation, and in some it may be optional. Used in conjunction, radiation and surgery may produce a higher cure rate than when either is used alone.

Radiation produces its effect by its energy colliding with atoms in tissue, releasing energy that causes ionization of water in cells. The result is to break chromosomes and DNA in cells, both normal and neoplastic. Normal cells appear to be able to repair themselves more adequately than tumor cells, a fortunate circumstance in planning treatment. Some cellular effects of radiation occur immediately, while others are delayed. Years may be required for gross changes to appear.

The penetration of roentgenograms depends upon the voltage of the machine and the distance from the source. Supervoltage machines (1000 to 50,000 kV) penetrate deeply and cause less skin damage than the 250kV machine formerly used.

The rad is the unit of measurement used to express the amount of absorbed radiation and a tumor dose of 3,000 rads refers to the average tumor dose within the whole field. By using rotational fields, shielding, and several treatment ports, it is often possible to deliver much higher doses to the tumor while sparing surrounding normal cells.

Tumors which are curable by radiation are radiosensitive, but radiosensitive tumors are not necessarily curable. In general, undifferentiated tumors and those showing large number of mitoses are more sensitive and radiosenstivity of malignant tumors usually parallels the radiosensitivity of the cell of origin. Epidermoid cells, lymphocytes, gonad germ cells, and hemopoietic cells are quite sensitive. The volume of tumor and its blood supply are important determinants of sensitivity and curability.

Radiation has been established to be superior to surgery in several common malignant tumors such as oat cell cancer of the lung, lymphomas, Ewing's sarcoma, locally advanced prostate cancer, and unresectable breast carcinoma. Cure rates with surgery and radiation are roughly equivalent in epidermoid carcinomas of the skin and anus and the squamous lined upper air and food passages, while surgery is clearly preferable in most gastrointestinal malignancies, melanoma, most sarcomas, and in tumors of the brain and spinal cord.

Postoperative radiation therapy is frequently indicated when surgical resection has not eradicated disease because of extension or if surgery would be unacceptably mutilating. Cancer of the ovary, Wilms' tumor, seminoma, and cancer of the bladder are almost routinely treated with radiation postoperatively. It is very useful in treating local recurrences and bone metastases in breast cancer.

The employment of surgery, radiation, and chemotherapy in combination is very useful in certain childhood malignancies such as Wilms' tumor, rhabdomyosarcoma, and retinoblastomas. The combination of the three modalities has not been shown to be useful in adults in most instances.

IMMUNOTHERAPY

There seems to be little doubt that neoplasia is deeply involved with immunity in man and the quest for effective immunotherapy is clearly worthwhile. Three approaches, active, passive and nonspecific, have been pursued but all have been relatively ineffective in the presence of advanced disease. At this time, immunotherapy used in conjunction with surgery or chemotherapy would seem to have the most potential. It is possible that the real future of cancer treatment lies in this area because of its focus on the malignant cell alone. The destruction of normal tissue associated with surgery, chemotherapy, and radiation is the limiting feature of these otherwise excellent treatment methods.

ORTHOPEDICS

Fractures and Dislocations

Most fractures result from trauma but pathologic processes such as osteoporosis, and metastatic tumor deposits may cause fractures with little or no evidence of injury. Fractures may be open (compound) or closed, the former being prone to infection. Treatment is based

upon return of fragments to approximately normal position (reduction) and immobilization until healing occurs. Some exceptions may be made when function may be restored quicker without anatomic reduction, such as upper humeral fractures in the aged. Reduction may be open or closed, depending upon requirements, and most open reductions are accompanied by some form of internal fixation (e.g., rods, plates, screws, etc.). Closed fractures usually require external immobilization such as casts, external fixation devices, or traction to maintain alignment and prevent movement. Closed reduction, where practicable, reduces risk of infection and usually shortens healing time because periosteal stripping is avoided.

Fractures in children tend to heal more rapidly than in adults, and anatomic reduction is less important because of the tendency for young bones to restore alignment. Open reductions are rarely necessary.

Pain after reduction and casting requires an immediate explanation, and cast removal or splitting is required. Patients with open fractures should be given tetanus prophylaxis and adequate debridement, when indicated, is mandatory ot avoid infection. Systemic antibiotics should be administered. A sterile dressing should be applied to all open fractures when first seen, and even "clean" open fracture wounds should not be closed after a delay of 6 to 8 hours.

Fractures of the spine are best classified as to whether or not neurologic deficits are present. Stability of spine fractures depends upon whether the anterior or posterior spinal ligaments are ruptured. Instability may be present if the pedicles or lamina are fractured. One of the catastrophes of management is the conversion of an injury with no neurologic deficit into a cord injury. Most notably, this occurs when the head is moved during resuscitation, often in patients not suspected of having a cervical spine injury. Cross-table lateral neck roentgenograms showing all seven cervical vertebrae usually identifies the injury. At the accident site, the application of a rigid cervical collar will protect during transport.

Complications of Fractures

Injury to adjacent blood vessels or nerves at the time of injury must be ruled out at initial evaluation. Neurologic deficits, absence or weakness of distal pulses, and significant discoloration or diminution of skin temperature are suggestive of vascular injury. Early arteriography is indicated since delay in diagnosis results in a high incidence of amputation. Manipulation may, in itself, injure vessels or nerves.

Delayed union, malunion, or nonunion may require further treatment, usually bone grafting. Avascular necrosis results from interruption of local blood supply at the time of injury. The bone becomes necrotic and is resorbed. The femoral head, talus, and carpal navicular are especially prone to this complication.

Fat embolism may result from major fractures, and signs usually appear in 1 to 3 days. It is poorly understood, but chylomicra appear to enter veins at the injury site and enter the pulmonary circulation to result in pulmonary insufficiency. Arterial oxygen falls; fat may be seen in retinal vessels; petechiae are common; dyspnea, restlessness, or even loss of consciousness may occur. Fat droplets in the urine, thrombocytopenia, right heart strain on ECG, and diffuse microatelectasis on chest roentgenogram go along with the clinical picture. Treatment centers about adequate oxygenation provided by volume-cycled ventilation by way of an endotracheal tube. Corticosteroids may be administered, but their efficacy is not proven.

Dislocations may be more serious than fractures, and vessel or nerve injuries may be more serious. Knee and spine dislocations are especiallly serious, with vascular compromise and spinal cord injuries being very common. Hip dislocations may result in late atrophy of the femoral head.

Pediatric Orthopedics

Many musculoskeletal disorders are seen only in children. Infants may present with congenital clubfoot (talipes equinovarus). Forefoot adduction and varus with plantar flexion characterize the deformity. Early treatment with correction and application of casts is indicated, and on occasion operation may be required. Congenital dislocation of the hip may exist at birth or occur in the first year. The femoral head lies superiorly and posteriorly. Early recognition and treatment are required to avoid permanent disability. Females are more prone to this disorder. Hip abduction and rotation are restricted, and with the hip flexed to 90 degrees the thigh cannot be abducted down to the examining table. Treatment consists of reducing the femoral head into the acetabulum and holding it there by plaster or other devices.

Osteogenesis imperfecta is a hereditary condition in which bone weakness results in fractures due to slight trauma. Many fractures may be present. Blue sclerae and otosclerosis accompany this disorder. Treatment of fractures as they occur is indicated.

Legg-Perthes disease is an osteochondrosis of the secondary ossification centers and represents a destruction of the capital femoral epiphysis (femoral head) due to loss of blood supply. Children ages 5 to 8 are most susceptible, and it is more common in males. Pain and limp usually are the presenting symptoms. Treatment consists of prohibiting weight-bearing and maintaining the femoral head in the acetabulum while the bone undergoes degeneration and subsequent healing.

Septic arthritis follows infection in other sites and is embolic in origin. Streptococci, staphylococci, *Hemophilus influenza,* and pneumococci are usual causes and the hip is a common site. Fever and irritability may be the only apparent signs, but limp and decreased motion usually supervene. Early drainage is mandatory to prevent joint destruction.

Scoliosis is a curvature of the spine in the coronal plane due to muscular weakness and neurologic or bony defect. Adolescent and teenage girls are prone to this disorder and the deformity ranges from slight to marked. Exercises, braces, and, in severe cases, casting and spinal fusion are required.

Adult Orthopedics

The skeletal system becomes involved in generalized processes in large numbers of patients. Rheumatoid arthritis is especially troublesome, and operative intervention may become necessary to relieve deformity and pain. Osteoarthritis may cause severe disability of the hip and knee, and joint replacement using prosthetic devices is commonly employed to relieve pain. Paget's disease is a metabolic disorder which may occasionally cause fractures or degenerative joint disease requiring operation. Usual treatment is conservative. Tuberculosis of bone and joints is usually part of a late generalized process. Fortunately rare, treatment consists of drug therapy and surgical debridement. The spine, hip, and knee seem predisposed. Osteoporosis is a decrease in bone mass which predisposes to fracture. Such fractures heal well when properly treated. Septic arthritis occurs in children and the staphylococcus predominates. Early open drainage is indicated if antibiotics are not promptly effective.

Herniated nucleus pulposus may affect the spine, predominantly in the lumbar and cervical region. Pressure upon the nerves from the spinal cord causes pain and motor dysfunction. Similarly, cervical radiculitis may result from arthritic osteophytes encroaching upon the neural foraminia. Both can usually be treated by conservative means. Operation may be required if symptoms are unrelenting. Laminectomy and/or fusion are the usual surgical procedures employed.

The thoracic outlet syndrome is the presence of pain in the upper extremity related to brachial plexus nerve roots as they pass from the thorax to the axilla. Nerves are impinged upon by either a cervical rib, scalenus muscle or clavicle. Sometimes abduction of the arm causes reduction or ablation of the radial pulse. Most can be treated by physiotherapy to strengthen shoulder elevators. Resection of the first rib is the preferred surgical procedure when conservative treatment fails.

The adult shoulder is subject to many disorders. Acute calcific tendinitis, chronic tendinitis of the rotator cuff, and rotator cuff tears are common. Most respond to local rest and injection of local anesthetics or steroids.

Tennis elbow results from repetitive forearm use, resulting in a tear of the extensor tendon at its lateral epicondyle origin. Tenderness over the epicondyle and pain on motion confirm the diagnosis. Local steroid injections or administration of anti-inflammatory agents are often effective. Ulnar neuritis may result from an old fracture or blunt trauma. Anterior transposition of the ulnar nerve is indicated to prevent atrophy of the hand muscles.

Infections and injuries of the hand are serious because of the importance of hand function in occupational competence. Penetrating injuries (i.e., bites, laceration, punctures) may disrupt tendons and nerves, causing serious dysfunction. Finger pulp deep space infections and space infections of the hand usually require surgical drainage. All should be given antibiotics.

Extensor tendon injuries are easily repaired. Flexor tendon injuries are more complicated. Nerve repair is indicated in clean wounds.

Ganglia are synovial joint herniations, and most occur on the dorsum of the wrist. Resection usually cures those that are bothersome but recurrence is common.

Contracture of the palmar fascia is called Dupuytren's contracture. It usually affects the fourth and fifth fingers. When disabling, removal of the diseased fascia is indicated.

A painful affliction of the hand is the carpal tunnel syndrome, which usually is idiopathic. Pain in the area served by the median nerve, often most prominent at night, characterizes the syndrome. Relief may be obtained by dividing the carpal tunnel, releasing pressure on the median nerve.

PEDIATRIC SURGERY

Benign Tumors of Childhood

The most common benign tumor is the hemangioma, predominantly in skin but occurring in liver and other organs. Large lymphangiomas may occur in the neck or axilla and are called cystic hygromas. They may appear in the tongue or mediastinum. "Juvenile" or adenomatous polyps of the intestine are common. Polyps associated with the Peutz-Jeghers' and Gardner's syndromes may undergo malignant degeneration.

Malignant Tumors of Childhood

Leukemia is the predominant malignancy of childhood. NonHodgkin's lymphomas, of both lymphocytic and histicytic types, are encountered, and Hodgkin's lymphoma has a significant incidence in late childhood.

About 40 percent of solid tumors of childhood affect the central nervous system. Retinoblastomas and rhabdomyosarcomas occur in the orbit. Neuroblastomas of the posterior mediastinum, teratomas of the anterior mediastinum, and lymphomas of the hilar regions are common.

Retroperitoneal Tumors

Wilms' tumor (nephroblastoma) and neuroblastomas are tumors of early childhood which may be massive and yet produce few clinical signs. They are to be differentiated from benign renal disease such as hydronephrosis and multicystic kidney. All may give rise to fever and anemia. Useful studies for differentiation are indicated (Table 14-6)

Treatment. Wilm's tumors are best treated by nephrectomy, radiotherapy, and chemotherapy. Dactinomycin and vincristine are both hightly effective and a survival rate of over 85 percent is achievable. Neuroblastomas are usually disseminated when diagnosed, but sometimes such tumors become resectable after vincristine and radiotherapy. Abdominal neuroblastomas have a much poorer outlook than those treated in the thorax.

Intestinal Obstruction

Gastrointestinal malformations occur in about 1.25 per 1,000 births. About a quarter of the mothers have hydramnios, presumably because the swallowed amni-

Table 14-6. Studies for Differentiation of Neuroblastoma and Wilm's Tumor

	IVP	Chest Roentgenogram	Liver Bone Scan	Urinary Catecholamine Excretion
Neuroblastoma	Extrinsic Distortion Pelvis	Often	Metastatic Lesions Common	Usually Positive
Wilm's Tumor	Intrinsic Distortion Pelvis	Rarely	Metastatic Lesions Rarely	Negative

otic fluid is regurgitated owing to the obstructed fetal gastrointestinal tract. Bile stained vomitus or the failure to pass meconium in 24 to 48 hours strongly suggests gastrointestinal obstruction. If a tube passed into the stomach at birth recovers more than 25 cc of fluid, obstruction probably exists. On upright and flat film, roentgenogram may show the "double bubble" of duodenal atresia and additional air-fluid levels will be present with lower levels of obstruction. If a low obstruction is suspected, a barium enema may show errors in rotation or the unused microcolon consistent with small bowel obstruction. The enema may dislodge a meconium plug if present.

Most obstructions are due to atresia. Incomplete colon rotation with insufficient fixation may cause volvulus. Cystic fibrosis, with its lack of pancreatic enzymes, leads to the formation of a sticky mass of meconium which may obstruct the distal ileum. The absence of ganglion cells in Auerbach's and Meissner's plexus results in diminished peristalsis of the involved segment, usually the distal colon and rectum, with resulting obstruction. Distension of the proximal colon may be massive, with marked constipation. This is Hirschsprung's disease.

All of the above forms of intestinal obstruction require operation, the choice of which depends upon the etiology of the obstruction. Operative corrections may be definitive or staged, depending upon the age and fitness of the patient. The obstruction must be relieved by whatever method is used. Intravenous hyperalimentation affords the opportunity for nutrition which "buys time" if prematurity or age considerations make major definitive operation inadvisable.

Inguinal hernia results from a failure of the peritoneal lining to close at the internal inguinal ring. If proximal closure occurs, fluid may build up on the distal sac causing a hydrocele. This very common defect may often be suspected by only the parents, who notice a groin bulge. The physician may only detect the "silk glove" sign which reflects thickening of the spermatic cord. Incarceration may occur and operation in indicated. Incarcerated hernias in infants usually reduce under sedation with elevation of the foot of the crib.

Infantile pyloric stenosis usually becomes apparent after three weeks of age. Vomiting may be projectile and does not contain bile. Weight loss and dehydration may ensue and peristaltic waves may be seen sweeping across the abdomen. The baby may suck eagerly and vomit shortly thereafter. Metabolic alkalosis with a rise in CO_2 and the passage of concentrated urine ensue. On examination an olive-shaped epigastric mass may be detected if gently examined. A "string-sign" on upper gastrointestinal roentgenogram examination is confirmatory.

Division of the hypertrophied circular muscle coat of the pylorus (Ramstedt procedure) after adequate rehydration and correction of acid-base balance, is curative.

PLASTIC SURGERY

Burns

Cutaneous burns occur with exposure to temperatures over 50°C. Burns are classified according to depth (i.e., first, second, and third degree). First-degree burns result in erythema with destruction of only the superficial epidermas. Sunburn is an example. Second-degree burns extend into the dermis but do not destroy all epithelial elements; consequently, skin regeneration is possible. These are "partial thickness" injuries. Third-degree burns are full thickness with destruction of all skin and dermal appendages.

The skin serves very important functions in controlling body temperature and conserving body water. Skin loss permits bacterial invasion and burn wound sepsis results. Fluid loss may be massive, and early therapy is structured to overcome these losses.

It is very important that the depth and extent of burns be estimated and recorded at first examination. A simple formula known as the Rule of Nine permits estimation of the extent of the burn and is calculated as follows. Each upper extremity accounts for 9 percent and 18 percent each for front and back of the thoracoabdominal area and each lower extremity. The head and neck comprise 9 percent of body area. Based upon the percentage of involvement, fluid requirements for the first 48 to 72 hours can be made with a maximum estimate of 50 percent burn in adults and 30 percent in children. One formula in common use is the Parkland formula in which Ringer's lactate 4 ml/kg body wt/percent burn is given intravenously during the first 24 hours. In the second 24 hours hydration and urine flow are maintained with dextrose/water solutions, and colloid is administered only if necessary to maintain urine output. Fluid administration sufficient to maintain a urine output of 50–100 ml/hr in adults and 30–50 ml/hr in children is the goal. Colloid administered during the second 24 hours may expand the plasma so much that pulmonary edema may occur. If it develops, diuretics and positive pressure ventilation are employed. Electrolytes, especially potassium, require careful monitoring. Intravenous potassium of about 80–120 mEq/L/day is required to cover losses due to the burn. Large urine volumes are required to combat the renal failure so commonly seen, and mannitol given as a single 25 g intravenous dose will usually assure prompt urine response if 300–500 ml of fluid is given over a 30 minute period.

Burn wound sepsis causes most deaths following extensive burns, and systemic antibiotics do little to change this. Topical sulfonamides and aqueous silver nitrate, when applied early after evaluation of the patient, are very effective in reducing wound sepsis. Systemic antibiotics are useful in combating pneumonia or cellulitis. Tetanus prophylaxis is mandatory.

Early debridement and coverage with homografts, pig skin, amnion and, now, synthetic "skin" are useful in getting burn wounds in condition for healing by skin grafting. Healing seems to be largely dependent upon reducing tissue bacterial counts below 10^5/g of tissue.

Renal failure, pneumonia, and gastrointestinal bleeding are common complications. Respiratory distress due to inhaled smoke may be fatal; early ventilatory support is indicated.

The Hand

Many occupations cannot be engaged in without good hand function. Consequently, this delicate tactile organ must be managed with great care when operated upon or when injured. Scars limit its usefulness, and incisions should not be made across skin creases.

Hand infections are especially serious, especially when neglected or treated improperly. Except for paronychia, drainage should be done under anesthesia unless contraindicated. Paronychia is an infection which starts between the nail and cuticle and may burrow under the nail. Drainage and antibiotics are appropriate. Felon is an infection of the pad of the fingertip which usually follows a puncture wound and is usually due to staphylococcus. Pain, tenderness, and swelling are usually marked. If neglected, osteomyelitis ensues, and treatment consists of prompt drainage and antibiotic administration. Human bites are especially prone to infection by multiple organisms including anaerobes. Prompt antibiotic administration in large doses is indicated.

Tumors of many types may affect the hand. About 10 percent are malignant. Melanomas, most of which arise from preexisting nevi, are especially serious. Ganglions are cystic swellings arising from a tendon sheath or joint capsule. When they interfere with function, excision is indicated.

Skin Grafting

A skin graft is a segment of epidermis and dermis which has been separated from its blood supply before being transplanted to a recipient site. Split thickness grafts consist of the epidermis and a portion of the dermis, while full thickness grafts include the complete thickness of both layers. When the donor receives the graft the term autograft is applied. Homografts are derived from another person, and xenografts are harvested from another species (e.g., porcine). Thin split grafts serve better but contract more than thick grafts.

Survival of skin grafts depends upon adequate blood supply and the presence of fewer than 100,000 (10^5) bacterial/g of tissue at the recipient site. Most areas which develop granulation tissue are potentially capable of supporting a graft, but grafts take well on vascular surfaces of fresh wounds as well. Only bone and cartilage lack the capability of developing granulation tissue.

Skin flaps provide another method of coverage in instances where bone is exposed or where durability of skin is a problem. Undermining of skin adjacent to the defect may permit moving skin into the defect by lateral or longitudinal advancement. For transfer to a remote location, the elevated skin and subcutaneous may be temporarily implanted in another location and, after the blood supply becomes secure at the recipient site, the flap is divided.

Free flaps require microsurgical technique but provide a means by which flaps from a distance may be translocated by reestablishing arterial and venous connections to vessels near the recipient site. The face, scalp, lower leg and hand are appropriate recipient areas.

MELANOMA

The etiology of malignant melanoma is obscure, but exposure to the sun and Celtic origin seem to predispose. They rarely occur in blacks. Three types, lentigo maligna, superficial spreading, and nodular malignant melanoma, are recognized. Nodular types respond least well to treatment.

Prognosis is related to depth of invasion and the presence of lymph node or hematogenous metastases. Treatment consists of local excision with a 5 cm margin except on the face, where necessity dictates a narrower margin. The underlying fascia should be removed, and when subungual lesions exist amputation of the digit is indicated. If nodes are palpable, regional lymphadenectomy should be done. The prophylactic resection of lymph nodes when no palpable nodes are present is controversial.

Five year survival in patients with no microscopically involved nodes is 80 percent or more, while node involvement is associated with a 50 percent or less survival.

ORGAN TRANSPLANTATION

Transplantation is the removal of living tissue from one individual and its implantation in the same or another person. As isograft is a transplant between genetically identical individuals, and an allograft is a transplant between genetically different individuals. A xenograft is a transplant between members of different species, and an autograft is one which is returned to the donor. Autografts and isografts are most compatible since they evoke no immunologic response. Commonly used autografts are skin to repair skin defects, saphenous vein for arterial obstruction bypass, and nerves to repair losses due to injury. Corneal allografts are effective because the cornea is isolated from the immune system. Allogeneic grafts otherwise require immunosuppressive treatment which may not be successful in warding off rejection except where, as in the case of bone, the graft acts merely as a framework for new tissue formation.

Success with homografts has been noteworthy with the kidney and, now, heart, lung, and liver. Intestine, pancreas, and endocrine organs have been transplanted but with very limited success.

Kidney transplantation has been quite successful in rehabilitating patients with irreversible kidney failure who would otherwise require dialysis. About half of the transplants acquired from cadavers survive one year; success with living related donors is about 80 percent. Donor and recipient should have at least one HLA haplotype in common with a living donor, and a cadaver kidney should be given to the recipient with the best HLA compatibility. Young adult brain-dead accident victims otherwise healthy are the preferred donors. Preservation of the kidney is required if the ischemic period is to exceed 30 minutes.

The recipient should have a firm diagnosis of irreversible renal failure with a creatinine above 10 mg/ml. He should be under 55 years old and should not have severe arteriosclerosis, juvenile diabetes, or other disorder likely to shorten life expectancy significantly. Bilateral nephrectomy is usually done to avoid a potential source of infection after transplantation and to assist in controlling hypertension.

Immunosuppression by azathioprine and corticosteroids is required, and antilymphocyte globulin (ALG), actinomycin, and thoracic duct cannulation are useful adjuncts. Hyperacute rejections may occur within hours of transplantation and are due to previous sensitization by antigens similar to those in the graft. Acute rejections often occur within the first few months and are manifested by a reduction in creatinine clearance. They usually may be reversed by increasing corticosteroid dosage. When chronic rejection occurs, it is usually experienced several months after transplantation and is characterized by arterial intimal proliferation with subendothelial thickening of glomerular capillaries and tubular atrophy.

REFERENCES

Davis C: Textbook of Surgery. 12th Ed. WB Saunders Co. Philadelphia, 1981
>An outstanding textbook written by many authors who are experts in their respective fields of interest.

Gibbon's Surgery of the Chest. 4th Ed. WB Saunders Co., Philadelphia, 1983
>This multiple author two volume text is the authoritative work on thoracic surgery. Very well illustrated.

Rhoads Textbook of Surgery. 5th Ed. JB Lippincott, Philadelphia, 1977
>A comprehensive multiple author textbook. An excellent source for more detailed information.

MULTIPLE CHOICE QUESTIONS

Each question below contains four suggested answers of which one or more is correct. Choose the answer:

> A if 1, 2, and 3 are correct
> B if 1 and 3 are correct
> C if 2 and 4 are correct
> D if 4 is correct
> E if 1, 2, 3 and 4 are correct

1. A 55 year old patient complains of episodes of diarrhea, anxiety, and "flushing," and a tentative diagnosis of carcinoid syndrome is made. The possible sites of the tumor responsible might be:
   1. Cecum
   2. Bronchus
   3. Ileum
   4. Thymus

2. Which of the following statements concerning appendicitis is (are) correct?
   1. The incidence of perforation is significantly less than that occurring in adults.
   2. Broad spectrum antibiotics should be administered intravenously preoperatively if perforation is suspected.
   3. Aspiration should always be carried out immediately after admission.
   4. Most intra-abdominal abscesses that form after appendectomy are located in the right lower quadrant.

3. Which of the following statements concerning the intravenous use of fat emulsions is (are) correct?
   1. Because the solution is hypertonic, severe diuresis may result.
   2. It is an ideal nutrient to be used in the presence of diabetes mellitus or coagulopathies.
   3. It is best not used simultaneously with amino acid solutions.
   4. May be infused through a peripheral vein.

4. Which of the following statements concerning parental hyperalimentation is (are) *not* correct?
   1. Impaired glucose tolerance becomes manifest in sepsis or shock.
   2. Adults can utilize about 0.5 g of glucose/kg/hr.

3. Parenteral hyperalimentation has proved useful in the treatment of small intestinal fistulas.

4. A significant advantage is the access of a large central line for the administration of blood should it become necessary.

5. The removal of lesions by major resections of the liver offers a reasonable opportunity for cure in which of the following under certain circumstances?
   1. Hepatocellular carcinoma
   2. Metastatic breast carcinoma
   3. Colorectal carcinoma
   4. Osteogenic sarcoma

6. Idiopathic scoliosis is a common disorder. Which of the following statements is (are) *not* correct?
   1. It is more frequently seen in females.
   2. Prognosis depends upon age at onset and the site of the curvature.
   3. Idiopathic scoliosis with an onset in infancy has a poor prognosis.
   4. Leg length must be determined during evaluation.

7. Which of the following statements concerning fractures of the hip is (are) *correct?*
   1. Most fractures of the hip can be suspected on examination when shortening and internal rotation of the lower extremity is noted.
   2. Most hip fractures in the elderly result from violent deceleration injuries.
   3. Operation is required in approximately 50 percent of patients.
   4. The female to male ratio in these patients exceeds 2 to 1.

8. Cervical bruits may be indicative of carotid artery stenosis. Under what circumstances should angiography be done?
   1. In all such patients in anticipation of prophylactic operation
   2. In the presence of amaurosis fugax
   3. In patients with a completed stroke of 96 hours standing
   4. In the presence of recent transient ischemic attacks (TIA)

9. Nipple discharge is a common cause for surgical consultation. Indicate which of the following are correct statements concerning it.
   1. It is never significant unless grossly bloody.
   2. A bloody discharge from a single duct on one side which is associated with a palpable mass is more significant than a bilateral discharge.

3. It is more commonly due to fibrocystic disease than any other entity.

4. Occult blood in the discharge should be tested for routinely.

10. Acute tubular necrosis is a frequent complication of inadequate renal blood flow. Which of the following is (are) appropriate in its management?
    1. Infusion of 10 percent glucose solution
    2. Infusion of amino acids to restore nitrogen balance
    3. Administration of sodium exchange resins
    4. Administration of albumin or plasma solutions

11. Below knee amputations are being done with increased frequency. Contraindication(s) for its use are recognized as:
    1. Diabetes with pedal gangrene
    2. Ischemic rigor of the calf muscles
    3. Absence of popliteal pulse
    4. The ability to provide only a two-inch length of tibia

12. Pancreatoduodenectomy performed for carcinoma of the head of the pancreas is associated with which of the following?
    1. A 5-year survival rate of approximately 25 percent
    2. A complication rate of 10 percent or less
    3. Postoperative radiation therapy is a useful adjunct.
    4. The residual pancreas is the major source of complication.

13. Which of the following statements concerning acid-base balance is (are) correct?
    1. When the cause of an acid-base imbalance is respiratory in origin, compensation is by way of the kidney.
    2. Respiratory acidemia is best managed by the administration of intravenous sodium bicarbonate.
    3. Addition of dead space is useful in overcoming respiratory alkalemia.
    4. Manipulations of ventilation are the most effective way to overcome metabolic acidosis.

14. Which of the following statements applies to small cell carcinoma of the lung?
    1. Most have metastasized to distant sites by the time of discovery.
    2. Radical pneumonectomy is indicated if hilar nodes are known to be involved.
    3. Chemotherapy using multiple chemotherapeutic agents is the preferred treatment mode.

4. The relationship with cigarette smoking is less than with adenocarcinoma.

15. All of the following concerning intra-abdominal abscesses are true *except:*
    1. Aerobic organisms are more frequently cultured than anaerobes.
    2. They develop spontaneously more often than following an abdominal operation.
    3. Treatment by laparotomy is contraindicated if ultrasound and CT scans are negative.
    4. Catheter drainage using imaging techniques is a practical method of treatment.

16. Which of the following features adversely affect(s) the prognosis in patients with melanoma?
    1. Ulceration on microscopic sections of lesion
    2. Depigmentation of lesion
    3. Polypoid lesions
    4. Lesion thickness over 4 mm

17. Recipients of human donor organ grafts have an increased incidence of neoplasia. Which of the following statements is (are) correct?
    1. The increased incidence is approximately 30 times that of a matched population.
    2. Most of the cancers which develop involve the skin.
    3. When lymphomas develop there is a high incidence of central nervous system involvement.
    4. Immunosuppression appears to be responsible for the increased incidence of neoplasia.

18. Air embolism is a serious complication of operation. Which of the following statements apply?
    1. Occurs primarily during operations requiring a head-down position.
    2. If discovered by the anesthetist, positive pressure should be maintained on the anesthetic bag.
    3. The patient should be monitored with right side down.
    4. A heart murmur usually develops in the presence of air embolism

19. A major transfusion reaction occurring during operation may become manifest by:
    1. A fall in blood pressure
    2. Increase in respiratory rate
    3. Excessive bleeding
    4. Thrombocytopenia

20. Which of the following statements concerning the gastric complications of the Zollinger-Ellison syndrome is (are) *not* correct?

1. Ninety-nine percent subtotal gastrectomy is established as the best surgical therapy.
2. Cimetidine has provided a method of treatment which has almost eliminated the need for operation.
3. Serum gastrin levels are reduced to normal in virtually all patients subjected to gastrectomy.
4. Total gastrectomy is no longer indicated in the management of the Zollinger-Ellison syndrome.

Choose the best answer.

21. A 20 year old male is admitted to the emergency department with a stab wound at the right sternal border. The knife is still in place. Blood pressure is 90/65, respirations are 24/min, the central venous pressure is found to be 26 cm water, and the chest roentgenogram shows a small right pleural effusion. The most useful therapeutic step to take would be:
    A. Give 1,000 ml of uncrossed type-specific blood immediately.
    B. Withdraw the knife blade and apply digital pressure to the wound.
    C. Insert a #30 chest tube into the right seventh interspace in the midclavicular line.
    D. Take the patient to the operating room for operation.
    E. Get a CT scan.

22. Peritoneal lavage is useful in diagnosis of abdominal injury requiring operation. In which of the following injuries is it least likely to be helpful?
    A. Knife stab wound in the right eighth interspace
    B. Rupture of the left kidney
    C. Tear of small intestinal mesentery
    D. Perforation of the sigmoid colon
    E. Patient with a blood pressure of 80/50 with fractures of 10th, 11th, and 12th ribs on left side

23. A 32-year-old lady develops Graves' disease in the first trimester of her pregnancy. Which of the following methods of treatment is preferred?
    A. Two weeks of iodine adminstration followed by thryroidectomy
    B. Radioactive iodine administration
    C. Administration of propylthiouracil
    D. A combination of propylthiouracil and iodine administration

24. The most frequent indication for pulmonary resection in children under 2 years of age is:
    A. Foreign body
    B. Lung abscess
    C. Lobar emphysema

D. Sequestration

E. Blunt traumatic rupture

25. Treatment of endometriosis in a 24-year-old woman may be treated by inhibition of ovulation, which is best accomplished by which one of the following?

A. Administration of an estrogen-progestin combination

B. Hypophysectomy

C. Administration of alkylating agents

D. Panhysterectomy

E. Radiation therapy to pelvis

26. Diethylstilbesterol (DES) has been used for prevention of spontaneous abortion. Which one of the following statements regarding patients receiving it is correct?

A. Their female offspring are prone to genital cancers.

B. Their female offspring show a striking increase in endometriosis

C. The female offspring are no longer at risk of developing side effects if asymptomatic at puberty.

D. Papanicolaou smears are abnormal in offspring.

27. Patients requiring operation for aortic valve disease do so for all of the following except:

A. Angina

B. Left ventricular failure

C. Ventricular tachycardia

D. To avoid risk of endocarditis

E. Syncope

28. Which one of the following statements concerning injury to the common bile duct is correct?

A. Blunt deceleration injuries are responsible for about one-third of common duct injuries.

B. Cholangiography is helpful in identifying the injury.

C. Dacron velour prosthetic grafts are excellent substitutes for long segments of injured common duct.

D. Despite the development of common duct stricture, biliary cirrhosis is a rare sequela.

29. Which one of the following statements concerning infections in vascular prostheses is correct?

A. The most common organism involved is *Streptococcus faecalis.*

B. Prophylactic antibiotics are contraindicated owing to the possibility of the development of resistant strains of bacteria.

C. A complete neo-intimal lining is a strong deterrent to infection.

D. If infection in a groin wound develops following insertion of a Gore-Tex prosthesis, the best approach is to irrigate the wound with Betadine solution and administer large doses of antibiotics intravenously.

30. Which one of the following statements concerning breast cancer patients is *not* correct?

A. Postmastectomy radiotherapy tends to decrease local and regional recurrence.

B. Postmastectomy radiotherapy tends to decrease overall relapse rate.

C. Patients with estrogen receptor negative tumors experience an increased recurrence rate.

D. Contralateral axillary lymph node involvement usually occurs only in patients having ipsilateral node involvement.

31. Which of the following may be associated with the topical application of silver nitrate to burns?

A. Hyponatremia

B. Hypochloremia

C. MET hemoglobinemia

D. Excessive cost

32. A victim of an auto crash sustains a closed displaced fracture of the proximal tibia and fibula. The entire extremity has a second degree burn. The best method of treating the fracture would be:

A. Open reduction of fracture and application of long leg cast.

B. Closed reduction with application of cast after skin had been treated with silver nitrate solution.

C. Steinman pin insertion and balanced traction.

D. Ignore the fracture and treat burn in conventional way. Treat fracture after skin healing occurs.

33. A 40-year-old man is admitted with a history of duodenal ulcer. He has been vomiting for two days. Laboratory data: BUN 60 mg/100 ml, serum creatinine 2.2 mg/100 ml, urine osmolality 710 mosm/kg, hematocrit 35 percent, electrolytes (mEq/l): Na^+ 125, K^+ 3.5, Cl^- 86, HCO_3^- 34. He was unable to provide a urine sample and when catheterized only 60 ml of urine was obtained. Of the following, which would be the preferred method of treatment?

A. Intravenous furosemide, 60 mg

B. Intravenous normal saline, 1,000 ml

C. Intravenous 3 percent saline, 700 ml

D. Intravenous 5 percent dextrose in water with KCl 40 mEq added, 600 cc
E. Hemodialysis

34. Which one of the following is the best answer concerning tumor cells found in venous blood in a cancer patient?
   A. They usually embolize in organs to form metastatic foci.
   B. They are almost never found in early cancers.
   C. Their presence precludes prolonged survival.
   D. Their presence usually indicates that a "no-touch" technique was not used at operation.
   E. They are usually destroyed by host defenses.

35. Surgery is the preferred treatment in all except which one of the following?
   A. Carcinoma of the stomach
   B. Level I melanoma
   C. Lymphoma
   D. Neuroblastoma
   E. Carcinoma of the colon

36. Currently accepted management of a patient with an acute dissecting aneurysm of the ascending thoracic aorta may include each of the following except:
   A. Reattachment of prolapsed aortic valve cusp
   B. Administration of guanethidine, chlorothiazide and reserpine
   C. Local restoration of flow to a compromised superior mesenteric artery
   D. Fenestration of the aneurysm into the thoracic aorta with closure of the distal channel
   E. Evacuation of secondary hemopericardium

37. Which of the following treatment modalities is the least likely to be effective in the treatment of a carbuncle?
   A. Kanamycin and local warm compresses

B. Amphotericin B administration
C. Excision
D. Incision and drainage
E. Penicillin G administration

38. Which of the following statements concerning testicular cancer is not true?
   A. Testicular cancer is the most common cancer in men between 15 and 35 years of age.
   B. The classical presentation is the presence of a painful enlargement of the testis.
   C. Alpha fetoprotein and chorionic gonadotrophin determinations are useful in the investigation of testicular tumors.
   D. Retroperitoneal lymph node dissection is usually not considered necessary if the tumor is a pure seminoma.

39. A 60 year old man experienced severe precordial pain radiating to the back and later shifting to the abdomen. His blood pressure is 200/130. His left leg is numb. Which of the following is most likely?
   A. Pancreatitis
   B. Myocardial infarction
   C. Arterial embolism
   D. Dissecting aneurysm
   E. Reflux esophagitis

Answers to Multiple Choice Questions

1 E	2 C	3 D	4 D	5 B
6 E	7 D	8 C	9 C	10 B
11 D	12 D	13 B	14 B	15 B
16 E	17 E	18 C	19 E	20 E
21 D	22 B	23 C	24 C	25 A
26 A	27 D	28 B	29 C	30 B
31 A	32 C	33 B	34 E	35 C
36 C	37 B	38 B	39 D	

INDEX

Page numbers followed by f represent figures; those followed by t represent tables.